W9-BUX-069

Vascular Brachytherapy

Third Edition

Edited by

Ron Waksman, MD

Associate Director of the Division of Cardiology
Washington Hospital Center
Clinical Professor of Medicine (Cardiology)
Georgetown University
Washington, DC

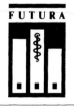

Futura Publishing Company, Inc.
Armonk, NY

Library of Congress Cataloging-in-Publications Data

Vascular brachytherapy / edited by Ron Waksman.—3rd ed.
    p. ; cm.
    Includes bibliographical references and index.
    ISBN 0-87993-489-1
        1. Coronary artery stenosis—Relapse—Radiotherapy. 2. Angioplasty—
Complications—Radiotherapy. 3. Radioisotope brachytherapy. I. Waksman, Ron.
    [DNLM: 1. Cardiovascular Diseases—therapy. 2. Brachytherapy—methods. WG
166 V331 2001]
    RC685.C58 .V37 2001
    616.1′0642—dc21

                                                          2001023946

Copyright © 2002
Futura Publishing Company, Inc.

Published by
Futura Publishing Company
135 Bedford Road
Armonk, NY 10504
www.futuraco.com

LC#: 2001023946
ISBN#: 0-87993-4891

Dedication

To my wife, Tali,
and my children,
Ori, Yarden, Jonathan, and Daniel
for their love and support.

Contributors

Harry Acquatella, MD Centro Medico de Caracas, Caracas, Venezuela

Andrew E. Ajani, MD Director of Clinical Pharmacology Trials, Cardiology Research Institute, Washington Cardiology Center, Washington, DC

Howard I. Amols, PhD Department of Physics, Memorial Sloan Kettering Cancer Center, New York, NY

Remo Albiero, MD Emo Centro Cuore Columbus, Milan, Italy

Marc Apple, MD Radiation Oncologist, Park View Memorial Hospital, Regional Oncology Center, Fort Wayne, IN

Stephen Balter, PhD Division of Invasive Cardiology, Lenox Hill Hospital, New York, NY

Billy G. Bass, PhD Radiation Safety Officer, Washington Hospital Center, Washington, DC

R. Bauernsachs, MD Department of Angiology, J.W. Goethe University, Frankfurt, Germany

Balram Bhargava, MD Department of Cardiology, Cardiothoracic Sciences Centre, New Delhi, India

Raoul Bonan, MD Vice President, Clinical Affairs, Medical Officer, Novoste Corporation, Norcross, GA

Heidi N. Bonneau, RN, MS Stanford University Medical Center, Stanford, CA

H.D. Böttcher, MD Department of Radiation Oncology, J.W. Goethe University, Frankfurt, Germany

Anthony J. Bradshaw, BS, ID Director of Product Development, Radiation Therapy, Guidant Corporation, Vascular Intervention Group, Santa Clara, CA

Kevin Browne, MD, FACC Watson Clinic, Lakeland, FL

Maurice Buchbinder, MD Foundation for Cardiovascular Medicine, Scripps Memorial Hospital, La Jolla, CA

Carlos Calderas, MD Department of Cardiology, Hospital Miguel Perez Carreño and Centro Médico de Caracas, Caracas, Venezuela

Richard V. Calfee, PhD Vice President and General Manager, Radiation Therapy, Guidant Corporation, Vascular Intervention Group, Santa Clara, CA

Allan R. Camrud, RN Division of Cardiovascular Diseases and Internal Medicine, Mayo Graduate School of Medicine, Mayo Clinic and Foundation, Rochester, MN

Stephane G. Carlier, MD, PhD Thoraxcenter, Erasmus Medical Center, Rotterdam, The Netherlands

Andrew J. Carter, DO, FACC Department of Cardiology, Heart Institute at Borgess Medical Center; Associate Professor of Medicine, Michigan State University, Kalamazoo, MI

Rosanna C. Chan, PhD Department of Radiation Oncology, Washington Hospital Center, Washington, DC

Changyi Chen, MD, PhD Division of Vascular Surgery, Surgery Research, Emory University School of Medicine, Atlanta, GA

Victor Chornenky, PhD Principal Scientist, XRT Corporation, St. Paul, MN

Guo Long Chu, PhD Division of Radiation Oncology, Scripps Clinic, La Jolla, CA

Jay P. Ciezki, MD Department of Radiation Oncology, The Cleveland Clinic Foundation, Cleveland, OH

Charles W. Coffey, II, PhD Division of Radiation Oncology, Vanderbilt University Medical Center, Nashville, TN

Antonio Colombo, MD Emo Centro Cuore Columbus, Milan, Italy

José A. Condado, MD Cardiologist, Centro Medico de Caracas, Caracas, Venezuela

Yves Cottin, MD, PhD Cardiovascular Research Institute, Washington Hospital Center, Washington, DC

Ian R. Crocker, MD, PhD Department of Radiation Oncology, Emory University School of Medicine, Atlanta, GA

Orlando Gurdiel, MD Centro Medico de Caracas, Caracas, Venezuela

Kartik J. Desai, MD Cardiovascular Research Foundation, Lenox Hill Heart and Vascular Institute and Leiden University Medical Center, Leiden, The Netherlands

Ivan DeScheerder, MD, PhD   Professor of Invasive Cardiology, University Hospital of Belgium, Gasthuisberg, Belgium

Richard DiMonda, MS, MBA   Vice President of Marketing, Novoste Corporation, Norcross, GA

Dennis M. Duggan, PhD   Division of Radiation Oncology, Vanderbilt University Medical Center, Nashville, TN

William D. Edwards, MD, FACC   Division of Pathology, Mayo Graduate School of Medicine, Mayo Clinic and Foundation, Rochester, MN

Kelly W. Elliott, RN, MS, CCRN   Global Product Training Manager, Novoste Corporation, Norcross, GA

Luis F. Fajardo L-G, MD   Professor of Pathology, Department of Pathology, Stanford University School of Medicine; Chief, Pathology and Laboratory Medicine Service, Veteran's Affairs Medical Center, Palo Alto, CA

Andrew Farb, MD   Department of Cardiovascular Pathology, Armed Forces Institute of Pathology, Washington, DC

David P. Faxon, MD   Chief, Division of Cardiology, University of Southern California School of Medicine, Los Angeles, CA

David R. Fischell, PhD   Isostent, Inc., Belmont, CA

Robert E. Fischell, ScD   Isostent, Inc., Belmont, CA

Tim A. Fischell, MD   Director of Cardiovascular Research, Heart Institute at Borgess Medical Center, Kalamazoo, MI

Peter Fitzgerald, MD, PhD   Center for Research in Cardiovascular Interventions, Stanford University Medical Center, Stanford, CA

Malcolm Foster, MD   Director of Peripheral Vascular Research, Heart Institute at Borgess Medical Center, Kalamazoo, MI

Tim Fox, PhD   Department of Radiation Oncology, Emory University School of Medicine, Atlanta, GA

Jean Gregoire, MD   Division of Cardiovascular Diseases and Internal Medicine, Mayo Graduate School of Medicine, Mayo Clinic and Foundation, Rochester, MN

Robert I. Grove, PhD   Miravant Cardiovascular, Inc., Santa Barbara, CA

Urs. O. Häfeli, PhD   Department of Radiation Oncology, The Cleveland Clinic Foundation

Eric J. Hall, DPhil, DSc, FACR, FRCR Higgins Professor of Radiology and Radiation Oncology, Director, Center for Radiological Research, College of Physicians and Surgeons of Columbia University, New York, NY

Janet M. Hampikian, PhD Associate Professor, School of Materials Science, Georgia Institute of Technology, Atlanta, GA

Christoph Hehrlein, MD Medizinische Klinik III, Abt. für Kardiologie, Ruprecht-Karls Universität Heidelberg, Heidelberg, Germany

David R. Holmes, Jr., MD, FACC Professor of Medicine, Division of Cardiovascular Diseases and Internal Medicine, Mayo Graduate School of Medicine, Mayo Clinic and Foundation, Rochester, MN

Yasuhiro Honda, MD Stanford University Medical Center, Stanford, CA

Gerard B. Huppe, BS Staff Physicist, Division of Radiation Oncology, Scripps Clinic, La Jolla, CA

Seung-Ho Hur, MD Stanford University Medical Center, Stanford, CA

Isabel Iturria, MD Centro Medico de Caracas, Caracas, Venezuela

Shirish K. Jani, PhD, FACR, FAAPM Director of Medical Physics, Division of Radiation Oncology, Scripps Clinic; Professor of Radiology, University of California San Diego, School of Medicine, La Jolla, CA

Myung Ho Jeong, MD, PhD Division of Cardiovascular Diseases and Internal Medicine, Mayo Graduate School of Medicine, Mayo Clinic and Foundation, Rochester, MN

Michael John, BA Department of Cardiovascular Pathology, Armed Forces Institute of Pathology, Washington, DC

Grzegorz L. Kaluza, MD, PhD The Methodist Hospital and Baylor College of Medicine, Houston, TX

Lisa R. Karam, PhD Physics Laboratory, National Institute of Standards and Technology, Gaithersburg, MD

Upendra Kaul, MD Professor of Cardiology, Batra Hospital and Medical Research Center, New Delhi, India

Michael H. Keelan, Jr., MD Professor of Medicine, Medical College of Wisconsin, Milwaukee, WI

Han-Soo Kim, MD Associate Professor, Department of Cardiology, Ajou University School of Medicine, Suwon, Korea

Nicholas N. Kipshidze, MD, PhD   Associate Professor of Medicine, Medical College of Wisconsin, Milwaukee, WI

Spencer B. King, III, MD   Fuqua Chair of Interventional Cardiology, The Fuqua Heart Center of Piedmont Hospital, Co-Director, Atlanta Cardiovascular Research Institute, Clinical Professor of Medicine, Emory University School of Medicine, Atlanta, GA

F.F. (Russ) Knapp, Jr., PhD   Nuclear Medicine Program, Life Sciences Division, Oak Ridge National Laboratory (ORNL), Oak Ridge, TN

Marc Kollum, MD   Cardiovascular Research Institute, Washington Hospital Center, Washington, DC

Gerhard Koning, MSc   Cardiovascular Research Foundation, Lenox Hill Heart and Vascular Institute and Leiden University Medical Center, Leiden, The Netherlands

Adalbert Kovacs, MS   Department of Radiochemistry, University of Heidelberg, Heidelberg, Germany

Thomas M. Koval, PhD   Division of Radiation Oncology, Mayo Graduate School of Medicine, Mayo Clinic and Foundation, Rochester, MN

Ken Kozuma, MD   Department of Interventional Cardiology, Thoraxcenter, University Hospital Dijkzigt, Rotterdam, The Netherlands

Michael J.B. Kutryk, MD, PhD, FRCPC   Thoraxcenter, University Hospital Dijkzigt, Rotterdam, The Netherlands

Alexandra J. Lansky, MD   Cardiovascular Research Foundation, Lenox Hill Heart and Vascular Institute and Leiden University Medical Center, Leiden, The Netherlands

Joerg Lehmann, PhD   Stanford University Medical Center, Stanford, CA

Ian Leitch, PhD   Miravant Cardiovascular, Inc., Santa Barbara, CA

Martin B. Leon, MD   Director and CEO, Cardiovascular Research Foundation, Lenox Hill Hospital, New York, NY

Peter C. Levendag, MD, PhD   Department of Radiotherapy, Daniel den Hoed Cancer Center, Rotterdam, Erasmus Medical Center, Rotterdam, The Netherlands

Dieter D. Liermann, MD   Department of Interventional Radiology, J.W. Goethe University, Frankfurt, Germany

Samuel F. Liprie, PD (Nuc)   Lake Charles, LA

Edgar G. Löffler, PhD   Business Development Manager, Nucletron BV, TX Vee-nendaal, The Netherlands

Alan B. Lumsden, MD   Division of Vascular Surgery, Surgery Research, Emory University School of Medicine, Atlanta, GA

M. Julia MacDonald, RN   Division of Vascular Surgery, Surgery Research, Emory University School of Medicine, Atlanta, GA

Monique M.H. Marijianowski, PhD   Assistant Professor of Medicine (Hematology), Department of Medicine, Division of Hematology, Emory University School of Medicine, Atlanta, GA

Louis G. Martin, MD   Vascular and Interventional Radiology Division, Emory University School of Medicine, Atlanta, GA

Vincent Massullo, MD   Radiation Oncologist, Division of Radiation Oncology, Scripps Clinic, La Jolla, CA

Erich Minar, MD   Department of Angiology, General Hospital Vienna, Vienna, Austria

Gary S. Mintz, MD   Cardiovascular Research Foundation, New York, NY

James B. Mitchell, PhD   Radiation Biology Branch, Division of Clinical Sciences, National Cancer Institute, Bethesda, MD

Shashadhar Mohapatra, PhD, DABR, DABSNM   Radiation Safety Office, Washington Hospital Center, Washington, DC

Jeffrey W. Moses, MD   Chief, Interventional Cardiology, Lenox Hill Hospital, New York, NY

Morris Mosseri, MD   Senior Cardiologist, Cardiology Department, Hadassah Medical Center; Senior Lecturer, Hadassah Hebrew University Medical School, Jerusalem, Israel; Medical Director, Medical Instruments Development Technologies, Ltd., Haifa, Israel

Ravinder Nath, PhD   Department of Therapeutic Radiology, Yale University School of Medicine, New Haven, CT

Victor Nikolaychik, MD, PhD   University of Wisconsin Medical School, Milwaukee Campus, Milwaukee, WI

Dattatreyudu Nori, MD, FACR   Professor and Chairman, Department of Radiation Oncology New York Hospital Medical Center of Queens and New York Hospital-Cornell Medical Center

Paul Okunieff, MD   Chair and Professor, Department of Radiation Oncology, University of Rochester Medical Center, Rochester, NY

Boris Pokrajac, MD   Department of Radiotherapy and Radiobiology, General Hospital Vienna, Vienna, Austria

Suhrid Parikh, MBBS, MS, MCh   Associate Professor of Radiology in Radiation Oncology, New York Hospital-Cornell Medical Center, New York, NY

Bogart Parra, MD   Centro Medico de Caracas, Caracas, Venezuela

Boris Pokrajac, MD Department of Radiotherapy and Radiobiology, General Hospital Vienna, Vienna, Austria

Youri Popowski, MD   Division of Radiation Oncology, University Hospital, Geneva, Switzerland

Richard Pötter, MD   Department of Radiotherapy and Radiobiology, General Hospital Vienna, Vienna, Austria

Albert E. Raizner, MD   Professor of Clinical Medicine, Baylor College of Medicine; Director, Cardiac Catheterization Laboratories, The Methodist Hospital, Houston, TX

Evelyn Regar, MD   Department of Interventional Cardiology, Thoraxcenter, Rotterdam, The Netherlands

Johan H.C. Reiber, PhD   Cardiovascular Research Foundation, Lenox Hill Heart and Vascular Institute and Leiden University Medical Center, Leiden, The Netherlands

Keith A. Robinson, PhD   Assistant Professor of Medicine (Cardiology), Director, Rich Cardiovascular Research Laboratories, The Andreas Gruentzig Cardiovascular Center, Emory University School of Medicine, Atlanta, GA

Marco Roffi, MD   Department of Cardiology, The Cleveland Clinic Foundation, Cleveland, OH

Philip Rubin, MD   Professor, Department of Radiation Oncology, University of Rochester Medical Center, Rochester, NY

Wilhelm Rutishauser, MD   Cardiology Service, Clinique de Genolier, Genolier, Switzerland

Tara A. Ryan, MS, MBA   Chief of Interventional Cardiology Devices Branch, Division of Cardiovascular, Respiratory, and Neurological Devices, Office of Device Evaluation, Center for Devices and Radiological Health, Food and Drug Administration, Rockville, MD

Steve Rychnovsky, PhD   Miravant Cardiovascular, Inc., Santa Barbara, CA

Manel Sabate, MD Department of Interventional Cardiology, Thoraxcenter, University Hospital Dijkzigt, Rotterdam, The Netherlands

Harry Sahota, MD Good Samaritan Hospital, Bellflower, CA

Jorge Saucedo, MD Director, Catheterization Laboratories, Department of Cardiology, University of Arkansas for Medical Sciences, and John L. McClellan Memorial Veterans Hospital, Little Rock, AR

Bernhard Schopohl, MD Department of Radiation Oncology, J.W. Goethe University, Frankfurt, Germany

Robert S. Schwartz, MD, FACC Professor of Medicine, Division of Cardiovascular Diseases and Internal Medicine, Mayo Graduate School of Medicine, Mayo Clinic and Foundation, Rochester, MN

Neal A. Scott, MD, PhD Vice President and Medical Director, RadioVascular Systems, Inc., Houston, TX

Jerome Segal, MD President and CEO, RadioVascular Systems, Inc., Houston, TX

Patrick W. Serruys, MD, PhD, FACC, FESC Thoraxcenter, Erasmus Medical Center, Rotterdam, The Netherlands

George Sianos, MD Department of Interventional Cardiology, Thoraxcenter, Rotterdam, The Netherlands

Christopher G. Soares, PhD Physicist, Ionizing Radiation Division, United States Department of Commerce, National Institute of Standards and Technology, Gaithersburg, MD

Gary Strathearn, PhD Radiance Medical Systems, Inc., Irvine, CA

Zvi Symon, MD Radiation Oncology, University of Michigan, Ann Arbor, MI

Allen J. Taylor, MD Department of Cardiovascular Pathology, Armed Forces Institute of Pathology, Washington, DC

Paul S. Teirstein, MD, FACC Director of Interventional Cardiology, Division of Interventional Cardiology, Scripps Clinic, La Jolla, CA

Attila Thury, MD Department of Interventional Cardiology, Thoraxcenter, University Hospital Dijkzigt, Rotterdam, The Netherlands

Brett Trauthen, MS Vice President of Clinical Affairs, Radiance Medical Systems, Inc., Irvine, CA

Prabhaker Tripuraneni, MD, FACR Head of the Division of Radiation Oncology, Scripps Clinic, La Jolla, CA

Joan Tuinenburg, MSc Leiden University Medical Center, Leiden, The Netherlands

E. Murat Tuzcu, MD Department of Cardiology, The Cleveland Clinic Foundation, Cleveland, OH

Frits M. van Krieken, MSc, PhD Product Manager, Endovascular Brachytherapy, Nucletron BV, TH Veenendaal, The Netherlands

Vitali Verin, MD Hôpital Cantonal, Department of Medicine, Cardiology Center, University Hospital, Geneva, Switzerland

Renu Virmani, MD Department of Cardiovascular Pathology, Armed Forces Institute of Pathology, Washington, DC

Ronald E. Vlietstra, MB, BCh, FACC Watson Clinic, Lakeland, FL

Yoram Vodovotz, PhD Cardiology Research Foundation and Medlantic Research Institute, Washington Hospital Center, Washington, DC

Ron Waksman, MD, FACC Associate Director of the Division of Cardiology, Washington Hospital Center, Clinical Professor of Medicine (Cardiology), Georgetown University, Washington, DC

Jeffrey Walker, MD Miravant Cardiovascular, Inc., Santa Barbara, CA

Robert P. Walsh, RN, BA, MBA Senior Director of Marketing, Novoste Corporation, Norcross, CA

Judah Weinberger, MD, PhD Director of Research, Cardiac Catheterization Laboratory, Associate Professor of Clinical Medicine, Columbia University, New York, NY

William S. Weintraub, MD Division of Cardiology, Department of Medicine, Emory University School of Medicine, Department of Health Policy and Management, Emory University School of Public Health, Atlanta, GA

Neil J. Weissman, MD Director of Cardiac Ultrasound and Ultrasound Core Laboratories, Cardiovascular Research Institute, Washington Hospital Center, Washington, DC

Patrick L. Whitlow, MD Department of Cardiology, The Cleveland Clinic Foundation, Cleveland, OH

Josiah N. Wilcox, PhD Associate Professor of Medicine, Department of Hematology/Oncology, Department of Medicine, Emory University School of Medicine, Atlanta, GA

Jacqueline P. Williams, PhD   Research Assistant Professor, Department of Radiation Oncology, University of Rochester Medical Center, Rochester, NY

Gerhard K. Wolf, PhD   Department of Radiochemistry, University of Heidelberg, Heidelberg, Germany

Roswitha Wolfram, MD   Department of Angiology, General Hospital Vienna, Vienna, Austria

Nai-Chuen Yang, PhD   Washington Cancer Institute, Washington Hospital Center, Washington, DC

Paul G. Yock, MD   Director, Center for Research in Cardiovascular Interventions, Stanford University Medical Center, Stanford, CA

Ning Yue, PhD   Department of Therapeutic Radiology, Yale University, New Haven, CT

Brian E. Zimmerman, PhD   Physics Laboratory, National Institute of Standards and Technology, Gaithersburg, MD

Preface

Vascular brachytherapy has become a standard of care for the treatment of in-stent restenosis. With the launch of the third edition of *Vascular Brachytherapy,* we have seen this technology disseminated to over 300 catheterization laboratories in the world, where patients are treated daily with this modality. In the United States, both gamma and beta systems have been approved, while one gamma and three beta systems are currently available and actively used in Europe. In the initial stages of vascular brachytherapy, we were confronted with issues related to the biology and physics of the field and the exploration of the optimal dose designing system, all while awaiting data from clinical trials. Since then, we have truly gained an advantageous knowledge of vascular brachytherapy, while discovering its limitations as well.

This edition is an on-going testimonial to the progress made in this field. Although brachytherapy is not a cure for restenosis, it substantially reduces its recurrence rate, and has saved thousands of repeat interventions and clinical events for our patients. During the past 10 years of research, we have learned to optimize results and minimize complications, as in the case of edge effect and late thrombosis. While vascular brachytherapy is a proven therapy for in-stent restenosis, expansion to other subsets of lesions is pending further clinical investigation.

Encompassing nearly a decade of experience, this edition boasts the contributions of leading experts in the field. As in the first two editions, the contributors of this book—cardiologists, scientists, radiation oncologists, radiobiologists, pathologists, vascular surgeons, radiation safety officers, regulators, engineers, and technicians—all experts and world-renowned in the field, present the latest data available from a multidisciplinary perspective. The basics are also incorporated for those who would like to embark on a journey to learn more about this promising therapy.

Although the first edition of this book was published only 3 years ago, enormous advances in the field have required extensive revisions to the text. This new edition includes twenty-one new and thirty revised chapters. A special attempt was made to maintain the balance and the depth of the variety of the multidisciplinary components of the field. For those who follow the fields of vascular intervention and radiation therapy, it is evident that vascular brachytherapy has moved from initial ideas and preclinical observations quite rapidly to clinical practice.

This edition is divided into ten parts: Part I reviews the mechanisms of restenosis and alternative treatments for the next millennium. Part II concerns the basic radiobiology of intravascular radiation, and discusses different mechanisms by which radiation prevents restenosis. In addition, Part II introduces the late effects of vascular radiation from a pathologist's perspective. Part III is dedicated to radiation physics –from basic principles to dosimetry planning for vascular brachytherapy for both beta and gamma sources, to health physics perspectives. Part IV summarizes the preclinical work that was conducted in animals; results from studies utilizing external radiation and endovascular radiation both with beta and gamma emitters are detailed. Part V reviews with radiation as adjunct therapy to intra-coronary stenting, from biology, physics, animal experiments, pathology, and clinical experiments. Part VI reports the data accumulated thus far from the use of vascular brachytherapy in the peripheral vascular system. The latest update is also provided on patients who were treated with radiation for superficial femoral artery lesions, and following intervention to arteriovenous dialysis shunts. Part VII concerns the imaging and analysis of vascular brachytherapy, including intravascular ultrasound observations. Part VIII provides the latest data from the clinical trials for coronary arteries that utilized both gamma and beta emitters, including those clinical trials with the radioactive stent. Part IX describes the various systems that are currently available for testing in the clinical trials for vascular brachytherapy. Descriptions of the system designs and their advantages for this technology are detailed. Part X, the final section, is dedicated to regulatory and health care milieu issues. Radiation safety issues and practical implementation of this technology for use in the catheterization laboratory, the U.S. Food and Drug Administration perspective, and the economic aspects of this field are detailed.

The rapid pace at which vascular brachytherapy continues to advance made it a challenge to provide a timely picture of this field in a traditional textbook. Still, the fundamentals for this field are presented for those who wish to introduce themselves to this fascinating field, which may change the approach to cardio-vascular intervention.

As in the first and second editions, we caution that the level of enthusiasm and expectation should be kept in perspective. Given the multifactorial and mechanistic nature of restenosis, it is perhaps too naïve to think that a single therapy of vascular brachytherapy will completely resolve this problem. It is the nature of every new technology to be driven by its own investigators, industry, and supporters to a high level of expectation. The real challenge of a technology is measured over time, and not by the initial positive results coming from feasibility trials. At the time of publication of the current, third edition of this book, new technologies are emerging that have enormous potential to nearly cure restenosis. The technology behind drug-eluting stents is waiting to be introduced clinically. Since the concept of this new modality is based on intervention in the cell cycle, the knowledge we have obtained with vascular brachytherapy can help to move this novelty forward. If successful, drug-eluting stents will eliminate restenosis and the need for brachytherapy. At best, drug-eluting stents will always be limited to a stent platform, while radiation is effective with balloons and other ablative devices. Yet as long as restenosis remains an unresolved problem, vascular brachytherapy will be an alternative technology to help to our patients. This should motivate us to persue, with intensive research efforts, improvements in the technology for better vascular brachytherapy treatment in patient care.

In closing, I must acknowledge the tremendous efforts of Jacques Strauss and his dedicated staff at Futura, who did not save any effort to bring this high quality and comprehensive edition to reality in a very timely manner. I would also like to thank Kathryn Coons for her assistance in the preparation and editing of this edition. Their dedicated work helped to turn this book from a pivotal document in the first edition, to a basic comprehensive textbook of vascular brachytherapy.

Ron Waksman, MD
Washington, DC

Preface
(Adapted and modified from the first edition)

More than 20 years ago, in 1977, the first coronary balloon angioplasty by Andreas R. Gruentzig introduced a new dimension to the field of interventional cardiology. The main concept was that the atherosclerotic plaque could be physically removed or ablated from within the vessel. This has lead to an evolution of new innovations, new devices, and prosthesis technologies all delivered within the vessel to treat arterial vasculopathies. However, it was learned very early that, subsequent to the intervention, a wound-healing process known as restenosis significantly limits the success of this new treatment modality. Restenosis modified the initial enthusiasm of balloon angioplasty and challenged scientists and clinicians to find a solution for a significant medical problem. Several therapeutic approaches have been suggested, including pharmaceutical agents, physical new devices, and, recently, gene therapy has been studied, but the problem of overexuberant cell proliferation after intervention leading to restenosis, although better understood, still remains the Achilles heel of this field.

Since the discovery of radium by Madame Curie in 1898, ionizing radiation has been well known as an antiproliferative agent for benign and malignant disorders; it is also documented that proliferative cells are radiosensitive to low doses of radiation. Therefore, several investigators have suggested that local treatment with radioactive sources placed nearby the angioplasty site (brachytherapy) will inhibit restenosis. This has led to the evolution of a new field in medicine called endovascular brachytherapy.

This book was conceived to introduce the field of endovascular brachytherapy from a multidisciplinary perspective. The contributors—cardiologists, interventional radiologists, radiation oncologists, medical physicists, radiobiologists, pathologists, vascular surgeons, as well as industry representatives in this field—have shared their experience in this new, exciting field. Thus this book is meant to serve all disciplines that need to collaborate in order to bring this therapy into clinical use. The integration of these many disciplines is reflected in the chapters of the book.

A word of caution is offered in regard to the enthusiasm and the eagerness to move forward into large clinical studies. Yet there is a lot to explore about the radiobiological mechanisms of endovascular brachytherapy and how they are contributing to the fight against restenosis. It is also to remember that very little is known about the long-term effects of this therapy in terms of safety to the patients. Thus, further work at the interface of physics, cell biology, science, and device engineering, as well as meticulous clinical work, should provide further progress and insight into the best way of treating diseases, and should help in patient care.

Ron Waksman, MD

Contents

Part I
Mechanisms of Restenosis and Alternative Treatments

Part II
Radiation Biology and Vascular Pathology

Part VI
Vascular Radiation and Peripheral Vascular Disease

Part VII
Imaging and Analysis

Part VIII
Endovascular Radiation Clinical Trials in Coronary Arteries

Part IX
Systems for Endovascular Radiation Therapy

Part X
Regulatory and Health Care Milieu Issues

Part I

Mechanisms of Restenosis and Alternative Treatments

## Chapter 1

Restenosis Following Angioplasty

Spencer B. King, III, MD

Introduction

Following a coronary intervention such as angioplasty, the artery may remain open or may reclose in the early phase due to thrombosis or dissection or a combination of the two, or the artery may close in the late phase due to a process of wound healing called restenosis. With the availability of modern techniques, the acute closure of arteries following angioplasty is relatively uncommon, and restenosis remains the major limitation of the technique. Although the size of the lumen decreases following almost all interventions, restenosis is defined as a compromise of the lumen which is felt to approach an obstruction that could result in hemodynamic compromise. This degree of narrowing is usually arbitrarily defined as a narrowing of the lumen that is equal to or exceeds 50% of the lumen diameter in the adjacent normal appearing segments.

In the early days of coronary angioplasty, Andreas Gruentzig predicted that restenosis would occur in approximately 30% of patients. This prediction proved to be correct for the first series of patients treated in Zurich. These patients, however, were primarily treated for proximal discrete lesions in relatively large arteries. As indications for angioplasty have been expanded, the restenosis rate has increased. Some trials of pharmacological therapy have reported restenosis rates ranging from 36% to 42%.[1–6] In the EAST Trial, the restenosis rate found on routine 1-year angiograms in a subset of patients with more diffuse multivessel disease was 44% per lesion dilated.[7] Since the introduction of coronary stents, the restenosis rate of patients treated with balloon angioplasty in randomized trials has ranged from 30% to 40%.[8,9]

What Produces Restenosis?

In order to understand the mechanism of restenosis, one must understand the mechanism by which arteries are opened. In balloon angioplasty, the balloon is inflated in a heavily diseased segment of the artery with thick eccentric or concentric plaque. The arterial lumen is narrowed, but the external dimensions of the artery may actually be wider than normal due to the radial growth of the space occupying plaque. When the balloon is inflated, the lumen is expanded and the external dimension of the artery is expanded as well. Cracks and splits develop in the plaque and arterial wall. Common sites of disruption are the juncture of the

From Waksman R (ed.). *Vascular Brachytherapy, Third Edition.* Armonk, NY: Futura Publishing Co., Inc.; © 2002.

plaque and the less involved arterial wall, especially at points where less compliant tissue such as calcified or densely fibrotic plaque interfaces with more compliant tissue components. Splits may extend into the plaque material, into the media, or through the media into the adventitial surface. Other technologies open arteries by this same mechanism, but there are special considerations for each and these will be discussed subsequently.

It is now understood that there are three components of restenosis. The first component is the elastic recoil that occurs promptly after the overstretch of the artery. This has been quantitated at approximately 50% of the cross-sectional area or one-third the lumen diameter on average. In other words, an artery dilated with a 3-mm balloon will commonly have a lumen in the dilated segment of 2 mm following balloon deflation and passage of a few minutes' time. This elastic recoil does not seem to progress much beyond the first few minutes after balloon deflation. Observations made the day following balloon angioplasty show little further decrease in lumen size. The second component of restenosis is intimal proliferation resulting in new tissue growth occupying the cracks and tears in the vessel wall and sometimes growing to produce very severe reobstruction of the artery. This process probably begins within days after angioplasty and continues for weeks or months. The mechanism by which this occurs will be discussed in subsequent chapters in this book.

The third mechanism for restenosis that has been recently elucidated is analogous to wound contracture. The entire artery may become contracted so that the external elastic lamina occupies a smaller circumference than it did following the procedure. It has been estimated by Mintz et al that this process may account for up to 60% to 65% of the lumen loss judged by intravascular ultrasound.[10] Other data from directional atherectomy samples and post-mortem histology would suggest a larger contribution from intimal proliferation.[11–13] However, each of these components certainly plays an important role in the restenosis process. The time course of angiographically observed restenosis also fits with the concept of a wound healing process. Nobuyoshi et al[14] studied patients with serial angiographic follow-up after angioplasty. This study showed little restenosis at 1 month and by 3 months the restenosis process was largely complete. We feel, based on rapidly accumulating data, that the process of restenosis is closely akin to wound healing following any type of tissue injury.[15]

Damage to the arterial wall and its surrounding tissues results in transformation of cells in the media and in the adventitia so that they are signaled to proliferate, migrate, and elaborate extracellular matrix. These same cells may then undergo phenotypic transformation and become cells capable of causing contracture, which is very familiar in wounds occurring in tissue such as the skin. An understanding of the relative contribution of these processes is important in planning methods to control the restenosis process.

Attempts to Control Restenosis

These mechanisms of restenosis have just recently been understood and therefore in the early stages of angioplasty, attempts to control the process were aimed at a wide array of targets. The first agents tested were anticoagulants and antiplatelet agents. The studies were carried out comparing coumadin to aspirin,[16] heparin of brief duration to longer term administration of heparin,[17] anti-platelet agents including aspirin,[18] aspirin versus persantine,[19] thromboxane synthetase inhibitors,[20] antispasmodics such as nifedipine[21] and diltiazem,[22] and agents felt to be important in the atherosclerotic process such as lipid-lowering agents including lovastatin[6] and omega-3 fatty acids.[23,24] Anti-inflammatory agents, including steroids,[1] were also tested.

Most of these were single center trials, although some were small multicenter attempts, and in the early 1990s a number of trials were initiated using agents that had been found to inhibit intimal proliferation in animal models. Some of the agents tested were angiotensin-converting enzyme (ACE) inhibitors including cilazipril,[2,3] the serotonin antagonist, ketanserin,[5] low molecular weight heparin, cholesterol-lowering agents including lovastatin[6] and pravastatin, and the somatostatin analog, angiopeptin.[4]

Although powerful effects in some animal models have been observed with these agents, common to the administration of many of them was the problem of dosing. The dose of the ACE inhibitor cilazipril, used in the rat experiments, was 10 mg per kilogram; however, the dose in the human trials was 10 mg or 20 mg per patient.

Some small systemic drug trials have proved interesting and are stimulating additional research. One example is the STARC Trial of trapidil[25] (a platelet-derived growth factor inhibitor), which showed a positive result; larger trials are being planned for such agents. The inflammatory component of restenosis has been addressed with the use of antioxidants. Probucol was shown to have an effect on vascular lumen size in our experimental laboratory using the porcine coronary angioplasty model.[26] Since there was no effect from lipid lowering in this model, the improved lumen size is felt to be due to the antioxidant properties of probucol. This approach was supported by two small clinical studies, one in Japan[27] and one at the Montreal Heart Institute.[28] In these studies, probucol was given for 1 month prior to the intervention. Despite the results from these trials, no drug has yet been recognized or generally used for restenosis prevention.

An observation from the Evaluation of C7E3 for the Prevention of Ischemic Complications (EPIC) Trial[29] was that, not only were acute complications decreased with this anti-platelet antibody, but late clinical events, especially repeat revascularizations, were also decreased. This has been interpreted by some as representing a decrease in clinical restenosis and may indeed correlate with improvement in angiographic restenosis. This concept, however, was not supported by other studies of IIb/IIIa blockers. The EPILOG Study[30] and the CAPTURE Study[31] did not show any reduction in clinical events occurring after the first month which would correlate with a restenosis effect. The RESTORE Trial contained an angiographic substudy which showed no difference in 6-month restenosis rates between patients treated with the IIb/IIIa blocker and placebo.[32,33]

Because of the problem of achieving adequate tissue concentrations in the local environment with systemic drug therapy, experimental efforts have concentrated on the delivery of drugs locally. Devices have ranged from porous balloons to methods of delivering compounds by ionophoresis.[34–37] Many types of local delivery catheters have developed since the original porous balloon[38] and some of them have gained approval by the Food and Drug Administration.

One of the most widely touted applications of local drug delivery has been in the transfer of antisense ologonucleitides directly into the vessel wall to signal the cells to stop replicating and thereby block neointimal formation after a vascular intervention. Although there is good evidence that genetic signals can be transported into the vessel wall, a number of problems regarding the mechanism of delivery, the agent to be used, and the time the agent must remain in the environment, are as yet unresolved. Several methods of retaining a drug, including the use of drug containing polymer-coated stents or other devices have been advocated. Recently acquired knowledge regarding the mechanism of restenosis may help in the targeting of these local agents, not only to the vessel wall, but also to the adventitia and surrounding structures.

Influence of New Interventional Devices on the Restenosis Problem

Methods for achieving increased arterial lumen size with new devices fall into two general categories: (1) atherectomy or tissue-removing techniques, and (2) stenting or vascular splinting techniques. Both of these methods are designed to provide a more complete arterial opening or lumen that is geometrically smoother with less pertubation of blood flow.

Atherectomy or Tissue Removing Techniques

In the first category fall the devices such as directional atherectomy, rotary ablation, transluminal extraction catheter atherectomy, and laser angioplasty. Directional atherectomy is designed to remove a large bulk of tissue and thereby create a greater lumen with perhaps less arterial dilatation. Directional atherectomy has been evaluated in controlled clinical trials compared to balloon angioplasty.

The CAVEAT 1 and C-CAT Trials[39,40] did not show a significant advantage as far as restenosis is concerned. This was an unexpected finding since creating a larger arterial lumen would seem intuitively beneficial and observational studies have shown some correlation between the final arterial lumen size achieved and the maintenance of that lumen, resulting in a lower restenosis rate for larger lumens. These trials of directional atherectomy, however, did not achieve a much larger lumen with atherectomy than with balloon angioplasty.

A subsequent trial, Balloon versus Optimal Atherectomy Trial (BOAT),[41] did show an improved restenosis rate from 40% with balloon angioplasty to 32% with optimal directional atherectomy. The other debulking devices, especially rotational atherectomy and laser, are designed to remove tissue without stretching the artery and thereby reducing arterial trauma. Both these types of devices have been tested against balloon angioplasty in trials,[42,43] but unfortunately no reduction in restenosis has been demonstrated. Further trials involving rotational ablation are currently under way (STRATAS) (DART), and those results are awaited.

Restenosis Following Stenting

Endovascular stenting aims to reduce restenosis by a very different mechanism. Endovascular stents, usually made of stainless steel, are placed in the artery either by a self-expanding mechanism or, more commonly, by expanding with balloons. The purpose of stenting is to maintain the arterial lumen by a scaffolding process, thus providing radial support. This technique results in the largest lumen and it obviously results in expansion of the artery to the greatest degree, as well.

Two trials, STRESS[8] and BENESTENT,[9] have shown significant reduction in the restenosis rates. This reduction is entirely due to the large initial lumen achieved since the late loss in lumen size, due to new tissue growth following the procedure is greater than that seen with balloon angioplasty alone. Nonetheless, the final minimal lumen diameter at 6 months and the percent diameter stenosis remain improved in the stented group. In the STRESS Trial, the rate of restenosis, judged by the 50% definition, was reduced from 42% in the balloon arm to 32% in the stent arm. In BENESTENT, the magnitude of reduction was from 32% to 22%.

Stenting technique has continued to evolve. Current approaches are to follow stent placement with high pressure inflations, from 14 to 20 atmospheres, in order to achieve very minimal stenosis and complete apposition of the stent to the vascular wall. BENESTENT II, using a heparin-coated stent and higher pressure balloon inflation techniques, resulted in a restenosis rate for the eligible lesions of 17%.[44] Interestingly, the restenosis rate in the balloon angioplasty group was also improved from historic controls. For patients with optimal balloon angioplasty results, the restenosis rate was as low as for those actually stented.

These studies, however, are confined to lesions in arteries greater than 3 mm in size and lesions that can be covered by one stent. Other lesions potentially suitable for stenting, such as ostial lesions, bifurcation lesions, lesions in small vessels, or lesions longer than 10 to 15 mm, have not undergone controlled trials with stenting as yet. Although stenting may result in an improvement in restenosis rates in some of these groups, the overall restenosis rate is likely to be significantly higher than in lesions evaluated in the previous clinical trials.[14]

The impact of stenting on restenosis in multivessel disease patients was seen in the recently completed ARTS Trial of coronary surgery versus percutaneous interventions. Using the surrogate endpoint of target vessel revascularization to represent restenosis, the rate of repeat procedures has been reduced by almost one half in the stent group compared to prior balloon angioplasty versus surgery trials. The need for repeat intervention in multivessel stented patients at 1 year was 17%. Although stents have reduced the restenosis rate for suitable lesions, restenosis within the stent remains a problem.[45] When it occurs, especially in a diffuse manner, retreatment is problematic with restenosis rates reported from 31% to 80%.[46–50] Since this narrowing is produced entirely by tissue growth within the stent, removal of this tissue would seem logical. However, debulking of in-stent lesions with atherectomy or laser or restenting has not been consistently effective in reducing restenosis in these patients.[51–54] Endovascular radiation has significantly reduced restenosis following treatment for in-stent restenosis in several randomized trials.[55,56]

Clinical Importance and Economic Impact of Restenosis

The restenosis process fortunately does not usually result in catastrophic clinical events. The principal adverse result of restenosis is economic. Patients must return for repeat procedures and surgery is required in 25% of multivessel angioplasty patients by 5 years as shown in the EAST[57] and BARI[58] Trials. After follow-up angiography, mortality was not shown to be different between patients who developed restenosis and those who did not in a large survey of the Emory University database.[59]

Likewise, the incidence of myocardial infarction was very small in this population although restenosis did emerge as a correlate of myocardial infarction. The rarity of myocardial infarction in restenotic patients can be explained by the lesions which are usually fibrotic and not lipid-rich or prone to thrombosis.

The economic impact of restenosis, however, was evident in the fact that those patients with restenosis were more likely to have angina (70.7%) than those patients without restenosis (38.7%). Because of this, repeat angioplasty was performed at 6 months in 56% of those with restenosis and only 4% of those without restenosis. The restenosis patients also required more bypass surgery by 6 years: 22% in the restenosis patients and 6% in the nonrestenosis patients.

Results of randomized trials of patients with multivessel disease also support the economic impact of restenosis. In the EAST Trial, the restenosis rate per lesion, observed by 1 year, totaled 44%.[7] This did not result in increased mortality in the percutaneous transluminal coronary angiography (PTCA) group compared to the patients randomized to surgery, but did result in a dramatic difference in the need for repeat PTCA and surgery by 3 years. The fact that over 50% of the patients required PTCA or coronary artery bypass graft by 3 years resulted in a nearly complete loss of the cost advantage of angioplasty over surgery by that time.[60]

A model based on several clinical trials was created by the Duke University group.[61] Calculating that a restenosis rate of 40% results in a 23% to 35% event rate, they projected savings from various reductions in restenosis. A cost savings from hospital and professional fees would be $1400 per patient for a 25% reduction in restenosis and $2000 per patient if restenosis rates were reduced by 33%. These figures do not reflect additional savings from lost productivity and medication costs.

Two new therapies to reduce late cardiac events have been analyzed for economic impact. Stenting in the STRESS Trial was more expensive than PTCA because of the high cost of the stent and the prolonged hospital stay mandated in that trial. Overall 1-year costs, however, were only a few hundred dollars more in the stent group because this strategy reduced restenosis.[62] The antiplatelet IIb/IIIa receptor blocker, Reopro, also showed a substantial post-discharge cost savings due to a reduction in clinical events.[63]

Conclusions

Restenosis following coronary interventions remains a major limitation to further application of these techniques. Despite progress against restenosis, especially in the form of coronary stenting, restenosis remains a major contributor to symptomatic limitation and medical resource utilization, although it is not a major contributor to cardiac mortality. Affordable new therapies, which could reduce restenosis by one fourth, one third, one half, or more, would have a profound effect on patient comfort and medical costs. Endovascular radiation is an exciting candidate therapy.

References

1. Pepine CJ, Hirshfeld JW, Macdonald RG, et al (M-HEART group). A controlled trial of corticosteroids to prevent restenosis after coronary angioplasty. Circulation 1990;81:1753–1761.

2. The Multicenter European Research Trial with Cilazapril after Angioplasty to Prevent Transluminal Coronary Obstruction and Restenosis (MERCATOR) study group. Does the new angiotensin converting enzyme inhibitor cilazapril prevent restenosis after PTCA? Circulation 1992;86:100–110.

3. Desmet WJ, Vrolix MC, de Scheerder IK, et al. Angiotensin-converting enzyme inhibition with fosinopril sodium in the prevention of restenosis after coronary angioplasty. 1994;Circulation 89:385–392.

4. Kent KN, Williams DO, Cassagneau B, et al. Double-blind, controlled trial of the effect of angiopeptin on coronary restenosis following coronary angioplasty [abstract]. Circulation 1993;88 (suppl 1):594.

5. Serruys PW, Klein W, Tijssen JPG, et al. Evaluation of ketanserin in the prevention of restenosis after PTCA. Circulation 1993;88:1588–1601.

6. Weintraub WS, Boccuzzi SJ, Klein JL, et al. Lack of effect of lovastatin on restenosis after coronary angioplasty. N Engl J Med 1994;331:1331–1337.

7. Zhao X-Q, Brown BG, Hillger LA, King SB III. One-year frequency of restenosis after PTCA in EAST [abstract]. J Am Coll Cardiol 1996;27:54A.

8. Fischman DL, Leon MB, Baim DS. A randomized comparison of stent placement and balloon angioplasty in the treatment of coronary artery disease. N Engl J Med 1994;331:496–501.

9. Serruys PW, de Jaegere P, Kiemeneij F, et al. A comparison of balloon-expandable stent implantation with balloon angioplasty in patients with coronary artery disease. N Engl J Med 1994;331:489–495.

10. Mintz GS, Popma JJ, Pichard AD, et al. Mechanisms of later arterial responses to transcatheter therapy: A serial quantitative angiographic and intravascular ultrasound study [abstract]. Circulation 1994;90:124.

11. Gravanis MB, Roubin GS. Histopathologic phenomena at the site of coronary angioplasty. Human Pathol 1989;20:477–485.

12. Waller BF. Morphologic correlates of coronary angiographic patterns at the site of coronary angioplasty. Clin Cardiol 1988;11:817–822.

13. Johnson DE, Hinohara T, Selmon MR, et al. Primary peripheral arterial stenoses and restenoses excised by transluminal atherectomy: Histopathologic study. J Am Coll Cardiol 1990;15:419–425.

14. Nobuyoshi M, Kimura T, Nosaka H, et al. Restenosis after successful PTCA: Serial angiographic followup of 229 patients. J Am Coll Cardiol 1988;12:616–623.

15. Karas SP, Gravanis MB, Santoian EC, et al. Coronary intimal proliferation after balloon injury and stenting in swine: An animal model of restenosis. J Am Coll Cardiol 1992;20:467–474.

16. Thornton MA, Gruentzig AR, Hollman J, et al. Coumadin and aspirin in the prevention of recurrence after transluminal coronary angioplasty: A randomized study. Circulation 1984;69:721–727.

17. Ellis SG, Roubin GS, Wilentz IJ, et al. Effect of 18 to 24 hour heparin administered for prevention of restenosis after uncomplicated coronary angioplasty. Am Heart J 1989;117:777–782.

18. Chesebro JH, Webster MWI, Reeder GS, et al. Coronary angioplasty antiplatelet therapy reduces acute complications but not restenosis [abstract]. Circulation 1989;80(suppl 2):64.

19. Schwartz L, Bourassa MG, Lesperance J, et al. Aspirin and dipyridamole in the prevention of restenosis after PTCA. N Engl J Med 1988;318:1714–1719.

20. Raizner AE, Hollman J, Abukhalil J, Demke D. Ciprostene for restenosis revisted: Quantitative analysis of angiograms [abstract]. J Am Coll Cardiol 1993;21:321A.

21. Whitworth HB, Roubin GS, Hollman J, et al. Effects of nifedipine on recurrent stenosis after PTCA. J Am Coll Cardiol 1986;8:1271–1276.

22. Corcos T, David PR, Val PG, et al. Failure of diltiazem to prevent restenosis after PTCA. Am Heart J 1985;109:926–931.

23. Dehmer GJ, Popma JJ, Egerton K, et al. Reduction in the rate of early restenosis after coronary angioplasty by a diet supplemented with w-3 fatty acids. N Engl J Med 1988;319:733–740.

24. Reis GJ, Boucher TM, Slipperly ME, et al. Randomized trial of fish oil for the prevention of restenosis after coronary angioplasty. Lancet 1989;2:177–181.

25. Maresta A, Balducelli M, Cantini L, Casari A, et al, for the STARC Investigators. Tra-

pidil (triazolopyrimidine), a platelet-derived growth factor antagonist, reduces restenosis after percutaneous transluminal coronary angioplasty: Results of the randomized double-blind STARC study. Circulation 1994;90:2710–2715.

26. Schneider JE, Berk BC, Gravanis MB, et al. Probucol decreases neointimal formation in a swine model of coronary artery balloon injury: A possible role for antioxidants in restenosis. Circulation 1993;88:628–637.

27. Lee YJ, Daida H, Yokoi H, et al. Effectiveness of probucol in preventing restenosis after percutaneous transluminal coronary angioplasty. Jpn Heart J 1996;37:327–332.

28. Tardif JC, Cote G, Lesperance J, et al. Probucol and multivitamins in the prevention of restenosis after coronary angioplasty: Multivitamins and Probucol Study Group. N Engl J Med 1997;337:365–372.

29. The EPIC Investigators. Use of a monoclonal antibody directed against the platelet glycoprotein IIb/IIIa receptor in high-risk coronary angioplasty. N Engl J Med 1994;330:956–961.

30. The EPILOG Investigators. Platelet glycoprotein IIb/IIIa receptor blockade and low-dose heparin during percutaneous coronary revascularization. N Engl J Med 1997;336:1689–1696.

31. The CAPTURE Investigators. Randomised placebo-controlled trial of abciximab before and during coronary intervention in refractory unstable angina: The CAPTURE Study. Lancet 1997;349:1429–1435.

32. The RESTORE Investigators. Effects of platelet glycoprotein IIb/IIIa blockade with tirofiban on adverse cardiac events in patients with unstable angina or acute myocardial infarction undergoing coronary angioplasty. Circulation 1997;96:1445–1453.

33. The RESTORE Investigators. Six month angiographic and clinical followup of patients prospectively randomized to either tirofiban or placebo during angioplasty in the RESTORE trial. J Am Coll Cardiol 1998;32:28–34.

34. Wolinsky H, Thung SW. Use of a perforated balloon catheter to deliver concentrated heparin into the wall of the normal canine artery. J Am Coll Cardiol 1991;15:475–481.

35. Santoian EC, Gravanis MB, Schneider JE, et al. Use of the porous balloon in porcine coronary arteries. Rationale for low pressure and volume delivery. Cathet Cardiovasc Diagn 1993;30:348–354.

36. Slepian MJ. Polymeric endoluminal paving and sealing: Therapeutics at the crossroads of biomechanics and pharmacology. In: Topol EJ (ed): Textbook of Interventional Cardiology. Philadelphia: Saunders; 1990:647–670.

37. Nabel EG, Plautz G, Nabel GJ. Gene transfer into vascular cells. J Am Coll Cardiol 1991;17:189B-194B.

38. Wolinsky H, King SB, Barbere MD. Catheter and method for locally applying medication to the wall of a blood vessel or other body lumen. United States Patent #5,087,244. February 11, 1992.

39. Topol EJ, Leya F, Pinkderton CA, et al. A comparison of patients with coronary artery disease. N Engl J Med 1993;329:221–227.

40. Adelman AG, Cohen EA, Kimball BP, et al. A comparison of directional atherectomy with balloon angioplasty for lesions of the left anterior descending coronary artery. N Engl J Med 1993;329:228–233.

41. Baim DS, Kuntz RE, Sharma SK, et al. Acute results of the ranadomized trial of the Balloon versus Optimal Atherectomy Trial (BOAT). Circulation 1995;91:1966–1974.

42. Bittl JA, Kuntz RE, Estella P, et al. Analysis of late lumen narrowing after excimer laser facilitated coronary angioplasty. J Am Coll Cardiol 1994;23:1314–1320.

43. Reifart N, Vandormael M, Krajcar M, et al. Randomized comparison of angioplasty of complex coronary lesions at a single center: Excimer Laser, Rotational Atherectomy, and Balloon Angioplasty Comparison (ERBAC) study. Circulation 1997;96:91–98.

44. Serruys PW, Emanuelsson H, van der Giessen W, et al. Heparin-coated Palmaz-Schatz stents in human coronary arteries: Early outcome of the Benestent-II Pilot Study. Circulation 1996;93:412–422.

45. Mehran R, Mintz GS, Popma JJ, et al. Mechanisms and results of balloon angioplasty for the treatment of in-stent restenosis. Am J Cardiol 1996;78:618–622.

46. Baim DS, Levine MJ, Leon MB, et al, for the U.S. Palmaz Stent Investigators. Management of restenosis within the Palmaz-Schatz coronary stent (The U.S. multicenter experience). Am J Cardiol 1993;71:364–366.

47. Gordon PC, Gibson M, Cohen DJ, et al. Mechanism of restenosis and redilation within coronary stents-quantitative angiographic assessment. J Am Coll Cardiol 1993;21:1166–1174.
48. Macander PJ, Roubin GS, Agrawal SK, et al. Balloon angioplasty for treatment of in-stent restenosis: Feasibility, safety, and efficacy. Cathet Cardiovasc Diagn 1994;32:125–131.
49. Schomig A, Kastrati A, Dietz R, et al. Emergency coronary stenting for dissection during percutaneous transluminal coronary angioplasty: Angiographic followup after stenting and after repeat angioplasty of the stented segment. J Am Coll Cardiol 1994;23:1053–1060.
50. Yokoi H, Kimura T, Nakagawa Y, et al. Long-term clinical and quantitative angiographic followup after the Palmaz-Schatz stent restenosis. J Am Coll Cardiol 1996;27:224.
51. Sharma SK, Duvvuri S, Dangas G, et al. Rotational atherectomy for in-stent restenosis. Acute and long-term results of the first 100 cases. J Am Coll Cardiol 1998;32:1358–1365.
52. Radke PW, Klues HG, Haager PK, et al. Mechanisms of acute lumen gain and recurrent restenosis after rotational atherectomy of diffuse in-stent restenosis: A quantitative angiographic and intravascular ultrasound study. J Am Coll Cardiol 1999;34:33–39.
53. Mehran R, Mintz GS, Satler LF, et al. Treatment of in-stent restenosis with excimer laser coronary angioplasty: Mechanisms and results compared with PTCA alone. Circulation 1997;96:2183–2189.
54. Sakamoto T, Kawarabayshi T, Taguchi H, et al. Intravascular ultrasound-guided balloon angioplasty for treatment of in-stent restenosis. Cathet Cardiovasc Intervent 1999;47:298–303.
55. Waksman R, White LR, Chan RC, et al. Intracoronary beta radiation therapy for patients with in-stent restenosis: The 6 months clinical and angiographic results. Circulation 1999;100(suppl I):I-75.
56. Leon MB, Moses JW, Lansky AJ, et al. Intracoronary gamma radiation for prevention of recurrent in-stent restenosis: Final results from the Gamma-1 Trial. Circulation 1999;100(suppl I):I-75.
57. King SB III, Lembo NJ, Weintraub WS, et al. A randomized trial comparing coronary angioplasty with coronary bypass surgery. N Engl J Med 1994;331:1044–1050.
58. The Bypass Angioplasty Revascularization Investigation (BARI) Investigators. Comparison of coronary bypass surgery with angioplasty in patients with multivessel disease. N Engl J Med 1996;335:217–225.
59. Weintraub WS, Ghazzal ZMB, Douglas JS, et al. Long term clinical followup in patients with angiographic restudy after successful angioplasty. Circulation 1993;87:831–840.
60. Weintraub WS, Mauldin PD, Becker E, King SB. The impact of additional procedures on the cost at 3 years of coronary angioplasty and coronary surgery in the EAST trial [abstract]. Circulation 1993;90(suppl I):I-480.
61. Mark DB, Gardner LG, Nelson CL, et al. Long-term cost of therapy for CAD: A prospective comparison of coronary angioplasty, coronary bypass surgery and medical therapy in 2,258 patients [abstract]. Circulation 1993;89 (suppl I):I-480.
62. Cohen DJ, Krumholz HM, Sukin C, et al, for the STRESS Investigators. Economic outcomes in the randomized stent restenosis study (STRESS): In-hospital and one year followup cost [abstract]. Circulation 1994;90(suppl I):I-620.
63. Mark DR, Talley JD, Lam LC, et al. Reduced restenosis from aggressive platelet inhibition reduces the cost of high risk angioplasty [abstract]. Circulation 1994;90(suppl I):I-44.

Restenosis and Remodeling

Robert S. Schwartz, MD, and
David R. Holmes, Jr., MD

Introduction

Restenosis remains a major problem in interventional cardiology. Most pharmacological and interventional devices have not decreased clinical restenosis rates despite much speculation and many studies, although the intracoronary stent improves long-term minimum luminal diameter and lowers restenosis rates.[1–6] Success of this device, however, is due to geometric considerations of achieving a larger postprocedural lumen and allowing more late loss without causing severe stenosis.[7,8] The stent possesses little biological activity against neointima, and does not limit neointimal thickening. Indeed, stenting is associated with increased neointima compared to balloon angioplasty.[9–11]

Ongoing failures to limit neointima raise questions about the prevailing idea of medial cell proliferation and neointimal hyperplasia as principal causes of restenosis.[12–15] Evidence suggests that coronary artery size changes (remodeling) following percutaneous revascularization may be responsible for much late lumen loss.[16–20] This is tempered however by confusion arising from a lack of consistent theory, definitions, and data analysis methods. The aim of this chapter is to summarize current data regarding remodeling and restenosis, and to enumerate a framework to analyze the impact of remodeling on the revascularized artery.

Compensatory Arterial Enlargement in Patients: Remodeling by a Different Name

In 1972 Mann et al[21] first reported coronary arterial size changes associated with atherosclerosis. African Masai tribesmen maintained large coronary artery lumina despite substantial atherosclerotic plaque size. With age, the coronary arteries developed thicker atherosclerotic plaque, but their coronary arteries also enlarged to accommodate plaque. The net result was actual luminal enlargement despite plaque formation. Despite equivalent plaque size, the Masai maintain larger lumina than their American counterparts.

Glagov concisely refined the principles of atherosclerotic artery growth, termed compensatory enlargement. A retrospective autopsy study of left main atherosclerosis documented compensatory enlargement with increased plaque

From Waksman R (ed.). *Vascular Brachytherapy, Third Edition.* Armonk, NY: Futura Publishing Co., Inc.; © 2002.

size, maintaining lumen size.[22–24] There was a poor relationship between lumen size and artery size until the histopathological stenosis reached 40%. Only after plaque volume increased above this threshold did lumen compromise occur, with lumen size inversely proportional to plaque volume.

Animal models show comparable effects. For example, Armstrong et al[25] measured lumen area, medial area, and intimal area in adult macaque monkeys consuming atherogenic diets. The relationship between these measurements demonstrated that lumen size was preserved, and no significant stenoses developed.

Arterial enlargement to accommodate atherosclerotic plaque is thus well established in the clinical and animal research literature. Lumen area changes only marginally with plaque growth, until a threshold plaque burden is reached. Arteries expand with plaque growth only in the early phases; expansion ceases after a threshold plaque size is reached. With further plaque growth the lumen narrows proportionally.

A New Cause of Coronary Restenosis: Remodeling

Artery size changes also occur following coronary angioplasty as neointimal hyperplasia forms; this phenomenon is termed remodeling.[26–31] Unfortunately, inconsistency by different groups investigating the problem has led to confusion.[32–36] Table 1 lists several terms applied in the literature to artery size changes and remodeling.

Kakuta et al[37] described arterial remodeling in atherosclerotic rabbit iliac arteries following balloon angioplasty. Remodeling (vessel enlargement) was more pronounced in animals without angiographic restenosis. Arterial expansion (or lack of it) was more important as a cause of restenosis than neointimal thickening. A strong relationship occurred between artery size and neointima, whereas none was found between neointima and lumen area.

Conversely, another group reported *loss* of arterial size in atherosclerotic rabbits after angioplasty.[38] Late lumen loss was larger than expected from neointimal size alone. Remodeling was defined as histologically measured neointima subtracted from late angiographic lumen loss. Post et al[20] reported similar arterial contraction in normal and hypercholesterolemic rabbit femoral and iliac arteries and also in normal pig coronary arteries. Conversely, with use of a porcine model, Waksman et al[39] concluded that luminal stenoses were not due to artery size changes, but were instead due primarily to neointimal formation. No formal or consistent definition has been applied to precisely define remodeling.

Table 1
Terms in the Literature for Remodeling
Compensatory enlargement Artery expansion Acute recoil Chronic recoil Chronic constriction Arterial shrinkage

Clinical Studies and Remodeling

Mintz and colleagues[19] first described coronary artery size changes after intervention in patients by use of intravascular ultrasound. In these clinical studies, coronary arteries contracted (here defined as remodeling), a phenomenon suggested to be a major cause of clinical restenosis. Further studies suggested that remodeling is limited in stenting, and that stent restenosis is principally a result of neointimal hyperplasia.[10]

Di Mario and colleagues[18] studied artery size changes associated with percutaneous transluminal coronary angioplasty (PTCA) and directional coronary atherectomy (DCA) and found that 92% of late lumen loss in the DCA group was primarily due to plaque increase from neointimal growth. Conversely, only 32% of the lumen loss in the PTCA group was due to plaque increase, with the remaining 68% from chronic reduction in total vessel area or from remodeling. This study concluded that in PTCA, remodeling is the dominant mechanism of late lumen loss.

The term remodeling is thus used inconsistently throughout the literature, variably referring to either enlargement or contraction of the internal or external elastic lamina following arterial injury. Further inconsistencies occur with the atherosclerosis literature, since remodeling here typically refers to enlargement rather than shrinkage.[35]

A Broad Definition of Remodeling

On the basis of the foregoing, arteries can enlarge, contract, or remain unchanged after balloon angioplasty in response to neointimal thickening. All size changes should be allowed in a broad remodeling definition. Since artery size changes may be favorable (adaptive) or unfavorable (pathological) in preserving lumen size (Fig. 1), neointima must be described in relation to artery size changes. Perfect remodeling occurs when the artery expands to equal or exceed neointimal growth. Lumen size is unchanged, and no angiographic stenosis occurs. Favorable remodeling occurs when an artery enlarges partially to compensate for neointimal thickness. Although lumen size decreases, it does so by less than the neointimal thickness, thus blunting the luminal effects of neointima.

Conversely, unfavorable (or pathological) remodeling occurs when an artery contracts. If artery size remains constant, the lumen is angiographically narrowed one-to-one with neointimal thickening. Worse, if the artery also contracts, the lumen is narrowed by more than neointimal thickness. Table 2 illustrates this principle, showing effects on lumen from all possibilities of remodeling.

A continuous spectrum thus exists between two outcomes of angioplasty: complete or partial compensatory enlargement at one extreme, and arterial contraction at the other. Any spectrum of size change may occur between these two responses. Remodeling is thus a continuously variable process that may have either beneficial or deleterious effects on the arterial lumen.

Remodeling and the Adventitia

We must conclude that the adventitia plays an important role in remodeling, since this connective tissue forms a ring around the artery. Important work has sug-

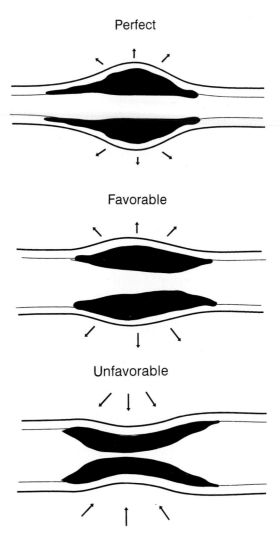

Figure 1. Perfect, favorable, and unfavorable remodeling are demonstrated in this figure. Perfect remodeling occurs when there is no lumen loss despite plaque or neointimal growth (line labeled 1:1). Favorable remodeling occurs when an artery partially expands in response to neointima or plaque. Unfavorable remodeling occurs when an artery either cannot expand, or shrinks after injury. Aneurysmal dilatation occurs if the artery expands greater than neointimal formation.

Table 2

Hypothetical Remolding Relationships Between
Neointima, Artery Size, and Net Lumen Size Effects

Neointima/plaque Size Change	Artery Size Change	Net Lumen Effect
Increase	Increase, greater than neointimal change	Increase
Increase	Increase, equal to neointimal change	No effect
Increase	Increase, less than neointimal change	Decrease
Increase	Decrease	Decrease

gested that cells of neointima may come from the adventitia.[40,41] Moreover, recent studies have shown that stenotic lesions can be produced in normal porcine coronary arteries by use of either heat or copper stent implantation.[42] Markedly different histopathological responses are found in the adventitia with these interventions. Heat injury causes dense collagen formation and little inflammation. Little remodeling occurs with this injury. Conversely, substantial remodeling occurs with copper stent lesions, where the adventitia is infiltrated by a dense inflammatory response. Adventitial inflammation from copper stent lesions has little structural integrity and cannot exert any force to prevent artery expansion. The artery expands easily as neointima forms, since there is little resistance to the process. Adventitial collagen formation in heat lesions provides significant structural strength that resists outward force as the artery attempts to expand from neointimal formation. This concept is quite attractive, as it relates to wound healing and contractures that form with many injuries involving dense collagen formation such as densely collagenous esophageal strictures. The ability of an artery to react to luminal tissue growth appears intimately related to cellular occurrences in the adventitia.

Figure 2 shows quantitative description of arterial expansion and neointima/plaque formation. The slope of the line relating neointimal growth with artery expansion is key to lumen size. If the slope is near 1.0, all neointimal growth is accommodated by artery expansion, whereas if the slope is zero (or less than zero in cases where the artery contracts), all neointimal thickening causes lumen loss. A key determinant of whether restenosis occurs in any lesion is the slope of the neointima-artery size line. Different lesions will presumably exhibit different slopes, if data from the porcine coronary injury studies are consistent. The slope is a continuous variable, and constitutes a spectrum of remodeling that may be useful for quantitating the artery size change.

A remarkable implication of this concept is that the degree of neointimal thickening following angioplasty (without stenting) may not be relevant to the

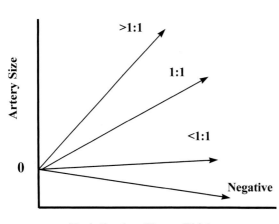

Neointimal or Plaque Thickness

Figure 2. Hypothetical graph indicating possible relationships between neointima or plaque formation and simultaneous artery size change. Cases of perfect (labeled 1:1), favorable (<1:1), and unfavorable (zero line, or negative) remodeling are shown. Better-than-perfect remodeling occurs when the artery expands by more than neointimal volume (>1:1, and slope >1.0), creating aneurysmal dilation. Conversely, a slope less than zero indicates constrictive remodeling where the artery shrinks despite neointimal growth. In this case the lumen is severely compromised, both from arterial shrinkage and from neointimal formation. Remodeling is a continuous variable, with varying degrees of expansion possible, and is determined by the relative slope in this relationship.

likelihood of restenosis. In some cases the artery expands appropriately to allow luminal preservation despite neointimal growth. More neointima simply causes more expansion to preserve lumen. In this situation a lesion moves along a single neointima-artery size line (Fig. 2) with neointimal growth. It is only when an artery is constrained to a low slope line that lumen compromise occurs from neointima. It is thus the ability (or lack thereof) of an artery to expand that determines its propensity for restenosis. With adequate expansion, neointimal thickness is not relevant. Conversely, with little expansion, or with contraction, neointimal size is crucial. Much work must be done to establish the nature of such relationships in human atherosclerosis and intervention.

Conclusions

Remodeling, geometry, and artery size changes are crucial to understanding restenosis. The exact role of remodeling and neointima in restenosis remains unclear despite much study. Ongoing studies and recent advances in stent technology will help delineate the impact of remodeling and neointima on clinical and angiographic restenosis. As this work proceeds, standardization of definitions and methods of analysis are essential toward a better understanding of this important pathophysiological process.

References

1. Serruys PW, de Jaegere P, Kiemeneij F, et al. A comparison of balloon-expandable stent implantation with balloon angioplasty in patients with coronary artery disease. N Engl J Med 1994;331:489–495.
2. Fischman DL, Leon MB, Baim DS, et al, for the Stent Restenosis Study Investigators. A randomized comparison of coronary-stent placement and balloon angioplasty in the treatment of coronary artery disease. N Engl J Med 1994;331:496–501.
3. Eeckhout E, Kappenberger L, Goy JL. Stents for intracoronary placement: Current status and future directions. J Am Coll Cardiol 1996;27:757–765.
4. Davis G, Roberts D. Articulation strut coronary restenosis in Palmaz-Schatz stents. Int J Cardiol 1996;54:266–271.
5. Moscucci M, Piana RN, Kuntz RE, et al. Effect of prior coronary restenosis on the risk of subsequent restenosis after stent placement or directional atherectomy. Am J Cardiol 1994;73:1147–1153.
6. Kuntz RE, Safian RD, Carrozza JP, et al. The importance of acute luminal diameter in determining restenosis after coronary atherectomy or stenting. Circulation 1992;86:1827–1835.
7. Dussaillant GR, Mintz GS, Pichard AD, et al. Small stent size and intimal hyperplasia contribute to restenosis: A volumetric intravascular ultrasound analysis. J Am Coll Cardiol 1995;26:720–724.
8. Mintz G, Pichard A, Kent K, et al. Endovascular stents reduce restenosis by eliminating geometric arterial remodeling: A serial intravascular ultrasound study. J Am Coll Cardiol 1995;95:36A.
9. Mintz GS, Popma JJ, Hong MK, et al. Intravascular ultrasound to discern device-specific effects and mechanisms of restenosis. Am J Cardiol 1996;78:18–22.
10. Mintz G, Pichard A, Kent K, et al. Endovascular stents reduce restenosis by eliminating geometric arterial remodeling: A serial intravascular ultrasound study [abstract]. J Am Coll Cardiol 1995;95:701–705.
11. Mintz G, Kent K, Satler L, et al. Dimorphic mechanisms of restenosis after DCA and stents: A serial intravascular ultrasound study. Circulation 1995;92:2610.
12. Schwartz RS, Edwards WD, Bailey KR, et al. Differential neointimal response to coro-

nary artery injury in pigs and dogs. Implications for restenosis models. Arterioscler Thromb 1994;14:395–400.

13. Schwartz SM, de Blois D, O'Brien ER. The intima. Soil for atherosclerosis and restenosis. Circ Res 1995;77:445–465.

14. Schwartz R, Holmes D Jr, Topol E. The restenosis paradigm revisited: An alternative proposal for cellular mechanisms. J Am Coll Cardiol 1992;20:1284–1293.

15. O'Brien E, Alpers CE, Stewart DK, et al. Proliferation in primary and restenotic coronary atherectomy tissue. Implications for antiproliferative therapy. Circ Res 1993;73:223–231.

16. Mintz GS, Kent KM, Pichard AD, et al. Contribution of inadequate arterial remodeling to the development of focal coronary artery stenoses. An intravascular ultrasound study. Circulation 1997;95:1791–1798.

17. Mintz GS, Kent KM, Pichard AD, et al. Intravascular ultrasound insights into mechanisms of stenosis formation and restenosis. Cardiol Clin 1997;15:17–29.

18. Di Mario C, Gil R, Camenzind E, et al. Quantitative assessment with intracoronary ultrasound of the mechanisms of restenosis after percutaneous transluminal coronary angioplasty and directional coronary atherectomy. Am J Cardiol 1995;75: 772–777.

19. Mintz G, Kovach J, Javier S, et al. Geometric remodeling is the predominant of late lumen loss after coronary angioplasty [abstract]. Circulation 1993;88:I654.

20. Post MJ, Borst C, Kuntz RE. The relative importance of arterial remodeling compared with intimal hyperplasia in lumen renarrowing after balloon angioplasty. A study in the normal rabbit and the hypercholesterolemic Yucatan micropig. Circulation 1994;89:2816–2821.

21. Mann G, Spoerry A, Gray M, Jarashow D. Atherosclerosis in the Masai. Am J Epidemiol 1972;95:26–37.

22. Glagov S, Weisenberg G, Zarins CK, et al. Compensatory enlargement of human atherosclerotic coronary arteries. N Engl J Med 1987;316:1371–1375.

23. Zarins C, Weisenberg E, Kolettis G, et al. Differential enlargement of artery segments in response to enlarging atherosclerotic plaques. J Vasc Surg 1988;7:386–394.

24. Zarins CK, Lu CT, Gewertz BL, et al. Arterial disruption and remodeling following balloon dilatation. Surgery 1982;92:1086–1095.

25. Armstrong M, Heistad D, Marcus M, et al. Structural and hemodynamic responses of peripheral arteries of macaque monkeys to atherogenic diet. Arteriosclerosis 1985;5:336–346.

26. Lafont A, Guzman L, Whitlow P, et al. Restenosis after experimental angioplasty. Intimal, medial, and adventitial changes associated with constrictive remodeling. Circ Res 1995;76:996–1002.

27. Guzman LA, Mick MJ, Arnold AM, et al. Role of intimal hyperplasia and arterial remodeling after balloon angioplasty: An experimental study in the atherosclerotic rabbit model. Arterioscler Thromb Vasc Biol 1996;16:479–487.

28. Geary RL, Williams JK, Golden D, et al. Time course of cellular proliferation, intimal hyperplasia, and remodeling following angioplasty in monkeys with established atherosclerosis. A nonhuman primate model of restenosis. Arterioscler Thromb Vasc Biol 1996;16:34–43.

29. Waller BF, Orr CM, Van Tassel J, et al. Coronary artery and saphenous vein graft remodeling: A review of histologic findings after various interventional procedures. Part V. Clin Cardiol 1997;20:67–74.

30. Waller BF, Orr CM, VanTassel J, et al. Coronary artery and saphenous vein graft remodeling: A review of histologic findings after various interventional procedures. Part I. Clin Cardiol 1996;19:744–748.

31. Zalewski A, Shi Y. Vascular myofibroblasts. Lessons from coronary repair and remodeling. Arterioscler Thromb Vasc Biol 1997;17:417–422.

32. Davies M. Remodeling, response to injury, and repair in the arterial wall. Curr Opin Cardiol 1990;5:387–391.

33. Cotton P. Restenosis trials suggest role for remodeling. JAMA 1994;271:1302–1303.

34. Dzau V, Gibbons G. Vascular remodeling: Mechanisms and implications. J Cardiovasc Pharmacol 1993;21(suppl 1):S1–S5.

35. Isner J. Vascular remodeling. Honey I think I shrunk the artery. Circulation 1994;89:2937–2940.

36. Post M, de Smet B, van der Helm Y, et al. Arterial remodeling contributes to restenosis after angioplasty, but is prevented by stenting in the atherosclerotic micropig. J Am Coll Cardiol 1995;Feb:303A.
37. Kakuta T, Currier JW, Haudenschild CC, et al. Differences in compensatory vessel enlargement, not intimal formation, account for restenosis after angioplasty in the hypercholesterolemic rabbit model. Circulation 1994;89:2809–2815.
38. Lafont A, Chisolm G, Whitlow P, et al. Postangioplasty restenosis in the atherosclerotic rabbit: Proliferative response or chronic constriction [abstract]? Circulation 1993;88 (suppl 1):521.
39. Waksman R, Robinson K, Sigman S, et al. Balloon overstretch injury correlates with neointimal formation and not with vascular remodeling in the pig coronary restenosis model [abstract]. J Am Coll Cardiol 1994;Feb:138A.
40. Scott NA, Cipolla GD, Ross CE, et al. Identification of a potential role for the adventitia in vascular lesion formation after balloon overstretch injury of porcine coronary arteries. Circulation 1996;93:2178–2187.
41. Scott RJ, Hall PA, Haldane JS, et al. A comparison of immunohistochemical markers of cell proliferation with experimentally determined growth fraction. J Pathol 1991; 165:173–178.
42. Staab M, Edwards W, Srivatsa S, et al. Adventitial injury and cellular response markedly affect arterial remodeling and neointimal formation [abstract]. Circulation 1995;92:I93.

## Chapter 3

Adventitial Remodeling Associated with Postangioplasty Restenosis

Josiah N. Wilcox, PhD, and Neal A. Scott, MD, PhD

Introduction

Postangioplasty restenosis is one of the major problems confronting cardiology today. More than 400,000 angioplasties are performed every year in the United States and 30% to 40% of these are subsequently affected by development of a postangioplasty restenosis lesion. While cellular proliferation after balloon injury is the most likely mechanism for the development of clinical postangioplasty restenosis, there is controversy regarding the degree of the proliferative response.[1,2] Endothelial denudation of peripheral vessels by use of a Fogarty catheter in combination with various degrees of smooth muscle cell damage in rats and rabbits induces smooth muscle cell proliferation and development of a neointima. This approach has been used extensively as a model for clinical postangioplasty restenosis. In this model, cell proliferation begins in the media within 48 hours after injury; after a week these cells migrate across the internal elastic lamina to form an intimal mass of actively proliferating cells.[3,4] Consequently, the major focus of efforts to prevent postangioplasty restenosis up to this time has been on regulating cell proliferation in the intima or media, with very little consideration about how other layers may contribute to the problem. This may be incorrect, and in this chapter we suggest that the adventitia may also play an important role in lesion formation after angioplasty.

Pigs have been used as models for postangioplasty restenosis with some success.[5-12] Since the coronary arteries of the pig and human are similar in size, the same clinical angioplasty catheters may be employed to perform balloon overstretch injury in the porcine angioplasty model as are used in the clinical interventional laboratory. This is important, since the characteristics of a Fogarty catheter and a clinical angioplasty catheter are very different. The clinical angioplasty catheter is a rigid, noncompliant balloon 2 to 4 cm in length that enlarges the lumen by causing a break in the medial wall. Fogarty catheters, which have been typically used for angioplasty studies in small animal models, are soft, compliant balloons which gently rub the endothelial cells off the surface of the artery with minimal medial

This work was supported by NIH grant HL47838 (JW) and a grant from the Gruentzig Center for Interventional Cardiology.
From Waksman R (ed.). *Vascular Brachytherapy, Third Edition*. Armonk, NY: Futura Publishing Co., Inc.; © 2002.

damage. These two types of injury are therefore very different, with the former possibly being closer to what occurs in human vessels after angioplasty.

Balloon overstretch injury of porcine coronary arteries by percutaneous angioplasty by use of a clinical catheter sized 1.3 times the vessel diameter tears the media wall, exposes the outer elastic lamina, and stimulates the formation of vascular lesions morphologically similar to that seen in human postangioplasty restenosis.[6,8,9] Vascular lesion formation occurs in the region between the broken ends of the media on the luminal side of the internal elastic lamina and is thought to consist of smooth muscle cells coming from the medial wall. Similar tearing of the intima and media occurs as a result of clinical percutaneous transluminal coronary angioplasty and is the primary mechanism for luminal enlargement by angioplasty.[13]

Human postangioplasty restenosis lesions are thought to consist of vascular smooth muscle cells, since the majority of cells in these lesions stain with α-smooth muscle actin.[14] In a similar fashion, it has been concluded that the cells in the porcine intima after balloon overstretch injury are smooth muscle cells, because these are also α-smooth muscle actin positive.[6,8,9] However, this does not necessarily mean that the intima is composed of smooth muscle cells, since there is evidence that many other nonmuscle cells may express α-smooth muscle actin as well with the appropriate stimulation.[15–20]

Myofibroblasts are specialized fibroblast-like cells that show induced expression of α-actin.[15] These cells have the ultrastructural features intermediate between a fibroblast and smooth muscle cell. Myofibroblasts typically lack markers of highly differentiated smooth muscle cells such as desmin, h-caldesmon, and smooth muscle myosin, but show induced expression of α-smooth muscle actin.[15,16,20–22] Recently, myofibroblasts have been identified at sites of healing human myocardial infarctions,[23] indicating that these cells are present in the heart.

Adventitial Responses after Injury of Porcine Coronary Arteries

Recent experiments suggest that myofibroblasts in the adventitia proliferate after angioplasty and may migrate into the neointima where they appear as smooth muscle actin-containing cells.[24–26] Domestic juvenile swine underwent injury to the left anterior descending and circumflex coronary arteries with standard clinical angioplasty balloon catheters. Proliferating cells were identified by injecting 5-bromo-2-deoxyuridine (BRdU) prior to sacrifice and localizing cells containing BRdU by immunohistochemistry. The time course of cell proliferation was not appreciably different to that seen previously in rats and rabbits,[3,27] with proliferation beginning between 24 and 48 hours after injury in the pig (Table 1). However, in the pig model the greatest number of proliferating cells 2 to 3 days after angioplasty was found primarily in the adventitia surrounding the injured artery and not in the medial wall. This proliferation was greatest in the adventitia at the site of the medial tear localized just beneath the external elastic lamina (Fig. l, panel A). Proliferating adventitial cells extended circumferentially around the entire vessel, even on the side opposite the medial tear furthest away from the injury site. One week after angioplasty, cell proliferation was reduced in the media and adventitia, with the greatest number of proliferating cells found in the neointima at this time. The adventitia was also the site of the greatest platelet-derived growth factor-A (PDGF-A) and PDGF receptor expression as determined

Table 1

The Time Course and Distribution of Cell Proliferation after Balloon Overstretch Injury of Porcine Coronary Arteries

		Mean Percent of Proliferating Cells ($\pm$SEM) BrDU-Positive Cells/(Hematoxylin Stained Nuclei + BrDU-Positive Cells) $\times$ 100				
		Compartment Number				
	# Animals	# Vessels	1	2	3	4	5
1 Day	2	3	0	0	0	0	NA
2 Days	1	2	3.41$\pm$0.90	1.95$\pm$0.65	26.37$\pm$1.59	20.08$\pm$4.63	NA
3 Days	3	4	11.25$\pm$2.05	5.35$\pm$1.02	32.53$\pm$1.40	23.71$\pm$4.11	NA
7 Days	5	5	2.61$\pm$0.59	1.31$\pm$0.22	8.60$\pm$3.02	4.78$\pm$3.10	17.00$\pm$3.72
14 Days	3	3	1.29$\pm$0.21	2.21$\pm$0.47	3.13$\pm$1.27	0.62$\pm$0.34	8.31$\pm$1.72

5-Bromo-2′-deoxyuridine (BrDU) was injected in three doses of 50mg/kg at 24, 16, and 8 h prior to necropsy. Proliferating cells were identified by BrDU immunohisto-chemistry and quantified using computer-assisted digital morphometry. Cell proliferation was analyzed in five regions in each vessel: 1) in the media adjacent to the me-dial tear; 2) in the media on the side opposite the medial tear; 3) in the adventitia adjacent to the medial tear; 4) in the adventitia on the side opposite the medial tear; and 5) in the intima defined as the luminal side of the internal elastic lamina between the torn ends of the media.

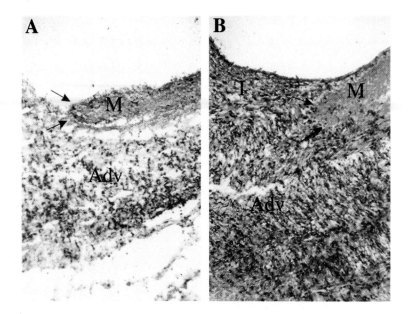

Figure 1. Localization of proliferating cells in the adventitia and their migration into the neointima using bromodeoxyuridine (BRdU) immunohistochemistry. **A.** Double-label immunohistochemistry for BRdU (dark spots), and α-smooth muscle actin (dark gray staining in the media) at the site of balloon overstretch injury of porcine coronary arteries. Animals received BRdU between days 2 and 3 and were sacrificed on day 3. Administration of BRdU between days 2 and 3 predominantly labeled adventitial cells when analyzed on day 3 (see Table 1). Double-label immunohistochemistry on these tissues indicated that the proliferating adventitial cells did not contain α-smooth muscle actin. **B.** To determine the fate of the cells proliferating on day 3, animals were injected with BRdU between days 2 and 3 and sacrificed on day 14 without subsequent BRdU administration. Numerous BRdU-positive cells were found remaining in the adventitia and 43.1±3.3% (mean±SEM) of the neointimal cells were positive as well. Double-label immunohistochemistry was performed to identify the BRdU-positive cells (labeled between days 2 and 3) on day 14. These cells stain uniformly with α-smooth muscle actin antibodies in both the adventitia and neointima. Comparison of the adventitial BRdU/α-smooth muscle actin staining in **A** and **B** suggests that the adventitial cells have changed phenotype and show increased production of contractile proteins by day 14. Many of the BRdU-positive neointimal cells also contained smooth muscle myosin antibody but not h-caldesmon (data not shown). The BRdU-positive adventitial cells did not stain with smooth muscle myosin or caldesmon on day 14. M = media; I = intima; Adv = adventitia; arrows indicate site of medial tear. Magnification = 32×. Reproduced from Reference 26, with permission.

by in situ hybridization. These data suggest that the adventitia may be important with respect to the first wave of growth after angioplasty of coronary arteries with later growth of the lesion occurring in the neointima.

Adventitial Cells May Migrate into the Restenosis Lesion

The finding of increased cell proliferation and growth factor synthesis in the adventitia relative to the medial wall at early times after angioplasty suggests that the adventitia may play a role in the formation of the subsequent vascular lesion. In order to determine the fate of the proliferating adventitial cells, we sought to label this cell population with BRdU at an early time point and then examine the distribution of these cells once the neointima was fully formed. Animals were injured on day 0, injected with BRdU between days 2 and 3, and the distribution of BRdU-positive cells was examined on day 14 without subsequent BRdU injection. Since the adventitial cells comprise the major population of proliferating cells on day 3, we expected that this would enable us to determine if these cells had migrated from their position in the adventitia and contributed to the cellular mass in the neointima. This approach had been used previously to follow the migration and subsequent proliferation of medial cells into the neointima in the rat-carotid injury model using ³H-thymidine labeling.[28] Two weeks after angioplasty a large number of cells labeled with BRdU between days 2 and 3 were still found in the adventitia surrounding the injured vessel; however 43.1±3.3% (mean±SEM) of the neointimal cells were BRdU-positive as well (Fig. 1, panel B). Since the largest proportion of cells incorporating BRdU at the time of BRdU injection between days 2 and 3 is in the adventitia, this suggests that some of the neointimal cells must be the daughter cells derived from the adventitial cells that incorporated BRdU and migrated into the lesion across the external elastic lamina. This is essentially the same experimental evidence that was used to prove that neointimal cells in the rat carotid injury model arise from the medial wall.[28] Additional work must be done in order to establish the exact percentage of cells migrating from the adventitia into the neointima.

The Proliferating Adventitial Cells are Myofibroblasts

Immunohistochemistry was performed to identify the proliferating adventitial cells as well as the cells that migrated to form the neointima. Single-label immunohistochemistry using antibodies against α-smooth muscle actin, smooth muscle myosin, h-caldesmon, or desmin consistently labeled smooth muscle cells in the medial wall of normal arteries but did not stain adventitial cells with the exception of a few smooth muscle cells surrounding small adventitial vessels. Consistent with previous work, vimentin staining of normal vessels was distributed throughout the adventitia and in the medial smooth muscle cells.[29] Single- or double-label immunohistochemistry with α-smooth muscle actin, smooth muscle myosin, h-caldesmon, desmin, or vimentin and the BRdU antibody on tissues from animals injected with BRdU 2 to 3 days after angioplasty and sacrificed on day 3 revealed a very similar pattern of staining, and indicated that the proliferating adventitial cells lacked smooth-muscle–specific markers (Fig. l, panel A).

Two weeks after angioplasty, smooth muscle α-actin staining was found to extend into the surrounding adventitial space well beyond the medial wall including regions where the proliferating cells had been found on day 3. Double-label immunohistochemistry with the α-actin and BRdU antibodies on vessels from animals that received BRdU between days 2 and 3 and were sacrificed on day 14 indicated that the previously actin-negative adventitial cells that had proliferated on day 3 now showed strong α-actin staining (Fig. 1, panel B). In the neointima, almost all of the BRdU-positive cells showed smooth muscle α-actin and vimentin staining. Staining with the other smooth muscle cell markers was much more limited and did not include the adventitial cells that had proliferated on Day 3: smooth muscle myosin was found in the media and neointima, and weakly stained some cells in the adventitia; h-caldesmon staining was restricted to the medial wall with some scattered positive intimal cells but did not stain the adventitial cells; and desmin staining was found in the medial smooth muscle cells alone. Segments of the coronary arteries proximal or distal to the injury site did not show similar changes in adventitial α-actin staining. Together, these data suggest a phenotypic switch of the adventitial cells that are responding to balloon injury by increasing α-actin content.

The observation of a phenotypic modulation of the adventitial cells with respect to actin expression between days 3 and 14 is similar to the phenotypic changes occurring in myofibroblasts associated with wound healing[30] or tumor formation.[21,31] Myofibroblast α-actin synthesis is stimulated in vitro and in vivo in response to a variety of stimuli including heparin,[22] γ-interferon,[32] and transforming growth factor-beta (TGF-β).[33] Expression of α-smooth muscle actin by myofibroblasts in healing skin wounds has been implicated in the process of scar contraction.[30,34] Recent data indicate that vascular remodeling, as indicated by a constriction of the external elastic lamina after angioplasty, may contribute to restenosis.[35–38] Experimental angioplasty studies in rabbits and pigs indicate that after balloon angioplasty the size of the intima does not explain the loss in luminal diameter measured morphometrically or by angiography.[36,37] Recent clinical data support these observations and suggest that clinical restenosis is associated with a constrictive remodeling occurring outside of the injured vessel.[38,39] Data derived from intravascular ultrasound measurements of the external elastic lamina before angioplasty, immediately after angioplasty, and at follow-up indicate that a decrease in the diameter of the external elastic lamina accounts for as much as 66% of late lumen loss.[39] The presence of myofibroblasts in the adventitial space surrounding injured coronary arteries and the upregulation of contractile proteins in these cells may play a role in vascular remodeling by constricting the vessels from the adventitial side, thus contributing to late lumen loss associated with postangioplasty restenosis.

Conclusions

The role of the adventitia in vascular lesion formation has been largely ignored despite numerous studies that have suggested its potential importance. Stripping of the adventitia stimulates vascular lesion formation and has been used as a model for atherosclerosis or postangioplasty restenosis research.[40–42] In addition, changes in the expression of genes like tissue factor[43] or angiotensinogen[44] have been observed in the adventitia after balloon catheter injury of rat aortas. Administration of drugs via the adventitia can stimulate vascular lesion formation. Antisense oligomers directed against c-myb,[45] heparin,[46,47] or calcium antagonists[48] placed in the adventitia have all effectively inhibited vascular lesion formation after denuding balloon catheter injury of rat carotid arteries. It has been assumed that these drugs acted directly on the medial smooth muscle cells, and the adventitia was simply a convenient route for administration. However, based on the current findings, it may be equally valid to hypothesize that these experiments worked through a direct action on adventitial cells rather than the medial smooth muscle cells.

The finding of adventitial proliferation after balloon angioplasty is not necessarily a new one. Balloon overstretch injury of the canine aorta has been shown to produce a medial wall rupture similar to what is seen in the porcine coronary artery system.[49] In these experiments the authors also noted a *marked proliferation of the adventitia which was most prominent at the areas of previous subtotal wall rupture.* They considered the adventitial proliferation to be similar to the formation of a neomedia containing smooth muscle cells and collagen fibers replacing the broken vessel wall. These authors also noted an increase in vasa vasorum development after injury, possibly to support this new tissue. These findings are very similar to what we have seen in the porcine coronary artery system.

The adventitia may be extremely important in regulating the growth of vascular lesions not only in the setting of angioplasty but also after arterial injury caused by vascular surgery. Removal or injury of the adventitia of large blood vessels may lead to endothelial loss on the luminal surface and may stimulate vascular lesion formation.[41,42] Vascular surgeons typically remove the adventitia and adherent vasa vasorum when preparing large vessels for surgery. This practice may not be recommended because clearly, such injury in itself will stimulate medial necrosis[50] and lesion formation. The mechanism by which removal of the adventitia leads to endothelial injury and vascular lesion formation is not clear. It is impossible to remove the adventitia without generating surgical trauma to the vessel wall. Furthermore, bleeding and hemorrhage into the adventitial space resulting from the surgery would be expected to generate thrombin. Thrombin is a potent mitogen for smooth muscle cells and fibroblasts[51–53] and may stimulate vascular lesion formation by initiating medial or adventitial cell proliferation. Alternatively, thrombin has been shown to cause endothelial injury and dysfunction,[54–56] which may contribute to lesion formation as well. Endothelial cell damage may also occur when the innervation extending into the medial wall from the adventitia is removed,[57] or possibly if the lymphatic ducts are damaged. Damage or removal of the vasa vasorum produces similar effects as removal of the adventitia and has been implicated in the process of vascular lesion formation in atherosclerosis[58–60] and experimental adventitial injury.[40,41,61–63] It is possible that injury to the vasa vasorum contributes to the stimulation of the proliferation of the adventitial myofibroblasts. Our work suggests that it may be necessary to consider the role that the adventitial fibroblasts may play in homeostatic regulation of vascular function and the effect of potential interventions on not only the medial cells but the adventitial cells as well.

The studies reported here suggest that the adventitia may play a role in vascular lesion formation after balloon overstretch injury of pig coronary arteries by contributing to the cellular mass of the neointima and the synthesis of growth factors. In addition, the adventitia may contribute to vascular remodeling and constriction of the external elastic lamina through an accumulation of myofibroblasts containing α-smooth muscle actin in the adventitia surrounding the injury site. Intravascular irradiation modifies these responses in the adventitia, inhibits early adventitial cell proliferation, and modifies the production of α-actin by the adventitial myofibroblasts at later times after injury. Thus, intravascular irradiation might be expected to reduce the growth of the restenosis lesion and has the potential to positively affect vascular remodeling through its action on adventitial cells. Clearly, additional work will have to be directed at a more detailed examination of the response of adventitial cells to balloon injury and intravascular irradiation in the setting of atherosclerosis to determine what role these cells might play in regulating vascular lesion development.

References

1. Pickering JG, Weir L, Jekanowski J, et al. Proliferative activity in peripheral and coronary atherosclerotic plaque among patients undergoing percutaneous revascularization. J Clin Invest 1993;91:1469–1480.
2. O'Brien ER, Alpers CE, Stewart DK, et al. Proliferation in primary and restenotic coronary atherectomy tissue. Implications for antiproliferative therapy. Circ Res 1993; 73:223–231.
3. Clowes AW, Reidy MA, Clowes MM. Kinetics of cellular proliferation after arterial injury. I. Smooth muscle growth in the absence of endothelium. Lab Invest 1983;49: 327–333.
4. Reidy MA, Fingerle J, Lindner V. Factors controlling the development of arterial lesions after injury. Circulation 1992;86(suppl 6):III43–III46.
5. Steele PM, Chesebro JH, Stanson AW, et al. Balloon angioplasty. Natural history of the pathophysiological response to injury in a pig model. Circ Res 1985;57:105–112.
6. Schwartz RS, Murphy JG, Edwards WD, et al. Restenosis after balloon angioplasty. A practical proliferative model in porcine coronary arteries. Circulation 1990;82: 2190–2200.
7. Schwartz RS, Huber KC, Murphy JG, et al. Restenosis and the proportional neointimal response to coronary artery injury: Results in a porcine model. J Am Coll Cardiol 1992;19:267–274.
8. Karas SP, Gravanis MB, Santoian EC, et al. Coronary intimal proliferation after balloon injury and stenting in swine: An animal model of restenosis. J Am Coll Cardiol 1992;20:467–474.
9. Schneider JE, Berk BC, Gravanis MB, et al. Probucol decreases neointimal formation in a swine model of coronary artery balloon injury. A possible role for antioxidants in restenosis. Circulation 1993;88:628–637.
10. Santoian ED, Schneider JE, Gravanis MB, et al. Angiopeptin inhibits intimal hyperplasia after angioplasty in porcine coronary arteries. Circulation 1993;88:11–14.
11. Weiner BH, Ockene IS, Jarmolych J, et al. Comparison of pathologic and angiographic findings in a porcine preparation of coronary atherosclerosis. Circulation 1985;72: 1081–1086.
12. Huber KC, Schwartz RS, Edwards WD, et al. Effects of angiotensin converting enzyme inhibition on neointimal proliferation in a porcine coronary injury model. Am Heart J 1993;125:695–701.
13. Morimoto S, Sekiguchi M, Endo M, et al. Mechanism of luminal enlargement in PTCA and restenosis: A histopathological study of necropsied coronary arteries collected from various centers in Japan. Jpn Circ J 1987;51:1101–1115.
14. Morimoto S, Mizuno Y, Hiramitsu S, et al. Restenosis after percutaneous transluminal coronary angioplasty: A histopathological study using autopsied hearts. Jpn Circ J 1990;54:43–56.
15. Skalli O, Schurch W, Seemayer T, et al. Myofibroblasts from diverse pathologic settings are heterogeneous in their content of actin isoforms and intermediate filament proteins. Lab Invest 1989;60:275–285.
16. Darby I, Skalli O, Gabbiani G. Alpha-smooth muscle actin is transiently expressed by myofibroblasts during experimental wound healing. Lab Invest 1990;63:21–29.
17. Kapanci Y, Burgan S, Pietra GG, et al. Modulation of actin isoform expression in alveolar myofibroblasts (contractile interstitial cells) during pulmonary hypertension. Am J Pathol 1990;136:881–889.
18. Leslie KO, Taatjes DJ, Schwarz J, et al. Cardiac myofibroblasts express alpha smooth muscle actin during right ventricular pressure overload in the rabbit. Am J Pathol 1991;139:207–216.
19. Tanaka Y, Nouchi T, Yamane M, et al. Phenotypic modulation in lipocytes in experimental liver fibrosis. J Pathol 1991;164:273–278.
20. Ronnov-Jessen L, Petersen OW, Koteliansky VE, et al. The origin of the myofibroblasts in breast cancer. Recapitulation of tumor environment in culture unravels diversity and implicates converted fibroblasts and recruited smooth muscle cells. J Clin Invest 1995;95:859–873.

21. Lazard D, Sastre X, Frid MG, et al. Expression of smooth muscle-specific proteins in myoepithelium and stromal myofibroblasts of normal and malignant human breast tissue. Proc Natl Acad Sci U S A 1993;90:999–1003.

22. Desmouliere A, Rubbia-Brandt L, Grau G, et al. Heparin induces alpha-smooth muscle actin expression in cultured fibroblasts and in granulation tissue myofibroblasts. Lab Invest 1992;67:716–726.

23. Willems IEMG, Havenith MG, De May JGR, et al. The alpha smooth muscle actin-positive cells in healing human myocardial scars. Am J Pathol 1994;145:868–875.

24. Scott NA, Martin F, Simonet L, et al. Contribution of adventitial myofibroblasts to vascular remodeling and lesion formation after experimental angioplasty in pig coronary arteries [abstract]. FASEB J 1995;9:A845.

25. Scott NA, Ross C, Subramanian R, et al. Characterization of the cellular response to coronary injury [abstract]. Circulation 1994;90:I392.

26. Scott NA, Ross CE, Dunn B, et al. Identification of a potential role for the adventitia in vascular lesion formation after balloon overstretch injury of porcine coronary arteries. Circulation 1996;93:2178–2187.

27. Hanke H, Strohschneider T, Oberhoff M, et al. Time course of smooth muscle cell proliferation in the intima and media of arteries following experimental angioplasty. Circ Res 1990;67:651–659.

28. Clowes AW, Schwartz SM. Significance of quiescent smooth muscle migration in the injured rat carotid artery. Circ Res 1985;56:139–145.

29. Osborn M, Debus E, Weber K. Monoclonal antibodies specific for vimentin. Eur J Cell Biol 1984;34:137–143.

30. Clark RA. Regulation of fibroplasia in cutaneous wound repair. Am J Med Sci 1993;306:42–48.

31. Ronnov-Jessen L, Van Deurs B, Nielsen M, et al. Identification, paracrine generation, and possible function of human breast carcinoma myofibroblasts in culture. In Vitro Cell Dev Biol 1992;28A:273–283.

32. Desmouliere A, Rubbia-Brandt L, Abdiu A, et al. Alpha-smooth muscle actin is expressed in a subpopulation of cultured and cloned fibroblasts and is modulated by gamma-interferon. Exp Cell Res 1992;201:64–73.

33. Desmouliere A, Geinoz A, Gabbiani F, et al. Transforming growth factor-beta 1 induces alpha-smooth muscle actin expression in granulation tissue myofibroblasts and in quiescent and growing cultured fibroblasts. J Cell Biol 1993;122:103–111.

34. Ehrlich HP. Wound closure: Evidence of cooperation between fibroblasts and collagen matrix. Eye 1988;2:149–157.

35. Abbadia Z, Clezardin P, Serre CM, et al. Thrombospondin (TSPl) mediates in vitro proliferation of human MG-63 osteoblastic cells induced by alpha-thrombin. FEBS Lett 1993;329:341–346.

36. Ohlstein EH, Douglas SA, Sung CP, et al. Carvedilol, a cardiovascular drug, prevents vascular smooth muscle cell proliferation, migration, and neointimal formation following vascular injury. Proc Natl Acad Sci U S A 1993;90:6189–6193.

37. Post MJ, Borst C, Kuntz RE. The relative importance of arterial remodeling compared with intimal hyperplasia in lumen renarrowing after balloon angioplasty. A study in the normal rabbit and the hypercholesterolemic Yucatan micropig. Circulation 1994;89:2816–2821.

38. Pasterkamp G, Wensing PJ, Post MJ, et al. Paradoxical arterial wall shrinkage may contribute to luminal narrowing of human atherosclerotic femoral arteries. Circulation 1995;91:1444–1449.

39. Mintz GS, Popma JJ, Pichard AD, et al. Mechanisms of later arterial responses to transcatheter therapy: A serial quantitative angiographic and intravascular ultrasound study [abstract]. Circulation 1994;90:I24.

40. Booth RF, Martin JF, Honey AC, et al. Rapid development of atherosclerotic lesions in the rabbit carotid artery induced by perivascular manipulation. Atherosclerosis 1989;76:257–268.

41. Barker SG, Tilling LC, Miller GC, et al. The adventitia and atherogenesis: Removal initiates intimal proliferation in the rabbit which regresses on generation of a 'neo-adventitia.' Atherosclerosis 1994;105:131–144.

42. Chignier E, Eloy R. Adventitial resection of small artery provokes endothelial loss and intimal hyperplasia. Surg Gynecol Obstet 1986;163:327–334.

43. Marmur JD, Rossikhina M, Guha A, et al. Tissue factor is rapidly induced in arterial smooth muscle after balloon injury. J Clin Invest 1993;91:2253–2259.
44. Rakugi H, Jacob HJ, Krieger JE, et al. Vascular injury induces angiotensinogen gene expression in the media and neointima. Circulation 1993;87:283–290.
45. Simons M, Edelman ER, DeKeyser JL, et al. Antisense c-myb oligonucleotides inhibit intimal arterial smooth muscle cell accumulation in vivo. Nature 1992;359:67–70.
46. Edelman ER, Adams DH, Karnovsky MJ. Effect of controlled adventitial heparin delivery on smooth muscle cell proliferation following endothelial injury. Proc Natl Acad Sci U S A 1990;87:3773–3777.
47. Okada T, Bark DH, Mayberg MR. Localized release of perivascular heparin inhibits intimal proliferation after endothelial injury without systemic anticoagulation. Neurosurgery 1989;25:892–898.
48. Hadeishi H, Mayberg MR, Seto M. Local application of calcium antagonists inhibits intimal hyperplasia after arterial injury. Neurosurgery 1994;34:114–121.
49. Zollikofer CL, Redha FH, Bruhlmann WF, et al. Acute and long-term effects of massive balloon dilation on the aortic wall and vasa vasorum. Radiology 1987;164:145–149.
50. Stefanadis C, Vlachopoulos C, Karayannacos P, et al. Effect of vasa vasorum flow on structure and function of the aorta in experimental animals. Circulation 1995;91:2669–2678.
51. Wilcox JN, Rodriguez J, Subramanian R, et al. Characterization of thrombin receptor expression during vascular lesion formation. Circ Res 1994;75:1029–1038.
52. Bar Shavit R, Benezra M, Eldor A, et al. Thrombin immobilized to extracellular matrix is a potent mitogen for vascular smooth muscle cells: Nonenzymatic mode of action. Cell Regul 1990;1:453–463.
53. McNamara CA, Sarembock IJ, Gimple LW, et al. Thrombin stimulates proliferation of cultured rat aortic smooth muscle cells by a proteolytical activated receptor. J Clin Invest 1993;91:94–98.
54. Malik AB, Lo SK, Bizios R. Thrombin-induced alterations in endothelial permeability. Ann N Y Acad Sci 1986;485:293–309.
55. Heaton JH, Dame MK, Gelehrter TD. Thrombin induction of plasminogen activator inhibitor mRNA in human umbilical vein endothelial cells in culture. J Lab Clin Med 1992;120:222–228.
56. Daniel TO, Gibbs VC, Milfay DF, et al. Thrombin stimulates c-sis gene expression in microvascular endothelial cells. J Biol Chem 1986;261:9579–9582.
57. Govyrin VA, Korneeva TE, Malovichko NA: [Disorders of the endothelial pavement of the vascular bed caused by denervation]. Fiziol Zh SSSR 1988;74:953–956.
58. Horn H, Finkelstein LE. Arteriosclerosis of the coronary arteries and the mechanism of their occlusion. Am Heart J 1940;19:655–682.
59. Gerlis LM. The significance of adventitial infiltrations in coronary atherosclerosis. Br Heart J 1956;18:166–172.
60. Martin JF, Booth RF, Moncada S. Arterial wall hypoxia following thrombosis of the vasa vasorum is an initial lesion in atherosclerosis. Eur J Clin Invest 1991;21:355–359.
61. Nakata Y, Shionoya S. Vascular lesions due to obstruction of the vasa vasorum. Nature 1966;212:1258–1259.
62. Sottiurai V, Fry WI, Stanley JC. Ultrastructural characteristics of experimental arterial medial fibroplasia induced by vasa vasorum occlusion. J Surg Res 1978;24:169–177.
63. Barker SG, Talbert A, Cottam S, et al. Arterial intimal hyperplasia after occlusion of the adventitial vasa vasorum in the pig. Arterioscler Thromb 1993;13:70–77.

## Chapter 4

Animal Models to Study Restenosis

Keith A. Robinson, PhD

Since the inception of modern biological scientific inquiry we have sought to understand normal physiological and disease states through the use of various animal species as experimental subjects. Observations from animal experimentation can be valuable to elucidate mechanisms of tissue, organ, system, and organism functions as well as to provide information about novel potential therapeutics. It is crucial, however, to comprehend and appreciate the limitations of data obtained from animal "models," particularly with respect to interpretation, and to view cautiously the extrapolation of results directly to human pathological conditions.

A classic case in point is the use of balloon catheter or stent arterial injury in other species as a means to test pharmaceuticals or new interventional devices (or a combination of these two entities as in local drug delivery) for potential efficacy against clinical postangioplasty or in-stent restenosis. At least partly because of inappropriate experimental protocols, unsuitable specimen preparation and measurement techniques, and overzealous data interpretation, premature or overtly misplaced enthusiasm regarding potential antirestenotic therapies has been generated. This has, in the wake of many failed clinical trials, led to a growing distrust of the animal models of restenosis.

Rather than abandoning preclinical studies entirely, it seems more reasonable to adjust our perception of the role of animal data and to improve and standardize our experimental and analytical techniques. In this chapter several of the animal pathophysiological preparations that have been used to reproduce one or more elements of the restenosis process are considered.

The Problem of Restenosis

Since its onset in the late 1970s by the Swiss cardiologist and radiologist Dr. Andreas R. Gruentzig, the revolutionary technique of percutaneous transluminal coronary angioplasty (PTCA), used for the treatment of obstructive coronary atherosclerosis, has undergone tremendous growth and development.[1,2] Now used in hundreds of centers and for hundreds of thousands of procedures annually worldwide, PTCA is an attractive, less invasive, and less expensive alternative to coronary artery bypass graft surgery.

However, the iatrogenic phenomenon of lesion recurrence or restenosis after PTCA continues to plague the technique, driving up long-term costs, usurping health care resources, increasing patient morbidity, and vexing the medical and

From Waksman R (ed.). *Vascular Brachytherapy, Third Edition.* Armonk, NY: Futura Publishing Co., Inc.; © 2002.

scientific communities. At a rate of about 35% overall, restenosis is a huge problem, and even reducing the rate by half would provide significant savings.[3]

To develop an effective strategy for the prevention of restenosis, the use of an appropriate animal preparation is important.[4] Techniques of mechanical arterial injury in animals have existed for decades and were initially developed to study the smooth muscle cell (SMC) proliferative component of atherosclerotic lesions.[5] Many forms of arterial injury, including adventitial insults, will provoke an intimal thickening.[6]

However, the histologic, cellular, and molecular pathways by which the injured artery is repaired may by quite specific to both the vessel type and the type of injury. Therefore, it seems appropriate to carefully consider the latter factors when designing a suitable animal model. At the same time, while a native atherosclerotic coronary artery would be the ideal substrate for angioplasty dilatation in producing such a model, economic constraints may limit the "perfect model" to only a final preclinical testing phase.[4] Initial screening and dose-response analysis could be performed in less expensive systems before proceeding to that phase.

Restenosis after Angioplasty in Humans

A number of autopsy studies as well as serial intravascular ultrasound analyses have helped define the mechanisms of restenosis in humans.[7–11] The two primary phenomena that contribute to late loss of lumen cross-sectional area (ie, the extent of restenosis) after a successful angioplasty procedure are intimal hyperplasia and chronic vessel constriction or shrinkage (negative remodeling). The degrees to which these processes contribute to the final outcome varies between individuals and perhaps even between arteries in the same individual.

It is important to first consider the process of the initial angioplasty dilatation when discerning the means by which the artery is subsequently healed and by which it may or may not experience restenosis. Stretch of the entire arterial wall appears to be the major means of luminal enlargement, as there is little compression of the atherosclerotic plaque or other structures.[8,10] Accompanying this stretch are variable degrees of dissection and dehiscence of the intima from the media, as well as fracture and separation of the media from the adventitia (Fig. 1, panel a). Stretch and dissection injury are inevitable consequences of successful PTCA.[8,10]

Subsequent to the injury there is a repair process that involves variable amounts of mural thrombosis and hemorrhage, inflammation, cellular migration and proliferation, and fibrosis. Fibrin and platelet thrombus is present within the first 2 weeks after angioplasty but replaced thereafter by a fibrocellular intimal proliferation (Fig. 1, panel b) that fills the dissection planes and circumscribes the lumen.[7–10]

In the later phases of healing there is radial constriction such that the overall vessel wall cross-sectional area is decreased.[11] Thus, the process of restenosis after balloon angioplasty parallels wound healing in other tissues; an initial phase of platelet aggregation and blood coagulation concomitant with leukocyte infiltration is followed by formation of granulation tissue, fibroplasia, and finally wound contraction.[12]

It seems plausible to consider restenosis as an aberrant or overexuberant form of wound healing analogous to hyperplastic scarring. Pharmacological or

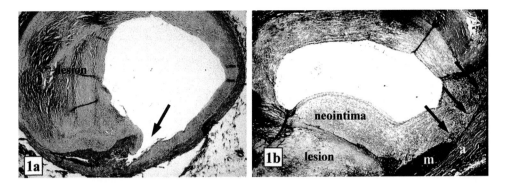

Figure 1. Light microscopy of human coronary arteries after angioplasty. Courtesy of Dr. Michael B. Gravanis. **a.** Six hours after angioplasty there is stretch and dissection injury to tunica media with dehiscence of atherosclerotic lesion from media (arrow). **b.** Four months after angioplasty, rupture of media from balloon expansion is still evident (arrows); proliferative neointima has also formed.

other therapeutic modulation of the healing response to produce a limited scar with minimal contraction should therefore yield lower rates of clinical restenosis. In several animal preparations information can be gained about the formation of balloon- or stent-induced neointima. The pig coronary artery preparation, in particular, provides a means to assess the efficacy of potential antirestenotic therapeutic strategies such as vascular radiotherapy by use of histopathological, histomorphometric, and immunocytochemical analysis of a wound-healing phenomenon similar to that observed in humans after PTCA, that is the formation of proliferative neointima as well as the chronic vessel shrinkage observed after stretch and dissection injury of the coronary artery.[13]

Animal Preparations

Mechanical or other injuries inflicted on the arterial luminal surface have long been used as means to invoke arteriosclerotic lesions in animals. Until after PTCA was introduced, however, the iatrogenic process of restenosis was not widely appreciated as the close clinical parallel to the previous observations of response to injury in the arteries of animals. A number of species including mice, rats, rabbits, dogs, pigs, and nonhuman primates are now employed in efforts to develop and test conventional pharmaceuticals, nucleotide-based compounds, interventional devices, and drug-device combinations designed toward thwarting the persistent problem of restenosis.

Animal models of angioplasty comprise some of the features of the clinical scenario, but none has attained perfect similitude. One of the most commonly employed models is deendothelialization and stretch injury of the carotid artery in the rat by embolectomy catheter. A cutdown to the external carotid artery is made and the catheter is introduced via arteriotomy and advanced retrograde into the common carotid artery. The balloon is inflated and withdrawn to the carotid bifurcation and the process is then repeated several times, after which the external carotid is ligated. An inexpensive and relatively uncomplicated undertaking, this model has value as an initial screening tool for potential antirestenotic therapies. It also has contributed substantially to our understanding of the basic cellular and molecular mechanisms involved in this form of wound healing.[14–16] However, it does not incorporate several of the histopathological features of balloon angioplasty in humans, especially medial dissection injury, separation of arterial layers, and hemorrhage within the dissection planes (Fig. 2). Furthermore, the relevance of injury to elastic, as opposed to muscular, arteries remains in question, and the positive effects of many therapies in this model have led to a number of failed clinical studies. Similar preparations have been developed in lagomorphs and in other rodents.

Another commonly used model involves balloon angioplasty of the atherosclerotic iliac artery in the rabbit. Atherosclerotic lesions are formed by initial balloon deendothelialization via the femoral artery, along with diet-induced hypercholesterolemia. After several weeks, stenotic lesions are formed amenable to balloon dilatation via the carotid artery under fluoroscopic guidance.[17,18] Subsequent restenosis is practically guaranteed with this preparation, making it somewhat unlike human coronary angioplasty, where approximately 65% of dilated lesions remain acceptably patent. Nevertheless, similar to the rat model, it has proved of value in screening antirestenotic compounds and elucidating restenosis mechanisms.[19] Furthermore, it has proved suitable for development and testing of new interventional devices such as lasers, atherectomy, and stents. One problem is that the restenosis lesions are sometimes difficult to distinguish histologically from the underlying atheroma, having a similar macrophage-foam cell-rich composition, unlike the almost exclusively SMC populace of the human restenotic tissue.

An animal model of clinical coronary restenosis used with increasing frequency involves the healing response to balloon overstretch injury in the normal coronary arteries of the juvenile pig.[13,20] Having a similar cardiac and coronary anatomy, collateral circulation, and closer phylogenetic proximity to humans, this species is also attractive due to a substantial intimal proliferative response to coronary injury unlike other large animal species such as the dog. In the standard balloon overdilatation injury, the tunica media is ruptured, leaving irregular craterlike defects which can be of considerable length (Figs. 3 and 4). The dissected media is also dehisced from the external lamina, thrombus accumulates in these tissue dissection planes, and there is hemorrhage and inflammation in the adventitia and perivascular space.

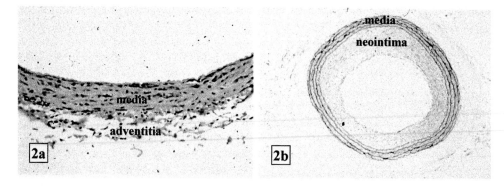

Figure 2. Light microscopy of rat carotid arteries after balloon deendothelialization. **a.** immunostaining for proliferating cell nuclear antigen shows high levels of cell proliferation (brown) in media and adventitia at 3 days. **b.** At 14 days there is a thick concentric neointima.

During a period of several weeks, the medial defect is replaced by a proliferative neointima quite similar by histologic appearance to the neointima of restenotic human coronary arteries after angioplasty (Figs 6 and 7), being composed primarily of stellate and spindle-shaped cells in an extensive extracellular matrix that contains proteoglycan and collagen.[13] The neointima appears to originate primarily by outgrowth from the torn edges of the tunica media (Fig. 6). This has been a consistent observation in time course histologic studies; only rarely are small tissue outgrowths from the region of the exposed external elastic lamina observed, and these are invariably associated with tears in the external lamina. Hence, the intact external lamina appears to be a substantial barrier to fibroblast migration from the adventitia to the lumen. Hemorrhage and mural thrombus is gradually resorbed concomitant with a resolution of the inflammatory reaction. During the same period, arterial wall cell proliferation declines and returns to near baseline by 2 to 4 weeks (Figs. 5 through 7).

Beginning at approximately 3 days after balloon overstretch injury, a curious phenomenon occurs in the tunica adventitia adjacent to the site of medial rupture. The fibroblasts in this region express SMC-specific α-actin filaments as detectable by immunocytochemistry (Figs. 5 and 6). This change lasts for several weeks and is restricted to the region subjacent to the medial damage; by 4 weeks the adventitial α-actin expression has subsided and it is largely absent by 8 weeks. This transient myofibroblastic differentiation in the adventitia suggests a chronic constrictive effect, in parallel to the changes in fibroblasts of the skin, which participate in scar contraction during wound healing.[21] Parallel vessel dimensional changes have not yet been confirmed by our group but studies by others have demonstrated a chronic vessel constriction component of luminal narrowing in similar medial rupture injury.[22] That we have not observed this change in our standard preparation is perhaps due the continued overall growth of the young animals used, with a consequent conflicting trend against vessel shrinkage.

Oversized stent placement in pig coronary arteries has also been used as a model of restenosis.[20,23] Neointimal lesions resulting from this injury are substantially larger than balloon-induced lesions.[20] This may be advantageous, but it appears that the healing response shows some distinct differences. Primarily,

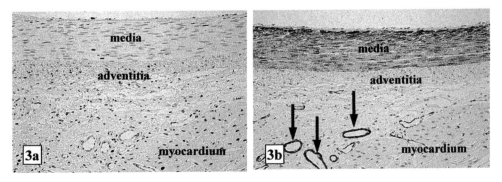

Figure 3. Light microscopic immunohistochemistry of normal pig coronary arteries. **a.** In uninjured artery of juvenile pig there is a low level of proliferating cell nuclear antigen staining (brown) with a few cells positive in media and endothelium, and higher levels in adventitia, perivascular space, and myocardium. **b.** Staining for smooth muscle α-actin (brown) appears only in media of epicardial artery and brach vessels of perivascular space (arrows).

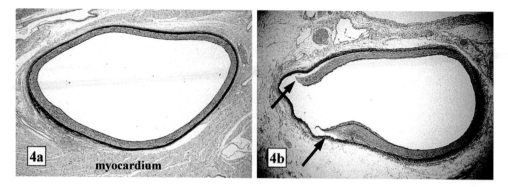

Figure 4. Light microscopy of pig coronary arteries. **a.** Normal coronary artery without balloon injury. **b.** Artery fixed immediately after balloon overstretch angioplasty injury; media is ruptured and edges of torn media (arrows) are dehisced from the external elastic lamina.

there appears to be more robust thrombotic and neointimal responses to metallic stents than to simple balloon injury.[20] Second, there appears to be a heightened inflammatory response to stents, including foreign-body giant-cell formation and granulomatosis.[13,20] Although balloon injuries invariably show inflammation also, in that case it is mostly in the form of a transient accumulation of neutrophils in the adventitia. With stent implantation, not only is the inflammation of a different character and more extensive but it is also more persistent. Finally, stents mechanically prevent chronic constriction or negative remodeling, thus excluding the possibility of studying this phenomenon in stent models in relation to its role in angioplasty restenosis. It is proposed that distinct phenomena may also lead to restenosis after angioplasty compared to stenting in humans, and that the study of these phenomena may comprise two separate disciplines. With the growing role of stents in coronary interventional procedures, however, the importance of a stent preparation is obvious. Although stenting does appear to attenuate resteno-

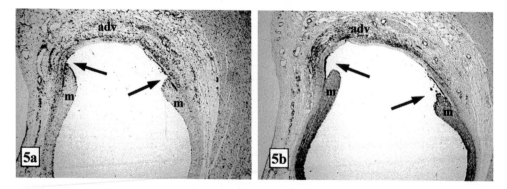

Figure 5. Light microscopic immunohistochemistry of pig coronary artery fixed 3 days after balloon injury. Torn edges of media (m) are indicated by arrows. **a.** Positive staining for proliferating cell nuclear antigen (brown) is seen at torn medial edges and in adventitia (adv) adjacent to rupture. **b.** Positive staining for smooth muscle α-actin (brown) is observed throughout arterial media and branch vessels, but now also appears in adventitia adjacent to rupture.

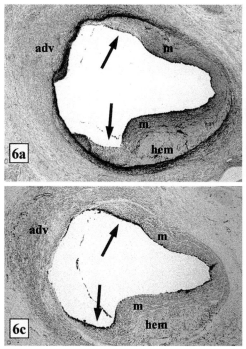

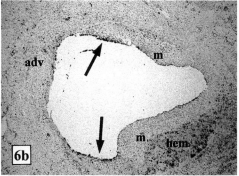

Figure 6. Light microscopy of pig coronary artery fixed 7 days after balloon injury. Neointimal tissue (arrows) has formed at edges of torn media (m) and a submedial hemorrhage (hem) is evident. **a.** Verhoeff-van Gieson stain; note neointimal tissue and expansion of adventitia (adv) adjacent to medial dissection. **b.** Proliferating cell nuclear antigen immunostain (brown) shows highest signal at luminal surface of neointimal tissue (arrows) and in submedial hemorrhage. Staining in adventitia (adv) adjacent to medial tear is decreased compared to 3 days. **c.** Immunostain for smooth muscle α-actin (brown) is positive throughout media and neointima (note higher intensity of luminal surface) and is extensive in adventitia (adv) subadjacent to medial rupture.

sis rates compared to angioplasty alone in "ideal" lesions, it is not clear that it is palliative for all types of lesions in all anatomic locations.

Nonhuman primates, in particular the cynomolgus monkey and the baboon, also have been used as restenosis models. In most instances the iliac or carotid arteries have been used for intervention, but in larger baboons it is possible to instrument the coronary arteries. The peripheral circulation is readily amenable to

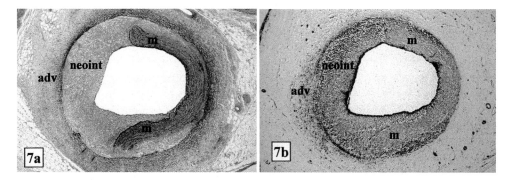

Figure 7. Light microscopy of pig coronary artery fixed 4 weeks after balloon injury; m = media. **a.** Verhoeff-van Gieson stain; neointima (neoint) has replaced the medial defect, and adventitia (adv) subadjacent to site of medial rupture has decreased in size compared to 7 days. **b.** Immunostain for smooth muscle α-actin (brown) is positive throughout media and neointima but is nearly absent in adventitia subadjacent to neointima at site of medial rupture.

surgical manipulation such as endarterectomy or to catheterization for balloon deendothelialization, balloon angioplasty, or stent implantation. The close phylogenetic proximity of these species to humans can be advantageous, particularly for testing of therapies with biochemical activity targeted against human proteins or nucleic acids which have poor cross-species homologies.[24]

Specimen Preparation and Analysis

A thorough treatise on specimen preparation, histologic staining, histochemistry and immunocytochemistry, and histomorphometry for arterial injury preparations is clearly beyond the scope of this chapter. However, there are certain specific caveats and guidelines regarding animal models of restenosis that are important to mention.

Specimen Preparation

First and foremost, for samples of blood vessels intended for histomorphometry and for most histopathological analysis as well, pressure perfusion fixation is essential and is best accomplished with the vessels in situ. Considerable shrinkage of all animal tissue during aldehyde fixation occurs due to extensive crosslinking of reactive groups on protein molecules; this effect is compounded when considering the dimensions of a tubular structure. Even stented arteries and grafts should be fixed at physiological pressure (mean arterial pressure is a good choice), because shrinkage can create artifacts at the stent ends or graft anastomoses. Furthermore, during immersion, fixative penetrates tissue by diffusion somewhat slowly. By fixing from within the lumen as well as the outside of the vessel and especially under physiological flow and pressure conditions, tissue penetration by fixative molecules is accelerated. For most arterial samples, maintenance of pressure for 10 to 15 minutes is adequate to thoroughly penetrate and preserve the sample close to its in vivo dimensions. The choice of fixative will depend on the desired analytical technique. We have found 10% neutral buffered formalin to be suitable for both routine histology as well as numerous immunostains.

It is necessary to further consider the means of analysis for determination of all steps of preparation. For ballooned arteries, standard paraffin embedding and microtomy is probably the best choice because it provides thinner sections and better staining than cryotomy, although in some instances immunostaining or in situ hybridization is not possible on paraffin sections. For the most part, however, modern antigen retrieval techniques permit a host of immunocytochemical and hybridization methods with excellent specificity. The preparation of stented arteries is a somewhat more complex issue. Removal of the metal prosthesis from the tissue after fixation enables standard paraffin embedding, but results in the worst artifactual distortion and outright tissue loss. Plastic embedding and use of the saw-and-grinding technique most faithfully preserves the specimen with the stent in place, but it is an exacting and laborious undertaking. A balance must be reached between the available resources in terms of manpower, expertise, equipment, and time on the one hand, with the desired analytical outcome on the other.

For routine histopathological examination, standard hematoxylin-eosin is still the stain of choice, and modified versions work well on frozen or plastic sections. For computerized histomorphometry, however, a connective tissue stain is superior to allow good visualization of elastic tissue components at low magnification. Verhoeff-van Gieson stain is suitable; others include Movat Pentachrome or Masson trichrome. For analysis of cell proliferation, PCNA immunocytochemistry can be performed; a better choice is to inject animals with bromodeoxyuridine (BrdU) prior to tissue harvest, then apply antibody staining for the brominated nucleic acid (although this adds considerably to the expense with large animals such as the pig). Other immunostains for a variety of tissue components, especially cytoplasmic filaments for cell characterization, are widely available.

Scanning electron microscopy (SEM) can be a valuable adjunct to light microscopy for the examination of arterial luminal surfaces, which allows for quick and accurate assessment of the extent of mural thrombosis, endothelialization, or other features. Additionally, it is an essential tool for the examination of biomaterials surfaces, before and after contact with blood or tissue. Transmission electron microscopy (TEM) can also be quite useful, particularly for cell typing and characterization of extracellular matrix. Specimens for SEM or TEM should be prepared in glutaraldehyde-based fixative.

Computer-Assisted Histomorphometry and Image Processing

An almost infinite variety of microscopic morphometry systems can be constructed, but the basic components are similar: a microscope; a video camera and monitor; a computer equipped with image digitizing card, processing software, and monitor; and a manual tracing tablet. For MacIntosh, NIH Image (developed at the National Institutes of Health) is a software package that enables most analytical techniques for planimetry and image densitometry. For PCs that run Microsoft Windows, Image ProPlus by Media Cybernetics (Silver Springs, MD) is a good choice.

Proper external calibration of magnification (should be checked at each measurement session if stored in the hard drive memory) and orientation of sections is clearly essential for accurate quantitation. Arterial lesions can be measured in a number of ways, but a guideline is to use all sections showing evidence of the type of injury and response of interest. Obviously, sections should also be measured by an experienced observer who is unaware of treatment assignment. These considerations substantially eliminate bias in the analytical process. Finally, if high-magnification images are analyzed, it is best to apply some type of consistent scheme involving multiple fields in a single section.

Restenosis models should also be evaluated with regard to the extent of injury and vessel size in individual sections. For histomorphometry of concentric lesions in a model of nondissecting-type injury such as the rat carotid, the commonly reported intima/media area ratio provides an index of the extent of lesion formation corrected for media size but not for overall vessel size or extent of injury. Other measurements, such as luminal area and external elastic lamina perimeter length, should perhaps also be reported. In the absence of outright medial dissection, it can be difficult to assess the extent of injury, but in the rat model fragmentation of the internal lamina is frequently seen. This can be evaluated at least semiquantitatively and compared between treatment groups. In the pig coronary model, the arc length of the medial fracture provides an index of injury that shows a positive linear relationship to neointima size.

Summary and Conclusions

Animal modeling of restenosis, when performed with special consideration to relevance and the scientific process, provides invaluable information for advancing medical practice and expanding the awareness of disease mechanisms. The intent of this chapter is not to exhaustively describe the cellular and molecular biology of restenosis; several excellent recent reviews of these subjects are available in the world literature.[25–28] Rather, a brief introduction and description of several animal preparations that have been used to study components of the restenosis process is provided. Each of these may prove useful for one or more features, including not only specific histopathological criteria but also ease of instrumentation and handling, expense, and other factors. It is incumbent on the individual researcher to weigh multiple factors, consider carefully among available options, and use animals only when necessary, and then only prudently with an approach to minimize both the numbers of animal subjects and their individual pain and stress. Furthermore, it is crucial to thoroughly review current literature, contact active researchers, and adopt the most thorough, objective, and standardized analytical techniques available. In this way scientific data of the greatest utility to the scientific and medical communities will be produced.

Acknowledgments: The author is grateful to the following individuals: Elisabeth Schieffer for immunohistochemical preparations and histomorphometry, Michael Gravanis for mentoring in cardiovascular histopathology, and Gus Cipolla for veterinary and cardiac catheterization expertise. Research fellows who have contributed to the development and analysis of the pig coronary artery preparation over the years include Steve Karas, Ed Santoian, Joel Schneider, Gilberto Nunes, Steve Sigman, Ron Waksman, and Nic Chronos. A special thanks also is extended to Spencer King without whose support, interest, knowledge, and expertise the development of the pig model would not have been possible.

References

1. Gruentzig AR, Senning A, Siegenthaler W. Non-operative dilatation of coronary artery stenoses: Percutaneous transluminal coronary angioplasty. N Engl J Med 1979; 301:61–63.
2. Holmes DR, King SB III. Percutaneous coronary revascularization for chronic coronary artery disease. In: Fuster V, Ross R, Topol EJ (eds.): Atherosclerosis and Coronary Artery Disease. Philadelphia, PA: Lippincott-Raven; 1996:1485–1503.
3. Califf RM, Ohman EM, Fried DJ. Restenosis: The clinical issues. In: Topol EJ (ed.): Textbook of Interventional Cardiology. Philadelphia, PA: WB Saunders Co.; 1990: 363–394.
4. Muller DWM, Ellis SG, Topol EJ. Experimental models of coronary artery restenosis. J Am Coll Cardiol 1992;19:418–432.
5. Murray M, Schrodt GR, Berg HF. Role of smooth muscle cells in healing of injured arteries. Arch Pathol 1966;82:138–146.
6. Booth RFG, Martin JF, Honey AC, et al. Rapid development of atherosclerotic lesions by perivascular manipulation. Atherosclerosis 1989;76:257–268.
7. Austin GE, Ratliff NB, Hollman J, et al. Intimal proliferation of smooth muscle cells as an explanation for recurrent coronary artery stenosis after percutaneous transluminal coronary angioplasty. J Am Coll Cardiol 1985;6:369–375.
8. Gravanis MB, Roubin GS. Histopathologic phenomena at the site of percutaneous transluminal coronary angioplasty: The problem of restenosis. Hum Pathol 1989; 20:477–485.
9. Waller BF, Pinkerton CA, Orr CM, et al. Restenosis 1 to 24 months after clinically successful coronary balloon angioplasty: A necropsy study of 20 patients. J Am Coll Cardiol 1991;17:58B–70B.

10. Farb A, Virmani R, Atkinson JB, et al. Plaque morphology and pathologic changes in arteries from patients dying after coronary balloon angioplasty. J Am Coll Cardiol 1990;16:1421–1429.
11. Mintz GS, Kovach JA, Pichard AD, et al. Geometric remodeling is the predominant mechanism of clinical restenosis after coronary angioplasty [abstract]. J Am Coll Cardiol 1994;23:138A.
12. Clark RAF. Overview and general considerations of wound repair. In: Clark RAF, Henson PM (eds.): The Molecular and Cellular Biology of Wound Repair. New York, NY: Plenum Press; 1998:3–23.
13. Gravanis MB, Robinson KA, Santoian EC, et al. The reparative phenomena at the site of balloon angioplasty in humans and experimental models. Cardiovasc Pathol 1993;24:263–273.
14. Clowes AW, Reidy MA, Clowes MM. Kinetics of cellular proliferation after arterial injury: I. Smooth muscle cell growth in the absence of endothelium. Lab Invest 1983; 49:327–333.
15. Fingerle J, Au YPT, Clowes AW, Reidy MA. Intimal lesion formation in rat carotid arteries after endothelial denudation in the absence of medial injury. Arteriosclerosis 1990;10:1082–1087.
16. Haudenschild CC, Schwartz SM. Endothelial regeneration: II. Restitution of endothelial continuity. Lab Invest 1979;41:407–418.
17. Block PC, Baughman KL, Pasternak RC, Fallon JT. Transluminal angioplasty: Correlation of morphologic and angiographic findings in an experimental model. Circulation 1980;61:778–785.
18. Faxon DP, Sanborn TA, Weber VJ, et al. Restenosis following transluminal angioplasty in experimental atherosclerosis. Arteriosclerosis 1984;4:189–195.
19. Wilentz JR, Sanborn TA, Haudenschild CC, et al. Platelet accumulation in experimental angioplasty: Time course and relation to vascular injury. Circulation 1987;75: 636–642.
20. Karas SP, Gravanis MB, Santoian EC, et al. Coronary intimal proliferation after balloon injury and stenting in swine: An animal model of restenosis. J Am Coll Cardiol 1992;20:467–474.
21. Gabbiani G, Ryan GB, Majno G. Presence of modified fibroblasts in granulation tissue and their role in wound contraction. Experientia 1971;27:459–460.
22. Andersen HR, Maeng M, Thorwest M, Falk E. Remodeling rather than neointimal formation explains luminal narrowing after deep vessel wall injury: Insights from a porcine coronary (re)stenosis model. Circulation 1996;93(9):1716–1724.
23. Schwartz RS, Murphy JG, Edwards WD, et al. Restenosis after balloon angioplasty: A practical proliferative model in porcine coronary arteries. Circulation 1990;82: 2190–2200.
24. Lumsden AB, Chen C, Hughes JD, et al. Anti-VLA-4 antibody reduces intimal hyperplasia in the endarterectomized carotid artery in nonhuman primates. J Vasc Surg 1997;26(1):87–93.
25. Nikol S, Huehns TY, Höfling B. Molecular biology and post-angioplasty restenosis. Atherosclerosis 1996;123(1–2):17–31.
26. Wilcox JN. Molecular biology: Insight into the causes and prevention of restenosis after arterial intervention. Am J Cardiol 1993;72(13):88E–95E.
27. Libby P, Schwartz D, Brogi E, et al. A cascade model for restenosis: A special case of atherosclerosis progression. Circulation 1992;86(6 suppl III):III47–III52.
28. Lee PC, Gibbons GH, Dzau VJ. Cellular and molecular mechanisms of coronary artery restenosis. Coron Artery Dis 1993;4(3):254–259.

## Chapter 5

Remodeling and Restenosis:

Observations from Intravascular Ultrasound Studies

Gary S. Mintz, MD

Restenosis continues to be the "Achilles' heel" of transcatheter interventions. The current review focuses on the contributions of remodeling to the restenosis process after non-stent interventions. Much of the evidence for remodeling as a mechanism of restenosis first came from serial intravascular ultrasound (IVUS) studies. Furthermore, IVUS substudies have now become routine in the investigation of any new approach to prevent restenosis.

Definitions

Several IVUS terms and concepts are important. During IVUS imaging of *non-stented lesions,* there are only two distinct boundaries that have consistent histologic correlates: the lumen-plaque interface and the media-adventitia interface. As a result, there are only two cross-sectional area (CSA) measurements that are reproducible: lumen CSA and external elastic membrane (EEM) CSA. Because the media cannot be quantified accurately, the cross-sectional measurement of athererosclerotic plaque is usually reported as plaque+media (P+M) CSA (calculated as EEM CSA minus lumen CSA). Two assumptions are made: (1) because the media has atrophied during atherogenesis, the contribution of media CSA to the P+M CSA is small; and (2) serial changes in media CSA are also minimal. The P+M CSA is often divided by the total arterial CSA to generate a measurement called plaque burden (which is also referred to as the cross-sectional narrowing, percent plaque area, or CSA obstruction). Serial IVUS analysis can only measure net changes in plaque mass; it cannot isolate the changes in the individual components of the plaque: thrombus, cellular proliferation, matrix deposition, atherosclerosis progression/regression, or plaque stabilization/apoptosis. Therefore, only net changes in P+M CSA can be reported. To reflect this, the term tissue growth or plaque is sometimes used. In stented lesions, there is an additional border—the stent CSA. The tissue that is deposited inside of a stent is typically measured as intimal hyperplasia (IH=stent minus lumen) CSA.

Remodeling is the term that has been applied to changes in EEM CSA. This

From Waksman R (ed.). *Vascular Brachytherapy, Third Edition.* Armonk, NY: Futura Publishing Co., Inc.; © 2002.

term has been applied to both de novo atherosclerosis and to the restenosis process. The ideal method to study remodeling is to perform serial IVUS studies. This has been done for restenosis, but obviously is more problematic in de novo atherosclerosis. In the absence of serial IVUS studies, *indirect* evidence of remodeling in de novo atherosclerosis can be inferred and/or defined in several ways. For example, lesion site EEM CSA can be compared to the reference EEM CSA. Positive remodeling can be defined as a lesion EEM CSA greater than the proximal reference; intermediate remodeling as a lesion EEM CSA smaller that the proximal reference, but greater than the distal reference; and negative remodeling as a lesion EEM CSA smaller than the distal reference.[1] A remodeling index can also be derived in which the lumen CSA (lesion versus reference) is compared to the EEM CSA (lesion versus reference) and P+M CSA (lesion versus reference). *Direct* evidence of remodeling can come only from serial changes in EEM CSA (or volume). While the term remodeling has been applied to both atherosclerosis and restenosis, this does not imply that remodeling in de novo atherosclerosis and remodeling in restenosis are the same process. Even using serial IVUS studies of restenosis, it is not possible to separate *primary* changes in arterial dimensions from *secondary* changes in EEM CSA due to an increase in adventitial thickness or peri-arterial scar formation. This has important implications in comparing serial IVUS studies in with histologic data.

Methodological Considerations

Certain methodological issues must be addressed in using serial IVUS to study restenosis, particularly using planar (single slice) analysis. These issues also apply to the assessment of brachytherapy.

1. The same anatomic slice must be identified and compared on serial studies. If image slices with different axial locations are compared, then the restenosis process cannot be separated from the axial variation in EEM, lumen, and P+M CSA. The axial locations of the image slice with the smallest pre-intervention, post-intervention, and follow-up lumen CSA are almost always different.
2. The axial location of the image slice selected for analysis should be at the smallest follow-up lumen CSA because this is the location of the restenosis process. If the axial location of the image slice selected for analysis is the smallest pre-intervention lumen CSA, then the restenosis lesion will often be missed.

To deal with some of these issues, it is necessary to develop a systematic approach to image acquisition and analysis. Only IVUS systems incorporating motorized transducer pullback through a stationary imaging sheath should be used. Motorized transducer pullback through a stationary imaging sheath permits the transducer to move at the same speed as the proximal end of the catheter. By using one or more reproducible axial landmarks (eg, the aorto-ostial junction, large proximal and/or distal side branches, or unusually shaped calcium deposits) and a known pullback speed, identical cross-sectional slices on serial studies can be identified for comparison. In practice, the following steps were performed: (1) The image slice with the smallest lumen CSA in the follow-up study was identified. (2) The distance from this image slice to the *closest* "unique" proximal axial landmark was measured (in seconds of videotape). (3) This axial landmark was identified on the post-intervention study. (4) The anatomic image slice on the post-intervention study corresponding to the image slice with the smallest follow-up lumen CSA was identified. (5) Finally, vascular and perivascular markings (eg, small side branches, venous structures, calcific and fibrotic deposits) were used to confirm image slice identification. If necessary, the post-intervention and follow-up studies were analyzed side-by-side and the imaging runs studied frame-by-frame to ensure that the same anatomic cross-section was measured.[2] While ECG-gating may improve on this methodology, evidence to support this contention is lacking.[3] Furthermore, it increases imaging time significantly, a problem in assessing long lesions.

Similar attention to detail is important in performing volumetric analyses. Once the studies are acquired, two general approaches have been used. Planar measurements can be made at fixed axial distances through the lesion – typically slices 1 mm apart. Volumes are then calculated as the sum of the CSA measurements (Simpson's Rule). Alternatively, automatic edge detection algorithms have been developed. Edge detection techniques are typically based on the interaction between longitudinal and cross-sectional contours throughout the length of the segment. A series of cross-sectional image slices are digitized, eg, 200 image slices (10 images/mm over a 20-mm long segment). Two longitudinal planes are then constructed and manually edited. Longitudinal tracings of the lumen and EEM borders facilitate automated contour detection on the cross-sectional IVUS images. A minimal cost algorithm is then used to identify the lumen and EEM borders. The longitudinal and cross-sectional images are compared, cross-referenced, visually checked, and again manually edited where necessary. The volumetric results are computed from the edited cross-sectional image data set.

Mechanisms of Restenosis in Non-Stented Lesions

Using IVUS, late lumen loss (lumen CSA) can be separated into two components: (1) remodeling (EEM CSA, whether positive, ie, an increase in EEM CSA; or negative, ie, a decrease in EEM CSA) and (2) tissue growth (P+M CSA). In our initial study of 221 non-stented lesions,[2] the change in lumen CSA correlated more strongly with the change in EEM CSA (r=0.751) than with the change in P+M CSA (r=0.284). Restenotic lesions had a greater decrease in EEM CSA ($P<0.0001$) and lumen CSA ($P<0.0001$) than nonrestenotic lesions, but only a trend towards a greater increase in P+M CSA ($P=0.0784$).

Twenty-two percent of the lesions in this series showed positive arterial remodeling (an *increase* in EEM CSA during follow-up). Lesions with positive remodeling showed a decreased incidence of restenosis and an increased incidence of late lumen gain *despite* a greater increase in P+M CSA. Thus, some patients can respond to the increase in P+M CSA by an increase in EEM CSA to prevent restenosis. This observation may also explain the finding that some lesions "look better" at follow-up than post intervention.

Diabetes Mellitus

There was one exception to these findings: diabetic patients.[4] In diabetic patients, remodeling appeared to be similar to nondiabetics ($P=0.6350$); but the increase in P+M CSA was exaggerated (P=0.0720). This was especially true when just the restenotic lesions were considered. Thus, while some nondiabetics were able to respond to the increase in P+M CSA with an increase in EEM CSA to limit the decrease in lumen CSA (see above), this was rare in diabetics. Of note, we also found a similar phenomenon during de novo atherogenesis in insulin-treated diabetics.[5] Some diabetic patients, ie, those treated with insulin, had less positive remodeling and more negative remodeling. While the pathophysiology of remodeling in atherogenesis versus restenosis may be different, diabetics (especially insulin-treated diabetics) appear to be different from nondiabetics in both diseases.

Confirmatory Studies in Humans

OARS

The Optimal Atherectomy Restenosis Study (OARS)[6] was a multicenter study of IVUS-guided directional coronary atherectomy (DCA) with angiographic and IVUS follow-up. One of the purposes of OARS was to understand the mechanism of restenosis after DCA. OARS confirmed the importance of remodeling as a mechanism of restenosis. In addition, 20% of the lesions in OARS had a late *increase* in EEM CSA (a number similar to our initial series). The unique finding in OARS was that remodeling extended into contiguous reference segments.[6] Reference segment remodeling paralleled that at the lesion site (r=0.608). The findings of OARS have been substantiated in one recent report,[7] but not in another.[8] The findings of reference segment negative remodeling may also explain the observation that some restenotic lesions are longer than the original lesion.

SURE

In the Serial Ultrasound REstenosis (SURE) Trial[9] patients were treated with percutaneous transluminal coronary angioplasty (PTCA) or DCA and studied pre intervention and immediately post intervention, 24 hours post intervention, after 1 month of follow-up, and after 6 months of follow-up (Fig. 1). Again, SURE confirmed the importance of remodeling as a mechanism of restenosis in non-stented lesions. There were no differences between the PTCA- and the DCA-treated lesions. The unique findings in the SURE Trial were: (1) an early (within 1 month) increase in EEM CSA (ie, early positive remodeling) and (2) that the early increase in EEM CSA was followed by a late (1 to 6 month) decrease in EEM CSA (ie, late negative remodeling). Critics of the previous studies suggested that remodeling was just passive elastic recoil that occurred in the first day post intervention, but was unrecognized until late follow-up. Because negative remodeling was a late event and was preceded by early positive remodeling, negative remodeling was proved to be distinct from early passive elastic recoil. Throughout the duration of the SURE Trial, the changes in lumen CSA correlated with the changes in EEM CSA (r=0.789), not with the changes in P+M CSA (r=0.176).

A secondary analysis from the SURE Trial (Fig. 1) looked at the relationship between lumen, P+M, and EEM CSA within and between the early (within 1 month) and late (5 to 6 months) time points.[10] In the first month post intervention, there was a measurable increase in P+M CSA; however, the early increase

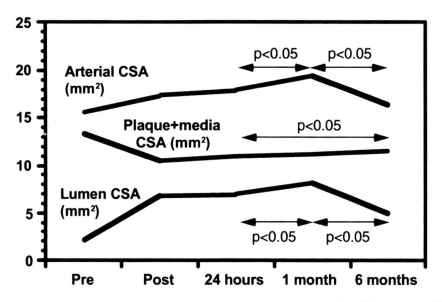

Figure 1. Serial IVUS changes in arterial, lumen, and plaque+media CSA from the SURE Trial are shown. Serial changes in lumen CSA closely parallel serial changes in arterial area. There was a significant increase in arterial CSA from 24 hours (17.9 ± 5.4 mm^2) to 1 month (19.4 ± 5.3 mm^2) and a significant decrease in arterial CSA from 1 month to 6 months (16.3 ± 5.5 mm^2). This was paralleled by a significant increase in lumen CSA from 24 hours (6.9 ± 2.5 mm^2) to 1 month (8.2 ± 2.8 mm^2) and a significant decrease in lumen CSA from 1 month to 6 months (4.9 ± 2.9 mm^2). There was an overall increase in plaque+media (P+M) CSA from 24 hours (11.0 ± 4.5 mm^2) to 6 months (11.5 ± 4.5 mm^2); however, this change was not significant at 1 month.

in EEM CSA was at least equal to this early increase in P+M CSA which prevented any decrease in lumen CSA. Then, the late decrease in EEM CSA correlated inversely with the early increase in P+M CSA. (Greater early increases in plaque area were associated with greater late decreases in arterial area.) One explanation is that a common trigger (ie, vessel injury during the intervention) caused both (1) the early increase in P+M CSA (resulting in early increase in EEM CSA) and (2) the late decrease in EEM CSA. Alternatively, the early increase in P+M CSA may have been the first step in a pathophysiologic process resulting directly in a late decrease in EEM CSA.

The early positive remodeling in SURE and the 20% to 25% frequency of late positive remodeling (which prevented restenosis) in previous studies[2,6] suggest that a therapy that can sustain the early positive remodeling will be beneficial in the long run regardless of the impact on neointimal hyperplasia.

Volumetric Analysis

There are two important criticisms of the previous studies: (1) some of these studies included multiple devices and (2) only planar analysis was performed. Planar analysis may be biased by decisions regarding lesion slice selection. Therefore, the DCA-treated lesions in OARS and SURE were submitted to independent volumetric IVUS analysis. Serial volumetric analysis using an automated contour detection algorithm confirmed the planar findings.[11] When 20-mm long segments were analyzed post intervention and at 1-month follow-up, lumen volume decreased from (P=0.0001) as a result of a decrease in EEM volume from (P=0.0003) with no change in P+M volume (P=0.5164). Lumen volume correlated with EEM volume (r=0.842), not with P+M volume (r=0.244).

Confirmatory Animal Studies

In general, animal studies supported both the general concept of remodeling and restenosis directly and indirectly. For example, O'Brien et al used proliferating cell nuclear antigen (PCNA) immunohistochemical labeling of human directional atherectomy specimens to show that proliferation in primary and restenotic lesions occurs infrequently,[12] as well as certain very specific observations (ie, that remodeling extends into reference segments and that remodeling is biphasic).[13–21]

Kakuta et al[13] compared histologic CSAs of vessels from animals sacrificed immediately after angioplasty with animals killed 4 weeks after angioplasty (when restenosis occurred) and showed that the total arterial cross-sectional area increased by 20% to accommodate nearly 60% of the neointimal tissue formation. The intimal areas in the restenotic versus nonrestenotic lesions were virtually identical. The difference between restenotic and nonrestenotic lesions was a significantly smaller internal elastic lamina (IEL) area in the restenotic group.

Similarly, Lafont et al[14] found that late stenosis correlated with histologic indices of chronic constriction (P=0.0003), but not with neointimal-medial growth. There was only a 33% increase in neointimal area following balloon injury, but a 52% decrease in lumen area as a result of a reduction in total arterial CSA compared to the reference site.

Guzman et al,[15] found that the most important independent predictor of lumen area 4 weeks after the second injury in a double injury model was the absolute EEM CSA. The intimal area was similar in restenotic and nonrestenotic lesions. In contrast, EEM CSA was significantly smaller (due to negative remodeling) in restenotic lesions.

Andersen et al[16] produced circumferential deep vessel wall injury by inflating and withdrawing an oversized chain-encircled angioplasty balloon in the left anterior descending coronary artery in pigs. Histology performed 3 weeks later revealed that the adventitia was markedly thickened as a result of neoadventitial formation. Lumen area did not correlate with neointima. Conversely, lumen area correlated strongly with vessel size (ie, remodeling, r=0.74, P=0.00005).

Post et al[17] used serial IVUS analysis to study restenosis in atherosclerotic iliac arteries of Yucatan micropigs. At 42 days, late lumen loss by IVUS correlated strongly with remodeling (R^2=0.843, P<0.001) and correlated weakly with intimal hyperplasia (R^2=0.214, P=0.02). Neointimal thickening accounted for only 11% of late lumen loss in normal pigs and 49% of late lumen loss in hypercholesterolemic pigs.

Labinaz et al[18] observed a biphasic time course to the remodeling process, similar to what was seen in SURE. In this same porcine coronary model, Pels et al[19] found that adventitial angiogenesis occurred within 3 days after balloon injury and that later regression of adventitial microvessels corresponded with arterial narrowing. Both Post et al[17] and Kakuta et al[20] found that remodeling extended to involve reference segments.

Last, recent *re*-examination of *original* animal experiments (using different quantitative analyses) now indicate that arterial remodeling (which was once ignored) is, in fact, an important part of the restenosis process.[21]

Confirmatory Human Necropsy Reports

There have also been several supportive human necropsy reports. Like the animal studies, the few human necropsy reports have proved useful in understanding how remodeling results in restenosis.

Nakamura et al[22] defined negative remodeling as PTCA site EEM CSA less than reference. According to this definition, negative remodeling occurred in all restenosis lesions, and in only one nonrestenotic. Dense caps of collagen fibers in the adventitia in the vicinity of the disrupted IEL (ie, scarring) were present in all of the negative remodeling lesions.

Sangiorgi et al[23] also compared the lesion site with the proximal reference. Histologically successful PTCA arteries (PTCA site lumen of 50% of the reference lumen, ie, nonrestenotic) demonstrated a larger lumen, smaller plaque size (normalized to the IEL area), and thinner adventitia compared with histologic failures. Relative to the reference sites, histologically successful PTCA showed expansion of the EEM. In contrast, histologic failures (ie, restenotic lesions) showed a reduced EEM, suggesting constrictive remodeling. Neointimal area correlated with the extent of internal elastic lamina disruption, but neither neointimal area nor IEL disruption was related to histologic success or failure.

It is important to note that any report comparing lesion site to reference segment EEM CSA is likely to underestimate the contribution of negative remodeling to restenosis. As shown in OARS and in two animal studies, the reference segment EEM CSA is also involved in the restenosis process (ie, it is smaller than baseline).

Predictors of Restenosis in Non-Stented Lesions

Two studies have shown that the residual plaque burden determined by IVUS is a predictor of restenosis. Our single center study used a multiplicity of devices[24] while the Guidance by Ultrasound Imaging for Decision Endpoints (GUIDE) Trial used only PTCA or DCA.[25] Comparison of restenosis rates and the residual plaque burdens in the Coronary Angioplasty Versus Excision Atherectomy Trial (CAVEAT), GUIDE, OARS, and Adjunct Balloon Angioplasty Coronary Atherectomy Study (ABACAS) substantiated this findings.

In another recent report from our group, pre-intervention remodeling also was identified as a predictor of target lesion revascularization after non-stent interventions.[26] Lesions with positive remodeling had more revascularization events despite a larger final (post intervention) IVUS lumen CSA. The probability of target lesion revascularization increased with increasing values of the remodeling index (lesion/reference EEM CSA). Positive remodeling during atherogenesis has been implicated in the pathogenesis of unstable coronary syndromes. Unstable angina and post-myocardial infarction lesions have a higher rate of clinical and angiographic restenosis. Lesions with positive remodeling may be more biologically active. This increased biological activity may cause both an unstable clinical presentation and more late revascularization events; as noted above, the late negative remodeling after non-stent interventions is quantitatively related to the early proliferative response. Conversely, lesions with intermediate/negative remodeling may not have the capacity to actively constrict ("negatively remodel") late post intervention; these lesions were unable to adapt to the initial growth of atherosclerotic plaque with a positive remodeling response.

There may also be a mechanical explanation for the observation that both the residual plaque burden and pre-intervention remodeling are predictors of restenosis. Arterial expansion is an important mechanism of lumen enlargement after all catheter-based interventions. Assuming that restenosis is, in part, a proportionate response to vascular and perivascular trauma, lesions with positive remodeling (which already have increased their arterial dimensions significantly) may have more trauma associated with the procedure-induced arterial expansion. Furthermore, baseline positive remodeling may be associated with a larger post-intervention plaque burden. It has been suggested that the residual plaque burden may act as an amplifier of the remodeling process.[21]

It is important to note that the predictive power of plaque burden was not confirmed in another study, Post-IntraCoronary Treatment Ultrasound Result Evaluation (PICTURE).[27] Using multivariate analysis, there were no IVUS predictors of restenosis. Unlike other studies assessing predictors of restenosis, PICTURE failed to identify *any* predictors of restenosis (ie, diabetes or the final angiographic minimum lumen diameter or diameter stenosis). It is also noteworthy that the relationship between pre-intervention remodeling and post-intervention remodeling and restenosis could not be substantiated in one recent animal study.[28]

Antirestenosis Therapies

Three therapies have been shown to reduce restenosis. It is noteworthy that all three appear to work by reducing late negative remodeling, thereby providing indirect evidence that remodeling is the main cause of restenosis after non-stent-based interventions.

Stents reduce restenosis by opposing late negative remodeling. The Palmaz-Schatz is the only stent that has been studied in detail using serial IVUS analysis. Serial IVUS studies have shown that Palmaz-Schatz stents almost never chronically recoil and that in-stent restenosis is almost solely the result of neointimal hyperplasia.[29,30] (This observation only applies to tubular-slotted or multicellular stents.) In an analysis of 115 stented lesions, lumen correlated more strongly with IH than with stent; this was true whether cross-sectional IVUS analysis was used (r=0.975 versus r=0.200) or whether volumetric IVUS analysis was used (r=0.990 versus r=0.028). Serial IVUS analysis also showed the impact of single Palmaz-Schatz stents on adjacent reference segments, similar to the observations in OARS. There appeared to be a continuum of changes beginning at the stent-vessel margin and continuing proximally and distally for 5 to 10 mm. At the stent edge, tissue proliferation and absence of chronic stent recoil were similar to the intra-stent analysis. There appeared to be a progressively more EEM CSA and progressively less P+M CSA at axial distances farther from the edge of the stent. The finding of an "edge effect" in stented lesions (in the absence of brachytherapy), and the finding that this edge effect involves a combination of neointimal hyperplasia and negative remodeling, provide important background information in understanding edge effects after brachytherapy. These findings, demonstrated most elegantly in the HIPS Study, are shown in Figure 2.

Comparison of stented and non-stented lesions have shown *more neointimal hyperplasia in stented lesions*.[31,32] As in non-stented lesions, in-stent neointimal tissue proliferation was exaggerated in diabetic patients.[4] Thus, it appears that by preventing chronic negative arterial remodeling, stents can accommodate increased amounts of neointima and still reduce restenosis. In addition, stents appear to abolish the influence that pre-intervention positive remodeling has on target lesion revascularization, supporting the concept that increased plaque burden or positive remodeling amplifies the late negative remodeling process.[33]

Probucol has been shown to reduce restenosis after balloon angioplasty. Serial planar IVUS analysis showed that the mechanism by which probucol reduced restenosis was by decreasing late negative remodeling.[34] In this study, lumen CSA correlated with EEM CSA (r=0.53, P=0.002), but not with P+M CSA (r=0.13, P=0.5). Probucol did not reduce P+M CSA compared to controls. These findings are shown in Figure 3.

While BERT, a beta-irradiation post-balloon angioplasty study, did not contain a control group, serial volumetric IVUS analysis indicated that late lumen loss was virtually eliminated. IVUS analysis also showed that beta-irradiation did not prevent an increase in lesion site P+M volume.[35] The findings from BERT are discussed elsewhere in this book.

Summary

Except in diabetic patients, late responses to non-stent coronary interventions are determined less by P+M CSA than by the direction and magnitude of EEM CSA (positive or negative remodeling). The decrease in EEM CSA is a late event, is often preceded by an early (nonsustained) increase in EEM CSA, and is

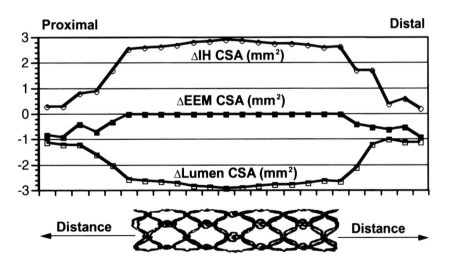

Figure 2. A millimeter by millimeter IVUS analysis of 151 patients from HIPS shows that in-stent lumen loss is entirely neointimal hyperplasia. This neointimal hyperplasia "spills over" into the adjacent reference segment. Beginning at the ends of the stents, lumen loss is progressively less neointimal hyperplasia and progressively more negative remodeling.

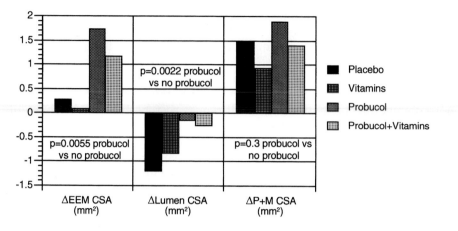

Figure 3. In one randomized trial, pre treatment with probucol reduced restenosis (lumen CSA) by promoting positive remodeling (increase in EEM CSA), not be reducing neointimal hyperplasia (increase in P+M CSA).

distinct from passive elastic recoil. *If* sustained, the early increase in EEM CSA may accommodate increased P+M CSA to prevent restenosis. Diabetics have both an exaggerated increase in P+M CSA as well as an impaired ability to mount a responsive increase in EEM CSA (positive remodeling). Plaque burden may play an important role in the restenosis process perhaps by amplifying late negative remodeling; the post-intervention plaque burden appears to predict restenosis in non-stented lesions. The pre-intervention remodeling characteristics of a lesion are also important; lesions with positive remodeling (lesion site EEM CSA greater than the reference) appear to be more biologically active and to have a higher rate of late revascularization. Stents do not exhibit chronic recoil; therefore, they reduce restenosis by opposing the late negative remodeling. This offsets a stent-related increase in neointimal hyperplasia, the dominant mechanism of in-stent restenosis. Both probucol and radiation appear to reduce late lumen loss after balloon angioplasty by promoting positive remodeling.

Conclusions

IVUS findings have been instrumental to the understanding of the restenosis process. These IVUS findings may reflect early scar formation and late scar retraction. In fact, the scar may actually be periadventitia. This concept is supported by a number of the animal and human necropsy studies that were cited above.

References

1. Nishioka T, Luo H, Eigler NL, et al. Contribution of inadequate compensatory enlargement to development of human coronary artery stenosis: An in vivo intravascular ultrasound study. J Am Coll Cardiol 1996;27:1571–1576.
2. Mintz GS, Popma JJ, Pichard AD, et al. Arterial remodeling after coronary angioplasty: A serial intravascular ultrasound study. Circulation 1996;94:35–43.
3. von Birgelen C, de Vrey E, Mintz GS, et al. ECG-gated three-dimensional intravascular ultrasound: Feasibility and reproducibility of the automated analysis of coronary

lumen and atherosclerotic plaque dimensions in humans. Circulation 1997;96:2944–2952.

4. Kornowski R, Mintz GS, Kent KM, et al. Increased restenosis in diabetes mellitus after coronary interventions is due to exaggerated intimal hyperplasia: A serial intravascular ultrasound study. Circulation 1997;95:1366–1369.

5. Kornowski R, Mintz GS, Lansky AH, et al. Paradoxic decreases in atherosclerotic plaque mass in insulin-treated diabetic patients. Am J Cardiol 1998;81:1298–1304.

6. Lansky AJ, Mintz GS, Popma JJ, et al. Remodeling after directional coronary atherectomy (±adjunct PTCA): A serial angiographic and intravascular ultrasound analysis from the Optimal Atherectomy Restenosis Study (OARS). J Am Coll Cardiol 1998;32:329–337.

7. Meine TJ, Bauman RP, Yock PG, et al. Coronary artery restenosis after atherectomy is primarily due to negative remodeling. Am J Cardiol 1999;84:141–146.

8. Suzuki T, Hosokawa H, Katoh O, et al. Effects of adjunctive balloon angioplasty after intravascular ultrasound-guided optimal directional coronary atherectomy: The result of Adjunctive Balloon Angioplasty After Coronary Atherectomy Study (ABACAS). J Am Coll Cardiol 1999;34:1028–1035.

9. Kimura T, Kaburagi S, Tamura T, et al. Remodeling of human coronary arteries undergoing coronary angioplasty or atherectomy. Circulation 1997;96:475–483.

10. Mintz GS, Kimura T, Nobuyoshi M, Leon MB. Intravascular ultrasound assessment of the relation between the early and late changes in arterial area and neointimal hyperplasia after percutaneous transluminal coronary angioplasty and directional coronary atherectomy. Am J Cardiol 1999;83:1518–1523.

11. de Vrey E, Mintz GS, von Birgelen C, et al. Arterial remodeling after directional coronary atherectomy: A serial volumetric (three-dimensional) intravascular ultrasound study. J Am Coll Cardiol 1998;32:1874–1880.

12. O'Brien ER, Alpres CE, Stewart DK, et al. Proliferation in primary and restenotic coronary atherectomy specimens: Implications for antiproliferative therapy. Circ Res 1993;73:223–231.

13. Kakuta T, Currier JW, Haudenschild CC, et al. Differences in compensatory vessel enlargement, not intimal formation, account for restenosis after angioplasty in the hypercholesterolemic rabbit model. Circulation 1994;89:2809–2815.

14. Lafont A, Guzman LA, Whitlow PL, et al. Restenosis after experimental angioplasty: Intimal, medial, and adventitial changes associated with constrictive remodeling. Circ Res 1995;76:996–1002.

15. Guzman LA, Mick MJ, Arnold AM, et al. Role of intimal hyperplasia and arterial remodeling after balloon angioplasty: An experimental study in the atherosclerotic rabbit model. Arterioscler Thromb Vasc Biol 1996;16:479–487.

16. Andersen HR, Maeng M, Thorwest M, Falk E. Remodeling rather than neointimal formation explains luminal narrowing after deep vessel wall injury: Insights from a porcine coronary (re)stenosis model. Circulation 1996;93:1716–1724.

17. Post MJ, de Smet BJ, van der Helm Y, et al. Arterial remodeling after balloon angioplasty or stenting in an atherosclerotic experimental model. Circulation 1997;96:996–1003.

18. Labinaz M, Pels K, Hoffert C, et al. Time course and importance of neoadventitial formation in arterial remodeling following balloon angioplasty of porcine coronary arteries. Cardiovasc Res 1999;41:255–266.

19. Pels K, Labinaz M, Hoffert C, O'Brien ER. Adventitial angiogenesis early after coronary angioplasty: Correlation with arterial remodeling. Arterioscler Thromb Vasc Biol 1999;19:229–238.

20. Kakuta T, Usui M, Coats WD Jr, et al. Arterial remodeling at the reference site after angioplasty in the atherosclerotic rabbit model. Arterioscler Thromb Vasc Biol 1998;18:47–51.

21. Currier JW, Faxon DP. Restenosis after percutaneous transluminal coronary angioplasty: Have we been aiming at the wrong target? J Am Coll Cardiol 1995;25:516–520.

22. Nakamura Y, Zhao H, Yutani C, et al. Morphometric and histologic assessment of remodeling associated with restenosis after percutaneous transluminal coronary angioplasty. Cardiology 1998;90:115–121.

23. Sangiorgi G, Taylor AJ, Carter AJ, et al. Histopathology of postpercutaneous transluminal coronary angioplasty remodeling in human coronary arteries. Am Heart J 1999;138:681–687.

24. Mintz GS, Popma JJ, Pichard AD, et al. Intravascular ultrasound predictors of restenosis following percutaneous transcatheter coronary revascularization. J Am Coll Cardiol 1996;27:1678–1687.
25. The GUIDE Trial Investigators. IVUS-determined predictors of restenosis in PTCA and DCA: Final report from the GUIDE Trial, phase II. J Am Coll Cardiol 1994;27:156A.
26. Dangas G, Mintz GS, Mehran R, et al. Pre-intervention arterial remodeling as an independent predictor of target lesion revascularization after non-stent coronary intervention: An analysis of 777 lesions with intravascular ultrasound imaging. Circulation 1999;99:3149–3154.
27. Peters RJG, Kok WEM, Di Mario C, et al. Prediction of restenosis after coronary angioplasty: Results of PICTURE (Post-IntraCoronary Treatment Ultrasound Result Evaluation), a prospective multicenter intracoronary ultrasound imaging study. Circulation 1997;95:2254–2261.
28. de Smet BJ, Pasterkamp G, van der Helm YJ, et al. The relation between de novo atherosclerosis remodeling and angioplasty-induced remodeling in an atherosclerotic Yucatan micropig model. Arterioscler Thromb Vasc Biol 1998;18:702–707.
29. Hoffmann R, Mintz GS, Dussaillant GR, et al. Patterns and mechanisms of in-stent restenosis: A serial intravascular ultrasound study. Circulation 1996;94:1247–1254.
30. Mudra H, Regar E, Klauss V, et al. Serial follow-up after optimized ultrasound-guided employment of Palmaz-Schatz stents: In-stent neointimal proliferation without significant reference segment response. Circulation 1997;95:363–370.
31. Mintz GS, Popma JJ, Hong MK, et al. Intravascular ultrasound to discern device-specific effects and mechanisms of restenosis. Am J Cardiol 1996;78(3A):18–22.
32. Tsuchikane E, Sumitsuji S, Awata N, et al. Final results of the Stent versus directional coronary Atherectomy Randomized Trial. J Am Coll Cardiol 1999;34:1050–10507.
33. Dangas G, Mintz GS, Mehran R, et al. Stent implantation neutralized the impact of pre-intervention arterial remodeling on subsequent target lesion revascularization. Am J Cardiol In press.
34. Cote G, Tardif JC, Lesperance J, et al. Effects of probucol on vascular remodeling after coronary angioplasty: Multivitamins and Protocol Study Group. Circulation 1999;99:30–35.
35. Sabate M, Serruys PW, van der Giessen WJ, et al. Geometric vascular remodeling after balloon angioplasty and beta-radiation therapy: A three-dimensional intravascular ultrasound study. Circulation 1999;100:1182–1188.

___ *Chapter 6* ___

Antirestenosis Alternatives in the New Millennium

Michael J.B. Kutryk, MD, PhD, and
Patrick W. Serruys, MD, PhD

The focus of the treatment of restenosis over the last two decades has been through the application of pharmacologically active agents and mechanical approaches with use of a host of different devices. Unfortunately, this frequent and costly complication of percutaneous revascularization techniques has proven refractory to all such therapies. Characteristic of the restenosis process is neointimal proliferation, which involves the migration of vascular smooth muscle cells from the media and the adventitia and their intraluminal proliferation, and vascular remodeling, which potentially involves all three layers of the vessel wall. The inciting stimuli involved in restenosis include disruption of the endothelial barrier layer, mechanical factors which disrupt the medial smooth muscle layer and serve as stimuli for smooth muscle cell proliferation and migration, and the contact of this disrupted layer with circulating blood factors and mitogens which serve as further stimuli to neointimal formation. Some of the major influences that contribute to the process of restenosis are summarized in Figure 1. Vascular injury sets into motion a cascade of events which result in the final hyperplastic response shown by the neointima. Early in our understanding of the pathophysiological processes involved in restenosis, attention was concentrated on factors that interact with smooth muscle cells through cell surface receptors. These include compounds like thrombin, platelet-derived growth factor (PDGF), angiotensin II, interleukin 1, insulin growth factor-1 (IGF-1), basic fibroblast growth factor (bFGF), and a whole host of other mitogenic factors. Initial treatments for restenosis targeted these receptors with pharmacological agents in an attempt to inhibit their effects. It soon became apparent, however, that none of these stimuli work through a unique pathway. Instead, these signals interact at an intracellular level through second messenger systems, which confers redundancy to the system. Ultimately, these second messenger systems converge on a final common pathway at the cellular DNA level known as the cell cycle (Fig. 2).

The life cycle of a normal cell can be considered in five different cell phases. G_0 (G = gap) is the quiescent state in which the cell is biologically active but is neither actively dividing or replicating. Under appropriate stimuli, the cell can enter the cell cycle at G_1, or interphase, in which biosynthetic activities of the cell

From Waksman R (ed.). *Vascular Brachytherapy, Third Edition.* Armonk, NY: Futura Publishing Co., Inc.; © 2002.

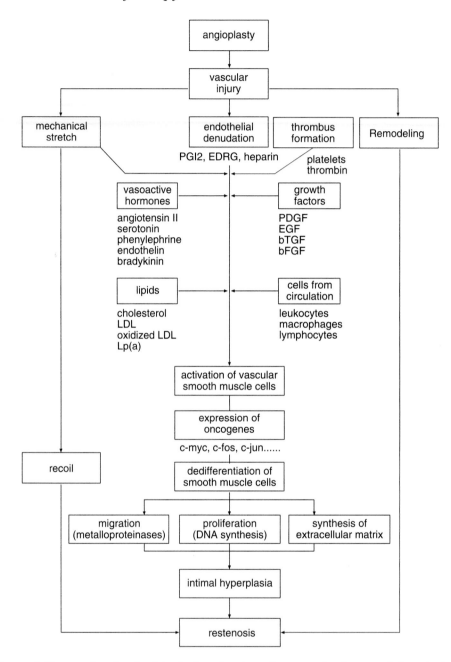

Figure 1. Proposed pathophysiological mechanism of restenosis after arterial angioplasty. The main mechanism for intimal hyperplasia is shown in the central pathway, which involves smooth muscle cell activation with subsequent proto-oncogene induction. Modified from Reference 19.

prepare the cell to enter into the next phase of the cell cycle, the S phase. The S phase begins when DNA synthesis starts, and ends when the DNA content of the nucleus has doubled and the chromosomes have replicated. The S phase is followed by G_2, which ends when mitosis starts, signalling the start of the M phase.

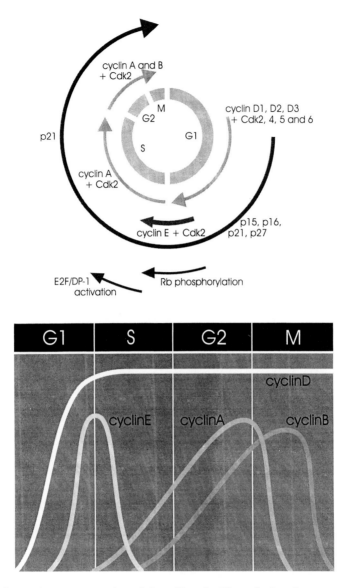

Figure 2. Schematic representation of the cell cycle. The relative time course of the oscillatory production of the major cyclin proteins is shown in the lower panel.

Activation of the cell cycle is responsible for normal physiological growth and cell division as well as for pathophysiological processes such as restenosis.

A large number of genes are involved in the control of cell cycle progression in eukaryotic cells. They can be divided into early G_1 genes (such as c-fos, c-myc, etc.), late G_1 genes (c-myb, retinoblastoma [rb], etc.), genes involved in G_1/S transition (cdc/ckd kinases, etc.), S phase genes involved in DNA synthesis (DNA polymerases, proliferating cell nuclear antigen [PCNA], etc.), genes involved in G_2/M transition (cdc/ckd kinases, etc.), and genes involved in mitosis (cytoskeletal proteins, mitosis-specific kinases, etc.) (Fig. 2). In theory, suppression of any one of these genes will lead to interruption of cell cycle progression, a strategy that is being explored for the prevention of restenosis as we approach the new millennium. Two different tactics are currently being tested. Brachytherapy bombards the nuclear material with ionizing radiation, disrupting the templates for the production of cell cycle regulatory proteins. With the correct radiation dose, the target smooth muscle cell remains viable but unable to replicate. The other approach depends on a biological attack on the cell regulatory machinery, using gene therapy technology for the introduction of foreign fragments of nuclear material to halt the pathophysiological processes typical of restenosis.

There are a number of different approaches using the basic techniques of gene therapy that are currently being tested for the prevention of neointimal hyperplasia. The most straightforward involve the transfer of a gene directly into the proliferating smooth muscle cells. This gene can encode for a cytotoxic protein (eg, herpes virus thymidine kinase), a cell cycle inhibitory protein (eg, p53, p21, Rb, cdk), angiogenic proteins (eg, vascular endothelial growth factor [VEGF], angiogenin, bFGF), or proteins with vasodilatory, antithrombotic, or antiproliferative properties (eg, NOS, cox-1, PAI-1). This type of approach has been shown to be effective in several animal models of restenosis. With use of adenovirus as a vector, herpes virus thymidine kinase has been successfully transfected into vascular smooth muscle cells at the site of balloon injury in the femoral arteries of swine.[1] This was followed by systemic administration of the nucleoside analogue ganciclovir, which, in the presence of the foreign thymidine kinase, can be incorporated into the cellular DNA. By use of this technique, both smooth muscle cell proliferation and luminal narrowing were shown to be inhibited.[1] Adenovirus-mediated transfer of the Rb gene, whose protein product inhibits cell cycle progression, has also been shown to be successful in a similar animal model.[2] Transfer of the gene coding for nitric oxide synthase by use of a protein/liposome hybrid vector,[3] as well as angiotensin II type 2 receptor[4] and the thrombin inhibitor hirudin[5] by use of adenovirus vectors, have also been shown to be effective for the prevention of restenosis in the rat carotid model of vessel injury.

It has recently been shown that vectors for the introduction of the DNA into the cell are not necessary. Introduction of naked DNA coding for the very potent angiogenic factor VEGF has been shown to be clinically effective for the treatment of peripheral vascular disease.[6] This unique approach is aimed at treating established disease rather than attempting to prevent neointimal formation, and targets the ischemic territory served by the stenotic vascular segment rather than the lesion itself. Neovascularization of the tissue surrounding the blockage can result in adequate perfusion of distal tissues. The effectiveness of this biological bypass in the cardiovascular system has also been recently demonstrated in animal models. Clinical trials for the treatment of myocardial ischemia with use of angiogenic factors are being planned in many centers around the world.

Another "nuclear weapon" that is being developed for the prevention of restenosis involves antisense oligonucleotide technology. Antisense oligodeoxynucleotides are short pieces of DNA with sequences that are complementary to specific regions of messenger RNA. The major mechanisms of action of these compounds are through the sequence-specific interaction with messenger RNA, although sequence-specific and sequence-nonspecific effects have also been demonstrated (Fig. 3). On binding to the target, the antisense compound sterically inhibits the interaction of ribosomes with the messenger RNA (Fig. 4). Another mech-

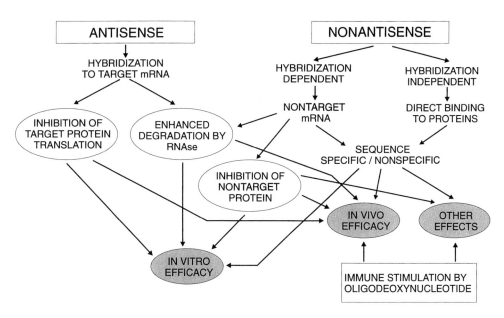

Figure 3. Intracellular interactions of antisense oligonucleotides. Some of the effects of antisense compounds may be due to non-antisense–specific events.

anism of action, which may be as important as the steric inhibition of ribosome binding, is a consequence of the DNA/RNA hybrid being more susceptible to degradation by intracellular RNAse than single-stranded messenger RNA. This results in a increased clearance of target mRNA from the cell. In principle, any gene may be selected for antisense suppression, but inhibition of certain genes will certainly be more biologically effective. Important in this regard are the abundance of the messenger RNA, the half-life of the protein product, and the existence of redundancy within the cell such that other proteins are capable of performing similar functions to that which is targeted. Given these considerations, it is not surprising that most of the attention of antisense technology has been focused on the short-lived regulators of the final common pathway of mitogenic stimuli, the cell cycle. Inhibition of the production of several of the mediators of the cell cycle with antisense oligonucleotides has been shown to be effective for the prevention of restenosis in several different animal models of vascular injury (Table 1).

With our increased understanding of vascular molecular biology, more sophisticated approaches which employ the basics of gene therapy are being investigated. For instance, cell-based vascular gene delivery techniques are now being explored as means to provide biologically relevant amounts of therapeutic agents to the site of vessel damage. This strategy involves the isolation of autologous endothelial or smooth muscle cells, ex vivo gene transfer, followed by the reintroduction of the genetically modified cells back to region selected for therapy. The disadvantages of this approach include the requirement to isolate and modify cells from each patient with the consequent delay in therapy and the failure to date, with few exceptions, to show a relevant expression of recombinant protein in vivo. In our laboratory, order to circumvent these problems, we are focusing our attention on the xenotransplantation of genetically modified endothelial cells for the

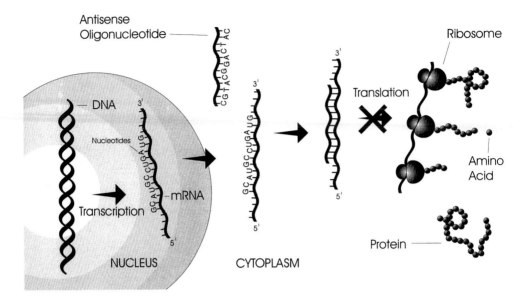

Figure 4. One of the proposed mechanisms of action of antisense deoxyribonucleotides. Normal gene transcription of DNA into mRNA is followed by translation into protein. Antisense oligonucleotides to a complementary portion of the mRNA prevent translation by the steric inhibition of ribosome binding.

prevention of restenosis. We have designed animals that are doubly transgenic in that they carry not only a human gene which can produce an agent for the prevention of restenosis, but also carry genes coding for human cell surface markers so that they may be effectively xenotransplanted into humans and therefore provide a local source of bioactive compounds. These animals provide a limitless sup-

Table 1

In Vivo Antisense Studies

Investigators	Experimental Model	Gene	Delivery Vehicle	% Intimal Suppression
Simons et al.[7]	rat	c-myb	Pluronic gel	84%
Edelman et al.[8]	rat	c-myb	EVav	80%
Azrin et al.[9]	pig	c-myb	Hydrogel catheter	NR
Gunn et al.[10]	pig	c-myb	None	65%
Bennet et al.[11]	rat	c-myc	Pluronic gel	53%
Edelman et al.[8]	rat	c-myc	EVac	90%
Shi et al.[12]	pig	c-myc	None	70%
Morishita et al.[13]	rat	cdc-2/PCNA	HVJ	68%
Abe et al.[14]	rat	cdc-2	Pluronic gel	47%
Abe et al.[14]	rat	cdk—2	Pluronic gel	55%
Morishita et al.[15]	rat	cdk-2	HVJ	40%
Simons et al.[16]	rat	PCNA	Pluronic gel	80%
Sirois et al.[17]	rat	PDFG-β receptor	EVac	70%

HVJ = Hemagglutinating virus of Japan; EVac = ethylenvinylacetate; NR = not reported.
Modified from Reference 18.

ply of endothelial cells, producing controllable levels of active compound, which can be used for xenotransplantation at the site of vessel injury in humans. These foreign cells act as a kind of Trojan horse, graciously accepted as self by the host organism, but capable of modifying the pathophysiological response to vessel damage typified by the process of restenosis. Once implanted, the production of the bioactive compound is under exogenous control by means of "designer" genes coding for modified cell surface receptors that are introduced with the transgene. In this system interaction of an orally administered compound with the modified cell receptor can switch on the transgene, while in its absence the transgene remains dormant. The feasibility of this type of approach has been demonstrated in other animal species, and it shows great potential for application to humans. The applicability of this type of therapeutic delivery systems to other pathophysiological conditions and the shortage of tissue for organ transplantation are the fuel for continued high research activity in this direction.

As our understanding of the molecular control of cellular function increases and our knowledge of the pathophysiology of restenosis expands, new types of gene therapy approaches will be developed for the treatment of this iatrogenic complication. An area of active investigation is the development of new techniques for the introduction of foreign DNA into whole cells. All of the currently available viral and nonviral vectors have significant limitations to their use. The introduction of an effective, nonimmunogenic delivery vehicle is on the horizon. As the last decade was the era of mechanical and pharmacological approaches to the prevention of restenosis, developments in the coming decade will be aimed at manipulating the genetic material of the proliferating cell.

References

1. Ohno T, Gordon D, San H, et al. Gene therapy for vascular smooth muscle cell proliferation after arterial injury. Science 1994;265:781–784.
2. Chang MW, Barr E, Seltzer J, et al. Cytostatic gene therapy for vascular proliferative disorders with a constitutively active form of the retinoblastoma gene product. Science 1995;267:518–522.
3. von der Leyen HE, Gibbons GH, Morishita R, et al. Gene therapy inhibiting neointimal vascular lesion: In vivo transfer of endothelial cell nitric oxide synthase gene. Proc Natl Acad Sci U S A 1995;92:1137–1141.
4. Nakajima M, Hutchison HG, Fujinaga M, et al. The angiotensin II type II receptor antagonizes the growth effects of the AT1 receptor: Gain-of-function study using gene transfer. Proc Natl Acad Sci U S A 1995;92:10663–10667.
5. Rade JJ, Schulick AH, Virmani R, Dichek DA. Local adenoviral-mediated expression of recombinant hirudin reduces neointima formation after arterial injury. Nat Med 1996;2:293–298.
6. Isner JM, Pieczek A, Schainfeld R, et al. Clinical evidence of angiogenesis after arterial gene transfer of phVEGF$_{165}$ in patient with ischaemic limb. Lancet 1996;348:370–374.
7. Simons M, Edelman ER, DeKeyser JL, et al. Antisense c-myb oligonucleotides inhibit intimal arterial smooth muscle cell accumulation in vivo. Nature 1992;359:67–70.
8. Edelman ER, Simons M, Sirois MG, Rosenberg RD. c-Myc in vasculo-proliferative disease. Circ Res 1995;76:176–182.
9. Azrin MA, Mitchel JF, Pedersen C. Inhibition of smooth muscle cell proliferation in vivo following local delivery of antisense c-myb oligonucleotide during angioplasty [abstract]. J Am Coll Cardiol 1994;23(suppl):396A.
10. Gunn J, Holt CM, Shepherd L, et al. Local delivery of c-myb antisense attenuates neointimal thickening in porcine model of coronary angioplasty [abstract]. J Am Coll Cardiol 1995;25(suppl):201A.

11. Bennet MR, Anglin S, McEwan JR, et al. Inhibition of vascular smooth muscle cell proliferation in vitro and in vivo by c-myuuc antisense oligodeoxynucleotides. J Clin Invest 1994;93:820–828.
12. Shi Y, Fard A, Galeo A, et al. Transcatheter delivery of c-myc antisense oligomers reduces neointimal formation in a porcine model of coronary artery balloon injury. Circulation 1994;90:944–951.
13. Morishita R, Gibbons GH, Ellison KE, et al. Single intraluminal delivery of antisense cdc2 kinase and proliferating-cell nuclear antigen oligonucleotides results in chronic inhibition of neointimal hyperplasia. Proc Natl Acad Sci U S A 1993;90:8474–8478.
14. Abe J, Zhou W, Taguchi J, et al. Suppression of neointimal smooth muscle cell accumulation in vivo by antisense cdc-2 and cdk-2 oligonucleotides in rat carotid artery. Biochem Biophys Res Commun 1994;198:16–24.
15. Morishita R, Gibbons GH, Ellison KE, et al. Intimal hyperplasia after vascular injury is inhibited by antisense cdk-2 oligonucleotides. J Clin Invest 1994;93:1458–1464.
16. Simons M, Edelman ER, Rosenberg RD. Antisense PCNA oligonucleotides inhibit intimal hyperplasia in a rat carotid injury model. J Clin Invest 1994;93:2351–2356.
17. Sirois MG, Simons M, Edelman ER, Rosenberg RD. Platelet release of platelet derived growth factor is required for intimal hyperplasia in rat vascular injury model [abstract]. Circulation 1994;90(suppl I):I–511.
18. Simons M. Endogenous expression modification: Antisense approaches. In: March KL (ed.): Gene Transfer in the Cardiovascular System. Experimental Approaches and Therapeutic Implications. Boston: Kluwer Academic Publishers; 1997.
19. Hamon M, Bauters C, McFadden P, et al. Restenosis after coronary angioplasty. Eur Heart J 1995;16(suppl I):33–48.

Part II

Radiation Biology and Vascular Pathology

## Chapter 7

The Basic Radiobiology of Intravascular Irradiation

Eric J. Hall, DPhil, DSc

Mechanisms of Restenosis

The improvement in blood flow resulting from balloon angioplasty is not always long lasting; restenosis—a subsequent re-obstruction in the artery—occurs in 30% to 50% of the cases within 6 to 12 months. Studies in humans and in animal models indicate that restenosis is a consequence of the combination of arterial remodeling and fibrocellular neointimal hyperplasia, with smooth muscle cell (SMC) proliferation beginning within a few days after injury. It is debatable which of these two mechanisms contributes predominantly to restenosis, but it is the intimal hyperplasia that is an inviting target for antiproliferative strategies.

The probable sequence of events is illustrated in Figure 1. The damage caused by balloon angioplasty causes the release of a host of cytokines and growth factors by platelets, leukocytes, and SMCs, which in turn leads to the synthesis of gene products that stimulate SMC migration and proliferation leading to intimal growth.[1,2] By use of bromodeoxyuridine labeling, it has been shown that 40% to 50% of SMCs are labeled in damaged segments of the artery, compared with less than 1% in the undamaged arterial wall.[3] SMCs pour in through the tear in the endothelial lining that was caused by the angioplasty as illustrated in Figure 1.

Following angioplasty, there is presumably a race between the invasion of SMCs through the tear in the endothelial lining and attempts to repair that tear by the migration of endothelial cells from outside the treated area. Restenosis occurs when the SMCs win that race.

It is a logical approach to use some local agent to inhibit cellular proliferation in order to delay or prevent restenosis. Strategies involving local delivery of cytotoxic drugs or suicide gene therapy have proved largely ineffective because, although conceived as site-specific approaches, in fact, much of the cytotoxic agent ends up in the surrounding tissue or in the systemic vasculature, with the potential for undesirable toxicity. An intravascular radiation source, emitting either β- or γ-rays truly localizes the antiproliferative effect to the necessary cells, as illustrated in the bottom panel of Figure 1.

From Waksman R (ed.). *Vascular Brachytherapy, Third Edition.* Armonk, NY: Futura Publishing Co., Inc.; © 2002.

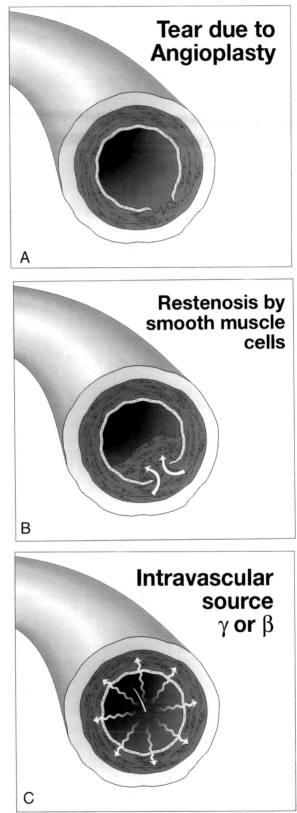

Figure 1. A: Balloon angioplasty causes a tear in the endothelial lining of the artery; **B:** Stimulated by cytokines and growth factors, smooth muscle cells proliferate and pour in through the tear in the endothelial lining; **C:** A γ- or β-emitting radionuclide source placed in the center of the artery irradiates the smooth muscle cells and inhibits their proliferation.

Modeling Restenosis

Two attempts have been made to model the process of cell proliferation that leads to restenosis in the human. As would be expected, the results vary to some extent according to the basic assumptions made, but the overall conclusion of both models is that comparatively few cell generations are required to produce sufficient neointima for arterial obstruction to occur. Schwartz and colleagues suggested about 10 doublings, while Brenner et al[6] estimated about 5. [4,5,6] Both of these models require an assumption to be made of the proportion of SMCs in a mature artery that retain the ability to proliferate, and this is a figure that is not known with any certainty.

Radiation Effects on Cells and Tissues

The effects of ionizing radiation on cells and tissues has been exhaustively studied for half a century. For differentiated cells that do not proliferate, such as nerve, muscle, or secretory cells, large doses of radiation in excess of 100 Gy are necessary to destroy cell function.[7] More modest doses of radiation do not affect cell function *per se* but produce DNA damage which causes the cell to die if and when it attempts to divide. Resting cells may be exposed to substantial doses of radiation (10 to 20 Gy) with no apparent ill effects, but when they attempt to divide days, months, or even years later, the damage to their DNA becomes apparent and they die. In other words, radiation can remove the proliferative potential, or reproductive integrity of a cell without destroying the ability of the cell to function during the interval before it is called upon to divide.

A survival curve is the relation between absorbed dose and the fraction of cells that retain their reproductive integrity. At the doses of interest here, the most important mechanism of radiation-induced death for the majority of cell types results from chromosomal damage, specifically the formation of exchange type aberrations such as dicentrics and rings which cause no problems when the cell is resting, but prove to be lethal if the complex process of cell division is attempted.[8,9] The basic lesion produced by radiation is a double-strand break (DSB).[10,11] If a DSB is produced in each of two chromosomes, they may interact and rejoin in an illegitimate way to form one of the lethal aberrations referred to above.[7]

The process of forming a dicentric aberration from DSBs in two different chromosomes is illustrated in Figure 2. Also illustrated in the figure is the possibility that the two DSBs may rejoin in such a way as to form a symmetrical translocation; this event is not lethal, but under certain circumstances, and at low probability, this can lead to the activation of an oncogene and the induction of a malignant change.

Cell death resulting from chromosomal aberrations is frequently referred to as "mitotic death" because it occurs if, and only if, the cell attempts to divide. This form of death leads to a dose-response relationship where the fraction of cells surviving (S) is a linear-quadratic function of dose (D), ie,

$$S = e^{-\alpha D - \beta D2}$$

Where α and β are constants which are characteristic of a given cell type.

At low doses, the linear component dominates, but at higher doses (such as

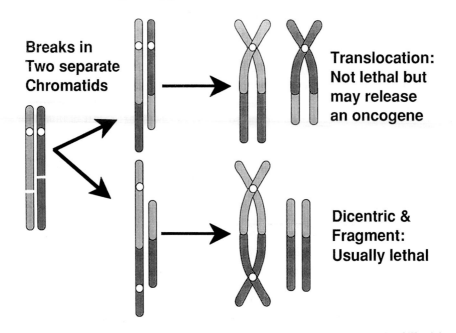

Figure 2. Illustrating the formation of chromosomal aberrations as a result of illegitimate rejoining of a double strand break in each of two different chromosomes. In the lower half of the figure, the pieces of broken chromosomes have rejoined to form a dicentric chromosome and an acentric fragment. This will prove to be lethal when the cell attempts to divide. In the top half of the figure, the pieces of broken chromosomes have rejoined to form a symmetrical translocation. This is compatible with viability, but if the breaks occurred in just the right places, this can result in the activation of an oncogene or the creation of a fusion gene that leads to a malignancy.

the single doses that are proposed for intravascular irradiation) the term that is quadratic in dose starts to dominate. This is illustrated in Figure 3.

For some cell types, particularly those of lymphoid origin, radiation-induced apoptosis may assume considerable importance.[12] In this model of cell death, survival is a linear function of dose—thus apoptotic cell death adds to the component of cell lethality from chromosome damage route. To date, there is no evidence that apoptosis is a dominant, or even an important, mechanism of radiation-induced cell death in either endothelial or SMCs.

Figure 4 shows in vitro cell survival data, generated in our laboratory, for SMCs of human origin. Their response to radiation and their radiosensitivity is unremarkable in that it falls within the range of that of most mammalian cells. For example, following a dose of 8 Gy, the fraction of cells surviving is about 10^{-2}, ie, approximately one in a hundred cells remain viable in the sense that it can proliferate indefinitely.

Early-Responding and Late-Responding Tissues

One of the major advances in radiation biology in the 1980s was the recognition that early- and late-responding normal tissues respond differently to radiation, in particular the survival curve is more "curvy" (ie, has a smaller α/β ratio)

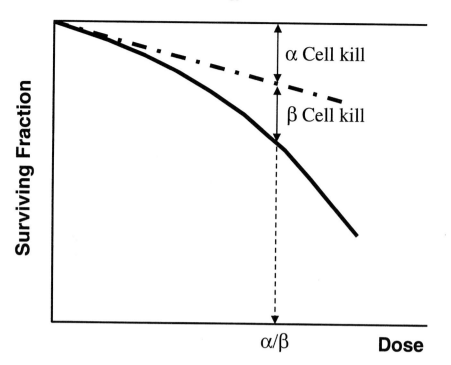

Figure 3. A typical survival curve for mammalian cells exposed to a single acute dose of radiation. The survival curve follows a linear-quadratic relationship with dose. The linear (α) component is derived from chromosomal aberrations formed through misrepair of pairs of double-strand breaks (DSB) produced by a single electron, set in motion by the absorption of a photon of x- or γ-rays. The quadratic (β) component is derived from aberrations formed through misrepair of pairs of DSB produced by two independent electrons.

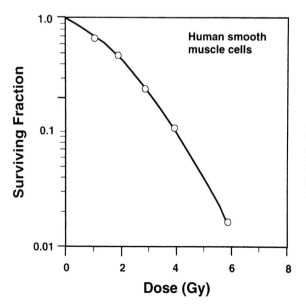

Figure 4. Survival data for smooth muscle cells of human origin exposed to graded doses of γ-rays. The curve represents a fit to the linear-quadratic formalism. The radiosensitivity of these cells is unremarkable and similar to many mammalian cells.

for late-responding tissues.[13] This is illustrated in Figure 5. While the mechanisms underlying this are not fully understood, the practical consequence is clear, namely that late-responding tissues are more sensitive to changes in fractionation schedules. In external beam radiotherapy (EBR) of malignant disease, the therapeutic ratio between tumor response and late-responding normal tissues is exaggerated by increasing the number of fractions. This important factor in opening the therapeutic window in the radiotherapy of cancer, between cells that we want to sterilize and those that we want to spare, is lost in endovascular irradiation because only a single dose can be delivered.

The Telomere Hypothesis

Telomeres cap and protect the ends of chromosomes.[14,15] Herman J. Muller coined the term telomere, which literally means end-part, coming from the two Greek roots, telos (meaning "end") and meros (meaning "part").[16] Mammalian telomeres consist of long arrays of the repeat sequence TTAGGG; most human telomeres range in size from 5 to 15 kb; however, some contain more. Each time a normal somatic cell divides 50 to 200 base pairs are lost from the terminal end of the telomere; successive divisions lead to progressive shortening and, after 40 to

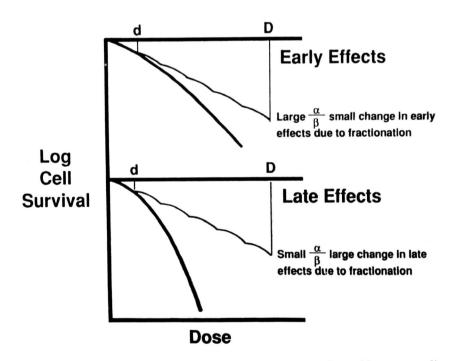

Figure 5. The difference in response to protraction between early- and late-responding tissues. Note that the more curvature that is shown by an acute dose-response curve, the greater will be its response to changes in protraction. Early-responding tissues (including, most likely, smooth muscle in arteries) exhibit relatively straight dose-response curves, and thus show only limited changes when a dose is fractionated. Dose-response relations for late-responding tissues, on the other hand, exhibit more curvature and hence show more sparing when the dose is protracted. Thus, overall, protraction increases the therapeutic ratio between early- and late-responding tissues.

60 divisions, vital DNA sequences are lost. At this point the cell cannot divide further and undergoes senescence. This is illustrated in Figure 6. Telomere length has been described as the "molecular clock," since it shortens with age in somatic tissue cells during adult life. Stem cells in self-renewing tissues, and cancer cells in particular, avoid this process of aging by activating the enzyme telomerase.[17,18] Telomerase is a reverse transcriptase which polymerizes TTAGGG repeats to offset the degradation of chromosome ends that occurs with successive cell divisions; in this way the cell becomes immortal. Since immortality and uncontrolled growth is the hallmark of cancer cells, the activation of telomerase would appear to be a vital step in carcinogenesis. In tissue culture, immortalization of cells, ie, cells that pass through a "crisis" and continue to be able to divide beyond the normal limit, is associated with telomere stabilization and activity of telomerase.

The important point in the present context is that telomeres shorten as a function of age in cells derived from normal human blood, skin, and colonic mucosa, and all somatic cells. Consequently, there is a marked reduction in telomere size in somatic cells from an adult compared to germ cells from the same individuals. As a consequence, since normal somatic cells lack telomerase, they have a limited proliferative potential and senesce after a predictable number of divisions.[19] Furthermore, proliferative potential decreases with age. In a newborn, a somatic cell may harbor the ability to divide 40 to 60 times, but in an adult of late middle age, cells may be capable of only half as many divisions. It is for this reason that doses of radiation sufficient to inhibit restenosis would not be adequate to control the smallest cancer, since the surviving cells have the ability to proliferate indefinitely. To control a cancer, every last malignant cell must be killed; this is not necessary to inhibit restenosis. Rather, it is only required to inhibit the proliferation of a suffi-

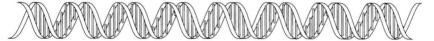

A) Telomeres are repeat sequences that cap chromosomes to protect their ends. TTAGGG is repeated for 1.5 to 30 kb.

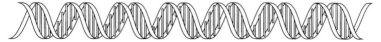

B) Each time a cell divides, the telmere of the progeny cells become shorter. Telomere length is the "molecular clock".

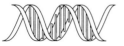

C) After 40-60 replications the telomeres are shortened dramatically; vital DNA sequences are lost, the cell cannot divide & dies.

Figure 6. Telomeres are the repeat sequences that cap the ends of chromosomes. Each time a normal somatic cell divides, part of the telomere cannot be replicated and it becomes shorter and shorter. After 40 to 60 divisions, important DNA is lost and the cell senesces. In a middle-aged adult, half of these divisions have already occurred, and thus somatic cells have a limited proliferation potential.

cient proportion of the cell population so that the survivors run out of proliferative ability before sufficient progeny are produced to cause restenosis.

Application of Radiobiological Principles to Restenosis

From our experimental data, we know the proportion of SMCs that preserve their ability to divide as a function of dose (see Fig. 4). A single acute radiation dose of 12 Gy results in a depopulation of about 10^{-3}, ie, only about 1 in 1000 cells would retain the ability to proliferate. These cells would need to go through 15 to 20 doublings to block the artery, made up of 10 doublings to overcome the depopulation caused by the radiation ($2^{10} \cong 1000$), and 5 to 10 more doublings to cause restenosis as estimated from the various modeling studies referred to earlier. This would take some months, and thus a 12-Gy dose would be expected to delay restenosis but not inhibit it permanently. By the same token, 15 Gy would result in a depopulation of 10^{-4}, ie, 1 in 10,000 cells would retain the ability to proliferate and these cells would require 18 to 23 doublings to block the artery. Twenty Gy would result in a depopulation to 5×10^{-6}, and the survivors would require 21 to 26 doublings to cause restenosis.

However, these SMCs are normal somatic cells; they are not malignant cancer cells and thus they have a limited potential to proliferate which decreases with age due to telomere shortening, as explained earlier. Lower doses might be expected to delay restenosis, with the length of the delay being dose-dependent. But a dose somewhere between 15 and 20 Gy might permanently inhibit the restenosis because cells surviving the radiation would not have the capability to proliferate enough to block the artery.

Overall, we can conclude that (a) the beneficial effect of endovascular irradiation is primarily related to the inhibition of proliferative ability of SMCs, which would otherwise initiate neointimal hyperplasia, and (b) there is not a large safety margin between the radiation dose required for the long-term control of restenosis (~20 Gy) and the radiation dose that might result in undesirable late sequelae due to damage to the artery wall (30 Gy).

Choice of Radioisotopes for Endovascular Brachytherapy

The few successful trials carried out to date in which radiation has been shown to inhibit restenosis in humans or pigs have all involved the γ-emitter iridium 192. The use of this radionuclide introduces two major problems.

1. Radiation safety. Because of the penetration of γ-rays involved, the patient must be in some sort of shielded room during treatment in order to protect staff.
2. Treatment time. Considerations of radiation safety also limit the activity of γ-emitting sources and, as a consequence, the treatment time to deliver a dose of 15 to 20 Gy at 3 mm from the source is about 20 minutes.

Both of these problems are solved instantly if a β-emitting radionuclide is used. Because of the limited range of β-rays, treatments could be carried out in the cardiology laboratory with minimal radiation protection, and treatment times could be on the order of a few minutes. For this reason, much commercial effort is focused on developing a practical system based on a β-emitting radionuclide. On the other hand, the short range of the β-rays makes them extremely sensitive to problems of source centering, which may well limit their eventual usefulness.

Dose-Rate Effect in Radiation Biology

The biological effect of a given dose of low linear energy transfer (LET), sparsely ionizing radiation, depends critically on the dose rate at which it is delivered or, put another way, on the total exposure time.[20] This has been known from clinical observations in brachytherapy since the 1940s, and was demonstrated in detail with cells in culture by Hall and Bedford in the 1960s.[21] This phenomenon has come to be known as the dose-rate effect and is one of the most important factors that determine the fraction of cells killed by a given dose of x-rays, γ-rays, or electrons.

The magnitude of the dose-rate effect depends on the cell type, and is largest for cells that characteristically die a mitotic death, and smallest for cells that die principally an apoptotic death.[22] The dose-rate range, or range of exposure times, over which the dose-rate effect is important, is determined by the rate of repair of sublethal damage, which is quantified by the half-time for sublethal damage repair ($T_{1/2}$). Brenner and Hall reviewed the literature for around 40 cell lines of human origin, cultured in vitro, and found a wide range of $T_{1/2}$ values, approximately log-normally distributed, with a geometric mean value of about 16 minutes.[23]

Dose-Rate Effect and its Influence on Vascular Brachytherapy to Prevent Restenosis

The beneficial effect of endovascular irradiation is related to inhibiting the proliferative potential of SMCs, which would otherwise initiate neointimal hyperplasia. There is not a large safety margin between the radiation dose required for the long-term control of restenosis (~20 Gy) and the radiation dose that might result in undesirable late sequelae (~30 Gy), so it is crucial to optimize the prescribed dose for restenosis prevention, and then to deliver the radiation dose that is iso-effective to this optimized dose, even when the dose rate changes significantly. The various techniques used or proposed for the delivery of the radiation dose include γ- and β-emitters, most of which have relatively short physical half-lives. The variation in exposure times over the practical lifetime of a given radioactive source are on the order of the half-time of repair of sublethal damage characteristic of human cells, so that the resultant biological effect will be critically dependent on the dose-rate/exposure time.

Thus, the dose-rate effect is a biological factor that will need to be taken into account on a daily basis in clinical practice, because almost all of the radionuclides proposed for use have relatively short half-lives. For example, iridium 192 has a half-life of 60 days and sources are usually replaced after about two half-lives; thus, the exposure times will vary by a factor of four during the practical lifetime of the sources, which will have a profound effect on the biological effectiveness of a given prescribed dose of about 20 Gy. As another example, a β-emitting source of [90]Y (radioactive half-life 64 hours) has a useful lifetime of about 1 week, during which the dose rate varies by a factor of six, with consequent significant impact on the biological effectiveness of a given prescribed dose. Figure 7 shows the results of calculations of the doses equivalent to 20 Gy delivered as an acute exposure lasting 2 minutes, for exposure times up to 25 minutes and for $T_{1/2}$ values of 15 to 45 minutes. A short exposure time of 1 or 2 minutes is possible with a β-emitting radionuclide. The longer and more variable exposure times up to 25 minutes are characteristic of γ-emitting radionuclides, such as iridium 192. It is evident that extending the exposure time has a substantial effect; 20 Gy delivered in 25 minutes is equivalent to only 17 to 19 Gy delivered in 1 minutes. If clinical results between patients are to be compared, particularly from institutions that use different radionuclides, this dose-rate effect must be taken into account.

Radiation Quality and its Influence on Vascular Brachytherapy to Prevent Restenosis

There is good radiobiological evidence that electrons in the megavoltage range are less effective biologically than kilovoltage x- or γ-rays. The microdosimetric analysis also suggests a relative biological effectiveness of less than unity, based on the different physical energy deposition properties associated with the two types of radiation.[24] Specifically, the average photon energy from a highly filtered 250 kVp x-ray beam is ~85 keV and the average electron energy set in motion by the interaction of these photons with tissue is ~20 keV.[25,26] These energies are much lower than those corresponding to either megavoltage photons or to β-rays emitted by radionuclides proposed for intravascular brachytherapy; those have an average electron energy of several hundred kilovolts and a maximum

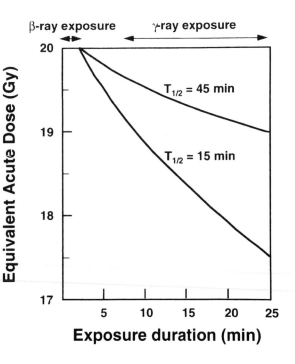

Figure 7. Equivalent acute doses to actual doses, delivered in exposure times up to 25 min. Two possible values are assumed for the half-time of repair of sub-lethal damage, namely 15 and 45 min. No experimental data are available for repair times in smooth muscle cells of human origin.

electron energy close to 1 MeV. This would imply a significant relative biological effectiveness difference, which could be 0.6 at very low doses and perhaps 0.85 at high therapeutic doses.

Conclusions

In summary, the early trials that have demonstrated the effectiveness of endovascular brachytherapy to inhibit restenosis have all involved the γ-emitter iridium 192. A great variety of systems are under development, driven largely by the technology. There is a lack of knowledge of the relative effectiveness of β-rays and γ-rays, and little knowledge of the influence of a time factor for overall treatment time between 60 seconds and 20 minutes, which is likely to be substantial when a single acute dose of 20 Gy is involved. Experimental data are urgently required to answer these questions and provide guidance for future clinical trials.

The limited radiobiological data available at the present time suggest the following conclusions:

- Doses of around 12 Gy may delay restenosis, possibly for a significant period of time, but are unlikely to produce long-term inhibition of restenosis.
- The dose required to permanently inhibit restenosis must be such that the proliferative potential of a sufficiently large proportion of SMCs is inhibited, so that the survivors are unable to divide enough times to result in restenosis. This dose may be around 20 Gy.
- The reason that much lower doses are adequate to inhibit restenosis than are needed to control the smallest cancer reflects the fact that SMCs are normal somatic cells that can only divide a limited number of times, especially in older persons.

There appears to be a relatively narrow window between the minimum dose needed to slow down the proliferation of SMCs and the maximum dose that can be tolerated before late sequelae occur in the vessel wall.

Successful trials of endovascular radiation completed to date involve γ-rays, whereas many systems being developed are based on β-emitting radionuclides. Experimental data are urgently needed so that allowances can be made for the difference in dose-rate and radiation quality between γ- and β-emitting radionuclides.

References

1. Epstein SE, Speir E, Unger EF, et al. The basis of molecular strategies for treating coronary restenosis after angioplasty. J Am Coll Cardiol 1994;23:1278–1288.
2. Ross R. The pathogenesis of atherosclerosis: A perspective for the 1990s. Nature 1993;362:801–809.
3. Wilcox JN, Crocker IR, Scott NA, et al. Mechanisms by which radiation may prevent restenosis: Inhibition of cell proliferation and vascular remodeling. In: Waksman R (ed.): Vascular Brachytherapy. Armonk, NY: Futura Publishing Co.; 1999:127–138.
4. Schwartz RS, Chu A, Myung HJ, et al. Vascular cell proliferation dynamic: Implications for gene transfer and restenosis. In: March KL (ed.): Gene transfer in the Cardiovascular System: Experimental Approaches and Therapeutic Implications. Boston: Kluwer Academic Publishers; 1995:293–306.
5. Schwartz RS, Chu A, Edwards WD, et al. A proliferation analysis of arterial neointimal hyperplasia. Int J Cardiol 1996;53:71–80.

6. Brenner DJ, Miller RC, Hall EJ. The radiobiology of intravascular irradiation. Int J Radiat Oncol Biol Phys 1996; 36:805–810.
7. Hall EJ. Radiobiology for the Radiologist. 4th Edition. Philadelphia: LB Lippincott Co.; 1994:30.
8. Revell SH. Relationship between chromosome damage and cell death. In: Ishihara T, Sasaki MS (eds.): Radiation-Induced Chromosome in Man. New York: Alan R. Liss; 1983:214–233.
9. Evans HJ. Chromosome aberrations induced by ionizing radiation. Int Rev Cytol 1962;13:221–321.
10. Ward JF. Some biochemical consequences of the spatial distribution of ionizing radiation produced free radicals. Radiat Res 1981; 86:185–195.
11. Ward JF. DNA damage produced by ionizing radiation in mammalian cells: Identities, mechanisms of formation and repairability. Prog Nucleic Acid Res Mol Biol 1988;35:95–125.
12. Kerr JFR, Searle J. Apoptosis: Its nature and kinetic role. In: Meyn RE, Withers HR (eds.): Radiation Biology in Cancer Research. New York: Raven Press; 1980:367–384.
13. Withers HR. Biologic basis for altered fractionation schemes. Cancer 1985;55(suppl 9):2086–2095.
14. McElligott R, Wellinger RJ. The terminal DNA structure of mammalian chromosomes. EMBO J 1997;16:3704.
15. Shay JW. At the end of the millennium, a view of the end. Nat Genet 1999;23:382.
16. Muller HJ. The making of chromosomes. The Collecting Net 1938;8:182.
17. Nugent CI, Lundbald V. The telomerase reverse transcriptase: Components and regulation. Genes Dev 1998;12:1073.
18. Bacchetti S, Wynford-Thomas D. Telomeres and telomerase in cancer. Special Issue: Eur J Cancer 1997;33:703.
19. Hayflick L. Aging, longevity and immortality in vitro. Exp Gerontol 1992;27:363–368.
20. Hall EJ, Brenner DJ. The dose-rate effect revisited: Radiobiological considerations of importance in radiotherapy. Int J Radiat Oncol Biol Phys 1991;21:1403–1414.
21. Hall EJ, Bedford JS. Dose-rate: Its effect on the survival of HeLa cells irradiated with gamma rays. Radiat Res 1964;22:305.
22. Hall EJ. The Weiss lecture: The dose-rate factor in radiation biology. Int J Radiat Biol 1991;59:595–610.
23. Brenner DJ, Hall EJ. Conditions for the equivalence of continuous to pulsed low dose rate brachytherapy. Int J Radiat Oncol Biol Phys 1991;20:181–190.
24. Bond VP, Meinhold CB, Rossi HH. Low-dose RBE and Q for x-ray compared to gamma-ray radiations. Health Phys 1978;34:433–438.
25. Johns HE. The Physics of Radiology. Springfield, IL: Charles C. Thomas; 1969.
26. Lea DE. Actions of Radiations on Living Cells. London: Cambridge University Press; 1946.

## Chapter 8

Radiation Injury to Blood Vessels

Luis F. Fajardo L-G, MD

Introduction

Injury to vessels is, unquestionably, one of the most common effects of therapeutic irradiation on normal tissues. In fact the alterations in capillaries and arterioles are pathological hallmarks of delayed damage in many mammalian tissues. Furthermore, many of the other delayed radiation effects, especially atrophy and fibrosis of organs such as the renal parenchyma, the alimentary tract, or the myocardium, can be explained by ischemia resulting from microvascular damage. Therefore for many years investigators have attributed the majority of delayed lesions in various parenchymatous organs and the skin to the initial blood vessel damage.

Although this is a well-proven mechanism for some tissues,[10] after more than 40 years of research there is still no definite proof that it is the mechanism for all tissues.[16] The concept that vascular damage is responsible for late effects has been challenged by Withers and collaborators.[20] Indeed, some delayed effects are mediated through mechanisms different from, or in addition to, ischemia. For instance, it has been shown recently that the release of fibrogenic cytokines such as TGFβ may be at least partially responsible for progressive fibrosis of the irradiated liver.[2]

In any case, the fact remains that alterations in blood vessels are markers for delayed radiation injury in many organs and tissues. Furthermore, the severity of the changes that occur in vessels is often dose-dependent, as demonstrated by experimental studies.[7,11,16]

The following is a description of such lesions as seen by the pathologists and as analyzed by epidemiologists, in various human organs subject to therapeutic irradiation. Experimental data are presented when applicable. The vascular alterations occasionally seen after radiation accidents or atomic warfare are not considered here. This chapter does not pretend to be a comprehensive review of the subject, but rather a description of the author's personal experience and a brief review of selected references. For more extensive information, readers are directed to papers by Fajardo and Berthrong[7] and by Reinhold et al.[16]

Morphology of Externally Irradiated Vessels

Acute Lesions

Few studies have been made of the immediate (minutes-to-hours) effects of ionizing radiations in blood vessels, and these are almost exclusively under ex-

From Waksman R (ed.). *Vascular Brachytherapy, Third Edition.* Armonk, NY: Futura Publishing Co., Inc.; © 2002.

perimental conditions. We have observed acute exudate of heterophils (the rabbit granulocytes) in the blood vessels of the heart including the subepicardial coronary arteries.[9] Such exudate appeared within 12 hours in some rabbits exposed to a single external x-ray dose of 2000 cGy in the cardiac area, and disappeared by 48 hours without leaving evidence of persistent lesions. Whether this acute, immediate vasculitis led eventually to permanent damage such as intimal proliferation is unknown. The latter was uncommon, mild, and in irradiated rabbits, observed for up to 1 year; intimal proliferation was no more frequent than in the controls.

Delayed Lesions

In humans and other mammals it appears that the segments of the vascular tree most easily and frequently damaged by ionizing radiation are the microvessels, especially the blood capillaries and the sinusoids. Experimental and human observations suggest that the endothelial cells (EC) may be the most radioresponsive cells in the mesenchyma. Thus the microvessels, whose wall consists mainly of endothelial cells, are the most vulnerable segments.

From the morphological point of view, the features of radiation-induced vascular damage are nonspecific because of the limited number of responses that the blood vessels, or any tissue for that matter, may have to multiple forms of injury. The following are the types of lesions that can be seen in the various segments of the vascular tree, starting from the smallest and most sensitive ones.

In capillaries and sinusoids there are alterations in the ECs that are best seen by electron microscopy. Initially there may be focal cytoplasmic degeneration, vacuolization, and irregular projections of the cytoplasm toward the lumen, with redistribution of organelles. Increased capillary permeability can be demonstrated early. Intracellular edema is a more severe alteration and may produce such swelling of the EC that vascular occlusion results. Then platelet and fibrin thromboses occur. EC may detach from their basement membrane. Further along there is necrosis of EC with wall rupture followed by permanent loss of a segment of a microvessel.[10] Less severe damage often results in permanent dilatation—telangiectasia. Compensatory EC proliferation may occur; presumably in minor lesions this proliferation can reestablish microvascular segments, but in severe lesions may be inadequate.[10]

Lesions of arterioles are also very frequent.[7] Most common is proliferation of the intima, which starts with medial smooth myocytes that migrate through the internal elastic membrane and proliferate in the intima, and thus is called myointimal proliferation. This proliferation may be concentric or eccentric and may vary in severity from minimal to severe with variable narrowing of the lumen from minimal to complete occlusion. In this intimal proliferation there may be foamy macrophages, ie, histiocytes that have phagocytized lipids. These accumulate at various levels of the intima and may also be present in the media. If this "foamy macrophage plaque" occurs in medium or large vessels, it cannot be distinguished from the far more common atheromatosis that characterizes radiation-unrelated atherosclerosis.

However, if this occurs in very small arterioles measuring less than 100 μm in diameter, such lesions are rarely the result of atherosclerosis and appear to be more characteristic, although still not specific, of radiation. Fibrin may accumulate in the media or in the intima of irradiated arteries and sometimes it replaces extensively the necrotic media (so-called fibrinoid necrosis). The media may also be replaced by dense collagen-rich tissue without nuclei which gives a uniform glassy appearance to the vascular wall (so-called hyalinization of the media).

Mural or occlusive thrombosis composed of platelets and fibrin in arterioles and larger arteries does occur at various stages after radiation, but its incidence is not known. Also unknown is the contribution of platelets to the atheromatous plaques associated with radiation. Some thromboses may result in permanent fibrous occlusion of the vessel, but this sequential evolution is difficult to prove in humans.[6,7]

We have observed several instances of delayed, acute lymphocytic vasculitis affecting the media, intima, and adventitia of medium-sized arteries, and accompanied by fibrinous exudate and occasionally thrombosis.[7] This vasculitis appears to be limited to the radiation field and, as far as we have been able to ascertain, is not part of a systemic vasculitis. Therefore, the finding of acute vasculitis in an irradiated tissue should be viewed as a probably localized event that does not require specific therapy. In fact, we have been able to observe what appeared to be scars of vasculitis in some delayed lesions of bloods vessels. The sites of this arteriolar vasculitis have been the breast, the mesentery, and in the wall of the small intestine.[7] However it is likely that it occurs in many other tissues, and this is supported by our recent discovery of a similar type of vasculitis in arterioles located around arteries of swine exposed to endovascular brachytherapy (see p. 85).

In arteries measuring more than 100 μm in external diameter (medium-sized and large-sized arteries) the lesions are observed less often than in the smaller vessels. These consist of lipid deposits (atheromas) and fibrosis, which are indistinguishable from those of the lesions that occur as a result of the general spontaneous process of arteriosclerosis (Fig. 1). In certain cases it can only be assumed that these are produced by radiation because of the young age of the patients, or unusual locations, or because of their sharp localization within a field of therapy. Thrombosis is also sometimes seen in these vessels, and also rupture (perforation) of the vessels may occur.[8]

Perforation of large vessels tends to occur mostly in the carotid artery, but also may take place in the femoral arteries, the pulmonary arteries, and the aorta. Initially we felt that such catastrophic vascular perforations resulted mainly from injurious agents other than radiation: surgical complications of operations such as radical neck dissection, with exposure and drying of the arteries, or leakage of digesting enzymes such as saliva were blamed for such ruptures.[8] However, one experimental study of canine carotid arteries exposed to ^{192}Ir or ^{125}I showed that at very high exposures rupture may be caused exclusively by radiation (see below).[11] In general, however, it can be said that lesions to large arteries are not common features of therapeutic radiation.

Even less common are injuries to large veins. We have only seen a few examples of damage to veins produced by therapeutic radiation, and those are mainly in small vessels. However, in some organs like the liver and the small intestine, damage to small-and medium-sized veins is common and, in the case of the liver, it is actually the main mechanism of symptomatic subacute injury.[6] Veno-occlusive disease of the liver is a characteristic lesion of the central veins, but may effect also sublobular veins and rarely some small portal veins. It produces a meshwork of collagen fibers that obstructs these vessels as well the afferent

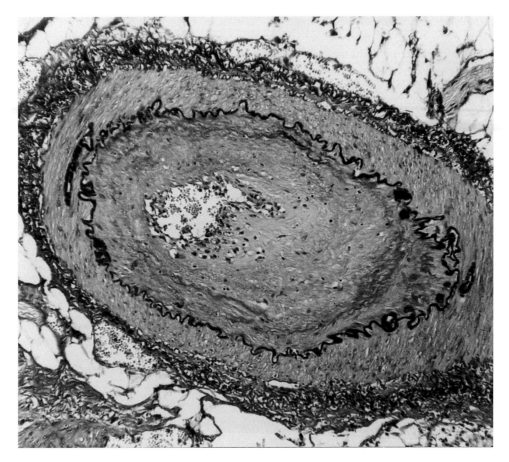

Figure 1. Artery in the submucosa of the small intestine, more than 1 year after exposure to a fractionated dose of 50 Gy. Notice severe, concentrical myointimal proliferation within the area delimited by the black, wavy, internal elastic membrane, which has reduced the lumen to a small orifice. Verhoeff-van Gieson stain x110. Reproduced from Reference 16 with permission from the authors and from Academic Press.

sinusoids and results in focal, severe congestion of the parenchyma, and necrosis of the central lobular hepatocytes. This unique lesion is typical of the liver, but not specific of radiation.[14] In fact today, in the U.S., it is seen most often in association with antineoplastic chemotherapy.

Coronary Artery Disease

In relation to large muscular vessels such as the coronary arteries, the effects of ionizing radiation are less well defined than in small vessels and there are less experimental data.

During the 1960s and 1970s we studied extensively in Stanford a population of patients with Hodgkin's disease and breast carcinoma who were irradiated using fields that included most or all of the heart. We followed a group of 318 patients treated for Hodgkin's disease who, in a prospective study, were examined for any evidence of heart disease prior to radiation. Then we expanded that series to include 93 Hodgkin's disease patients from the University of California in San Francisco.[18] Most of the Hodgkin's patients received a total dose of 42.8 Gy to a large volume of the heart.[18]

These patients were then followed for at least 1 year after radiation therapy. This prospective study showed an important incidence of pericardial disease which was overall 6.6%, but increased considerably at the higher doses (in re-treated individuals), up to 50%. There was also severe myocardial fibrosis, particularly in individuals that had been re-treated.[18] However, we did not detect an increase in coronary artery disease (CAD). Furthermore, in the autopsies of some of these patients we were not impressed by coronary artery lesions.[18]

Ten years later, Boivin and Hutchison[3] analyzed retrospectively the histories of 957 patients that had been treated for Hodgkin's disease in various hospitals in the Boston area and who had been followed for at least 2 years: several patients were followed for up to 10 years. This review also showed no significant increase in CAD.[3]

The belief that CAD was not an important complication of irradiation to the heart was supported by experimental studies performed in our laboratories during the 1960s and 1970s. In order to study the pericardial and myocardial disease that occurs in humans, we irradiated more than 600 New Zealand white rabbits, in the heart, using single doses between 16 Gy and 82 Gy, or fractionated radiation schemes up to 108 Gy. These animals were studied histologically and by other techniques from minutes to more than 1 year after exposure.[9]

The rabbit is a splendid model to reproduce the pericardial disease and the myocardial fibrosis that occurs in humans and indeed we were able to demonstrate the mechanism of myocardial fibrosis by following the sequence of events after a single exposure, with light and electron microscopy, and by incorporation of tritiated thymidine (to detect compensatory cellular proliferation).[10] However, in these many rabbits we were not able to ascertain evidence of CAD up to 1 year of follow-up. Most hearts were examined carefully, and the coronary arteries were usually in the areas reviewed histologically. Nevertheless, some cases of CAD might have escaped our detection.[9]

Therefore, by the mid 1980s, the impression was that external radiation of the heart did not increase the risk of CAD, and we stated so in several publications including an editorial.[5,18] However, we cautiously mentioned that a large population of patients irradiated for lymphomas and particularly for Hodgkin's disease was only beginning to be followed and that we did not know what would happen to these patients many years later.

It should be noted that even at that time there had been a number of isolated observations of what appeared to be CAD produced by radiation. Most of those publications referred to individuals that had developed CAD with ischemia, often fatal, at an age in which spontaneous coronary atherosclerosis and myocardial infarcts would be expected. Most of those CAD cases were statistically more likely to be the result of the spontaneous disease than of radiation. A few of those cases did suggest strongly the possibility of a radiation etiology.

As an example, in the early 1960s a 14-year-old boy was treated for Hodgkin's disease at Stanford, receiving a total dose of 4000 cGy in the mediastinum. Six months later, while recovering from the lymphoma, he died suddenly. He had developed severe myointimal proliferation of the left anterior descending coronary artery with more than 95% narrowing, and died of an acute myocardial infarct.[5] This boy did not have history of familial CAD, hyperlipidemia, or any other important risk factor for spontaneous atherosclerosis at such young age. Cases such as this suggested the possibility that radiation could play a role in some cases of CAD.

Recently, three lines of evidence have indicated that in fact CAD is an important delayed manifestation of therapeutic radiation to the heart. In a second retrospective study, Boivin et al[4] reviewed 4665 Hodgkin's patients from several hospitals in the Boston area who had been irradiated in the heart (precise doses not stated). The patients were followed this time for 7 years on average. This study did show an excess number of deaths due to myocardial ischemia. The relative risk (RR) for myocardial infarct after mediastinal irradiation was 2.56 with 95% confidence intervals of 1.11 to 5.93. There was no increase in myocardial infarct associated with chemotherapy.[4]

Another retrospective study, performed by Rutqvist et al in Stockholm,[17] compared postoperative therapy with surgery alone in breast carcinoma and showed an excess mortality due to CAD in the women who had received high-dose radiation to the heart as postoperative treatment for carcinoma of the left breast, and found a relative hazard of 3.2.

The most compeling study was the one performed by Hancock and collaborators[13] in our institution and published in 1993. They reviewed retrospectively 2232 Hodgkin's patients, 79% of whom had received greater than or equal to 40 Gy (most often 44 Gy to the mantle field) at Stanford. The patients were followed for 9.5 years on average. They compared this population with controls matched for age, sex, and race. Fatal myocardial infarct occurred in an unexpectedly large number of patients: 55 versus 17.3 expected for all treated patients; 35 versus 8.4 expected in patients treated by radiation alone.

The overall RR for myocardial infarct in patients treated by radiation alone was 3.8 (95% CI: 2.8 to 4.8). This relative risk increased consistently with the latency period and was particularly high in individuals who had been treated by radiation (with or without chemotherapy) prior to age 20. In fact, the RR of myocardial infarct for such patients was 44 (95% CI: 17.8 to 91.8).

This finding differs from that of Boivin et al,[4] who found that the RR for people treated at 60 years of age or older was greater than for those irradiated at a younger age, although the age distribution in their population was not specified.

In summary, current epidemiological studies show that indeed CAD is a significant risk of radiation to the heart in the course of treatment to adjacent neoplasms. The risk increases within the first 5 years and probably remains high for 10 years or more. Because of the narrow range of doses used in the therapy of Hodgkin's disease it is not possible to determine if there is a relation between dose and risk of coronary disease.[13]

Although no dose effect was observed, a serendipitous change provided two groups for comparison. As a result of studies on radiation-induced pericardial and myocardial disease, there were some modifications in the treatment for mediastinal neoplasms at Stanford. After 1972 the exposure to the heart was limited to 30 to 35 Gy (versus 40 to 45 Gy prior to 1972) by the use of subcarinal blocks. Also, both anterior and posterior fields were treated daily (versus only one daily). and the daily fractions were reduced from greater than or equal to 2.2 Gy per day to less than or equal to 1.8 Gy per day.[13]

These alterations in therapy decreased significantly the risk of pericardial disease and myocardial fibrosis but did not alter significantly the risk for fatal myocardial infarct: RR was 3.7 prior to subcarinal blocking and 3.4 after.[13]

Experimental Radiation-Induced Vascular Disease

Many experimental observations in various mammals have confirmed the great radiosensitivity of EC and microvessels.[6] Less consistent are the lesions produced in larger vessels. In relation to the coronary arteries, only a few models reproduce the lesions that occur in humans. This is mainly due to the fact that in humans radiation-induced CAD is multifactorial: ie is caused by radiation and other factors—particularly those that produce spontaneous atherosclerosis. It is quite possible that if the patients being treated for Hodgkin's disease by radiation were individuals with nonatherogenic diets and without any genetic abnormalities predisposing to atherosclerosis, the incidence of CAD associated with radiation would be much lower than that described in the above studies.

As indicated in the preceding section, heart-irradiated rabbits, which are splendid models for radiation pericardial and myocardial disease, do not develop coronary artery atherosclerosis ordinarily. However, rabbits treated with fractionated schemes totaling 25 Gy and receiving a high-cholesterol fat diet do develop coronary atherosclerosis.[1] On the other hand, fibrosis of the intima and media (sclerosis, deposition of collagen) does develop in animals that have a normal diet and receive large local doses of radiation.[6] Such lesions can be produced segmentally in the aorta but their clinical importance is probably limited and, in the majority of cases, would not result in ischemic events.

All of the above refers to external irradiation. Until recently[15,19] there has been little information about the effects of brachytherapy on arteries in general and specifically on coronary arteries. Some data from the mid 1960s are available on the effects of implants of radioactive isotopes on rabbit aortas.[12] In one study performed in the mid 1980s, we explored the effects of various doses of ^{192}Ir and ^{125}I implanted near the external carotid artery of dogs.[11] The purpose was to determine the effects on the carotid arteries of a radical neck dissection followed by brachytherapy to treat metastatic tumors to the neck.[11]

Seeds containing permanent implants of ^{125}I or transient implants of ^{192}Ir were placed a few millimeters from the carotid artery after a simulated radical neck dissection. That study showed that doses of up to 225 Gy using ^{125}I or up to 90 Gy using ^{192}Ir were safe and did not result in any significant damage to the arteries that could be demonstrated up to 2 years of follow-up by sequential arteriography or by final histology. However, doses above these levels (eg, 300 Gy with ^{125}I or 120 Gy with ^{192}Ir) did cause several carotid lesions including complete obstruction. In fact three dogs receiving the higher doses had rupture of the carotid with exsanguination.[11]

My experience with the topic of endovascular radiation to prevent restenosis stems from a project performed in collaboration with researchers of Baylor University.[15] The purpose of that project was to explore the possibility that intense but brief intraluminal radiation exposures at the time of transluminal coronary angioplasty (TCA) would prevent the high rate of restenosis that occurs with TCA. Thirty-four Hanford miniature swine were used. In each animal, each of the major three coronary arteries was treated in a different manner using special intra-arterial catheters. Segments of these vessels were exposed using ^{192}Ir to doses of 1000 cGy, 1500 cGy, and 2500 cGy or mock irradiation (control).

Immediately after, the treated segments of the arteries were subject to mechanical injury: stent implantation in the left anterior descending and in the right coronary artery, and balloon overstretch in the circumflex artery. The controls received the same mechanical injury but no irradiation. Coronary angiography was performed prior to treatment and immediately before euthanasia 28 days later. The coronary arteries were perfusion-fixed with 10% buffered formalin at the pressure of 100 mm Hg, widely excised, and examined histologically at consistent levels.

The perpendicular sections of the arteries at several specified distances from the ostium were examined morphometrically by digitizing the circumference of the artery as well as the area of intimal proliferation. Semiquantitative histologic evaluation of the sections of the vessels stained by H&E and trichrome was performed by a pathologist (LFF) unaware of the treatment of each animal.

The morphometry indicated that the irradiated segments (of the left arteries) had significantly less intimal proliferation after injury by stent or balloon overstretch than the unirradiated controls. This was confirmed by angiography. This short treatment of 4 to 10 minutes, particularly in the 1000 cGy and 1500 cGy groups appears to be a satisfactory method to prevent at least short-term restenosis after TCA. In addition to confirming the above, the histopathological evaluation of these vessels showed miscellaneous alterations such as stromal fibrin in most of the irradiated vessels, thinning of the (overstreched) media, and adventitial fibrosis often with leukocyte infiltration. Medial and adventitial hemorrhage was seen, especially in the 2500 cGy group. The latter may be important for patients receiving intensive anticoagulation.

Mural thrombosis was a common finding (these animals were not anticoagulated and did not receive aspirin) but occlusive thrombosis was not a problem. In addition, there was intimal proliferation in the small arteries adjacent to the treated artery. None of the vessels showed evidence of aneurysmal dilatation or rupture.[15]

At the time of preparation of this 3rd edition of *Vascular Brachytherapy,* other experiments in swine, rabbits, dogs, etc., by numerous researchers, including us, have investigated the effects of endovascular radiation from isotopic sources in coronary and other arteries. Many of these experiments have shown promising results, usually in the short term. Some—especially long term—have been disappointing. Robinson et al. have recently commented on the long-term data of various researchers.[21] A few of our own studies are discussed below.*

In one series of experiments, swine coronary arteries were given 3500 cGy (at 0.5 mm depth) from a ^{32}P endovascular source after balloon angioplasty or stent. The animals were followed for 6 months. The balloon-treated animals tended to have larger lumina. However, 5 of 10 animals had occlusive thrombosis at the treated site, resulting in deaths at 5 days, 7 days, 3 months (two), and 4 months.[22]

One study was designed to assess the effects of beta radiation (35 Gy at 0.5 mm from an endovascular ^{32}P source) without the trauma of balloon dilatation or stenting. The coronary arteries showed only mild, healing or healed, vascular injury by 28 days, and an ample lumen, often larger than in controls (Fajardo LF, Ali N, Raizner A, unpublished observations). This short-term result suggests that the negative outcomes described in the preceding paragraph may not necessarily result from radiation alone, but from the mechanical trauma (with or without added radiation) inherent to angioplasty.

In more recent experiments, we have observed an additional effect associated

*These studies have been supported by Guidant Co.

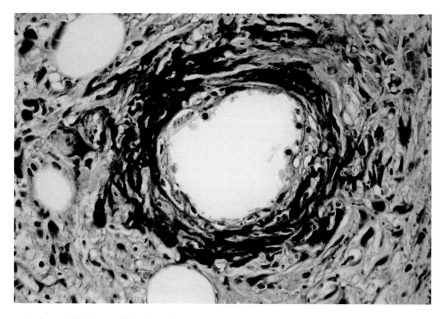

Figure 2. Arteriole located in the adventitia of porcine left anterior descending (LAD) coronary artery that was exposed to an endovascular ^{32}P source. The LAD received 35 Gy at a depth of 0.5 mm into the coronary arterial wall and at a rate of 25 to 45 cGy/sec and was not subjected to mechanical trauma (stent or angioplasty). Twenty-eight days after exposure this small vessel shows severe necrosis of most myocytes in the media and extensive deposition of fibrin (the purple concentric material that extends into the adventitia). The intima in this arteriole has a few lymphocytes; in other arterioles similarly treated there is proliferation of endothelial cells—sometimes occluding the lumen—and heavier inflammatory exudate; thrombi may be present. Trichrome-elastic × 400.

with endovascular beta radiation of porcine coronary and iliac arteries: acute necrotizing vasculitis.

This lesion is characterized by "fibrinoid necrosis" in arterioles (and very rarely in venules) measuring 50 to 250 μm in diameter (average 132 μm). These vessels are located in the adipose tissue, outside of the adventitia of the treated coronary artery, and approximately 0.38 to 2.05 mm (average 0.75 μm) from the endothelial surface of such artery (as measured in trichrome-stained paraffin sections of hearts fixed by formalin perfusion at 150 mm Hg). In plastic sections of iliac artery specimens, the affected arterioles measure 30 to 380 mm in diameter and are located at 0.72 mm from the lumenal surface of the arteries.

The involved arterioles show replacement of the medial muscle cells by concentric layers of fibrin. Intact muscle cells are difficult to find in the affected segments (Fig. 2). The fibrin deposits extend into the adventitia. In some of the necrotic vessels the intima shows proliferation of endothelial cells and infiltration by lymphocytes and neutrophils. Thrombi are uncommon. A few lymphocytes may be present around the affected artery but in most cases there is no perivascular cellular inflammatory exudate. This lesion is usually seen in only 1 arteriole at a given section plane, although occasionally 2, or even 3 arterioles are affected; around a few iliac arteries as many as 6 involved vessels have been counted.

At least three experiments have shown this phenomenon. In each one, porcine arteries have been exposed to endovascular sources of ^{32}P, receiving single doses of 35 Gy at 0.5-mm tissue depth and at dose rates varying between 25 and 150 cGy/sec. All arteries were harvested 28 days after exposure.

1. In one study, coronary arteries were exposed only to endovascular radiation (neither angioplasty nor stent were used (Protocol 0016). Vasculitis occurred in 6 of 18 irradiated vessels. Two additional samples were suggestive, but not diagnostic, of vasculitis. None of the 6 control vessels had vasculitis.
2. One experiment was designed to study the edge effect (Protocol 0024). Right coronary arteries were balloon-injured and irradiated; left anterior descending coronary arteries were only irradiated. All 12 vessels showed arteriolar vasculitis and only in the irradiated segments.
3. One study involved iliac arteries subject to stenting and radiation (Protocol 0025). Each of the irradiated vessels in 6 animals showed arteriolar vasculitis. No vasculitis was seen in the unirradiated samples.

Interestingly enough, this type of acute (active) necrotizing vasculitis was not detected in our early coronary artery experiments using endovascular gamma sources, which obviously deposited higher doses in the periarterial tissues than did the beta sources used in the current experiments. However, around the gamma-treated porcine arteries we observed occasional arterioles totally occluded by old, organized thrombi that could have resulted from this type of acute vasculitis. It is possible that a few specimens did have acute vasculitis but it was not detected because of different sampling technique. In the early experiments fewer levels of the vascular segments were prepared than in the current experiments, which may have as many as 25 levels available from each vessel.

It is too early to speculate on the mechanism of this vasculitis, although it is clearly related to radiation. Acute lymphocytic vasculitis has been observed in human tissues, months to years after exposure,[7] but there is no definite evidence that it is radiation-induced. Except for the fact that they are localized to the radiation site, those lesions are reminiscent of polyarteritis nodosa. We are correlating the vasculitis in these experiments with the various repetitive alterations detected in the main coronary arteries. We are also in the process of calculating the radiation dose received by the affected arterioles.

The physiological impact of the vasculitis is not clear: we have not detected ischemic lesions in the immediate areas, but we have not systematically examined the hearts of these pigs. Finally, the natural history of these lesions is unknown because of the time limit (28 days) of these experiments. Examination of samples from long-term experiments (3 and 6 months, and longer) may give us some information about the ultimate fate of these lesions.

Conclusions

As the result of therapeutic *external* irradiation, blood vessels of various organs and tissues suffer and reveal significant injury. This is particularly important in microvessels: capillaries and sinusoids. Larger vessels suffer also with external radiation, but the exposure is often less critical to the major arteries and veins.

External irradiation of human coronary arteries in the course of therapy for mediastinal neoplasms, such as lymphomas or for breast carcinoma, is associated with an increase in the risk of fatal CAD that appears within 5 years of exposure and increases with time of observation. In the setting of brachytherapy for lesions of the neck, perivascular implants with gamma-emitting isotopes are ordinarily safe and produce only minimal lesions in the carotid artery.

Endovascular brachytherapy is a promising approach for the prevention of arterial restenosis after angioplasty, especially in the coronary vessels. It is the subject of multiple current studies and is discussed in many of the chapters of this book. The results of human trials with 7 or more years of observation (in femoral arteries) are encouraging. The experiments in swine were quite satisfactory at 1 month, but subsequent observations at 6 months have revealed unexpected fatal coronary thrombosis in some animals at the sites of mechanical injury. A role for radiation in this complication has not been established. We have detected acute necrotizing vasculitis in small branches of the coronary and iliac arteries of swine after endovascular beta radiation; these lesions appear to be radiation-related, but their mechanism and clinical implications are not clear.

References

1. Amromin GD, Gildenhorn HL, Solomon RD, et al. The synergism of x-radiation and cholesterol-fat feeding on the development of coronary artery lesions. *J Atheroscler Res* 1964;4:325–334.
2. Anscher MS, Crocker IR, Jirtle RL. Transforming growth factor-b$_1$ expression in irradiated liver. *Radiat Res* 1990;122:77–85.
3. Boivin J-F, Hutchison GB. Coronary heart disease mortality after irradiation for Hodgkin's disease. *Cancer* 1982;49:2470–2475.
4. Boivin J-F, Hutchison GB, Lubin JH, Mauch P. Coronary artery disease mortality in patients treated for Hodgkin's disease. *Cancer* 1992;69:1241–1247.
5. Fajardo LF. Radiation-induced coronary artery disease [editorial]. *Chest* 1977;71:563–564.
6. Fajardo LF. *Pathology of Radiation Injury.* New York, NY: Masson Publishing; 1982.
7. Fajardo LF, Berthrong M. Vascular lesions following radiation. *Pathol Annu* 1988;23:297–330.
8. Fajardo LF, Lee A. Rupture of major vessels after radiation. *Cancer* 1975;36:904–913.
9. Fajardo LF, Stewart JR. Experimental radiation-induced heart disease. I. Light microscopic studies. *Am J Pathol* 1970;59:299–316.
10. Fajardo LF, Stewart JR. Pathogenesis of radiation-induced myocardial fibrosis. *Lab Invest* 1973;29:244–257.
11. Fee WE Jr, Goffinet DR, Fajardo LF, et al. Safety of [125]Iodine and [192]Iridium implants to the canine carotid. Long-term results. *Acta Otolaryngol (Stockh)* 1987;103:514–518.
12. Friedman M, Felton L, Byres S. The antiatherogenic effect of ^{192}Ir upon the cholesterol-fed rabbit. *J Clin Invest* 1964;43:185–192.
13. Hancock SL, Tucker MA, Hoppe RT. Factors affecting late mortality from heart disease after treatment of Hodgkin's disease. *JAMA* 1993;270:1949–1955.
14. Lawrence TS, Robertson JM, Anscher MS, et al. Hepatic toxicity resulting from cancer treatment. *Int J Radiat Oncol Biol Phys* 1995;31:1237–1248.
15. Mazur W, Ali MN, Khan MM, et al. High dose-rate intracoronary radiation for inhibition of neointimal formation in the stented and balloon-injured porcine models of restenosis: Angiographic, morphometric and histopathologic analyses. *Int J Radiat Oncol Biol Phys* 1996;36:777–788.
16. Reinhold HS, Fajardo LF, Hopewell JW. The vascular system. In: Altman KI, Lett JT (eds.): *Advances in Radiation Biology, Vol 14, Relative Radiation Sensitivities of Human Organ Systems, Part II.* San Diego, CA: Academic Press; 1990:177–226.
17. Rutqvist LE, Lax I, Fornander T, Johansson H. Cardiovascular mortality in a randomized trial of adjuvant radiation therapy vs surgery alone in primary breast cancer. *Int J Radiat Oncol Biol Phys* 1992;22:887–896.

18. Stewart JR, Fajardo LF. Radiation-induced heart disease. Clinical and experimental aspects. *Radiol Clin North Am* 1971;9:511–531.
19. Waksman R, Robinson KA, Crocker IR, et al. Endovascular low-dose irradiation inhibits neointima formation after coronary artery balloon injury in swine. A possible role for radiation therapy in restenosis prevention. *Circulation* 1995;91:1533–1539.
20. Withers HR, Peters LJ, Kogelnik HS. The pathobiology of late effects of irradiation. In: Meyn RE, Withers HR (eds.): *Radiation Biology in Cancer Research*. New York, NY: Raven Press; 1980:439–448.
21. Robinson KA. Long-term effects of endovascular brachytherapy: Non-issue or imminent catastrophe? Vasc Radiother Monitor 2000;3:9–13.
22. Kaluza G, Raizner AE, Mazur W, et al. Long-term effects of intracoronary beta-radiation in balloon- and stent-injured porcine coronary arteries. Circulation In press.

## Chapter 9

Radiation Biology Concepts for the Use of Radiation to Prevent Restenosis

James B. Mitchell, PhD

Introduction

The effective therapeutic use of ionizing radiation in cancer treatment has always required a delicate balancing act. This is particularly true since the response of the majority of normal tissues within a given treatment field may be similar to or greater than that of the target tissue, ie, the tumor. To achieve a therapeutic gain (greater effects in target tissue than the normal tissue), a complex interplay of physical and biological factors are required; these include total radiation dose, dose fractionation, treatment time, inherent radiosensitivity of the respective tissues, proliferation status of the tissues, and numerous physiological factors that have yet to be defined. An enormous body of knowledge, much of it empirical, has emerged over the past 100 years regarding the effective use of ionizing radiation in cancer treatment. Despite the collective experience of many outstanding radiation oncologists, physicists, and radiobiologists who strive to explain and define biological factors important in treatment, there is still much room for improvement.

Over the past few years there has been an increased interest in the use of ionizing radiation to control restenosis that can arise following percutaneous transluminal coronary angioplasty (PTCA).[1,2] On the surface it would seem that using radiation to inhibit restenosis would represent a more simple challenge than encountered in cancer treatment; however, the response of the blood vessel to radiation treatment may be quite complex. It is known that radiation treatment can damage blood vessels. For example, radiation treatment in certain settings (arteriovenous malformation) is used to close or obliterate blood vessels.[3] Likewise, an untoward effect of radiation treatment to the mediastinum in Hodgkin's disease is coronary artery disease.[4,5] These two examples point out that radiation can and does have the potential to destroy blood vessels. Even though early reports of radiation treatment to control restenosis are encouraging, the effective use of radiation in this setting is likely to also require a delicate balancing act. The challenge is to treat the blood vessels to a point where restenosis is inhibited, yet the vessel is not irreparably damaged.

This chapter focuses on the basics of radiobiology as they relate to vascular irradiation. The aim is to equip the cardiologist with necessary background in-

From Waksman R (ed.). *Vascular Brachytherapy, Third Edition*. Armonk, NY: Futura Publishing Co., Inc.; © 2002.

formation to comprehend and evaluate the use of radiation to control restenosis. This chapter is not intended to be an exhaustive treatise on the entire field of radiobiology. Many fine textbooks and reviews fulfill this need and the reader who requires a more detailed review is encouraged to review these texts.[6-9]

The Chemistry of Ionizing Radiation

The transfer of ionizing radiation energy to an absorbing medium causes either excitation or ionization of the component molecules. If the energy of the incident radiation is sufficient to eject an electron from the outer orbital of an atom or molecule, then the incident radiation is defined as ionizing radiation. Ionizing radiation can transfer energy in excess of the typical bond energies of molecules (5 eV) and thereby has the potential to break them. Radiation that causes excitation without ionization has wavelengths in the ultraviolet (UV)/visible region.

Both electromagnetic radiation and particulate radiation such as alpha particles, protons, and neutrons can cause ionization. X-rays, which are produced extranuclearly, and γ-rays, which are produced intranuclearly, are two forms of electromagnetic radiation that have sufficient energy to ionize atoms or molecules.

Direct and Indirect Effects

When x- or γ-rays are absorbed in biological material, they can directly ionize a critical site (direct effect) or interact with other molecules to produce reactive free radicals, which can subsequently damage critical biological molecules (indirect effect). Indirect effects account for approximately 80% of the damage rendered by a given exposure of radiation. The chemical nature of the free radicals produced by indirect effects depends on the abundance of chemical species in the absorbing material. Since biological matter is composed of approximately 80% water, the effect of radiation on water molecules is important. Free radical species formed from water radiolysis result in damage to critical molecules. Damage to critical molecules eventually leads to biological damage. The two major effects of radiation on water molecules are described below.

$$H_2O \longrightarrow H_2O^+\cdot + e^- \text{ (ionization)} \tag{1}$$

$$H_2O \longrightarrow H_2O^* \text{ (excitation)} \tag{2}$$

The electron e^- becomes solvated by the surrounding water molecules and is called the solvated electron (eqation 3), which can also produce H atoms (equation 4).

$$e^- + (H_2O)_n \longrightarrow e_{aq}^- \tag{3}$$

$$e_{aq}^- + H^+ \longrightarrow H\cdot \tag{4}$$

The $H_2O^+\cdot$ produced by ionization (eq. 1) is strongly acidic and loses a proton to the surrounding water molecules to give the hydroxyl radical $\cdot OH$.

$$H_2O^+\cdot + H_2O \longrightarrow \cdot OH + H_3O^+ \tag{5}$$

The water molecule in the excited state (H_2O^*) can also homolytically split to produce H atoms and $\cdot OH$ radicals.

$$H_2O^* \longrightarrow H\cdot + \cdot OH \tag{6}$$

The H atoms and OH radicals should be distinguished from the protons (H^+) and the hydroxide ion ($-OH$). H^+ has no outer orbital electrons and ^-OH orbital electrons are completely paired up without any free electrons. This is not the case for H atoms and $\cdot OH$ radicals.

The initially produced free radical species can react with each other within regions of high local concentrations of ionization products called a spur, or diffuse into the bulk of the solution. Recombination reaction of all of the water radiolysis products in the spur are described below.

$$H\cdot + H\cdot \longrightarrow \quad H_2 \tag{7}$$

$$e_{aq}^- + e_{aq}^- \longrightarrow \quad H_2 + 2\ ^-OH \tag{8}$$

$$\cdot OH + \cdot OH \longrightarrow \quad H_2O_2 \tag{9}$$

The primary radicals can also be back-converted into water in the spurs.

$$H\cdot + \cdot OH \longrightarrow \quad H_2O \tag{10}$$

$$e_{aq}^- + \cdot OH \longrightarrow \quad ^-OH \tag{11}$$

The initial ionizing events leading to primary lesions in cells and tissues are completed in less than 10^{-10} seconds. The transfer of energy from the primary species to cause damage to biologically important molecules such as DNA that can result in genetic or metabolic alterations is completed in less than 10^{-6} seconds (1 microsecond). Thus, all of the chemical recombination reactions of highly reactive species occur rapidly and inflict damage through chemical modification of critical molecules within the cell. It should be emphasized that even though radiation exposure deposits energy into a biological system, the actual damage exerted is not through the dissipation of heat, but through ionizations and free radical processes.

Cellular Targets of Radiation Damage

While radiation is capable of damaging a variety of intracellular molecules, DNA is considered the critical target damaged by ionizing radiation by both direct or indirect processes.[10,11] The OH radical is considered the most damaging to DNA. The damage rendered to DNA consists of DNA-DNA crosslinks, base damage, DNA single- and double-strand breaks, and base release. Unrepaired DNA double-strand breaks lead to chromosome aberrations which may be lethal, result in mutations, or unmask tumor suppressor genes. There is a strong correlation between cell survival after radiation exposure and the average number of lethal chromosome aberrations.[12,13] Lethal chromosome aberrations include dicentrics and rings.

Cell Death and Viability

Biological tissue must possess the ability to either repair itself or reproduce itself in order to maintain function and the health of the organism throughout its natural life span. One of the most important consequences of exposure of biological tissue (and its component cells) to ionizing radiation is the loss of the cell's ability to reproduce, which results in the ultimate death of the cell. Cell death is the main cause of the early and late toxic effects of radiation on normal tissues, and the most likely reason that radiation has the potential to control restenosis.

Cell death should be distinguished from the intuitive concept we have of death: that is, complete, instantaneous, and irreversible loss of all function. While it is true that super-high doses of radiation (in the region of several hundred gray) will certainly cause such a death to occur as surely as though the cell were physically crushed, lower radiation doses (several hundred centigray) exert no such obvious effect. In fact, the vast majority of such irradiated cells appear morphologically normal and continue to perform complex biological functions including protein and DNA synthesis. They may even be able to pass through a limited number of mitoses and give rise to some progeny. However, in terms of the continued health of that biological tissue, a proportion of these cells will lose their ability to sustain reproduction and will die at the next or subsequent mitosis or give rise to progeny incapable of reproduction. The cell's ability to reproduce itself and form "clones" of itself, is referred to as its clonogenic potential. For many tissues, the greater the proportion of clonogenic cells damaged by ionizing radiation, the greater the perturbation on the function of that tissue. In normal tissues, the general rule is that a variable proportion of cells may be clonogenic; their number is decreased by ionizing radiation.

Another means by which cells die has been termed apoptosis, or programmed cell death.[14] Apoptosis has been reported to be a consequence of a bewildering variety of stimuli, including ionizing radiation, and may be important in a number of disease states.[15,16] Apoptosis is a highly active process requiring energy (ATP) and signaling factors (including calcium),[17] both of which are essential for the activation of specific endonucleases.[18] A burst of cellular protein and RNA synthetic activity always precedes apoptosis, and inhibition of endonuclease activity, such as by protein inhibitors (actinomycin-D, cycloheximide), blocks apoptosis. Apoptosis has been shown following irradiation in a number of systems.[19–22] The intriguing phenomenon of interphase death in lymphocytes following irradiation suggests a role for apoptosis.[23–25] The rapidity of onset of apoptosis (6 to 7 hours)[19] offers a possible explanation for some early acute reactions in normal tissues exposed to radiation.

It is particularly important to be able to determine a cell's sensitivity to loss of reproductive or clonogenic potential. Several methods have been devised to assess cell viability in vitro and in vivo. These are potent tools not only in radiation biology, but in the study of the effects of other cytotoxic agents such as chemotherapy.

Radiation Dose-Response Curves

A single cell that has retained its clonogenic viability is capable of reproducing multiple clones of itself that may be visualized as discrete colonies in tissue culture flasks or Petri dishes. This type of assay, first described by Puck and Marcus in 1956,[10] provides in vitro evidence of clonogenic viability. Cells from normal tissues (such as smooth muscle or endothelial cells) can be disaggregated physically and treated with proteolytic enzymes such as trypsin, to produce single-cell suspensions. These cells can then be seeded into culture flasks under aseptic conditions at 37°C with medium appropriate to support growth. Viable cells will attach to the plate and grow to form colonies which may be stained and counted. The number of single cells seeded may be counted with use of an automated cell counter, and therefore the plating efficiency (PE) for each cell suspension may be calculated. PEs may therefore be compared, in the absence of any cytotoxic agent (controls) and in the presence of various doses of the cytotoxic agent to be tested. A cell undergoing apoptosis after treatment will not form a colony. Therefore, it is important to note that this clonogenic assay, which measures the ability of a cell to multiply and form colonies, also takes into account any cell that may die as a result of apoptosis.

An example of a radiation dose-response curve for rat and human smooth muscle cells is shown in Figure 1. The survival curves are characteristic of the radiation response of most mammalian cells exposed to ionizing radiation. The shape and slope of the curve are important parameters, defining the response of these cells to radiation and by inference, the biological tissues from which they derive. As can be clearly seen, as the radiation dose is increased, there is progressively more cell kill. Notice that for low radiation doses the response is not exponential. Mammalian cells irradiated with x- or γ-rays generally show some curvature or "shoulder" in the initial (or low dose) segment of the survival curve. Often, though not invariably, at higher radiation doses, the curve becomes

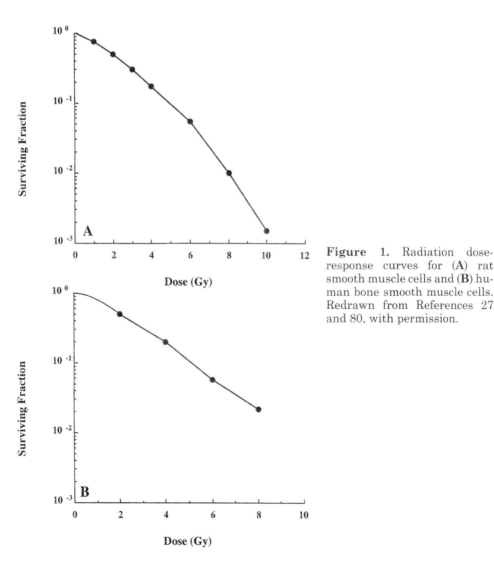

Figure 1. Radiation dose-response curves for **(A)** rat smooth muscle cells and **(B)** human bone smooth muscle cells. Redrawn from References 27 and 80, with permission.

straight with a constant exponential slope downward as shown in Figure 1. The shoulder region of the dose-response curve implies that for low radiation doses, cells have the capacity to repair radiation damage (discussed below). For higher radiation doses, the dose-response curve is essentially exponential. Several mathematical models have been proposed to fit such shouldered survival curves,[6,26] and are quite useful when comparing the radiosensitivity of different cell types.

Considering the survival curves shown in Figure 1 and assuming that smooth muscle cells are the cells responsible for restenosis, it is clear that a single dose of 12 to 15 Gy to the blood vessel following PTCA will result in significant cell kill. Using cell survival data similar to that shown in Figure 1, Brenner et al[27] have estimated that in the radiation treatment volume of the blood vessel, there are approximately 5×10^7 potentially clonogenic cells. They further suggested that radiation doses greater than 20 Gy would completely eliminate the smooth muscle cell population from the treated area and possibly present a problem of late complications. Doses less than 20 Gy, however, will result in significant cell kill, but some cells will remain that will have the capability of re-populating, in effect, simply delaying the restenosis process for some time (perhaps 1 to 3 years).[27] The likelihood that 12 to 15 Gy is sufficient to permanently prevent restenosis depends largely on the capacity of smooth muscle cells to proliferate, since cells from normal tissue have a limited capacity to proliferate.[28] The vast majority of preclinical studies using experimental animals have not evaluated the success of intravascular radiation treatment beyond a few months. Because of the potential to induce significant late effects, there is a definite need for long-term studies.

Radiosensitivity Varies as Function of Cell Cycle Position

As mammalian cells proliferate and multiply, individual cells traverse through distinct phases: mitosis, G1, S, and G2.[29] The time required for a cell to divide, traverse through Gl, S, and G2, and reach mitosis again is called the cell cycle time. The survival curve shown in Figure 1 is derived from cells in exponential cell growth, where cells are distributed in different proportions among these phases. Elegant studies in the 1960s showed that cells vary in radiosensitivity as a function of their position in the cell cycle.[30–32] Cells in G2 and mitosis are the most radiosensitive, while cells in late S phase are the most resistant to a given dose of radiation. Cells in G1 have an intermediate radiosensitivity. The difference in radiosensitivity between a cell in mitosis and one in S phase (DNA synthesis phase) is approximately threefold. Cells comprising many normal tissues that are not actively proliferating are arrested in a substage of G1 called G_o. The radiosensitivity of cells in G_o is similar to that of cells in the G1 phase. It is impressive that the same cell would vary so much in radiosensitivity as it simply traverses the cell cycle. Little is known about why this happens. Possible explanations may be differential repair capacities, inability to appropriately arrest in critical phases of the cell cycle for repair, or changes in the biophysical nature of DNA as cells progress through the cell cycle. Presently this is a very fruitful area of research now that a number of molecules (in particular, the cyclins) that are quite important in controlling movement through the cell cycle have been discovered.[33–36]

Repair of Radiation Damage

Biological tissues possess a differential ability to accumulate and repair radiation damage. Two operationally defined terms, sublethal damage and potentially lethal damage, have been coined to account for the observation that cells can survive radiation under certain conditions. While these terms were originally defined in an abstract way, without reference to the molecular or subcellular entities experiencing the actual radiation damage, a wealth of experimental data now exists to support the concepts, and perhaps to allow for the design of therapeutic strategies.[37]

Potentially Lethal Damage (PLD)

Alteration of a cell's environment following radiation has been found to obviate a proportion of the radiation injury. This phenomenon was observed in normal tissues and tumors; it suggested that a component of radiation damage is repairable under certain environmental conditions and irreparable in others. In vitro, allowing cells to remain in a density inhibited state (plateau phase) for several hours post irradiation or incubating them in a balanced salt solution instead of culture medium leads to improved survival, which is indicative of PLD repair. Similar conditions may be mimicked in vivo. For example, mouse thyroid or mammary cells may be irradiated in situ, then transplanted into a fat pad for survival assay. If the transplant is delayed several hours, enhanced survival is seen. The enhanced survival is thought to be due to PLD repair.[38] The hypothesis underlying such observations of PLD is that a proportion of radiation damage may be repaired if, for a period of time following the radiation, cells are somehow prevented from attempting the complex process of mitosis and cell division. Normal cells within tissues are frequently in a resting (nondividing) state that is akin to plateau phase cell cultures in vitro.

Sublethal Damage

As discussed above, the survival curve for mammalian cells irradiated in vitro has a characteristic shape (see Fig. 1). The initial portion of the curve is shallower, sweeping downward in a continuously curving shoulder of varying magnitude and extent. The terminal portion has a steeper slope, and falls "exponentially." The general interpretation of the initial shoulder region is that a proportion of the radiation damage is being repaired and therefore not producing lethality. After sufficient radiation damage has been accumulated, each additional dose causes exponential cell kill. Although lower radiation doses do not produce exponential cell kill, such doses do cause sublethal damage, which the cell appears capable of repairing under appropriate conditions. The association between the initial shoulder on the survival curve and the repair of sublethal damage has been well established.[39] Mammalian cells exposed to smaller doses of radiation (ie, in the initial shoulder region) can repair a proportion of the radiation damage (sublethal damage) given sufficient time and nutrients, etc. A proportion of the cells irradiated, however, will sustain lethal damage and will not survive. The addition of a second small dose of radiation will reproduce exactly the same initial curve and kill the same proportion of the remaining cells (Fig. 2). The survival curve for multifractionated irradiation can be generated by joining these curves as shown. Theoretically, the curve approaches an exponential decline, with a uniform albeit shallower slope than seen with acute single-dose exposures. The broader the shoulder, the greater the capacity for repair. In general, the survival curves of late-reacting normal tissues have such shoulders. Thus, multifractionated radiation schedules, using small doses per fraction, tend to spare late reactions in normal tissues.

Evidence for this important phenomenon of sublethal repair was first provided in the classic studies of Elkind and Sutton.[40] In a series of experiments comparing the lethality of a large single dose of radiation with the same total dose that was split into two smaller fractions separated by a time interval (fractionated irradiation), it was shown that the split dose produced less lethality.[41] The

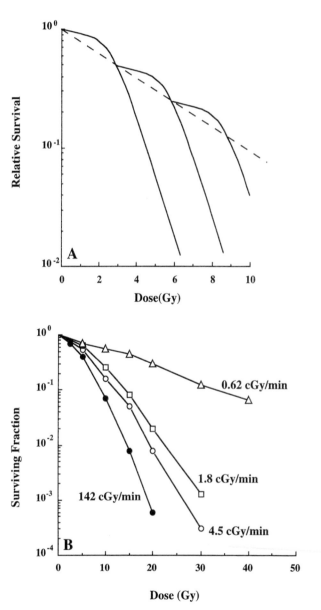

Figure 2. A. Theoretical survival curves illustrating the effect of repeated administration of 3-Gy doses of radiation to a population of mammalian cells. Because of the cells' capacity to repair sublethal damage caused by these doses, a proportion of the cells survives each time, giving rise to the shoulder. The net effect of such fractionation yields an exponentially falling curve (dotted line) much shallower than when single doses are used (solid lines). Thus, the "sparing" effect of radiation dose fractionation. **B.** Radiation dose-response curve for Chinese hamster V79 cells exposed to different dose rates of ionizing radiation. As the dose rate decreases there is an increase in cell survival for a given total dose. Redrawn from Reference 44, with permission.

interval between the two fractions allows repair of sublethal damage. The half-time for such repair has been estimated at 0.5 to 1 .5 hours depending on the cells studied.[39] It is generally accepted that a time interval of at least 6 hours between radiation fractions is required in order to avoid severe late normal tissue reactions in fractionated radiotherapy.[42]

Dose-Rate Effect

The sparing effect of fractionating a dose of radiation over time has been explained by the repair of sublethal damage in those cells whose survival curve is characterized by an initial shoulder (eg, late-reacting normal mammalian tissues). Stated a different way, a given single dose of radiation will tend to spare normal tissues if it is protracted over time. Dose fractionation is one example of protracting the treatment time to spare such tissue. A second example is provided by slowing the rate at which a single continuous dose is given. This is referred to as the dose-rate effect. Dose-rate effects have been demonstrated in vitro as well as in vivo. The dose-rate effect is an important radiobiological tenet underlying effective administration of radiation. Reduction of the dose rate at which certain cell lines are irradiated in vitro shows a progressive sparing effect that is most marked between 1 and 100 cGy/min as shown in Figure 2, panel B.[43–45] A tremendous variability exists between differing cell lines irradiated at varying dose rates in vitro, depending on their ability to accumulate and repair sublethal damage.[38] Furthermore, there is little if any additional effect seen at rates above 100 cGy/min. However, over a range of dose rates between 0.3 and 1.6 cGy/min, a paradoxical "inverse" dose-rate effect is observed (Fig. 3); the survival curve becomes steeper once again, as cell cycle effects increase the radiation sensitivity and outweigh the effect of repair of sublethal damage.[44] The reason for the inverse dose-rate effect is that continuous irradiation over this dose rate range effectively blocks cells in the radiosensitive phase of the cell cycle (G2).[44] Once this occurs, the low dose rate treatment becomes much more efficient with respect to cell killing.

Different approaches to treat the intravascular treatment volume presently under evaluation will result in the delivery of radiation at different dose rates to the tissue. It must be appreciated that not only is the total dose of radiation delivered important, but also that the time interval over which radiation is delivered (dose rate) is equally important because of repair of radiation damage between fractionated radiation doses or during the exposure (dose-rate effect). This concept is particularly important when comparing results of intravascular treatments in which high dose rates are used with those that use radioactive stents that deliver radiation doses over extended times (low dose rates).

External Beam versus Intravascular Radiation Treatment

There is presently considerable controversy regarding the use of external beam radiation treatment to prevent restenosis. Some studies suggest that external beam treatment does not work and, in fact, makes the restenosis problem worse.[46,47] This particular study used doses of 4 or 8 Gy which, because of inadequate cell killing, are much too low to effectively prevent restenosis (see Fig. 1).

Figure 3. Radiation dose-response curves for human HeLa cells exposed to different dose rates of continuous radiation. Notice that 0.6 cGy/min is more effective for cell killing than 0.2 or 2.6 cGy/min (inverse dose-rate effect). This is due to cell cycle blockade. At this dose rate, the cells are selectively blocked at G2/M, a more radiosensitive phase of the cell cycle. Redrawn from Reference 44, with permission.

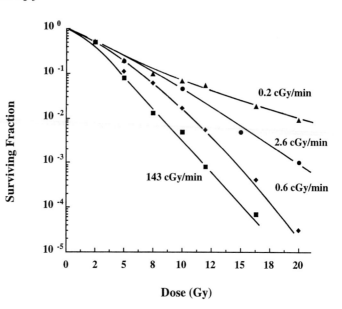

In fact, low doses such as these may stimulate repopulation as has been observed previously in normal tissues at the beginning of fractionated radiotherapy.[48,49] Other studies where higher external beam doses (15 to 22.5 Gy) were used have reported satisfactory prevention of restenosis.[50]

There is a need to evaluate this issue more carefully in preclinical trials. Presently, intravascular delivery of radiation by ^{192}Ir sources delivers a total dose of ~15 Gy in 15 minutes (dose rate = 1.0 Gy/min). Delivery of the same dose at the same dose rate by use of external beam should yield the same results with respect to preventing restenosis. The major difference in the two techniques is dose distribution. Intravascular delivery results in extremely high doses to the lumen with a fall-off in dose as a function of distance from the source; whereas, external beam would deliver a uniform dose over the entire volume of tissue treated. It would be beneficial to compare these two approaches, given that the technology of precise external beam delivery to vessels is available.[51]

Radioactive Stents

An important and central theme in radiation oncology is the fact that cells (and tissues) can repair radiation damage between acute fractions and during continuous low dose rate irradiation. Likewise, the issue of repair is also important in the use of radiation to prevent restenosis by using radioactive stents that may be placed in the vessel following PTCA. The selection of the appropriate isotope and the activity to use (ie, the total dose to deliver and the dose rate of delivery) are extremely important variables in considering this approach to prevent restenosis with acceptable toxicity. Issues such as cell cycle redistribution during continuous low dose rate irradiation, possible inverse dose-rate effects, and the minimum dose rate required to stop cell division must be explored. An example of the complexity of the response obtained from using radioactive stents in preclinical models of restenosis is demonstrated in the study by Carter et al.[52] In this study, different activities of ^{32}P-containing stents were used in a porcine coronary restenosis model. The doses delivered by the different activities of ^{32}P were divided into three categories: low (<2000 cGy), intermediate (4000 cGy), and high (>10,000 cGy). Based on these values, the average dose rates to the tissue over the 25-day period of the study were: low (~3 cGy/h), intermediate (6 cGy/h), and high (15 cGy/h). It is interesting that both the high and low doses and dose rates were effective in reducing the extent of restenosis, whereas, the intermediate dose/dose rate was ineffective if not worse than the control.[52] These findings do not conform to the findings that would be expected as dose and dose rate are reduced. One might expect the high dose/dose rate to be effective, and perhaps the intermediate and low dose/dose rate to be ineffective. The fact that the low dose/dose rate treatment was effective in this study suggests that perhaps an inverse dose-rate effect is operative over a narrow range of dose rates in this model.

Modifiers of Radiation Response

The inherent radiosensitivity of cells and tissues can be influenced by a number of chemical approaches and manipulations. This is important for at least two reasons. Modification of the radiosensitivity by specific agents of known mechanisms of action can provide information about how radiation damage is registered and repaired. Second, selective modification of radiosensitivity (eg, in the cell population responsible for restenosis) would allow for a lower radiation dose to be used. For example, if a tumor-specific radiation sensitizer enhanced the effectiveness of radiation by a factor of 1.5, a delivered dose of 10 Gy would actually be equivalent to 15 Gy. The major goal is to develop a treatment that affords a therapeutic gain; that is, enhanced response with respect to preventing restenosis, without increased damage to surrounding normal tissue. Selected modifiers of the radiation response are discussed below.

Oxygen

Perhaps the most efficient radiation sensitizer is molecular oxygen. As shown in panel A of Figure 4, oxygen has long been known to enhance the effectiveness of radiation (x-rays) in killing cells in culture by a factor of 2 to 3 when compared to irradiation conducted under oxygen-free conditions.[53] In other words, if cells are irradiated in an hypoxic (<0.5% oxygen) as opposed to aerobic (~20% oxygen) environment they are two to three times more resistant to the cytotoxic effects of radiation. When comparing the radiosensitivity of cells in aerobic versus hypoxic conditions, radiobiologists use the term oxygen enhancement ratio (OER). Thus the OER for mammalian cells exposed to x-rays is 2.0 to 3.0. As discussed above, it has been postulated that radiation produces carbon centered radicals (most likely in the cellular DNA) that can react with molecular oxygen (a diradical molecule) to yield a lesion that is toxic and, if not repaired, will result in death of the cell.[7] Under hypoxic conditions, very few, if any, oxygen-related lesions are formed and hence there is less cell killing.

A major research effort has been directed toward the potential problem of the presence of viable hypoxic cells within tumors. Does hypoxia play a role in the use of radiation to prevent restenosis? At present the answer to this question is not

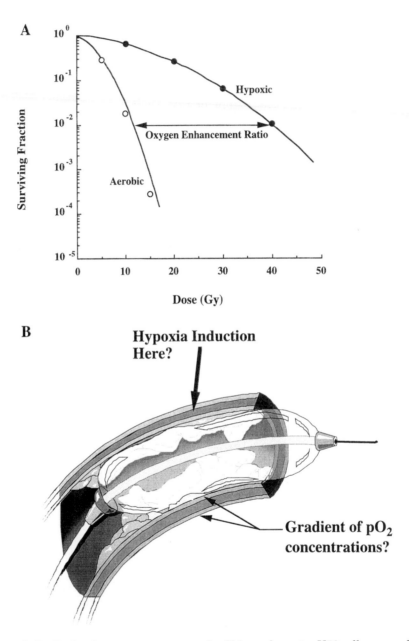

Figure 4. A. Radiation dose-response curves for Chinese hamster V79 cells exposed under aerobic and hypoxic conditions (<10 ppm oxygen). Notice that cells under hypoxic conditions are much more resistant to radiation than cells exposed under aerobic conditions. The oxygen enhancement ratio (OER) is the ratio of hypoxic to aerated radiation doses required to achieve the same level of survival. For mammalian cells the OER values range between 2.0 and 3.3. **B.** Graphic representation of a blood vessel with balloon in place. Does the percutaneous transluminal coronary angioplasty (PTCA) procedure produce transient hypoxia in tissue in the vessel wall? If it does, these tissues may be resistant to radiation treatment. Image modified by J.B. Mitchell. Original image ©1994 by TechPool Studios Corp., USA. Used with permission from Williams and Wilkins.

known; however, one could envision the possibility that PTCA might induce hypoxia as depicted in Figure 4, panel B. Because of the mechanical force used in PTCA, it is possible that blood flow to tissue surrounding the vessel is disrupted temporally, which would render it hypoxic. If radiation exposure were to follow soon after PTCA, target cells could be hypoxic and hence more resistant to radiation treatment than fully oxygenated tissue. Likewise, if balloons were used to center the radiation source in the vessel during treatment, one could envisage hypoxia induction in tissue surrounding the vessel because of the force exerted on the vessel wall by the balloon. Whether hypoxia is induced by PTCA is not known. There are several ways to address the problem that would arise if hypoxia was induced.

For the past 30 years radiobiologists and radiotherapists have actively pursued a variety of approaches to sensitize hypoxic cells to radiation. The goal of such research is to identify an approach that will reduce the OER from ~3.0 to 1.0, that is, hypoxic cells will have the same response to radiation as aerobic cells. The use of high linear energy transfer radiation and hyperbaric oxygen has been explored in radiation therapy; however, neither of these approaches would be practical for consideration in intravascular radiation treatments. Another approach that has received much attention is the development of chemicals that would not be metabolized like oxygen but could diffuse into hypoxic regions in tumors and sensitize hypoxic cells to radiation.[54] A class of compounds known as nitroimadazoles was identified to have such characteristics.[54] These compounds were shown not to radiosensitize aerobic cells; however, at concentrations of ~1 mmol/L hypoxic cells were radiosensitized (OER = 1.6). Two nitroimadazoles, misonidazole and SR-2508, have been introduced into clinical radiotherapy trials.[55,56] Another approach at radiosensitizing hypoxic cells is the use of nitric oxide.[57,58] Technological advances in the area of tumor oxygen measurements in tissues will allow for the evaluation of whether hypoxia is induced in vessel walls following PTCA and whether treatment with hypoxic cell radiosensitizers is warranted.

Radiation Sensitizers

A number of drugs have been identified as radiation sensitizers, including many chemotherapeutic agents such as cisplatin, adriamycin, mitomycin C, 5 fluorouracil, paclitaxel, and halogenated pyrimidines (HPs). These agents can radiosensitize cells by a variety of mechanisms, including increase of radiation damage, inhibition of radiation repair, imposition of cell cycle blocks, etc. The ideal use of radiation sensitizers should allow for a lower radiation dose to be used to achieve the same level of response. Two examples of radiation sensitizers are discussed in order to demonstrate the importance of knowing the mechanism(s) of radiation-induced cell killing and drug action.

Paclitaxel

Paclitaxel binds to microtubules, possibly at a site on β-tubulin,[59] and interferes with normal microtubule structure and function. In order for paclitaxel to exert cytotoxicity, cells must be *moving* through the cell cycle, as cells in plateau phase are resistant to paclitaxel.[60] Long-term treatment of cells with relatively low concentrations of paclitaxel results in radiosensitization of log phase cells but no radiosensitization is observed for cells that are exposed to paclitaxel and immediately irradiated.[61] The radiosensitization observed after prolonged treatment with paclitaxel is most likely due to the paclitaxel-mediated G2/M block in the cell cycle.[62,63] For most cell lines in culture, paclitaxel treatment is required for at least 24 hours for a G2/M block to occur. Thus, this particular type of radiation sensitizer would not be expected to have utility in intravascular radiation treatments presently used because the target cells do not divide prior to the radiation treatment. In order for paclitaxel to have utility for this particular application, the radiation treatment must be delivered some time after PTCA, when cells are induced into the division cycle. Paclitaxel treatment would have to commence soon after PTCA and continue for perhaps 1 to 2 days before radiation treatment in order for this approach to be effective. This might be impractical for the placement of a radioactive implant several days after PTCA; however, external beam radiotherapy could be easily administered. On the other hand, paclitaxel impregnated within a radioactive stent and placed in the vessel after PTCA might afford high/continuous local concentrations of paclitaxel to the dividing target cells. Cell cycle blockage in the radiosensitive G2/M phases by paclitaxel plus continuous low dose rate irradiation might be an effective means to radiosensitize. These ideas must be explored in a preclinical setting; however, they illustrate the necessity of understanding the mechanism of action of a particular drug as radiosensitizer before it can be effectively used.

Halogenated Pyrimidines

HPs were synthesized in the early 1960s. The structure of HP mimics that of thymidine, a normal base required for DNA synthesis. The difference in structure resides in a replacement of 5′ methyl group of thymidine with a halogen (iodine, bromine, chlorine, or fluorine). Because of the similarity of the van der Waal radius of the methyl group to that of the halogen, cells are capable of readily incorporating iodo-, bromo-, and chloro-deoxyuridine into DNA. An exception is fluorodeoxyuridine, whose van der Waal radius is significantly smaller than that of the methyl group of thymidine. As a result, fluorodeoxyuridine actually blocks cells at the Gl/S phase interface, inhibits DNA synthesis, and has been used as a cell cycle-specific chemotherapy agent.

When cells are grown for several generations in the presence of HP (iodine, bromine, chlorine), they become sensitized to both ultraviolet light[64] and ionizing radiation.[65,66] In order for HP to sensitize cells to radiation they must be incorporated into cellular DNA.[67] The major requirement is an adequate concentration of the HP for extended periods, as cells undergo DNA synthesis to compete with thymidine pools for incorporation into DNA. HP, which are incorporated into cellular DNA, can exhibit significant radiosensitization (enhancement ratio ~2.0) when replacement of thymidine is greater than 10% to 15%.[68–71] As the percentage of replacement of thymidine bases with HP bases increases, so does the extent of radiosensitization.[67,72]

How might HPs be used in the setting of PTCA? PTCA stimulates smooth muscle cells to proliferate in response to the mechanical stress. In fact, Wilcox et al[73] have demonstrated this with use of HP labeling. The fact that smooth muscle cells incorporate HP for labeling studies indicates that given a long enough exposure time to sufficient concentrations of HPs, smooth muscle cells can be significantly radiosensitized. The pharmacology of HP delivery to patients has already been worked out in clinical trials for tumor radiosensitization.[74] A proposed protocol for the use of HPs as radiation sensitizers for restenosis is shown in Figure 5, panel A. The protocol would require continuous infusion of HP immediately following PTCA. Smooth muscle cells that are normally out of the cell cycle (G_o) would be stimulated to proliferate by the PTCA procedure and would incorporate HPs into their DNA in sufficient amounts for radiosensitization. A radiation treatment would be administered (either external beam of intravascular source) 1 to 3 days after PTCA. There are several possible advantages to this approach. First, the radiation sensitizer used would be specific to the proliferating cell population

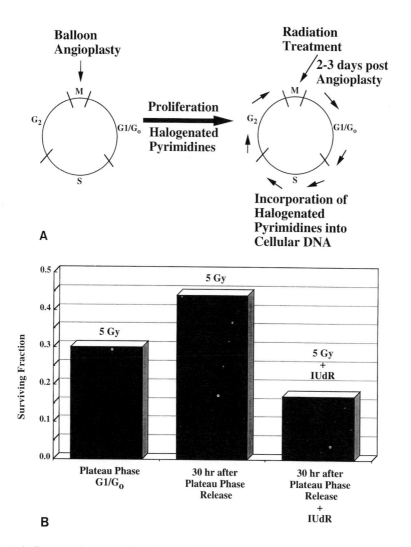

A

B

Figure 5. A. Proposed protocol for the use of halogenated pyrimidines to radiosensitize proliferating smooth muscle cells following percutaneous transluminal coronary angioplasty (PTCA). **B.** Survival of Chinese hamster V79 following a 5-Gy dose of radiation in plateau phase, 30 hours after release from plateau phase, or 30 hours after release from plateau phase + IUdR (cells were grown in medium containing 10 μmol/L IUdR for the entire time after release from plateau phase; 30 h).

(smooth muscle cells). Other cells/tissues within the radiation treatment volume would not be radiosensitized. Second, if adequate concentrations of HPs are incorporated into smooth muscle cells, inhibition of restenosis can be achieved with use of a much lower dose of radiation. Finally, use of a lower dose of radiation to achieve an acceptable inhibition of restenosis would mean that other normal tissues within the radiation treatment volume would be at a lower risk for potential late effects. To demonstrate the feasibility of this approach, results from a cell study to simulate the protocol described above are shown in Figure 5, panel B. In this study, Chinese hamster cells in plateau phase (Gl/G_o) were subcultured to low cell density into medium containing iododeoxyuridine (IUdR). When plateau cells are subcultured, they immediately reenter the cell cycle and in the process incorporate IUdR into their DNA. A 5-Gy dose given 30 hours after subculture shows that cells that have incorporated IUdR have approximately threefold more sensitivity than control cells. The study serves to demonstrate yet another use of selective radiosensitizers and how they might be used in the restenosis area. As an aside, the use of UV light might also be considered since it has been shown that incorporation of HP into the DNA of cells sensitizes cells to UV.[64] Of course, preclinical animal studies would have to be conducted to determine if this approach works in vivo.

Late Effects

From a radiotherapy point of view, when considering the radiotolerance of tissue, the critical targets may be thought of as functional subunits and the tolerance of the tissue is related to the number, as well as to the radiosensitivity, of such units. Biological tissue is composed of a heterogenous population of living cells, interacting in a complex fashion. Clinical effects of radiation are not predictable solely on the basis of cell kill, but on a host of interrelated variables which may be difficult to accurately quantitate. It is recognized, however, that death of critical cells or functional subunits may contribute significantly to loss of function of the tissue or organ. This is particularly dramatic in tissues composed of cells that are proliferating rapidly as part of their normal function (bone marrow, gastrointestinal mucosa, testis, skin, hair follicles). The dose required in order to see a measurable effect on the function of such a tissue is termed the threshold dose and may be quite low depending on the intrinsic radiosensitivity of the individual cells. Late effects differ in time course and natural history from acute reactions following radiation treatment. The onset of late effects usually occurs several months following completion of therapy, and they are generally irreversible. The pathological hallmarks are fibrosis, atrophy, vascular damage, and, less frequently, necrosis. Although there has been debate as to the exact cause of late effects, it seems likely that a combination of direct cytotoxicity on tissue stem cells, allied with indirect effects from damage to microenvironmental supporting tissues (eg, vascular and lymphatic systems), is important. Tissues particularly at risk for late reactions are generally those with slow cellular renewal and long cell cycle times. Reduction in the number of stem cells and loss of reproductive ability in those remaining have both been implicated in the genesis of late reactions.[75] The slower proliferation rate and longer cell cycle times (months to years) account for the delayed onset and gradual manifestation of these effects. For example, it has been shown that the turnover time of normal tissue endothelium in the mouse is estimated to be 20 to 2000 times longer (47 to 23,000 days) than tumor cells derived from the same animal (2.4 to 13 days).[76] In addition, loss of vascular endothelial cells and other supporting stromal cells, along with growth and regulatory factors, may also play a role.[77] Although the latent interval between radiation and late effects shortens with increasing total radiation dose,[78] the severity of these effects worsens with increasing radiation dose-fraction size. Myocardial dysfunction occurs due to vascular damage and progressive fibrosis and thickening of the myocardium. Coronary artery stenosis and occlusion is a particularly significant component of radiation injury to the heart. With mature follow-up now available from earlier studies that used radiation therapy in diseases such as Hodgkin's disease and breast cancer comes the realization of the importance of cardiac toxicity due to radiation in clinical practice. Long-term follow-up of patients treated with radiation for Hodgkin's disease is now showing markedly increased rates of various cardiac injuries including myocardial infarctions.[4,79]

While these examples come from the use of radiation in cancer treatment, they serve as reminders that radiation can kill cells and damage tissue. The use of radiation to prevent restenosis should be weighed against possible late effects that may follow the procedure. It is imperative, therefore, that long-term studies in animals be conducted to determine not only the radiation dose-response relationship to effectively inhibit restenosis, but also the extent and severity of late complications. Identifying a "therapeutic window" for use of radiation in restenosis will be, as it has in radiation oncology, a delicate balancing act.

References

1. Condado JA, Gurdiel O, Espinoza R, et al. Percutaneous transluminal coronary angioplasty (PTCA) and intracoronary radiation therapy (ICRT): A possible new modality for the treatment of coronary restenosis: A preliminary report of the first 10 patients treated with intracoronary radiation therapy. J Am Coll Cardiol 1994;23:288A.
2. Teirstein PS, Massullo V, Jani S, et al. Catheter-based radiotherapy to inhibit restenosis after coronary stenting. N Engl J Med 1997;336:1697–1703.
3. Flickinger JC, Pollock BE, Kondziolka D, Lunsford LD. A dose-response analysis of arteriovenous malformation obliteration after radiosurgery. Int J Radiat Oncol Biol Phys 1996;36:873–879.
4. Hancock SL, Tucker MA, Hoppe RT. Factors affecting late mortality from heart disease after treatment of Hodgkin's disease. JAMA 1993;270:1949–1955.
5. King V, Constine LS, Clark D, et al. Symptomatic coronary artery disease after mantle irradiation for Hodgkin's disease. Int J Radiat Oncol Biol Phys 1996;36:881–889.
6. Hall EJ. Radiobiology for the Radiologist. Philadelphia, PA: J.B. Lippincott Co.; 1994.
7. von Sonntag C. The Chemical Basis of Radiation Biology. London: Taylor and Francis; 1987.
8. Tubiana M, Dutreix J, Wambersie A. Introduction to Radiobiology. London: Taylor and Francis; 1990.
9. Steel GG, Adams GE, Peckham MJ. The Biological Basis of Radiotherapy. Amsterdam: Elsevier Science Publishers, 1983.
10. Puck TT, Marcus PI. Action of x-rays on mammalian cells. J Exp Med 1956;103:653–666.
11. Munro TR. The relative radiosensitivity of the nucleus and cytoplasm of the Chinese hamster fibroblasts. Radiat Res 1970;42:451–470.
12. Cornforth MN, Bedford JS. A quantitative comparis n of potentially lethal damage repair and the rejoining of interphase chromosome breaks in low passage normal human fibroblasts. Radiat Res 1987;111:385–405.
13. Bedford JS, Cornforth MN. Relationship between the recovery from sublethal x-ray damage and the rejoining of chromosome breaks in normal human fibroblasts. Radiat Res 1987;111:406–423.

14. Kerr JF, Wyllie AH, Currie AR. Apoptosis: A basic biological phenomenon with wide-ranging implications in tissue kinetics. Br J Cancer 1972;26:239–257.

15. Alnemri ES, Fernandes TF, Haldar S, et al. Involvement of BCL-2 in glucocorticoid-induced apoptosis of human pre-B-leukemias. Cancer Res 1992;52:491–495.

16. Shaw P, Bovey R, Tardy S, et al. Induction of apoptosis by wild-type p53 in a human colon tumor-derived cell line. Proc Natl Acad Sci U S A 1992;89:4495–4499.

17. Whitfield JF. Calcium signals and cancer. Crit Rev Oncog 1992;3:55–90.

18. Arends MJ, Morris RG, Wyllie AH. Apoptosis. The role of the endonuclease. Am J Pathol 1990;136:593–608.

19. Sellins KS, Cohen JJ. Gene induction by gamma-irradiation leads to DNA fragmentation in lymphocytes. J Immunol 1987;139:3199–3206.

20. Ijiri K. Cell death (apoptosis) in mouse intestine after continuous irradiation with gamma rays and with beta rays from tritiated water. Radiat Res 1989;118:180–191.

21. Stephens LC, Ang KK, Schultheiss TE, et al. Apoptosis in irradiated murine tumors. Radiat Res 1991;127:308–316.

22. Warters RL. Radiation-induced apoptosis in a murine T-cell hybridoma. Cancer Res 1992;52:883–890.

23. Okada S. Radiation induced death. In: Altman KI, Gerber GB, Okada S (eds.): *Radiation Biochemistry*. New York: Academic Press Inc.; 1970:247–307.

24. Duvall E. Death and the cell. Immunol Today 1986;7:115–119.

25. Yamada T, Ohyama H. Radiation-induced interphase death of rat thymocytes is internally programmed (apoptosis). Int J Radiat Biol 1988;53:65–75.

26. Fowler JF. Dose response curves for organ function or cell survival. Br J Radiol 1983;56:497–500.

27. Brenner DJ, Miller RC, Hall EJ. The radiobiology of intravascular irradiation. Int J Radiat Oncol Biol Phys 1996;36:805–810.

28. Hayflick L. Aging, longevity, and immortality in vitro. Exp Gerontol 1992;27:363–368.

29. Howard A, Pelc S. Synthesis of deoxyribonucleic acid in normal and irradiated cells and its relation to chromosome breakage. Heredity 1953;6:261–273.

30. Terasima T, Tolmach LJ. Changes in x-ray sensitivity of HeLa cells during the division cycle. Nature 1961;190:1210–1211.

31. Terasima R, Tolmach LJ. X-ray sensitivity and DNA synthesis in synchronous populations of HeLa cells. Science 1963;140:490–492.

32. Sinclair WK. Cyclic x-ray responses in mammalian cells in vitro. Radiat Res 1968;33:620–643.

33. Murray AW. Cell biology. Cyclins in meiosis and mitosis. Nature 1987;326:542–543.

34. Hanley-Hyde J. Cyclins in the cell cycle: An overview. Curr Top Microbiol Immunol 1992;182:461–466.

35. Sherr CJ. Mammalian Gl cyclins. Cell 1993;73:1059–1065.

36. Bernard EJ, Maity A, Muschel RJ, McKenna WG. Effects of ionizing radiation on cell cycle progression. A review. Radiat Environ Biophys 1995;34:79–83.

37. Bedford JS. Sublethal damage, potentially lethal damage, and chromosomal aberrations in mammalian cells exposed to ionizing radiations. Int J Radiat Oncol Biol Phys 1991;21:1457–1469.

38. Hall EJ. Repair of radiation damage and the dose-rate effect. In: *Radiobiology for the Radiologist*. Philadelphia, PA: J.B. Lippincott Co.; 1994:107–131.

39. Tubiana M, Dutreix J, Wambersie A. Cellular effects of ionizing radiation. Cell survival curves. In: *Introduction to Radiobiology*. London: Taylor and Francis; 1990:86–125.

40. Elkind MM, Sutton H. X-ray damage and recovery in mammalian cells in culture. Nature 1959;184:1293–1295.

41. Elkind MM, Sutten-Gilbert H, Moses WB, et al. Radiation response of mammalian cells in culture V. Temperature dependence of the repair of x-ray damage in surviving cells (aerobic and hypoxic). Radiat Res 1965;25:359–376.

42. Fowler JF. Intervals between multiple fractions per day. Differences between early and late radiation reactions. Acta Oncol 1988;27:181–183.

43. Bedford JS, Hall EJ. Survival of HeLa cells cultured in vitro and exposed to protracted gamma irradiation. Int J Radiat Biol 1963;7:337–383.

44. Mitchell JB, Bedford JS, Bailey SM. Dose-rate effects in mammalian cells in culture

III. Comparison of cell killing and cell proliferation during continuous irradiation for six different cell lines. Radiat Res 1979;79:537–551.

45. Bedford JS, Mitchell JB, Fox MH. Variations in responses of several mammalian cell lines to low dose-rate irradiation. In: Meyn RE, Withers HR (eds.): *Radiation Biology in Cancer Research*. New York, NY: Raven Press; 1980:251–262.

46. Schwartz RS, Koval TM, Edwards WD, et al. Effect of external beam irradiation on neointimal hyperplasia after experimental coronary artery injury. J Am Coll Cardiol 1992;19:1106–1113.

47. Schwartz RS, Koval TM, Gregoire J, et al. External beam irradiation, stent injury and neointimal hyperplasia: Results in a porcine coronary model. In: Waksman R, King SB, Crocker IR, Mould RF (eds.): *Vascular Brachytherapy*. Veenendaal, The Netherlands: Nucletron B.V.; 1996:119–132.

48. Denekamp J. Changes in the rate of repopulation during multifraction irradiation of mouse skin. Brit J Radiol 1973;46:381–387.

49. Fowler JF. Fractionated radiation therapy after Strandqvist. Acta Radiol 1884;23: 209–216.

50. Shimotakahara S, Mayberg MR. Gamma irradiation inhibits neointimal hyperplasia in rats after arterial injury. Stroke 1994;25:424–428.

51. Koh WJ, Mayberg MR, Chambers J, et al. The potential role of external beam radiation in preventing restenosis after coronary angioplasty. Int J Radiat Oncol Biol Phys 1996;36:829–834.

52. Carter AJ, Laird JR, Bailey LR, et al. Effects of endovascular radiation from a b-particle-emitting stent in a porcine coronary restenosis model. Circulation 1996;94: 2364–2368.

53. Hall EJ. The oxygen effect and reoxygenation. In: *Radiobiology for the Radiologist*. Philadelphia, PA: J.B. Lippincott Co.; 1994:133–152.

54. Adams GE, Flockhart IR, Smithen CE, et al. Electron-affinic sensitization. VII. A correlation between structures, one-electron reduction potentials, and efficiencies of nitroimadizoles as hypoxic cell radiosensitizers. Radiat Res 1976;67:9–20.

55. Phillips TL, Wasserman T. Promise of radiosensitizers and radioprotectors in the treatment of human cancer. Cancer Treat Rep 1984;68:291–301.

56. Coleman CN, Wasserman TH, Urtasun RC, et al. Phase I trial of the hypoxic cell radiosensitizer SR-2508: The results of the five to six week drug schedule. Int J Radiat Oncol Biol Phys 1986;12:1105–1108.

57. Mitchell JB, Wink DA, DeGraff W, et al. Hypoxic mammalian cell radiosensitization by nitric oxide. Cancer Res 1993;53:5845–5848.

58. Mitchell JB, Cook JA, Krishna MC, et al. Radiation sensitization by nitric oxide releasing agents. Br J Cancer 1996;74:S181–S184.

59. Rao S, Horwitz SB, Ringel I. Direct photoaffinity labeling of tubulin with taxol. J Natl Cancer Inst 1992;84:785–788.

60. Liebmann IE, Cook JA, Lipschultz C, et al. Cytotoxic studies of paclitaxel (Taxol®) in human tumour cell lines. Br J Cancer 1993;68:1104–1109.

61. Liebmann JE, Cook JA, Fisher J, et al. In vitro studies of paclitaxel (Taxol®) as a radiation sensitizer in human tumor cells. J Natl Cancer Inst 1994;86:441–446.

62. Cook JA, DeGraff W, Teague D, Liebmann JE. Radiation sensitization of Chinese hamster V79 cells by paclitaxel. Radiat Oncol Invest 1993;l:103–110.

63. Liebmann JE, Cook JA, Fisher J, et al. Changes in radiation survival curve parameters in human tumor and rodent cells exposed to paclitaxel (Taxol®). Int J Radiat Oncol Biol Phys 1994;29:559–564.

64. Greer S. Studies on ultraviolet irradiation of Escherichia coli containing S-bromouracil in its DNA. J Gen Micro 1960;22:618–634.

65. Djordjevic B, Szybalski W. Genetics of human cell lines. III. Incorporation of 5-bromo and 5-iododeoxyuridine into the deoxyribonucleic acid of human cells and its effect on radiation sensitivity. J Exp Med 1960;112:509–531.

66. Szybalski W. X-ray sensitization by halopyrimidines *Cancer Chemother Rep* 1974;58: 539–557.

67. Erikson RL, Szybalski W. Molecular radiobiology of human cell lines. V. Comparative radiosensitizing properties of 5-halodeoxycytidines and 5-halodeoxyuridines. Radiat Res 1963;20:252–262.

68. Mitchell JB, Russo A, Cook JA, et al. Radiobiology and clinical application of halo-genated pyrimidine radiosensitizers. Int J Radiat Biol 1989;56:827–836.
69. Lawrence TS, Davis MA, Maybaum J, et al. The dependence of halogenated pyrimidine incorporation and radiosensitization on the duration of drug exposure. Int J Radiat Oncol Biol Phys 1990;18:1393–1398.
70. Uhl V, Phillips TL, Ross GY, et al. Iododeoxyuridine incorporation and radiosensitization in three human tumor cell lines. Int J Radiat Oncol Biol Phys 1992;22:489–494.
71. Miller EM, Fowler JF, Kinsella TJ. Linear-quadratic analysis of radiosensitization by halogenated pyrimidines. I. Radiosensitization of human colon cancer cells by iodo-deoxyuridine. Radiat Res 1992;131:81–89.
72. Kinsella TJ, Dobson PP, Mitchell JB, Fornace AJJ. Enhancement of x-ray induced DNA damage by pre-treatment with halogenated pyrimidine analogs. Int J Radiat Oncol Biol Phys 1987;13:733–739.
73. Wilcox JN, Waksman R, King SB, Scott NA. The role of the adventitia in the arterial response to angioplasty: The effect of intravascular radiation. Int J Radiat Oncol Biol Phys 1996;36:789–796.
74. Russo A, Gianni L, Kinsella TJ, et al. Pharmacological evaluation of intravenous delivery of 5-bromodeoxyuridine to patients with brain tumors. Cancer Res 1984;44:1702–1705.
75. Williams MV. The cellular basis of renal injury by radiation. Br J Cancer Suppl 1986;7:257–264.
76. Hobson B, Denekamp J. Endothelial proliferation in tumours and normal tissues: Continuous labelling studies. Br J Cancer 1984;49:405–413.
77. Tubiana M, Dutreix J, Wambersie A. Effects on normal tissues. In: *Introduction to Radiobiology*. London: Taylor and Francis; 1990:126–173.
78. Wheldon TE, Michalowski AS. Alternative models for the proliferative structure of normal tissues and their response to irradiation. Br J Cancer 1986;53(suppl VII):155–171.
79. Cosset JM, Henry-Amar M, Pellae-Cosset B, et al. Pericarditis and myocardial infarctions after Hodgkin's disease therapy. Int J Radiat Oncol Biol Phys 1991;21:447–449.
80. Rosen EM, Goldberg ID, Myrick KV, Levenson S. Radiation survival properties of cultured vascular smooth muscle cells. Radiat Res 1984;100:182–191.

## Chapter 10

A Paradigm Shift for the Radiation Prophylaxis of Arterial Restenosis

Philip Rubin, MD, Jacqueline P. Williams, PhD, and Paul Okunieff, MD

Introduction

A precise identification of the target cell(s) that are responsible for the induction of restenosis and/or vascular remodeling following injury has proved to be elusive, despite active research into their pathogenesis. In recent years, this particular goal has become a major radiobiological issue in the determination of the rationale for the use of radiation to inhibit vascular restenosis, and a critical determinant of whether a therapeutic window exists. The apparent success of moderate doses of irradiation to inhibit the restenotic proliferative process has been demonstrated by a number of investigators in a variety of laboratory animal models—the rat,[1–3] the rabbit,[4–6] and the pig[7–9]—using a wide variety of radiation delivery systems and sources, both external and endovascular, the latter via catheters or radioactive stents. However, there exists a real concern with respect to the possibility of a late induction of radiation vascular effects and, therefore, this risk needs to be balanced against enthusiasm for radiation's potential for inhibiting restenosis, which has been demonstrated post angioplasty with both immediate and persistent benefits.

The paradox found clinically is: How can an injurious modality, such as radiation, be effective therapeutically when it can induce the very process (stenosis of the arterial wall) that it is being used to prevent? The underlying emphasis of previously held classic concepts of the cellular origins of late radiation damage lay in specific target cells and their ability to account for injury. With the introduction of increasingly sophisticated molecular biological techniques, our group has extended the original paradigm of the clinical pathological course of late events,[10] induced by both irradiation and chemotherapy, from a single target cell to involve all of the cell types in the milieu, together with the intercellular communication, ie, the "molecular" conversation between cells. This inclusion has resulted in a series of paradigm shifts, ultimately leading to a clearer explanation of the mechanisms underlying cytotoxic-induced late effects.[11]

In our currently held paradigm on the induction of radiation late effects, the emphasis has moved from the target cells themselves to the autocrine, paracrine and, possibly, endocrine mRNA messages and related proteins which are passed

From Waksman R (ed.). *Vascular Brachytherapy, Third Edition.* Armonk, NY: Futura Publishing Co., Inc.; © 2002.

between cells. The irradiation of a target organ, with its multiple cellular components, results in the development of cytokine cascades, and we believe it is the incremental sustenance of these messages that allows surviving cells to recover or express late effects.[11] A cytokine cascade (Fig. 1) is initiated after a primary cell injury, and, over time, provokes a series of downstream events as other cells receive and respond to the mRNA message(s). Furthermore, we, and others, have demonstrated the importance of the macrophage as a key manufacturer of numerous cytokines, eg, transforming growth factor-β (TGF-β),[12] interleukin-6 (IL-6), and platelet-derived growth factor (PDGF).[13,14] All of these factors have been shown to induce fibroblast proliferation, either directly or indirectly,[15,16] leading ultimately to the altered elaboration of collagen I and III proteins.[17,18] Thus, based on over a decade of our group's experimental radiobiological concepts in the late effects of fibrogenesis, we have developed a cellular and molecular model of the fibrogenic process, based on multicellular communication via cytokine cascades, in which a critical role is played by the monocyte-derived macrophage.[11]

By extrapolating these multicellular radiation late effect concepts to vascular restenosis, we have postulated that activation of either the smooth muscle cell or adventitial fibroblast-derived myofibroblast by radiation, at the doses being used therapeutically, would not lead to a luxuriant fibrogenic response, and that the monocyte-derived macrophage is required to co-activate and promote the myofibroblast proliferation (Fig. 2). Therefore, it is the effect of radiation on the macrophage, in the therapeutic dose range being used, that is the determining factor for the inhibition of restenosis.

Unified Hypothesis for Vascular Restenosis

We propose a new and unified hypothesis for arterial stenosis and restenosis, ie, that the critical cell responsible for restenosis post angioplasty is the same as the cell that initiates the atherosclerotic plaque, namely the monocyte-derived

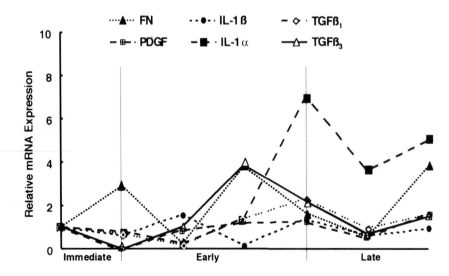

Figure 1. The cytokine cascade initiated after irradiation of the lung. Modified from Reference 11.

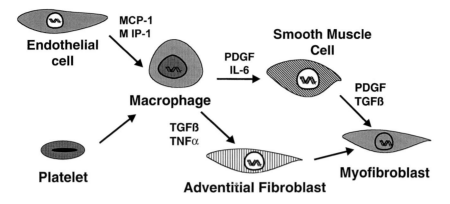

Figure 2. Cartoon illustrating the cellular sequence of events from initial injury to activation of the myofibroblast.

macrophage. By extension, therefore, we believe the macrophage is also responsible for initiating external vascular remodeling. However, of most relevance to this discussion is that these cells, when activated, are the most radiosensitive family of cells in the arterial wall and, we believe, act as the trigger mechanism for myofibroblast proliferation (Table 1).

This central hypothesis is illustrated in Figure 3 as a sequence of cellular and cytokine events; there is both experimental and clinical data to support this postulate. We hypothesize that subsequent to vascular injury, the following series of events occurs:

1. Endothelial cell injury triggers the release of chemokines[19,20] either at the luminal surface or, in the case of a more widespread trauma, in the vasovasorum on the adventitial side. Endothelial cells are of intermediate radiosensitivity.
2. Platelets, which respond to hemorrhagic injury, are highly radioresistant, but can release a large number of factors, including PDGF,[21,22] and induce the secretion of monocyte chemotactic protein-1 (MCP-1),[23] attracting monocyte/macrophages and T cells.
3. Monocytes/macrophages/T cells are primary expressors of cytokines and

Table 1		
Order of Radiosensitivity of Cells Present in the Arterial Wall		
Very sensitive	< 10 Gy	
• T cell		
• Monocyte macrophage		
Intermediate radiosensitivity	10–20 Gy	
• Endothelial cell		
Radioresistant	> 20 Gy	
• Fibroblast		
• Smooth muscle cell		
Very radioresistant	> 1000 Gy	
• Platelets		

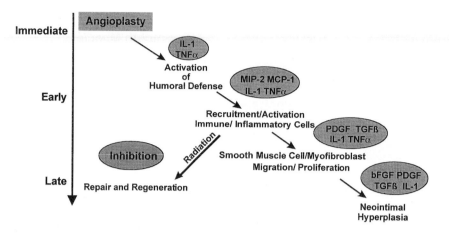

Figure 3. A generalized, hypothetical pathway illustrating the chain of events following vascular injury, eg, angioplasty, and their associated cytokines, chemokines, and growth factors.

chemokines and are recruited directly from the circulation or from the vasovasorum, along a cytokine/chemokine gradient, with an associated expression of adhesion molecules. These cells, once activated, are exquisitely sensitive to radiation.

4. Later in the temporal sequence, the adventitial fibroblasts and/or medial smooth muscle cells are stimulated to migrate and proliferate, undergoing phenotypic conversion to myofibroblasts. These cells are more radioresistant than endothelial cells, except when proliferating, at which point they become of comparable radiosensitivity.[24]

The demonstrated radiosensitivity of the restenotic process has led numerous authors to suggest that the proliferating smooth muscle cell is the target cell population in vascular radiation injury.[25–27] However, effective endovascular irradiation is applied immediately post angioplasty, while the proliferative response of smooth muscle cells requires days to week(s) to occur[28,29]; neither quiescent smooth muscle cells nor fibroblasts are considered to be particularly radiosensitive[10] and, in addition, in vitro studies have shown that irradiated smooth muscle cells do not undergo apoptosis and that radiation does not inhibit smooth muscle cell migration.[30] Of the other cells within the vascular milieu, it is well known that platelets are relatively radioresistant, withstanding large radiation doses for sterilization purposes prior to platelet transfusion,[21,22] while the endothelial cell is of intermediate radiosensitivity[10] and not a source of PDGF. By exclusion, therefore, we propose that it is the inflammatory/immune cells, involved in a variety of the ongoing pathophysiological processes, which lead to intimal thickening and vascular remodeling. It is the radiation ablation of the monocyte/macrophage cells that halts the resultant luminal narrowing of arteries by interrupting the cascade of cytokine and chemokine messages.

Evidence for Unified Hypothesis

The following vascular conditions, known for their induction of luminal narrowing, are examined as evidence for the central role of the monocyte-derived macrophage. These entities include atherogenesis, angioplasty, surgical bypass (at the artery to artery or artery to vein anastomoses), external vascular remodeling, accelerated arteriosclerosis associated with cardiac transplant rejection, stents, and radiation-induced arterial stenosis. In all of these situations, there is a role played by intimal hyperplasia as part of the "response to injury"; that is, although the injury varies, the response is consistent.

"Response-to-Injury" Thesis of Atherogenesis

The "response-to-injury" hypothesis of atherogenesis, first introduced by Virchow[31] and discussed in detail by Ross et al,[32] has been repeatedly revised over the past two decades. Current evidence essentially demonstrates the adherence of clusters of monocytes and lymphocytes, which migrate into the arterial wall in an inflammatory response, presumably to a local accumulation of modified lipoproteins[33]; activation of these cells leads to an induction of cytokines which stimulate the smooth muscle cells to migrate and proliferate.[34,35] Investigators have, through special staining in hyperlipemic nonhuman primates with atherosclerosis, identified the dominant cell initiating and stimulating the proliferative process as the foamy macrophage/monocyte, which is followed, days to weeks later, by the myofibroblast.[36]

Some investigators[37] have shown the full potential of the macrophage in atherogenesis, and stressed the interactions between macrophages, lymphocytes, smooth muscle cells, and endothelial cells with a large variety of cytokines, which act as growth agonists, antagonists, and powerful chemoattractants (Fig. 4). Evidence indicates that in atheromatous plaque formation, macrophage replication may exceed smooth muscle cell proliferation and, in fact, plays a key role in the in-

Figure 4. Cartoon illustrating potential roles played by the monocyte-derived macrophage in atherogenesis, with the reverse arrows between the T cell and the macrophage suggesting a form of immune response. Of note, all of the cells with which macrophages can interact can present CSF to the macrophages, maintaining cell viability and preventing apoptosis. On activation, macrophages can produce a large number of biologically relevant molecules, only some of which are listed. Adapted from Reference 37.

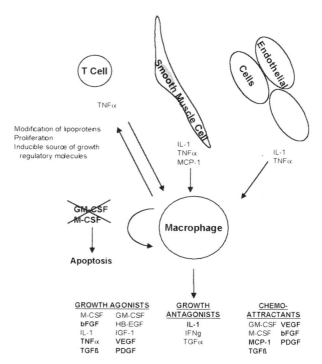

duction of smooth muscle cell proliferation and connective tissue formation; smooth muscle cells, in turn, produce M-CSF and GM-CSF,[38,39] resulting in more monocyte-derived macrophage proliferation in the lesions. A number of investigators have identified pathologically this sequence of events; for example, Ross has used dual immunohistochemical techniques and has identified, using monoclonal antibodies for monocyte-derived macrophages (HAM-56) and smooth muscle cells (HHF-35), each of these cells in human tissue.[37] Similarly, our group has used Ox42 and α-smooth muscle actin, respectively, to distinguish these two classes of cells.[40,41] Libby et al[34] noted that human atheromata contain variable numbers of macrophages, and that the macrophage content of a particular lesion could determine its propensity for restenosis after angioplasty, explaining why not all lesions develop this process. Once the macrophages are activated, the expression of the interleukins (eg, IL-1), tumor necrosis factor-α (TNF-α), PDGF, TGF-β, and basic fibroblast growth factor (bFGF), among others, could provide a cytokine cascade and lead to neointimal hyperplasia. However, no experimental evidence was offered and their hypothesis rested mainly on atheromatous lesional macrophage activation.

Nonetheless, the monocyte is ubiquitous, and is the precursor of macrophages in all tissues as well as in every phase of atherogenesis. Modified low-density lipoproteins (LDLs) are a major cause of the initiating injury in vessels,[42,43] but also are chemotactic for monocytes through regulation of M-CSF and MCP.[44,45] This sets up a cycle that expands the inflammatory response to the LDLs by attracting new circulating monocyte/macrophages and stimulating their replication. The removal and sequestration of the modified LDL particles by macrophages are important components of the initial protective role in atherogenesis.[46,47] However, the internalization of the modified lipid particles by the macrophages ultimately leads to the formation of foam cells.[48,49] In addition, although at one time it was thought that the expansion of arterial sclerotic lesions was due to the replication of smooth muscle cells only, however, it has now been shown that the proliferation of macrophages and T cells is of equal importance.[50]

"Response to Injury" Thesis for Angioplasty

The "response-to-injury" thesis can clearly be applied to both angioplasty and vascular surgical reconstruction, either of which may provoke restenosis, in addition to any underlying atherosclerotic process. The disruption of the tunicae intima and media following percutaneous transluminal coronary angioplasty (PTCA) has been shown to lead to an inflammatory cell infiltrate of mononuclear macrophages and lymphocytes.[34,51] In the particular case of neointimal hyperplasia, whether due to atherogenesis or angioplasty, it has been demonstrated that platelets may be activated within thrombi or hemorrhage into the wall,[32,52] releasing various cytokines, eg, PDGF, a powerful chemoattractant for recruiting more monocytes/macrophages[53] and that has been identified also as a potent stimulator of smooth muscle cell migration and proliferation.[54,55]

A number of molecular mechanistic models have been postulated in which cytokine expression has been identified as the basis of restenosis.[34,56,57] For instance, in Klagsbrun's model following vascular angioplasty[58] (Fig. 5A), there is endothelial cell disruption, platelet adhesion, and an inflammatory cell infiltrate of monocyte/macrophages and T cells from the luminal side. A cytokine cascade mechanism has been proposed by Libby et al[34] (Fig. 5B) as a novel model for restenosis patho-

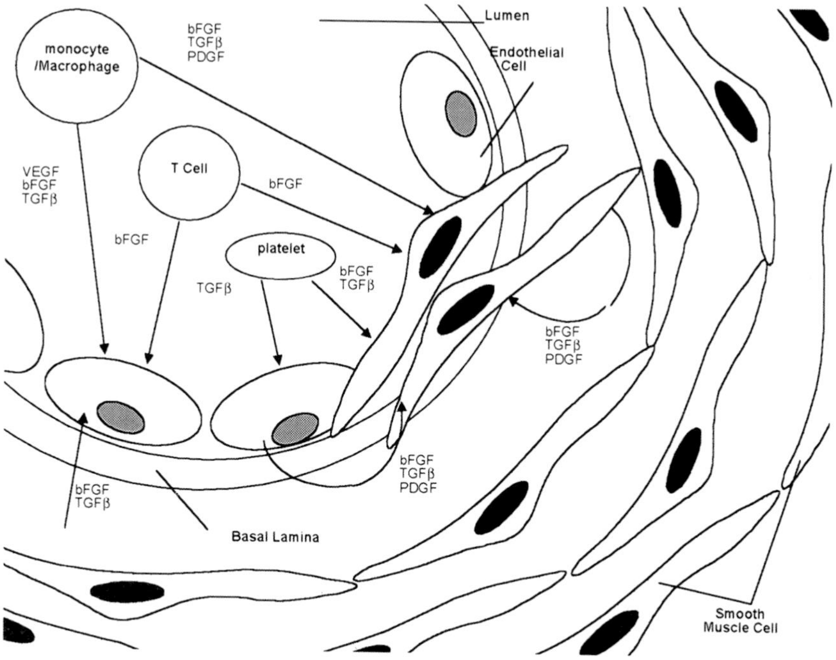

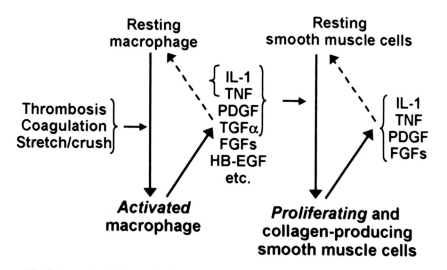

Figure 5A. Diagram representing a denuded blood vessel wall into which smooth muscle cells are migrating. Possible pathways are indicated for some of the more important growth factors and their cellular sources, notably the monocyte/macrophage, the T cell, and the platelet. Adapted from Reference 58.

Figure 5B. Schematic of a hypothetical pathway leading to the activation of smooth muscle cells, illustrating the proposed central and critical role played by the monocyte/macrophage. From Reference 34.

biology, which reconciles the disparities observed in initiating events. These investigators suggested that acute local thrombosis, blood coagulation, and/or a mechanical injury initiate cytokine expression through macrophages and/or smooth muscle cells within the plaque. This acute expression would lead to continuing autocrine and paracrine growth factor and cytokine expression.

An important, but neglected, observation is that macrophage infiltrates exist at the site of trauma, induced by angioplasty or surgical manipulation during bypass surgery,[59] in addition to the migratory and proliferating smooth muscle cells. The accumulation of macrophages in the arterial vessel wall following experimental balloon angioplasty in the rabbit carotid wall has been shown by Hanke et al.[59] Based on histologic and immunochemical markers for monocyte-derived macrophages (RAM-11), a significant increase of macrophages was found in the intima on days 14 to 21 post injury (repeat electrical stimulation with a cholesterol diet), after which levels returned to baseline values. The percentage increase was 9.1±4.3% as compared to 2.0±1.7% in controls. There is also some clinical evidence to support this concept, which can be found in a small series of 7 patients who died within 20 days of PTCA with autopsy pathological analysis by Ueda et al.[51] They noted an early tissue response was characterized by fibrin platelet deposition, a proliferation of macrophages and spindle-shaped cells, and referred to the cellular interaction as an exposure of "trigger-happy" cells within plaque morphology. In addition, in patients with unstable angina, a biassociation has been found in atherosclerotic plaques between thrombus and macrophages that suggested episodic disruption and healing.[60]

An interesting histologic study was recently performed on tissue samples available from patients treated for restenotic carotid plaque with carotid endarterectomy.[61] Twenty-nine tissue specimens were available, in addition to 14 original specimens from the same patients. Although, in general, the proliferative activity was low (1% to 3%), activity was nonetheless seen in 41% of the recurrent lesions, compared to only 14% of the primaries. The proliferation rate (measured by proliferating cell nuclear antigen [PCNA]) was found to be most pronounced in the macrophages associated with either thrombus or atheroma, but not in the smooth muscle cells. The investigators urged further investigation into the role of inflammatory cells in restenosis.

Surgical Bypass and Reconstruction Procedures

A variety of vascular and endovascular procedures for revascularization of stenosing lesions have been described, and include percutaneous angioplasty, endarterectomy, vein grafts, and synthetic grafting. In a recent editorial review by Pauletto et al,[62] the importance of smooth muscle cell proliferation and differentiation was noted for myointimal hyperplasia after vascular grafting or vein bypass, but an initial accumulation of inflammatory cell infiltrates and macrophages was also noted, preceding smooth muscle cell activation. They particularly noted that nondividing, but migrating, smooth muscle cells appeared for 2 weeks within the intima before proliferation began. Experimental observations of leukocytes and cytokine gene expression in vein graft intimal hyperplasia also can be found in a report by Hoch et al.[63] Neointimal hyperplasia was studied serially in arterialized vein grafts showing the importance of adventitial inflammatory cells starting on day 4, but with greater adventitial cellular infiltration at 1 week. Media infiltration of macrophages started at 2 weeks and there was a melding of cellular infiltrates occurring at 4 weeks in the adventitia, media, and intima. These authors emphasized that the graft-infiltrating macrophages and T cell lymphocytes furnished an additional potential source of cytokines and growth factors.

More recently, Hoch and his team have demonstrated convincingly that macrophage depletion alters the induction of intimal hyperplasia in vein grafts.[64] Using a rodent model, the investigators depleted both circulating monocytes and splenic and hepatic macrophages using liposome-encapsulated dichloromethylene bisphosphonate (L-Cl$_2$MBP). Administration of L-Cl$_2$MBP 48 hours prior to surgery induced a significant reduction in the numbers of macrophages observed in the vein grafts at 1 to 2 weeks post surgery compared to controls, and was accompanied by a trend towards a reduction in intimal hyperplasia. At 4 weeks, the macrophage numbers returned to control levels, and intimal hyperplasia was similarly resumed. Administration of a second dose of L-Cl$_2$MBP at 2 weeks post surgery induced a persistent reduction of macrophage numbers at 4 weeks, and there was a significant attenuation in intimal hyperplasia. The authors concluded that the differentiation of adventitial fibroblasts to myofibroblasts leading to neointimal hyperplasia was regulated by the infiltrating macrophages.

External Vascular Remodeling

In addition to luminal narrowing due to neointimal hyperplasia, numerous investigators have documented "constrictive vascular remodeling" as a predominant mechanism[65,66]; that is, the vessel wall thickens with myofibroblasts or adventitial fibroblasts, constricting the vessel in a similar fashion to a tourniquet. The relationship between arterial lumen and arterial wall or vessel size suggests that some species, including humans, will maintain an adequate lumen despite an increase in wall thickness. We postulate that vascular remodeling, which can be constrictive in nature, has a similar basis to neointimal hyperplasia; that is, where the angioplasty injury tears the smooth muscle cell media (type III injury) leading to an excess stimulus, there also could be adventitial fibroblastic hyperplasia due to a stimulus from the macrophage/monocyte cells before they migrate to the luminal side, piling up in some cases within the adventitia.

Recent studies based on serial intravascular ultrasound (IVUS) by Mintz et al have demonstrated that the restenosis occurring post angioplasty is due more often to external remodeling than to intimal hyperplasia (72% versus 28%, respectively).[67] The use of stents, as compared to other devices, has been shown to maintain larger acute luminal dimensions by withstanding the arterial remodeling and elastic recoil, therefore balancing against the neointimal hyperplasia that would lead to late luminal loss. Of note, diabetic patients do not appear to demonstrate vascular remodeling and lose lumen size mainly due to neointimal thickening.[68]

Morphological observations of the smooth muscle cell component of restenosis were based on the rat carotid model of Clowes et al,[69,70] but increasingly, this has been challenged by the work of a number of other investigators including Nabel,[71] Marzocchi et al,[72] and Wilcox et al,[73] who, using different animal models, have implicated other cells as the primary initiators, including the adventitial fibroblast. However, as observed in our work, it is not unreasonable to postulate that macrophages could infiltrate the arterial wall from the adventitia and become localized in the intima[40]; the subsequent release of specific factors, eg, PD GF, would lead to phenotypic conversion of fibroblasts and/or smooth muscle cells to myofibroblasts. Such a mechanism may result in either positive or negative remodeling depending on the compensatory hemodynamic physiological response to alterations in blood pressure and flow.

Recently, following similar work in humans, Frangogiannis et al examined the characteristics of resident cardiac inflammatory cells in the dog.[74] The group identified two groups of perivascular cells, macrophages and mast cells; the larger population was the macrophages (60%) and these were found to be predominantly periarteriolar. Both populations of inflammatory cells were recognized for their ability to release cytokines and growth factors, and it was suggested that their strategic perivascular location might account for their importance in the pathological processes of inflammation and fibrosis.

Accelerated Arteriosclerosis Associated with Cardiac Transplant Rejection

Observers have noted a difference between transplant-associated arteriosclerosis and typical atherosclerosis; specifically, that a concentric narrowing versus an eccentric stenosis[75] and lipid deposition, as described during typical atherosclerosis, does not appear to be an essential mechanism of graft arteriosclerosis.[76] The lesions, when examined histologically, exhibit large numbers of T cells, both CD4 and CD8,[77,78] and variable numbers of macrophages throughout the expanded intima[76]; the symmetrical annular pattern is reflected in the uniform subendothelial location of lymphocytes surrounding the lumen.[77,78] Such observations have led Libby et al to hypothesize that the pathogenesis of transplantation-associated arteriosclerosis is based on an allogenic immune response model.[76,79]

The sequence of events is believed to be an initial allogenic stimulus of T cells with a subsequent recruitment of mononuclear phagocytes and penetration of the intimal vascular wall cells, which precede and lead to the chronic fibroproliferative stage.[76,80] Libby et al have hypothesized that helper T cells of the recipient engage the foreign class II antigens on the surface of engrafted endothelial cells and direct the expression of vascular and intracellular adhesion molecules (VCAM and ICAM).[79] After recruitment of T cells, release of IL-2 leads to proliferation and amplification of alloreactive clones of T cells which, once activated, produce interferon-gamma (IFN-γ), which further stimulates macrophages into inducing a cytokine cascade of TGF-α and -β, TNF-α, and IL-1. Additional support for this view can be found in laboratory modeling with rodent heart allografts, where the persistent expression of specific inflammatory cytokines, eg, IL-6, IL-10, TNF-α, and IL-1β, has suggested an association between chronic inflammation and the promotion of graft coronary artery disease.[81] Further clinical support for the allogenic reactive model leading to a chronic, delayed hypersensitivity response is the ability of small doses of total body irradiation to lead to selective immunosuppression of lymphocytes and improved long-term survival of heart transplants by avoiding accelerated arteriosclerosis.[82,83]

Stents

A number of major clinical trials (eg, Benestent[84,85] and STRESS[86]) have used stents post angioplasty and demonstrated that the rates of restenosis could be significantly, although modestly, reduced[87,88]; a large percentage of interventional cardiologists have now adopted this procedure as standard, although some still have reservations.[89] The mode of action of stents is to create an advantage in the acute therapeutic gain through a further widening of the lumen, countering the elastic recoil and external vascular remodeling. However, it is apparent that neointimal hyperplasia is still a problem, leading to in-stent restenosis in 20% of cases.[90,91] In the swine model, the degree of injury, ie, whether the internal elastic lamina (Grade II) or the external elastic lamina (Grade III) is injured, will lead to increasing neointimal hyperplasia as compared to simple compression of the media without disruption of internal elastic laminae.[92]

The initial event after injury differs between angioplastied and stented arteries,[93,94] with the formation of platelet-rich thrombi in between stent struts acting as a scaffold into which inflammatory cells are recruited.[95] Numerous investigators have commented that the inflammatory cell components play a greater role in stented lesions than in PTCA,[96,97] and the degree of neointimal hyperplasia formation due to smooth muscle cell migration and proliferation is proportional to the early inflammatory cell involvement.[98] The persistent nature of stents results in a chronic stimulus, as determined histologically, with progressive changes from 1 to 12 weeks post implantation. These inflammatory changes were not seen in angioplasty alone, which acts as an acute injury; however stents are foreign bodies, and depending on their design, geometry, and composition, act as a chronic stimulus.[99]

Coronary vessels from patients who died shortly after stent implantation have been systematically studied by a Japanese group using serial histologic and immunohistochemical techniques to identify the cells involved.[100] At 9 and 12 days post implantation, the stent sites showed the formation of thrombus and early neointimal hyperplasia, which was composed of abundant macrophages together with smooth muscle actin-α *negative* spindle cells. By 64 days, the neointima contained macrophages, but was composed predominantly of smooth muscle actin-α *positive* cells. These observations strongly support an early temporal role for macrophages with a later, staged redifferentiation of smooth muscle cells.

Hehrlein's group in Germany have looked at the relative roles of apoptosis and proliferation following angioplasty versus stent implantation.[101] They showed that macrophage accumulation and apoptosis were considerably higher in the early phase (1 to 4 weeks) after stent implantation compared to angioplastied vessels. Kollum et al suggested that these two processes, macrophage accumulation and apoptosis, played a role in extracellular matrix secretion, and led to the increased intimal hyperplasia formation observed, in their model, in the stented animals after 4 and 12 weeks.

Radiation-Induced Arterial Stenosis

Using the analogy of the heart as a large artery, the most radiosensitive of its layers, as measured by the frequency of complications, is the pericardial surface, which is lined by endothelial-type cells and is akin to the fine vasculature of the vasovasorum. The response of the heart to single doses of radiation has been studied extensively by Fajardo and Stewart et al in a rabbit model,[102,103] and subsequently confirmed by other investigators in other models.[104,105] They meticulously scored the events following a radiation injury of 20 Gy[102,106]: within the first few days, pericardial and myocardial capillary endothelial lesions appeared, with swelling of the cytoplasm and a scarcity of pinocytotic vesicles. Progressive myocardial fibrosis began at 3 months and could increase up to 1 year post injury. Subsequent animal studies, using a range of single doses of radiation, have confirmed 15 Gy as the threshold dose for cardiac injury in a recent review on the subject of cardiac tolerance to re-irradiation by Trott[107]; endocardial lesions are less common and less persistent.

We have hypothesized, based on our work in the rat carotid model, that radiation injures the vasovasorum of large uninjured arteries causing an inflammatory infiltrate of monocyte-derived macrophages that invades the vessel wall, releasing a cytokine cascade which in turn induces myofibroblast migration and proliferation. This process is similar to events seen post angioplasty, but is capable of repair at 6 months reflecting the radioresistance of larger arteries. Our group has shown that large arteries in the rabbit are tolerant to single doses of up to 30 Gy at 6 months post irradiation,[108] however, at longer times, perhaps years later, endothelial loss both from vasovasorum and luminal surfaces could lead to neointimal hyperplasia. Another supportive observation of the vasovasorum inflammatory response is in analyzing the work by Mazur et al using swine coronary arteries post angioplasty and post-catheter irradiation, where vessels adjacent to the irradiated arteries showed these changes as described by Fajardo (Table 2).[109]

Unified Pathogenesis Model: The Role of the Monocyte/Macrophage in Restenosis Induction

The literature provides a background for the role of the monocyte-derived macrophage in the induction of both arterial stenosis and restenosis. The trigger involves some form of endothelial cell injury, followed by the release of chemokines, eg, macrophage inflammatory protein (MIP), monocyte chemoattractant protein

Table 2

Histological Findings in Irradiated Coronary Arteries

Histologic Feature	Control n=125 #	10 Gy n=126 #	15 Gy n=156 #	25 Gy n=140 #
Intima				
Thrombus	0%	25%	39%	48%
Stromal fibrin exudate	5%	70%	72%	62%
Media				
Fibrosis	**42%**	**44%**	**27%**	**29%**
Thinning	46%	54%	53%	55%
Hypertrophy	14%	17%	10%	9%
Adventitia				
Fibrosis (G3 or 4)	**16%**	**47%**	**38%**	**51%**
Hemorrhage (G3 or 4)	0%	7%	4%	15%
Leukocyte infiltration	10%	21%	19%	13%

= percent of histologic sections with feature. Note the reduction in neointimal hyperplasia, ie, fibrosis and hypertrophy of adventitia, as a function of dose. From Reference 109.

(MCP), and/or RANTES, which attract the monocyte/macrophages and T cells. There are two sites for the inflammatory/immune cells to be attracted to the arterial wall: the luminal lining of intimal endothelial cells, and/or the endothelium of the vasovasorum. Depending on the type of injury and the state of disease in the vessel, either or both of the above may be involved.

In our proposed unified hypothesis, the sequential phase leading to myofibroblast proliferation and the polarization of events in the intima or the adventitia followed by neointimal hyperplasia or external vascular remodeling, respectively, are driven by similar cytokine cascades, which only vary by degree or intensity between each scenario. Arteries can undergo positive or negative remodeling: with positive remodeling, an adequate lumen is maintained despite neointimal hyperplasia; in negative remodeling, a constrictive process can narrow the artery with minimal intimal proliferation and leads to late lumen loss. Through a series of diagrams (Fig. 6a–d), the source and direction of infiltration of the monocytes/macrophages will be indicated under the above proposed conditions and discussed in the previous section:

1. Atherogenesis: The atheromata are multifocal, the neointimal hyperplasia is eccentric, and external vascular remodeling, if positive, can lead to an increase in arterial size, but if negative, hastens the restenotic process.

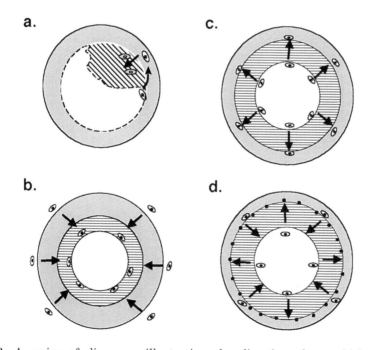

Figure 6. A series of diagrams illustrating the direction along which monocyte/macrophages may infiltrate under a series of vascular conditions. **a.** Atherogenesis. Monocyte/macrophages present within the luminal atheromatous plaque move from the lumen into the media. **b.** Post angioplasty. Activation of the monocyte/macrophages in the vasovasorum with migration towards the lumen forms the major direction of infiltration. This can be supplemented, if plaque is present, by the addition of macrophages from the lumen. **c.** Accelerated arteriosclerosis. The major direction of monocyte/macrophage infiltration is from the lumen. **d.** Stents. This chronic injury prompts monocyte/macrophage infiltration from both the lumen and the vasa vasorum. The stent struts are represented by the solid circles.

The direction of monocyte/macrophage infiltration is from the luminal side to the adventitia (Fig. 6a).

2. Angioplasty: Angioplasty disrupts the endothelial lining and tears the media, leading to rapid infiltration of monocyte/macrophages from the adventitial vasovasorum to the intima (Fig. 6b). If atheromata are present, monocytes/macrophages in the intimal plaque can be activated,[34] with additional recruitment from the luminal side.

3. Arteriovenous bypass: This is a typical wound-healing model with inflammatory cells entering from the vasovasorum on the adventitial side, resembling the angioplasty model, and leads to both neointimal hyperplasia and external vascular remodeling (Fig. 6b). The predominant direction is from the adventitia to the intima.

4. Accelerated arteriosclerosis: The concentric, generally uniform arterial lumen narrowing is from subendothelial infiltration of monocyte/ macrophages/T cells from the luminal side (Fig. 6c).

5. Stents: Stents post angioplasty provide a chronic injury model, since the expanded vessel wall and lumen have a stimulant wire enmeshed. There is a monocyte/macrophage infiltrate from both the luminal and adventitial sides depending on the degree of injury to the internal and external elastic laminae, leading to in-stent restenosis (Fig. 6d).

6. Radiation-induced neointimal hyperplasia: This is due to a slow infiltration of monocyte/macrophages from the adventitial vasovasorum since the endothelial cells of the vasovasorum are affected over a longer period of time, ie, 6 months to 1 year.

In Table 3, we summarize whether monocyte/macrophages are recruited from the luminal surface and/or adventitial vasovasorum. When the stimulus is bidirectional, the loss of lumen may be accelerated as both neointimal hyperplasia and external vascular remodeling are induced simultaneously.

The Puzzle and the Paradox

The puzzle that remains is the determination of the radiosensitive target cell. There are two hypotheses put forward: one is based on the myofibroblast, and is

Table 3

Presence of Monocyte-Derived Macrophage as Stimulus for Myofibroblast Proliferation

	Lumen	Vasa vasorum
Atherogenesis	+ +	Ø
Angioplasty (normal)	Ø	+ +
Angioplasty (diseased)	+ +	+ +
Arteriovenous bypass	Ø	+ +
Accelerated arteriosclerosis	+ +	Ø
Stents	+ +	+ +
RT-induced stenosis	Ø	+ +

RT = radiation therapy.

explained elsewhere in this book, and the other is based on the monocyte-derived macrophage. Our experimental evidence in a rat carotid model supports the monocyte/macrophage as the primary target or radiosensitive cell in the process of restenosis,[40] and is as follows:

1. Endovascular irradiation is usually given at the time of angioplasty or within an hour of trauma to the arterial wall when there would be no proliferating myofibroblasts or smooth muscle cells present. When the angioplastied walls were immunochemically stained for macrophages (mac-1, CD11b), they were found to be present in the adventitia within 24 hours of injury, and were associated in matching sections with PDGF expression. At this time, the endothelial cell surface had not regenerated, and neointimal changes were not in evidence. However, in many microsections, mononuclear inflammatory cells were seen streaming in from the vasovasorum. No macrophages were seen in the tunicae media or intima.

2. Dramatic changes occurred within 1 week of injury, where macrophages were seen in all layers of the arterial wall. Macrophage-specific stains identified macrophages in a highly nucleated intimal region as well as in the media. Platelet-derived growth factor expression also corresponded to these zones of macrophage infiltration. No α-smooth muscle actin was in evidence in these intimal cells, but was present in the tunica media. Other investigators have shown that at this time GM-CSF and M-CSF are released by smooth muscle cells and myofibroblasts which will further recruit additional inflammatory cells. The role of chemokines, such as MIP, MCP, and RANTES, and their importance in monocyte/macrophage recruitment is currently under investigation.

3. As the neointimal hyperplasia thickened and progressed from 3 weeks to 6 months, smooth muscle cells and/or myofibroblasts migrated and proliferated with an accompanying accumulation of PDGF protein. Through actin-staining, smooth muscle cells were identified in the tunica media at 1 week and in the zone of neointimal hyperplasia from 3 weeks to 6 months post injury. However, infiltrated among the myofibroblast cells were monocyte/macrophages, which were more scattered and intermixed. The PDGF expression in the intima would act as a stimulus for smooth muscle cell and fibroblast migration and proliferation.

4. Following irradiation, angioplastied vessels were inhibited from forming restenotic lesions, and in turn, very few to no inflammatory monocyte/macrophage cells were detected in the walls; there was a relative absence of PDGF.

5. A delay in the timing of the irradiation, 24 to 48 hours after angioplasty, has been shown to be more effective in inhibiting restenosis,[25,110] reflecting the greater accumulation of inflammatory cells just prior to smooth muscle cell migration and proliferation usually detected at days 2 and 3 post-PTCA.

6. Similar processes involving inflammatory cells, particularly macrophages, are in evidence in arterial venous anastomoses with infiltration of the media and intima.[63,111]

7. We postulate, based on our reported experimental evidence,[1,40,41] that the following sequence of events occurs after angioplasty and irradiation of an atheromatous plaque: a resident macrophage population, normally pres-

ent in the intimal atheromatous plaque is augmented by an induced population of adventitial monocytes/macrophages in the immediate 24 to 48 hours post angioplasty, and both are eliminated with moderate doses of irradiation. Since the dysregulated cytokine cascades are not generated, primary stimulants (eg, PDGF) are no longer elaborated to act as chemoattractants for more monocytes and T cells and, without an inflammatory response, the PDGF stimulus for smooth muscle cells and/or fibroblasts to migrate and proliferate does not occur, inhibiting the restenotic processes – neointimal hyperplasia and external vascular remodeling.

An important part of the puzzle is the myofibroblast proliferative process and many authors now regard the myofibroblast, whether derived from smooth muscle cells of the tunica media or the adventitial fibroblasts, as the critical target cell of restenosis. Radiobiological experiments, looking at the effects of radiation on cells at different points of the cell cycle, have demonstrated that actively dividing cells are more radiosensitive and that smooth muscle cells are vulnerable to moderate doses in culture when at, or close to, mitosis.[112] Brenner et al,[113] using a simple radiobiological model, have assumed that there are $\sim 10^7$ clonogenic cells in a 2-cm segment of arterial wall, while a subsequent population of only 5×10^7 cells would cause complete restenosis of a vessel with a 1.5- to 3-mm lumen. By applying different doses (12 to 20 Gy), different degrees of log cell kill would occur, delaying the onset of restenosis accordingly. Radiation, therefore, may be used as a cytostatic agent since the aim of treatment in benign disease, unlike oncology, is not to kill every potential clonogenic cell. However, the major limitation with this view is the widely used application of endovascular radiation immediately post angioplasty (within hours), whereas myofibroblasts are not in evidence for days to weeks later.

Apoptosis may be important post radiation as a mechanism of cell killing in smooth muscle cells and fibroblasts. Investigators have, in different animal models, attempted to define whether this form of cell killing may be more critical to controlling restenosis than radiation-induced mitotic cell death,[114,115] and Waksman et al have identified apoptosis 3 to 7 days after irradiation. At issue is which cell is undergoing apoptosis. Monocyte-derived macrophages, T lymphocytes, and inflammatory/immune cells typically die in interphase, although smooth muscle cells and fibroblasts may be candidates for accelerated apoptosis. However, if this were a primary mode of cell death for these cell types, one would expect more immediate evidence of positive remodeling of arteries, aneurysms, and focal rupture or dissections shortly after endovascular irradiation.

One explanation that would link the roles played by the monocyte/macrophage and the myofibroblast is an important mechanism of radiation cell killing, related to cell recruitment into active cycle from the resting state, and this mechanism may well apply to restenosis. That is, radiation applied prior to the application of a stimulus forces entry of a resting quiescent cell into cell cycle and division, causing a cryptic injury to unfold. For example, the liver hepatocyte is not considered to be radiosensitive. However, if the liver is irradiated and then a subsequent hepatectomy is performed, chromosomal damage can be unmasked resulting in early hepatocyte death.[116,117] Similarly, small to moderate doses of radiation prior to estrogen therapy in male prostate cancer patients will prophylax against estrogen-induced gynecomastia.[118,119] However, once gynecomastia is induced, the effectiveness of irradiation is lost and fractionated doses of 50 to 60 Gy will not produce breast atrophy.

In laboratory in vitro experiments, cells irradiated during the quiescent phase appear to be more radiosensitive (by dying) if forced to divide immediately post radiation compared to those stimulated after a delay of hours or days, which has allowed time for repair.[120–122] Conceivably, the normally quiescent smooth muscle cell or fibroblast could be more vulnerable if irradiated immediately prior to the stimulus to divide. Therefore, if angioplasty is followed by irradiation, the resultant monocyte/macrophage stimulus would trigger smooth muscle cell and fibroblast recruitment into cycle, and at the time of mitosis, as they pass through S phase into G_2/M, chromosomal injury would be unmasked. Experimental evidence suggesting that smooth muscle cells and/or fibroblasts are more radiosensitive when cycling rather than in the normal state[112,123] is, however, contradicted by in vivo experimental studies when single-dose radiation immediately following balloon angioplasty showed that irradiation was less effective when applied later than 2 days post injury,[124] when smooth muscle cells and myofibroblasts would be proliferating. Thus, the application of radiation prior to cell recruitment may affect a more "radiosensitive" phase than when cells are actively cycling and dividing.

The New Paradigm

In summary, the paradox presented by radiation's ability to both inhibit and induce fibrosis in the form of restenosis has a resolution in identification of the pivotal roles played by monocyte-derived macrophages and/or T cells and their interaction in myofibroblast recruitment. The monocyte/macrophage, once induced by angioplasty, is radiosensitive and readily eradicated by modest doses of radiation. In contrast, the ability of radiation to injure normal arteries and induce the same inflammatory processes and reactive proliferative responses as neointimal hyperplasia fortunately requires large doses and longer times to be manifested as clinically significant restenosis. This differential accounts for the therapeutic window.

A new paradigm is needed to fully understand the biological complexity of the various vascular entities leading to luminal narrowing. The modeling of restenosis by Brenner et al[113] is based on oncological parameters where clonogenic cell kill is essential; however, when extrapolated to benign proliferative processes, it provides an oversimplification of a complex pathophysiology. The basis for a new paradigm is Ross's final review article entitled "Atherosclerosis: An Inflammatory Disease."[125] This article presented compelling evidence supporting the view that the cellular mechanisms of atherogenesis are fundamentally no different from those of other chronic inflammatory-fibroproliferative diseases, such as cirrhosis, rheumatoid arthritis, glomerulosclerosis, pulmonary fibrosis, and chronic pancreatitis. In the majority of conditions, granulocytes may appear, but the monocyte/macrophages and T cells predominate. The initial inflammatory protective phase develops into chronic injury if the injurious agent is not removed, and each tissue attempts to repair the damage through a fibroproliferative response; this can overshoot and be excessive, reducing the function of the tissue/organ. Atherosclerosis is thus considered to be an inflammatory disease, leading eventually to a fibrogenic phase, and arteries respond the same as the other major tissues and organs.

Wound injury is not "a simple linear process of phylogistic events activating parenchymal cell proliferation and migration, but rather an integration of dynamic interactive processes involving soluble mediators, formed blood elements, extracellular matrix and parenchymal cells."[126] Clark, in his introduction to "The

Molecular and Cellular Biology of Wound Repair"[126] provides an excellent parallel model for arterial restenosis in the three phases of cutaneous wound healing (Fig. 7): the first wave of proinflammatory events is immediate, ie, within hours of injury with monocyte-derived macrophages entering immediately after neutrophils, triggering cytokine cascades and, depending on the severity of the injury, is often coupled with some hemorrhage and thrombus formation. The second wave of reendothelialization follows within days 1 to 3 post injury and represents a regenerative phase of events. The third wave of events (1 to 3 weeks post injury) leads to an active and proliferative phase for fibroblasts, with the concurrent production and upregulation of profibrotic cytokines. There is considerable overlap of these phases, creating both cellular and cytokine expression leading to cicatrization, which in arteries can result in restenosis and remodeling.

In extending the paradigm from wound healing to angioplasty, we now view the restenosis process as involving *all of the cells normally present in the arterial wall,* each with a different role to play. Endothelial cell injury is the initial event, both experimentally and clinically, followed by recruitment of platelets and the monocyte/macrophage/T cells, with the accompanying induction of cytokines. The subsequent myofibroblast activity is aborted if the recruited monocyte/macrophages are exposed to irradiation and thereby eliminated, since they are responsible for triggering the dysregulated cytokine and chemokine cascades. This paradigm attempts to provide a unified hypothesis for a variety of vascular lesions and injuries that all lead, ultimately, to a hyperplastic response.

It is difficult to accept the view that each of the processes noted above has

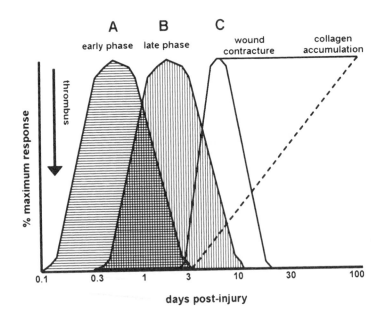

Figure 7. A series of "wave" events that constitute cutaneous wound repair following injury. As thrombus formation occurs, neutrophils enter the field (**A**), immediately followed by the monocyte/macrophages. The second wave of repair (**B**) consists of reendothelialization, which is followed by the final phase (**C**), consisting of the migration and proliferation of the smooth muscle cells/fibroblasts/myofibroblasts followed by collagen accumulation. Modified from Reference 126.

its own unique mechanism of induction since there is an economy in nature not to reinvent itself. There may be differences in the inflammatory component of the fibroproliferative response due to variations in timing and/or levels of cytokine/chemokine gene expression, but, fundamentally, similar cellular and molecular processes occur under each of the different conditions and circumstances. Therefore, we believe it is time to rethink the pathogenesis of restenosis as a dynamic interactive process of cells, cytokines, and chemokines—and not due to an enigmatic "target" cell or tissue, but part of a spectrum of inflammatory responses in which radiation could play a major therapeutic role.[127]

References

1. Sarac TP, Riggs PN, Williams JP, et al. The effects of low-dose radiation on neointimal hyperplasia. J Vasc Surg 1995;22:17–24.
2. Mayberg MR, London S, Rasey J, et al. Inhibition of rat smooth muscle proliferation by radiation after arterial injury: Temporal characteristics in vivo and in vitro. Radiat Res 2000;153:153–163.
3. Williams JP, Eagleton M, Hernady E, et al. Effectiveness of fractionated external beam radiation in the inhibition of vascular restenosis. Cardiovasc Radiat Med 1999;1:257–264.
4. Friedman M, Felton L, Byers S. The antiatherogenic effect of iridium192 upon the cholesterol-fed rabbit. J Clin Invest 1964;43:185–192.
5. Hehrlein C, Gollan C, Donges K, et al. Low-dose radioactive endovascular stents prevent smooth muscle cell proliferation and neointimal hyperplasia in rabbits. Circulation 1995;92:1570–1575.
6. Hirai T, Korogi Y, Harada M, et al. Prevention of intimal hyperplasia by irradiation: An experimental study in rabbits. Acta Radiol 1996;37:229–233.
7. Wiedermann JG, Marboe C, Amols H, et al. Intracoronary irradiation markedly reduces restenosis after balloon angioplasty in a porcine model. J Am Coll Cardiol 1994;23:1491–1498.
8. Waksman R, Robinson KA, Crocker IR, et al. Intracoronary low-dose beta-irradiation inhibits neointima formation after coronary artery balloon injury in the swine restenosis model. Circulation 1995;92:3025–3031.
9. Carter AJ, Laird JR, Bailey LR, et al. Effects of endovascular radiation from a β-particle-emitting stent in a porcine coronary restenosis model: A dose-response study. Circulation 1996;94:2364–2368.
10. Rubin P, Casarett GW. Clinical Radiation Pathology. Philadelphia: WB Saunders; 1968.
11. Rubin P, Johnston CJ, Williams JP, et al. A perpetual cascade of cytokines postirradiation leads to pulmonary fibrosis. Int J Radiat Oncol Biol Phys 1995;33:99–109.
12. Finkelstein JN, Johnston CJ, Baggs R, et al. Early alterations in extracellular matrix and transforming growth factor beta gene expression in mouse lung indicative of late radiation fibrosis. Int J Radiat Oncol Biol Phys 1994;28:621–631.
13. Brody AR, Bonner JC, Overby LH, et al. Interstitial pulmonary macrophages produce platelet-derived growth factor that stimulates rat lung fibroblast proliferation in vitro. J Leuk Biol 1992;51:640–648.
14. Brody AR. Control of lung fibroblast proliferation by macrophage-derived platelet-derived growth factor. Ann NY Acad Sci 1994;725:193–199.
15. Pierce GF, Mustoe TA, Lingelbach J, et al. Platelet-derived growth factor and transforming growth factor-beta enhance tissue repair activities by unique mechanisms. J Cell Biol 1989;109:429–440.
16. Shahar I, Fireman E, Topilsky M, et al. Effect of IL-6 on alveolar fibroblast proliferation in interstitial lung diseases. Clin Immunol Immunopathol 1996;79:244–251.
17. Amento EP, Ehsani N, Palmer H, et al. Cytokines and growth factors positively and negatively regulate interstitial collagen gene expression in human vascular smooth muscle cells. Arterioscler Thromb 1991;11:1223–1230.
18. Tang WW, Ulich TR, Lacey DL, et al. Platelet-derived growth factor-BB induces renal

tubulointerstitial myofibroblast formation and tubulointerstitial fibrosis. Am J Pathol 1996;148:1169–1180.

19. Mantovani A, Sozzani S, Vecchi A, et al. Cytokine activation of endothelial cells: New molecules for an old paradigm. Thromb Haemost 1997;78:406–414.
20. Wakefield TW, Strieter RM, Prince MR, et al. Pathogenesis of venous thrombosis: A new insight. Cardiovasc Surg 1997;5:6–15.
21. Ebbe S, Phalen E, Yee T. Postirradiation thrombocytopoiesis: Suppression, recovery, compensatory states, and macromegakaryocytosis. Prog Clin Biol Res 1986;215:71–89.
22. Kalovidouris AE, Papayannis AG. Effect of ionizing radiation on platelet function in vitro. Acta Radiol Oncol 1981;20:333–336.
23. Gawaz M, Neumann FJ, Dickfeld T, et al. Activated platelets induce monocyte chemotactic protein-1 secretion and surface expression of intercellular adhesion molecule-1 on endothelial cells. Circulation 1998;98:1164–1171.
24. Hall EJ, Marchese M, Rubin J, et al. Low dose rate irradiation. Front Radiat Ther Oncol 1988;22:19–29.
25. Mayberg MR, Luo Z, London S, et al. Radiation inhibition of intimal hyperplasia after arterial injury. Radiat Res 1995;142:212–220.
26. Rosen EM, Goldberg ID, Myrick KV, et al. Radiation survival properties of cultured vascular smooth muscle cells. Radiat Res 1984;100:182–191.
27. Shimotakahara S, Mayberg MR. Gamma irradiation inhibits neointimal hyperplasia in rats after arterial injury. Stroke 1994;25:424–428.
28. Tanaka H, Sukhova G, Schwartz D, et al. Proliferating arterial smooth muscle cells after balloon injury express TNF-alpha but not interleukin-1 or basic fibroblast growth factor. Arterioscler Thromb Vasc Biol 1996;16:12–18.
29. Wilensky RL, March KL, Gradus-Pizlo I, et al. Vascular injury, repair, and restenosis after percutaneous transluminal angioplasty in the atherosclerotic rabbit. Circulation 1995;92:2995–3005.
30. Rasey JS, Gajdusek CM, Mayberg MR. Radiation effects on intimal hyperplasia after endothelial injury in a rat restenosis model [abstract]. Proc Radiat Res Soc 1998;S15–23.
31. Virchow R. Phlogose und Thrombose im Gefasssystem. Gesammelte Abhandlugen zur Wissenschaftlichen Medizin. Frankfurt-am-Mein: Meidinger Sohn Co.; 1856.
32. Ross R, Glomset J, Harker L. Response to injury and atherogenesis. Am J Pathol 1977;86:675–684.
33. Simionescu M, Simionescu N. Proatherosclerotic events: Pathobiochemical changes occurring in the arterial wall before monocyte migration. FASEB J 1993;7:1359–1366.
34. Libby P, Schwartz D, Brogi E, et al. A cascade model for restenosis: A special case of atherosclerosis progression. Circulation 1992;86:III47-III52.
35. Jang IK, Lassila R, Fuster V. Atherogenesis and inflammation. Eur Heart J 1993;14(suppl K):2–6.
36. Geary RL, Williams JK, Golden D, et al. Time course of cellular proliferation, intimal hyperplasia, and remodeling following angioplasty in monkeys with established atherosclerosis: A nonhuman primate model of restenosis. Arterioscler Thromb Vasc Biol 1996;16:34–43.
37. Ross R. Arteriosclerosis: An overview. In: Haber E (ed.): Molecular Cardiovascular Medicine. New York: Scientific American; 1995:11–30.
38. Clinton SK, Underwood R, Hayes L, et al. Macrophage colony-stimulating factor gene expression in vascular cells and in experimental and human atherosclerosis. Am J Pathol 1992;140:301–316.
39. Filonzi EL, Zoellner H, Stanton H, et al. Cytokine regulation of granulocyte-macrophage colony stimulating factor and macrophage colony-stimulating factor production in human arterial smooth muscle cells. Atherosclerosis 1993;99:241–252.
40. Rubin P, Williams JP, Riggs PN, et al. Cellular and molecular mechanisms of radiation inhibition of restenosis. Part I: Role of the macrophage and platelet-derived growth factor. Int J Radiat Oncol Biol Phys 1998;40:929–941.
41. Williams JP, Rubin P, Soni A, et al. Comparability of the external vs. internal location of radiation in inhibiting neointimal hyperplasia. Cardiovasc Radiat Med 1999;1:55–63.
42. Navab M, Berliner JA, Watson AD, et al. The Yin and Yang of oxidation in the development of the fatty streak: A review based on the 1994 George Lyman Duff Memorial Lecture. Arterioscler Thromb Vasc Biol 1996;16:831–842.

43. Griendling KK, Alexander RW. Oxidative stress and cardiovascular disease. Circulation 1997;96:3264–3265.
44. Quinn MT, Parthasarathy S, Fong LG, et al. Oxidatively modified low density lipoproteins: A potential role in recruitment and retention of monocyte/macrophages during atherogenesis. Proc Natl Acad Sci USA 1987;84:2995–2998.
45. Rajavashisth TB, Andalibi A, Territo MC, et al. Induction of endothelial cell expression of granulocyte and macrophage colony-stimulating factors by modified low-density lipoproteins. Nature 1990;344:254–257.
46. Han J, Hajjar DP, Febbraio M, et al. Native and modified low density lipoproteins increase the functional expression of the macrophage class B scavenger receptor, CD36. J Biol Chem 1997;272:21654-21659.
47. Diaz MN, Frei B, Vita JA, et al. Antioxidants and atherosclerotic heart disease. N Engl J Med 1997;337:408–416.
48. de Villiers WJ, Smart EJ. Macrophage scavenger receptors and foam cell formation. J Leuk Biol 1999;66:740–746.
49. Maor I, Kaplan M, Hayek T, et al. Oxidised monocyte-derived macrophages in aortic atherosclerotic lesion from apolipoprotein E-deficient mice and from human carotid artery contain lipid peroxides and oxysterols. Biochem Biophys Res Comm 2000;269:775–780.
50. Rosenfeld ME, Ross R. Macrophage and smooth muscle cell proliferation in atherosclerotic lesions of WHHL and comparably hypercholesterolemic fat-fed rabbits. Arteriosclerosis 1990;10:680–687.
51. Ueda M, Becker AE, Fujimoto T, et al. The early phenomena of restenosis following percutaneous transluminal coronary angioplasty. Eur Heart J 1991;12:937–945.
52. Harker LA, Ross R, Glomset J. Role of the platelet in atherogenesis. Ann NY Acad Sci 1976;275:321–329.
53. Taubman MB, Rollins BJ, Poon M, et al. JE mRNA accumulates rapidly in aortic injury and in platelet-derived growth factor-stimulated vascular smooth muscle cells. Circ Res 1992;70:314–325.
54. Bowen-Pope DF, Ross R, Seifert RA. Locally acting growth factors for vascular smooth muscle cells: Endogenous synthesis and release from platelets. Circulation 1985;72:735–740.
55. Grotendorst GR, Chang T, Seppa HE, et al. Platelet-derived growth factor is a chemoattractant for vascular smooth muscle cells. J Cell Physiol 1982;113:261–266.
56. Crowley ST, Ray CJ, Nawaz D, et al. Multiple growth factors are released from mechanically injured vascular smooth muscle cells. Am J Physiol 1995;269:H1641-H1647.
57. Ross R. The pathogenesis of atherosclerosis: A perspective for the 1990s. Nature 1993;362:801–809.
58. Klagsbrun M. Vascular cell growth factors and the arterial wall. In: Haber E (ed.): Molecular Cardiovascular Medicine. New York: Scientific American; 1995:63–78.
59. Hanke H, Hassenstein S, Ulmer A, et al. Accumulation of macrophages in the arterial vessel wall following experimental balloon angioplasty. Eur Heart J 1994;15:691–698.
60. Mann JM, Kaski JC, Pereira WI, et al. Histological patterns of atherosclerotic plaques in unstable angina patients vary according to clinical presentation. Heart 1998;80:19–22.
61. Marek JM, Koehler C, Aguirre ML, et al. The histologic characteristics of primary and restenotic carotid plaque. J Surg Res 1998;74:27–33.
62. Pauletto P, Sartore S, Pessina AC. Smooth-muscle-cell proliferation and differentiation in neointima formation and vascular restenosis. Clin Sci 1994;87:467–479.
63. Hoch JR, Stark VK, Hullett DA, et al. Vein graft intimal hyperplasia: Leukocytes and cytokine gene expression. Surgery 1994;116:463–470.
64. Hoch JR, Stark VK, van Rooijen N, et al. Macrophage depletion alters vein graft intimal hyperplasia. Surgery 1999;126:428–437.
65. Lafont A, Guzman LA, Whitlow PL, et al. Restenosis after experimental angioplasty: Intimal, medial, and adventitial changes associated with constrictive remodeling. Circ Res 1995;76:996–1002.
66. Post MJ, Borst C, Kuntz RE. The relative importance of arterial remodeling compared with intimal hyperplasia in lumen renarrowing after balloon angioplasty: A study in the normal rabbit and the hypercholesterolemic Yucatan micropig. Circulation 1994;89:2816–2821.

67. Mintz GS, Kent KM, Pichard AD, et al. Intravascular ultrasound insights into mechanisms of stenosis formation and restenosis. Cardiol Clin 1997;15:17–29.
68. Kornowski R, Mintz GS, Kent KM, et al. Increased restenosis in diabetes mellitus after coronary interventions is due to exaggerated intimal hyperplasia: A serial intravascular ultrasound study. Circulation 1997;95:1366–1369.
69. Clowes AW, Reidy MA, Clowes MM. Mechanisms of stenosis after arterial injury. Lab Invest 1983;49:208–215.
70. Clowes AW, Reidy MA, Clowes MM. Kinetics of cellular proliferation after arterial injury. I. Smooth muscle growth in the absence of endothelium. Lab Invest 1983;49:327–333.
71. Nabel EG. Biology of the impaired endothelium. Am J Cardiol 1991;68:6C-8C.
72. Marzocchi A, Marrozzini C, Piovaccari G, et al. Restenosis after coronary angioplasty: Its pathogenesis and prevention. Cardiologia 1991;36:309–320.
73. Wilcox JN, Waksman R, King SB, et al. The role of the adventitia in the arterial response to angioplasty: The effect of intravascular radiation. Int J Radiat Oncol Biol Phys 1996;36:789–796.
74. Frangogiannis NG, Burns AR, Michael LH, et al. Histochemical and morphological characteristics of canine cardiac mast cells. Histochem J 1999;31:221–229.
75. Billingham ME. Cardiac transplant atherosclerosis. Transplant Proc 1987;19:19–25.
76. Libby P, Schoen FJ, Pober JS. Arteriosclerosis of cardiac transplantation. In: Haber E (ed.): Molecular Cardiovascular Medicine. New York: Scientific American; 1995:311–324.
77. Hruban RH, Beschorner WE, Baumgartner WA, et al. Accelerated arteriosclerosis in heart transplant recipients is associated with a T-lymphocyte-mediated endothelialitis. Am J Pathol 1990;137:871–882.
78. Salomon RN, Hughes CC, Schoen FJ, et al. Human coronary transplantation-associated arteriosclerosis: Evidence for a chronic immune reaction to activated graft endothelial cells. Am J Pathol 1991;138:791–798.
79. Libby P, Salomon RN, Payne DD, et al. Functions of vascular wall cells related to development of transplantation-associated coronary arteriosclerosis. Transplant Proc 1989;21:3677–3684.
80. Libby P, Friedman GB, Salomon RN. Cytokines as modulators of cell proliferation in fibrotic diseases. Am Rev Respir Dis 1989;140:1114–1117.
81. Furukawa Y, Matsumori A, Hwang MW, et al. Cytokine gene expression during the development of graft coronary artery disease in mice. Jpn Circ J 1999;63:775–782.
82. Strober S, Modry DL, Hoppe RT, et al. Induction of specific unresponsiveness to heart allografts in mongrel dogs treated with total lymphoid irradiation and antithymocyte globulin. J Immunol 1984;132:1013–1018.
83. Koretz SH, Gottlieb MS, Strober S, et al. Organ transplantation in mongrel dogs using total lymphoid irradiation (TLI). Transplant Proc 1981;13:443–445.
84. Macaya C, Serruys PW, Ruygrok P, et al. Continued benefit of coronary stenting versus balloon angioplasty: One-year clinical follow-up of Benestent trial. Benestent Study Group. J Am Coll Cardiol 1996;27:255–261.
85. Serruys PW, Emanuelsson H, van der Giessen W, et al. Heparin-coated Palmaz-Schatz stents in human coronary arteries: Early outcome of the Benestent-II Pilot Study. Circulation 1996;93:412–422.
86. Slota PA, Fischman DL, Savage MP, et al. Frequency and outcome of development of coronary artery aneurysm after intracoronary stent placement and angioplasty. STRESS Trial Investigators. Am J Cardiol 1997;79:1104–1106.
87. Foley DP, Melkert R, Umans VA, et al. Differences in restenosis propensity of devices for transluminal coronary intervention: A quantitative angiographic comparison of balloon angioplasty, directional atherectomy, stent implantation and excimer laser angioplasty. CARPORT, MERCATOR, MARCATOR, PARK, and BENESTENT Trial Groups. Eur Heart J 1995;16:1331–1346.
88. Masotti M, Serra A, Betriu A. Stents and de novo coronary lesions: Meta-analysis. Rev Espanola Cardiol 1997;50(suppl 2):3–9.
89. Dietz R, Waigand J, Uhlich F, et al. Stents: New studies – new trends. Zeitsch Kardiol 1997;86:65–70.
90. Hoffmann R, Mintz GS, Dussaillant GR, et al. Patterns and mechanisms of in-stent restenosis: A serial intravascular ultrasound study. Circulation 1996;94:1247–1254.

91. Kearney M, Pieczek A, Haley L, et al. Histopathology of in-stent restenosis in patients with peripheral artery disease. Circulation 1997;95:1998–2002.
92. Schwartz RS, Murphy JG, Edwards WD, et al. Restenosis occurs with internal elastic lamina laceration and is proportional to severity of vessel injury in a porcine coronary artery model [abstract]. Circulation 1990;82:III656.
93. van Beusekom HM, van der Giessen WJ, van Suylen R, et al. Histology after stenting of human saphenous vein bypass grafts: Observations from surgically excised grafts 3 to 320 days after stent implantation. J Am Coll Cardiol 1993;21:45–54.
94. van Beusekom HM, Serruys PW, Post JC, et al. Stenting or balloon angioplasty of stenosed autologous saphenous vein grafts in pigs. Am Heart J 1994;127:273–281.
95. Rogers C, Welt FG, Karnovsky MJ, et al. Monocyte recruitment and neointimal hyperplasia in rabbits: Coupled inhibitory effects of heparin. Arterioscler Thromb Vasc Biol 1996;16:1312–1318.
96. Karas SP, Gravanis MB, Santoian EC, et al. Coronary intimal proliferation after balloon injury and stenting in swine: An animal model of restenosis. J Am Coll Cardiol 1992;20:467–474.
97. Rogers C, Edelman ER. Endovascular stent design dictates experimental restenosis and thrombosis. Circulation 1995;91:2995–3001.
98. Schwartz RS, Huber KC, Murphy JG, et al. Restenosis and the proportional neointimal response to coronary artery injury: Results in a porcine model. J Am Coll Cardiol 1992;19:267–274.
99. Murphy JG, Schwartz RS, Edwards WD, et al. Percutaneous polymeric stents in porcine coronary arteries: Initial experience with polyethylene terephthalate stents. Circulation 1992;86:1596–1604.
100. Komatsu R, Ueda M, Naruko T, et al. Neointimal tissue response at sites of coronary stenting in humans: Macroscopic, histological, and immunohistochemical analyses. Circulation 1998;98:224–233.
101. Kollum M, Kaiser S, Kinscherf R, et al. Apoptosis after stent implantation compared with balloon angioplasty in rabbits: Role of macrophages. Arterioscler Thromb Vasc Biol 1997;17:2383–2388.
102. Fajardo LF, Stewart JR. Pathogenesis of radiation-induced myocardial fibrosis. Lab Invest 1973;29:244–257.
103. Stewart JR, Fajardo LF, Gillette SM, et al. Radiation injury to the heart. Int J Radiat Oncol Biol Phys 1995;31:1205–1211.
104. Gillette SM, Gillette EL, Shida T, et al. Late radiation response of canine mediastinal tissues. Radiother Oncol 1992;23:41–52.
105. Lauk S, Trott KR. Endothelial cell proliferation in the rat heart following local heart irradiation. Int J Radiat Biol 1990;57:1017–1030.
106. Fajardo LF. The unique physiology of endothelial cells and its implications in radiobiology. Front Radiat Ther Oncol 1989;23:96–112.
107. Trott KR. Retreatment tolerance of the heart. Int J Radiat Oncol Biol Phys 1996;36:985–986.
108. Tallman MP, Williams JP, Eagleton MJ, et al. Tolerance of normal rabbit femoral arteries to single high dose external beam irradiation. Cardiovasc Radiat Med 1999;1:131–137.
109. Mazur W, Ali MN, Khan MM, et al. High dose rate intracoronary radiation for inhibition of neointimal formation in the stented and balloon-injured porcine models of restenosis: Angiographic, morphometric, and histopathologic analyses. Int J Radiat Oncol Biol Phys 1996;36:777–788.
110. Waksman R, Robinson KA, Crocker IR, et al. Endovascular low-dose irradiation inhibits neointima formation after coronary artery balloon injury in swine: A possible role for radiation therapy in restenosis prevention. Circulation 1995;91:1533–1539.
111. Stark VK, Hoch JR, Warner TF, et al. Monocyte chemotactic protein-1 expression is associated with the development of vein graft intimal hyperplasia. Arterioscler Thromb Vasc Biol 1997;17:1614–1621.
112. Hall EJ (ed.). Radiobiology for the Radiologist, 4th Edition. Philadelphia: JB Lippincott Co.; 1994.
113. Brenner DJ, Miller RC, Hall EJ. The radiobiology of intravascular irradiation. Int J Radiat Oncol Biol Phys 1996;36:805–810.

114. Gajdusek CM, Tian H, London S, et al. Gamma radiation effect on vascular smooth muscle cells in culture. Int J Radiat Oncol Biol Phys 1996;36:821–828.
115. Waksman R, Rodriguez JC, Robinson KA, et al. Effect of intravascular irradiation on cell proliferation, apoptosis, and vascular remodeling after balloon overstretch injury of porcine coronary arteries. Circulation 1997;96:1944–1952.
116. Geraci JP, Mariano MS. Radiation hepatology of the rat: The effects of the proliferation stimulus induced by subtotal hepatectomy. Radiat Res 1994;140:249–256.
117. Bossola M, Merrick HW, Eltaki A, et al. Rat liver tolerance for partial resection and intraoperative radiation therapy: Regeneration is radiation dose dependent. J Surg Oncol 1990;45:196–200.
118. Cook S, Rodriguez-Antunez A. Pre-estrogen irradiation of the breast to prevent gynecomastia. Am J Roentgenol 1973;117:662–663.
119. Alfthan OS. The inhibiting effect of irradiation on gynecomastia induced by estrogen hormone stimulation: An experimental study. J Urol 1969;101:905–908.
120. Malaise EP, Deschavanne PJ, Fertil B. The relationship between potentially lethal damage repair and intrinsic radiosensitivity of human cells. Int J Radiat Biol 1989;56:597–604.
121. Cheng X, Pantelias GE, Okayasu R, et al. Mitosis-promoting factor activity of inducer mitotic cells may affect radiation yield of interphase chromosome breaks in the premature chromosome condensation assay. Cancer Res 1993;53:5592–5596.
122. van der Meer Y, Huiskamp R, Davids JA, et al. The sensitivity of quiescent and proliferating mouse spermatogonial stem cells to X irradiation. Radiat Res 1992;130:289–295.
123. Hirst DG, Denekamp J, Hobson B. Proliferation studies of the endothelial and smooth muscle cells of the mouse mesentery after irradiation. Cell Tiss Kinet 1980;13:91–104.
124. Herbaux B, Bethouart M, Rohart J, et al. Effets des irradiation sur les sutures microchirurgicales vasculaires. J Chir (Paris) 1983;120:115–123.
125. Ross R. Atherosclerosis: An inflammatory disease. N Engl J Med 1999;340:115–126.
126. Clark RAF. Wound repair. In: Clark RAF (ed.): Molecular and Cellular Biology of Wound Repair. New York: Plenum Press; 1996:3–50.
127. Rubin P, Soni A, Williams JP. The molecular and cellular biologic basis for the radiation treatment of benign proliferative diseases. Semin Radiat Oncol 1999;9:203–214.

## Chapter 11

Mechanisms by Which Radiation May Prevent Restenosis:

Inhibition of Cell Proliferation and Vascular Remodeling

Josiah N. Wilcox, PhD, Ian R. Crocker, MD,
Neal A. Scott, MD, PhD, Keith A. Robinson, PhD,
Spencer B. King, MD, and
Ron Waksman, MD

Introduction

There are a number of studies that indicate that radiation treatment reduces vascular lesion formation after balloon overstretch injury of porcine coronary arteries. A significant reduction in the size of the neointima has been observed when balloon angioplasty is immediately preceded or followed by intracoronary ionizing radiation with use of both gamma- and beta-emitting radioactive sources including iridium 192,[1-3] strontium 90/yttrium 90, and yttrium 90.[4-6] Similar results have been reported on the prevention of lesion development in stented vessels either by intravascular irradiation at the time of stent placement[7] or in studies using radioactive stents.[8,9] The effect on lesion development appears stable and long-lasting and at least two of the pig studies has been carried out to 6 months with good results.[2,4] Currently there are several clinical trials in progress which will assess the effect of intravascular irradiation on clinical restenosis.

Many different mechanisms have been proposed to explain the sequence of events leading to arterial narrowing or restenosis after angioplasty. Previously, the major focus was on the medial smooth muscle cells, which were thought to give rise to a restenosis lesion. It is well documented in the rat and rabbit injury models that balloon injury stimulates the proliferation of medial smooth muscle cells, which migrate to the intima where they continue to proliferate and produce matrix proteins forming a neointima.[10-13] However such injuries rarely produce a narrowing of the arterial lumen that is associated with clinical restenosis. It was suggested that geometric remodeling may be more important than neointima formation in the restenosis process. This is supported by intravascular ultra-

This work was supported by NIH grant HL47838 (JW) and a grant from the Gruentzig Center for Interventional Cardiology.
From Waksman R (ed.). *Vascular Brachytherapy, Third Edition.* Armonk, NY: Futura Publishing Co., Inc.; © 2002.

sound studies in patients[14–17] and a number of animal studies,[14,15,18] all of which indicate that there is a reduction in the diameter of the external elastic lamina after angioplasty and that this decrease in the overall vessel size is a better correlate with the degree of luminal narrowing than the size of the intimal mass.

Angioplasty of porcine coronary arteries stimulates adventitial myofibroblast proliferation, leading to a fibrotic response in the adventitia.[19] These cells show increased synthesis of α-smooth muscle actin[19] and nonmuscle myosin heavy chain,[20] and accumulate in the adventitia surrounding the injury site. In healing dermal wounds, similar cells are involved in the process of scar contraction.[21,22] We hypothesize that the adventitial myofibroblasts may constrict the injured vessel in a similar fashion, thus contributing to the process of geometric remodeling and late lumen loss after angioplasty.[19] We have recently completed a series of experiments which examined the effect of ionizing radiation on vascular lesion formation after angioplasty of porcine coronary arteries. These studies indicate that radiation at the time of angioplasty inhibits cell proliferation in both the media and adventitia at early times after injury, inhibits vascular lesion formation, and prevents constrictive arterial remodeling associated with restenosis.[23]

Radiation Reduces Cell Proliferation in Both the Media and the Adventitia

Balloon injury was performed on porcine coronary arteries as previously described,[23–25] followed immediately by ionizing radiation using either a source train of ^{90}Sr/Y or ^{192}Ir seeds designed to deliver 14 or 28 Gy at a depth of 2 mm into the artery wall. The animals were killed 3 or 7 days after injury. Bromodeoxyuridine (BRdU) was administered 24 hours prior to sacrifice to label proliferating cells, which were detected by immunohistochemistry by use of a BRdU-specific antibody (Fig. 1). The number of proliferating (BRdU-positive) cells relative to the total number of cells was determined by computer-based image analysis (Fig. 2).

In agreement with our previous observations,[19] cell proliferation in the control vessels 3 days after angioplasty was greatest in the adventitia at the site of the medial tear (region 3, 30.14±2.21%, mean±SEM) compared to the medial wall in the same region (region 1, 14.9±2.23%). Intravascular irradiation significantly reduced the number of proliferating cells compared to controls in both the adventitia (region 3, 14 Gy=15.5±2.6%, $P<0.001$; 28 Gy=4.9±1.0%, $P<0.001$) and medial wall (region 1, 14 Gy=5.0±1.4%, $P<0.05$; 28 Gy=3.8±1.6%, $P<0.01$) at this time. The higher 28-Gy dose resulted in a much greater inhibition of cell proliferation in the adventitia compared to 14 Gy (region 3, $P<0.05$). While not significant, there was a tendency for the higher 28-Gy dose to produce a greater inhibition of cell proliferation than 14 Gy in the other regions analyzed as well.

Seven days after angioplasty no differences in cell proliferation in the media or adventitia between the irradiated and control arteries were detected, although there was an apparent reduction in the degree of intimal development at this time (Fig. 1). Morphometric analysis indicated that the average intimal area per cross section was significantly smaller in the 14 G (0.073±0.016 mm^2) and 28 G (0.057±0.007 mm^2) groups compared to controls (0.144±0.014 mm^2) ($P<0.05$ and $P<0.01$, respectively), although there was no difference in the den-

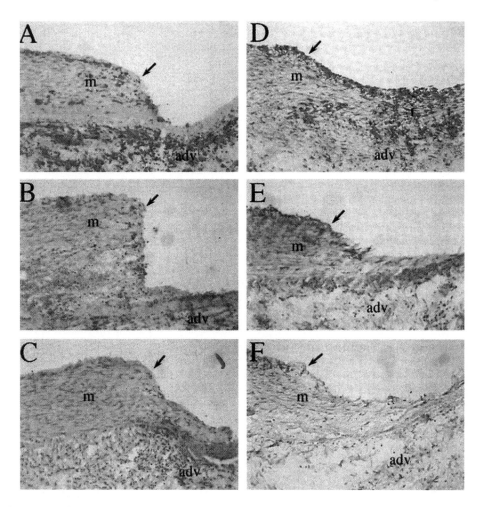

Figure 1. Distribution of Bromodeoxyuridine (BRdU)-positive cells in control (**A, D**), 14-Gy (**B, E**), and 28-Gy (**C, F**) irradiated vessels 3 days (**A** through **C**) or 7 days (**D** through **F**) after balloon overstretch injury of porcine coronary arteries. Three days after injury BRdU-positive proliferating cells were localized primarily in the adventitia and the broken end of the media in control vessels while fewer proliferating cells were seen in the irradiated vessels. Seven days after injury intimal proliferation dominated in the control vessels while little proliferation was seen in the vessels treated with 14 or 28 Gy. Less intimal formation is apparent in the irradiated vessels, which tended to artificially increase the percent of proliferating cells in region 5 of these tissues. (Magnification=50×.) From Reference 23, with permission.

sity of intimal cells (number of hematoxylin-stained nuclei per mm^2) between the three groups.

Radiation Has No Effect on Apoptosis Measured 3 and 7 Days after Angioplasty

Apoptosis was estimated by terminal transferase-mediated UTP nick-end labeling (TUNEL) at 3 and 7 days after balloon injury and the number of apoptotic cells was counted by computer-based image analysis (Fig. 3). These studies sug-

Figure 2. Determination of the percent of BRdU-positive cells in control (open bars), 14-Gy (hatched bars), and 28-Gy (solid bars) irradiated vessels 3 (**A**) and 7 (**B**) days after balloon overstretch injury of porcine coronary arteries. The number of BRdU-positive proliferating cells was determined by computer-assisted image analysis as previously described (References 23–25) in five regions of the vessel wall after angioplasty as follows: Region 1–in the media adjacent to the medial tear; Region 2–in the media on the side opposite the medial tear; Region 3–in the adventitia adjacent to the medial tear; Region 4–in the adventitia on the side opposite the medial tear; and Region 5–in the intima defined as the luminal side of the external elastic lamina between the torn ends of the media (counted only of day 7 when the intima was formed). Data are presented as the mean percent of BRdU-positive cells±SEM (*$P<0.05$, **$P<0.01$, ***$P<0.001$ compared to controls; # $P<0.05$ compared to 14 Gy).

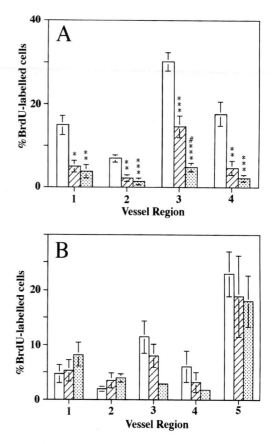

gested that there was histochemical evidence of apoptosis in all of the injured vessels. However, there were no quantitative differences in the amount of labeling among irradiated and control vessels in any region examined on either day 3 or day 7. Three days after angioplasty, the number of TUNEL-labeled cells was greatest along the luminal surface of the external elastic lamina, which was exposed by the tearing of the medial wall at the time of angioplasty (region 5). Morphological examination of these cells suggests that these were neutrophils which had accumulated at the injury site. A great number of TUNEL-labeled cells were also detected in the adventitia beneath the external elastic lamina between the broken ends of the media and in the torn ends of the medial wall. These are all sites of the greatest amount of cell proliferation at this time, as determined by BRdU immunohistochemistry.

Cell density, calculated as the mean number of hematoxylin-stained nuclei per mm², was examined in control and irradiated vessels to determine if radiation caused a loss of medial cells in the first few days after treatment. There were no significant differences in cell density between the control, 14-Gy, or 28-Gy arteries 3 days after injury in any portion of the media or adventitia. Seven days after angioplasty there appeared to be significantly more cells per mm² in region 2 (normal media on the side opposite the break) of the 28-Gy–treated vessels compared to either control or 14 Gy treatment ($P<0.01$), but no other significant differences in cell number in the intima, media at the break site, or adventitia were found.

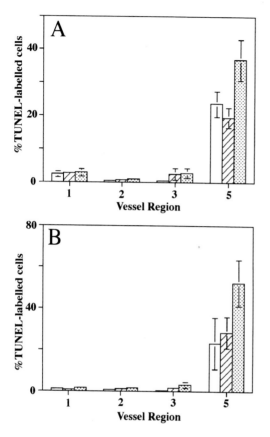

Figure 3. Comparison of TUNEL labeling in control (open bars), 14-Gy (hatched bars), and 28-Gy (solid bars) irradiated vessels 3 (**A**) and 7 (**B**) days after angioplasty determined by computer-assisted image analysis. TUNEL labeling was performed on irradiated and control vessels to estimate apoptosis in these tissues. TUNEL-positive cells in the five regions (see Fig. 2 legend) of the injured vessels were counted wuth use of computer-assisted image analysis as previously described (References 23–25). There were no significant differences in the percent of TUNEL-positive cells in any region examined. Data are presented as the mean percent of TUNEL-positive cells±SEM.

Radiation Inhibits Constrictive Vascular Remodeling Associated with Angioplasty

The recruitment of adventitial myofibroblasts to the injury site was assessed by immunohistochemistry for α-smooth muscle actin on days 3, 7, and 14 after injury. There was a clear difference in the extent of adventitial α-actin staining in the irradiated vessels compared to control vessels at all timepoints (Fig. 4), suggesting an inhibition of adventitial fibrosis by the radiation treatment. Morphometric analysis among 18 specimens 2 weeks after balloon injury with and without radiation confirmed that there was a larger vessel perimeter in the irradiated vessels (Table 1).

Radiation Reduces the Number of Adventitial Cells Expressing Nonmuscle Myosin

Previous work indicated that the expression of NMMHC-B, as determined by in situ hybridization, was increased in the adventitial myofibroblasts recruited to the area surrounding the porcine coronary artery after balloon angioplasty.[26] These studies indicated that the expression of NMMHC-B could be used as a marker for the adventitial myofibroblasts that are recruited to the injury site. Re-

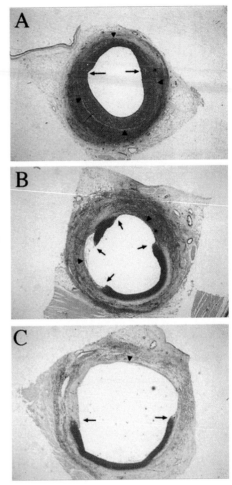

Figure 4. Effect of intravascular irradiation on the recruitment of α-actin–positive myofibroblasts in the adventitia 14 days after balloon overstretch injury of porcine coronary arteries. Alpha actin staining (red) was performed on pressure perfusion fixed paraffin embedded segments of coronary arteries from control animals (**A**) and animals receiving 14-Gy (**B**) or 28-Gy (**C**) intravascular irradiation at the time of injury. Note the reduction in α-actin staining in the 14-Gy and 28-Gy irradiated vessels as well as the larger lumen of the irradiated vessels compared to the controls. Arrows indicate breaks in the medial wall; arrowheads indicate the border of the external elastic lamina. (Magnification=50×.) From Reference 23, with permission.

Table 1

Effect of Intravascular Irradiation at the Time of Angioplasty on Vascular Remodeling in Porcine Coronary Arteries

	Control (n=20)	14 Gy (n=19)	28 Gy (n=4)	P Value
Vessel perimeter (mm)	7.2±1.3	7.4±1.3	9.2±0.9*	<0.01
Lumen perimeter (mm)	5.6±1.5	6.3±1.6	8.5±0.9*	<0.003
Lumen area (mm)	2.1±1.2	2.6±1.2	3.8±0.8*	<0.001

Animals were subjected to balloon overstretch injury as described in the text and tissues were harvested on day 14 after injury. Computer-based morphometric analysis was performed and the vessel perimeter, lumen perimeter, and luminal area measured. Results are expressed as the mean±SD and were analyzed by one-way analysis of variance (ANOVA).

cent studies from our laboratories examined the expression of NMMHC-B mRNA using in situ hybridization in irradiated and control vessels (J. Wilcox and R. Waksman, unpublished observations). Radiation treatment at the 28-Gy dose reduced the number of NMMHC-B–expressing cells seen by in situ hybridization in the adventitia surrounding the injured porcine coronary arteries 3 days after angioplasty. This is further evidence that intravascular irradiation at the time of angioplasty reduced the recruitment and/or proliferation of adventitial myofibroblasts. We hypothesize that the inhibition of adventitial myofibroblasts by radiation prevents the fibrotic changes in the adventitia and thereby improves vascular remodeling after angioplasty.

Conclusions

In the present series of experiments we have shown that intravascular irradiation administered at the time of angioplasty effectively reduces cell proliferation 3 days after balloon injury in both the medial wall and adventitia. Radiation did not affect cell proliferation in the intima or media 7 days after angioplasty. These findings are correlated with the effect of radiation on the extent of lesion development assessed 2 weeks or 6 months after angioplasty.[2,4] There were no significant differences in the percent of TUNEL-positive cells in irradiated and control vessels in any region examined either 3 or 7 days after injury, suggesting that radiation did not increase apoptosis in the media or adventitia at these times. A positive effect of radiation treatment was seen on vascular remodeling, as the irradiated vessels had a larger vessel perimeter when measured 2 weeks after angioplasty. In addition, there was a reduction in adventitial α-smooth muscle actin staining and cells expressing NMMHC-B in the irradiated vessels after angioplasty. We hypothesize that this represents a reduction in the distribution of myofibroblasts in the adventitia surrounding the injury site. Together these results suggest that radiation treatment inhibits vascular lesion formation by reducing the first wave of cell proliferation in the media and adventitia and reducing the adventitial fibrosis, which may be the underlying cause of geometric remodeling associated with clinical restenosis.

There are a number of studies that support the hypothesis that cell proliferation is the key contributor to vascular narrowing after angioplasty,[27–30] but agents that inhibit cell proliferation do not necessarily reduce the size of the ultimate vascular lesion that develops. Proliferation in the arterial wall after angioplasty can be broken down into two components: early, or first-wave, proliferation occurs in the medial wall within 24 to 72 hours after injury; late, or second wave of, cell proliferation occurs in the intima and may continue for as long a 2 months after injury. Previous studies have shown successful reduction in first-wave proliferation (ie, by treatment with fibroblast growth factor [FGF] antibodies), but such treatment did not reduce the size of the neointima.[31] It has been hypothesized that there are multiple pathways that stimulate the growth of the neointima such that inhibition of one pathway for growth stimulation may be replaced by another. Thus, the few cells that proliferated in the media in the presence of the FGF antibody migrated to the intima and continued to grow there, independent of FGF, giving rise to the lesion. Presumably, this ensures that proper repair mechanisms remain in place after vascular injury. In contrast, intravascular irradiation at the time of angioplasty effectively reduced first-wave proliferation 3 days after injury but had no effect on the second wave of growth, measured on day 7, in the intima. Yet this treatment successfully reduced lesion size measured not only at an early timepoint 2 weeks after angioplasty,[2,5] but at 6 months later as well.[2,4] This could mean one of two things, either intimal proliferation is not important in generating the final lesion or radiation may have caused an earlier termination of intimal proliferation sometime after day 7, the timepoint examined in this study. Given the present knowledge about radiation's effect on cell growth in other systems, the latter hypothesis seems more tenable. Additional work must done in order to determine if intimal proliferation is suppressed at an earlier timepoint in irradiated versus nonirradiated vessels.

There was some variability in cell proliferation within the adjacent segments of an individual irradiated artery. These occurred primarily when radiation with the pure beta emitter ^{90}Sr/Y was applied, and may be related to the lower penetration properties of the beta compared to the gamma combined with heterogeneous distribution of radiation emanating from the source train. It is possible that inhomogeneous packing of the radioactivity in the seeds caused some of this variability. Alternatively, the thick end caps placed on the seeds used in the first prototype version of the device resulted in spaces between the radioactive sources in the train such that a lower dose was delivered to the tissues positioned at these junctions. Consequently, some segments of the vessel did not receive a sufficient radiation dose to inhibit cell proliferation. Alternatively, malpositioning of the source train at the injury site may also have spared a portion of the vessel from exposure to radiation. An examination of the Lucite block in which the source train was stored for several weeks suggests that the former hypothesis is correct. This has been corrected in latter versions of the radiation sources. These findings stress the importance of accuracy in positioning the source at the angioplasty site and the need to design the delivery device in such a way as to assure the even distribution of radiation into the surrounding tissues. These results also indicate that intravascular radiation therapy using ^{90}Sr/Y produces highly localized effects in the surrounding vessel. This may be important such that in clinical use, the radiation should not damage deep adventitial structures. Thus, a large population of resident adventitial cells will not have been exposed to high doses of radiation and should be capable of responding to maintain vessel integrity in the setting of a subsequent injury or cellular loss at that site. We hypothesize that this may reduce the potential for aneurysmal dilation of the vessel over long periods.

These studies suggest that it is important that a sufficient dose of radiation be delivered to the adventitial structures at the injury site to prevent arterial remodeling and restenosis. We have previously presented data which suggest that adventitial myofibroblasts may migrate into the developing neointima across the external elastic lamina and contribute to the mass of the lesion that develops after balloon overstretch injury of porcine coronary arteries.[19] In addition, the proliferation of adventitial cells produces a fibrotic response around the injured vessel and probably contributes to the geometric remodeling associated with balloon injury. In the present study we directed our dose not to the intimal surface (ideally calculated 1.5 mm from the center of the source train), but to a depth sufficient to ensure an adequate dose to the adventitia surrounding the injury site (2.0 mm). This reduced the proliferation of the adventitial myofibroblasts and the recruitment of α-smooth muscle actin positive cells around the vessel. We hypothesize that the reduction of adventitial fibrosis prevented negative arterial remodeling, resulting in a larger vessel perimeter of the irradiated vessels. This may also have had the favorable secondary effect of inhibiting migration of adventitial myofibroblasts across the external elastic lamina into the neointima.

Apoptosis is also known as programmed cell death and is distinct from necrosis or other forms of cellular death.[32] Radiation therapy of tumors has been reported to cause signs of apoptotic death within 3 hours. If a tumor responds rapidly to a relatively low dose of radiation, it generally means that apoptosis is involved since the process peaks at 3 to 5 hours after irradiation. Susceptibility to the induction of apoptosis may also be an important factor determining radiosensitivity, as apoptosis appears to be prominent early in radiosensitive mouse tumors and essentially absent in radioresistant tumors. It has been suggested that apoptosis is the dominant form of cell death in lymphoma cells treated with photodynamic therapy, and that process occurs more rapidly than after x-irradiation.[33–35]

Apoptosis is also a feature of human vascular pathology, including restenotic lesions.[36] Coronary arterial specimens of patients with restenotic lesions retrieved via atherectomy demonstrated a high level of apoptosis and it was suggested that apoptosis may modulate the cellularity of lesions that produce vascular obstruction. Balloon injury of rat carotid arteries also stimulates apoptosis in the medial wall and neointima in regions of greatest cell proliferation.[37] These observations are similar to our finding of TUNEL-positive cells at the sites of greatest cell proliferation in the media and adventitia of the injured porcine coronary arteries. However radiation did not increase TUNEL labeling either 3 or 7 days after injury compared to control vessels. While this suggests that radiation may not work through an induction of apoptosis, these studies do not eliminate the possibility that radiation may induce an increase in apoptosis much earlier, within hours of treatment. Furthermore, it should be pointed out that TUNEL labeling alone is not a perfect measure of apoptosis and tends to overestimate actual rates of apoptosis in normal and atherosclerotic vessels.[38] Additional studies will have to be done with additional markers of apoptosis at earlier timepoints to determine what proportion of the TUNEL-positive cells are beginning programmed cell death as a result of the radiation therapy.

Arterial remodeling has a major role in wound healing repair mechanism and has been described as a major contributor to the restenosis process. Several authors have suggested that vascular remodeling post injury is more important than neointima formation in late luminal narrowing.[14,15] Others relate vascular remodeling to the device used for the arterial dilation.[39,40] In the present study we observed an increase of the vessel perimeter and the luminal area of irradiated vessels compared to controls, with a positive relationship between the dose and vessel size. This morphometric observation is supported by the reduction in α-smooth muscle actin staining of adventitial myofibroblasts in the irradiated vessels. Therefore, we hypothesize that intravascular irradiation had a positive effect on vascular remodeling due to the reduction in the recruitment of adventitial myofibroblasts in the adventitia at the injury site which prevented constriction. Intravascular irradiation may be a substitute to intracoronary stenting if chronic vascular constriction after angioplasty is diminished by radiation.

These results suggest that intracoronary radiation prevents vascular lesion formation after coronary intervention by reducing cell proliferation in the media and adventitia 3 days after injury. In addition, intravascular radiation may contribute to positive remodeling and reduction of vessel constriction by reduction of α-smooth muscle actin containing in the adventitia. Additional work is needed to determine the effect of radiation on cell migration from the media or adventitia to the neointima, and to determine the effects of radiation on normal and atherosclerotic vessels.

References

1. Wiedermann JG, Marboe C, Amols H, et al. Intracoronary irradiation markedly reduces restenosis after balloon angioplasty in a porcine model. J Am Coll Cardiol 1994;23:1491–1498.
2. Waksman R, Robinson KA, Crocker IR, et al. Endovascular low-dose irradiation inhibits neointima formation after coronary artery balloon injury in swine. A possible role for radiation therapy in restenosis prevention. Circulation 1995;91:1533–1539.
3. Mazur W, Ali NM, Dabaghi SF, et al. High dose rate intracoronary radiation suppresses neointimal proliferation in the stented and ballooned model of porcine restenosis [abstract]. Circulation 1994;90:I652.
4. Wiedermann JG, Marboe C, Amols H, et al. Intracoronary irradiation markedly reduces neointimal proliferation after balloon angioplasty in swine: Persistent benefit at 6-month follow-up. J Am Coll Cardiol 1995;25:1451–1456.
5. Waksman R, Robinson KA, Crocker IR, et al. Intracoronary low-dose beta-irradiation inhibits neointima formation after coronary artery balloon injury in the swine restenosis model. Circulation 1995;92:3025–3031.
6. Verin V, Popowski Y, Urban P, et al. Intra-arterial beta irradiation prevents neointimal hyperplasia in a hypercholesterolemic rabbit restenosis model. Circulation 1995;92:2284–2290.
7. Waksman R, Robinson KA, Crocker IR, et al. Intracoronary radiation before stent implantation inhibits neointima formation in stented porcine coronary arteries. Circulation 1995;92:1383–1386.
8. Hehrlein C, Gollan C, Donges K, et al. Low-dose radioactive endovascular stents prevent smooth muscle cell proliferation and neointimal hyperplasia in rabbits. Circulation 1995;92:1570–1575.
9. Laird JR, Carter AI, Kufs WM, et al. Inhibition of neointimal proliferation with low-dose irradiation from a beta-particle-emitting stent. Circulation 1996;93:529–536.
10. Clowes AW, Reidy MA, Clowes MM. Kinetics of cellular proliferation after arterial injury. I. Smooth muscle growth in the absence of endothelium. Lab Invest 1983;49:327–333.
11. Schwartz RS, Holmes DR Jr., Topol EJ. The restenosis paradigm revisited: An alternative proposal for cellular mechanisms. J Am Coll Cardiol 1992;20:1284–1293.
12. Gravanis MB, Roubin GS. Histopathologic phenomena at the site of percutaneous transluminal coronary angioplasty: The problem of restenosis. Human Pathol 1989;20:477–485.
13. Johnson DE, Hinohara T, Selmon MR, et al. Primary peripheral arterial stenoses and restenoses excised by transluminal atherectomy: A histopathologic study. J Am Coll Cardiol 1990;15:419–425.
14. Post MJ, Borst C, Kuntz RE. The relative importance of arterial remodeling compared with intimal hyperplasia in lumen renarrowing after balloon angioplasty. A study in the normal rabbit and the hypercholesterolemic Yucatan micropig. Circulation 1994;89:2816–2821.
15. Andersen HR, Maeng M, Thorwest M, et al. Remodeling rather than neointimal formation explains luminal narrowing after deep vessel wall injury. Circulation 1996;93:1716–1724.
16. Mintz GS, Kovach JA, Pichard AD, et al. Geometric remodeling is the predominant mechanism of clinical restenosis after coronary angioplasty [abstract]. J Am Coll Cardiol 1994;23:138A.
17. Mintz GS, Popma JJ, Pichard AD, et al. Arterial remodeling after coronary angioplasty: A serial intravascular ultrasound study. Circulation 1996;94:35–43.
18. Kakuta T, Currier JW, Haudenschild CC, et al. Differences in compensatory vessel en-

largement, not intimal formation, account for restenosis after angioplasty in the hyper-cholesterolemic rabbit model. Circulation 1994;89:2809–2815.

19. Scott NA, Ross CE, Dunn B, et al. Identification of a potential role for the adventitia in vascular lesion formation after balloon overstretch injury of porcine coronary arteries. Circulation 1996;93:2178–2187.

20. de Leon H, Scott NA, Martin F, et al. Expression of nonmuscle myosin heavy chain-B isoform in the vessel wall of porcine coronary arteries after balloon angioplasty. Circ Res 1997;80:514–519.

21. Clark RA. Regulation of fibroplasia in cutaneous wound repair. Am J Med Sci 1993; 306:42–48.

22. Ehrlich HP. Wound closure: Evidence of cooperation between fibroblasts and collagen matrix. Eye 1988;2:149–157.

23. Waksman R, Rodriguez JC, Robinson KA, et al. Effect of intravascular irradiation on cell proliferation, apoptosis and vascular remodeling after balloon overstretch injury of porcine coronary arteries. Circulation 1997;96:1944–1952.

24. Karas SP, Gravanis MB, Santoian EC, et al. Coronary intimal proliferation after balloon injury and stenting in swine: An animal model of restenosis. J Am Coll Cardiol 1992;20:467–474.

25. Schwartz RS, Huber KC, Murphy JG, et al. Restenosis and the proportional neointimal response to coronary artery injury: Results in a porcine model. J Am Coll Cardiol 1992;19:267–274.

26. de Leon H, Scott NA, Martin F, et al. Expression of nonmuscle myosin heavy chain-B isoform in the vessel wall of porcine coronary arteries after balloon angioplasty. Circ Res 1997;80:514–519.

27. Gertz SD, Gimple LW, Banai S, et al. Geometric remodeling is not the principal pathogenetic process in restenosis after balloon angioplasty. Evidence from correlative angio-graphic- histomorphometric studies of atherosclerotic arteries in rabbits. Circulation 1994;90:3001–3008.

28. Clowes AW, Reidy MA, Clowes MM. Mechanisms of stenosis after arterial injury. Lab Invest 1983;49:208–215.

29. O'Brien ER, Alpers CE, Stewart DK, et al. Proliferation in primary and restenotic coronary atherectomy tissue. Implications for antiproliferative therapy. Circ Res 1993;73:223–231.

30. Gordon D, Reidy MA, Benditt EP, et al. Cell proliferation in human coronary arteries. Proc Natl Acad Sci U S A 1990;87:4600–4604.

31. Lindner V, Reidy MA. Smooth muscle proliferation after vascular injury is inhibited by an antibody against basic FGF [abstract]. J Cell Biochem 1991;(suppl 15C):118.

32. Kerr JF, Wyllie AH, Currie AR. Apoptosis: A basic biological phenomenon with wide-ranging implications in tissue kinetics [review]. Br J Cancer 1972;26:239–257.

33. Kerr JF, Winterford CM, Harmon BV. Apoptosis. Its significance in cancer and cancer therapy [published erratum appears in Cancer 1994 Jun 15;73(12):3108] [review]. Cancer 1994;73:2013–2026.

34. Arends MJ, McGregor AH, Wyllie AH. Apoptosis is inversely related to necrosis and determines net growth in tumors bearing constitutively expressed myc, ras, and HPV oncogenes. Am J Pathol 1994;144:1045–1057.

35. Reinhold HS. Quantitative evaluation of the radiosensitivity of cells of a transplantable rhabdomyosarcoma in the rat. Eur J Cancer 1966;2:33–42.

36. Isner JM, Kearney M, Bortman S, et al. Apoptosis in human atherosclerosis and restenosis. Circulation 1995;91:2703–2711.

37. Bochaton-Piallat ML, Gabbiani F, Redard M, et al. Apoptosis participates in cellularity regulation during rat aortic intimal thickening. Am J Pathol 1996;146:1059–1064.

38. Geng YJ, Libby P. Evidence for apoptosis in advanced human atheroma. Colocalization with interleukin-1 beta-converting enzyme (see comments). Am J Pathol 1995;147: 251–266.

39. Mintz GS, Popma JJ, Pichard AD, et al. Mechanisms of later arterial responses to transcatheter therapy: A serial quantitative angiographic and intravascular ultrasound study [abstract]. Circulation 1994;90:I24.

40. Isner JM. Vascular remodeling. Honey, I think I shrunk the artery [editorial; comment]. Circulation 1994;89:2937–2941.

## Chapter 12

Nitric Oxide and Intracoronary Radiation:

Thrombosis, Vasoreactivity, and Restenosis

Yoram Vodovotz, PhD, Balram Bhargava, MD,
Marc Kollum, MD, Yves Cottin, MD, PhD,
Han-Soo Kim, MD, Rosanna C. Chan, PhD,
and Ron Waksman, MD

Introduction

Although interventions such as percutaneous transluminal coronary angioplasty (PTCA) and stenting have helped in the treatment of coronary artery disease, an exaggerated wound healing response (restenosis) accompanies them. The restenotic process may be divided into the initial inflammatory response to the balloon or stent injury, the subsequent migration and proliferation of smooth muscle cells and/or myofibroblasts which results in the formation of a neointima, and finally, fibrosis and matrix deposition which may eventually lead to negative arterial remodeling.[1,2] Thus, therapies may be directed at components of the inflammatory, proliferative, or fibrotic responses, with the ideal therapy modulating all three. Numerous groups have been examining the endovascular administration of ionizing radiation and it has been determined that this therapeutic modality reduces neointimal thickening, at least in part by suppressing the proliferative response.[3,4]

The profound antirestenotic effect of intracoronary radiation (IR) may be due solely to a direct antimitotic effect of radiation on smooth muscle cells, mediated through the production of free radicals which damage DNA irreparably; such a process could be initiated even in cells that are quiescent and not replicating, and be triggered upon entry into the cell cycle.[5] As described below, we have elucidated some effects of IR that cannot be explained solely through cell killing; we hypothesize that IR may exert at least part of its effects through the modulation of the expression and/or activity of various genes.[6] Furthermore, the effect of IR on the inflammatory response and the modulation of signaling molecules by IR have not been examined previously; we have concentrated on these issues, and also on the roles of the free radical molecule nitric oxide (NO).[7]

Proinflammatory cytokines such as interferon-γ (IFN-γ), tumor necrosis fac-

From Waksman R (ed.). *Vascular Brachytherapy, Third Edition.* Armonk, NY: Futura Publishing Co., Inc.; © 2002.

tor-α (TNF-α), and interleukin-1 (IL-1), as well as anti-inflammatory cytokines such as transforming growth factor-β1 (TGF-β1) can be induced by radiation.[6] In turn, these cytokines modulate the expression of the enzyme inducible NO synthase (NOS2; iNOS), positively in the case of IFN-γ, TNF-α, and IL-1, and negatively in the case of TGF-β1.[8,9] Ionizing radiation delivered by external beam is associated with increased production of NO.[6,10–17] The evidence for the beneficial effects of NO following balloon overstretch injury (BI) is abundant: administration of the precursor for NO production, L-arginine[18,19]; chemical NO donors[20–24]; or delivery of isoforms of NOS through gene therapy techniques[25–27] all reduce neointimal proliferation in cells, animals, and humans. Nitric oxide also enhances the proliferation and viability of endothelial cells,[28–30] and enhances the reendothelialization of denuded arteries and suppresses platelet aggregation in various settings including PTCA.[31–33] In addition to the antiproliferative effects of NO mentioned above, this free radical can also cause apoptosis under certain conditions.[34,35] These findings led us to hypothesize a role for NO derived from NOS2 in the beneficial effects of IR on suppression of neointima formation, as well as an association of NO with some of the effects of this therapy on thrombosis. Furthermore, we investigated whether IR affected vasoreactivity in any way, since several studies had suggested a possible negative effect of radiation on the vasculature.[36,37]

Radiation, Thrombosis, and Neointima: Effects of Nitric Oxide

One of the parameters considered key for the inflammatory process that precedes the formation of neointima is the presence of platelet thrombi.[2,38] Previous studies on the vascular effects of external beam radiation have suggested that increased thrombosis is an adverse late effect,[36,39] and there have been reports of acute thrombosis following IR despite treatment with antithrombotic agents in the feasibility clinical trials.[40–43] This finding is paradoxical, since thrombosis has been linked to increased neointimal hyperplasia,[2,38] while IR reduces neointimal hyperplasia.[2,44–47] We performed a retrospective study in order to address this paradox and to study this phenomenon in detail, examining porcine coronary arteries 14 days post treatment with BI followed by IR at doses of 0 to18 Gy of either β- or γ-radiation, as determined by dosimetry calculated at the vessel wall.[48] This timepoint was chosen since it occurs sufficiently late after BI to have a statistically increased neointima, yet it is early enough after BI that thrombi are still present.[49] The parameters we examined were the overall thrombosis rate (TR), the luminal thrombosis rate (LT), the mural thrombosis rate (MT), and the thrombus area (TA). Furthermore, we examined the intimal area (IA) corrected for medial fracture length (IA/FL)[49] following BI alone or with subsequent IR. We found that the overall TR increased dose-dependently from 0 to18 Gy. Our results were confirmed by in vitro studies of Salame et al,[50] who demonstrated that arteries subjected to BI followed by IR exhibited increased ^{111}In-labeled platelet deposition between 1 day and 1 month post irradiation. The authors showed increases in platelet recruitment both at 15 and 30 Gy as compared to 0 Gy.[50]

We further observed that LT and TA decreased with increasing radiation dose, while MT increased. The decrease in TA correlated very highly with decreased IA/FL ($r^2 = 1.00$). Furthermore, LT present after IR tended to consist mostly of fibrin and thus were less organized than in controls.[48] These findings again demonstrated the striking relationship between TA and IA, but also suggested that some mechanism had been set in motion by IR that acts to reduce TA despite the presence of a larger number of nascent thrombi.

In a subsequent study,[51] we examined the possible mechanisms that might account for the increase in TR and MT.[48] In this study, we examined porcine coronary arteries subjected to BI alone or with subsequent IR (18 Gy of ^{90}Y). Significant differences were observed between irradiated and control arteries with regard to the presence of mural thrombi, 1/11 (9%) versus 11/14 (78%) ($P<0.001$). However, mural TA was larger in the 18-Gy group as compared to the control group, respectively (0.44±0.08 mm^2 versus 0.07 mm^2[only one case]), similar to our previous findings.[48] We next examined the surface of the internal elastic lamina (IEL), both qualitatively and quantitatively through analysis of the roughness index (RI).[52] The RI was determined as follows: the length of the surface profile of the IEL (SP) and the length of the straight line of the IEL (L) were measured between both edges of the medial break, adapted from the analysis of luminal thrombosis carried out by Fernández-Ortiz et al.[52] The RI of the IEL was calculated as follows: [(SP–L)/L] * 100=RI (%). To evaluate the difference between the break segment and the uninjured segment of the IEL, we obtained the RI in a particular length (450 μm) at the break edges and on the opposite site of the injury.

The straight length of the IEL was significantly shorter in the irradiated group. Histologic examination of the injured arteries showed that the surface of the IEL was more irregular after IR, particularly at the sites of medial break. In the irradiated group, we also observed more disruption of the IEL at both edges of the break as compared to the control group. When mural thrombi were present, there was a positive relation between mural TA and medial α-actin density, as well as between TA and RI. Furthermore, in the irradiated group, we found a positive correlation between RI and medial α-actin density, and no correlation between RI and neointima formation.[51] We interpreted these findings to suggest that vessel irregularity and changes in medial structure following IR are associated with the process of arterial healing, which indirectly affects thrombosis, but not with intimal hyperplasia or remodeling. This lack of healing has also been demonstrated in arteries treated with radioactive stents.[37] It is our hypothesis that these profound changes in the architecture of injured vessels subjected to IR leads to the late thrombosis described clinically.[42,43]

The studies mentioned above were all conducted in swine that received both aspirin and ticlopidine, standard antithrombotic medications. Thrombi were still observed in these animals following IR; we have therefore sought to find novel means of reducing this thrombosis. We focused our attentions on NO: the production of NO should be beneficial in the early period after arterial injury, since NO is a potent suppressor of platelet aggregation whether delivered in drug form,[31–33] or more interestingly, through the induction of NOS2 in injured arteries.[53] We have tested this hypothesis directly in two ways: by infusing the chemical NO donor S-nitrosoglutathione (GSNO)[32,33] and observing its effects on thrombosis as analyzed above, and by examining the effect of IR on the expression of NOS2 in porcine arteries subjected to BI.

We treated domestic swine with GSNO and quantified various parameters related to thrombosis and restenosis in tissue sections from injured arteries. We found that GSNO reduced the thrombosis rate at every dose of radiation administered (0, 5, and 15 Gy) without altering the efficacy of IR for prevention of restenosis. Furthermore, thrombi present despite treatment with GSNO appeared better organized upon histologic examination than thrombi present in arteries subjected to IR without GSNO.[54] While these effects of NO are beneficial, some of its possible negative effects include hypotension[55,56] and negative inotropic effects.[57–60] While swine treated with GSNO indeed became hypotensive, this was reversed shortly after cessation of the infusion.[54] Furthermore, we observed a slight increase in heart rate following treatment with GSNO,[54] in agreement with the reported positive inotropic effects of low levels of NO.[61,62] It is possible that BI may interfere with the production of NO by endothelial cells, and this effect may explain why an NO donor can reduce the rate of thrombosis despite the presence of antiplatelet agents such as aspirin and ticlopidine used in the above experiments.[54] Our findings suggest that NO delivered during in the early period after BI can reduce the extent of thrombosis. However, our results indicated no reduction of restenosis by this short-term infusion of GSNO.[54]

Effects of Intracoronary Radiation on Inflammation and Apoptosis after Balloon Injury

Though studies on the mechanistic effects of IR are few, several have focused on the suppression of proliferation of intimal smooth muscle cells by IR, as well as a possible role for apoptosis. This area of investigation has been controversial. Some cells, such as lymphocytes, respond to radiation by undergoing apoptosis.[63] Numerous studies, however, have indicated that ionizing radiation does not increase directly the rate of apoptosis of smooth muscle cells in vitro,[64] nor was increased apoptosis observed 3 or 7 days following treatment with either 14 or 28 Gy of ^{90}Sr/Y.[65] However, we observed that 14 days following treatment with 18 Gy of ^{90}Y, approximately threefold more apoptotic cells were observed in the media and adventitia of balloon-injured porcine coronary arteries as compared to arteries treated with 0 Gy (Y. Vodovotz and R. Waksman, submitted). While at first glance these findings appeared to suggest a late proapoptotic effect of IR on medial and adventitial smooth muscle cells and/or myofibroblasts,[66] a closer examination utilizing a panel of antibodies directed against cell surface markers of inflammatory cells demonstrated that the cells undergoing apoptosis appeared to be T cells rather than smooth muscle cells (see below).

Our recent studies have suggested that delayed healing and increased thrombosis occur as a consequence of IR,[48,51] and that this delayed healing brings with it increased T cell and macrophage infiltration (Table 1). Our findings therefore suggest that, following BI and subsequent IR, there is an increase in cytokines and other proteins involved in inflammation, as a consequence of the impaired healing of these arteries. Interestingly, we observed an approximately threefold higher number of apoptotic cells in the media and adventitia of irradiated arteries as compared to controls. A further examination of the TUNEL-positive cells suggested that they were in fact the infiltrating T cells, since they were positive for the T cell marker CD3 but not for smooth muscle α-actin (Fig. 1). Radiation can cause apoptosis in T cells,[63] but we do not believe that this is the likely explanation for the results we observe since the T cells likely infiltrate the injured media after the radiation source has been removed. We believe that our results represent the feedback response, which suppresses the T cell-mediated inflammation.[63]

It is likely that the inflammation we observe at the site of medial fracture and

Table 1

Analysis of Immunocytochemistry for Macrophages and T Cells in Balloon-Injured Porcine Coronary Arteries Subjected to Intracoronary Radiation

| | Control | | | γ-Radiation | | | |
	3 days	7 days	14 days	3 days	7 days	14 days	ANOVA
N	8	7	9	7	5	8	
Macrophage Staining							
Adventitia	54±11	3±2*	17±17*	41±9	48±18	7±1*$	<0.01
Media	13±9	0±0	0±0	2±2	4±4	0±0	NS
Neointima	60±20	29±10	0±0*	52±18	115±270	35±11*$	<0.01
TCell Staining							
Adventitia	0±0	0±0	2±1*$	3±2	0±0	227±73*$	<0.05
Media	0±0	0±0	0±0	0±0	0±0	0±0	NS
Neointima	0±0	22±10*	0±0	3±2	129±55	63±50	<0.05

Porcine coronary arteries were subjected to balloon injury and subsequent intracoronary radiation with 15 Gy of ^{192}Ir delivered to 2 mm from the source. The animals were euthanized at the indicated timepoints, and arterial cross-sections stained with antibodies to macrophages (LN-5) or T cells (CD3) were analyzed microscopically in adventitia, the media, and the neointima around the whole cross-section. Positive cells were scored using a computerized PC-compatible image analysis program (Optimas 6; Optimas, Inc., Bothell, WA) after being digitized and stored in a frame-grabberboard (DAGE-MTI, Michigan City, IN). The cell densities are given as cell per 0.1 mm″.

*$P < 0.005$ vs. 14 d, radiation and vs. 3d, no radiation.

$$P < 0.05 vs. 7d, no radiation.

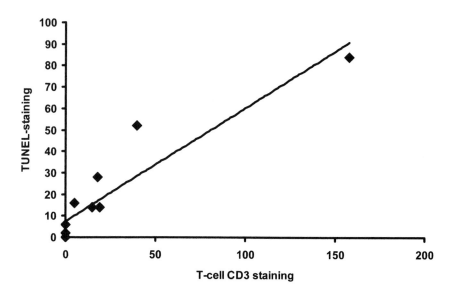

Figure 1. Apoptotic cells in injured and irradiated porcine arteries are T cells. Apoptotic cells (TUNEL-positive) and T cells (CD3-positive cells) were assessed by immunocytochemistry in injured and irradiated (18 Gy ^{90}Y) arteries 14 days post treatment. A positive correlation was obtained between these two markers ($r^2=0.82$; $P<0.001$) in the media and adventitia adjacent to the medial tear.

irradiation results from a combination of these two injuries. It has been established that inflammation is associated with increased neointima formation following angioplasty or stenting.[67–69] It appears that IR is able to overcome the proliferative stimulus derived from this inflammation, hence the antirestenotic efficacy of this therapy. However, numerous studies have demonstrated that ionizing radiation modulates the expression of inflammatory genes.[6] These genes include proinflammatory cytokines such as IFN-γ, TNF-α, and IL-1.[6] Additionally, the cytokine TGF-β1 is also modulated by radiation.[6] This cytokine is often thought of as anti-inflammatory, but in fact is a potent chemoattractive agent for inflammatory cells.[70] Thus, the combined inflammation from both the initial injury and subsequent IR may drive the increased inflammation we observe, at least in animal models, and may suggest that certain anti-inflammatory treatments could be used as adjunct therapies for this side effect of IR.

Expression of NOS2 Following Balloon Injury: Effect of Intracoronary Radiation

Our findings on the effects of IR on neointima, thrombosis, and apoptosis were in agreement with a possible role for NO. Indeed, the presence of large numbers of inflammatory cells and the increased production of inflammatory cytokines can often lead to increased production of NO. Recent studies further suggest that cells and tissues subjected to radiation express higher levels of NOS2.[6]

We have recently characterized the expression of NOS2 in porcine coronary arteries that were subjected to BI and then either placebo or IR. Our findings suggest that the expression of NOS2 is associated with decreased IA/FL (Fig. 2), whether in irradiated arteries or controls.[71] These findings are exciting for several reasons. First, they suggest that IR increases the expression of NOS2. Since, as summarized above, the expression of NOS2 following BI has been considered beneficial, our findings may suggest a mechanism independent of a direct antimitotic effect of ionizing radiation by which to explain the antirestenotic efficacy of IR. Furthermore, the expression of NOS2 has been also suggested to reduce platelet aggregation in balloon-injured arteries[53]; this observation may explain why TA was lower in arteries treated with IR following BI.[48] Finally, the expression of NOS2 is consistent with the proposed roles for NO and NOS2 in apoptosis of T cells.[34,35]

Effects of Intracoronary Radiation on Vasoreactivity after Balloon Injury

While the studies described above are consistent with the increased expression of NOS2 following treatment with IR, it is still formally possible that other isoforms of NOS may be involved in this process.[72] Furthermore, it is imperative to note that radiation may cause detrimental effects on the vasculature, including impairment of endothelialization.[36,37,50] In our own experiments, we observed increased endothelialization from 3 to 14 days post-BI in porcine arteries (Fig. 3, open circles), confirming previous observations in the porcine BI model.[49] The reendothelialization process was impaired in arteries subjected to BI and subsequent 15 Gy of [192]Ir (Fig. 3, filled circles).

Theoretically, the reduced endothelial coverage should reduce the presence of

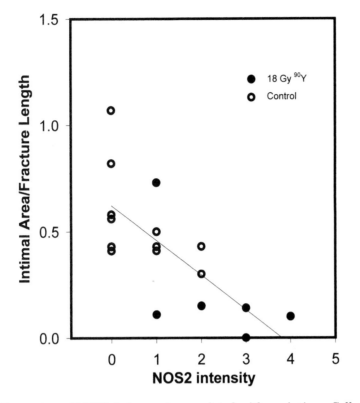

Figure 2. Expression of NOS2 is inversely correlated with neointima. Cells expressing NOS2 were assessed by immunocytochemistry in injured and irradiated (18 Gy ^{90}Y) arteries 14 days post treatment. An inverse correlation was obtained between these two markers (r^2=0.53, $\alpha_{(P<0.05)}$=0.95) in the media and adventitia. The expression of NOS2 was higher in irradiated arteries (filled circles) than in controls (open circles).

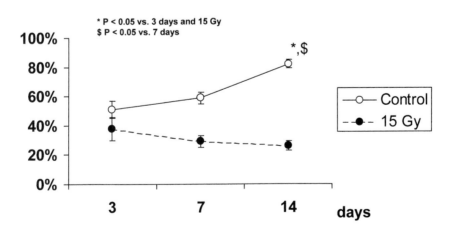

Figure 3. Intracoronary radiation impairs reendothelialization at 14 days. Endothelial cells were assessed by Factor VIII immunocytochemistry in injured and irradiated (15 Gy ^{192}Ir) arteries 3, 7, and 14 days post treatment. The number of factor VIII-positive endothelial cells was higher in irradiated arteries (filled circles) than in controls (open circles). *$P<0.005$ versus 14 days, radiation and versus 3 days, no radiation. $^{\$}P<0.05$ versus 7 days, no radiation.

endothelial-derived NO, and this reduction should impact the ability of these arterial segments to vasodilate. The question remains, though, as to whether this reduced regional endothelialization post-BI has functional consequences. Wiedermann et al have reported that arteries treated with IR alone (no BI) dilated normally in response to acetylcholine (an agent which activates endothelial cells expressing NOS3 to produce NO[55,73]) but not to nitroglycerin (an NO donor that acts directly on smooth muscle cells).[40] We studied the vasoreactive properties of porcine arteries subjected to BI alone or with subsequent IR, thereby assessing not only the possible safety issue of reendothelialization following IR, but also, indirectly, the expression or activity of NOS3 in response to this treatment. We carried out this study in porcine arteries subjected to BI alone or with subsequent IR, using [186/188]Re at a dose of 15 Gy.[74] We found no statistical differences in vasodilatation among three treatment groups (group I–no BI, no radiation group; group II–BI, radiation group; group III–BI, no radiation group), either in response to acetylcholine (an endothelium-dependent vasodilator that acts by inducing NO production from NOS3[31,55]) or nitroglycerin (an NO donor that acts directly on smooth muscle cells). These findings suggest that the endothelium is reconstituted following catheter-based IR, at least in the porcine overstretch BI model and using [186/188]Re as the isotope. These findings also suggest that IR does not alter the expression or activity of the endothelial isoform of nitric oxide synthase (ecNOS; NOS3), that is generally expressed constitutively in endothelial cells but whose expression and activity can be modified under certain circumstances.[75]

Conclusions and Future Directions

The studies described above shed new light on the possible roles of NO in the effects of IR, at least in the porcine model. They suggest that the pharmacological or genetic modulation of NO production may be beneficial adjunct therapies for increased thrombosis due IR. Further studies in animal models, especially studies designed to test the durability of the effect of short-term administration of NO donors, are necessary in order to determine whether modulation of NO will be of benefit in conjunction with IR.

Acknowledgments: The authors would like to acknowledge the technical help of Rufus Seabron, Sara Collins, and Anthony Pierre, as well as the contributions of Dr. Won Ho Kim, all of the Cardiovascular Research Foundation, Washington, D.C., without whose help the studies described in this chapter would not have been possible.

References

1. Schwartz SM, Reidy MA, O'Brien ERM. Assessment of factors important in atherosclerotic occlusion and restenosis. Thromb Haemost 1995;74:541–551.
2. Dangas G, Fuster V. Management of restenosis after coronary intervention. Am Heart J 1996;132:428–436.
3. Bhargava B, Vodovotz Y, Waksman R. Intracoronary radiation therapy for prevention of restenosis. Indian Heart J 1998;50(suppl I):120–129.
4. Teirstein PS. Prevention of vascular restenosis with radiation. Tex Heart Inst J 1998;25:30–33.
5. Mitchell JB. Radiation biology concepts for the use of radiation to prevent restenosis. In: Waksman R (ed.): Vascular Brachytherapy, 2 Edition. Armonk, NY: Futura Publishing Co.; 1999:83–102.

6. Vodovotz Y, Mitchell JB, Lucia MS, et al. Modulation of protein expression and activity by radiation: Relevance to intracoronary radiation for the prevention of restenosis. Cardiovasc Radiation Med 1999;1:336–343.

7. Vodovotz Y, Waksman R. Potential roles for nitric oxide and transforming growth factor-β1 in endovascular brachytherapy. In: Waksman R, Serruys PW (eds.): Handbook of Vascular Brachytherapy, 2nd Edition. London: Martin Dunitz; 1998:139–146.

8. Nathan C, Xie Q-W. Regulation of biosynthesis of nitric oxide. J Biol Chem 1994;269:13725-13728.

9. Vodovotz Y. Control of nitric oxide production by transforming growth factor-β1: Mechanistic insights and potential relevance to human disease. Nitric oxide. Biol Chem 1997;1:3–17.

10. Voevodskaya NV, Vanin AF. Gamma-irradiation potentiates L-arginine-dependent nitric oxide formation in mice. Biochem Biophys Res Commun 1992;186:1423–1428.

11. Mikoyan VD, Voevodskaya NV, Kubrina LN, et al. Exogenous iron and γ-irradiation induce NO-synthase synthesis in mouse liver. Biochemistry (Moscow) 1994;59:732–738.

12. Ibuki Y, Goto R. Augmentation of NO production and cytolytic activity of Mphi obtained from mice irradiated with a low dose of γ-rays. J Radiat Res 1995;36:209–220.

13. Cohen EP, Fish BL, Moulder JE. The role of nitric oxide in radiation nephropathy. Arch Biochem Biophys 1996;104:200–206.

14. Hatjikondi O, Ravazoula P, Kardamakis D, et al. In vivo experimental evidence that the nitric oxide pathway is involved in the X-ray-induced antiangiogenicity. Br J Cancer 1996;74:1916–1923.

15. Ibuki Y, Goto R. Enhancement of NO production from resident peritoneal macrophages by in vitro γ-irradiation and its relationship to reactive oxygen intermediates. Free Rad Biol Med 1997;22:1029–1035.

16. McKinney LC, Aquila EM, Coffin D, et al. Ionizing radiation potentiates the induction of nitric oxide synthase by interferon-g and/or lipopolysaccharide in murine macrophage cell lines: Role of tumor necrosis factor-α. J Leukoc Biol 1998;64:459–466.

17. Vodovotz Y, Coffin C, DeLuca AM, et al. Induction of nitric oxide production in infiltrating leukocytes following in vivo irradiation of tumor-bearing mice. Radiat Oncol Inv 1999;7:86–97.

18. McNamara DB, Bedi B, Aurora H, et al. L-arginine inhibits balloon catheter-induced intimal hyperplasia. Biochem Biophys Res Commun 1993;193:291–296.

19. Wang B-Y, Candipan RC, Arjomandi M, et al. Arginine restores nitric oxide activity and inhibits monocyte accumulation after vascular injury in hypercholesterolemic rabbits. J Am Coll Cardiol 1996;28:1573–1579.

20. Guo J, Milhoan KA, Tuan RS, Lefer AM. Beneficial effect of SPM-5185, a cysteine-containing nitric oxide donor, in rat carotid intimal injury. Circ Res 1994;75:77–84.

21. Kolpakow V, Kulik TJ. Nitric oxide-generating compounds inhibit total protein and collagen synthesis in cultured vascular smooth muscle cells. Circ Res 1995;76:305–309.

22. Marks DS, Vita JA, Folts JD, et al. Inhibition of neointimal proliferation in rabbits after vascular injury by a single treatment with a protein adduct of nitric oxide. J Clin Invest 1995;96:2630–2638.

23. Mooradian DL, Hutsell TC, Keefer LK. Nitric oxide (NO) donor molecules: Effect of NO release rate on vascular smooth muscle cell proliferation in vitro. Am J Physiol 1995;25:674–678.

24. Lablanche J-M, Grollier G, Lusson J-R, et al. Effect of the direct nitric oxide donors linsidomine and molsidomine on angiographic restenosis after coronary balloon angioplasty: The ACCORD study. Circulation 1997;95:83–89.

25. von der Leyen H, Gibbons GH, Morishita R, et al. Gene therapy inhibiting neointimal vascular lesion: In vivo transfer of endothelial cell nitric oxide synthase gene. Proc Natl Acad Sci USA 1995;92:1137–1141.

26. Tzeng E, Shears LL, II, Robbins PD, et al. Vascular gene transfer of the human inducible nitric oxide synthase: Characterization of activity and effects on myointimal hyperplasia. Mol Med 1996;2:211–225.

27. Varenne O, Pislaru S, Gillijns H, et al. Local adenovirus-mediated transfer of human endothelial nitric oxide synthase reduces luminal narrowing after coronary angioplasty in pigs. Circulation 1998;98:919–926.

28. Ziche M, Morbidelli L, Masini E, et al. Nitric oxide promotes DNA synthesis and cyclic

GMP formation in endothelial cells from postcapillary venules. Biochem Biophys Res Commun 1993;192:1198–1203.

29. Guo J, Siegfried MR, Lefer AM. Endothelial preserving actions of a nitric oxide donor in carotid arterial intimal injury. Meth Find Exp Clin Pharmacol 1994;16:347–354.
30. De Caterina R, Libby P, Peng H-B, et al. Nitric oxide decreases cytokine-induced endothelial activation: Nitric oxide selectively reduces endothelial expression of adhesion molecules and proinflammatory cytokines. J Clin Invest 1995;96:60–68.
31. Moncada S, Higgs A. Mechanisms of disease: The L-arginine-nitric oxide pathway. N Engl J Med 1993;329:2002–2012.
32. Radomski MW, Rees DD, Dutra A, Moncada S. S-nitroso-glutathione inhibits platelet activation in vitro and in vivo. Br J Pharmacol 1992;107:745–749.
33. Langford EJ, Brown AS, Wainwright RJ, et al. Inhibition of platelet activity by S-nitrosoglutathione during coronary angioplasty. Lancet 1994;344:1458–1460.
34. Nicotera P, Bonfoco E, Brüne B. Mechanisms for nitric oxide-induced cell death: Involvement of apoptosis. Adv Neuroimmunol 1995;5:411–420.
35. Dimmeler S, Zeiher AM. Nitric oxide and apoptosis: Another paradigm for the double-edged role of nitric oxide. Nitric oxide: Biol Chem 1997; 1:275–281.
36. Stewart JR, Fajardo LF, Gillette SM, Constine LS. Radiation injury to the heart. Int J Radiat Oncol Biol Phys 1995;31:1205–1211.
37. Farb A, Tang AL, Virmani R. Neointima is reduced but endothelialization is incomplete 3 months after ^{32}P β-emitting stent placement [abstract]. Circulation 1998;98:I-779.
38. Fingerle J, Johnson R, Clowes AW, et al. Role of platelets in smooth muscle cell proliferation and migration after vascular injury in rat carotid artery. Proc Natl Acad Sci USA 1989;86:8412–8416.
39. Gillette EL, LaRue SM, Gillette SM. Normal tissue tolerance and management of radiation injury. Semin Vet Med Surg (Small Anim) 1995;10:209–213.
40. Wiedermann JG, Leavy JA, Amols H, et al. Effects of high-dose intracoronary irradiation on vasomotor function and smooth muscle histopathology. Am J Physiol 1994;267:H125–H132.
41. Condado JA, Waksman R, Gurdiel O, et al. Long-term angiographic and clinical outcome after percutaneous transluminal coronary angioplasty and intracoronary radiation therapy in humans. Circulation 1997;96:727–732.
42. Costa MA, Sabate M, van der Giessen W, et al. Late coronary occlusion after intracoronary brachytherapy. Circulation 1999;100:789–792.
43. Waksman R, Bhargava B, Leon MB. Late thrombosis following intracoronary brachytherapy. Catheter Cardiovasc Interv 2000;49:344–347.
44. Wiedermann JG, Marboe C, Amols H, et al. Intracoronary irradiation markedly reduces restenosis after balloon angioplasty in a porcine model. J Am Coll Cardiol 1994;23:1491–1498.
45. Waksman R, Robinson KA, Crocker IR, et al. Intracoronary radiation before stent implantation inhibits neointima formation in stented porcine coronary arteries. Circulation 1995;92:1383–1386.
46. Waksman R, Robinson KA, Crocker IR, et al. Intracoronary low-dose β-irradiation inhibits neointima formation after coronary artery balloon injury in the swine restenosis model. Circulation 1995;92:3025–3031.
47. Anonymous. Vascular Brachytherapy, 1 Edition. Veenendaal, The Netherlands: Nucletron B.V.; 1996.
48. Vodovotz Y, Waksman R, Kim WH, et al. Effects of intracoronary radiation on thrombosis following balloon injury in the porcine model. Circulation 1999;100:2527–2533.
49. Robinson KA. Pig coronary artery model of post-angioplasty restenosis. In: Waksman R, King SB, Crocker IR, Mould RF (eds.): Vascular Brachytherapy. 1996:30–40.
50. Salame MY, Verheye S, Mulkey SP, et al. The effect of endovascular irradiation on platelet recruitment at sites of balloon angioplasty in pig coronary arteries. Circulation 2000;101:1087–1090.
51. Cottin Y, Kollum M, Kim HS, et al. Surface profile of the internal elastic lamina may modulate thrombosis following intracoronary radiation in balloon-injured porcine arteries. J Intervent Cardiol In press.
52. Tatemichi M, Ogura T, Nagata H, Esumi H. Enhanced expression of inducible nitric oxide synthase in chronic gastritis with intestinal metaplasia. J Clin Gastroenterol 1998;27:240–245.

53. Yan Z, Yokota T, Zhang W, Hansson GK. Expression of inducible nitric oxide synthase inhibits platelet adhesion and restores blood flow in the injured artery. Circ Res 1996;79:38–44.
54. Vodovotz Y, Waksman R, Cook JA, et al. S-nitrosoglutathione reduces non-occlusive thrombosis rate following balloon overstretch injury and intracoronary irradiation of porcine coronary arteries. Int J Radiat Oncol Biol Phys In press.
55. Ignarro LJ. Biosynthesis and metabolism of endothelium-derived nitric oxide. Annu Rev Pharmacol Toxicol 1990;30:535–560.
56. Moncada S, Palmer RMJ, Higgs EA. Nitric oxide: Physiology, pathophysiology, and pharmacology. Pharmacol Rev 1991;43:109–142.
57. Roberts AB, Vodovotz Y, Roche NS, et al. Role of nitric oxide in antagonistic effects of transforming growth factor-β and interleukin-1β on the beating rate of cultured cardiac myocytes. Mol Endocrinol 1992;6:1921–1930.
58. Finkel MS, Oddis CV, Jacob TD, et al. Negative inotropic effects of cytokines on the heart mediated by nitric oxide. Science 1992;257:387–389.
59. Schulz R, Nava E, Moncada S. Induction and potential biological relevance of a Ca^{2+}-independent nitric oxide synthase in the myocardium. Br J Pharmacol 1992;105:575–580.
60. Brady AJB, Poole-Wilson PA, Harding SE, Warren JB. Nitric oxide production within cardiac myocytes reduces their contractility in endotoxemia. Am J Physiol (Heart Circ Physiol) 1992;263:H1963-H1966.
61. Amrani M, O'Shea J, Allen NJ, et al. Role of basal release of nitric oxide on coronary flow and mechanical performance of the isolated rat heart. J Physiol (London) 1992;456:681–687.
62. Klabunde RE, Kimber ND, Kuk JE, et al. N^G-methyl-L-arginine decreases contractility, cGMP and cAMP in isoproterenol-stimulated rat hearts in vitro. Eur J Pharmacol 1992;223:1–7.
63. Crompton NE. Programmed cellular response to ionizing radiation damage [see comments]. Acta Oncol 1998;37:129–142.
64. Gajdusek CM, Tian H, London S, et al. Gamma radiation effect on vascular smooth muscle cells in culture. Int J Radiat Oncol Biol Phys 1996;36:821–828.
65. Wilcox JN, Waksman R, King SB, Scott NA. The role of the adventitia in the arterial response to angioplasty: The effect of intravascular radiation. Int J Radiat Oncol Biol Phys 1996;36:789–796.
66. Wilcox JN, Waksman R, King SB, Scott NA. Role of the adventitia in the arterial response to angioplasty. In: Waksman R, King SB, Crocker IR, Mould RF (eds.): Vascular Brachytherapy. Veenendaal, The Netherlands: Nucletron B.V.; 1996:17–29.
67. Miller DD, Karim MA, Edwards WD, Schwartz RS. Relationship of vascular thrombosis and inflammatory leukocyte infiltration to neointimal growth following porcine coronary artery stent placement. Atherosclerosis 1996;124:145–155.
68. Kornowski R, Hong MK, Tio FO, et al. In-stent restenosis: Contributions of inflammatory responses and arterial injury to neointimal hyperplasia. J Am Coll Cardiol 1998;31:224–230.
69. Kornowski R, Hong MK, Virmani R, et al. Granulomatous foreign body reactions contribute to exaggerated in-stent restenosis. Coron Artery Dis 1999;10:9–14.
70. Wahl SM, McCartney-Francis N, Mergenhagen SE. Inflammatory and immunomodulatory roles of TGF-Beta. Immunol Today 1989;10:258–261.
71. Vodovotz Y, Chan R, Collins S, et al. Intracoronary radiation decreases expression of active transforming growth factor-β1 and increases expression of inducible nitric oxide synthase following balloon injury in porcine coronary arteries [abstract]. Circulation 1998;98:I-112.
72. Cooke JP, Dzau VJ. Nitric oxide synthase: Role in the genesis of vascular disease. Annu Rev Med 1997;48:489–509.
73. Lüscher TF, Noll G. Endothelial function as an end-point in interventional trials: Concepts, methods and current data. J Hypertens 1996;14(suppl 2):S111-S121.
74. Bhargava B, Waksman R, Vodovotz Y, et al. Intracoronary irradiation with [186/188]Rhenium following balloon overstretch injury reduces neointima but does not impair vasoreactivity of porcine coronary arteries. J Intervent Cardiol 1999;12:263–270.
75. Sase K, Michel T. Expression and regulation of endothelial nitric oxide synthase. Trends Cardiovasc Med 1997;7:28–37.

## Chapter 13

Endovascular Radiation and Vasoreactivity

Attila Thury, MD, Ken Kozuma, MD, Manel Sabate, MD, and Patrick W. Serruys, MD, PhD

This chapter will provide a review of the basic current literature on endothelial function and its assessment; the possible role of endothelial dysfunction in restenosis and the impact of intracoronary brachytherapy on vasoreactivity is also discussed.

Introduction to Endothelial Dysfunction

The healthy endothelium has multiple functions:

1. It forms a highly selective barrier by separating blood from medial smooth muscle cells (SMCs)[1] and prevents blood contact with the subendothelial matrix, causing antithrombotic effect.[2]
2. The intact endothelium possesses anti-inflammatory properties by inhibiting infective agents and a variety of substances to penetrate the subintimal structures.[3,4]
3. It is also a highly active metabolic tissue, capable of forming several vasoactive substances[5] and connective tissue macromolecules.[6]
4. The endothelium is able to sense and respond to stimuli from outside, resulting in either vasoconstriction or vasodilatation, mediated by numerous transmitting substances. Local vascular control depends on a balance between these dilators and constrictors. Endothelium-dependent vasodilatation is an important adaptive response of the healthy vasculature to an increase in oxygen demand, eg, during exercise. Most of the vasodilatory stimuli induce the release of nitric oxide (NO), which has received substantial scientific attention.[7,8] By controlling vasomotion, the endothelium maintains optimal shear stress of the vessel wall,[9] which in the longer term might prevent remodeling process of the vessel.[10]

The term "endothelial dysfunction" refers to an impaired endothelium, which results in ineffective endothelium-dependent vasodilatation. When it manifests in the coronary arteries it may cause exercise-induced ischemia.[11] It is not a static

Attila Thury, MD, is a recipient of Hungarian Postgraduate Fellowship Eotvos and Soros Foundation. The Wenckebach Prize was awarded to P.W. Serruys, MD, by the Dutch Heart Foundation for brachytherapy research.

condition of a particular vessel but rather a dynamic and systemic process,[12] occurring in the presence of atherosclerosis[13] or its risk factors.[14,15] Recent study established its prognostic value for long-term atherosclerotic disease progression and cardiovascular event rates in patients with coronary heart disease.[16] It has been associated with many other cardiac and noncardiac conditions, such as hypertension, diabetes mellitus, active and passive smoking, homocystinuria, and after cardiac transplantation.[17–22]

In the first stage of endothelial dysfunction, signal transduction processes, mediated by G-protein pathways are damaged[23] (Fig. 1). At this early phase, NO production is decreased due to impaired NO synthase activity,[24] which is followed by a decrease in prostacyclin biosynthesis.[25] These processes will ultimately lead to an altered response to vasodilatory stimuli. Due to its powerful vasoconstrictory property, increased endothelin activity also appears to play a role in endothelial dysfunction.[26] In the early stages, functional alterations precede the morphological changes of the vessel wall,[15] but later structural damage may occur due to shift in phenotype of SMCs into a proliferative form and their consequent migration to the intima.[27] Persistent decrease in NO level is the major factor for the deteriorating atherosclerotic state of the vessel.[28]

Methods to Assess Endothelial Function

During recent decades, different techniques have been implemented to assess endothelial function of both peripheral and coronary arteries:

- Impedance plethysmography: the direct measurement of blood flow of an extremity. It has low reproducibility,[29] however, and thus it has not been extensively used.
- Positron emission tomography: an accurate but expensive noninvasive technique to assess basal and hyperemic flow.[30, 31] It is also dependent on oper-

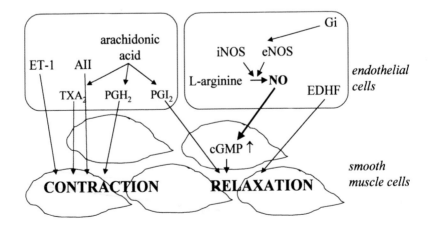

Figure 1. Basic mechanisms and factors involved in the development of endothelial dysfunction. ET-1 = endothelin-1; AII = angiotenzin II; TXA_2 = thromboxane-A_2; PGH_2 = prostaglandin-H_2; PGI_2 = prostaglandin-I_2 (prostacyclin); NO = nitric oxide; iNOS = inducible nitric oxide synthase; eNOS = endothelium-specific nitric oxide synthase; Gi = Gi subclass of G proteins; cGMP = cyclic GMP.

ator expertise and time consuming, hence it is not frequently used in clinical studies.

- Brachial ultrasound: a noninvasive method to measure the change of vessel diameter during reactive hyperemia, which causes flow-mediated vasodilatation (FMD) after a short period of obstruction of the forearm.[32] It is routinely applied in many laboratories due to its excellent feasibility and good reproducibility.[33]

Intracoronary Administration of Vasoactive Agents (Table 1)

The basal release of NO level is enhanced by acetylcholine (ACh), which was first demonstrated to administer safely into coronary vessels selectively.[34] Its effect on coronaries is two-faceted: acting on muscarinic receptors, it constricts the smooth muscle layer due to its cholinergic property and it mediates the release of NO,[23] and endothelium-derived hyperpolarizing factor[35] with signal transduction through G proteins. If stimulation of NO release prevails, it will result in endothelium-dependent vasodilatation in normal individuals. ACh-induced paradoxical vasoconstriction is one of the earliest manifestations of endothelial dysfunction.[36] One can detect the exact change of vessel diameter after ACh infusion by quantitative coronary angiography and the extent is related to the functional condition of that particular vessel segment.

Coronary blood flow, which could be reproducibly assessed by intracoronary Doppler wire,[37] increases in response to agonists, such as ACh or adenosine, and the magnitude of this increase can be used as a quantitative measure of endothelial function.

Endothelial Dysfunction after Balloon Angioplasty and Stent Implantation

Percutaneous transluminal coronary angioplasty (PTCA) has been an accepted treatment for coronary artery disease for many years.[38] There is experimental evidence[39] of the augmented production of endothelin immediately after balloon angio-

---

Table 1

Vasodilator Stimuli to Assess Endothelial Function

Endothelium-Dependent Pathway	Endothelium-Independent Pathway

Activating a receptor:
  Acetylcholine
  Bradykinin
  Substance P
"Flow-mediated vasodilation":
  Reactive hyperemia
  Exercise
  Cold pressor test
  Adenosine(?)
	Nitroglycerine
	Nitroprusside
	Papaverine
	Adenosine

plasty (BA); this peptide may cause vasoconstriction and also enhance the formation of neointima at the site of injury due to its mitogenic property.[40] In addition to this, angiotensin-converting enzyme and angiotensin II receptors are also up-regulated in the neointima[41]; possibly resulting in a long-lasting hypercontractile state of the vessel. Biochemical factors such as oxidative stress may also contribute to endothelial dysfunction due to persistent vasoconstriction by enhancing the breakdown of NO.[42] Table 2 lists important observations of studies investigating endothelial dysfunction after BA in animals and humans.

After the injury, endothelial cells regenerate and the lesion is covered by neoendothelium. Endothelial regrowth depends upon the extent of the lesion and the degree of intimal injury.[43] This process has the opposite effect on vascular healing: (1) Release of platelet-derived growth factor (PDGF) and PDGF-like proteins from these injured cells may further increase vasoconstriction[44] and contribute to the large intimal thickening observed after BA.[45] (2) In contrast, an increased expression of the endothelial NO synthase during proliferation has been demonstrated in cultured endothelial cells, which could have an impact on the inhibition of the proliferation of SMCs. Whether NO release may also occur in vivo remains to be investigated. However, porcine coronary arteries demonstrated progressive worsening of endothelium-dependent relaxation during the regeneration

Table 2

Studies Investigating Endothelial Dysfunction after Balloon Angioplasty

	Author	Set-up of the Study	Findings
Animal	Wang et al, 1996[39]	Rat carotid artery BA PCR to measure mRNA	ET-converting enzyme-1, ET-1,3 and their receptor expression↑
	Azuma et al, 1994[40]	Balloon denudation of carotid artery, plasma level of ET, and histology evaluation	ET level ↑ during 4 weeks of regeneration, associated with neointima formation
	Shimokawa et al, 1989[47]	Respective weeks after removal of coronary endothelium, serotonin, and platelet-induced relaxation	Endothelium-dependent relaxation worsened after regeneration of endothelium
	De Meyer et al, 1991[56]	Neointima formation induced, isometric tension, bioassay of NO	Dysfunctional segments at 7 days, ACh-induced NO-release↓
Human	Kruger et al, 1998[51]	Blood samples from the CS and a peripheral vein before and minute(s), and some hours after BA	ET levels↑, remained↑ during 3 hours of post-PTCA period and returned to normal at 6 hours
	el-Tamimi et al, 1993[54]	ic. ACh 8 days after BA, diameter of angioplasty and distal segment	Degments distal to the dilated site showed hyperreactivity to ACh
	Vassanelli et al, 1994[55]	3–6 months after BA luminal diameter changes after ic. ACh at proximal, distal, and angioplasty site	All the segments showed ↓ dose-related vasodilatation

BA = balloon angioplasty; PCR = polymerase chain reaction; ET = endothelin; NO = nitric oxide; Ach = acetylcholine; CS = coronary sinus.

process 4 to 24 weeks after removal of the endothelium.[46,47] This is also supported by the observations in animals[48,49] that regenerated endothelium was associated with persistent dysfunction manifesting in depressed vasoreactivity. Both the degree and the duration of the endothelial dysfunction appeared to be proportional to the severity of the injury.[48]

In the human, BA is mere damage impacted to the vessel wall causing denudation of the endothelial layer. It has been demonstrated that soon after balloon-induced injury, there is a release of von Willebrand factor[50] and endothelin.[51] This could be implicated as a mechanism for abnormal endothelium-dependent vasomotion, which has frequently been observed both immediately[52,53] and 8 days after PTCA.[54] Endothelial function still remained impaired at 3 to 6 months after BA at the site of remote injury in vivo.[55] In contrast, endothelium-independent vasodilatation by nitroglycerin was maintained. Although sufficient data are not available, the possible mechanisms for this long-lasting phenomena could be the persisting release of contracting factors[46] or impairment of endothelial muscarinic receptors.[56] Persisting endothelial dysfunction was also described following stent implantation.[57] Additionally, a recent report[58] described the micromorphological changes after BA and stenting; much of the described changes may contribute to the development of impaired vasomotion after BA. Contrary to these observations, only Suter et al reported that in some patients coronary vasomotion could normalize 4 to 30 months after BA.[59]

The Possible Link Between Endothelial Dysfunction and Restenosis

Endothelial dysfunction, one of the first changes in the etiology of atherosclerosis itself, may promote tissue growth.[1] After numerous investigations, it has been concluded that restenosis after BA is dictated by the interplay of constrictive remodeling (vessel shrinkage) and tissue growth.[60–62] Arterial remodeling in uninjured blood vessels has been established to be endothelium-dependent.[63] Flow alteration is also a major factor controlling remodeling.[64] However, the association between endothelial dysfunction and the development of restenosis has not yet been clearly clarified. In a report by Lafont et al,[65] a strong association between endothelial dysfunction and the presence of unfavorable remodeling has been described at 4-weeks follow-up after BA. In their rabbit coronary angioplasty model they found that functional (endothelium-dependent relaxation to ACh) and structural alterations (collagen accumulation) were both correlated with the severity of restenosis. Endothelium-independent vasodilator sodium nitroprusside was not associated with restenosis, underlying the pivotal role of endothelium in this process. The capacity to vasodilate in response to ACh was significantly more decreased in arteries with constrictive remodeling than in those with positive remodeling. Neointimal collagen density was also larger in a group with vessel shrinkage. Endothelial function and collagen density was an independent predictor of restenosis in this study.[65] In vitro studies have emphasized the possible role for NO in controlling SMC growth.[66, 67] Tronc et al[68] have shown that nitro-L-arginine methyl ester, by counteracting NO production, inhibits vessel enlargement. Chronic administration of NO donors was associated with a decreased restenosis rate in humans.[69] This observation would further support the hypothesis that decreased generation of NO in dysfunctional endothelium might be involved in restenosis. Thus, it is conceivable that the static decrease or the impaired capacity to raise concentration of NO is the major contributor to the link between endothelial dysfunction and restenosis, as demonstrated in Figure 2. We must add that whether endothelial dysfunction is a cause or a consequence of restenosis remains to be clarified.

Biological Response to Intracoronary Brachytherapy

Since radiotherapy had proven to be effective in treating the exuberant fibroelastic activity of keloid scar formation,[70] it was assumed that this adjunctive therapy would also inhibit coronary restenosis after BA. The first experimental study in this field was carried out in 1964 by Friedman and Byers, by the use of ^{192}Ir in the cholesterol-fed rabbit.[71] Since then, several clinical trials have been initiated with intracoronary ionizing radiation and it appears to be a promising new technique to prevent restenosis.[72–74] When radiation is absorbed into a tissue it can cause direct damage to DNA by ionization or indirectly by interacting with other molecules to produce free radicals. The affected cells lose their ability to proliferate, which will ultimately lead to their death.[75] Endothelial nuclear swelling was described in dogs[76] within 48 hours; intimal thickening subsequently occurred but reendothelialization was still not completed at 4 months.

After angioplasty, myofibroblasts in the adventitia proliferate and may migrate into the intima where they appear as smooth muscle actin-containing cells.[77,78] The effects of radiation on myofibroblast proliferation in the adventitia as well as on the vessel remodeling have been recently reported.[79] On the other hand, monocyte/macrophage/T cell populations, normally present in the adventitia are augmented in the immediate hours post angioplasty, and could be eliminated with moderate doses of radiation.[80] Thus, without an inflammatory response, the PDGF stimulus for inducing SMCs and/or fibroblasts to migrate and proliferate does not occur. Unlike intraluminal therapies, radiation is able to pen-

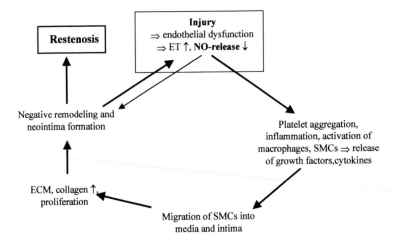

Figure 2. Processes linking endothelial dysfunction to the development of restenosis. ET = endothelin; NO = nitric oxide; SMCs = smooth muscle cells; ECM = extracellular matrix.

etrate the arterial wall and to reach and ablate the adventitial inflammatory cells.[81] Investigators from our center concluded that the beneficial effect of radiation in preventing restenosis might be partially explained by the positive influence of brachytherapy on the remodeling process.[82, 83]

Effect of Irradiation on Coronary Vasoreactivity

A number of studies have investigated the impact of radiation therapy on vasomotor function on peripheral arteries or using external, broadly focused sources. As early as 1970, Phillips reported[84] that after 10 Gy whole-body x-irradiation impaired the cold (-17 °C) tolerance of rats, probably due to damaged vasoconstrictor response. Endothelium-dependent (ACh) and endothelium-independent (nitroglycerin) dilator responses were both reported to be depressed in rat aortic segments 6 months after 15-Gy irradiation.[85] Other animal studies also showed dose- and time-dependent impairment of endothelial function after irradiation of peripheral arteries.[86, 87] On endothelium-denuded porcine coronaries, x-irradiation caused enhanced constriction to serotonin, histamine,[88] and also to ergonovine.[89]

The first study to evaluate coronary vasoreactivity in response to endovascular irradiation was performed by Wiedermann et al[90] in 1994. These investigators assessed vasomotor function of porcine coronary arteries acutely and 32 days after the delivery of high-dose (20 Gy) intracoronary γ-irradiation, with pathological analysis at follow-up. Changes in luminal area were measured by intravascular ultrasound. Irradiated segments acutely displayed vasoconstriction to ACh, with loss of smooth muscle response to nitroglycerin. Paradoxically, restudy revealed restoration of vasodilatory response to ACh but persistent loss of response to nitroglycerin (Fig. 3). Histopathology at 32 days detected minor neointima formation without luminal compromise and diffuse fibrosis of the SMC layer (Fig. 4). The authors concluded that medial fibrosis without significant endothelial dam-

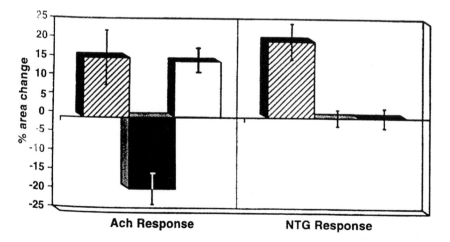

Figure 3. Vasomotor responses to graded infusions of intracoronary ACh (10^{-6} to 10^{-4} M) and bolus nitroglycerin (NTG; 200 μg) as assessed by intravascular ultrasound. Response is measured pre irradiation (hatched bars), immediately after irradiation (solid bars), and at follow-up (open bars; mean 32 days), in % area change. Error bars, SD. Reprinted with permission from Reference 90.

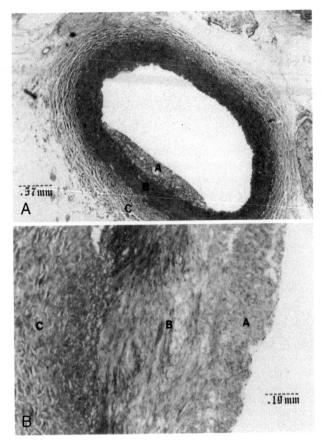

Figure 4. Masson's trichrome staining of irradiated segment of mid-LAD. Bottom: enlarged neointimal zone. **A:** neointima; **B:** smooth muscle layer with fibrosis; **C:** adventitia. Smooth muscle cells appear red; collagen is blue. Scale as indicated on photomicrograph. Reprinted with permission from Reference 90.

age could be achieved via this technique, and suggested that "intracoronary irradiation, therefore, may be an effective way of impairing the restenosis process."[90]

A recent publication[91] reported that PTCA and intracoronary irradiation altered the passive mechanical properties of porcine coronary arterial wall. Furthermore, at 6 weeks, receptor-operated release of endothelium-derived NO and hyperpolarizing factor was reduced by intracoronary irradiation and PTCA alone, respectively, and was prevented by their combination.

However in humans, the only observation available about the effect of brachytherapy on vasomotor function after BA is from the study by Sabate et al.[92] Patients enrolled in the Beta Energy Restenosis Trial (BERT-1.5) were included who underwent β-irradiation using $^{90}Sr/^{90}Y$-source receiving calculated mean dose of 5.2 ± 1.9 Gy at 90% of the adventitial and 8.2 ± 3.8 Gy at the luminal layer. Endothelial dysfunction was defined as a significant vasoconstriction detected by quantitative coronary angiography after the maximal dose of intracoronary ACh (10^{-6} mmol/l) at the scheduled 6-month follow-up. Surprisingly, as many as 89.5% of the irradiated segments demonstrated normal endothelial function (an example is shown in Fig. 5), in contrast to only 53% of the distal nonirradiated segments and 45% of that of control patients who had not received brachytherapy. Also, mean percentage of change in minimal luminal diameter after ACh was significantly higher in irradiated segments (3.8 ± 7.1% versus -6.6 ± 10% and -3.2 ± 7%, respectively [$P=0.01$], Fig. 6). Thus, this study demonstrated for the first time

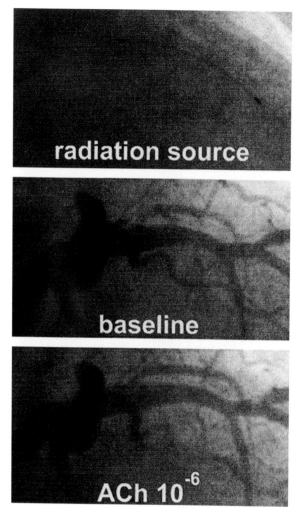

Figure 5. Coronary angiogram showing mild vasodilation in irradiated segment at 6-month follow-up. Reprinted with permission from Reference 92.

that the endothelium-dependent vasomotor function of coronary segments treated with BA followed by moderate dose (mean 5.2 Gy at the adventitia and 8.2 Gy at the luminal layer) of β-radiation could be improved in the majority of patient at 6-month follow-up. Moreover, this functional response observed in irradiated segments appeared to be better than in the control segments. These findings have confirmed the previous experimental observations by Wiedermann et al[90] in terms of restoration of endothelium-dependent vasomotion.

The Possible Mechanisms of Improvement of Endothelial Dysfunction after Brachytherapy

Finding a possible mechanism to explain the restoration of coronary function after intracoronary brachytherapy is still puzzling. As Sabate et al discussed,[92] the lack of paradoxical vasoconstriction was not likely due to damaged muscular media since it showed unaltered vasomotor response to nitroglycerin suggesting an absence of radiation-induced impairment of the medial layer. One of the plau-

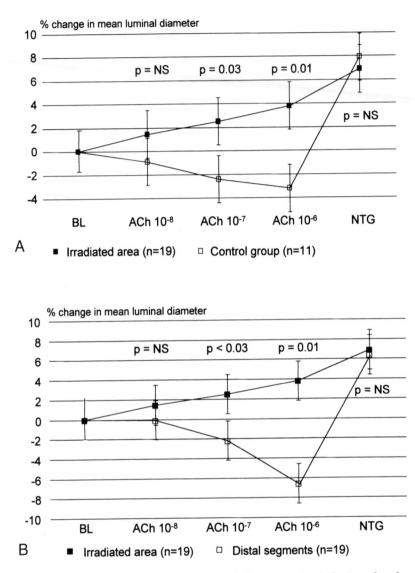

Figure 6. Percentage of change in mean luminal diameter after infusion of each substance in irradiated segments versus in control group **(A)** and versus distal segments **(B)**. BL indicates baseline. Modified with permission from Reference 92.

sible explanations is that, in a human cell culture model[93] endothelial cells appeared to be more radioresistant than vascular SMCs to the similarly moderate range of β-particle delivery which was also delivered in this study.

Wiedermann et al[90] interpreted their results that medial fibrosis interferes with the diffusion of nitroglycerin in such a way as to blunt its direct effects, whereas endothelial cells activated by ACh act through preferential anatomic or functional pathways on adjacent SMCs to produce vasodilatation. Alternatively, the irradiated SMCs may have an augmented sensitivity to ACh. Moreover, the existence of an NO-independent, endothelium-dependent mechanism for coronary vasodilatation has also been demonstrated,[94] and hence may serve as a basis for the observed characteristics of vasoreactivity in this study. Another possible mechanism for how radiation alters endothelial function, was shown in a porcine model of balloon overstretch injury after 18 Gy irradiation.[95] Expression of cytokine transforming growth factor-β_1 (TGF-β_1) was suppressed, which would enhance intimal hyperplasia and fibrosis by negatively modulating the expression of enzyme-inducible nitric oxide synthase (iNOS). It has been demonstrated that low dose radiation would induce an anti-inflammatory reaction through specific dose-dependent modulation of the NO pathway.[96]

As a conclusion, one might hypothesize that irradiation restores the capability of endothelium to response to NO, possibly permitting penetration of this to media, by inhibiting medial and intimal hyperplasia after BA. But to entirely elucidate the possible mechanism of improvement of endothelial function after brachytherapy would require further investigations. It remains to be investigated whether this chain reaction after radiation would result in a late reduction in restenosis rate. However, normalization of endothelial function may play an important role in this regard.

Future Perspectives

There are some directions indicated for future investigation. First, further histologic study could reveal details of alteration to the structure of irradiated segments. It was postulated that modification of the endothelial muscarinic receptors[56] was responsible for persistent impaired endothelium-dependent relaxation to ACh; therefore, it is possible that complete evaluation of cholinergic receptors affected by irradiation may confirm this concept. Second, further experimental studies are needed to clarify the influence of different doses of radiation on vasoreactivity, as there is growing information about intracoronary brachytherapy delivering various doses to different depth of coronaries may result in different clinical consequences.[97] Third, Doppler-tipped angioplasty guidewire allows the reliable measurement of adenosine-induced coronary flow velocity reserve (CFR),[98] and it has also correlated with long-term angiographic restenosis rate.[99] Since adenosine-induced vasodilatation has recently been suggested to be partly NO-dependent,[100,101] CFR may also carry information about endothelial function besides macro- and microvascular alterations. It is conceivable, that further study with intracoronary adenosine may clarify whether radiation improves CFR, revealing a possible way in which it ultimately modifies the restenotic process.

Summary

Endothelial dysfunction may play a role in the restenotic process after angioplasty and its normalization by means of intracoronary radiation therapy could be of utmost clinical importance. Providing more results in this respect and explaining the underlying mechanisms require further investigations.

References

1. Ross R. The pathogenesis of atherosclerosis: An update. N Engl J Med 1986;314:488–500.
2. Moncada S, Herman AG, Higgs EA, et al. Differential formation of prostacyclin (PGX

or PGI2) by layers of the arterial wall: An explanation for the anti-thrombotic properties of vascular endothelium. Thromb Res 1977;11:323–344.

3. Granger DN, Kubes P. Nitric oxide as antiinflammatory agent. Methods Enzymol 1996;269:434–442.

4. Ross R. Atherosclerosis: An inflammatory disease. N Engl J Med 1999;276:H663–H670.

5. Gimbrone MA Jr, Alexander RW. Angiotensin II stimulation of prostaglandin production in cultured human vascular endothelium. Science 1975;189:219–220.

6. Jaffe EA, Minick CR, Adelman B, et al. Synthesis of basement membrane by cultured human endothelial cells. J Exp Med 1976;144:209.

7. Furchgott RF, Zawadzki JV. The obligatory role of endothelial cells in the relaxation of smooth muscle by acetylcholine. Nature 1980;288:373–376.

8. Quyyumi AA, Dakak N, Andrews NP, et al. Nitric oxide activity in the human coronary circulation: Impact of risk factors for coronary atherosclerosis. J Clin Invest 1995;95:1747–1755.

9. Lie M, Sejersted OM, Kiil F. Local regulation of vascular cross section during changes in femoral arterial blood flow in dogs. Circ Res 1970;27:727.

10. Maatsson EJ, Kohler TR, Vergel SM, Clowes AW. Increased blood flow induces regression of intimal hyperplasia. Arterioscler Thromb Vasc Biol 1997;17:2245–2249.

11. Zeiher AM, Krause T, Schachinger V, et al. Impaired endothelium-dependent vasodilation of coronary resistance vessels is associated with exercise-induced myocardial ischemia. Circulation 1995;91:2345–2352.

12. Anderson TJ. Assessment and treatment of endothelial dysfunction in humans. J Am Coll Cardiol 1999;34:631–638.

13. Zeiher AM, Drexler H, Wollschlager H, Just H. Endothelial dysfunction of the coronary microvasculature is associated with impaired coronary blood flow regulation in patients with early atherosclerosis. Circulation 1991;84:1984–1992.

14. Vita JA, Treasure CB, Nabel EG, et al. Coronary vasomotor response to acetylcholine relates to risk factors for coronary artery disease. Circulation 1990;81:491–497.

15. Reddy KG, Nair RN, Sheehan HM, Hodgson JM. Evidence that selective endothelial dysfunction may occur in the absence of angiographic or ultrasound atherosclerosis in patients with risk factors for atherosclerosis. J Am Coll Cardiol 1994;23:833–843.

16. Schachinger V, Britten MB, Zeiher AM. Prognostic impact of coronary vasodilator dysfunction on adverse long-term outcome of coronary heart disease. Circulation 2000;101:1899–1906.

17. Panza JA. Endothelial dysfunction in essential hypertension. Clin Cardiol 1997;20(11 suppl 2):II-26–33.

18. Johnstone MT, Creager SJ, Scales KM, et al. Impaired endothelium-dependent vasodilation in patients with insulin-dependent diabetes mellitus. Circulation 1993;88:2510–2516.

19. Celermajer DS, Sorensen KE, Georgakopoulos D, et al. Cigarette smoking is associated with dose-related and potentially reversible impairment of endothelium-dependent dilation in healthy young adults. Circulation 1993;88(5 Pt 1):2149–2155.

20. Celermajer DS, Adams MR, Clarkson P, et al. Passive smoking and impaired endothelium-dependent arterial dilatation in healthy young adults. N Engl J Med 1996; 334:150–154.

21. Celermajer DS, Sorensen K, Ryalls M, et al. Impaired endothelial function occurs in the systemic arteries of children with homozygous homocystinuria but not in their heterozygous parents. J Am Coll Cardiol 1993;22:854–858.

22. Anderson TJ, Meredith IT, Uehata A, et al. Functional significance of intimal thickening as detected by intravascular ultrasound early and late after cardiac transplantation. Circulation 1993;88:1093–1100.

23. Flavahan N. Atherosclerosis or lipoprotein induced endothelial dysfunction: Potential mechanisms underlying reduction in EDRF/NO activity. Circulation 1992;85:1927–1938.

24. Oemar BS, Tschudi MR, Godoy N, et al. Reduced endothelial nitric oxide synthase expression and production in human atherosclerosis. Circulation 1998;97:2494–2998.

25. Beetens JR, Coene MC, Verheyen A, et al. Biphasic response of intimal prostacyclin production during the development of experimental atherosclerosis. Prostaglandins 1986;32:319–334.

26. Hasdai D, Holmes DR Jr, Garratt KN, et al. Mechanical pressure and stretch release

endothelin-1 from human atherosclerotic coronary arteries in vivo. Circulation 1997;95:357–362.

27. Ross R. The pathogenesis of atherosclerosis: A perspective for the 1990s. Nature 1993;362:801–809.

28. Cooke JP, Singer AH, Tsao P, et al. Antiatherogenic effects of L-arginine in the hypercholesterolemic rabbit. J Clin Invest 1992;90:1168–1172.

29. Creager MA, Cooke JP, Mendelsohn ME, et al. Impaired vasodilation of forearm resistance vessels in hypercholesterolemic humans. J Clin Invest 1990;86:228–234.

30. Gould KL. Clinical cardiac positron emission tomography: State of the art. Circulation 1991;84(suppl 3):I22–I36.

31. Uren NG, Melin JA, De Bruyne B, et al. Relation between myocardial blood flow and the severity of coronary artery stenosis. N Engl J Med 1994;330:1782–1788.

32. Celermajer DS, Sorensen KE, Gooch VM, et al. Non-invasive detection of endothelial dysfunction in children and adults at risk of atherosclerosis. Lancet 1992;340:1111–1115.

33. Uehata A, Lieberman EH, Gerhard MD, et al. Noninvasive assessment of endothelium-dependent flow-mediated dilation of the brachial artery. Vasc Med 1997;2:87–92.

34. Ludmer PL, Selwyn AP, Shook TL, et al. Paradoxical vasoconstriction induced by acetylcholine in atherosclerotic coronary arteries. N Engl J Med 1986;315:1046–1051.

35. Cohen RA, Vanhoutte PM. Endothelium-dependent hyperpolarization: Beyond nitric oxide and cyclic GMP. Circulation 1995;92:3337–3349.

36. Zeiher AM, Drexler H, Wollschlager H, Just H. Modulation of coronary vasomotor tone in humans: Progressive endothelial dysfunction with different early stages of coronary atherosclerosis. Circulation 1991;83:391–401.

37. Di Mario C, Gil R, Serruys PW. Long-term reproducibility of coronary flow velocity measurements in patients with coronary artery disease. Am J Cardiol 1995;75:1177–1180.

38. Mabin TA, Holmes DR Jr, Smith HC, et al. Follow-up clinical results in patients undergoing percutaneous transluminal coronary angioplasty. Circulation 1985;71:754–760.

39. Wang X, Douglas SA, Louden C, et al. Expression of endothelin-1, endothelin-3, endothelin-converting enzyme-1, and endothelin-A and endothelin-B receptor mRNA after angioplasty-induced neointimal formation in the rat. Circ Res 1996;78:322–328.

40. Azuma H, Hamasaki H, Niimi Y, et al. Role of endothelin-1 in neointima formation after endothelial removal in rabbit carotid arteries. Am J Physiol 1994;267(6 Pt 2):H2259–H2267.

41. Janiak P, Pillon A, Prost JF, Vilaine JP. Role of angiotensin subtype 2 receptor in neointima formation after vascular injury. Hypertension 1992;20:737–745.

42. Gryglewski RJ, Palmer RM, Moncada S. Superoxide anion is involved in the breakdown of endothelium-derived vascular relaxing factor. Nature 1986;320:454–456.

43. Lindner V, Reidy MA, Fingerle J. Regrowth of arterial endothelium: Denudation with minimal trauma leads to complete endothelial cell regrowth. Lab Invest 1989;61:556–563.

44. Berk BC, Alexander RW, Brock TA, et al. Vasoconstriction: A new activity for platelet-derived growth factor. Science 1986;232:87–90.

45. Jackson CL, Raines EW, Ross R, Reidy MA. Role of endogenous platelet-derived growth factor in arterial smooth muscle cell migration after balloon catheter injury. Arterioscler Thromb 1993;13:1218–1226.

46. Shimokawa H, Flavahan NA, Vanhoutte PM. Natural course of the impairment of endothelium-dependent relaxations after balloon endothelium removal in porcine coronary arteries: Possible dysfunction of a pertussis toxin-sensitive G protein. Circ Res 1989;65:740–753.

47. Shimokawa H, Flavahan NA, Shepherd JT, Vanhoutte PM. Endothelium-dependent inhibition of ergonovine-induced contraction is impaired in porcine coronary arteries with regenerated endothelium. Circulation 1989;80:643–650.

48. Weidinger FF, McLenachan JM, Cybulsky MI, et al. Persistent dysfunction of regenerated endothelium after balloon angioplasty of rabbit iliac artery. Circulation 1990;81:1667–1679.

49. Cox RH, Haas KS, Moisey DM, Tulenko TN. Effects of endothelium regeneration on canine coronary artery function. Am J Physiol 1989;257(5 Pt 2):H1681–H1692.

50. Blann A, Midgley H, Burrows G, et al. Free radicals, antioxidants, and endothelial cell damage after percutaneous transluminal coronary angioplasty. Coron Artery Dis 1993;4:905–910.

51. Kruger D, Giannitsis E, Sheikhzadeh A, Stierle U. Cardiac release and kinetics of endothelin after uncomplicated percutaneous transluminal coronary angioplasty. Am J Cardiol 1998;81:1421–1426.
52. Fischell TA, Nellessen U, Johnson DE, Ginsburg R. Endothelium-dependent arterial vasoconstriction after balloon angioplasty. Circulation 1989;79:899–910.
53. Fischell TA, Bausback KN, McDonald TV. Evidence for altered epicardial coronary artery autoregulation as a cause of distal coronary vasoconstriction after successful percutaneous transluminal coronary angioplasty. J Clin Invest 1990;86:575–584.
54. el-Tamimi H, Davies GJ, Crea F, Maseri A. Response of human coronary arteries to acetylcholine after injury by coronary angioplasty. J Am Coll Cardiol 1993;21:1152–1157.
55. Vassanelli C, Menegatti G, Zanolla L, et al. Coronary vasoconstriction in response to acetylcholine after balloon angioplasty: Possible role of endothelial dysfunction. Coron Artery Dis 1994;5:979–986.
56. De Meyer GR, Bult H, Van Hoydonck AE, et al. Neointima formation impairs endothelial muscarinic receptors while enhancing prostacyclin-mediated responses in the rabbit carotid artery. Circ Res 1991;68:1669–1680.
57. Caramori PR, Lima VC, Seidelin PH, et al. Long-term endothelial dysfunction after coronary artery stenting. J Am Coll Cardiol 1999;34:1675–1679.
58. van Beusekom HM, Whelan DM, Hofma SH, et al. Long-term endothelial dysfunction is more pronounced after stenting than after balloon angioplasty in porcine coronary arteries. J Am Coll Cardiol 1998;32:1109–1117.
59. Suter TM, Buechi M, Hess OM, et al. Normalization of coronary vasomotion after percutaneous transluminal coronary angioplasty? Circulation 1992;85:86–92.
60. Post MJ, Borst C, Kuntz RE. The relative importance of arterial remodeling compared with intimal hyperplasia in lumen renarrowing after balloon angioplasty: A study in the normal rabbit and the hypercholesterolemic Yucatan micropig. Circulation 1994;89:2816–2821.
61. Mintz GS, Pichard AD, Kent KM, et al. Intravascular ultrasound comparison of restenotic and de novo coronary artery narrowings. Am J Cardiol 1994;74:1278–1280.
62. Di Mario C, Gil R, Camenzind E, et al. Quantitative assessment with intracoronary ultrasound of the mechanisms of restenosis after percutaneous transluminal coronary angioplasty and directional coronary atherectomy. Am J Cardiol 1995;75:772–777.
63. Langille BL, Bendeck MP, Keeley FW. Adaptations of carotid arteries of young and mature rabbits to reduced carotid blood flow. Am J Physiol 1989;256(4 Pt 2):H931–H939.
64. Guyton JR, Hartley CJ. Flow restriction of one carotid artery in juvenile rats inhibits growth of arterial diameter. Am J Physiol 1985;248(4 Pt 2):H540–H546.
65. Lafont A, Durand E, Samuel JL, et al. Endothelial dysfunction and collagen accumulation: Two independent factors for restenosis and constrictive remodeling after experimental angioplasty. Circulation 1999;100:1109–1115.
66. Scott-Burden T, Vanhoutte PM. The endothelium as a regulator of vascular smooth muscle proliferation. Circulation 1993;87(suppl IV):V51–V55.
67. Garg UC, Hassid A. Nitric oxide-generating vasodilators and 8-bromo-cyclic guanosine monophosphate inhibit mitogenesis and proliferation of cultured rat vascular smooth muscle cells. J Clin Invest 1989;83:1774–1777.
68. Tronc F, Wassef M, Esposito B, et al. Role of NO in flow-induced remodeling of the rabbit common carotid artery. Arterioscler Thromb Vasc Biol 1996;16:1256–1262.
69. Lablanche JM, Grollier G, Lusson JR, et al. Effect of the direct nitric oxide donors linsidomine and molsidomine on angiographic restenosis after coronary balloon angioplasty: The ACCORD Study. Circulation 1997;95:83–89.
70. Kovalic JJ, Perez CA. Radiation therapy following keloidectomy: A 20-year experience. Int J Radiat Oncol Biol Phys 1989;17:77–80.
71. Friedman M, Felton L, Byers S. The antiatherogenic effect of iridium192 upon the cholesterol-fed rabbit. J Clin Invest 1964:43.
72. Wiedermann JG, Marboe C, Amols H, et al. Intracoronary irradiation markedly reduces restenosis after balloon angioplasty in a porcine model. J Am Coll Cardiol 1994;23:1491–1498.
73. Waksman R, Robinson KA, Crocker IR, et al. Intracoronary low-dose beta-irradiation inhibits neointima formation after coronary artery balloon injury in the swine restenosis model. Circulation 1995;92:3025–3031.

74. Verin V, Popowski Y, Urban P, et al. Intra-arterial beta irradiation prevents neointimal hyperplasia in a hypercholesterolemic rabbit restenosis model. Circulation 1995;92:2284–2290.
75. Hall EJ MR, Miller RC, Brenner DJ. The basic radiobiology of intravascular irradiation. In: Waksman R (ed.): Vascular Brachytherapy, 2nd Edition. Armonk, NY: Futura Publishing Co.; 1999:63–72.
76. Fonkalsrud EW, Sanchez M, Zerubavel R, Mahoney A. Serial changes in arterial structure following radiation therapy. Surg Gynecol Obstet 1977;145:395–400.
77. Willems IE, Havenith MG, De Mey JG, Daemen MJ. The alpha-smooth muscle actin-positive cells in healing human myocardial scars. Am J Pathol 1994;145:868–875.
78. Scott NA, Cipolla GD, Ross CE, et al. Identification of a potential role for the adventitia in vascular lesion formation after balloon overstretch injury of porcine coronary arteries. Circulation 1996;93:2178–2187.
79. Waksman R, Rodriguez JC, Robinson KA, et al. Effect of intravascular irradiation on cell proliferation, apoptosis, and vascular remodeling after balloon overstretch injury of porcine coronary arteries. Circulation 1997;96:1944–1952.
80. Rubin P, Williams J. The paradox and puzzle of radiation to inhibit vascular restenosis. Cellular and molecular mechanisms of radiation inhibiton of restenosis: Is there a therapeutic window? Vascular Brachytherapy: New Perspectives. Remedica Publishing; 1999:26.
81. Wilcox JN, Waksman R, King SB, Scott NA. The role of the adventitia in the arterial response to angioplasty: The effect of intravascular radiation. Int J Radiat Oncol Biol Phys 1996;36:789–796.
82. Sabate M, Serruys PW, van der Giessen WJ, et al. Geometric vascular remodeling after balloon angioplasty and beta-radiation therapy: A three-dimensional intravascular ultrasound study. Circulation 1999;100:1182–1188.
83. Costa MA, Sabate M, Serrano P, et al. The effect of 32P beta-radiotherapy on both vessel remodeling and neointimal hyperplasia after balloon angioplasty and stenting: A three-dimensional intravascular ultrasound investigation. J Invas Cardiol 2000;12:113–120.
84. Phillips RD. Mechanisms of injury for radiation-induced decrease in cold tolerance. J Appl Physiol 1970;28:821–825.
85. Menendez JC, Casanova D, Amado JA, et al. Effects of radiation on endothelial function. Int J Radiat Oncol Biol Phys 1998;41:905–913.
86. Qi F, Sugihara T, Hattori Y, et al. Functional and morphological damage of endothelium in rabbit ear artery following irradiation with cobalt 60. Br J Pharmacol 1998;123:653–660.
87. Bourlier V, Diserbo M, Joyeux M, et al. Early effects of acute gamma-radiation on vascular arterial tone. Br J Pharmacol 1998;123:1168–1172.
88. Mitsuoka W, Egashira S, Tagawa H, et al. Augmentation of coronary responsiveness to serotonin at the site of X-ray-induced intimal thickening in miniature pigs. Cardiovasc Res 1995;30:246–254.
89. Egashira S, Mitsuoka W, Tagawa H, et al. Mechanisms of ergonovine-induced hyperconstriction of coronary artery after x-ray irradiation in pigs. Basic Res Cardiol 1995;90:167–175.
90. Wiedermann JG, Leavy JA, Amols H, et al. Effects of high-dose intracoronary irradiation on vasomotor function and smooth muscle histopathology. Am J Physiol 1994;267(1 Pt 2):H125–H132.
91. Thorin E, Meerkin D, Bertrand OF, et al. Influence of postangioplasty beta-irradiation on endothelial function in porcine coronary arteries. Circulation 2000;101:1430–1435.
92. Sabate M, Kay IP, van der Giessen WJ, et al. Preserved endothelium-dependent vasodilation in coronary segments previously treated with balloon angioplasty and intracoronary irradiation. Circulation 1999;100:1623–1629.
93. Fareh J, Martel R, Kermani P, Leclerc G. Cellular effects of beta-particle delivery on vascular smooth muscle cells and endothelial cells: A dose-response study. Circulation 1999;99:1477–1484.
94. Cowan CL, Cohen RA. Two mechanisms mediate relaxation by bradykinin of pig coronary artery: NO-dependent and -independent responses. Am J Physiol 1991;261(3 Pt 2):H830–H835.

95. Vodovotz Y, Waksman R. Potential roles for nitirc oxide and transforming growth factor-β1 in endovascular brachytherapy. In: Waksman R (ed.): Vascular Brachytherapy, 2nd Edition. Armonk NY: Futura Publishing Co.; 1999:139–146.

96. Hildebrandt G, Seed MP, Freemantle CN, et al. Mechanisms of the anti-inflammatory activity of low-dose radiation therapy. Int J Radiat Biol 1998;74:367–378.

97. Carlier SG, Crocker I, Sabate M, et al. Correlation between dose deposited to the vessel wall and outcomes following intracoronary beta-radiation. Circulation 1999;100(I):516.

98. de Bruyne B, Bartunek J, Sys SU, et al. Simultaneous coronary pressure and flow velocity measurements in humans: Feasibility, reproducibility, and hemodynamic dependence of coronary flow velocity reserve, hyperemic flow versus pressure slope index, and fractional flow reserve. Circulation 1996;94:1842–1849.

99. Serruys PW, di Mario C, Piek J, et al. Prognostic value of intracoronary flow velocity and diameter stenosis in assessing the short- and long-term outcomes of coronary balloon angioplasty: The DEBATE Study (Doppler Endpoints Balloon Angioplasty Trial Europe). Circulation 1997;96:3369–3377.

100. Jones CJ, Kuo L, Davis MJ, et al. Role of nitric oxide in the coronary microvascular responses to adenosine and increased metabolic demand. Circulation 1995;91:1807–1813.

101. Smits P, Williams SB, Lipson DE, et al. Endothelial release of nitric oxide contributes to the vasodilator effect of adenosine in humans. Circulation 1995;92:2135–2141.

Late Total Occlusion Following Intracoronary Brachytherapy

Ron Waksman, MD

Introduction

Vascular brachytherapy is effective in preventing restenosis. Pre-clinical studies utilizing both beta and gamma emitters have shown a reduction of smooth muscle proliferation, prevention of late contraction, and a delayed healing response following vascular injury.[1-4]

An important clinical application of vascular brachytherapy is an adjunct therapy for the treatment of in-stent restenosis. Several studies, including three randomized trials, have shown a reduction in recurrent in-stent restenosis of 50 to 70% compared to conventional therapy.[5-9] However, radiation has been reported to induce thrombosis. Previous studies on the vascular effects of external beam radiation have suggested that increased thrombosis is a complication of delayed healing.[10,11]

Thrombotic occlusion following balloon angioplasty usually occurs either immediately or within 24 hours following intervention. Stents are more often associated with subacute thrombosis (within 30 days of implantation) which is well controlled using antiplatelet therapy for 15 days.[12-15] Among the complications associated with vascular brachytherapy is the phenomenon of late coronary thrombosis (>30 days).[16-18]

Definition and Nomenclature

Acute thrombosis occurs during the early post-intervention period, and subacute thrombosis occurs within the subsequent 30 days; both usually present with unstable symptoms and angiographic evidence of thrombus. However, the definition of late thrombosis may be problematic; it may not present with symptoms or visible thrombus and may be detected only by follow-up angiogram as late total occlusion, which could be attributed to progressive intimal hyperplasia (a different mechanism of action). Therefore, we cannot differentiate between late thrombosis to late total occlusion without a clinical event or evidence of angiographic thrombus. Late total occlusion/thrombosis is usually defined as any angiographically documented total occlusion more than 30 days after the procedure. For pa-

From Waksman R (ed.). *Vascular Brachytherapy, Third Edition.* Armonk, NY: Futura Publishing Co., Inc.; © 2002.

tients who have a patent treatment site at 6 months and subsequently develop thrombosis, we propose the term "late late thrombosis."

Is Late Thrombosis a Known Phenomenon Post Conventional PTCA or Stenting?

The literature identifies high risk patients who presented with late reocclusion following conventional percutaneous transluminal coronary angioplasty (PTCA) as: (1) total occlusions treated with stenting are reported to have 7% recurrence rate of late total occlusion at 6 months[19]; and (2) treatment of an infarcted related vessel is associated with 30% reocclusion rate following thrombolytic therapy at 3 months[14] and up to 17% of reocclusion after PTCA at 6 months.[15] The majority of these events were clinically silent and the proposed etiologies were rethrombosis or progressive narrowing. Patients treated with stents and ticlopidine rarely present with late thrombosis. Colombo et al reported 0.6% late thrombosis rate 3 to 6 months following stenting.[12] However, greater than 7% of patients presented to the Washington Hospital Center with in-stent restenosis also had total occlusion of the stented segment prior to the intervention.

Late Thrombosis in Clinical Radiation Trials

The first question is, "Does late thrombosis occur in other radiation clinical trials?" Feasibility trials typically include highly selective small cohorts of patients, usually lack control groups, and have nonuniform anticoagulation/antithrombotic drug regimens; thus, complications that occur in less than 10% of patients can be easily missed.

We reviewed the reported cases of late thrombosis/occlusion for each of the completed and published feasibility radiation studies. A discussion of this review follows.

Condado et al treated 21 patients with gamma radiation (iridium 192 following balloon angioplasty with doses that exceeded 55 Gy to the near wall) and discharged all patients with aspirin and coumadin for a period of 3 months. Two patients developed silent thrombosis (at 30 and 38 days post treatment) without electrocardiographic evidence of myocardial infarction (MI). One of these patients had primary total occlusion and the other had a severe post-PTCA dissection prior to radiation.[5] None of the other 19 patients had late total occlusion at 2-year angiographic follow-up.[20]

Verin and coworkers treated 15 patients applying β-radiation (yttrium 90) following balloon angioplasty of de novo lesions. Patients were discharged with aspirin as the sole antiplatelet therapy. At 6 months, none of the patients had clinical or angiographic evidence of thrombosis; but one asymptomatic patient had total occlusion.[21]

In BERT, 23 patients with de novo lesions who were treated with balloon angioplasty alone were assigned to intracoronary radiation therapy with 90-strontium/yttrium (a pure beta emitter). Patients were discharged with no antiplatelet agent other than aspirin. At 6 months, only one patient presented with a late total occlusion.[7] Conversely, in the middle of the Beta Cath Study[22]–a randomized study which utilized the same radiation system, the same prescription dose, and the same antiplatelet regimen as BERT–the data safety monitoring committee advised a change in the antithrombotic regimen of the provisional stent arm to 3 months of ticlopidine due to an excess of late thrombosis in one of the treated groups.

In the SCRIPPS Trial, 55 patients with restenosis were randomized to placebo (n=29) versus iridium 192 (n=26) and were discharged with ticlopidine and aspirin for 3 months *only* if new stents were implanted.[6] At 2 years there were two MIs associated with deaths at the placebo group while only one patient from the irradiated group developed stent thrombosis and MI at day 18 due to early cessation of ticlopidine.[21]

In the WRIST Study (Table 1), patients with in-stent restenosis were randomized to either placebo or radioactive iridium 192 seeds after conventional treatment of in-stent restenosis. The anticoagulation protocol for all patients was aspirin and ticlopidine for 1 month. Late total occlusion (at 6 months) was documented in 5 of 65 (7.7%) patients in the irradiated group (2 were asymptomatic) versus 3 of 65 (4.6%) in the control group (all symptomatic).[8]

In BETA WRIST, 50 patients with in-stent restenosis in native arteries were treated with β-radiation (yttrium 90) and discharged with the same anticoagulation as in WRIST. At 6-month angiographic follow-up, late total occlusion was documented in 5 patients (10%); 2 were asymptomatic.[23]

Information from other radiation trials (ie, GAMMA1, LONG WRIST, SVG WRIST, PREVENT) suggest that late occlusion is present as well, and that the rate varied from 6% to 10%. In the study by Costa et al,[17] the late thrombosis in a cohort of 105 patients from the Thoraxcenter, Rotterdam, The Netherlands, was 6.6%.

In reviewing records of 473 patients at the Washington Hospital Center, Washington, D.C., who presented with in-stent restenosis and who were enrolled in various radiation protocols, whether randomized to placebo versus radiation or entered into registries, there were 165 placebo and 308 radiated patients, including both γ and β emitters. Maximum dose to the vessel wall was 30 to 55 Gy. Following radiation, all patients received antiplatelet therapy with aspirin and either ticlopidine or clopidogrel for 1 month. All patients completed at least 6-months angiographic follow-up. Late total occlusion was documented in 28 pa-

Table 1

Rate of Late Total Occlusion by Studies, Emitters, and Doses

Study	Emitter	Dose (Gy)	Late Total Occlusion Rate	
			Treated	Control
WRIST	[192]Ir	15 at 2 mm	10/104 (9.6%)	2/65 (3.1%)
GAMMA 1	[192]Ir	8–30 by IVUS	3/20 (15%)	0/20 (0%)
ARTISTIC	[192]Ir	15 at 2 mm	2/24 (8.3%)	0/8 (0%)
SVG WRIST	[192]Ir	15 at 2 mm	1/27 (3.7%)	0/27 (0%)
LONG WRIST	[192]Ir	15 at 2 mm	4/45 (8.8%)	0/45 (0%)
High Dose WRIST	[192]Ir	15 at 2.4 mm	2/29 (6.9%)	*
BETA WRIST	[90]Y	20.6 at 1 mm	4/49 (8.1%)	*
PREVENT	[32]P	20–24 at 1mm	2/10 (20.0%)	0/5 (0%)
Total	All	**Any**	**28/308 (9.1%)**	**2/165 (1.2%)**

*Registries in which all patients received radiation.

tients (9.1%) from the irradiated group versus 2 placebo patients (1.2%, $P<0.0001$). Late total occlusion (LTO) rates were similar across studies and emitters. LTO in the irradiated group presented as acute MI in 12 patients (43%), unstable angina in 14 (50%), and asymptotic in 2 (7%). Mean time to LTO was 5.4 ± 3.2 months in the irradiated group versus 4.5 ± 2.1 in placebo patients ($P=$NS). The overall rate of re-stenting for the entire study group at the time of radiation was 48.6%. Importantly, new stents were placed in 82% of the irradiated and in 100% of the placebo patients *who presented with LTO*. Multivariate logistic regression analysis was performed for the patients in the various WRIST studies. New stenting (odds ratio=2.55, 95% confidence interval=1.0 to 5.1, $P=0.04$) and long lesions (odds ratio=1.15, confidence interval=1.0 to 1.2, $P=0.04$) were found to be the predictors for late thrombosis.[18]

Delayed Healing and /or Platelet Recruitment

The second question is, "Why does late thrombosis occur?" Is it the patient, the stent, the operator, or the radiation? Potential causes for late thrombosis are listed in Table 2.

Late thrombosis, not neointimal hyperplasia, is probably the major etiology for late total occlusion following intracoronary radiation therapy. While not absolutely conclusive, the evidence is as follows.

Ionizing radiation inhibits neointima formation following vascular injury as shown in numerous studies in the porcine model of restenosis.[24,25] Most cases of radiation treatment failure are focal (ie, edge stenosis), not diffuse progressive occlusive disease.

The majority of patients with late total occlusion following radiation therapy presented with acute events similar to subacute thrombosis.

There is increased evidence from the animal studies that radiation *induces* thrombosis and that the thrombosis rate is related to the dose. Our studies showed luminal thrombi after radiation consisting mostly of fibrin and less organized than thrombus found in nonirradiated arteries after vascular injury. Furthermore, thrombi present in irradiated arteries lacked cells thought to be involved in the healing response to arterial injury (monocytes, lymphocytes, and macrophages) may prolong the platelet residence and delay thrombus organization.[24] Others demonstrated that thrombosis is a dose-dependent recruitment of platelets at the site of injury and irradiation.[25]

Stents may increase the risk of late thrombosis by being more thrombogenic and radiation may further delay compete reendothelialization. Delayed healing

---

Table 2

Potential Causes of Late Thrombosis Following Radiation

- Delayed reendothelialization
- Fibrin deposition and platelet recruitment
- Impaired vasoreactivity and spasm
- Tissue erosion around the stent
- Unhealed dissection

---

was seen at 12 weeks with the radioactive stent. It is possible that the new endothelium may be dysfunctional, causing arterial spasm and flow impairment.

Unhealed dissections were also seen (both angiographically and by intravascular ultrasound at 6-months follow-up) in some patients who were treated with balloon angioplasty and intracoronary radiation.[26]

A different explanation is required for the striking phenomenon of late late thrombosis seen many months after a patent artery was documented at 6-month angiographic follow-up. At this time we do not know the incidence, time, or mechanism of this new phenomenon, nor how to prevent it.

Is it possible that there is gradual erosion of tissue surrounding the stent, leaving the stent unopposed to the vessel wall, which will serve as a nidus for thrombosis. The intravascular ultrasound studies of patients who underwent radiation in the WRIST studies demonstrated reduction of in-stent neointimal tissue at follow-up in more than 50%. This could be paralleled by a reduction in the peri-stent tissue causing the stents to become unopposed to the vessel wall.

Clinical Implications and Therapeutic Strategy

The immediate solution to the problem of late thrombosis is prolonged antiplatelet therapy (minimum of 3 months). Adjunct antiplatelet therapy with ticlopidine proved to be effective in reducing the acute and subacute thrombosis in the Stent Arterial Anticoagulation Regimen Study (STARS).[27] Now, the important questions are: (1) whether prolonged antiplatelet therapy for patients treated with intracoronary radiation will be effective; and (2) what will be the duration of prolonged antiplatelet therapy? The recent beta clinical trials, START[28] and INHIBIT,[29] (Table 3) for patients with in-stent restenosis, have used at least 3 months of clopidogrel and demonstrated that this therapy is effective in reducing the thrombosis rate to background levels. Three gamma studies for patients with in-stent restenosis were designed to test the effectiveness of prolonged antiplatelet therapy with 6 to 12 months of clopidogrel and demonstrated a reduction in the late thrombosis event rate. SCRIPPS III enrolled 500 patients and reported no late thrombosis with this regimen. WRIST PLUS, with 6 months of clopidogrel, included 120 consecutive patients with diffuse in-stent restenosis in native

Table 3

Rate of Late Thrombosis with the Use of Prolonged Antiplatelet Therapy (>3 months) after Radiation Therapy for In-Stent Restenosis

Study	Emitter	Dose (Gy)	Late Total Occlusion Rate	
			Treated	Control
START	^{90}Sr/Y	16–20 at 2mm	0/232 (0.0%)	0/244 (0.0%)
INHIBIT	^{32}P	20 at 1.0mm	3/166 (1.8%)	1/166 (0.6%)
WRIST PLUS	^{192}Ir	14 at 2 mm	3/120 (2.5%)	
SCRIPPS III	^{192}Ir	14 at 2 mm	0/500 (0.0%)	
START 40/20	^{90}Sr/Y	16–20 at 2mm	2/137 (1.5%)	
BRITE	^{32}P	20 at1.0 mm	0/27 (0.0%)	

coronaries and vein grafts with lesions less than 80 mm in length who underwent PTCA, laser ablation, and rotational atherectomy. Additional stenting was placed in 34 (28.3%) patients. Patients were followed clinically and angiographically at 6 months. The late total occlusion and thrombosis rates were compared with the γ-treated and the placebo groups (250 patients) of the WRIST and LONG WRIST studies. Clopidogrel was tolerated well except for one patient and there was no report of leukopenia. At 6 months, the overall rate of total occlusion was 5.6%, and the late thrombosis rate of 2.5% with prolonged antiplatelet therapy was significantly lower compared to the active γ group of the WRIST studies, and similar to the historical placebo groups. Gamma V has completed enrollment of 600 patients treated with iridium 192 for in-stent restenosis who received Plavix (clopidogrel) for either 6 to 12 months after percutaneous coronary intervention without stent or if a new stent was placed during the intervention. So far, the results of these studies suggest that prolonged antiplatelet therapy has a protective effect and prevents the late thrombosis phenomenon. The question that requires further follow-up is, "Is 6 months enough, or should these patients take clopidogrel for life?" Also, should we use other strategies to minimize the late thrombosis effect, such the use of IIB/ IIIA inhibitors, heparin-coated stents, or other protective agents?

Nevertheless, the risk of thrombosis after radiation has been proven. The immediate solutions are to minimize re-stenting and to administer prolonged antiplatelet therapy, which will add cost to the overall procedure.

References

1. Wiedermann JG, Marboe C, Amols H, et al. Intracoronary irradiation markedly reduces restenosis after balloon angioplasty in a porcine model. J Am Coll Cardiol 1994;23:1491–1498.
2. Waksman R, Robinson KA, Crocker IR, et al. Endovascular low-dose irradiation inhibits neointima formation after coronary artery balloon injury in swine: A possible role for radiation therapy in restenosis prevention. Circulation 1995;91:1533–1539.
3. Waksman R, Robinson KA, Crocker IR, et al. Intracoronary low-dose β-irradiation inhibits neointima formation after coronary artery balloon injury in the swine restenosis model. Circulation 1995;92:3025–3031.
4. Waksman R, Rodriquez JC, Robinson KA, et al. Effect of intravascular irradiation on cell proliferation, apoptosis and vascular remodeling after balloon overstretch injury of porcine coronary arteries. Circulation 1997;96:1944–1952.
5. Condado JA, Waksman R, Gurdiel O, et al. Long-term angiographic and clinical outcome after percutaneous transluminal coronary angioplasty and intracoronary radiation therapy in humans. Circulation 1997;96:727–732.
6. Teirstein PS, Massullo V, Jani S, et al. Catheter-based radiotherapy to inhibit restenosis after coronary stenting. N Engl J Med 1997;336:1697–1703.
7. King SB, Williams DO, Chougule P, et al. Endovascular beta-radiation to reduce restenosis after coronary balloon angioplasty: Results of the beta energy restenosis trial (BERT). Circulation 1998;97:2025–2030.
8. Waksman R, White RL, Chan RC, et al. Intracoronary gamma radiation therapy after angioplasty inhibits recurrence in patients with in-stent restenosis. Circulation 2000;101:2165–2171.
9. Leon MB, Teirstein PS, Lansky AJ, et al. Intracoronary gamma radiation to reduce in-stent restenosis: The multicenter GAMMA 1 randomized clinical trial [abstract]. J Am Coll Cardiol 1999;33:56A.
10. Stewart JR, Fajardo LF, Gillette SM, Constine LS. Radiation injury to the heart. Int J Radiat Oncol Biol Phys 1995;31:1205–1211.

11. Grollier G, Commeau P, Mercier V, et al. Post-radiotherapeutic left main coronary ostial stenosis: Clinical and histological study. Eur Heart J 1988;9:567–570.
12. Colombo A, Hall P, Makamura S, et al. Intracoronary stenting without anticoagulation accomplished with intravascular guidance. Circulation 1995;91:1676–1688.
13. Wilson SH, Rihal CS, Bell MR, et al. Timing of coronary stent thrombosis in patients treated with ticlopidine and aspirin. Am J Cardiol 1999;83:1006–1011.
14. Meijer AS, Verheugt FWA, Werter CJPJ, et al. Aspirin versus coumadin in the prevention of reocclusion and recurrent ischemia after successful thrombolysis: A prospective placebo-controlled angiographic study. Circulation 1993;87:1524–1530
15. Bauters C, Delomez M, Van Belle E, et al. Angiographically documented late reocclusion after successful coronary angioplasty of an infarct related lesion is a powerful predictor of long-term mortality. Circulation 1999;99:2243–2250.
16. Waksman R. Late thrombosis after radiation: Sitting on a time bomb. Circulation 1999;100:780–782.
17. Costa MA, Sabate M, van der Giessen WJ, et al. Late coronary occlusion after intracoronary brachytherapy. Circulation 1999;100:789–792.
18. Waksman R, Bhargava B, Mintz GS, et al. Late total occlusion after intracoronary brachytherapy for patients with in-stent restenosis. J Am Coll Cardiol 2000;36:65–68.
19. Rau T, Schofer J, Schluter M, et al. Stenting of nonacute total coronary occlusions: Predictors of late angiographic outcome. J Am Coll Cardiol 1998;31:275–280.
20. Condado JA, Waksman R, Calderas C, et al. Two-year follow-up after intracoronary gamma radiation therapy. Cardiovasc Radiat Med 1999;11:30–35.
21. Verin V, Urban P, Popowski Y, et al. Feasibility of intracoronary beta-irradiation to reduce restenosis after balloon angioplasty: A clinical pilot study. Circulation 1997;95:1138–1144.
22. Teirstein PS, Massullo V, Jani S, et al. Two-year follow-up after catheter-based radiotherapy to inhibit coronary restenosis. Circulation 1999;99:243–247.
23. Waksman R, White RL, Chan RC, et al. Intracoronary beta radiation therapy inhibits recurrence of in-stent restenosis. Circulation 2000;101:1895–1898.
24. Vodovotz Y, Waksman R, Kim WH, et al. Effects of intracoronary radiation on thrombosis following balloon overstretch injury in the porcine model. Circulation 1999;100:2527–2533.
25. Salame M, Lampkin J, Mulkey P, et al. Effects of endovascular irradiation on platelet recruitment at site of balloon angioplasty in pig coronary arteries [abstract]. J Am Coll Cardiol 1999;33:44A.
26. Meerkin D, Tardif JC, Crocker IR, et al. Effects of intracoronary beta-radiation therapy after coronary angioplasty: An intravascular ultrasound study. Circulation 1999;99:1660–1665.
27. Leon MB, Baim DS, Popma JJ, et al. A clinical trial comparing three antithrombotic-drug regimens after coronary artery stenting. N Engl J Med 1998;339:1665–1671.
28. Lansky AJ, et al. START 40/20. Late Breaking Clinical Trial: Oral Presentation. Transcatheter Cardiovascular Therapeutics Symposium. October 2000.
29. Waksman R, Raizner A, Lansky AJ, et al. Beta radiation to inhibit recurrence of in-stent restenosis: Study design, device and dosimetry details of the multicenter randomized double blind study. Circulation 2000;102:II-667.

## Chapter 15

Effects of External Beam Radiation on the Human Heart and Great Vessels

Renu Virmani, MD, and Andrew Farb, MD

Introduction

Interest in the effects of external beam radiation therapy on the human heart and great vessels following treatment for thoracic malignancies has been rekindled because of the use of β- and γ-radiation delivered via catheter-based systems to treat coronary artery atherosclerosis and restenosis. To date, intravascular brachytherapy has shown promise in reducing restenosis rates at 6-months to 3-years follow-up in a limited number of patients.[1,2] However, several problems associated with intravascular radiation therapy have emerged from experimental and clinical studies. Animal studies utilizing coronary artery brachytherapy via source wires or stents have demonstrated delayed intimal healing and accelerated atherosclerosis.[3,4] Early reports from two β-radiation trials show a higher rate of subacute arterial thrombosis in vessels treated with radiation (6.6% and 9.1%) than in nonradiated vessels (<1%).[5,6] Patients treated with low dose ^{32}P β-emitting stents have little in-stent neointimal formation, but significant luminal narrowing proximal and/or distal to the stent (candy wrapper effect) has been observed. Therefore, more work is needed to define optimal isotopes, dosimetry, and delivery systems before intravascular brachytherapy can be endorsed for widespread application in coronary interventions.

Pathology of Radiation-Induced Pericardial, Myocardial, Endocardial, and Valvular Heart Disease

Since the 1960s, radiation-induced heart disease has been known to occur following therapeutic irradiation of adjacent neoplasms.[7,8] It has been well documented in humans that the pericardium, myocardium, endocardium, valves, conduction system, coronary arteries, and aorta and its major branches may be affected by mediastinal radiation.[7,9–12] The pericardium is the most frequent car-

The opinions or assertions contained herein are the private views of the authors and are not to be construed as official or reflecting the views of the Department of the Army, the Department of the Air Force, or the Department of Defense.
From Waksman R (ed.). *Vascular Brachytherapy, Third Edition.* Armonk, NY: Futura Publishing Co., Inc.; © 2002.

diac structure involved in radiation cardiotoxicity, and pathological findings are observed in 70% of cases evaluated at autopsy.[9] The sequence of pericardial damage advances from pericardial effusion, to fibrinous pericarditis, pericardial fibrosis, and finally constrictive pericarditis. The pericardial effusion is typically protein-rich,[13] and fluid accumulation may be abundant leading to pericardial tamponade.[8,13,14] In fibrinous pericarditis, fibrin layers are deposited on the mesothelial surfaces and within the stroma of the pericardium.[8,13,15] In late stages of post-radiation pericardial damage (Fig. 1), there are always pericardial adhesions, but the mechanisms underlying the fibrosis are poorly understood.[7,16] The mean radiation dose leading to constrictive pericarditis reported in one study was 4400 rads, and the mean time from radiation treatment to symptoms was 58 months.[9] Patients with pericardial effusion present within 15 months, whereas patients with constriction usually present after 48 months.[9]

Radiation-associated myocardial toxicity is less frequently seen than pericardial involvement and consists of patchy fibrosis usually involving the anterior left ventricular wall.[7,13] The myocardial fibrosis (Fig. 2A) is often diffuse with areas of interstitial fibrosis surrounding individual myocytes or groups of myocytes,[7,11,13] but neither myocyte hypertrophy nor transmural fibrosis occur secondary to radiation injury.[13] Myocardial necrosis is usually not observed.[9] Myocardial damage following radiation is dose-dependent and is greatest in patients who received greater than 3000 rads (>30 Gy); it is typically detected after a latency period of greater than 36 months.[9,13]

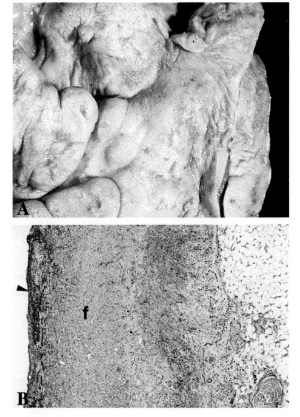

Figure 1. Fibrous and fibrinous pericarditis in a 26-year-old male treated with mediastinal radiation therapy for Hodgkin's disease 6.5 years prior to death. The anterior surface of the heart received 4185 rads and the posterior surface 3000 rads. At autopsy, a 200-mL pericardial effusion was present. Grossly, the visceral pericardial surface of the heart **(A)** was diffusely thickened. A histologic section **(B)** shows pericardial fibrin deposition (arrowhead) with underlying marked fibrosis **(f)** of the epicardium. Reproduced with permission from Reference 48.

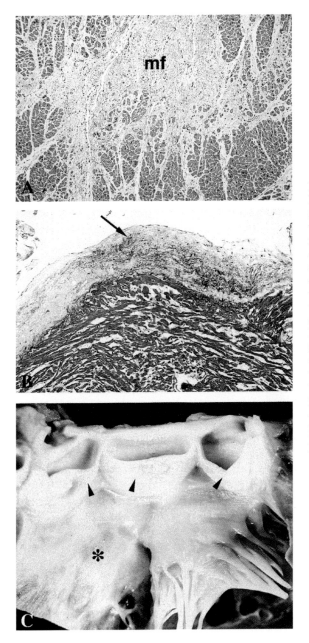

Figure 2. Panel **A** shows a histologic section of the left ventricular mid-myocardium from a patient with radiation-induced myocardial fibrosis **(mf).** Right ventricular endocardial thickening with elastosis (panel **B,** arrow) found in a 49-year-old woman with breast carcinoma treated with surgery and radiation therapy 9 years prior to the development of constrictive pericarditis. Panel **C** shows marked endocardial fibrosis (*) of the left ventricular outflow tract with aortic valve thickening (arrowheads) secondary to radiation. The patient was a 25-year-old male who received mediastinal radiation therapy (3600 rads) at the age of 15 years for non-Hodgkin's lymphoma. Reproduced with permission from Reference 48.

Radiation-Induced Changes in Capillaries, Arterioles, and Muscular Arteries

Radiation-induced myocardial disease is said to be secondary to intramyocardial muscular artery, arteriolar, and capillary damage.[17] In humans, various organs such as the brain, kidney, uterine vessels, and the heart have demonstrated vascular damage, especially of the capillary endothelium, which ranges from endothelial swelling to intraluminal platelet thrombi. Similar vascular changes have been observed in the rabbit at 40 days following a single dose of 20 Gy consisting of endothelial swelling, platelet and fibrin thrombi, capillary wall rupture, microhemorrhages, and progressive capillary damage with macrophage infiltration.[18] By 70 days, there is a decrease in the capillary network area associated with diffuse myocardial fibrosis.[18] Single dose or fractionated doses cause similar changes in the rabbit.

Small-sized arterioles (≤300 μm in diameter) show necrotizing "arteriolitis" and phlebitis, with loss of cellular details and hyaline medial change as early as 20 days following radiation.[18] Late changes following radiation mostly consist of intimal thickening and medial fibrosis with an intact or a partially destroyed internal elastic lamina. Muscular arteries and arterioles (100 to 500 μm in diameter) show foam cell infiltration in the subendothelial and intimal regions with or without fibrin deposition around foam cells. This change was first reported by Sheehan in 1944 as characteristic of vascular radiation injury.[19]

In muscular arteries, it has been thought that foam cells, and cholesterol clefts are unusual and they have not been reported in animals following radiation.[17,18] In these vessels, injured endothelial cells show edema and hyperchromatic nuclei; normal appearing endothelial cells may nonetheless have abnormal endothelial junctions with increased permeability allowing lipids to gain access into subendothelial spaces. Although it has been reported that foam cells are not seen in muscular arteries of experimental animals following radiation unless there is hypercholesterolemia, the most likely reason for the absence of foam cells is related to the short duration radiation experiments (≤6 months). We have observed atherosclerotic changes in rabbit iliac arteries 6 and 12 months following implantation of high activity ^{32}P β-emitting radioactive stents (24 and 48 μCi). These animals were on a normal diet, indicating that hypercholesterolemia is not a prerequisite for the development of atherosclerotic change following radiation.

Vasculitis has also been reported in muscular arteries, and is more commonly observed after radiation. The vasculitis is characterized by fibrinoid change, predominantly lymphohistiocytic inflammation, and luminal thrombosis. Concentric or eccentric intimal thickening are very common in patients following radiation. Foam cell infiltration is reported to be less frequent in larger muscular arteries in humans and this change has not been observed in animals except in the presence of hypercholesterolemia, at least in animals.[17]

Large caliber arteries are relatively resistant to radiation injury, but like small arteries, endothelial cells may suffer extensive damage associated with platelet deposition. Myointimal proliferation with histocyte infiltration is reported in animals as well as in humans, but lipid accumulation and cholesterol crystal formation are reported to be less frequent in large arteries exposed to radiation compared to typical atherosclerotic lesions.[17] However, in humans, the changes of typical atherosclerosis and those of radiation-associated atherosclerosis may be difficult to distinguish. In general, radiation-induced atherosclerosis is characterized by adventitial fibrosis, medial atrophy, and hemorrhage into plaque with a large number of macrophages within the plaque; these features can be often seen in nonradiation associated atherosclerosis.

Radiation-Induced Endocardial and Valvular Changes

Post radiation, the endocardium of the heart may become thickened, by accumulated fibroblasts, collagen, and proteoglycans with increased elastic fiber de-

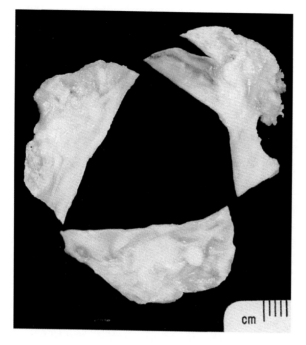

Figure 3. A 54-year-old man with coronary atherosclerosis and mixed aortic valve stenosis and regurgitation underwent coronary bypass surgery and aortic valve replacement. The patient had a history of Hodgkin's disease treated with 4000 rads mediastinal radiation 24 years prior to valve replacement. The aortic valve is tricuspid with focal fibrosis and calcification in the sinus of the valve.

position (Fig. 2B).[7] Marked radiation-induced endocardial fibrosis is uncommon, but when present, involves the right ventricle more frequently than the left ventricle. While valvular fibrosis is not uncommon and more often involves left-sided valves, symptomatic radiation-associated valve disease is unusual (Fig. 2C).[20–23] Only limited valvular morphological data are available. In one series of radiation-induced heart disease from the Mayo Clinic, valve thickening was present in greater than 50% of autopsy cases consisting of diffuse fibrosis, with or without calcification, and an absence of inflammation.[9] A review of the available literature reveals that the mitral valve (42%) is more frequently involved than the aortic valve (37%), and the most common physiological disturbances are pure mitral or aortic regurgitation with or without aortic stenosis (Fig. 3).[9]

Few clinical studies have shown a definite link between fatal valvular heart disease and therapeutic radiation. In a study by Hancock et al, patients treated with radiation for Hodgkin's disease (mean age 15.4 years), with a follow-up duration of 10.3 years, 12 patients died of cardiac causes (relative risk [RR] 29.6, 95% confidence interval [CI] 16.0 to 49.3), 7 from acute myocardial infarction, 3 from valvular heart disease, and 2 from radiation pericarditis/pancarditis.[24]

Radiation and Coronary Heart Disease

Reports of radiation-induced heart disease in patients treated with external beam radiation for malignancies such as Hodgkin's disease, breast cancer, seminoma, or lung cancer began to appear in the literature in the 1960s.[7] The early reports emphasized the involvement of the pericardium, myocardium, and endocardium.[7,25,26] Although initial case reports of radiation-induced coronary artery disease were published in the 1960s to 1970s, it was not until the 1980s that it was widely recognized that radiation therapy increased the incidence of premature coronary atherosclerosis.[27–29] In 1976, McReynolds et al described 2 patients (aged 33 and 42 years) with severe coronary heart disease who had received mediastinal radiation for Hodgkin's disease 8 and 6 years antemortem. The latter patient had an acute myocardial infarction. The 33-year-old patient had sudden cardiac death, and post-mortem examination showed severe 3-vessel coronary atherosclerosis; coronary artery adventitial and intimal fibrosis were present.

Prior to the 1990s, there was controversy as to whether mediastinal radiation was responsible for accelerated coronary artery atherosclerosis leading to increased mortality or morbidity. Multiple studies suggested an association,[28–34] but others did not.[35,36] Support for the hypothesis of radiotherapy-induced accelerated coronary atherosclerosis was shown in studies that encompassed longer patient follow-up and survival following radiation, and included data on the delivered radiation dose and the type of radiation used. The two malignancies with the longest survival and the best-documented association of radiation therapy with accelerated coronary disease are Hodgkin's disease and breast cancer. King et al noted a 5.5% incidence of cardiac morbidity in 326 patients with Hodgkin's disease treated with radiation therapy who survived more than 3 years. The mean radiation dose was 44.3 Gy; all patients had coronary artery disease with a similar distribution of radiation-induced pathology among the epicardial coronary arteries.[37,38] Rutqvist et al reported long-term follow-up (mean 16 years, range 13 to 19 years) of patients with breast cancer who were treated with mastectomy and radiation (45 Gy over 5 weeks) versus those treated with surgery alone. Radiation-treated patients had a better overall survival. However, those that received the highest radiation doses and those treated with tangential ^{60}Co fields for left-sided tumors were found to have a significantly increased risk of death due to ischemic heart disease compared to surgical controls (relative hazard 3.2, $P<0.05$).[39]

Boivin and Hutchison reported that the mortality from coronary heart disease was higher in patients with Hodgkin's disease treated with radiation compared to those treated with chemotherapy; the relative risk of death from coronary disease after mediastinal radiation and after chemotherapy was 1.87 (95% CI, 0.92 to 3.80) and 1.28 (CI, 0.77 to 2.15), respectively. A significantly increased risk of death from acute myocardial infarction was observed following mediastinal radiation (RR 2.56; CI 1.11 to 5.93) but not after chemotherapy (RR 0.97; CI 0.53 to 1.77).[28] Similarly, Hancock et al reported a higher death rate (3.9%) from heart disease in patients treated with mediastinal radiation for Hodgkin's disease with the relative risk 3.1 times than expected for an aged-matched general population. This resulted in an absolute risk of 28 excess deaths per 10,000 person-years of observation. The relative risk for heart disease was similar for men and women (3.1 versus 2.7, respectively); however, the absolute risk was higher for men than women (40.0 versus 11.9). Mediastinal radiation of less than 30 Gy did not increase risk, but for an accumulated dose of greater than or equal to 30 Gy, the relative risk was 3.5 (CI 2.7 to 4.3). Shielding to limit cardiac exposure (used after 1972) reduced the relative risk of radiation-induced cardiac disease from 4.3 (CI 3.1 to 5.5) to 2.6 (CI 1.7 to 3.6), but did not reduce the risk of acute myocardial infarction. Further, the relative and absolute risk for acute myocardial infarction increased with increasing duration of post-radiation treatment (RR 2.0 at 0 to 4 years and 5.6 at ≥20 years).[24] The relative risk for acute myocardial infarction was highest when radiation therapy was administered before age 20 years and decreased with increasing age at the time of treatment. Taken together, these studies strongly suggest a cause and effect relationship between radiation and accelerated coronary atherosclerosis.

Pathology of Radiation-Induced Coronary Disease

There are relatively few studies that have documented the morphological changes in the coronary arteries of patients who had received mediastinal radiation therapy.[7,9,10,27,40] In 1981, Brosius et al described 16 young patients (mean age 26 years, range 15 to 33 years, 13 men and 3 women) who had received greater than 3500 rads to the heart 5- to 144-months antemortem.[10] Most patients were treated for Hodgkin's disease (13 patients). These radiated patients were compared to 10 age- and sex-matched control subjects who died of noncardiac causes and had never received radiation. Coronary arteries were carefully examined, and 6 of the 16 radiation patients had greater than 75% cross-sectional area luminal narrowing of one or more coronary arteries, whereas only one of the 10 controls had a similar degree of narrowing. After sectioning all major coronary arteries at 5 mm intervals, 6% of the segments examined from the radiation group were narrowed 76 to 100% (versus 0.2% in controls, $P=0.06$) and 22% were narrowed 50 to 75% (versus 12% of controls). The proximal portion of the coronary arteries from the radiation group was more severely narrowed than the distal segments. Further, the adventitia was more densely fibrotic, and the media was more frequently replaced by fibrous tissue in the radiated group compared with the nonradiated controls. Thus, radiation resulted in a greater degree of atherosclerosis and luminal narrowing along with increased adventitial and medial fibrosis. Importantly, the total cholesterol was greater than 200 mg/dL in only 2 of the 16 radiated patients and 1 of 10 control patients.[10]

The clinical aspects of radiation-induced accelerated coronary atherosclerosis were examined by McEniery et al in 15 patients (mean age 48 years, range 26 to 63 years) who developed coronary disease following radiation (mean duration after radiation 16 years, range 3 to 9 years). Ten patients had angina, 3 had acute myocardial infarction, 1 had syncope, and 1 had dyspnea.[41] Only 2 had risk factors for the development of premature atherosclerosis. Most remarkable was that 8 of 15 patients had at least 50% diameter narrowing of the left main coronary artery, and 4 had severe ostial stenosis of the right coronary artery.[41]

In our laboratory, we have examined 10 patients (age range 33 to 67 years) who died of coronary artery disease and had received mediastinal radiation therapy (3- to 25-years antemortem); our findings are very similar to those of Brosius et al.[10] The malignancies treated were Hodgkin's disease, lung cancer, breast cancer, seminoma, and embryonal carcinoma. At autopsy, all patients had severe coronary atherosclerosis, and 5 of 10 had coronary artery thrombosis. Two patients had healed myocardial infarction, and 3 had acute myocardial infarction. We also noted marked adventitial fibrosis and medial atrophy and replacement with fibrous tissue, especially involving the proximal right and the left anterior descending coronary arteries (Fig. 4).

A causal link between radiation therapy and coronary disease is difficult to prove unless atherosclerosis is evident at a young age, since the prevalence of coronary artery disease in patients over 50 years of age is high. Patients with Hodgkin's disease or seminoma that receive radiation therapy are usually in their second to third decade at the time of diagnosis, while those with breast and lung neoplasms are typically older than the fourth to fifth decade. Coronary artery complications develop on average more than 10 years following radiation, and the radiation dose received is an important variable. Many patients with breast cancer

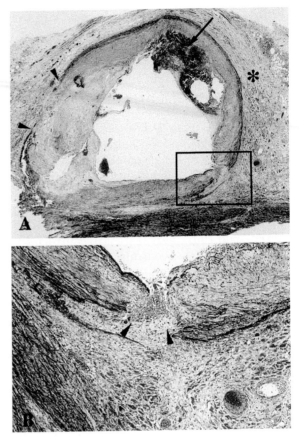

Figure 4. Right coronary artery from a 62-year-old man with mediastinal radiation therapy for Hodgkin's disease 25-years antemortem. At autopsy, there was 70% lumen area narrowing (panel **A**) with intraplaque hemorrhage (arrow), marked adventitial fibrosis (*), and focal destruction of the arterial media (arrowheads). The boxed-in area in panel A is shown at higher magnification in panel **B**; note medial disruption (arrowheads) and replacement by smooth muscle cells in a collagenous matrix. Reproduced with permission from Reproduced with permission from Reference 48.

and most individuals with lung cancer do not live beyond 10 years after their diagnosis; therefore, it is not surprising that coronary artery complications may not be seen. If coronary atherosclerosis develops in a person older than age 50, one should be cautious in concluding that the coronary disease was radiation-induced.

Extracardiac Arterial Complications of Radiation

Radiation therapy has also been linked to the development of arterial disease involving the aorta and its major branches and other large arteries in the radiation field.[12,42] The most commonly involved vessels are the carotid arteries, and less common are the aorta, pulmonary artery, iliac arteries, and femoral arteries.[42] It has been reported that there is an increased risk of arterial rupture and development of atherosclerotic disease following radiation.

Of 9 cases (aged 47 to 63 years) of arterial rupture associated with radiation therapy reported by Fajardo and Lee,[42] 7 had squamous cell carcinoma (involving the esophagus in 2, tonsil in 2, larynx in 1, pyriform sinus in 1, and the penis in 1) and 2 had lung carcinoma. All patients had received radiation between 5,000 to 11,000 rads, and the interval from radiation to vessel rupture varied from 25 days to 60 months (mean 20 months). All patients had surgery prior to radiation. The ruptured artery was the carotid in 3, aorta in 2, femoral in 1, pulmonary in 1, innominate in 1, and branch of left internal maxillary artery in 1. The rupture site length varied from 0.5 mm to 2.0 cm. The vessels were not calcified, and atherosclerosis was present in half the cases with the other half demonstrating myo-intimal hyperplasia. Morphologically, necrosis of the vessel wall was noted along with fragmentation of the elastic fibers at the borders of the rupture site. Half of the cases had acute inflammatory infiltrates associated with bacterial colonies. Fajardo and Lee postulated that the surgical procedure itself, rather than radiation therapy, plays a more important role in the occurrence of arterial rupture.[42] They proposed that the mechanism of arterial rupture involves surgically induced adventitial damage, leading to compromise of the vasa vasorum and necrosis of the vessel wall, ultimately resulting in vessel wall weakness and rupture. In support of their argument, the authors note that the radiation dose was not related to the incidence of rupture whereas more extensive surgery appeared to increase the frequency of rupture.

We believe that radiation-induced arterial damage augments that produced by surgery and increases the risk of arterial rupture. We have recently had the opportunity to review a case of ascending aortic rupture in a 25-year-old male who had radical surgical resection of the chest wall for Ewing's sarcoma of the rib followed by external beam radiation (2300 rads). The interval between radiation therapy and aortic rupture was 17 days. At autopsy, there was a discreet rupture of the aorta with massive hemorrhage into the chest cavity (Fig. 5). Histologically, smooth muscle cells at the borders of the rupture site were absent, and elastic fibers were fragmented. Hyperchromatic and hyperplastic smooth muscle nuclei were present in the adjoining areas of smooth muscle cell loss within the aortic wall. There was marked luminal narrowing of the adventitial arteries (vasa vasorum) associated with hyperplastic endothelial cells and smooth muscle cells. We believe that these changes represent radiation effects, and we have not observed similar findings from other causes of acute aortic rupture.

Carotid and Intracranial Vascular Disease Following Radiation Therapy

Most cases of symptomatic carotid artery disease following radiation of head and neck tumors have been reported in older patients.[43–45] However, occlusive carotid disease following radiation for neck neoplasms was reported by Silverberg et al in 9 patients who were younger and had fewer risk factors for atherosclerosis compared to 40 control subjects.[44] An elevated serum cholesterol level increased likelihood of developing radiation-induced carotid disease. The distribution of the post-radiation carotid atherosclerotic disease differs from typical atherosclerosis by its extension proximally into the common carotid artery, and distally beyond the bulb; peri-adventitial inflammation, adventitial, and medial sclerosis have been reported.[45] The increased adventitial fibrosis in arteries exposed to radiation causes difficulty in separating the media from the plaque during surgical endarterectomy.[44]

Subsequent to reports of post-radiation carotid artery disease in older patients, several studies of patients younger than age 40 have now been published. King et al performed carotid ultrasonography in 42 survivors of childhood or early adult Hodgkin's lymphoma, aged 18 to 37 years, who had undergone radiation

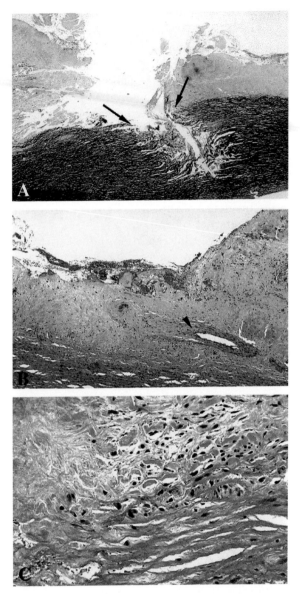

Figure 5. Ascending aortic rupture in a 25-year-old male with Ewing's sarcoma of the rib treated with radical surgery and radiation (2300 rads) 17 days prior to death. A histologic section (panel **A**) of the ascending aorta at the rupture site demonstrates a focal tear (arrows) with adventitial fibrosis and hemorrhage. Adventitial fibrosis and marked vasa vasorum thickening (arrowhead) are shown in panel **B**. In panel **C**, the aortic wall close to the tear is located on the left. In the adjoining aortic wall to the right, the smooth muscle cells are hyperplastic, bizarrely shaped, and hyperchromatic secondary to radiation injury. Reproduced with permission from Reference 48.

therapy (dose 2250 to 4000 cGy delivered in 15 to 25 fractions) more than 5 years earlier (range 5.1 to 22.8 years) and compared the findings to 33 control subjects.[46] They identified significantly greater abnormal scans (26%) in the radiated patients compared to nonradiated controls (3%). Post-radiation patients had a significantly greater intimal/medial thickness (0.51) than control subjects (0.43 mm; $P<0.005$). Of the 11 patients with abnormal scans, 10 had nonsignificant stenosis and 1 patient had 70% stenoses of both carotid arteries. Patients with radiation therapy alone and radiation plus chemotherapy had no significant differences in the prevalence of carotid disease.[46]

In patients treated with cranial radiation for acute lymphoblastic leukemia, there is a significantly higher incidence of vascular and other abnormalities (43%)

on magnetic resonance imaging of the brain and magnetic resonance angiography compared to control patients (17%) with malignancies elsewhere.[47]

Summary

The pericardium, myocardium, endocardium, valves, and coronary arteries may be affected by external beam radiation. There is now little doubt that external beam radiation to the mediastinum is associated with an increased incidence of atherosclerotic coronary disease compared to an age- and sex-matched population. The factors that predict the development of coronary disease are individuals who receive radiation at a young age, a radiation dose greater than 30 Gy, and survival more than 10 years following radiation. The morphological characteristics that distinguish radiation-induced coronary disease from nonradiation-induced atherosclerosis are adventitial fibrosis and medial atrophy. Two complications of extracardiac arterial radiation exposure are carotid and aortic rupture and occlusive carotid disease. There is controversy whether, in the absence of surgery, radiation can induce arterial rupture. Evidence suggests that arterial rupture occur from the synergistic weakening of the arterial wall from surgery and radiation.

References

1. Teirstein PS, Massullo V, Jani S, et al. Two-year follow-up after catheter-based radiotherapy to inhibit coronary restenosis. Circulation 1999;99:243–247.
2. Condado JA, Waksman R, Gurdiel O, et al. Long-term angiographic and clinical outcome after percutaneous transluminal coronary angioplasty and intracoronary radiation therapy in humans. Circulation 1997;96:727–732.
3. Carter AJ, Scott D, Bailey LR, et al. High activity 32P stents promote developmemt of atherosclerosis at six months in a porcine model. Circulation 1997;96:I-607.
4. Farb A, Tang A, Virmani R. Neointima is reduced but endothelialization is incomplete 3 months after 32P β-emitting stent placement. Circulation 1998;98:I-779.
5. Costa MA, Sabat M, van der Giessen WJ, et al. Late coronary occlusion after intracoronary brachytherapy. Circulation 1999;100:789–792.
6. Waksman R. Late thrombosis after radiation: Sitting on a time bomb. Circulation 1999;100:780–782.
7. Fajardo LF, Stewart JR, Cohn KE. Morphology of radiation-induced heart disease. Arch Pathol 1968;86:512–519.
8. Cohn KE, Stewart JR, Fajardo LF, Hancock EW. Heart disease following radiation. Medicine (Baltimore) 1967;46:281–298.
9. Veinot JP, Edwards WD. Pathology of radiation-induced heart disease: A surgical and autopsy study of 27 cases. Hum Pathol 1996;27:766–773.
10. Brosius FC, Waller BF, Roberts WC. Radiation heart disease: Analysis of 16 young (aged 15 to 33 years) necropsy patients who received over 3,500 rads to the heart. Am J Med 1981;70:519–530.
11. Schultz-Hector S. Radiation-induced heart disease: Review of experimental data on dose response and pathogenesis. Int J Radiat Biol 1992;61:149–160.
12. Arsenian MA. Cardiovascular sequelae of therapeutic thoracic radiation. Prog Cardiovasc Dis 1991;33:299–311.
13. Stewart JR, Fajardo LF, Gillette SM, Constine LS. Radiation injury to the heart. Int J Radiat Oncol Biol Phys 1995;31:1205–1211.
14. Applefeld MM, Cole JF, Pollock SH, et al. The late appearance of chronic pericardial disease in patients treated by radiotherapy for Hodgkin's disease. Ann Intern Med 1981;94:338–341.

15. Stewart JR, Fajardo LF. Radiation-induced heart disease: An update. Prog Cardiovasc Dis 1984;27:173–194.
16. Applefeld MM, Slawson RG, Hall-Craigs M, et al. Delayed pericardial disease after radiotherapy. Am J Cardiol 1981;47:210–213.
17. Fajardo LF, Berthrong M. Vascular lesions following radiation. Pathol Annu 1988;23(Pt 1):297–330.
18. Fajardo LF, Stewart JR. Pathogenesis of radiation-induced myocardial fibrosis. Lab Invest 1973;29:244–257.
19. Sheehan JF. Foam cell plaques in intima of irradiated small arteries. Arch Pathol 1944;37:297–325.
20. Carlson RG, Mayfield WR, Normann S, Alexander JA. Radiation-associated valvular disease. Chest 1991;99:538–545.
21. Perrault DJ, Levy M, Herman JD, et al. Echocardiographic abnormalities following cardiac radiation. J Clin Oncol 1985;3:546–551.
22. Warda M, Khan A, Massumi A, et al. Radiation-induced valvular dysfunction. J Am Coll Cardiol 1983;2:180–185.
23. Gottdiener JS, Katin MJ, Borer JS, et al. Late cardiac effects of therapeutic mediastinal irradiation: Assessment by echocardiography and radionuclide angiography. N Engl J Med 1983;308:569–572.
24. Hancock SL, Donaldson SS, Hoppe RT. Cardiac disease following treatment of Hodgkin's disease in children and adolescents. J Clin Oncol 1993;11:1208–1215.
25. Stewart JR, Fajardo LF. Radiation-induced heart disease: Clinical and experimental aspects. Radiol Clin North Am 1971;9:511–531.
26. Morton DL, Kagan AR, Roberts WC, et al. Pericardiectomy for radiation-induced pericarditis with effusion. Ann Thorac Surg 1969;8:195–208.
27. McReynolds RA, Gold GL, Roberts WC. Coronary heart disease after mediastinal irradiation for Hodgkin's disease. Am J Med 1976;60:39–45.
28. Boivin JF, Hutchison GB. Coronary heart disease mortality after irradiation for Hodgkin's disease. Cancer 1982; 49:2470–2475.
29. Annest LS, Anderson RP, Li W, Hafermann MD. Coronary artery disease following mediastinal radiation therapy. J Thorac Cardiovasc Surg 1983;85:257–263.
30. Lederman GS, Sheldon TA, Chaffey JT, et al. Cardiac disease after mediastinal irradiation for seminoma. Cancer 1987;60:772–776.
31. Pohjola-Sintonen S, Totterman KJ, Salmo M, Siltanen P. Late cardiac effects of mediastinal radiotherapy in patients with Hodgkin's disease. Cancer 1987;60:31–37.
32. Donaldson SS, Kaplan HS. Complications of treatment of Hodgkin's disease in children. Cancer Treat Rep 1982;66:977–989.
33. Host H, Brennhovd IO, Loeb M. Postoperative radiotherapy in breast cancer: Long-term results from the Oslo study. Int J Radiat Oncol Biol Phys 1986;12:727–732.
34. Jones JM, Ribeiro GG. Mortality patterns over 34 years of breast cancer patients in a clinical trial of post-operative radiotherapy. Clin Radiol 1989;40:204–208.
35. Strender LE, Lindahl J, Larsson LE. Incidence of heart disease and functional significance of changes in the electrocardiogram 10 years after radiotherapy for breast cancer. Cancer 1986;57:929–934.
36. Willan BD, McGowan DG. Seminoma of the testis: A 22-year experience with radiation therapy. Int J Radiat Oncol Biol Phys 1985;11:1769–1775.
37. King SB. Intravascular radiation for restenosis prevention: Could it be the holy grail? [editorial] Heart 1996;76:99–100.
38. King V, Constine LS, Clark D, et al. Symptomatic coronary artery disease after mantle irradiation for Hodgkin's disease. Int J Radiat Oncol Biol Phys 1996;36:881–889.
39. Rutqvist LE, Lax I, Fornander T, Johansson H. Cardiovascular mortality in a randomized trial of adjuvant radiation therapy versus surgery alone in primary breast cancer. Int J Radiat Oncol Biol Phys 1992;22:887–896.
40. Fajardo LF. Radiation-induced coronary artery disease. Chest 1977;71:563–564.
41. McEniery PT, Dorosti K, Schiavone WA, et al. Clinical and angiographic features of coronary artery disease after chest irradiation. Am J Cardiol 1987;60:1020–1024.
42. Fajardo LF, Lee A. Rupture of major vessels after radiation. Cancer 1975;36:904–913.
43. Levinson SA, Close MB, Ehrenfeld WK, Stoney RJ. Carotid artery occlusive disease following external cervical irradiation. Arch Surg 1973;107:395–397.

44. Silverberg GD, Britt RH, Goffinet DR. Radiation-induced carotid artery disease. Cancer 1978;41:130–137.
45. Cormier JM, Brisset D, Speir Y, et al. Fifty-three atherosclerotic carotid stenoses in an irradiated environment. J Mal Vasc 1993;18:269–274.
46. King LJ, Hasnain SN, Webb JA, et al. Asymptomatic carotid arterial disease in young patients following neck radiation therapy for Hodgkin lymphoma. Radiology 1999;213:167–172.
47. Laitt RD, Chambers EJ, Goddard PR, et al. Magnetic resonance imaging and magnetic resonance angiography in long term survivors of acute lymphoblastic leukemia treated with cranial irradiation. Cancer 1995;76:1846–1852.
48. Virmani R, Farb A. Effects of external beam radiation on the human heart and great vessels. J Invasive Cardiol 1999;11:703–708.

Part III

Radiation Physics and Dosimetry for Vascular Brachytherapy

## Chapter 16

Dosimetry of Sealed Beta-Particle Sources

Christopher G. Soares, PhD

Scope

This chapter is a discussion of the methods used at the National Institute of Standards and Technology (NIST) to characterize sealed beta-particle sources and to measure the radiation fields produced by these sources in tissue-equivalent media. The sources considered are limited to sealed beta-particle emitters in the form of small (<1 mm diameter) cylinders, either in loose form referred to as seeds (or seed trains) or attached to the end of wires. The techniques used are generally applicable to any such source capable of producing an absorbed dose rate of 3 Gy/min (50 mGy/s) at a distance of 2 mm from the source center in a tissue-equivalent medium. For the beta-particle isotopes considered ($E_{max}>1.5$ MeV), this dose rate corresponds to contained activities of the order of 40 MBq/mm (1 mCi/mm) of length. Characteristics of some isotopes which fulfill the energy requirements of these sources and which are suitable for use in medical therapy are shown in Table 1.

Background

The need for accurate beta-particle dosimetry measurements first arose with the use of beta-particle-emitting eye plaques for the treatment of ocular diseases.[1–3] In the 1950s, Loevinger[4,5] developed techniques for contact dosimetry measurements of these sources by modifying an instrument invented by Failla[6] in the late 1930s. This instrument, the extrapolation ionization chamber, became and remains the standard measurement device for beta-particle dosimetry.

In the area of protection-level dosimetry, rudimentary efforts to design personnel monitors sensitive to beta particles were begun during the Manhattan Project because of the high skin doses possible in the processing of weapons-grade material. Calibration of these dosimeters was performed either with contact measurements with depleted uranium slabs, or at distances in air from ^{90}Sr/Y. The poor irradiation geometry of the slab, and the widely varying characteristics of ^{90}Sr/Y fields with source construction and encapsulation led to the development of standardized sources at the National Physical Laboratory (NPL) in Great

From Waksman R (ed.). *Vascular Brachytherapy, Third Edition*. Armonk, NY: Futura Publishing Co., Inc.; © 2002.

Table 1

Properties of Beta-Particle Emitting Isotopes Appropriate for Intravascular Brachytherapy

Isotope	Half-Life (Days)	Maximum Energy (MeV)	Average Energy (MeV)
P	14.262	1.71	0.695
[88]W+	69.4	0.35	0.10
[188]Re	0.71	2.12	0.77
Sr+	10636	0.55	0.20
[90]Y	2.67	2.28	0.93
[144]Ce+	284.9	0.32	0.082
[144]Pr	0.012	3.00	1.21
[106]Ru+	371.63	0.04	0.01
[106]Rh	0.000345	3.54	1.415

+ Indicates a long-lived parent of the more energetic daughter listed in the line below.

Britain in the 1970s.[7,8] This work was extended and coupled with fundamental work on the extrapolation chamber at the Physikalisch-Technische Bundesanstalt (PTB) in Germany,[9,10] which led to an International Organization for Standardization (ISO) standard[11] for the production and dosimetry of reference beta-particle fields for personnel dosimeter calibration. This work is important for the dosimetry of medical beta-particle sources because it provides solid underpinnings to all the dosimetry methods which will be discussed in the remainder of this chapter.

Dose rate to radiation workers from very small radioactive fragments was first identified as a radiation protection dosimetry problem in the 1980s. These sources, known as hot particles, are usually beta-particle emitters that have dimensions on the order of less than 0.1 mm and activities of the order of a few MBq. When in contact or near contact with the skin for prolonged periods (hours), these sources produce small burns, which, except for the fact that they are produced by radiation, are not medically significant. Because the injury is radiation induced, dosimetry for reporting purposes is necessary. Techniques have been developed to perform this dosimetry,[12–14] which at first were confined to the rather unimportant problem of hot particles. However, with the advent of intravascular brachytherapy using beta-particle sources, it was realized that many of the dosimetry techniques developed for hot particle dosimetry were immediately applicable to the dosimetry of these new sources.

Measurement Techniques

Before specific methods are discussed, some general remarks about the desired characteristics of beta-particle detectors are made below. The most important characteristic of a beta-particle detector is its thickness; for energy independence, as well as for vertical spatial resolution it should be as thin as possible. For good lateral spatial resolution it should also have as small an area as possible. Both these requirements come at the expense of sensitivity, however, and compromises must be made for real-world detectors.

The Extrapolation Ionization Chamber

The extrapolation chamber has long been the standard instrument for measuring absorbed-dose rate from beta-particle sources. Of critical importance is the effective area of the collecting electrode used, since accurate knowledge of this area is needed for determining the dose rate from the measured currents, and this is the area that the measured dose rate will be averaged over. It is also important that the area of the collecting electrode be smaller than the radiation field being measured, so that the measurement averaging area is determined by the collecting electrode rather than the radiation field.[15] Also, very often the construction of the source or the distribution of the activity within the source causes the radiation field being measured to be nonuniform in the measurement plane. Thus, it must be kept in mind that the measured dose rate in such a field with an extrapolation chamber will be a function both of the collecting area and the location of the collector within the radiation field.

The dose rate is determined from current measurements at a series of air gaps; the current versus air gap data are fitted to determine the slope of these data at the limit of zero air gap. The dose rate is then given by:

$$\dot{D} = \frac{(\overline{W}/e)S_{air}^{water}}{\rho_a A} (\Delta I/\Delta d)_{d\to 0}\, k_{back} k_{foil} \tag{1}$$

where $\overline{W}/e$ is the average energy in joules needed to produce one coulomb of ions of either sign in air; S_{air}^{water} is the ratio of the mean mass stopping power of water to that of air; ρ_a is the density of air at the reference temperature and pressure (22°C and 1 standard atmosphere); A is the area of the collecting electrode; $(\Delta I/\Delta d)_{d\to 0}$ is the rate of change of current (corrected to the reference temperature and pressure) with extrapolation chamber air gap thickness as the thickness approaches zero; k_{back} is a correction for reduced backscatter from the collecting electrode; and k_{foil} is a correction for attenuation by the high-voltage electrode. Each measured current I_c is given by:

$$I_c = \left(\frac{VC}{t}\right) k_{recom} k_{di} k_{Tp} k_{decay} \tag{2}$$

where V is the measured voltage, C is the capacitance, and t is the integration time. The raw currents are also corrected for ion recombination (k_{recom}), source field divergence (k_{di}), temperature and pressure (k_{Tp}), and decay between the measurement date and the reference date (k_{decay}).

Because of the contribution to the measured current by beta particles stopped in the collecting electrode, current measurements are made at both positive and negative polarities. The difference of these divided by two is the current due to ionization in the air gap; the sum of these divided by two is the current due to beta particles stopped in the collecting electrode and electrode leakage.

The various corrections to the measured ionization current are described below.

Recombination

When ions are lost due to recombination before they can be collected, the resulting current losses are dominated by the diffusion of ions against the electric field for the small air gaps used for near surface dose rate measurement. This correction can be adequately made by:

$$k_{recom} = \frac{1}{1 - \frac{0.04554}{\sqrt{(Xd^2)}}} \quad (3)$$

where X is the voltage gradient in V/mm, and d is the air gap in mm.[5]

Divergence

At close-to-surface geometries, or with the small sources encountered in brachytherapy, the current versus air gap data is seen to exhibit curvature. This curvature is stronger for larger air gaps, smaller fields, and smaller collecting electrodes.[12] It can be minimized by selecting air gaps as small as possible, but without corrections, it can never be entirely removed. The curvature can largely be explained by geometrical considerations of the measurement of an extended source with a parallel plate chamber.[16,17] Traditionally it is ignored when the air gaps can be made small enough.[15] At large distances, the correction reduces to simple inverse-square dependence.[18]

Temperature and Pressure

Corrections for changes in air density from ambient conditions at the time of measurement to reference conditions take the form of:

$$k_{Tp} = (T / 295.15 \text{ K})(760 \text{ mm Hg} / p) \quad (4)$$

where T is the ambient temperature in K and p is the ambient pressure in mm Hg.

Decay

Corrections of measurements to a reference time are made using:

$$k_{decay} = \exp[(0.693 \, t / T_{1/2})] \quad (5)$$

where t is the elapsed time interval between the measurement time and the reference time, and $T_{1/2}$ is the half-life of the isotope being measured.

Backscatter Correction

Strictly speaking, the correction k_{back} is not independent of air gap, because the amount of the current due to backscattered electrons is a function of the number and directional distribution of the beta particles incident on the collecting plane. In its most general form, the backscatter correction should be analyzed similarly to the divergence correction above. This has not as yet taken place. For now, it is considered to be independent of air gap, and to only account for the difference in backscatter between the material of the collecting electrode and water. In this form, k_{back} can be estimated from published formulae of backscatter probability as a function of effective atomic number and electron energy. For energetic beta particles such as those from ^{90}Sr/Y and ^{32}P, the estimated correction relative to water is k_{back}=1.010 for A150 plastic[19] and k_{back}=1.005 for carbon.[15]

High-Voltage Electrode/Window Attenuation

Measurements with the extrapolation chamber must be made with a foil to provide both the high-voltage electrode for the electric field within the air gap, and to define that air gap. The foil must be both conducting and as thin as possible. Usually aluminized or carbonized polyethylene terephthalate (PET) of mass-density thickness of less than 1 mg/cm² is used. For an 0.8 mg/cm² aluminized PET foil, the correction k_{foil} has been estimated to be 1.003 for ^{90}Sr/Y beta particles.[15]

Measurement Uncertainties

For the extrapolation chamber used with the small collecting electrodes ($\leq$4-mm diameter), the measurement uncertainty is dominated by the uncertainty in the effective area of the collecting electrode. While the physical area can be determined with accuracy using a traveling microscope, the amount of the area of the small ring which isolates the collecting electrode from the guard ring, which should be included in the effective collecting electrode area, is not known. Usually, it is assumed that the collecting area extends halfway into the insulating gap.[20]

The combined uncertainty in a calibration performed with an extrapolation chamber equipped with a 1-mm-diameter graphite collection electrode is estimated to be ±7.5% at the equivalent of one standard deviation (Table 2). The random uncertainty components are calculated as standard deviations of the mean of replicate readings; other components are estimated so that they can be assumed to have the approximate character of standard deviations. The total uncertainty is the square root of the quadratic sum of all the component uncertainties. Use of smaller collecting electrodes increases this uncertainty because of increased relative uncertainty in electrode area, and possibly less precision in the current measurements.

Table 2

Estimated Uncertainties in Source Calibration Using an Extrapolation Chamber with a 1-mm Collecting Electrode

Component	Uncertainty(%)
Instrumental	0.3
Average energy per ion pair	0.4
Stopping-power ratio	3
Rate of change of current, $(\Delta I/\Delta d)_{d\rightarrow 0}$	3
Backscatter correction, k_{back}	1
Attenuation correction, k_{foil}	<0.1
Electrode area, A	6
Combined uncertainty (quadratic sum)	7.5

Radiochromic Film

Radiosensitive films fulfill many of the requirements of an ideal beta-particle detector. Of extremely fine grain size, they are able to be read with high-resolution densitometry at spacings of tens of micrometers. Radiochromic film consists of a thin layer of radiosensitive emulsion on the order of 6 to 30 μm thick (depending on type), coated onto a PET backing of 60 to 100 μm. The film sensitivity is a nearly linear function of the emulsion thickness. The initially nearly colorless emulsion darkens with irradiation and requires no processing. Films are read out using conventional densitometry. The absorbance spectrum of a commonly used film emulsion, GAFChromic™ (Nuclear Associates, Carle Place, NY), exhibits a major peak at about 660 nm and a minor peak at 610 nm. Thus, the film is most sensitive at these wavelengths. The absorption properties of radiochromic film allow an He-Ne laser densitometer, with a wavelength of 633 nm, to be used effectively for optical density measurements. For radiation field mapping, such a scanning densitometer, which as a translational device measures density point by point over the film surface, may be used, or an imaging system that digitizes a uniformly backlit image of a film can be employed at any wavelength for which a wide-area uniform light source can be made. The combination of the dosimeter and densitometer must be calibrated, and density versus dose nonlinearities are often due to limitations in the densitometry. The film is calibrated by contact exposures with an ophthalmic applicator calibrated at NIST; comparisons with calibrations done with ^{60}Co gamma-rays and ^{90}Y protection-level beta-particle fields show no difference for absorbances below about 1.5, within the film measurement uncertainties.[14] Users may also calibrate film with clinical electron beams from therapy linacs with known absorbed-dose rates.

Advantages of this material include good tissue equivalence for electrons and higher energy photons (flat energy response); insensitivity to visible light; high resolution (about 1200 line pairs/mm), self-processing with optical density increasing approximately linearly with dose (subject to the caveats mentioned above) over several orders of magnitude; and availability of large sheets (up to 20 by 25 cm). Disadvantages include rather high cost; low sensitivity (when read at a wavelength of 633 nm, the bulk sensitivity of the emulsion is approximately 0.6 mAU/μm/Gy); poor tissue equivalence for photons below 100 keV due to excess carbon relative to tissue in the emulsion; sensitivity variations from sample to sample of 5% or more due to nonuniformities in the sensitive emulsion layer thickness; and a complicated dependence of time and temperature on the shape of the absorbance spectrum which causes the need to control the time between irradiation and readout as well as the storage temperature for optimal reproducibility. An excellent review of this dosimetric technique is available in the literature.[21]

Dosimetry Measurements

General Procedure

The dosimetry and characterization of the catheter-based beta-particle—emitting brachytherapy sources can be accomplished in three distinct steps. The first step involves a characterization of the sources to determine the axial and transaxial uniformity of each source, as determined by measurements near contact, and at 3 mm in a cylindrical plastic phantom. These measurements are an essential preliminary to the second and third steps, since these latter steps involve multiple insertions of sources in phantoms. Since there are no axial orientation markings on these very small sources, uniformity of dose rate perpendicular to the seed axis is crucial to obtaining reproducible results. Once a source has demonstrated suitable axial and transaxial uniformity, it can be used in the second step, which involves the measurement of the absorbed-dose rate at a depth of 2 mm in a tissue-equivalent medium. A150 tissue-equivalent plastic (a conductor) is used at NIST to avoid possible charge buildup problems which would distort the depth-dose profile in a good insulator. Once the reference dose rate is established, the source can be used in the third step, which involves radiochromic film measurements at several depths in A150 plastic; the information resulting from these irradiations can be used to construct tables of data to determine the dose rate at any arbitrary point in A150 plastic. Finally, guidance is given for determining the dose rate in media other than A150 plastic. Each of these topics will be discussed in turn below.

Uniformity

The first step in the calibration procedure is to make measurements with radiochromic films in near contact and cylindrical geometries. For the near contact measurements, the source can be placed on a piece of radiochromic dye film to make an autoradiograph. The film can be covered with a thin (1 mg/cm^2 or less) layer of PET, and a 1-cm layer of A150 plastic placed over the source to hold it in contact with the film and to provide backscatter. The results of this irradiation can be used to assess uniformity of the source along its axis, and to assess the effective length of the source. For these measurements, the effective length can be defined as the full width at 70% of the dose rate maximum.

The second irradiation geometry is cylindrical, and the source is used to irradiate radiochromic film which is wrapped around a 6-mm diameter cylinder of A150 plastic; the source is placed in a hole in the center of the cylinder, and the film-wrapped cylinder is then placed inside an A150 block with a hole drilled in it. A150 plastic is placed on both sides of the block holding the film cylinder, totally imbedding the source and film combination. All air gaps should be kept to a minimum by careful machining of the plastic pieces. Irradiation times are on the order of 1 hour. The results of these irradiations allow the determination of the average dose rate at a depth of 3 mm in a water-equivalent medium, as well as the uniformity of the radiation field perpendicular to the seed axis (transaxial uniformity). The data can be analyzed by averaging the dose interpretations in a 1-mm band about the seed center. Relative standard deviations of 5% or less about this average are considered suitable to allow sources to be used in random orientations, both in the extrapolation-chamber calibrations and the other measurements described below.

Reference Point Dosimetry

Single sources must be calibrated in terms of the absorbed-dose rate in a tissue-equivalent medium. Absorbed-dose rate at a depth near 2 mm, averaged over a 1-mm diameter area, can be determined from current measurements with an extrapolation ionization chamber that has a graphite electrode.[19] The construction of this electrode is described elsewhere.[20] The effective area is assumed to extend halfway into the 0.15-mm thick insulator separating the collecting electrode from the guard electrode. This lack of information on the validity of this assumption causes the uncertainty of the effective collecting area to be the major component of the overall measurement uncertainty with the extrapolation chamber method (see below and Table 2). For this measurement, the seed is inserted into an A150 plastic phantom block of dimensions of the order of 25 mm on a side. The source axis is parallel to the surface of the block. To keep the electric field within the extrapolation chamber collecting volume free of distortions, the phantom is held at the same high voltage as the entrance window/high-voltage electrode. The contact point of the phantom surface and the extrapolation chamber entrance window is determined by moving the phantom toward the window and noting the position where the current begins to decrease due to window deformation. A traveling microscope should be used to determine the thickness of A150 plastic above the source surface, and the source diameter can be determined using a micrometer. The calibration distance, taken as the distance between the entrance window of the extrapolation chamber and the seed axis can be determined from these measurements. For consistency with proposed protocols, a depth of approximately 2 mm should be used. For the calibration, the rate of change of current with air-gap thickness is measured with a 1-mm diameter graphite collecting electrode. Currents should be measured at several air gaps of less than 0.10 mm and corrected to the reference temperature and pressure and for recombination losses; these data should yield a nearly linear relation between corrected current and air gap. An example of such a measurement for a 12-seed ^{90}Sr/Y train is shown plotted in Figure 1. The location of the center of the dose distribution in the plane of the A150 phantom surface above the seed axis can be determined by mapping the dose rate across this surface with the 1-mm diameter collecting electrode at a fixed air gap of 0.15 mm. In addition, a two-dimensional scan of a calibrated radiochromic dye film should be made at this surface. The results of this scan can be used to confirm the extrapolation chamber dosimetry; an iso-dose rate contour map constructed from one of these films for a single ^{90}Sr/Y seed is shown in Figure 2. The dashed line on this plot represents the area averaged over by the extrapolation chamber equipped with the 1-mm diameter collecting electrode.

The uncertainty in this measurement is estimated to be ∀7.5% (see Table 2). The Type A uncertainty components are calculated as standard deviations of the mean of replicate readings; other components are estimated so that they can be assumed to have the approximate character of standard deviations.

Depth Dose and Off-Axis Measurements

The third step of the calibration process involves measurements made with the source inserted at various depths (measured from the seed axis to the block surface) between 0.5 and 5.0 mm in tissue-equivalent material. For beta-particle sources, an electrically conducting material such as A150 plastic is recommended to avoid possible charge build-up problems. At each of these depths, several radiochromic films should be exposed for a range of times to gain a good image of the radiation field. These films are read out and converted to absorbed-dose rate using

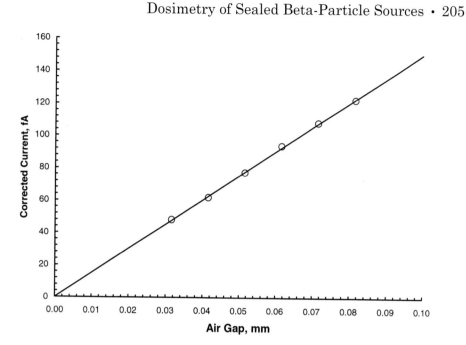

Figure 1. Extrapolation chamber data obtained from a sealed beta-particle source (a 12-seed ^{90}Sr/Y train) imbedded in A150 plastic at a depth of about 2 mm measured with a 1-mm-diameter collecting electrode.

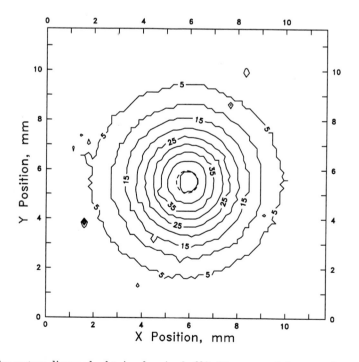

Figure 2. An autoradiograph obtained a single ^{90}Sr/Y source of the type shown measured in Figure 1. The contour lines are at 5 mGy/s intervals, and the dashed line indicates the position of the 1-mm-diameter collecting electrode of the extrapolation chamber.

the calibration curve and the known exposure time. The resulting images can be combined for each depth using the centering method described below. When the film absorbance is read at a wavelength of 633 nm, it is only possible to achieve at most about one and a half decades (a factor of about 30) in dynamic range from a single exposure. Absorbances below about 0.1 cause poor signal-to-noise characteristics, while films exposed to total doses causing absorbances above about 3 are of too high a density to be read reliably due to low light transmission. To extend the film dynamic range, it is necessary to make several different exposures for widely different times. Although films exposed for long times will exhibit saturation for areas close to the source, areas farther away will receive more dose and hence yield dose-rate information for larger radii. By properly combining and editing the images, it is possible to obtain a radial dose profile for any desired radius.

Centering Method

The method described here may be used for any symmetric source such as a point or line source. The shortest exposure made should image the source without saturation. Additional films are then exposed for powers of 3 to 10 times the initial exposure; sufficient numbers are made to obtain a clear image at the desired maximum radius. An example of such a series of films, exposed with a 27-mm-long ^{32}P source at a depth of 0.5 mm in A150 plastic, is shown in Figure 3. After a suitable delay period, the films are read with a high resolution densitometer. Since the films must be read separately, it is not possible to preserve a source-centered coordinate system common to each film. To overcome this difficulty, each film is analyzed to find the central point of the distribution. This central location is determined in the following manner. For the vertical center position, the y coordinates of the locations of the two half-maximum points (above and below the central maximum) are determined by interpolation for each x column; these are then averaged for each column; finally the y center is calculated from the average over all the x columns containing data larger than the half maximum. The analogous

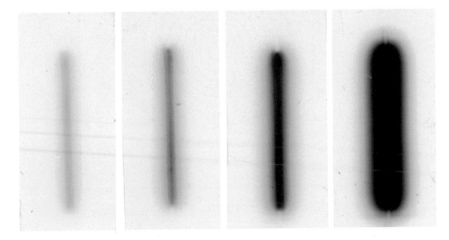

Figure 3. Autoradiographs obtained from a 27-mm-long ^{32}P wire source imbedded in A150 plastic at a depth of about 0.5 mm. Shown are exposures of 1, 3, 10, and 100 minutes.

procedure is used for the horizontal center position. Algebraically they are obtained from:

$$x_c = \left[\frac{1}{n} \right] \sum_{i=1}^{n} \frac{x50^-_i + x\,50^+_i}{2} \tag{6}$$

and

$$y_c = \left[\frac{1}{m} \right] \sum_{j=1}^{m} \frac{y\,50^-_j + y\,50^+_j}{2} \tag{7}$$

where x_c and y_c are the determined center coordinates, n is the number of rows and m is the number of columns containing data larger than the half maximum, $x50_i$ and $y50_j$ are the x or y positions of the half-maximum point determined by linear interpolation for the ith row or the jth column, above or right of (+) and below or left of (−) the center.

The combined images are then edited to remove saturated and low optical density pixels. The resulting images, when combined with the known depths, can then be used to generate tables of data that can be used to determine the absorbed dose at any arbitrary point in A150 plastic. An example of such a combination is shown in Figure 4, where a profile for a 27-mm long ^{32}P wire source was generated from 20 films (including the four films shown in Fig. 3) exposed at depths of between 0.5 and 5 mm in A150 plastic. Points perpendicular to the source axis on the film images are used to generate data at depths greater than the block hole depth.

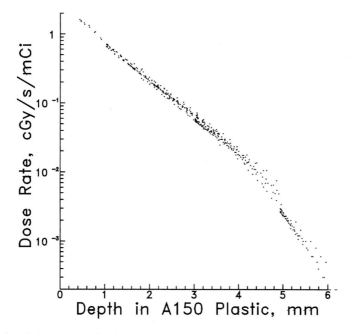

Figure 4. A depth dose curve for the same source as was used in Figure 3, constructed from 20 radiochromic film exposures at depths between 0.5 and 5 mm in A150 plastic. Off-axis film data were used to extend the range of depths available.

Scaling of Dose Distributions to Other Media

Finally, some guidance is proposed for converting from dose in A150 plastic to dose in water or some other medium. For point sources in infinite media, the dose at a distance r_m corresponding to an areal density of $r_m\rho_m$ (in g/cm^2) in the medium, $D_m(r_m\rho_m)$, can be related (to a good approximation) to the dose in water, D_w at the same areal density, $r_w\rho_w$, but scaled,[22] by:

$$D_m(r_m\rho_m) = \eta^3 (\rho_m/\rho_w)^2 D_w(\eta r_w\rho_w) \tag{8}$$

where 0 is the scaling factor of the medium relative to water, and ρ_w and ρ_m are the densities of water and the medium respectively. For A150 plastic, $\theta=0.968$ (see Reference 22) and $\rho_m=1.127$ g/cm^3. While the seed sources considered in this chapter are not true point sources, treating them as such is a reasonable approach to the problem. If this assumption is made, then to obtain the dose rate in water at a distance of 2 mm from a seed, we require (1) $\theta r_w=2$ mm; and (2) $r_m\rho_m=r_w\rho_w$. Combining these indicates that the dose rate in A150 plastic at a distance of (2 mm)/(0.968×1.127 g/cm^3)=1.83 mm should be divided by the factor $\theta^3(\rho_m/\rho_w)^2=1.152$ to yield the dose rate in water at 2 mm.

Theoretical Modeling

It is possible to predict the dose distribution in an irradiated medium through a knowledge of the properties of the radiation source and the probabilities of the various interactions of radiation with matter. This knowledge, coupled with a determination of the contained activity in the source, allows an independent check of the dosimetry methods outlined in this chapter. There are at least two ways, discussed below, to approach this calculational problem.

Monte Carlo Method

In the 1960s a method was developed by which dose distributions could be determined by following individual emissions from a source and "rolling the dice" to determine statistically how each emitted photon or electron would interact with matter at any given point. This technique is referred to as the Monte Carlo method, and is becoming more attractive as a tool with the advent of faster and more powerful computers. The accuracy of the method is limited by (1) the accuracy with which the source and surrounding media are modeled; (2) the accuracy with which the various interaction probabilities are known as a function of energy; and (3) the number of emissions tracked. Typically, 1 million or more emissions (histories) are followed as they interact with the surrounding media, loosing energy which is scored as dose at the location where it occurs, generating secondary radiations which are also followed and scored, until their energy is at some low energy limit where it is assumed that all remaining energy is deposited locally. The advantage of this method is that quite complicated geometries can be modeled, for which measurements would be difficult or impossible to perform. The disadvantage is that the calculations are time consuming, usually taking on the order of hours even on the fastest computers, to achieve statistical accuracy levels of less than a few percent.

Point Dose Function

A less computationally demanding approach to the prediction of dose distributions from extended source geometries is to use determinations of dose distributions of point sources. These distributions, called point kernels or point dose functions, can be calculated by Monte Carlo techniques or constructed from the results of measurements. By integrating (summing) the functions over the extended source volume, one can predict the dose distribution. The advantage of this approach is that the calculation can be performed quite quickly, usually on the order of seconds. The disadvantage is that point dose functions are only known for near water-equivalent media, and thus errors can occur when geometries containing modest amounts of non–water-equivalent material are modeled. For brachytherapy applications, the approach is quite successful because the amount of non-water material is usually minimal due to the very light encapsulation of these sources. Excellent reviews of both these techniques are available in the literature.[23]

Radiation-Field Parameterization

A full description of the radiation field produced by a source imbedded in a tissue-equivalent medium would require a specification of the absorbed-dose rate at every point in the medium. Rather than maintaining this very large array of data, certain parameterization schemes have been developed over the years. The representation recommended in this chapter is that of the American Association of Physicists in Medicine (AAPM) Task Group 43 (TG-43), described below.

Task Group 43 Approach

This representation of the radiation field from a brachytherapy source is described in the Report of AAPM TG-43 on the dosimetry of interstitial brachytherapy sources.[24] The formalism states that the dose rate at any point (r,θ) in a two-dimensional plane containing the source axis is given by:

$$D(r,\theta) = D(r_0,\theta_0)[G(r,\theta)/G(r_0,\theta_0)]g(r)F(r,\theta) \qquad (9)$$

where (r_0,θ_0) is the reference position, for which the recommended value[25] for encapsulated beta-particle sources is $r_0=2$ mm and $\theta_0=90°$; $G(r,\theta)$ is a geometry factor; $g(r)$ is the radial dose function; and $F(r,\theta)$ is the source anisotropy function. The coordinate system for this protocol is shown in Figure 5. The geometry factor accounts for the geometric fall off of dose rate with distance and is calculated using the line source approximation as:

$$G(r,\theta) = (\theta_2-\theta_1)/(L\,r\,\sin\theta) \qquad (10)$$

where L is the active source length (see Fig. 5). The radial dose function describes the effects of absorption and scatter along the transverse axis of the source and is defined as:

$$g(r) = D(r,\theta_0)G(r_0,\theta_0)/D(r_0,\theta_0)G(r,\theta_0) \qquad (11)$$

where $D(r,\theta_0)$ refers to the dose at radius r and $\theta_0=90°$. Finally, the anisotropy factor is defined as:

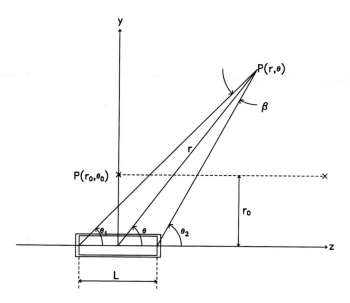

Figure 5. The geometrical conventions of the TG-43 Protocol for the representation of the absorbed-dose profile of a brachytherapy source in a tissue-equivalent medium.

$$F(r,\theta) = D(r,\theta)G(r,\theta_0)/D(r,\theta_0)G(r,\theta) \qquad (12)$$

where again, $D(r,\theta)$ refers to the dose at (r,θ). Values for the reference dose rate for a source can be determined from extrapolation chamber measurements as described above. Values for the active length, L, of a source can be determined from film measurements, also as described above. The meaning of these quantities are described further in the TG-43 protocol.[24]

Transfer of Calibrations

In order for calibrations to be transferred from a standards laboratory to a user, a mechanism must be defined. It is proposed that, similar to the case of photon-emitting brachytherapy sources, secondary-standard well-type ionization chambers be used to affect this transfer. To calibrate the secondary standard ionization chambers, sources that have been calibrated in terms of reference absorbed-dose rate to water at the primary standards laboratory are used to establish a relationship to instrument reading. Such a calibrated instrument can then be used to determine reference absorbed-dose rate for other sources of exactly the same type (isotope, construction, encapsulation) in exactly the same geometry (source holding jig, position within chamber). It must be understood that each source type has a unique calibration factor for each instrument type, and that variation in calibration factors for the same source type among different instruments of the same type should not be unexpected. This is because well-type ionization chambers respond mainly to the bremsstrahlung photons created by the primary beta-particle emissions, and the bremsstrahlung production is strongly dependent on the material immediately surrounding the source and the ionization chamber wall material.

References

1. Lentino W, Zaret MM, Rossignol B, et al. Treatment of pterygium by surgery followed by beta radiation. Am J Roentgenol 1959;81:93–98.
2. van den Brenk HAS. Results of prophylactic postoperative irradiation in 1300 cases of pterygium. Am J Roentgenol 1968;103:723–768.
3. Cooper JS. Postoperative irradiation of pterygia: Ten more years of experience. Radiology 1978;128:753–756.
4. Loevinger R. Extrapolation chamber for the measurement of beta sources. Rev Sci Inst 1953;24:907–914.
5. Loevinger R, Trott NG. Design and operation of an extrapolation chamber with removable electrodes. Int J Appl Radiat Isot 1966;17:103–111.
6. Failla G. The measurement of tissue dose in terms of the same unit for all ionising radiations. Radiology 1937;29:202–215.
7. Owen B. The beta calibration of radiation survey instruments at protection levels. Phys Med Biol 1972;17:175–186.
8. Owen B. Factors for converting beta-ray dose rates measured in air to dose rates in tissue. Phys Med Biol 1973;18:355–368.
9. Böhm J. Saturation corrections for plane-parallel ionization chambers. Phys Med Biol 1976;21:754–759.
10. Böhm J. The perturbation correction factor of ionization chambers in β-radiation fields. Phys Med Biol 1980;25:65–75.
11. International Organization for Standardization. Reference Beta Radiations for Calibrating Dosimeters and Doseratemeters and for Determining their Response as a Function of Beta Radiation Energy, International Standard ISO 6980. Geneva: International Organization for Standardization; 1984, revised 1995.
12. Soares CG, Darley, PJ, Charles MW, et al. Hot particle dosimetry using extrapolation chambers and radiochromic foils. Rad Prot Dosim 1991;39:55–59.
13. McWilliams FF, Scannell MJ, Soares CG, et al. Hot particle dosimetry using ^{60}Co spheres. Rad Prot Dosim 1992;40:223–234.
14. Soares CG, McLaughlin WL. Measurement if radial dose distributions around small beta particle emitters using high resolution radiochromic foil dosimetry. Rad Prot Dosim 1993;47:367–372.
15. Soares CG. Calibration of ophthalmic applicators at NIST: A revised approach. Med Phys 1991;18:787–793.
16. Darley PJ, Charles MW, Hart CD, et al. Dosimetry of planar and punctiform beta sources using an automated extrapolation chamber and radiochromic dye films. Rad Prot Dosim 1991;39:61–66.
17. Deasy JO, Soares CG. Extrapolation chamber measurements of ^{90}Sr+^{90}Y beta-particle ophthalmic applicator dose rates. Med Phys 1994;21:91–99.
18. Pruitt JS, Soares CG, Ehrlich M. Calibration of Beta-Particle Radiation Instrumentation and Sources. NBS Special Publication 250–21. Gaithersburg, MD: National Institute of Standards and Technology; 1988.
19. Soares CG, Halpern DG, Wang C-K. Calibration and characterization of beta-particle sources for intravascular brachytherapy. Med Phys 1998;25:339–346.
20. Pruitt JS. Calibration of Beta-Particle Emitting Ophthalmic Applicators. NBS Special Publication 250–9. Gaithersburg, MD: National Institute of Standards and Technology; 1987.
21. Niroomand-Rad A, Blackwell CR, Coursey BM, et al. Radiochromic dosimetry: Recommendations of the AAPM Radiation Therapy Task Group 55. Med Phys 1998;25:2093–2115.
22. Cross WG. Variation of beta dose attenuation in different media. Phys Med Biol 1968;13:611–618.
23. International Commission on Radiation Units and Measurements. Dosimetry of External Beta Rays for Radiation Protection. ICRU Report 56. Bethesda, MD: International Commission on Radiation Units and Measurements; 1997.
24. Nath R, Anderson LL, Luxton G, et al. Dosimetry of interstitial brachytherapy sources: Recommendations of the AAPM Radiation Therapy Task Group No. 43. Med Phys 1995;22:209–234.
25. Nath R, Amols H, Coffey C, et al. Intravascular brachytherapy physics: Report of the AAPM Radiation Therapy Task Group No. 60. Med Phys 1999;26:119–152.

## Chapter 17

The Physics and Dosimetry of Gamma and X-Ray Emitting Isotopes

Shirish K. Jani, PhD

Introduction

Radioactivity is the process in which atomic nuclei spontaneously change their configuration and energy content. This event normally brings a change in the basic element itself and is known as radioactive disintegration or radioactive decay. This process is usually associated with the emission of particulate or electromagnetic radiation. The particulate radiation is either alpha emission or beta emission. Alpha particles are heavy charged particles and have a short range in tissues. Beta particles are lightweight particles and possess positive or negative charge. They travel finite distances within tissues. A third type of emission, known as gamma emission, is in the form of electromagnetic radiation. Most often, an atomic nucleus with excess energy will emit a particle followed by gamma radiation. There are very few radioisotopes that emit only particles. An example of a pure beta emitter is phosphorus 32.

An alternate way for an unstable nucleus to reach a stable state (often called ground state) is to capture an electron orbiting just outside the nucleus. This process is called electron capture. The nucleus may reach a stable state by capturing the electron but the outer shell where electrons are orbiting becomes unstable. To fill the void of the swallowed electron, other electrons from nearby orbits jump to the inner most orbit (closest to the nucleus). This leads to emission of x-rays which are characteristic to the electron configuration. An example of the electron capture process is iodine 125.

The emission of a particle (α or β) or the capture of an orbital electron may not be sufficient to bring the nucleus to the ground energy level. In this case, the nucleus relieves itself of the excess energy by radiating it in the form of one or more gamma photons. An example of gamma emission is cobalt 60.

The γ-rays emitted by nucleus may have one or two discrete energy values or they may have a very complicated spectrum consisting of many energy values. The γ-ray is the same as an x-ray photon of the same energy. The only distinction between the two terms lies in their origins. X-rays are electromagnetic waves (pockets of energy) that originate in the outer shell of atoms or due to slow-down of charged particles. The gamma rays, on the other hand, are electromagnetic radiation that arise in the atomic nuclei. Figures 1 through 5 illustrate decay schemes

From Waksman R (ed.). *Vascular Brachytherapy, Third Edition.* Armonk, NY: Futura Publishing Co., Inc.; © 2002.

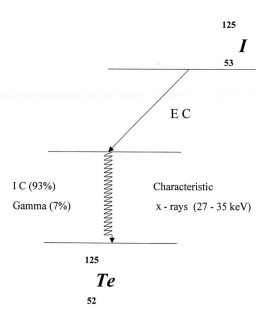

Figure 1. Disintegration scheme for ^{125}I nuclei. See references for more detailed information on this decay process.

of commonly used radioisotopes in brachytherapy. Further details of this subject are given in several books.[1–3]

Iodine (atomic number Z=53; atomic mass A=125) nuclei decay via electron capture to excited state of tellurium 125 (Z=52). The ^{125}Te reaches its ground state by either internal conversion (93% of the time) or gamma emission. As shown in

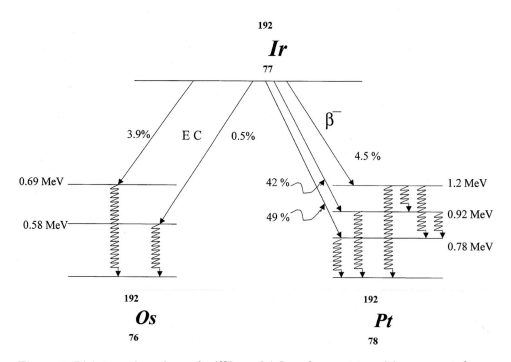

Figure 2. Disintegration scheme for ^{192}Ir nuclei. Less frequent transitions are not shown. The gamma spectrum is very complex with emission ranging in energy from 0.1 to 1.06 MeV. Average number of gammas per decay is 2.2.

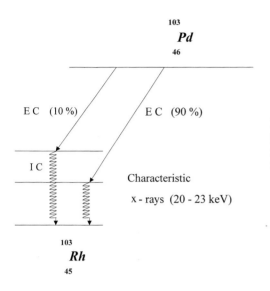

Figure 3. Disintegration mode for [103]Pd nuclei. Only a few of the characteristic x-ray energies are shown here. Average number of photons per decay is 0.8.

Figure 1, both of these processes lead to the production of characteristic x-rays, mainly in the range of 27.4 to 35 keV.

Iridium (atomic number Z=77; atomic mass A=192) nuclei decay via negative beta emission (95.6% of the time) to platinum 192 (Z=78) and via electron capture (4.4%) to osmium 192 (Z=76). The excited nuclei of [192]Pt and [192]Os emit a number of gamma rays in the energy range of 0.136 to 1.06 MeV; the primary emission being in the 0.3 to 0.6 MeV range (Fig. 2).

Palladium (atomic number Z=46; atomic mass A=103) nuclei decay via electron capture, largely to the first (90%) and second (10%) excited states of rhodium 103 (Z=45). The characteristic x-rays from [103]Rh are mainly in the range of 20 to 23 keV (Fig. 3).

Samarium (atomic number Z=62; atomic mass A=145) nuclei decay via electron capture to promethium 145 (Z=61), which, in turn, decays to stable neodymium 145 (Z=60) by the same mechanism. As shown in Figure 4, the x-rays in the energy range of 38 to 61 keV are emitted from a sealed [145]Sm source.

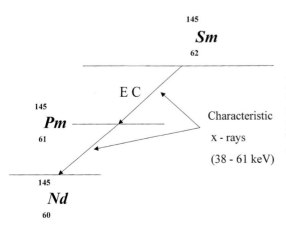

Figure 4. Decay mode of [145]Sm nuclei. Characteristic x-rays resulting from the two successive electron capture processes have more than 10 energy values. Average number of photons per decay is 2.29.

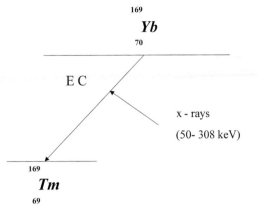

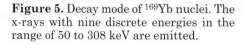

Figure 5. Decay mode of ^{169}Yb nuclei. The x-rays with nine discrete energies in the range of 50 to 308 keV are emitted.

Ytterbium (atomic number Z=70; atomic mass A=169) nuclei decay via electron capture to stable thulium 169 (Z=69), emitting x-rays in the engery range of 50 to 308 keV. The principal x-ray energies are 50, 51, 57, 63, 178, and 198 keV (Fig. 5).

Radioactive Decay

The process of radioactive decay is a spontaneous, random event; therefore, it must be studied statistically. In a sample with a large number of atoms (which happens to be the case in the practical world!), the decay process follows the exponential behavior. The radioactivity (or simply activity) of a sample is defined as the number of disintegrations occurring per unit time. The units in which activity has been conventionally measured are:

1 becquerel (Bq) = 1 disintegration/second
1 curie (Ci) = 3.7×10^{10} Bq
1 millicurie (mCi) = 3.7×10^7 Bq

As the nuclei of radioactive material disintegrate (ie, decay), the number of nuclei available for decay decreases. In other words, the activity of a sample material decreases with time. The rate of decrease varies quite a bit among radioisotopes. Its value is unique to each isotope. This rate of decay follows the exponential formula:

$$A(t) = A(o) \, e^{-0.693*t/T_{1/2}}$$

a where A (o) is the known activity of the isotope at certain time, we call zero; A (t) is the activity remaining in the sample material at time t; and $T_{1/2}$ is a constant called half-life. The half-life of an isotope is the time during which its activity reduces to half its original value. For example, let us consider 10 mCi of an iridium 192 seed source on a certain day. The half-life of ^{192}Ir is 74.2 days. Therefore, 74.2 days later, the source activity will decrease to 5 mCi. After 148.4 days (ie, two half-life time spans), the remaining activity will be 2.5 mCi. The above equation shows that decay process follows an exponential, and not linear, curve. Thus, the activity of a source approaches zero over time, but does not ever become zero. Table 1 lists the decay of activity over time for five γ- or x-ray emitting isotopes.

Table 1

Decay Characteristics of Some Gamma Isotopes

Time (Days)	% of Remaining Activity (mCi)				
	^{125}I	^{192}Ir	^{103}Pd	^{145}Sm	^{169}Yb
0	100	100	100	100	100
1	98.8	99.1	96.0	99.8	97.9
2	97.7	98.1	92.2	99.6	95.8
4	95.4	96.3	84.9	99.2	91.7
6	93.3	94.6	78.3	98.8	87.8
8	91.1	92.8	72.2	98.4	84.1
10	89.0	91.1	66.5	98.0	80.5
20	79.2	83.0	44.2	96.0	64.8
30	70.6	75.6	29.4	94.1	52.2
40	62.8	68.8	19.6	92.2	42.0
50	55.9	62.7	13.0	90.3	33.9
60	49.8	57.1	08.7	88.5	27.3

Interaction of Gamma and X-Rays with Tissues

It is important to understand how gamma rays deliver their radiation energy to tissues during vascular brachytherapy. This helps us study the effects of tissue inhomogeneity like calcified plaque or metallic stent on the dose perturbations during arterial irradiation.

Gamma rays interact with medium (like tissues) in one of three ways:

1. Photoelectric effect (PE)
2. Compton scattering (CS)
3. Pair production (PP)

In each of these interactions, a γ-ray imparts its energy to the medium and sets an electron in motion. Thus, the energy transfer (or radiation dose delivery) for γ-rays is a two-step process: in the first step, a γ-ray produces a high-speed electron, and in the second step, this electron imparts all its kinetic energy to tissues through the process of ionization. This is an important feature of gamma that sets it apart from beta radiation.

The probability of each of the above interactions depends mainly on two factors: energy E of gamma and atomic number Z of the medium it travels through. The probability of PE interaction is directly proportional to Z^3 and inversely proportional to E^3. In other words, PE is strongly dependent on E and Z. As Z of a medium is increased, the likelihood of a gamma interacting with it goes up. As the gamma energy increases, PE probability falls rapidly. For example, a 10 keV photon is 8 times more likely to have PE interaction in water than a 20 keV photon. On the other hand, a 20 keV photon (ie, a γ-ray) is 4.4 times more likely to interact with bone (Z≈12.3) compared to soft tissues (Z≈7.5). This is the reason why bone casts a very clear shadow on a diagnostic x-ray radiograph where bone/soft tissue contrast is enhanced by PE interaction due to their differing Z values.

The CS interaction is independent of atomic number Z of the medium. Its

Table 2

Physical Properties of Gamma and X-Ray Emitting Isotopes

			Isotope		
Property	^{125}I	^{192}Ir	^{103}Pd	^{145}Sm	^{169}Yb
Average gamma energy (keV)	28	370	21	41	93
Half-life (days)	60	74.2	17	340	32
Half-value layer in mm of lead	0.025	3	0.01	0.06	0.2
Commercially available source size (mm)	0.8 × 4.5	0.5 × 3	0.8 × 4.5	0.8 × 4.5*	0.8 × 4.5*
Exposure rate constant $\dfrac{R\ cm^2}{mCi \cdot hr}$	1.45	4.69	1.48	0.88	1.80
Dose rate constant (cGy/mCi hr)	1.16	4.55	0.95	1.1	—

*Not available commercially.

probability decreases with increase in gamma energy. Above 100 keV gamma energy, CS interaction is predominant because PE probability is negligible.

The PP interaction increases with energy as well as Z. However, it occurs at energies above 1.022 MeV. Therefore, it is not of interest to discuss it for vascular brachytherapy application where low-energy gamma is preferred due to radiation safety concerns.

Table 2 gives important physical properties of the γ- and x-ray emitting isotopes discussed in this chapter. Half-value layer (HVL) for an isotope is defined as the thickness of a material required to reduce the isotope's radiation exposure by 50%. Exposure rate constant of an isotope is defined as the exposure rate in roentgen per hour at a 1-cm distance from a 1-mCi source. Dose rate constant is defined as the dose rate in cGy/hr at 1 cm from a 1-mCi source in water.

Table 3 describes the relative importance of PE and CS interactions for the gamma- and x-ray emitting isotopes. The f-factor given here is defined as the amount of dose delivered (cGy) per unit exposure (roentgen, or simply R). As such, it is a mea-

Table 3

Process of Energy Absorption for Gamma and X-Ray Emitting Isotopes

		^{125}I	^{192}Ir	^{103}Pd	^{145}Sm	^{169}Yb
% Energy transferred in water* (Relative importance of interactions)	PE	93%	0%	99%	81%	15%
	CS	7%	100%	1%	19%	85%
f-factor in (cGy/R)† (See text for details)	Water	0.88	0.97	0.89	0.89	0.95
	Muscle	0.92	0.96	0.92	0.93	0.95
	Bone	4.44	0.93	4.3	4.2	1.7

PE = photoelectric effect; CS = Crompton scattering.
*Page 163 of Reference 1. †Page 739 of Reference 1.

sure of the amount of energy absorbed in various media for same amount of radiation exposure offered to the medium. As shown in Table 3, for example, the absorption of energy in bone for 125I gammas is 4.44/0.92=4.82 times more than in muscle. This is because PE interaction is very dominant here due to lower gamma energy and high Z difference between bone and muscle. In vascular brachytherapy, a calcified plaque (with calcium having Z=20 compared to water with $Z \approx 7.5$) is highly likely to absorb low-energy gamma from iodine or palladium compared to surrounding muscle cell layers in arterial walls. As a result, a calcified plaque could cast a dose shadow behind a plaque with calcium. If the intent of vascular radiotherapy is to deliver a certain dose to treat media, then portions of media shadowed by plaque could receive decreased doses. This is an unwanted feature of low-energy gammas in vascular brachytherapy.

The above-described feature may be very helpful in radiation protection aspects of gamma brachytherapy. As shown in Table 2, a very thin foil of lead (less than a tenth of a millimeter) is sufficient in stopping all gammas from 125I, 103Pd, or 145Sm isotopes. This is because PE interaction probability is very high at these low energies for a material-like lead (Pb, Z=82). At high gamma energy, for example, 192Ir emission, the HVL is 3 mm of lead which is a lot more than the beam values of most diagnostic and interventional procedures.

The energy absorbed by tissues from gamma radiation is called dose. The radiation dose is defined as the amount of energy absorbed per unit mass of tissue. The unit of radiation absorbed dose is gray or rad and is defined as follows:

1 gray (Gy) = 1 joule/kg
1 gray (Gy) = 100 centigray (cGy)
1 centigray (cGy) = 1 rad (old unit)

Dose Distribution Near Gamma Sources

The radiation dose at any point around a small gamma-emitting source depends primarily on its distance away from the source. Energy of gamma plays a very little, if any, role in affecting dose distribution close to a source. For a point source (ie, a source small enough to be considered a point source), the dose intensity around it is proportional to the inverse of the square of distance. For example, the dose at 2 cm away from a small 125I source will be 4 times less than the dose at 1 cm. In other words, the dose drops off very fast with distance around a point source. In practice, there is no such thing as a perfect point source. However, the sources developed for conventional radiotherapy have been very small in size. As shown in Table 2, these gamma sources are available in the form of sealed seeds a few millimeters in size. For conventional brachyradiotherapy where point of interest is greater than or equal to 10 mm away, these sources may be safely assumed as a point source for dose computation. However, for vascular brachytherapy, the tissues of interest for dose delivery may be 2 to 4 mm away from a source. In this instance, the sources are not small enough to be considered a point source.

In practice, we need to employ a line source to treat a finite (2 to 8 cm) length of an arterial wall during vascular brachytherapy.[4] Theoretically, the dose intensity around a line source is proportional to the inverse of distance. However, in close proximity of the source, the dose depends on a variety of factors such as oblique filtration of gammas through source wall (ie, source geometry), scatter of gammas within tissues from the source itself and possible contribution from betas for some isotopes. The dose within a few millimeters of a line source is a complex issue that has not yet been fully explored by medical physics community.

The dose rate around a source depends primarily on its strength, ie, activity. Table 2 lists the dose rate constants (dose rate in cGy/hr at a 1-cm distance from a 1-mCi source strength) for the gamma isotopes of interest. It can be seen that for every mCi of activity, ^{192}Ir isotope offers 3 times greater dose rate than ^{125}I or [103]Pd source. This is important in vascular brachytherapy where short treatment times are desirable.

Dose to Surrounding Normal Tissues from Gamma Sources

Dose distribution around sealed sources depend, in general, on four factors: distance, source size and make, absorption in tissues, and scattering by tissues.[5] Absorption decreases the dose at a point whereas scatter increases it. At distances very close to a source, the absorption and scattering in tissues have opposite and equal effects and therefore nullify each other's effects. Therefore, at distances of less than about 10 mm, the dose depends primarily on distance and secondarily on source size and housing. Further away from the source, the dose begins to be influenced by absorption and scatter phenomena which are not equal in magnitude. Since these two depend on gamma energy, the dose at several centimeters is energy-dependent. For low-energy gammas, the absorption by tissues is greater than scatter; hence, dose drops off faster than the inverse square effect. For high-energy gammas this effect is not as pronounced.

The dosimetric parameter that accounts for absorption and scatter within the medium is called radial dose function (g[r]). It is defined as the ratio of dose at distance r to dose at 1 cm in tissues with the effect of the inverse square law removed; both points being on the transverse axis of the source. The g(r) has conventionally been obtained experimentally from the depth dose data of *small* sealed sources. It is unity at 1 cm by definition. Table 4 lists the radial dose function for five gamma

Table 4

The Radial Dose Function of *Small* Gamma and X-Ray Emitting Sealed Sources

Radial Distance r (cm)	Radial Dose Function, g(r)*				
	[125]I	[192]Ir	[103]Pd	[145]Sm	[169]Yb
1	1.00	1.00	1.00	1.00	1.00
2	0.86	1.03	0.54	1.02	1.10
3	0.68	1.00	0.29	0.97	1.18
4	0.53	0.97	0.16	0.92	1.21
5	0.38	0.97	0.09	0.87	1.23
6	0.29	0.97	—	0.78	1.23
7	0.23	0.95	—	0.69	1.20
8	0.20	0.94	—	0.61	1.17
9	—	0.91	—	0.52	1.14
10	—	0.87	—	0.44	1.10

*Page 161 of Reference 2.

Table 5

Estimated Dose to Surrounding Normal Tissues from Gamma
and X-Ray Emitting Sealed Sources

Distance from Source (cm)	Relative Dose (%)				
	125I	192Ir	103Pd	145Sm	169Yb
1	100	100	100	100	100
2	22	26	14	26	28
3	8	11	3	11	13
4	3	6	1	6	8
5	2	4	0.4	4	5

isotopes of interest to us for vascular application. Variation of dose with distance beyond 1 cm for small (point-like) sealed sources is given in Table 5. These depth dose data show that dose beyond 1 cm is still greatly influenced by distance. Also, the dose at these distances is very little. It is important to note that dose values given in Table 5 are normalized to 1-cm distance. For vascular brachytherapy, the dose may be prescribed at, let us say, 3-mm distance. The values relative to this dose prescription would be much smaller than those of Table 5. Furthermore, the data given here are for small sources. In clinical applications where linear sources of several centimeters in length are utilized, it would be necessary to employ the measured depth dose data.

Dose to Other Body Organs from Gamma Sources

Dose to tissues within 5 cm from irradiated artery was described in the previous section. The gamma source that is widely used in many brachytherapy procedures is 192Ir. It is used in manually loaded implants as well as remotely loaded high dose rate (HDR) units, such as the Micro-Selectron machine by Nucletron Corporation in the use of a peripheral vascular irradiation study. At present, this isotope happens to be the most frequently used gamma source in coronary irradiation studies as well. Since it is a medium- to high-energy gamma emitter, it may be of interest to examine dose to peripheral tissues and organs from an 192Ir brachytherapy.

Measurements made in humanoid phantom show that tissue attenuation begins to affect the dose as the point of interest moves further away from a source.[6] This is partly because the influence of the inverse square law is not as dominant as it is at close distances. Using calculated dose gradient from an 192Ir linear source,[7] for up to 1 cm distance and measured values beyond this distance,[6] we have estimated the dose to tissues which may be tens of centimeters away from a vascular brachytherapy site. Table 6 shows that doses to far away tissues within a patient are small. In fact, the dose to body tissues may be significantly higher from a standard interventional procedure the patient must undergo during balloon angioplasty and/or stenting than these 192Ir values. The issue of the biological effect of these small doses is beyond the scope of this chapter.

Table 6

Estimated Dose to Peripheral Organs fom an Iridium 192 Vascular Application. A Dose of 800 cGy Is Assumed to be Delivered at 0.3 cm from a 5-cm Linear Source

Distance from Source (cm)	Estimated Dose* (cGy)
0.3	800
1.0	179
—	—
10	2.5
20	0.44
30	0.12
40	0.04
50	0.01

*Values derived from data of References 5 and 6.

Acknowledgments: The author would like to acknowledge the help of Marcia Straile of Scripps Clinic, and Ashish Jani and Shyam Jani in the preparation of this manuscript.

References

1. Johns HE, Cunningham JR. The Physics of Radiology. Springfield, IL: Charles C. Thomas Publishers; 1983:71–99.
2. Jani SK. Handbook of Dosimetry Data for Radiotherapy. Boca Raton, FL: CRC Press; 1993:137–167.
3. Selman J. The Basic Physics of Radiation Therapy. Springfield, IL: Charles C. Thomas Publishers; 1990:396–437.
4. Nath R. Physical properties and clinical uses of brachytherapy radionuclide. In: Williamson JF, Thomadsen BR, Nath R (eds.): Brachytherapy Physics. Madison, WI: Medical Physics Publishing Co.; 1995:7–38.
5. Jani SK. Physics of vascular brachytherapy. J Invas Cardiol 1999;11:517–523.
6. Venselaar JLM, van der Giessen PH, Dries WJF. Measurement and calculation of the dose at large distances from brachytherapy sources: Cs-137, Ir-192 and Co-60. Med Phys 1996;23:537–543.
7. Kline RW, Gillin MT, Grimm DF, et al. Computer dosimetry of ^{192}Ir wire. Med Phys 1985;12:634–638.

## Chapter 18

Intravascular Brachytherapy Physics:

Review of Radiation Sources and Techniques

Howard I. Amols, PhD

Introduction

Over the past 8 years intravascular brachytherapy (IVB) has gradually evolved from an investigational device to an accepted clinical procedure. Of the numerous radioactive isotopes and delivery systems that have been proposed or tested, several have emerged as the "most likely" to achieve widespread clinical use (at least in the foreseeable future). This chapter will focus on these more common systems, although alternate isotopes and delivery systems will also be discussed, as IVB is likely to remain an evolving field for several years to come.

Most commonly, radiation is administered immediately after coronary balloon angioplasty by inserting high-activity radioactive seed or wire sources for several minutes into the target artery, via conventional or slightly modified catheters, after which the sources and catheters are removed. Although there is still no consensus on the "ideal isotope," a "short list" of most commonly used isotopes has emerged,[1–8] which includes almost exclusively ^{192}Ir, ^{90}Sr/^{90}Y, and ^{32}P. Isotopes such as ^{188}W\$^{188}$Re, ^{186}Re, ^{133}Xe, ^{99m}Tc, ^{103}Pd, and others, have also seen limited use in small experimental protocols, but do not appear to be likely candidates for widespread clinical use in the immediate future. The most widely tested source to date (based on number of trials, and total number of patients treated) has been the gamma isotope ^{192}Ir, followed by the beta isotopes ^{90}Sr/^{90}Y, and ^{32}P. The "Glossary" at the end of this chapter provides a review of basic terms in radiation physics, and a list of isotopes is included in Table 1.

Alternate isotope and delivery systems (on the horizon, vis-à-vis widespread clinical use) continue to be explored such as:

1. Inflation of the angiographic balloon with radioactive liquid or gas[9,10] (^{188}Re, ^{186}Re, ^{133}Xe);
2. Infusion of radioactive liquids into the vessel walls via infusion catheters[11] (^{99m}Tc);
3. The use of balloons with radioactive walls[12] (^{32}P);
4. Development of miniature x-ray tubes small enough to be inserted through angiographic catheters[13];

From Waksman R (ed.). *Vascular Brachytherapy, Third Edition.* Armonk, NY: Futura Publishing Co., Inc.; © 2002.

Table 1

Possible Sources for Intraluminal Brachytherapy: Temporary Implants and Stents

Isotope	Energy (keV)		Half-life	Comment
	Maximum	Average		
^{192}Ir	612	378	74 d	High-energy gamma, some radiation safety concerns, used in many clinical trials.
^{32}P	1710	690	14 d	Beta energy lower than optimal. Used in several clinical trials, and also for radioactive stents.
^{90}Sr/Y	2270	970	28 yr	Beta emitter with better range than ^{32}P. Parent-daughter pair provides acceptable energy and long half-life. Used in clinical trials.
^{90}Y	2270	970	64 hr	Beta emitter, but half-life lower than optimal. Wire source used in limited clinical trial.
^{188}W/Re	2130	780	69 d	Parent-daughter beta source combining acceptable half-life and high energy. Limited testing of wire source prototype. Also emits gammas.
^{188}Re	2130	780	17 hr	Short-lived beta source produced from long-lived ^{188}W generator. Used for radioactive liquid-filled balloon. Also emits gammas.
^{103}Pd	21	21	19 d	Low-energy x-ray emitter. Cannot be produced at high enough activity yet for catheter use, but being tested for permanent radioactive stent.
^{99m}Tc	140	140	6 hr	Prototype infusion catheter. Gamma emitter.
x-ray tube	30	10	NA	Prototype miniaturized (1.25-mm diameter) tube for catheter use.
^{106}Ru/Rh	3540	1180	1 yr	High-energy parent-daughter beta emitter, but hard to produce and also emits gammas.
^{48}V	690	230	16d	Positron emitter proposed for radioactive stents. Also emits 511 keV gammas.
^{133}Xe	340	115	5.3 d	Prototype gas-filled balloon. Very low-energy beta with limited range.
^{125}I	35	28	60 d	Low-energy x-ray emitter. Cannot be produced at high enough activity yet.

5. Delivery of radiation using pulsed or gated external photon or electron beams[14,15] from a linear accelerator (such as those used in conventional cancer radiation therapy); and

6. Permanently implanted radioactive stents[16–18] (^{32}P, ^{103}Pd, ^{48}V).

Of these alternate systems, only radioactive stents have had significant clinical testing, and as such appear to be the only alternate system likely to see "routine" clinical application in the near future.

While the target cells and radiobiological mechanisms by which radiation inhibits restenosis are still not clearly understood, enough radiobiological and clinical data has been accumulated to enable us to define "reasonable" constraints on the source and dosimetry requirements for catheter-based, high dose rate, IVB. In particular, we know or strongly suspect that the following dosimetric parameters will result in good clinical outcome:

1. A minimum dose of 8 to 10 Gy to the media, internal elastic lamina, and/or adventitia;

2. An average dose of 15 to 20 Gy to "most" of the vessel wall;
3. A maximum dose of 30 to 40 Gy to the internal elastic lamina;
4. A maximum dose of 40 to 60 Gy to the innermost lumen wall.

The exact dose values are still somewhat uncertain. Conditions 1 and 3 are based on the dosimetry protocol and positive clinical findings of the SCRIPPS Trial (Tierstein et al[1,2]). Condition 2 is based on the WRIST trial (Waksman et al[3]), and condition 4 on the Venezuelan experience (Condado et al[4,5]). It is important to recognize that the radiation dose delivered to *any* coronary artery via *any* radiation isotope or delivery system will be extremely inhomogeneous (for reasons discussed below). The goal of any patient treatment is therefore to deliver an adequate dose to all target tissues, while at the same time ensuring that normal tissue dose tolerance (which could cause long-term biological damage to the treated artery) is not exceeded. This "biological dose window" is believed to be in the range of a mininum dose of 8 or 10 Gy, to a maximum dose of 40 or 60 Gy. That is, a minimum dose of 8 to 10 Gy is required to inhibit hyperplasia and restenosis, but a maximum dose of 40 to 60 Gy should not be exceeded.

As we discuss more fully below, doses from all radioactive sources decrease by at least 30 to 50% per millimeter, with the dose being very high near the source, but decreasing rapidly with increasing distance.[19] Thus, if the arterial wall is more than a few millimeters in thickness (which is true in many clinical scenarios), delivering the radiation dose to all required tissues in the vessel wall within the above hypothesized dose window may not be possible. In such situations clinical outcome may be compromised.

With this in mind, we present a review of the dosimetric requirements for the irradiation of coronary arteries, and the physical and dosimetric characteristics of the various irradiation techniques. For effective treatments, the dose distribution must be confined to the region of the angioplasty, with reduced doses to normal vessels and myocardium. Irradiation times should ideally be no more 5 to 30 minutes to reduce the risk of thrombosis, ischemia, and other possible complications during treatment. Treatment times significantly shorter than 3 to 5 minutes, however, may increase the risk of dosimetry errors due to the fact that source transit time in and out of the catheter becomes a significant fraction of the total treatment time. To deliver radiation doses of 8 to 60 Gy at distances of 1 to 4 mm from a radioactive catheter or balloon in a time period of 5 to 30 minutes requires source activities on the order of hundreds of millicuries (mCi) to several curies (Ci) for gamma sources, or 10 to 100 mCi for beta sources. These are significant quantities of radioactive material, the use of which introduces radiation safety issues for both patients and staff, particularly so when using gamma sources.

In all countries, the possession and use of radioactive materials for therapeutic use is strictly regulated. In the United States, regulations originate from the Nuclear Regulatory Commission (NRC), or in so-called "Agreement States" (ie, states in which the NRC permits state agencies to perform these functions) with various state agencies. For IVB in particular, the U.S. Food and Drug Administration has issued additional legal constraints on the use of radioisotopes. Similar guidelines on the therapeutic use of radioactive materials are given by both the International Commission on Radiological Protection (ICRP) and Euratom. Most European and other countries have their own regulatory requirements, but all are based (generally) on ICRP guidelines.

Dosimetry of Gamma-Emitting Seeds and Wires

We consider first the physical and dosimetric requirements of IVB with radio-active seeds or wires, which can be summarized as follows:

1. Single fraction dose of 8 to 60 Gy to a length of 2 to 5 cm of arterial wall, approximately 2- to 5-mm inner diameter, 0.5- to 3-mm wall thickness;
2. High dose volume confined to the region of angioplasty, with minimum dose to normal vessels and myocardium;
3. Dose rates less than 2 Gy/min (to keep treatment times <30 min);
4. The radioactive source must have dimensions, stiffness, and flexibility compatible for use with angiographic catheters. Source diameter must therefore be less than 0.5 to 1.0 mm, yet stiff enough to be pushed through greater than 100 cm of artery, and flexible enough to negotiate multiple bends in the coronary tree. Source integrity is of great importance as dislodgment into a coronary artery could be fatal.

Any gamma- (or x-ray-, or photon-) emitting source with energy greater than approximately 30 keV and activity greater than 1 Ci would ideally meet these requirements. The radial dose fall-off from any gamma source (ie, the rate at which dose decreases with increasing distance from the source) is determined by two factors; geometry and attenuation:

1. Geometry factors have the most impact on the dose distribution. For a "point source" of radiation, the dose decreases approximately as the square of the distance from the source. That is, if the distance from the source is doubled, eg, from 2 mm distance to 4 mm, the dose decreases by a factor of 4. If the distance is tripled, eg, from 2 mm to 6 mm, the dose decreases by a factor of 9, etc. Radioactive sources used for IVB, however, are not "point sources," but are more typically 20 to 30 mm in length. For these linear sources the geometric decrease in dose is slightly less severe, falling more nearly as the first power of the distance, rather than the square of the distance.
2. In addition to the geometric decrease, the dose rate also decreases with increasing distance from the source because of attenuation of the gammas by the intervening tissues. That is, gammas are physically removed from the beam via absorption by tissue, thus decreasing the dose.

For gammas greater than 30 keV energy attenuation over the first 4 to 5 mm of tissue is negligible, and the dose fall-off with distance is determined almost entirely by the geometry. For lower energy gammas or x-rays, such as ^{103}Pd (21 keV energy) attenuation of photons by intervening tissue amounts to less than 5% additional dose fall-off, although this can be significantly higher if the intervening tissue has high density or high atomic number (such as calcified plaque). In general, so long as the photon energy is greater than 20 to 30 keV, the "near field" dosimetry will have the similar ideal properties, independent of energy. At larger distances, however, such as several centimeters from the source, one would ideally like the dose to decrease as rapidly as possible to spare normal tissues outside the treatment region from unnecessary dose. At distances of several centimeters, both high- and low-energy photon sources still have identical geometric dose fall-off, but tissue absorption now becomes more significant for the lower energy sources. For example, with ^{192}Ir (average gamma energy of 378 keV) tissue attenuation at a distance of 5 cm from the source amounts only to approximately 1%. For ^{125}I (average x-ray energy of 28 keV), tissue attenuation at a distance of 5 cm from the source exceeds 60%, and for ^{103}Pd, attenuation exceeds 90%. Thus, in terms of radiation safety, lower energy photon sources have advantages over higher energy sources. Lower energy photon sources have, in fact, radiation safety features similar to betas (discussed further below).

Unfortunately, most lower energy photon sources (including ^{125}I and ^{103}Pd) cannot at present be fabricated into very high-activity seeds or wires, and the dose rates from such sources are, at present, too low for IVB. The only readily available gamma source to date has been ^{192}Ir. Table 1 lists the properties of most isotopes used in IVB. We see that ^{192}Ir has an average gamma energy of 378 keV, which is significantly higher than optimum. Although other potentially more suitable isotopes exist, practical considerations with other isotopes, such as low specific activity, production logistics, high cost, chemical form, toxicity, or short half-life have rendered ^{192}Ir the gamma isotope of choice, at least at the present time. It has therefore become the "work horse" isotope in experiments and clinical trials thus far reported.[1-5] Most IVB studies to date have used an array of ^{192}Ir seeds of total activity 200 to 700 mCi. Each seed is typically 33-mCi activity, 0.5-mm diameter and 3-mm length. A linear array of 4 to 22 seeds can be encased inside a 1-mm diameter plastic catheter to yield an "active length" of approximately 2 to 8 cm. Although higher activity (>10 Ci) ^{192}Ir sources are available for use with high dose rate afterloading devices used in radiation oncology, such sources are too large for intracoronary use. They are however, being used for restenosis treatments in larger peripheral vessels, and could, in theory, be miniaturized for use in coronary-based IVB.

Dose distributions for point- or line-source gamma- and x-ray emitters have been well studied theoretically and experimentally, although measurements at distances less than several millimeters are difficult due to the extremely large dose gradients and other technical considerations. At small distances from the source, dose perturbations caused by scatter and self-absorption make theoretical calculations difficult. The American Association of Physicists in Medicine (AAPM) Task Groups 43[20] and 60[21] have reviewed this problem and recommended that the dose be calculated according to the following formula:

$$\text{Dose}(r,\theta) = S * \Gamma * G(r,\theta) * g(r) * F(r,\theta) \tag{1}$$

where S = air kerma strength; Γ = dose rate constant; r = radial distance from source; θ = angle from point of interest to center of source, as measured from the axial dimension of the source; $F(r,\theta)$ = anisotropy factor describing dose variation versus angle. This function is normalized to unity at $\theta = 90°$; $G(r,\theta)$ = "geometry factor" resulting from spatial distribution of the radioactivity within the source. For a 3- to 5-mm long line source, $G(r,\theta) \approx 1/r^2$ for $\theta \approx 90°$, $g(r)$ = radial dose function which corrects for tissue attenuation. It is given as $\Sigma a_i * r^i$, where a_i = fitted parameters to a fifth order polynomial. $g(r) \approx 1$ for $r < 1$ cm (ie, negligible attenuation).

The formalism of equation 1 was first presented in AAPM Task Group No. 43 (TG-43) as a technique for specifying radiation doses in "conventional" cancer brachytherapy, where dose prescriptions are typically specified at distances greater than 5 to 10 mm from the radiation source. For IVB, where dose prescriptions are required at distances less than 5 mm, many of the functions in equation 1, including the "anisotropy factor" $F(r,\theta)$, the "geometry factor" $G(r,\theta)$, and the radial dose function $g(r)$, are not accurately known. More generally, neither experimental nor theoretical formalisms for determining brachytherapy doses at such short distances are well developed. This issue, and recommendations for future improvements, have been addressed by TG-60.

In Figure 1, we demonstrate that even though some of the terms in equation 1 are not accurately known at distances less than 1 cm, linear extrapolation of data given by TG-43 for larger distances yields reasonably good agreement with experimental results. In Figure 1, we compare calculated (using equation 1) and measured values of dose versus radial distance from a single ^{192}Ir source of 0.5-mm diameter, and 3-mm length.[19] The measured data were obtained by "sandwiching" a 1.1 mCi ^{192}Ir seed between multiple slices of GAFChromic[TM] film (Nuclear Associates, Carle Place, NY) in a water-equivalent plastic phantom for several hours. GAFChromic has become a standard medium for IVB dosimetry measurements[22,23] because it is nearly tissue equivalent, has a near linear response to dose, and requires no post-irradiation processing. Its relative insensitivity and large dynamic range (doses of several Gy are required to obtain optical densities between 0.5 and 2.5) make it particularly useful for measurements of brachytherapy sources where dose rates and dose gradients are large. Doses in Figure 1 are plotted on an absolute scale of cGy/hr/mCi. Agreement at distances from 1.5 to 5.0 mm (typical arterial radii) is seen to be within ±7%, which is quite adequate considering the uncertainties of the measurement technique, the use of extrapolated data, and the high dose gradients involved. More recently, Monte Carlo (MC) calculations and more extensive dosimetry measurements

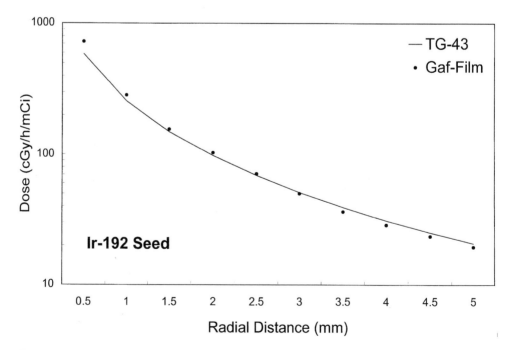

Figure 1. Calculated (using equation 1) and measured (using GAFChromic film) radial dose versus distance for 0.5-mm diameter × 3.0-mm long ^{192}Ir source. Doses are plotted on an absolute scale of cGy/hr/mCi.

have been reported on the dosimetric properties of the radioactive sources for IVB.[24–26]

In Figure 2, we depict calculated isodose distribution in the axial plane around a linear array of 5 ^{192}Ir seeds with 2.0-mm spacing between 3.0-mm long seeds. This source configuration, and resulting dose distributions, are similar to both the SCRIPPS[1,2] and WRIST[3] Trials. The dose distribution at the internal surface of the arterial wall (typically at radial distance=1.5 mm) is seen to be relatively uniform (±10%) with a rapid dose fall-off radially and axially beyond the implant volume (noted schematically in Fig. 2 by the dashed seed locations). The highest dose at a radial distance of 1.5 mm is normalized to 100%. Only half of the implant zone of 23-mm axial length is plotted (because the dose distribution is symmetric about the axial center of the implant).

Dosimetry of Beta-Emitting Seeds and Wires and Comparison with Gamma Sources

While the use of high-energy ^{192}Ir gamma sources results in the most uniform possible dose distribution for IVB, the relative difficulties in shielding these sources has caused concern vis-à-vis radiation safety. In particular, questions regarding whole body doses to patients, and doses to cath lab staff have been raised. Quality assurance programs for "conventional" brachytherapy are well developed,[27] and doses to staff and patients are, in general, kept well below legal lim-

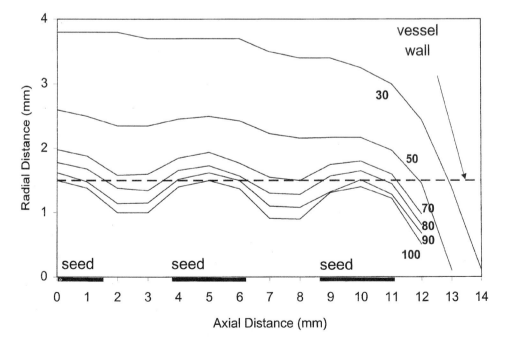

Figure 2. Calculated isodose distribution in the axial plane for a linear array of 5 ^{192}Ir seeds (2.0-mm spacing between 3.0-mm-long seeds as indicated by thick solid lines; total length is approximately 23 mm). The highest dose at a radial distance of 1.5 mm (dashed line) was normalized to 100%, and only half of the implant zone is plotted (the implant is symmetric about the axial center).

its. Special precautions for gamma-based IVB have also been developed, and it has been shown that a careful quality assurance program designed for IVB can reduce patient and staff doses to levels that are comparable to, or even less than, doses attributable to fluoroscopy, cineangiography, and even conventional brachytherapy.[28,29] Despite this, a less penetrating radiation source for IVB applications would clearly be desirable. Since "safer" (ie, easier to shield), low-energy gamma sources are not available at this time (and will be difficult to manufacture), much effort has been directed towards the development of beta sources for IVB. The major difference between gamma and beta particle dosimetry vis-à-vis IVB is that, whereas gammas are merely attenuated (but never completely stopped) by tissue, betas have relatively short, finite ranges. Thus, even though both gamma and beta sources exhibit relatively rapid dose fall-off versus distance because of identical geometric factors (described above for gammas), there is an additional dose fall-off for betas because of their finite range.

Whereas dose for gammas never decreases to zero (because tissue absorption is only a few percent per centimeter), the finite range of betas (typically 1 to 2 cm, depending on energy) results in zero dose delivered beyond this maximum range. Thus, an isotope emitting only beta-minus particles (note that many beta-emitting isotopes also emit some gammas or x-rays) will deliver a large dose to tissues within a few millimeters of the source, and essentially zero dose beyond a 1 to 2 cm distance. The lower the energy of the betas, the more severe the tissue attenuation, and the shorter the range. Like gamma emitters, different beta isotopes emit different energy radiation, and a minimum transition energy of approximately 2 MeV is required for a beta isotope to have a range that is useful for IVB. Three beta isotopes, ^{90}Sr/^{90}Y, and ^{32}P, have emerged as "the most useful" for IVB, and have received the greatest amount of clinical testing.[6–8] The properties of these isotopes are given in Table 1. A comparison of the dose fall-off as a function of distance for different beta and gamma isotopes is given in Figure 3 (discussed more fully later in this section).

The dose calculation formalism presented in equation 1 for gamma isotopes cannot readily be applied to beta isotopes because a beta equivalent of a "dose rate constant" (Γ in equation 1) cannot be physically defined. We can, however, in an analogous fashion, determine dose versus radial distance from a beta source as[30,31]:

$$\text{Dose}(r) = \int_{E=E_{min}}^{E=E_{max}} F(E) * A * k * S(E') * dE / (4\pi\rho r^2) \qquad (2)$$

where r = distance; $F(E)dE$ = electrons emitted per decay in the energy interval $(E+dE)$; A = activity; $S(E')$ = mean restricted stopping power for electron of energy E'; E' = energy at distance r from the source of electron with initial energy E; ρ = density; E_{min} = minimum energy of electron with range $\geq r$; k = units conversion factor of 21.31 (for r=cm, E=MeV, A=mCi, S=MeV/cm, and ρ=gm/cm^3).

Electron ranges and stopping powers using the "continuous slowing down approximation" (CSDA) have been tabulated[32] and $F(E)$ spectra are well known for most isotopes.[33] Dose calculations based on CSDA ranges, however, may introduce errors due to electron "range straggling." More accurate dose determination based on MC calculations are available in the form of dose kernel functions,[22] which give directly the dose per beta decay as a function of distance from the source. More details on beta dose calculations can also be found in Chapter 16 of this book.

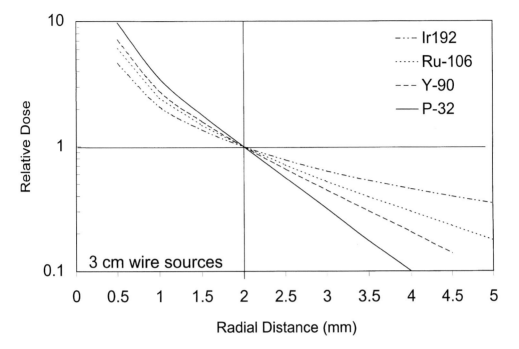

Figure 3. Radial dose versus distance for photon isotope ^{192}Ir, and beta isotopes ^{32}P, ^{90}Sr/^{90}Y, and [106]Ru/[106]Rh. All sources are of a 0.5-mm diameter and 30.0-mm length. Doses are normalized to 1.0 at a radial treatment distance of 2.0 mm.

Depth Dose Comparisons Between Beta and Gamma Sources

In Figure 3, we plot the radial dose fall-off for several gamma and beta sources as calculated using equations 1 and 2. For the beta dose calculations, equation 2 has been simplified via the application of dose kernel functions[33] described above, which "pre-calculate" radial dose distributions using the MC technique. All doses plotted in Figure 3 were calculated for 0.5-mm diameter by 30-mm long wire sources. While the actual dimensions of most commercial sources differ slightly from these values, the dose distributions are relatively insensitive to small changes in source dimensions. For comparative purposes, all doses are normalized to unity at a radial distance of 2 mm, which represents the radial distance to the vessel wall in an artery with a (typical) diameter of 4 mm. It is seen that the beta emitters have a more rapid dose fall-off versus distance than the ^{192}Ir gamma source because of the larger tissue attenuation factors. Also effecting the dose fall-off of the betas is the fact that beta-emitting isotopes actually emit a spectrum of different energy betas rather than monoenergetic betas, and the transition energies quoted in Table 1 represent the maximum beta energy. In fact, the average energy of any beta emitter is approximately one third of the maximum energy. The low-energy electrons in the spectra have very short ranges in tissue (several millimeters, or even fractions of a millimeter). As these low-energy electrons are absorbed in the tissue, the dose rate decreases even more rapidly than the "geometric only" decrease of gamma sources. [32]P with the lowest transition energy (1.71 MeV maximum) has the "poorest" radial dose penetration, while

^{90}Sr/^{90}Y (maximum transition energy of 2.21 MeV) has significantly better radial penetration. We also see in Figure 3 that energy has a large effect on beta dose distributions. For gammas, dose distributions are only slightly effected by energy. Other gamma depth dose curves, such as ^{125}I and ^{103}Pd are not plotted in Figure 3, as their depth dose curves would, essentially, be identical to ^{192}Ir.

The greater variability in beta dose verses distance from source has additional ramifications vis-à-vis dose uniformity to the arterial wall, which may be of clinical importance. In particular, for asymmetrically shaped vessels, the radial distance from the source to the vessel wall, and consequently the dose, will vary. For betas, which have larger dose fall-off, this dose variability will be greater. Even in a symmetric vessel, dose asymmetry will exist if the source is not perfectly centered within the artery. The dose asymmetry resulting from inaccurate source centering can be calculated from the depth dose curves in Figure 3. As an example, we note that centering errors as small as 0.5 mm in a 5-mm diameter vessel will produce dose asymmetries (defined as the ratio of maximum dose at the closest distance divided by minimum dose at the furthest distance) of 1.6 for ^{192}Ir, and 2.1 for ^{90}Sr/^{90}Y.

Dose uniformity can be improved if the balloon catheter automatically centers the source, and several such catheters are now available.[8] Even with a centered source, dose asymmetries will always result in a noncylindrical artery, or even in a curved section of an otherwise symmetric artery. One can show, for example, that for an artery having a 1-cm radius of curvature, the dose along the "inner track" of the curve will be 10 to 15% higher than along the "outer track" due to the fact that the "inner track" is at a smaller average distance from the source. Further, even a "symmetric" artery is unlikely to have a uniform diameter or shape along the entire axial length of a lesion, resulting in nonuniform doses in the axial as well as the radial directions. Thus, if complete isodose information is desired, intravascular ultrasound (IVUS), or similar type measurements, will have to be performed at multiple axial positions along the lesion length. Some, but not all IVB clinical protocols, require such measurements,[1,2] and one must bear in mind that all dose prescriptions quoted for IVB protocols represent, at best, only average doses. Dose variations within the vessel wall are, by nature, unavoidably large for all IVB treatments, and more so for beta sources than for gammas.

The variation of beta dose penetration with beta energy, and the depth dose differences between different energy gammas and betas may be particularly relevant when treating in-stent restenosis (as opposed to de novo lesions). An increasing number of angioplasty patients now receive stent implants to reduce vascular remodeling and the ensuing restenosis rate. In-stent restenosis, however, continues to be a major clinical problem, and many of the IVB clinical trials have especially focused on this issue. Thus, IVB is frequently prescribed for patients who already have metal stents implanted in the arterial wall. It has been shown[34] that because stent struts have higher atomic number and physical density than soft tissue they can cause significant perturbations in the radiation dose, particularly for beta sources. In particular, stents with very dense, thick struts attenuate the short-ranged betas and can reduce the average dose by up to 15%. The strut wires may also produce local cold spots in the dose distribution of up to 35%. Thus, the choice of radioactive isotope and the determination of treatment dose may require consideration of stent properties as well as other geometric factors.

A few additional points need be made with regard to beta sources and dose distributions. First, the doses in Figure 3 have been normalized at 2 mm, and do not reflect the different absolute dose rates (expressed in cGy/min/mCi) for the different isotopes. Dose rate depends on the type of emission (beta or gamma), the energy of the radiation, and the details of the radioactive decay scheme. Many isotopes emit multiple particles of different energies per nuclear decay, and many emit both betas and gammas. Thus, the dose delivered to the patient *per nuclear decay* is highly variable. In general, however, the dose delivered per decay is significantly higher for beta emitters than for gamma sources. For IVB, therefore, the source activities required (to deliver approximately 1 to 2 Gy/min at a 2-mm radial distance) are typically 0.4 to 1.0 Ci for gamma sources, but only 10 to 50 mCi for betas.

For gammas, we discussed the radiation safety advantages that could be achieved with lower energy sources. Analogously improved radial dose distributions could be achieved with *higher* energy beta isotopes. Such isotopes do exist, but most higher energy beta isotopes either have a very short half-life, or also emit significant amounts of gamma radiation. The only pure beta emitter with both reasonable half-life and reasonable energy is ^{32}P, with a half-life of 14 days and maximum energy of 1.7 MeV (see Table 1). Because of these properties, this isotope has been used in several IVB protocols. The other commonly used beta isotope, ^{90}Sr/^{90}Y achieves the combination of long half-life and high energy) via a "quirk" of radioactive decay known as radioactive equilibrium.

Radioactive equilibrium refers to the physical phenomenon wherein one radioactive isotope (called the "parent"), such as ^{90}Sr, decays via *low*-energy beta decay (in the case of ^{90}Sr, 540 keV) but with a long half-life (28 years), into a second, or "daughter" isotope (in this case ^{90}Y) which decays with a *short* half-life (2.4 days for ^{90}Y) but with higher energy (2.21 MeV). The parent and daughter isotopes remain physically together, in "radioactive equilibrium" such that it appears as if the short-lived daughter is decaying at the same rate as the longer lived parent, with the isotope pair emitting the higher energy betas of the daughter. At least one manufacturer has utilized this parent-daughter pair to produce an IVB delivery system consisting of a chain of ^{90}Sr/^{90}Y pellets which provide a long-lived, high-energy beta source.[7] Another manufacturer has produced a wire[6] consisting of pure ^{90}Y (ie, without ^{90}Sr). Although this source has a shorter than optimum half-life, there are some advantages to the use of a wire source rather than a string of pellets, and ^{90}Sr cannot be easily fabricated into flexible wires.

The second parent-daughter pair which has found use in IVB is ^{188}W/^{188}Re. Use of this isotopic pair has thus far been limited primarily to the radioactive liquid-filled balloon technique (described later), although attempts at fabricating a wire source have also been discussed. Other possible isotope pairs (some with significantly higher energy) can be found in the periodic table, although the two pairs discussed here are the only ones that appear feasible at present. Unfortunately, most higher energy beta isotopes (and, in fact, even ^{188}W/^{188}Re) also emit some gammas during the decay process. Although the gammas contribute negligible therapeutic dose to the patient as compared to the betas, they create radiation safety concerns that are similar to those of "real" gamma sources.

Alternate Radiation Delivery Systems

One alternative delivery system for intraluminal irradiation of arterial walls is to inflate the balloon dilation catheter with a radioactive liquid.[9] This may have advantages over wires and seeds in that accurate source positioning and uniform dose to the vessel wall is virtually assured. In addition, radioactive liquids can be used in conjunction with existing catheters. Specific concentrations of less than 50 mCi/mL yield dose rates less than 400 cGy/min at the surface of the balloon, and such concentrations are achievable for several isotopes including ^{90}Y, ^{32}P, and ^{188}Re. While this technique may yield more symmetric dose distributions, the chemical and radiological toxicity of the radioactive liquid must be considered, as there is always a small risk of balloon rupture. Several available beta emitters including ^{32}P and ^{90}Y are bone-seeking compounds which, if released into the bloodstream would result in unacceptably high (1 to 10 Gy) whole body and bone marrow doses in the event of balloon rupture. More recently, however, a liquid ^{188}Re delivery system has been shown to be biologically safer to use,[35] and several small clinical trials have been attempted.

Other alternate dose delivery systems have been proposed, and/or tested on a very limited basis, but due to space constraints we mention them only for completeness. One such technique involves inflating the angiographic balloon with radioactive ^{133}Xe gas.[10] Advantages of this system are similar to the liquid balloon, although the ^{133}Xe is a very low-energy beta emitter which will, at best, be suitable only for very small, thin lesions. Infusion of the radioactive liquid ^{99m}Tc into the vessel walls via infusion catheters has also been proposed,[11] although uniform absorption of the liquid by the vessel wall is problematic. To date, both of these techniques have seen only limited use in small animal trials.

Another alternate delivery system that has been proposed is the use of angiographic balloons with radioactive ^{32}P impregnated into the walls of the balloon.[12] This system has advantages similar to the liquid balloon in terms of dose uniformity and avoids the risk of a radioactive liquid spill. Finally, the use of miniature x-ray tubes for insertion directly into angiographic catheters has been proposed.[13] Prototype designs of 30 kVp x-ray tubes as small as 1.25-mm diameter have been presented, which should have depth dose profiles comparable to ^{32}P, but without (virtually) any radiation safety problems because there is no radiation from such a device unless the high voltage is activated. Higher voltage tubes could provide depth dose distributions comparable to low-energy gamma isotopes such as ^{103}Pd or ^{125}I, but at present higher tube voltages present difficult cooling and shielding problems with the x-ray tubes. Space does not permit a more detailed description of these devices.

Dosimetry of External Beam Irradiation

External beam irradiation has also been proposed for the treatment of coronary arteries.[14,15] A combination of two or more megavoltage x-ray beams from a conventional linear accelerator could provide a uniform dose coverage of a 2- to 3-cm length of targeted arterial wall, although a significant amount of normal tissues would have to be included in the treatment field. A minimum field size of at least 2×5 cm^2 would be required, not counting the effects of coronary motion during treatment which would necessitate significantly larger treatment fields and a concomitant increase in the volume of normal tissues being irra diated. This might necessitate fractionating the treatments (to reduce normal tissue damage) which then raises the additional complications of target localization and treatment reproducibility, as coronary arteries cannot be visualized on standard radiation oncology type simulation films or portal images.

One possibility that is technically feasible is to synchronize the radiation pulse from the linear accelerator with the cardiac cycle. This would enable treatment with smaller field sizes and reduce normal tissue complications. External beam irradiation may also prove feasible for the treatment of peripheral vessels, and in particular for superficially located hemodialysis shunts. Here, a single *en face* 6 MeV electron beam could be tailored to ideally match the desired treatment volume with rapid dose fall-off beyond the field edges. External electron beam treatments would, in fact, provide a more uniform dose distribution than an intraluminal insertion. Since the shunts are superficial, simple palpation could enable accurate field alignment, even for fractionated treatments.

Dosimetry of Permanent Radioactive Stents

The implantation of permanent stents in conjunction with balloon angioplasty has become a common clinical procedure in recent years. Stent placement creates a "physical barrier" which reduces vascular remodeling and provides a larger final lumen diameter, thus reducing the rate of restenosis. Neointima formation, however, is still a significant problem with stents, and the presence of a stent may in fact exacerbate neointima formation. The use of radioactive impregnated or radioactive coated stents has been suggested.[16–18] To date, most trials with radioactive stents have been limited to the use of beta emitters (mostly ^{32}P). The radioactive stent has dosimetry advantages similar to the radioactive liquid-filled balloon and also the ^{32}P impregnated balloon in that the radioactive source is in intimate contact with the vessel walls. The dose distribution however for radioactive stents is extremely nonuniform[36,37] because of the gridded structure of the stent, and the concomitant inhomogeneous distribution of the radioactive source. Some improvements in dose uniformity can be achieved via better stent design[37] and also via the use of low-energy photon emitters (such as ^{103}Pd).[37,38]

Unlike catheter-based IVB where beta source activities greater than 20 mCi are required, permanent radioactive stents containing only a few microcuries activity have been reported to be effective in reducing restenosis, although there is still uncertainty as to the optimum activity for a radioactive stent. ^{32}P has thus far been the isotope of choice for use in radioactive stents principally because its half-life of 14 days is very convenient. This half-life is long enough for the stent to have a reasonable "shelf life," but short enough so that the radiation dose is delivered in a beneficially short time. A 1-μCi ^{32}P stent, for example, yields approximately the same total dose as does a 5-minute exposure to a 6-mCi intraluminal source. This is because the total dose delivered is equal to the product of the total activity (corrected for radioactive decay) and the total treatment time. Thus, the total doses delivered by stents and by catheter-based wire or seed sources are quite similar; only the time sequence is different. A complete dosimetric description of radioactive stents is beyond the scope of this report, but has been discussed in detail elsewhere,[36–38] and also in Chapter 28 of this book.

AAPM TG-60

Task Group-60 of the AAPM has recently published a report entitled "Intravascular Brachytherapy Physics: Report of the AAPM Radiation Therapy Committee Task Group No. 60."[21] The purpose of the report was to summarize existing physics and dosimetry techniques for IVB, and to make recommendations for standardization of dosimetry and calibration procedures, dose prescription criteria, and quality assurance and radiation safety procedures. The group recognized the need for a uniform system of prescription definition. A summary of the groups recommendations are as follows:

1. For catheter-based systems, the dose at 2-mm distance from the source should be clearly specified. Three-dimensional dosimetry information, such as that obtained from IVUS, should be given in at least three planes if available.
2. Dose calculations for gamma sources should be made according to the formalism presented in AAPM Report TG-43,[20] wherein dose is determined from the air kerma strength of the source, plus anisotropy, radial, and geometric factors which should be determined for each individual source design by the manufacturer. The penetrating ability of the source should be specified in terms of a radial dose function from 0.5- to 10-mm distances.
3. Dosimetry data should be traceable to a National Institute of Standards and Technology (NIST) standard source.
4. Source strength for beta sources should be expressed in terms of dose rate in water. Dose calibrations should be performed using an extrapolation ionization chamber according to procedures developed at the NIST.
5. For radioactive stents, the dose should be specified at a distance of 0.5 mm from the surface of the stent. The activity, deployed diameter, length, type, and model stent should be clearly specified for each patient. Radial and axial dose calculations should be made according to the procedures quoted in the report. The activity of each stent should be independently determined by measurement of bremsstrahlung photons with a NaI(Ti) detector and multichannel analyzer.
6. A comprehensive quality assurance program should be in place which includes accurate records of radiation safety, source receipt and disposal, dosimetry, leak tests, calibration, and emergency procedures.
7. A working team for intravascular brachytherapy must include an interventional cardiologist or radiologist, radiation oncologist, radiotherapy physicist, radiation safety staff, and nurse/coordinator.

Conclusions

IVB currently being performed with high-energy gamma or beta emitters. The ideal source will have a high specific activity, long half-life, uniform dose over treatment distances of at least 2 to 3 mm, and low cost. No available isotope is ideal. Beta emitters such as ^{32}P, ^{90}Sr/^{90}Y, and ^{188}We/^{188}Re have advantages in terms of high specific activity, dose rate, and radiation safety; while gamma emitters such as ^{192}Ir have advantages in terms of radial dose uniformity. Lower energy gamma isotopes such as ^{103}Pd and ^{125}I may combine the depth dose advantages of ^{192}Ir with the safety advantages of beta. Over a dozen different clinical trials have either been completed or are under way using a variety of isotopes and delivery systems. There is a trade-off between the increased radial range of gamma emitters, and the safety advantages of beta emitters. Both beta and gamma emitters will be safer and easier to use with semi-automated and/or computer-controlled high dose rate type delivery systems, which are now currently under development by several manufacturers.

The choice of source and ultimate success of treatment, however, may well depend on a "biological window." It is known for example that a minimum dose on the order of 8 to 10 Gy is required to prevent restenosis. Maximum vessel tolerance dose is not well known but is hypothesized to be on the order of 40 to 60 Gy. Dose uniformity within the target region must therefore be within a factor of 4 to 7.5 (ie, 40 Gy/10 Gy or 60/8). Vessel wall thickness is on the order of 0.5 mm in a normal artery, but may be significantly larger in a diseased vessel. The ideal radiation source should have no worse than a 3 to 7.5 factor of dose fall-off over that distance. Thick vessel walls and inaccurate source centering will produce dose asymmetries that may make this dose window even more difficult to achieve. The introduction of a radioactive liquid or gas directly into the angioplasty balloon, radioactive liquid infusion, miniaturized x-ray tubes, implantation of radioactive stents, or external beam irradiation have all been proposed as alternate radiation delivery systems. All of these proposals offer both advantages and disadvantages as compared to catheter-based IVB with radioactive seeds and wires. Other radioactive sources with better physical dose properties than those currently being used do exist and could possibly be developed in future.

Glossary

Activity   Used to quantity the amount of radioactive material based upon the number of radioactive decays per second. Any physical mass or quantity of radioactive material that produces 3.7×10^{10} decays per second has an activity of 1 curie (Ci). 1/1000 Ci = 1 millicurie (mCi). Typical activities used to treat restenosis are 10 to 100 mCi for beta sources, or 200 to 1000 mCi for gamma sources, or 10 microcuries (μCi) for permanently implanted beta stents. The new unit (MKS system) of activity is the becquerel (Bq) which is equal to 1 decay/sec (1 Ci=3.7×10^{10} Bq). Activity is directly proportional to the number of radioactive nuclei present, and inversely proportional to the half-life. Historically, the unit derives from the fact that 1 gram of radium has an activity of 1 curie.

Beta   Type of radioactive emission which is really a high-energy electron emitted by a radioactive nucleus during the decay process. All beta particles have a finite range, proportional to their energy. Beta decay can be characterized by the maximum energy of the beta particles (which is a property of the radioisotope undergoing decay) and the half-life. Usually each decaying nucleus emits one beta particle, which can have any energy between zero and the maximum energy, with an average energy of approximately one third of the maximum. Sources being used for prevention of restenosis have maximum beta energies of at least several hundred keV, but more ideally 2 to 3 MeV.

Curie   See "Activity."

Decay (radioactive decay)   All radioactive materials decay as a function of time. The rate of decay is characterized by the half-life, which is the time required for the activity of the source to be reduced to one half of its initial value. Sources being used for prevention of restenosis have half-lives varying from several hours to many years.

Depth dose distribution   The dose absorbed from any radioactive source decreases as the distance from the source increases. The rate of decrease depends on the type of radioactive source (gamma or beta), energy, composition of the absorbing medium, and geometry of the source.

Dose   Energy absorbed per unit mass of material from ionizing radiation. The unit of dose is the gray (Gy) defined as 1 joule of energy absorbed per kilogram of material. Centigray (cGy) or rad is used to denote 10^{-2} gray. Note that radiation dose is defined by the energy absorbed by the patient, NOT by the physical amount or quantity of radioactive materials (this latter quantity is defined by "activity").

Electron volt   Unit of energy used specifically for ionizing radiation such as beta, gamma, and x-ray. keV and MeV are used to denote 10^3 and 10^6 electron volts (or eV), respectively. One eV is the energy of an electron which has been accelerated by a voltage potential of 1 volt.

Energy   When a radioisotope decays it may emit γ-rays, x-rays, beta particles, or positrons, or a combination. Each emitted particle or ray has an energy that determines its range or penetration, and the dose that is deposited. Energy is measured in units of eV (or keV, or MeV).

Gammas   High-energy electromagnetic radiation emitted when a nucleus decays. Basically gammas are very high-frequency light capable of producing ionization damage in tissue. See also "Photon."

Gray   See "Dose."

Half-life   The time it takes any for radioactive material to decay to the point where only half of the original nuclei remain. Every radioactive isotope has a specific half-life.

Half value layer (HVL)   The amount of absorbing material (usually measured in millimeters) required to reduce the dose rate of a radioactive source by one half. Gammas typically have an HVL of several millimeters (or more) of lead. X-rays have an HVL of 1-mm lead or less. Theoretically, neither gammas nor x-rays can ever be completely stopped by any finite thickness of material, but, in reality, 10 HVL of material absorb 99.9% of the radiation. Beta particles, on the other hand, are always completely absorbed by only a fraction of a millimeter of lead, and the concept of HVL has no real meaning.

Isotope   Nuclear "species" of a specific element, defined by the atomic weight. All isotopes of the same element have the same atomic number (ie, number of protons in the nucleus), and hence the same chemical properties, but different numbers of neutrons in the nucleus. Some isotopes of a particular element are stable, while others may be radioactive.

Photon   Literally "particles" or "quantized energy packets" of electromagnetic radiation produced by the motion of high-energy charged particles such as electrons and nuclei. Photons have no charge or mass, but can be specified by their frequency or energy (which are proportionally related). We recognize low-energy, or low-frequency photons as radiowaves, or visible light; and higher energy photons as x-rays and gammas.

Radioisotope   Any unstable isotope. Radioisotopes are characterized by the type of radiation they emit (beta or gamma), the energy of the emissions, and the half-life.

X-ray   Type of radioactive emission which is really a high-energy photon, usually emitted from electrons in atomic orbitals. X-rays that emanate from the nucleus are given the special designation of γ-ray. See also "Photon."

References

1. Tierstein PS, Massullo V, Jani S, et al. Catheter based radiotherapy to inhibit restenosis after coronary stenting. N Engl J Med 1997;336:1697–1703.
2. Tierstein PS, Massullo V, Jani S, et al. Two-year follow-up after catheter-based radiotherapy to inhibit coronary restenosis. Circulation 1999;99:243–247.
3. Waksman R, White RI, Chan RC, et al. Localized intracoronary radiation therapy for patients with in-stent restenosis: Preliminary results from a randomized clinical study. Circulation 1997;96:I-219, 1212.
4. Condado JA, Gurdiel O, Espinoza R, et al. Percutaneous transluminal coronary angioplasty (PCTA) and intracoronary radiation therapy (ICRT): A possible new modality for the treatment of coronary restenosis. A preliminary report of the first 10 patients treated with intracoronary radiation therapy. J Am Coll Cardiol 1995;(special issue): 228A.
5. Condado JA, Waksman R, Gurdiel O, et al. Long-term angiographic and clinical outcome after percutaneous transluminal coronary angioplasty and intracoronary radiation therapy in humans. Circulation 1997;96:927–932.
6. Verin V, Urban B, Popowski Y, et al. Feasibility of intracoronary β-irradiation to reduce restenosis after balloon angioplasty: A clinical pilot study. Circulation 1997;97:1138–1144.
7. King SB, Williams DO, Chougule P, et al. Endovascular beta-radiation to reduce restenosis after coronary balloon angioplasty: Results of the beta energy restenosis trial (BERT). Circulation 1998;97:2025–2030.
8. Raizner A, Calfee RV, Nadir M, et al. The guidant coronary source wire system. In: Waksman R (ed.): Vascular Brachytherapy, 2nd Edition. Armonk, NY: Futura Publishing Co.; 1998:505–519.
9. Amols HI, Reinstein LE, Weinberger J. Dosimetry of a radioactive coronary balloon dilation catheter for treatment of neointimal hyperplasia. Med Phys 1996;23:1783–1788.
10. Apple M, Waksman R. Xenon-133 gas-filled balloon. In: Waksman R (ed.): Vascular Brachytherapy, 2nd Edition. Armonk, NY: Futura Publishing Co.; 1998:569–578.
11. Waksman R. The irradiator. In: Waksman R, Serruys P (eds.): Handbook of Vascular Brachytherapy, 2nd Edition. London: Martin Dunitz Publishers; 2000:139–143.
12. Buchbinder M, Strathearn G, Tam LA, et al. RDX™ radiation delivery system: Balloon based radiation therapy. In: Waksman R, Serruys P (eds.): Handbook of Vascular Brachytherapy, 2nd Edition. London: Martin Dunitz Publishers; 2000:145–152.
13. Chornenky V. Intravascular soft x-ray therapy. In: Waksman R (ed): Vascular Brachytherapy, 2nd Edition. Armonk, NY: Futura Publishing Co.; 1998:561–567.
14. Schwartz RS, Koval TM, Edwards WD, et al. Effect of external beam irradiation on neointimal hyperplasia after experimental coronary artery injury. J Am Coll Cardiol 1992;19:1106–1113.
15. Abbas MA, Afshari NA, Standius ML, et al. External beam irradiation inhibits neointimal hyperplasia following balloon angioplasty. Cardiology 1994;44:191–202.
16. Fischell TA, Abbas MA, Kallman RF. Low-dose radiation inhibits clonal proliferation of smooth muscle cells: A new approach to restenosis [abstract]. Arterioscler Thromb 1991;11:1435.
17. Bottcher HD, Schopohl B, Liermann D, et al. Endovascular irradiation-a new method to avoid recurrent stenosis after stent implantation in peripheral arteries: Technique and preliminary results. Int J Rad Onc Biol Phys 1994;29:183–186.
18. Hehrlein C, Zimmermann J, Metz J, et al. Radioactive coronary stent implantation inhibits neointimal proliferation in nonatherosclerotic rabbits. Circulation 1993;88:1–651.
19. Amols HI, Zaider M, Weinberger J, et al. Dosimetric considerations for catheter based beta and gamma emitters in the therapy of neointimal hyperplasia in human coronary arteries. Int J Rad Onc Biol Phy 1996;36:913–921.
20. Nath R, Anderson L, Luxton G, et al. Dosimetry of interstitial brachytherapy sources: Recommendations of the AAPM radiation therapy committee task group No 43. Med Phys 1995;22:209–234.
21. Nath R, Amols H, Coffey C, et al. Intravascular brachytherapy physics: Report of the AAPM radiation therapy task group no. 60. Med Phys 1999;26:119–152.
22. Niroomand A, Blackwell CR, Coursey BM, et al. Radiochromic film dosimetry: Recom-

mendations of AAPM radiation therapy committee task group 55. Med Phys 1998; 25: 2093–2115.

23. McLaughlin WL, Chen YD, Soares CG, et al. Sensitometry of the response of a new radiochromic film dosimeter to gamma radiation and electron beams. NIM Phys Res 1991;A302:165–176.

24. Williamson J. Comparison of measured and calculated dose rates in water near I-125 and Ir-192 seeds. Med Phys 1991;18:776–786.

25. Bambynek M, Fluhs D, Quast U, et al. A high-precision, high-resolution and fast dosimetry system for beta sources applied in cardiovascular brachytherapy. Med Phys 2000;27:662–667.

26. Stabin MG, Konijnenber M, Knapp FF, Spencer RH. Monte Carlo modeling of radiation dose distributions in intravascular radiation therapy. Med Phys 2000;27:1086–1092.

27. Nath R, Anderson L, Meli J, et al. Code of practice for brachytherapy physics: Report of the AAPM radiation therapy committee task group 56. Med Phys 1997;24:1557–1598.

28. Jani S, Massullo V, Tierstein P, et al. Physics and safety aspects of a coronary irradiation pilot study to inhibit restenosis using manually loaded Ir-192 ribbons. Semin Intervent Cardiol 1997;2:119–124.

29. Balter S. Endovascular brachytherapy safety tips. In: Waksman R, Serruys P (eds.): Handbook of Vascular Brachytherapy, 2nd Edition. London: Martin Dunitz Publishers; 2000:217–226.

30. Loevinger R. Distribution of absorbed energy around a point source of beta radiation. Science 1950;112:530–531.

31. Loevinger R, Berman M. A schema for absorbed-dose calculations for biologically-distributed radionuclides, MIRD Pamphlet #1. J Nucl Med 1968;9(suppl 1):7–14.

32. Berger MJ, Seltzer SM. Stopping powers and ranges of electrons and positrons, 2nd Edition. US Dept Commerce Publication NBSIR 82-2550-A, 1983.

33. Simpkin DJ, Mackie TR. EGS4 Monte Carlo determination of the beta dose kernel in water. Med Phys 1990;17:179–186.

34. Amols HI, Trichter F, Weinberger J. Intracoronary radiation for prevention of restenosis: Dose perturbations caused by stents. Circulation 1998;19:2024–2029.

35. Knapp FF, Callahan AP, Beets AL, et al. Processing of reactor-produced 188W for fabrication of clinical scale alumina-based 188W/188Re generators. Appl Radiat Isot 1994;45:1123–1128.

36. Prestwich WV, Kennet TJ, Kus FW. The dose distribution produced by a P32-coated stent. Med Phys 1995;22:313–320.

37. Amols HI. Methods to improve dose uniformity for radioactive stents in endovascular brachytherapy. Cardiovasc Radiat Med 1999;1:270–277.

38. Sioshansi P, Bricault RJ. Low-energy 103Pd gamma (x-ray) source for vascular brachytherapy. Cardiovasc Radiat Med 1999;1:278–287.

## Chapter 19

Vascular Brachytherapy:

A Health Physics Perspective

Stephen Balter, PhD

Introduction

Vascular brachytherapy safety is an adaptation of conventional radiation safety measures associated with radioactive materials (RAM). Because vascular brachytherapy is an add-on to an interventional vascular procedure, overall safety management includes attention to the patient's medical status. Treatments are typically administered in the interventional laboratory using strong (relative to nuclear scanning agents) removable sources of radiation. This chapter focuses on various safety issues associated with this environment.

In any therapeutic use of RAM, technology and process are combined to minimize the probability of a significant safety failure. It is prudent to exceed minimums so that minor lapses of attention do not cause a loss of safety. The keys are preplanning and redundant checks.

Safety management requires that the risks be reduced to socially acceptable levels. Radiation and RAM risk management is influenced by an almost unique public anxiety. Incidents involving even trivial amounts of radioactivity often attract adverse media attention. Coping with the public relations consequences of unwanted events can be difficult. Thus, regulatory policy and safety limits are very conservative.

This chapter addresses some the consequences of unwanted events without regard to their frequency. Significant events are rare. The objective is simply to prepare the reader to react appropriately when they do occur.

Patient Safety

For the purposes of this chapter, a safe treatment is the delivery of the prescribed dose of radiation to an identified anatomic target. It also implies the minimization of unwanted irradiation. We assume that the dose distribution around the source is known and factored into the dose prescription. Thus, major issues affecting clinical results and potential long-term complications, such as the choice of radionuclide and device centering are not considered here.

From Waksman R (ed.). *Vascular Brachytherapy, Third Edition.* Armonk, NY: Futura Publishing Co., Inc.; © 2002.

There is an unfortunate history of cancer brachytherapy misadministration. Over time, the radiation oncology and medical physics communities have developed standard operating procedures intended to minimize the frequency and severity of such incidents. Despite this knowledge, there has been an unexpectedly high frequency of reported vascular brachytherapy misadministrations. These events have encouraged additional regulatory oversight. Events are accessible on the Nuclear Regulatory Commission's website (*www.nrc.gov.*).

Proper Utilization of the Proper Source

A variety of vascular brachytherapy sources and devices will be available in the clinic. The best way to assure that the correct device is used is to conduct redundant cross checks between team members.

Another predictable mistake is an improper calculation of the treatment time. Possible errors include using radioactive decay factors for the wrong radionuclide, calculations for the wrong treatment date, and calculations for the wrong device. There will be an increased frequency of such errors if the calculation is made under the pressure of an imminent treatment. *It is inappropriate to start vascular brachytherapy calculations (or secondary safety calculations) while the treatment is in progress.*

As an example, our laboratory has several ^{192}Ir ribbons of different lengths available for treatment on any given day. An additional label has been applied to each container as part of the initial quality assurance process (Fig. 1). The same clip art is applied to all paperwork associated with that source. Figure 1 also illustrates a portion of the worksheet used for treatment with that source on a particular day. Details and format of the worksheet will vary depending on the nature of the individual device. In some cases, the "worksheet" is built into the device's software.

The medical physicist prepares the requested source and selects the matching worksheet. When the source is brought into the laboratory, the interventionalist visually inspects the source to ascertain that this is actually the requested device and that the source and the worksheet match. The authorized user verifies the calculations, and confirms the match and the setting of the two treatment timers. Both the authorized user and the medical physicist agree on the dwell time before the treatment is started.

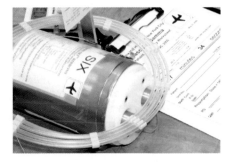

Figure 1. A gamma source container and its associated worksheet. For this protocol, a separate worksheet is prepared for each source, for each treatment day. Note that the clipart provides an immediate visual match between the source and its worksheet.

Dwell Time

Reducing that time that the source is in the treatment position (dwell time) has many clinical and operational benefits. Most removable beta and gamma vascular brachytherapy sources can be manufactured with enough activity to reduce dwell time to less than 1 minute.

Long dwell times have not proven to be a medical risk for the patient. We have had to interrupt treatment three times in our experience of over 300 procedures using dwell times in the range from 13 to 30 minutes. Both interruptions occurred in the first moments of dwell. Two were attributed to drug reactions; the other one might be attributable to an ischemic incident. In all three cases, we were able to resume treatment in less than 5 minutes.

Decreasing the dwell time increases the dose delivered to tissues along the path from the entrance point to the treated segment. Reduced dwell time can increase relative staff dose when using any vascular brachytherapy source. This is because the transit time is determined by the mechanical design of the treatment device. Stronger sources used in any given system emit more radiation during this fixed time. Redesigning the device to reduce transit time might require measures such as a stiffer treatment catheter to minimize the risk of mechanical malfunction.

A significant disadvantage of too short a dwell time is catheter motion relative to the target. Catheters can be displaced from their ideal treatment position for a variety of reasons. When this happens, it usually occurs in the time between initial catheter positioning and active source delivery. With any system, it will take some time for the operator to detect the problem, determine a corrective action, and appropriately reposition the source. Such processes typically take a few tens of seconds.

For completeness, the influence of dwell time if a source-transfer malfunction occurs needs to be mentioned. During such an event, the source could be temporarily "stuck" somewhere in the vascular tree. It will locally irradiate tissue in its vicinity. Retrieval procedures such as removing the source and treatment catheter into the bail-out box can be expected to take several tens of seconds. Issues include recognition of the problem, probable exchange of position between the authorized user and interventionalist, and actual device removal.

Practical issues of normal laboratory operations, vascular interventions brachytherapy technology, patient safety, and comfort need to be considered. Human response to normal treatment variations and emergencies also enters the equation. Given all of these factors, the optimum dwell time seems to be in the range of 10 to 15 minutes.

Custodianship of Radioactive Materials

Therapeutic quantities of RAM needed for vascular brachytherapy are a significant hazard. Formal policies and procedures are appropriately designed to avoid problems. A portion of the formality is similar to the procedures used to manage narcotics. Additional items are intended to protect people and the environment against specific radiation hazards.

Handling of RAM involves items such as specific safety training, familiarity with applicable regulations, and access to calibrated instrumentation. In most hospitals, individuals who handle RAM include: authorized users, medical physicists, nuclear medicine technologists, radiation safety staff members, radiopharmacists, or radiation therapists. The list of involved persons at a particular institution will depend on staffing patterns, hospital policy, and local regulatory requirements.

Sources must pass a quality assurance procedure before they are used. The nature of the procedures is too source- and device-specific to review here at any level of detail. The manufacturer's labeling and calibration is often only a starting point. In most cases, the license specifies that the integrity and calibration of RAM is the institution's responsibility.

Storage and Staging Areas

It is inappropriate, as well as illegal, to store any quantity of RAM with normal interventional laboratory inventory. RAM must be placed in a secure storage area unless it is under the positive control of a RAM handler.

A staging area near the laboratory is helpful. This may or may not be the approved radionuclide storage area. If it is not, sources are positioned in the staging area at the start of the treatment day and returned to storage when the day's treatments are concluded. Leaving RAM "temporarily" unattended in a corner of the laboratory or in the corridor is not acceptable.

The paths used for moving sources within the hospital need to be well defined for both safety and public-relations purposes. Visitor areas and elevators should be avoided whenever possible. Vertical transport can be achieved using either patient or clean-utility elevators.

Radioactive Waste Disposal

Outdated sources are often returned to the supplier (or another authorized recipient) for disposal of the RAM. There are specific packaging and package labeling requirements for such shipments.

RAM can be also disposed of by inclusion in the institution's radioactive waste stream, or it can be held in secure storage until radioactive decay has run its course. Direct release of any level of RAM to the environment is highly discouraged. The choice of disposal method depends on the identity of the radionuclide and its initial activity. Table 1 reviews in-place decay times.

Staff and Facility Safety

The goal is to deliver optimum treatment to the patient without any risk of staff harm. There are two limitations to this process. The first limitation involves inherent differences between sources and delivery systems during routine treatments. The second relates to system characteristics under accident or emergency conditions.

The beta-gamma "debate" is ultimately little more than an evaluation of the relative efficacy of different radionuclides in comparison to staff radiation risk associated with delivering the therapy. There are ethical considerations in this risk-benefit balance. Benefits accrue to the patient; risks are borne by both patient and staff.

Table 1

Time Required for a Source to Decay to 37 Bq (1 nCi)

Nuclide Half-Life	^{99m}Tc 0.25 Days	^{90}Y 2.7 Days	^{133}Xe 5.2 Days	^{32}P 14.3 Days	^{103}Pd 17 Days	^{192}Ir 74 Days	^{90}Sr 28 years
Initial Activity	Days	Months				Years	
370 GBq 10 Ci	8.3	3.0	5.8	15.8	18.8	6.7	930
370 MBq 10 mCi	5.8	2.1	4.0	11.1	13.2	4.7	651
370 KBq 10 µCi	3.3	1.2	2.3	6.3	7.5	2.7	372

Under normal circumstances, staff risk is stochastic. Thus, one would like to reduce the risk to a level As Low As Reasonably Achievable (ALARA). When working with sealed sources, the risk is attributable to external radiation received both outside and inside the laboratory. Opportunities for staff irradiation "outside" the laboratory include: source shipping, quality assurance, device preparation and cleaning, and transportation of sources within the institution.

There are two parts to the risk of irradiation "inside" the laboratory. The first is that attributable to brachytherapy. The second is attributable to the radiation used to guide angioplasty. A full optimization includes considerations of both factors over time. Vascular brachytherapy may eventually reduce the staff's collective dose by reducing the total number of angioplasties.

There are both stochastic and deterministic risk components under emergency conditions. If an event occurs, some of these risks will be borne by the patient and other risks will be borne by the staff. Minimizing response time is usually the best way to minimize risk. It is essential to plan and rehearse responses to several levels of emergencies.

Source Handling

Dwell time is the best single indicator of the hazard associated with handling a source. Sources that deliver the treatment with shorter dwell times are more dangerous. Other important factors are the identity of the radionuclide, its physical and chemical form, and its packaging for treatment. The activity of a source (Bq or Ci) does not directly reflect the degree of hazard. Longer half-life sources are potentially more dangerous than shorter half-life radionuclides.

Touching any removable vascular brachytherapy source can cause an immediate radiation burn. Depending on the radionuclide and construction of the source, contact dose rates range from 2 to 10 times as high as that at the typical 2-mm prescription point (Geometry Factor). Table 2 gives estimates of the time needed to deliver 5 Gy in contact with the source. Simplifying assumptions may make these estimates optimistic; burns might occur in shorter times.

Standard techniques for minimizing hand dose while working with radionuclides include the use of long instruments. Minimum instrument lengths for vascular brachytherapy sources are about 10 cm. Longer instruments (15 to 25 cm) are desirable. Appropriate instruments need to be immediately available wherever sources are handled.

Emergency Response and the Bail-Out Box

It is human nature is to attempt to solve problems. Protocol and rehearsals can modify this behavior to initiate immediate normal source retraction if any abnormal situation arises. This should be sufficient to deal with most medical emergencies and many technical difficulties.

A bail-out box is an appropriately shielded emergency container that is available at the tableside in the laboratory. The first line of defense if the source cannot be advanced is to withdraw it into its container. If the source cannot be withdrawn normally, then the source and treatment catheter are withdrawn from the patient as a unit and placed in the bail-out box. Figure 2 illustrates beta and gamma bail-out boxes.

Rapidly pulling a catheter with an unshielded source from a patient can be medically and mechanically hazardous to the patient. Events that require recourse to the bail-out box should never be regarded as a routine part of the treatment protocol. Each event should be investigated with the objective of eliminating its recurrence.

Staff Safety

Beta Sources

The radiations emitted from beta sources are almost entirely attenuated by a few centimeters of tissue or plastic. Air is not an efficient attenuator of beta particles. The range of high-energy beta particles in air is several meters. Unshielded therapeutic beta sources are a significant radiation hazard.

A lead apron is not a good shield for beta particles. X-rays are produced when high-energy electrons, such as beta particles, interact with metal. This same physical process produces x-rays in an x-ray tube. Thin layers of lead convert a fraction of the energy carried by "nonpenetrating" beta particles into "penetrating" x-rays.

Paradoxically, the excellent attenuation of beta radiation by tissue is a patient safety hazard. Post-treatment radiation measurements of the patient may

Table 2

Time to Produce a 5-Gy Radiation Burn (Prescription is 15 Gy at 2 mm)

Geometry Factor	Dwell Time (Minutes)			
	2	5	10	20
	Burn Time (Minutes)			
10	0.07	0.17	0.33	0.67
5	0.13	0.33	0.67	1.33
2	0.33	0.83	1.67	3.33

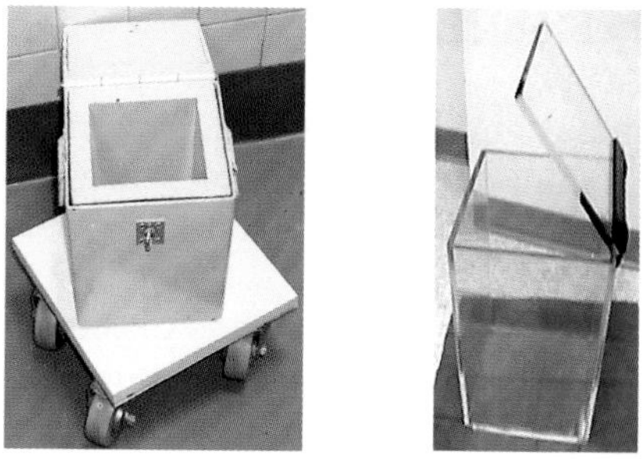

Figure 2. Examples of gamma (left) and beta (right) bail-out boxes. The appropriate box should be immediately available. Its use should never be regarded as routine.

fail to detect a retained source. Positive checks of the treatment device are needed to assure retrieval of all of the sources. These checks can be mechanical, radiological, or visual.

Gamma Sources

The principle additional hazard of high-energy gamma sources is the presence of a radiation field outside of the patient during the treatment. Therefore staff should stay away from the patient whenever the source is deployed. In addition, source strengths are limited (prolonging dwell time) and auxiliary shielding is often deployed for "gamma" treatments.

Conventional angiographic lead aprons or portable shields offer no real protection from high-energy gamma rays, but they are still required for protection during the fluoroscopic and cinefluorographic portions of the procedure.

Contamination

Sealed beta or gamma sources have virtually zero risk of producing radiation contamination of the patient, laboratory, or work areas. Indeed, this lack of contamination hazard is a major part of the definition of a sealed source.

Liquid or gas sources have significant contamination potential. RAM spills can be toxic to the patient. Areas that can be contaminated include storage areas, preparation areas, transportation paths, and the interventional laboratory itself.

After a spill, decontamination of facilities is required before they can be used again. Decontamination measures cover a spectrum, ranging from simply diluting and venting radioactive gasses to more complex measures. Gas venting has special rules and public relations challenges. Allowing radioactive decay to run its course is an option for RAM with half-lives in the range of hours to a few days. One such incident (during a live course demonstration) resulted in a week's closure of an interventional lab.

Significant contamination with long half-life radionuclides is a major cleanup problem. Contaminated supplies, equipment, and other materials may have to be physically removed from the lab and sent to a radioactive waste dump. This is very expensive and time consuming.

For completeness, patients treated with removable sealed sources are not contaminated once the sources are removed from the patient. This lack of hazard has to be communicated to the patient, family, and clinical staff.

Facility Shielding

The patient's tissues usually provide adequate shielding for beta- and low-energy gamma-emitting sources. Very superficial source placement is an exception. Therefore, this section on facility shielding will focus on high-energy gamma sources.

A conservative approach is to consider all spaces outside the procedure room itself as fully occupied, noncontrolled areas (eg, this permits a secretary to work full time in the angiographic control room.) The applicable regulatory guideline is no more than 20 μSv (2 mrem) in any 1 hour or 1000 μSv (100 mrem) in any 1 year.

The most intense source that can be used in a lab is limited by the rule that there can be no more than 20 μSv in any 1 hour. The 1000 μSv/y corresponds to the difference in natural background radiation between New York and Denver. The risk is minimal even under these extremely conservative assumptions.

Auxiliary radiation shields may be used to reduce environmental levels (Fig. 3). These shields may be required in architecturally small laboratories but they should be used in all laboratories in the interest of ALARA. Relatively small shields provide large radiation shadows when they are placed close to the patient. Larger shields may be placed further from the angiographic table, which can facilitate access to the patient.

Auxiliary shields serve their purpose when they block the line-of-sight between the source and the protected point. Design considerations for the shields include positions of the treatment team and architecture of the control room. Staff, standing or sitting in control rooms with raised floors, should not be able to see the patient's chest over the top of the shields.

Personnel Monitoring

The use of appropriate personnel monitors should not be ignored. These include both finger and body dosimeters. Factors influencing the effective dose received by an individual include the nature of the radionuclide, and the characteristics of the treatment device and the lead apron worn in the interventional lab.

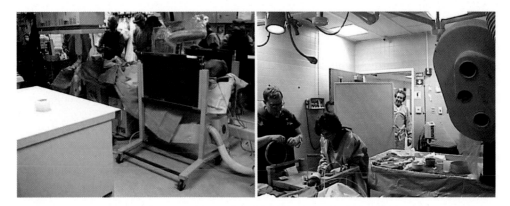

Figure 3. Examples of large (left) and small (right) gamma shields. Smaller shields provide equivalent protection when they are placed closer to the patient's chest.

There should be a minimum of hand exposure in normal use anywhere in the vascular brachytherapy cycle. Dosimeter rings are worn to document hand exposure in an emergency situation.

Based on our experience with ^{192}Ir, the medical physicist is the most highly exposed individual. Dosimeter readings indicate effective doses of less than 10 μSv per case in the laboratory and less than 20 μSv per case for the entire vascular brachytherapy treatment cycle. The irradiation of other individuals occurs during the procedure; the maximum is less than 10 μSv per case. The overall collective dose from the vascular brachytherapy treatment portion of the procedure is estimated to be comparable to the dose attributable to the angioplasty.

Long-Term Safety

At the time of this writing, a large variety of vascular brachytherapy sources and devices are progressing through various stages of basic science investigations and clinical trials. The initial clinical results have offered very positive results in treating the otherwise intracticable process of in-stent restenosis.

A word of caution needs to be introduced into the discussion. Currently available long-term follow-up is 4 years or less; however, complications of radiation therapy are known to occur later than this. Thus, this uncertainty should to be taken into consideration during the patient selection process for vascular brachytherapy.

As the technology improves, it is almost certain that better understanding of the underlying biology, along with technical improvements in the apparatus, will yield increased margins of safety for both patients and staff.

## Chapter 20

Dosimetry of Clinical Trials:

Beta and Gamma

Rosanna C. Chan, PhD, and Nai-Chuen Yang, PhD

Introduction

Intravascular brachytherapy (IVBT) has been viewed as a potential cure for restenosis. Clinical data gathered over the last 5 years have shown very promising results in terms of both safety and efficacy.[1–5] Failure of the GENEVA trial,[6,7] radioactive stents,[8] the edge effect phenomenon,[9,10] geographic miss,[11,12] and the dose rate finding studies,[13,14] all demonstrated that an adequate dose to the target area is essential. Although the long-term effects have yet to be determined, the fact that clinical dosimetry plays a vital part in the success of IVBT cannot be denied.

As in all radiation therapy procedures, the effectiveness is based on the precision with which the target area is localized and how accurately the dose is delivered. Late complications are definitely something that should be avoided. However, reducing the dose levels may not be the ultimate solution since radiation levels are not the only contributing factor for complications.[15] In addition, a low dose to the target area has been reported to have a stimulating effect on surrounding tissues.[16]

Target Definition

There is yet to be a consensus regarding the most ideal anatomic tissue to target. Most experts believe that the target lies somewhere in the arterial wall: the intima, media, and/or adventitia,[17] which spans between 2 to 5 mm in diameter for coronary arteries. Although the tolerance dose for the lumen wall has not been well established, this innermost lining is normally used as the limiting factor for dose delivery and prescription.

In early clinical trials, treatment length was restricted to a very tight margin within the stenotic or restenotic area in the vessel. Subsequently, intervened or injured tissue caused by angioplasty, new stent placement, or other debulking procedures that were outside the stenotic area did not receive treatment. The rationale was to minimize late effect. As a result, most patients who failed IVBT had recurrent restenosis at the edges of the radiated area, which has been described as the "candy wrapper effect,"[9] "edge effect," and "geographic miss" (Fig. 1). Now, it is gen-

From Waksman R (ed.). *Vascular Brachytherapy, Third Edition.* Armonk, NY: Futura Publishing Co., Inc.; © 2002.

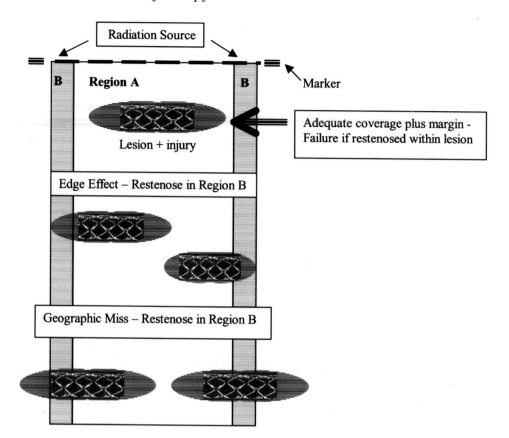

Figure 1. Definition of edge effect and geographic miss.

erally agreed upon that, to ensure proper coverage, the clinical target area needs to include the segment injured during angioplasty. In addition, the safety margin is extended to account for both the movement of the heart and the penumbra effect of the radiation source used. This margin varies depending on the source type and design.

Dose Specifications

Depending on the protocol, the prescription dose may largely vary according to the isotope used and the design of the delivery system. Table 1 lists the prescription dose for some of the clinical trials. Animal studies and clinical trials have indicated that a dose between 8 to 20 Gy to the adventitia wall will yield positive results.[4–6,18] A basic requirement of dosing is that an adequate dose be delivered to the right depth. The American Association of Physicists in Medicine (AAPM) Task Group 60 recommended that, for gamma and noncentered beta sources, the dose prescription point should be at 2 mm from the center of the source; and 1 mm from the surface of the centering balloon for centered beta sources.[19] The only studies that show drastic deviations from these recommendations are the original SCRIPPS and GAMMA 1 Trials. Dose prescription for these two studies is based on intravascular ultrasound (IVUS) measurements over the axial length of the stented segment. These trials called for a minimum dose of 8 Gy to the external

Table 1

List of Clinical Trial Prescriptions

Trial	Sponsor	Isotope	Dose (Gy) Prescription
ARTISTIC	US Surgical	^{192}Ir Wire	12 Gy to depth of 1.8 mm from source center for vessels with ≥2.5 to ≤3.0 mm diameter. 15 Gy to depth of 2.0 mm from source center for vessels with >3.0 to ≤4.0 mm diameter. 18 Gy to depth of 2.2 mm from source center for vessels with >4.0 to ≤5.0 mm diameter.
Beta-Cath	Novoste	Sr/^{90}Y Seeds	14 Gy to depth of 2 mm from source center for vessels ≥ 2.7 but ≤3.35 mm in diameter. 18 Gy to depth of 2 mm from source center for vessels with >3.35 but ≤4.0 mm diameter.
BetaWRIST	Schneider	^{90}Y Wire	20.6 Gy to depth of 1 mm beyond the surface of the centering balloon.
BRITE	Radiance	^{32}P Balloon	20 Gy to depth of 1 mm beyond the surface of the treatment balloon.
INHIBIT	Guidant	^{32}P Wire	20 Gy to depth of 1 mm into the arterial wall based on the average of the proximal and distal reference lumen diameters.
PARIS	Nucletron	^{192}Ir HDR	14 Gy to depth of 2 mm from source center (peripheral arteries).
PRVENT	Guidant	^{32}P Wire	28, 35, or 42 Gy to depth of 0.5 mm beyond surface of the centering balloon catheter diameter used. (Randomized dose finding study.)
SCRIPPS GAMMA 1	Cordis	^{192}Ir Seeds	8 Gy to the longest distance between the center of catheter and the leading edge of the media based on IVUS measurements along the stent vessel segment, but not to exceed 30 Gy to the shortest distance measured.
SMART	AngioRad	^{192}Ir Wire	12 Gy to depth of 1.3 mm from source center with 4 atm balloon inflation for vessels <2.5mm in diameter.
START	Novoste	Sr/^{90}Y Seeds	12 Gy to depth of 2.0 mm from core center with 11 atm balloon inflation. 16 Gy to depth of 2 mm from source center for vessels ≥ 2.7 but ≤3.35 mm in diameter. 20 Gy to depth of 2 mm from source center for vessels with >3.35 but ≤4.0 mm diameter.
WRIST SVG WRIST Long WRIST	Washington Hospital Center	^{192}Ir Seeds	15 Gy to depth of 2 mm from source center for vessels with diameter <4 mm. 15 Gy to depth of 2.4 mm from source center for vessels with diameter ≥4 mm.

IVUS Pull-back

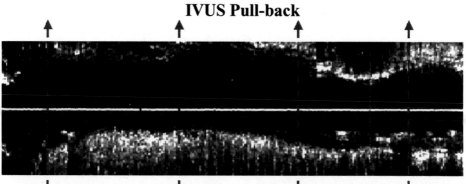

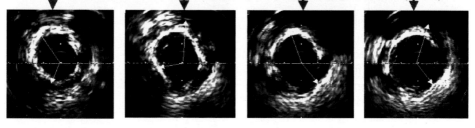

Search for minimum distance (Pt. A) and maximum distance (Pt. B)

Figure 2A. SCRIPPS dosimetry method. Select a minimum of three slices along the treatment length. Measure the maximum and minimum distance from the center of the IVUS catheter to the external elastic membrane (EEM) for each slice. The longest and shortest distance found among those cuts would be the limiting factor for the prescribed dose.

elastic lamina (EEL) without exceeding 30 Gy to the internal elastic lamina (IEL) (Figs. 2A and B). Regardless of the variation, all prescription schematics used at the present time are based on the point dose method. This method is straightforward and does not take into account any real life irregularities. To ensure proper dose comparison between studies and institutions, it is highly recommended that the dosage to different areas and volumes be recorded.

Figure 2B. Schematic representation of the SCRIPPS dosimetry.

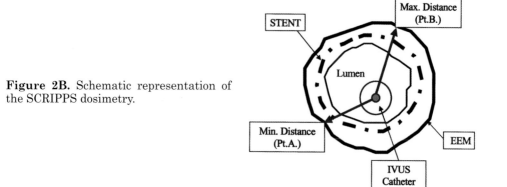

Point Dose Method

By definition, point dose method is the delivery of a dose to one point in space or depth. This point is taken along the perpendicular bisector of the source. Dose calculation using this method is relatively simple. Radial dose rate at a depth for each source train can be established in advance and, by knowing the source activity at treatment time, one can easily calculate the delivery time.

$$t = TD(r) / A(t) * D(A,r)$$

where t = treatment time in minutes; TD(r) = prescribed dose to depth r in Gy; A(t) = source activity in mCi at treatment time; D(A,r) = radial dose rate at prescribed depth of r in (Gy/min/mCi source).

For all IVBT protocols, the prescription dose (except for SCRIPPS and Gamma 1 which assumed that dose uniformity existed along the axial length of the source train) D(A,r) is along the perpendicular bisector of the source with no heterogeneity correction. In general, this method is acceptable because most of the earlier studies are for focal lesions. With a source length of 3 to 5 cm, curvature of the artery can be ignored.

The dose limiting factor lies in the lumen wall, which receives the highest dose. Although the actual tolerance dose for the lumen has yet to be determined, the Food and Drug Administration, to be on the safe side, has restricted this dose, under all circumstances, to less than 4 times the prescription dose. Gamma sources, which are more penetrating by nature, deposit less energy per unit area, thus delivering a lower dose to the lumen surface.[20] Figure 3A compares the relative dose of two commercially available sources, a Best [192]Ir (gamma) seed and a Novoste Sr/[90]Y (beta) source, as a function of depth. By the same reasoning, less time is required for a beta source to deliver a therapeutic dose in an IVBT procedure, than a gamma source with the same activity (Fig. 3B). The use of a center-

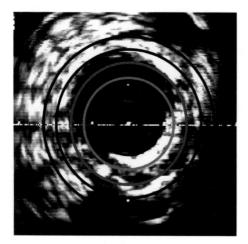

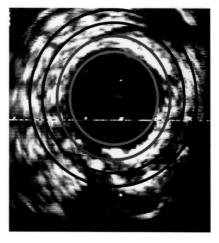

Isodose Distribution with a
Non-centered Source

Isodose Distribution with a
Centered Source

Figure 3. Effect of source centering on an eccentric vessel.

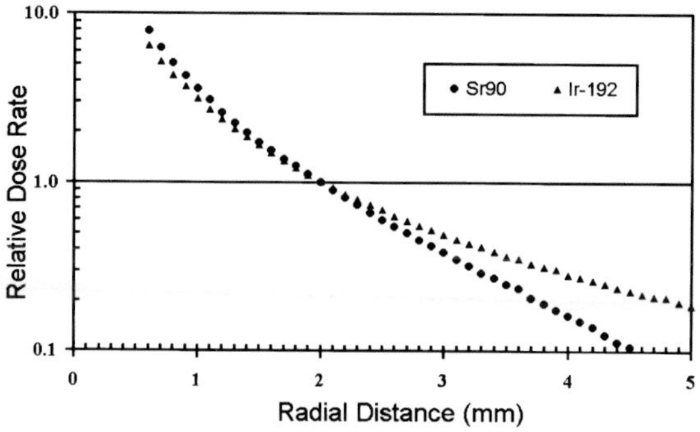

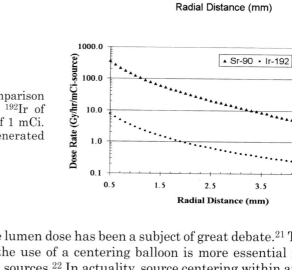

Figure 4A. Relative dose of a single ^{192}Ir (gamma) seed and a single Sr/^{90}Y (beta) seed. (Based on MCNP4B generated data.)

Figure 4B. Dose rate comparison between ^{90}Sr source and ^{192}Ir of equal contained activity of 1 mCi. (Based on MCNP4B generated data.)

ing balloon to reduce the lumen dose has been a subject of great debate.[21] The general consensus is that the use of a centering balloon is more essential for beta sources than for gamma sources.[22] In actuality, source centering within an eccentric vessel can achieve dose uniformity for the lumen only, but not necessarily the vessel wall (Fig. 4). In addition, the material used for the filling of the centering balloon can drastically alter the output of the beta source. Figure 5 shows the effect that a carbon dioxide-filled balloon catheter has on the dose rate of an ^{90}Y (beta) source. Thus, special care must be taken when inflating the centering balloons with saline as contrast material and/or air bubbles inside the balloon can induce dose variation along the treatment area.

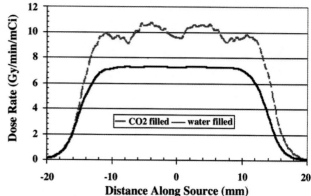

Figure 5. Effect of CO_2 on output of ^{90}Y source wire. (MCNP4B generated data.)

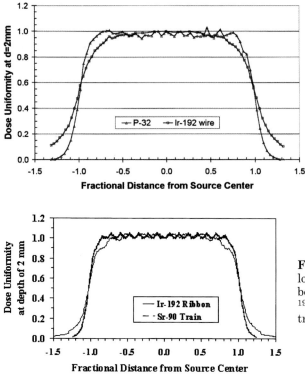

Figure 6A. Dose fall-off along the longitudinal axis of two wire sources. (MCNP4B modeled Angiorad ^{192}Ir wire and Guidant ^{32}P wire data.)

Figure 6B. Dose fall-off along the longitudinal axis of two source ribbons. (MCNP4B modeled Cordis ^{192}Ir ribbon and Novoste Sr/^{90}Y train.)

Two-Dimensional Isodose Planes

A low dose in an injured zone can instigate the onset of edge effect. To ensure proper coverage along the treatment length, it is pertinent to know the isodose distribution of the source. Dose distribution is a function of source design and can be altered, especially for beta sources, by the design of the centering catheter and other heterogeneity materials. The dose fall-off along the longitudinal axis of two different source types and configurations is shown in Figures 6A and B. Beta emitters that lack forward scatter deposit their energy more locally, resulting in a useful length that is longer than that produced by a gamma source of similar design. In addition, longitudinal dose uniformity can be improved to some extent (limited by the isotope) with the use of a multiple seed train as depicted in Figure 7.

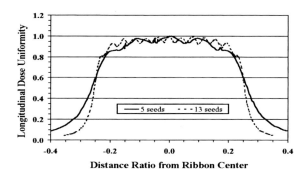

Figure 7. Longitudinal dose uniformity increases with number of seeds in ribbon. Variations shown here are at depth of 2 mm from the source center.

Three-Dimensional Treatment Planning

At the present time, the use of three-dimensional treatment planning is limited to post-treatment dose analysis[23–27] in an attempt to improve local control and to lower the probability of complications. For IVBT treatment planning, images from IVUS pullback studies are used for structure definition and three-dimensional volumetric dose reconstruction. IVUS is a diagnostic tool and therefore, the images lack the accuracy expected for radiation treatment planning. Geometric distortions caused by the position of the ultrasound catheter within the artery are generally ignored.[28–30] These artifacts, together with organ motion and curvature of the artery, can greatly affect the accuracy in qualitative and quantitative analyses of the wall structures. Another deficiency is that the center of the ultrasound catheter is interpreted to be the center of the radiation catheter (3.2–5F). When replacing the IVUS catheter with the radiation catheter for treatment, the likelihood that the two catheters' centers will be at the same location decreases as the vessel's lumen increases. Thus, care must be taken when using these images for dose calculation.

Despite the limitations, IVUS is still the best tool available for measuring the extent of restenosis. The use of an electrocardiogram (ECG)-gated IVUS[31] and a three-dimensional geometric model[29,32] can help minimize some of these problems. Further development is needed to make IVUS more effective for treatment planning. In addition, more data is required for near-field dosimetry of IVBT sources. The ultimate goal for the radiation therapy community is to develop a three-dimensional real-time treatment planning system that would account for heterogeneity effects due to the presence of stents and calcification plaque in the arterial wall.

Dosimetry Data

Traditional brachytherapy formalism treats all radioactive seeds as idealized point sources. Dose rate approximation follows the inverse square law as a simple function of distance. No consideration was made for the anisotropy correction which could affect the dose distribution drastically. For close vicinity use, such as eye plaques, the effect becomes more prominent. The new TG-43 formalism, introduced in 1995, was designed to account for the absorption and scatter due to source design and tissue media.[33]

$$D(r,\, \theta) = S_k \times \Lambda \times \frac{G(r,\theta)}{G(r_0,\theta_0)} \times g(r) \times F(r,\theta)$$

where $D(r,\theta)$ = dose rate at point (r,θ) (cGy/hr); S_k = air-kerma strength of source (U); Λ = dose rate constant at $r_0,\ \theta_0$ (cGy/hr/U) $G(r,\theta)$ = geometry function; $g(r)$ = radial dose function; $F(r,\theta)$ = two-dimensional anisotropy function; and (r_0,θ_0) = reference point for dose measurement (1 cm , $\pi/2$).

At the time of publication in 1995, TG-43 was intended for interstitial implants. The seed sources available were limited and no data was taken to the near-field zone (less than 5 mm away from the source), the prime region of interest for IVBT. In order to determine the dose to the near field, a lined source approximation has to be used for analyzing the source data. In addition, each new source design has to have its own geometry functions.

With the increased success of IVBT and the development of beta sources for the procedure, TG-60[19] recommended that the reference depth for TG-43 formalism be changed from 10 mm to 2 mm. Since national standards for air kerma strength do not exist for beta-emitting sources, the following formula was recommended:

$$D(r,\theta) = D(r_0, \theta_0) \times \frac{G(r,\theta)}{G(r_0,\theta_0)} \times g\,(r) \times F(r,\theta)$$

where $D(r_0,\theta_0)$ = Dose rate in water at r = 2 mm and $\theta_0 = \pi/2$ (cGy/hr);

However, for beta sources longer than its particle range, the TG-60 formalism fails. Inaccuracy in the interpolation of anisotropy function increases with angle θ, and thus compromises the accuracy in treatment planning. To overcome this problem, Patel et al[34] proposed the adaptation of the cylindrical coordinates system and three new parameters. These parameters are analogous to those used in TG-60, and therefore preserve the original formalism.

Dose Measurement

It is the responsibility of the physicist to verify that the dose delivered to the patient is correct. For most sources that are commercially available, National Institute of Standards and Technology (NIST) or ADCL traceable calibration factors are available. However, this is not a requirement and there are different ways for specifying source strength. Care must be taken to ensure that the "correct" parameter is used with the right formalism.

Traditionally, source strength is specified by the activity contained in the source. The basic SI unit Becquerel, (1 Bq = 1 disintegration per second), denotes the rate of spontaneous disintegration of the source. Because the SI unit Becquerel does not take into account self-absorption and encapsulation, the term "apparent activity," A_{app}, was introduced to measure the relative output of a source to that of a standard source. In 1991, TG-32[35] recommended a new quantity, air kerma strength, which is a measurable quantity for use with gamma radiation thereby eliminating the use of the dummy variable, exposure rate constant. With TG-43 formalism, all data are then normalized to the dose rate constant, Λ, which is defined as the absolute dose rate to water at a distance of 1 cm in water, on the transverse axis of a unit air kerma strength source in a water phantom:

$$\Lambda = D(r_0,\theta_0)/S_k$$

This factor includes the effect of source geometry, self-absorption, and encapsulation. Since the dose rate constant is a measured quantity, and S_k is measurable and traceable to NIST, a crosscheck program can be established in house to ensure accurate dose delivery.

Source Calibration

Accuracy in the delivery of the prescribed dose is a prerequisite for the success of any radiation therapy treatment schema. The TG-40[36] report recommended that each institution independently verify the source strength provided by the manufacturer. For short half-life single sources, the agreement between in-

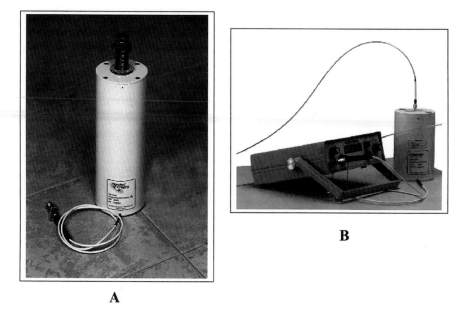

A

B

Figure 8. A. New IVB 1000 Chamber. Courtesy of Standard Imaging, Inc. **B.** 32P Wire Chamber. Courtesy of Guidant Company.

Figure 9A. Sweet spot axial response of standard imaging chamber HDR1000 Plus.

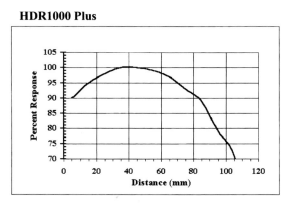

Figure 9B. Sweet spot axial response of standard imaging chamber IVB100. Reprinted with permission from Standard Imaging, Inc.

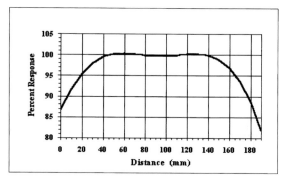

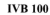

stitution and manufacturer should be within 3%, and for individual source in a batch, within 5%. Although there is no federal requirement to calibrate low dose rate brachytherapy sources, it is a requirement for high dose rate (HDR) sources. Because IVBT delivers high doses to the near-field target, both strength and uniformity of the source should be verified before use in a clinical setting. A reentrant well-type ionization chamber used for HDR can be calibrated for use in a consistency check for both gamma and beta sources. Length and uniformity of the chamber's "sweet spot" will limit the length of the source ribbon it can measure. A correction factor has to be established for each individual chamber to compensate for the geometry effect. A new IVB 1000 chamber (Fig. 8A) was specially designed by Standard Imaging, Inc. for the Cordis/Best ribbon. This chamber has a long uniform sweet spot that can accommodate source trains up to 100 mm without a sweet spot correction factor.[37] Figures 9A and B compare the axial sweet spot of the two chambers HDR 1000 Plus and IVB1000. A similar chamber has also been modified for the Guidant P-32 beta source (Fig. 8B). This chamber was calibrated by NIST using a destruction method[38,39] enabling the S_k calibration factor to reflect the contained activity of the source.

Well-type ionization chambers provide a simple way for source verification and consistency checks. However, care must be taken to ensure source positioning and repositioning within the sweet spot. Source holder material is also very important especially for beta sources. A slight change in catheter thickness (mm) can and will vary the output of a beta source by a few percentage points. It is important to preserve the same calibration set-up for each subsequent measurement. Any modification to the source design and or holder material would require a calibration check.

Autoradiography

Linear activity and dose uniformity are very crucial for IVBT. Visual inspection of autoradiographs can quickly review any irregularities in the seed or the ribbon assembly provided that proper exposure and set-up geometry are used. Figure 10 shows a defective seed inside a 23 seed ribbon. This seed that was only partially activated could not have been detected through calibration alone (<2%

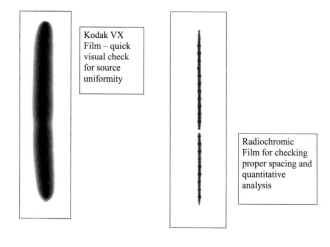

Kodak VX Film – quick visual check for source uniformity

Radiochromic Film for checking proper spacing and quantitative analysis

Figure 10. Autoradiography.

difference). For quality analysis, regular VX film with a very short exposure time would be appropriate to detect any irregularities. However, for quantitative analysis, it is necessary to use radiochromic film.[40]

With the use of an automated source delivery system, the source and dummy positions need to be within 1 mm. Depending on the usage and design of the system, this could be a daily quality assurance procedure. Figure 11 shows a special jig designed by one company for verifying source uniformity and position accuracy. This jig has an adapter for attachment to the automated IVBT devices. The dummy source is first sent to the marker position under the magnifying window. A piece of radiochromic film is then placed directly under the catheter and the active source is sent to the same position. The difference between the dummy source and the active source positions should be less than 1 mm. Positioning becomes more critical if multiple steps will be used for treatment of long lesions. Using a similar method, any overlapping or gapping between source steps can be easily spotted (Fig. 12).

Dosimetry Parameters

TG-43 lacks data for near-field dosimetry and beta sources. Physical measurements of these parameters is tedious and can give rise to large experimental

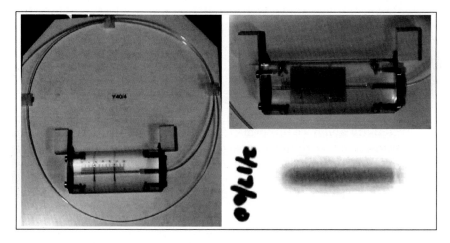

Figure 11. Special jig designed for source positioning and uniformity verification with automated device. Courtesy of Schneider.

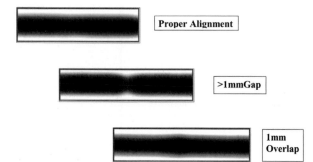

Figure 12. Overlap and gap of a ^{32}P wire source as shown by autoradiography. Reprinted with permission from Guidant.

Proper Alignment

>1mmGap

1mm Overlap

uncertainties. Monte Carlo modeling is viewed as an alternative method. To ensure accuracy, attention to greater detail of the source design is very critical. Figure 13 shows the difference between isodose curves generated with an air gap between seeds as opposed to using unit density material between seeds. Table 2 lists the dose rate and percent depth dose of some of the sources generated using MCNP4B. At near field, the parameters that are generated are very source-specific and results should be verified experimentally before they are used in a clinical setting. Source design, special delivering catheter, plaque, and stent can alter the dose dramatically and should be taken into consideration in determining the prescription.

Conclusion

Dosimetry plays a very crucial part in the success and long-term safety of IVBT. There is an immediate need for dosimetry parameters in the near-field zone as well as standardization of source activity. New formalism for long beta sources will help in the development of an IVUS-based three-dimensional treatment planning system. When new data is established and the real target is revealed, there will be an adjustment of doses. Until then, consistency is more important than accuracy.

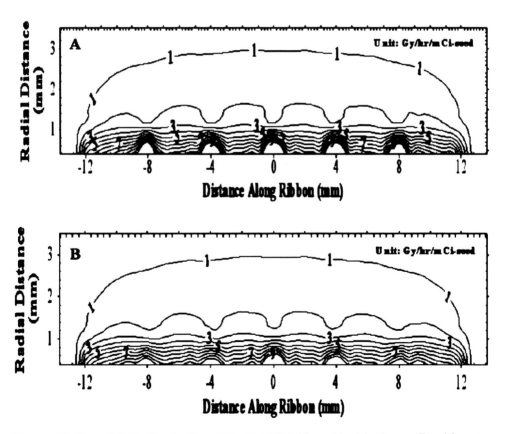

Figure 13. Dose distribution for 6 seed Cordis IRT Ribbon. **A)** with air gap; **B)** with water gap. (MCNP4B generated data.)

Table 2

Depth Dose Table based on MCNP4B Modeling for Various Commercially Available Sources*

Depth from Source Center (mm)	Cordis/Best Ribbon			Angiorad	90Y Wire with CO₂-Filled Balloon				32P Wire with Saline-Filled Balloon			
	6 seeds	10 seed	14 seed	^{192}Ir wire	2.5 mm balloon dia.	3.0 mm balloon dia.	3.5 mm balloon dia.	4.0 mm balloon dia.	2.5 mm balloon dia.	3.0 mm balloon dia.	3.5 mm balloon dia.	4.0 mm balloon dia.
0.6	5.01	4.85	4.80	10.09								
0.7	3.69	3.58	3.54	7.11								
0.8	2.99	2.91	2.88	5.12								
0.9	2.55	2.48	2.46	4.09								
1.0	2.20	2.15	2.13	3.23								
1.1	1.92	1.88	1.87	2.46								
1.2	1.72	1.69	1.68	2.08								
1.3	1.56	1.54	1.53	1.82								
1.4	1.43	1.41	1.41	1.60	1.79				2.61			
1.5	1.33	1.31	1.30	1.44	1.66				2.35			
1.6	1.24	1.23	1.22	1.28	1.56	1.79			2.07	2.80		
1.7	1.17	1.16	1.16	1.20	1.46	1.66			1.86	2.52		
1.8	1.11	1.10	1.10	1.12	1.36	1.58			1.63	2.21		
1.9	1.05	1.05	1.05	1.05	1.26	1.48	1.65		1.48	2.00	2.57	
2.0	1.00	1.00	1.00	1.00	1.19	1.40	1.55		1.34	1.81	2.34	
2.1	0.95	0.96	0.96	0.96	1.11	1.28	1.44	1.61	1.19	1.61	2.08	3.03
2.2	0.91	0.92	0.92	0.91	1.03	1.18	1.36	1.50	1.05	1.42	1.84	2.68
2.3	0.87	0.88	0.88	0.86	0.96	1.11	1.29	1.42	0.95	1.28	1.65	2.41
2.4	0.83	0.84	0.85	0.82	0.90	1.05	1.22	1.36	0.85	1.14	1.48	2.16
2.5	0.80	0.81	0.81	0.78	0.82	1.00	1.14	1.26	0.74	1.00	1.29	1.89
2.6	0.77	0.78	0.78	0.75	0.76	0.91	1.07	1.23	0.68	0.92	1.19	1.74
2.7	0.74	0.75	0.75	0.72	0.73	0.86	1.02	1.15	0.63	0.85	1.09	1.60
2.8	0.71	0.72	0.73	0.69	0.68	0.84	0.96	1.11	0.54	0.73	0.94	1.37
2.9	0.68	0.70	0.70	0.67	0.63	0.79	0.90	1.05	0.45	0.61	0.79	1.15
3.0	0.65	0.67	0.68	0.64	0.60	0.71	0.87	1.00	0.39	0.53	0.68	1.00
3.1	0.63	0.65	0.66	0.62	0.57	0.68	0.82	0.94	0.36	0.49	0.63	0.92

3.2	0.61	0.63	0.63	0.59	0.53	0.64	0.75	0.88	0.32	0.43	0.56	0.82
3.3	0.59	0.61	0.61	0.57	0.50	0.60	0.71	0.82	0.29	0.39	0.50	0.73
3.4	0.57	0.59	0.59	0.55	0.47	0.56	0.67	0.77	0.24	0.33	0.42	0.62
3.5	0.55	0.57	0.58	0.54	0.44	0.53	0.62	0.71	0.20	0.27	0.35	0.51
3.6	0.53	0.55	0.56	0.52	0.40	0.49	0.58	0.69	0.19	0.25	0.32	0.47
3.7	0.51	0.54	0.55	0.50	0.38	0.47	0.54	0.65	0.17	0.22	0.29	0.42
3.8	0.50	0.52	0.53	0.49	0.36	0.44	0.51	0.62	0.14	0.19	0.25	0.36
3.9	0.49	0.51	0.52	0.47	0.33	0.41	0.48	0.59	0.13	0.17	0.22	0.32
4.0	0.47	0.50	0.51	0.46	0.31	0.39	0.46	0.55	0.10	0.13	0.17	0.25
4.1	0.46	0.48	0.49	0.45	0.28	0.36	0.43	0.51	0.09	0.12	0.15	0.22
4.2	0.45	0.47	0.48	0.43	0.27	0.35	0.41	0.48	0.09	0.12	0.15	0.22
4.3	0.44	0.46	0.47	0.42	0.26	0.32	0.39	0.46	0.07	0.09	0.11	0.17
4.4	0.42	0.45	0.46	0.41	0.23	0.29	0.37	0.42	0.05	0.07	0.09	0.13
4.5	0.41	0.44	0.45	0.40	0.22	0.27	0.35	0.40	0.04	0.06	0.08	0.11
4.6	0.40	0.43	0.44	0.39	0.21	0.25	0.32	0.37	0.04	0.05	0.06	0.09
4.7	0.39	0.42	0.43	0.38	0.19	0.24	0.30	0.35	0.03	0.04	0.05	0.08
4.8	0.38	0.41	0.42	0.37	0.18	0.22	0.27	0.33	0.02	0.03	0.04	0.06
4.9	0.37	0.40	0.41	0.36	0.17	0.21	0.25	0.32	0.02	0.03	0.04	0.06
5.0	0.36	0.39	0.40	0.35	0.16	0.20	0.24	0.30	0.02	0.03	0.03	0.05

*All doses are normalized to their respective prescription point, which is along the perpendicular bisector of the source.

References

1. Condado JA, Waksman R, Gurdiel O, et al. Long-term angiographic and clinical outcome after percutaneous transluminal coronary angioplasty and intracoronary radiation therapy in humans [see comments]. Circulation 1997;96:727–732.
2. Waksman R. Radiation catheter-based therapy for prevention of restenosis. Cardiologia 1996;41:849–854.
3. Waksman R, Bhargava B, White L, et al. Intracoronary beta-radiation therapy inhibits recurrence of in-stent restenosis. Circulation 2000 Apr 25 101;1895–1898.
4. Waksman R. Response to radiation therapy in animal restenosis models. Semin Interv Cardiol 1997;2:95–101.
5. Waksman R. Vascular brachytherapy: Update on clinical trials. J Invas Cardiol 2000 Feb 1912;18A–28A.
6. Urban P, Verin V, Popowski Y, Rutishauser W. Feasibility and safety of beta irradiation in human coronary arteries. Semin Interv Cardiol 1997 Jun 1902;125–131.
7. Verin V, Popowski Y. Intraarterial beta irradiation to reduce restenosis after PTCA: Experimental and clinical experience. Herz 1998 Sep 1923;347–355.
8. Wardeh AJ, Kay IP, Sabate M, et al. Beta-particle-emitting radioactive stent implantation: A safety and feasibility study. Circulation 1999;100:1684–1689.
9. Albiero R, Nishida T, Adamian M, et al. Edge restenosis after implantation of high activity (32)P radioactive beta-emitting stents. Circulation 2000;101:2454–2457.
10. Albiero R, Adamian M, Kobayashi N, et al. Short- and intermediate-term results of (32)P radioactive beta-emitting stent implantation in patients with coronary artery disease: The Milan Dose-Response Study [see comments]. Circulation 2000;101:18–26.
11. Giap H, Teirstein P, Massullo V, Tripuraneni P. Barotrauma due to stent deployment in endovascular brachytherapy for restenosis prevention. Int J Radiat Oncol Biol Phys 2000;47:1021–1024.
12. Tripuraneni P, Parikh S, Giap H, et al. How long is enough? Defining the treatment length in endovascular brachytherapy. Catheter Cardiovasc Interv 2000;51:147–153.
13. Verin V, Popowski Y, Bochaton-Piallat ML, et al. Intraarterial beta irradiation induces smooth muscle cell apoptosis and reduces medial cellularity in a hypercholesterolemic rabbit restenosis model. Int J Radiat Oncol Biol Phys 2000;46:661–670.
14. Albiero R, Colombo A. European high-activity (32)P radioactive stent experience. J Invas Cardiol 2000;12:416–421.
15. Perez CA, Purdy JA. Rationale for treatment planning in radiation therapy. In: Levitt SH, Khan FM, Potish RA (eds.): Technological Basis of Radiation Therapy. Philadelphia: Lea & Febiger; 1992:14–26.
16. Weinberger J, Amols H, Ennis RD, et al. Intracoronary irradiation: Dose response for the prevention of restenosis in swine. Int J Radiat Oncol Biol Phys 1996;36:767–775.
17. Wilcox JN, Waksman R, King SB, Scott NA. The role of the adventitia in the arterial response to angioplasty: The effect of intravascular radiation. Int J Radiat Oncol Biol Phys 1996;36:789–796.
18. Popowski Y, Verin V, Urban P. Endovascular beta-irradiation after percutaneous transluminal coronary balloon angioplasty. Int J Radiat Oncol Biol Phys 1996;36:841–845.
19. Nath R, Amols H, Coffey C, et al. Intravascular brachytherapy physics: Report of the AAPM Radiation Therapy Committee Task Group No. 60. American Association of Physicists in Medicine. Med Phys 1999;26:119–152.
20. Waksman R, Bhargava B, White L, et al. Intracoronary beta-radiation therapy inhibits recurrence of in-stent restenosis. Circulation 2000;101:1895–1898.
21. Waksman R, Bhargava B, Saucedo JF, et al. Yttrium-90 delivered via centering catheter and afterloader, given both before and after stent implantation, completely inhibits neointimal formation in swine coronary arteries [abstract]. J Am Coll Cardiol 1999;33:20A.
22. Waksman R, Abizaid A, Chan R, Osaki S. The importance of centering for intracoronary radiation therapy: an ultrasound-dosimetry analysis for gamma and beta emitters [abstract]. Adv Cardiovasc Radiat Ther 11, 26; 3800.
23. Ahmed JM, Mintz GS, Waksman R, et al. Safety of intracoronary gamma-radiation on uninjured reference segments during the first 6 months after treatment of in-stent restenosis: A serial intravascular ultrasound study. Circulation 2000;101:2227–2230.

24. Carlier SG, Marijnissen JP, Coen VL, et al. Guidance of intracoronary radiation therapy based on dose-volume histograms derived from quantitative intravascular ultrasound. IEEE Trans Med Imag 1998;17:772–778.
25. Limpijankit T, Waksman R, Yock PG, Fitzgerald PJ. Intravascular ultrasound volumetric assessment of intimal hyperplasia in stents treated with intracoronary radiation. Am J Cardiol 1999;84:850–854.
26. Mintz GS, Kent KM, Pichard AD, et al. Contribution of inadequate arterial remodeling to the development of focal coronary artery stenoses: An intravascular ultrasound study [see comments]. Circulation 1997;95:1791–1798.
27. Costa MA, Sabate M, Serrano P, et al. The effect of 32P beta-radiotherapy on both vessel remodeling and neointimal hyperplasia after coronary balloon angioplasty and stenting: A three-dimensional intravascular ultrasound investigation. J Invas Cardiol 2000;12:113–120.
28. Roelandt JR, di Mario C, Pandian NG, et al. Three-dimensional reconstruction of intracoronary ultrasound images: Rationale, approaches, problems, and directions. Circulation 1994;90:1044–1055.
29. Delachartre P, Cachard C, Finet G, et al. Modeling geometric artefacts in intravascular ultrasound imaging. Ultrasound Med Biol 1999;25:567–575.
30. Finet G, Cachard C, Delachartre P, et al. Artifacts in intravascular ultrasound imaging during coronary artery stent implantation. Ultrasound Med Biol 1998;24:793–802.
31. Carlier SG, Marijnissen JP, Coen VL, et al. Guidance of intracoronary radiation therapy based on dose-volume histograms derived from quantitative intravascular ultrasound. IEEE Trans Med Imaging 1998;17:772–778.
32. Finet G, Maurincomme E, Reiber JH, et al. Evaluation of an automatic intraluminal edge detection technique for intravascular ultrasound images. Jpn Circ J 1998;62:115–121.
33. Nath R, Anderson LL, Luxton G, et al. Dosimetry of interstitial brachytherapy sources: Recommendations of the AAPM Radiation Therapy Committee Task Group No. 43. American Association of Physicists in Medicine [see comments] [published erratum appears in Med Phys 1996;9:1579]. Med Phys 1995;22:209–234.
34. Patel NS, Chiu-Tsao ST, Tsao HS, Harrison LB. A new treatment planning formalism for catheter-based beta sources used in intravascular brachytherapy. Submitted for publication.
35. Nath R, Anderson L, Luxton G, et al. Dosimetry of interstitial brachytherapy sources: Recommendations of the AAPM Radiation Therapy Committee Task Group No. 43. American Association of Physicists in Medicine. Med Phys 1995;22:209–234.
36. Kutcher GJ, Coia L, Gillin M, et al. Comprehensive QA for radiation oncology: Report of AAPM Radiation Therapy Committee Task Group 40. Med Phys 1994;21:581–618.
37. DeWerd LA, Micka JA, Schmidt D, Reavis RJ. Calibration of Well-type Chambers for Intravascular Ir-192 Source Trains. CIRMS meeting, Gaithersburg, MD, Oct 30-Nov 1, 2000. (Poster.)
38. Colle R. On the radioanalytical methods used to assay stainless-steel-encapsulated, ceramic-based 90Sr-90Y intravascular brachytherapy sources. Appl Radiat Isot 2000;52:1–18.
39. Colle R. Chemical digestion and radionuclidic assay of TiNi-encapsulated 32P intravascular brachytherapy sources. Appl Radiat Isot 1999;50:811–833.
40. Niroomand-Rad A, Blackwell CR, Coursey BM, et al. Radiochromic film dosimetry: Recommendations of AAPM Radiation Therapy Committee Task Group 55. American Association of Physicists in Medicine. Med Phys 1998;25:2093–2115.

Part IV

Radiation for Restenosis in Animal Models

## Chapter 21

External Beam Irradiation, Stent Injury, and Neointimal Hyperplasia:

Results from the Porcine Model

Robert S. Schwartz, MD,
Thomas M. Koval, PhD, Jean Gregoire, MD,
Myung Ho Jeong, MD, PhD,
William D. Edwards, MD,
Allan R. Camrud, RN, Kevin Browne, MD,
Ronald E. Vlietstra, MB, BCh, and
David R. Holmes, MD

Introduction

The causes of restenosis following percutaneous transluminal coronary angioplasty (PTCA) are complex, but principally include remodeling, or size changes of the artery wall, and neointimal hyperplasia that forms in response to vessel injury. Clinical trials of drugs, including antiplatelet agents, anticoagulants, corticosteroids, and calcium channel blockers, have proven unsuccessful in reducing restenosis rates.[1] Only the coronary stent, and now potentially intravascular radiation, appear promising for reducing the restenosis rates.[2,3] The mechanisms involved with stenting are mechanically and geometrically based alone. A larger initial lumen is achieved, but the stent does not have effect in reducing neointimal hyperplasia, and in fact has the opposite effect of stimulating neointimal growth.[4–6] It will thus be necessary for the solution to restenosis, especially within stents, to inhibit neointimal formation.

The early excitement from animal trials has progressed into early clinical results.[7–9] Current technologies use intravascular radiation in the form of gamma or beta radiation for inhibiting neointima.

In early studies, we examined *external* beam radiation as a pilot to examine its vascular effects.[10] This approach was selected because it is used extensively in the treatment of proliferative neoplastic and non-neoplastic disease. The hypothesis was that external x-radiation might reduce the amount of neointima fol-

From Waksman R (ed.). *Vascular Brachytherapy, Third Edition.* Armonk, NY: Futura Publishing Co., Inc.; © 2002.

lowing coronary artery injury through inhibition of neointimal growth by reducing smooth muscle cell proliferation. The porcine coronary injury model was used because it accurately mimics the amount and character of human restenotic neointima. This model used an intracoronary stent, making for clinical relevance since a major goal of interventional therapy today is to limit stent restenosis.[11] In this model, the amount of hyperplastic neointima is proportional to the severity of injury, providing a quantitative mechanism for direct comparison of treated and untreated animals.[12]

External Beam Radiation in Stented Pig Coronary Arteries: Methods of Study

All studies were performed in accordance with the guidelines of the Mayo Clinic Institutional Animal Care and Use Committee.

Juvenile domestic crossbred pigs (weight 25 to 35 kg) were fed a normal laboratory chow diet without lipid or cholesterol supplementation. Heparin (10,000 units) was administered as an arterial bolus. The method of stent injury has been described previously. All stents were placed in the left anterior descending (LAD) coronary arteries of 37 animals.

The stent:artery oversize ratio was 1.5–2.0, resulting in reliable, significant coronary artery injury. The LAD artery was used because it could be given a calibrated x-ray dose reliably, being directly beneath the sternum. The coil location beneath the sternum was externally identified fluoroscopically, and the skin was marked at this site with an indelible ink marker, for later x-ray window location.

Calibration of the x-ray beam was accomplished as follows. A pig carcass was placed in the position used for irradiation, with a radiation dosimeter on the LAD to verify that delivered doses were in agreement with calculated doses. Doses reaching the artery were also estimated with use of a phantom of the pig chest. Estimated accuracy of the dose reaching the coronary artery was within ±5%.

Four groups of animals were used: three treatment, and one control group, shown in Table 1. These groups were chosen for a variety of radiation doses and timing following arterial injury, and doses were consistent with radiation doses for nonmalignant disease. Interestingly, these doses are somewhat lower than those typically used in transvascular brachytherapy today. The dose schedule was chosen soon after coronary artery injury because of studies showing smooth muscle cell proliferation within 48 hours of arterial injury.[13] The control group obviously received no radiation. Group I received 400 cGy 1 day following coronary injury. Group II received a split radiation dose consisting of 400 cGy at 1 and 4 days after arterial injury. Group III received 800 cGy 1 day after coronary artery injury.

A 300-kV General Electric Maxitron x-ray machine was used for all radiation treatments. The machine was operated at 300 kV and 20 ma. The x-ray beam was filtered by 2 mm of copper (Cu) for a half-value layer slightly greater than 1.8 mmCu. X-rays were delivered to a 25-cm^2 field centered on the external skin mark for coil location, at a dose rate of approximately 100 cGy/min. Except for this 25 cm^2 field, the animal was shielded with about 3 to 4 mm of lead, and backscatter was minimized. The port size was thus minimized. The animals were returned to quarters for recovery after irradiation (treated groups). With use of this radiation

Table 1

Radiation Assignment

		Time After Coronary Injury	
Control	Group I	Group II	Group III
No radiation	400 cGy 24 hours	400 cGy 24 hours 400 cGy 4 days	800 cGy 24 hours

protocol, no noticeable ill effects on the general well-being of the animals was expected. Careful attention was paid to animals for illness or untoward effects following radiation.

The pigs were euthanized 28 days after coronary artery injury, the hearts were removed and perfusion fixed. The coronary arteries were sectioned in 2-mm increments. Each 2-mm histologic section of a given artery was examined, without knowledge of group, to determine the section showing maximal luminal narrowing.

An injury score was assigned to each wire site, and neointimal thickness was measured.[12] For each section, the mean neointimal thickness for all wire sites was calculated, as was the mean injury score (Table 2). This injury-response normalization is important due to the strong relationship between these two parameters. For each arterial segment in this study, there was thus a mean injury score and a mean thickness of neointimal response.

Data analysis was done using two approaches. The first modeled the relationship between injury and thickness for untreated and treated groups separately. The second compared the groups separately. This was accomplished by use of three linear models, as described previously.[14]

Table 2

Assignment of Vessel Injury Score

Description of Assigned Weight	Injury
0	Internal elastic lamina intact; endothelium typically denuded, media may be compressed but not lacerated.
1	Internal elastic lamina lacerated; media typically compressed but not lacerated.
2	Internal elastic lamina lacerated; media visibly lacerated. External elastic lamina intact but may be compressed.
3	External elastic lamina lacerated. Typically large lacerations of media extending through the external elastic lamina. Coil wires sometimes residing in adventitia.

Results of Radiation and Neointimal Growth

Thirty-seven animals successfully completed the protocol, shown in Table 3. Not all animals survived the expected 28 days. Sudden death occurred in four pigs, as shown in Table 3. All sudden and unexpected deaths were in pigs that underwent radiation. Histopathological examination of the coronary arteries in these animals showed severe stenoses consisting of organized neointima, but also with fresh thrombus at those injury sites.

No adverse clinical or behavioral effects were apparent in any irradiated animal surviving until sacrifice. This was expected based on results in humans with comparable radiation doses. Gross examination of the hearts after death was also negative for radiation effect. Figure 1 is a series of representative gross photographs of the neointimal proliferation found in A) the control group; B) group I; C) group II; and D) group III. Progressively more neointimal formation and greater stenosis is seen in this series of photographs as radiation dose increases. Figure 2 shows coronary artery photomicrographs which are similarly representative of radiated animals.

Microscopic examination revealed neointimal responses and luminal stenoses of varying magnitude in all groups. The character of this neointima has been previously described.[11] In group III there were a few giant cells, a finding associated with irradiated tissue in humans. In this highest radiation dose group, medial edema was routinely observed. There was moderate to severe myocardial and adventitial fibrosis in all three radiation groups (Fig. 3). No fibrosis was noted in any control animal. The areas of fibrosis were typical of those seen following radiation, being hypocellular and patchy. Segments of coronary arteries that were not injured by the coil, yet were in the radiation field, showed essentially no reaction to the radiation, and appeared entirely normal.

Table 4 shows mean arterial injury scores and percent-area stenosis for each vessel in each group. Table 5 shows the results of the linear regression modeling performed for each group separately. For group III, a meaningful regression line could not be generated because there were no low-level injuries. Figure 4 shows the data graphically. It is evident that the regression lines for the treated groups are higher than the control lines, with roughly equivalent slope but differing intercepts. Overall, these results are similar to those of prior studies wherein the degree of neointimal proliferation was proportional to vessel injury. Figure 5 shows the percent-area stenosis measured histologically. It clear that the percent stenosis increases with increased radiation dose.

Table 3

Demographic Data for all Groups

Group	Number of Animals	Number of Unexpected Deaths	Days to Unexpected Death
Control	8	0	–
I 400 cGy	10	2	Days 5,9
II 400/400 cGy	10	1	Day 4
III 800 cGy	9	1	Day 15

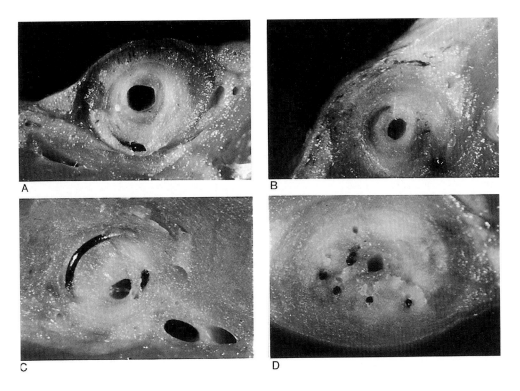

Figure 1. Gross photographs of representative coronary artery segments at 28 days following injury in the **A)** control group, **B)** group I (400 cGy), **C)** group II (400/400 cGy), and **D)** group III (800 cGy). Wires from the injuring coils are shown. The degree of proliferation increases with groups receiving higher doses of radiation.

Uncertainty remains about the use of external beam therapy after coronary artery angioplasty.[15] A study in nonatherosclerotic rabbits examined external beam radiation using 600 or 1200 cGy following iliac balloon jury.[16] The authors found no difference in neointimal cross-sectional area between control and radiated segments in the 600 cGy group, but did note a significant reduction in the 1200 cGy group. The authors concluded that in the rabbit model, external beam may be useful.[16]

Interestingly, a major cardiac interventional center performed an unpublished pilot study of external beam radiation in patients following coronary artery with stenting. The data were reported to show a restenosis rate higher than expected from stenting alone. These data, suggesting an enhanced restenosis rate, by implication also suggest a stimulation of neointimal hyperplasia, since the stent should eliminate remodeling as a factor in restenosis. Whether these results would hold true had this been a larger study is unclear. Regardless, it suggests caution about external beam therapy and restenosis.

The restenosis problem remains a major limitation of percutaneous interventions for coronary artery disease, even with the advent of stents. Early and recent stent animal trials found lower restenosis rates (Table 6), but these were selected lesions.[2,3] Recent estimates of "non-STRESS/non-BENESTENT" restenosis rates are higher (Table 6, part B).

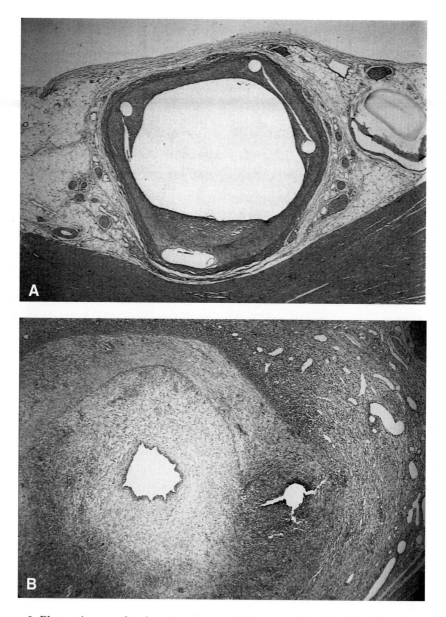

Figure 2. Photomicrographs showing representative control and radiated coronary arteries. Severe stenoses are shown along with mechanical injury resulting from the stents (all panels hematoxylin-eosin, x10). **A.** Control group, no irradiation; **B.** group III, 800 cGy.

Since smooth muscle cell proliferation and neointimal hyperplasia may play a major role in the genesis of obstructive lesions after balloon angioplasty and with stenting, it is reasonable to consider radiation therapy as a potential solution. The usefulness and safety of x-irradiation for the treatment of both malignant and nonmalignant proliferative conditions is well established.[17–20] Clinical studies appear to confirm this hypothesis.[21–24]

It remains unclear whether external radiation can be made to give effective

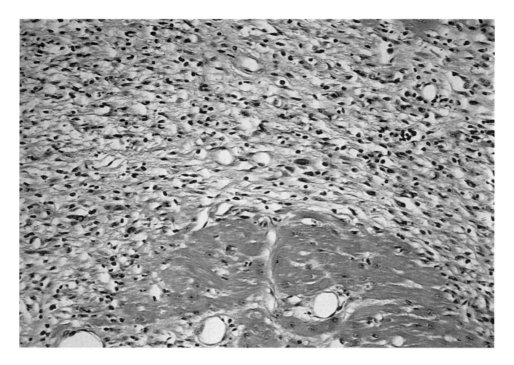

Figure 3. Patchy areas of myocardial fibrosis were found in the radiated groups. This figure shows a region of extensive myocardial fibrosis in a pig that received 800 rads 24 hours after injury. A small area of residual myocardial cells is noted. (Hematoxylin-eosin, × 50)

Table 4

Treatment Groups

Injury, Neointimal Thickness, and Percent Stenosis

Group	Mean Injury Score	Mean Neointimal Thickness	Percent Stenosis
Control	2.0±0.7	0.66±0.23	58±20%
400 cGy	1.9 0.7	.79±.23	67±31%
400/400 cGy	2.2±0.7	.90±.22	81±11%
800 cGy	2.6±0.2	.99±17	91±9%

Table 5

Individual Linear Regression Results:
Mean Neointimal Thickness versus Mean Arterial Injury Score

Group	Slope	P	Intercept	P	r
Control Group	0.21	0.03	0.25	ns	0.73
Group I 400 cGy	0.26	0.04	0.30	ns	0.73
Group II 400/400 cGy	0.25	0.005	0.37	0.03	0.84
Group III* 800 cGy	–	–	–	–	–

*For Group III, there were no low level injuries; thus a meaningful regression line could not be derived.

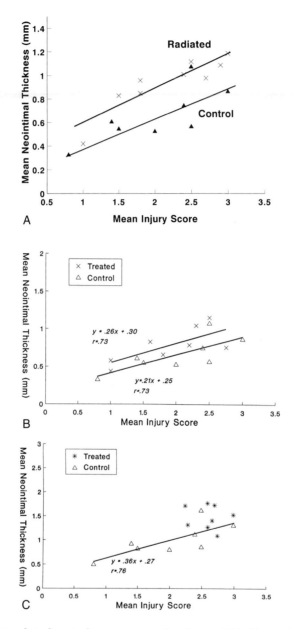

Figure 4. A. Scatterplot of control versus group I animals (400 cGy) and respective regression lines. Mean neointimal thickness in millimeters is the dependent variable, plotted as a function of mean arterial injury score. Animals in the treated groups had significantly more neointimal thickness than control animals. The slopes of the regression lines are not significantly different but the y-intercepts differ significantly. The regression line expressions and Pearson correlation coefficients are shown for each group. **B.** Same as in **A,** except for control versus group II animals (400 cGy at 24 hours and 400 cGy at 4 days following coronary injury). The difference in intercepts is again statistically significant while slope is not. **C.** Mean neointimal thickness versus mean injury score is plotted for group III animals (800 cGy at 24 hours following coronary artery injury). There were not enough data points with low values of injury score to make a meaningful linear regression model. The lack of low injury values may either be a coincidence or might imply that the higher dose of radiation exacerbated the mechanical injury from the metal coil.

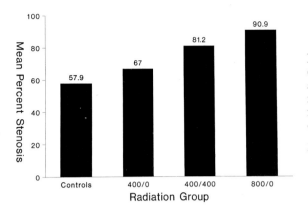

Figure 5. Percent-area stenosis (measured histologically) of control and radiated groups. It is clear that radiation resulted in progressively increased neointima as dose was escalated. The 400/400 and 800/0 groups were significantly different than control ($P<0.05$).

clinical results, especially given the apparent problems of the animal and pilot clinical studies. The mechanisms for these results are unclear, and the differences between this study and other similar studies are similarly unclear. Potential reasons are summarized in Table 7.

One obvious difference was the use of *external* beam radiation. It is possible that the intraluminal approach compared to external beam radiation may explain this difference. The adventitia has recently been implicated in restenosis, and it is possible that differential effects on the adventitia by an external, more widely ap-

Table 6

Part A

Stress and Benestent Restenosis Results

	PTCA		Stenting		
	Restenosis Rate	6 mo MLD	Restenosis Rate	6 mo MLD	Difference in 6 mo MLD
BENESTENT	32%	1.73 mm	22%	1.82 mm	.09 mm
STRESS	41%	1.56 mm	32%	1.74 mm	.18 mm

Part B

Estimated Restenosis Rates non-STRESS and non-BENESTENT Lesions (from Nobuyoshi, unpublished)

Lesion Type	Estimated Stent Restenosis Rate
Small arteries (<2.6 mm)	30%
Long lesions	32%
Ostial lesions	40%
Vein graft lesions	34%

PTCA = Percutaneous transluminal coronary angioplasty;
MLD = Minimal luminal diameter

Table 7

Possible Reasons for Outcome Differences

External versus intraluminal radiation
Control for vessel degree of injury
Radiation dose
Stents, more severe arterial injury

See text for discussion.

plied, beam may explain the observed differences. A point against this reason is that transluminal gamma radiation has been shown effective. However, penetrating effects of gamma radiation, even if intraluminal, should penetrate the small distance from lumen to adventitia.

Another difference may lie in the appropriate doses. Doses have been chosen that are comparable to those used in other nonmalignant conditions such as heterotopic bone formation—comparatively low by standards used in malignant disease; yet other groups have used comparably low doses and shown efficacy. Moreover, escalating doses in this study caused increasing amounts of neointima, not less. Splitting the dose in our external beam study (400 cGy/400 cGy) made no difference in outcome.

The degree of injury was accounted for in this study, while it was not in other stent studies. This is not likely to be a reason for the observed differences, since it would then be necessary that in other studies, the radiated arteries were selectively injured more severely, an unlikely possibility. Moreover the balloon injury studies of Waksman and colleagues did control for injury, and found significant differences.[7]

Additional animal studies include work by Shimotakahara and Mayberg, which showed an inhibition of neointimal hyperplasia in the rat carotid artery model using gamma radiation exposure of only one carotid artery with use of a ^{137}Cs source.[25] These authors delivered single fraction exposures of 7.5, 15, and 22.5 Gy at either 1 or 2 days following the carotid artery injury by overstretch balloon. At 21 days after the injury, there was substantial inhibition of neointima, but the two higher doses had the greatest effect. The receiving doses delivered 1 day after injury had greater inhibition than those of 2 days. These studies and methods were repeated by the same group with use of a broader range of doses: 1-, 2.5-, 5-, 7.5-, 10-, 12.5-, 15-, and 20-Gy gamma delivered in a single fraction.[26] As expected, there was a similar dose response found. A subset of the rats were allowed to survive for 6 months and a lasting effect was found.

These results are interesting in relation to the known inaccuracies of the rat carotid artery injury model. Many agents and therapies shown effective in this model have failed to replicate results of clinical trials, the most notorious being those of the ACE inhibitor cilazapril.[27–29] This drug was markedly effective in the rat carotid model, but completely failed when applied to the porcine model,[14] and in human clinical trials showed no effect whatsoever.

These apparent disparate findings suggest questions regarding the model and also whether stenting is indicated with the radiation effects. It has been suggested that a clinical trial of external beam therapy might be warranted.[15] In light of the disappointing clinical pilot trial results, this may not be well advised. Doses may be a factor in the potential use of external beam therapy, since the most significant radiation toxicity to coronary arteries may occur in the younger patient. Regardless, the external beam delivery route may provide for more homogeneous therapy of an angioplasty site. Despite what some have written, a trial of external beam therapy should not be undertaken lightly in view of enhanced proliferation in stented porcine arteries, apparently corroborated by the noted clinical pilot trial.

The most likely reason for observed differences in animal and patient studies is that the stent study was oversized and caused severe, ongoing coronary artery injury. This is manifest by the ongoing inflammatory response around the stent wires, even late in the course after injury. Other published studies using stents indicate substantially less arterial injury by the devices. The anomalous results from the 800 cGy group are suggestive in this regard. The injury scores here were substantially higher than in all other groups. It is distinctly unusual in this model to have such a lack of overall variation in injury, since the amount of injury is generally difficult to standardize. The lack of lower mean injury scores was thus either a strange coincidence or else higher doses enhance the mechanical damage done by stents. How well this finding translates to human studies and how much injury results from stenting remains to be seen. If stenting in patients causes severe injury, clinical results may show that radiation is not as effective as the preclinical animal work.

There are other possible reasons for the observations of this study. Endothelial cells are more radiation-sensitive than medial smooth muscle cells. Radiation may have enhanced the endothelial damage done by the wire coil alone. Alternatively, radiation may have prolonged the time required for endothelialization of the injury site. The result would be prolonged exposure of subintimal elements to flowing blood, or possibly, prolonged exposure in a larger area of damaged endothelium. Permeability of the internal elastic lamina has been shown to result from radiation damage,[30] as has arterial spasm,[31] both of which might also have contributed to the observed proliferative response.

Limited data are available on the effects of x-irradiation on arterial structure and function. Normal, uninjured coronary arteries are resistant to radiation in small and moderate doses.[32] However, radiation-induced coronary artery disease from larger doses of radiation given for noncoronary neoplasia is well documented; for example, there was an early report in 1967,[33] showing fatal myocardial infarction in a 15-year-old boy who received 40 Gy for Hodgkin's disease. The association between arterial stenosis for both muscular coronary arteries and larger elastic vessels has been known for more than 30 years.[18,19,32–42] Patients who have received large doses of radiation are reported to have unusable internal mammary arteries if coronary artery bypass grafting is contemplated.[43]

Human coronary artery lesions resulting from radiation are substantially different from those in atheromatous coronary disease.[36,40] They typically exhibit dense fibrotic reactions, and generally affect vessels in the more proximal portions.[44,45] The human coronary lesions present late, typically 6 to 12 years following radiation exposure.[35,38,46,47]

One study using hypercholesterolemic rabbits with iliac artery lesions showed strong synergism between lipids and the radiation for inducing atheromatous-like lesions.[48] Others have found similar potentiation of radiation injury by hyperlipidemia.[49]

Conclusions

Clinical trials to date that have used pharmacological methods and have been aimed at reducing or eliminating restenosis after coronary intervention have largely failed. The widespread application of radiation, either beta-emitting stents or intracoronary gamma radiation, to patients will have two important outcomes. The obvious will be to understand how radiation will fit into the armamentarium of the interventional cardiologist in combating restenosis. The second, and less obvious, will be to understand how current animal model technologies translate to patient data. Diametrically opposite differences across animal model studies will have a single resolution, and will teach how to better apply those models in order to better understand the restenosis problem.

References

1. Faxon DP, Currier JW. Prevention of post-PTCA restenosis. Ann N Y Acad Sci 1995;748:419–427.
2. Fischman DL, Leon MB, Baim DS, et al, for the Stent Restenosis Study Investigators. A randomized comparison of coronary-stent placement and balloon angioplasty in the treatment of coronary artery disease. N Engl J Med 1994;331:496–501.
3. Serruys PW, de Jaegere P, Kiemeneij F, et al. A comparison of balloon-expandable stent implantation with balloon angioplasty in patients with coronary artery disease. N Engl J Med 1994;331:489–495.
4. Mintz G, Pichard A, Kent K, et al. Endovascular stents reduce restenosis by eliminating geometric arterial remodeling: A serial intravascular ultrasound study. J Am Coll Cardiol 1995;Feb:36A.
5. Mintz G, Kent K, Satler L, et al. Dimorphic mechanisms of restenosis after DCA and stents: A serial intravascular ultrasound study. Circulation 1995;92:2610.
6. Mintz G, Pichard A, Kent K, et al. Endovascular stents reduce restenosis by eliminating geometric arterial remodeling: A serial intravascular ultrasound study [abstract]. J Am Coll Cardiol 1995;95:701–705.
7. Waksman R, Robinson KA, Crocker IR, et al. Intracoronary radiation before stent implantation inhibits neointima formation in stented porcine coronary arteries. Circulation 1995;92:1383–1386.
8. Wiedermann JG, Marboe C, Amols H, et al. Intracoronary irradiation markedly reduces restenosis after balloon angioplasty in a porcine model. J Am Coll Cardiol 1994;23:1491–1498.
9. Wiedermann JG, Marboe C, Amols H, et al. Intracoronary irradiation markedly reduces neointimal proliferation after balloon angioplasty in swine: Persistent benefit at 6-month follow-up. J Am Coll Cardiol 1995;25:1451–1456.
10. Schwartz R, Koval T, Edwards W, et al. Effect of external beam irradiation on neointimal hyperplasia after experimental coronary artery injury. J Am Coll Cardiol 1992;19:1106–1113.
11. Schwartz RS, Murphy JG, Edwards WD, et al. Restenosis after balloon angioplasty: A practical proliferative model in porcine coronary arteries. Circulation 1990;82:2190–2200.
12. Schwartz R, Huber K, Murphy J, et al. Restenosis and the proportional neointimal response to coronary artery injury: Results in a porcine model. J Am Coll Cardiol 1992;19:267–274.
13. Webster MWI, Chesebro JH, Heras M. New nonisotropic in vivo technique of quantitating cellular proliferation in arterial media and intima [abstract]. Circulation 1989;80:II-523.
14. Huber KC, Schwartz RS, Edwards WD, et al. Effects of angiotensin converting enzyme inhibition on neointimal hyperplasia in a porcine coronary injury model. Am Heart J 1993;125:695–701.

15. Koh WJ, Mayberg MR, Chambers J, et al. The potential role of external beam radiation in preventing restenosis after coronary angioplasty [review]. Int J Radiat Oncol Biol Phys 1996;36:829–834.

16. Fischell T, Carter A, Laird J. The beta-particle-emitting radioisotope stent (isostent): Animal studies and planned clinical trials. Am J Cardiol 1996;78:45–50.

17. Anthony P, Keys H, Evarts CM, et al. Prevention of heterotopic bone formation with early post operative irradiation in high risk patients undergoing total hip arthroplasty: Comparison of 10 Gy vs 20 Gy schedules. Int J Radiat Oncol Biol Phys 1986;13:365–369.

18. Carmel RJ, Kaplan HS. Mantle irradiation in Hodgkin's disease. Cancer 1976;37:2813–2825.

19. Hirst DG, Denekamp J, Hobson B. Proliferation studies of the endothelial and smooth muscle cells of the mouse mesentery after irradiation. Cell Tissue Kinet 1980;13:91–104.

20. Sylvester JE, Greenberg P, Selch MT, et al. The use of postoperative irradiation for the prevention of heterotopic bone formation after total hip replacement. Int J Radiat Oncol Biol Phys 1988;14:471–476.

21. Waksman R, Robinson KA, Crocker IR, et al. Intracoronary low-dose beta-irradiation inhibits neointima formation after coronary artery balloon injury in the swine restenosis model. Circulation 1995;92:3025–3031.

22. Waksman R, Robinson KA, Crocker IR, et al. Endovascular low-dose irradiation inhibits neotima formation after coronary artery balloon injury in swine. A possible role for radiation therapy in restenosis prevention. Circulation 1995;91:1533–1539.

23. Wiedermann JG, Leavy JA, Amols H, et al. Effects of high-dose intracoronary irradiation on vasomotor function and smooth muscle histopathology. Am J Physiol 1994;267:H125–H132.

24. Fischer JJ. Proliferation of rat aortic endothelial cells following x-radiation. Radiat Res 1982;92:405–410.

25. Shimotakahara S, Mayberg MR. Gamma irradiation inhibits neointimal hyperplasia in rats after arterial injury. Stroke 1994;25:424–428.

26. Mayberg M, Luo Z, London S, Rasey J. Radiation inhibition of intimal hyperplasia after arterial injury. Radiat Res 1995;142:212–220.

27. Powell JS, Muller RK, Baumgartner HR. Suppression of the vascular response to injury: The role of angiotensin-converting enzyme inhibitors. J Am Coll Cardiol 1991;17(6 suppl. B):137B–142B.

28. Serruys P, Hermans R. The new angiotensin converting enzyme inhibitor cilazapril does not prevent restenosis after coronary angioplasty: The results of the MERCATOR trial [abstract]. J Am Coll Cardiol 1992;19:258A.

29. Faxon DP. Effect of high dose angiotensin-converting enzyme inhibition on restenosis: Final results of the MARCATOR Study, a multicenter, double-blind, placebo-controlled trial of cilazapril. The Multicenter American Research Trial With Cilazapril After Angioplasty to Prevent Transluminal Coronary Obstruction and Restenosis (MARCATOR) Study Group. J Am Coll Cardiol 1995;25:362–369.

30. Hampton JC, Rosario B. Permeability of arterial internal elastic laminae in irradiated mice. Exp Mol Pathol 1972;17:307–316.

31. Miller DD, Waters DD, Dangiosse V, David PR. Symptomatic coronary artery spasm following radiotherapy for Hodgkin's disease. Chest 1983;83:284–285.

32. Niemtzow RC, Reynolds RD. Radiation therapy and the heart. In: Kapoor AS (ed.): Cancer and the Heart. New York: Springer-Verlag; 1986:232–237.

33. Cohn KE, Stewart JR, Fajardo LF, Hancock EW. Heart disease following radiation. Medicine 1967;46:281–298.

34. Annest LS, Anderson RP, Li W, Haferman MD. Coronary artery disease following mediastinal radiation therapy. J Cardiovasc Surg 1983;85:257–263.

35. Applefeld MM, Wiernik PH. Cardiac disease after radiation therapy for Hodgkin's disease. Analysis of 48 patients. Am J Cardiol 1983;51:1679–1681.

36. Brosius FC, Waller BF, Roberts WC. Radiation heart disease: Analysis of 16 young (aged 15 to 33 years) necropsy patients who received over 3500 rads to the heart. Am J Med 1981;70:519–530.

37. Dollinger MR, Lavine DM, Foye LV Jr. Myocardial infarction due to post-irradiation fi-

brosis of the coronary arteries. Case of successfully treated Hodgkin's disease with lower esophageal involvement. JAMA 1966;195:316–319.

38. Gottdiener JS, Katin MJ, Borer JS, et al. Late cardiac effects of therapeutic mediastinal irradiation. Assessment by echocardiography and radionuclide angiography. N Engl J Med 1983;308:569–572.

39. Huff H, Sanders EM. Coronary artery occlusion after radiation. N Engl J Med 1972; 286:1660–1662.

40. McReynolds RA, Gold GL, Roberts WC. Coronary heart disease after mediastinal irradiation for Hodgkin's disease. Am J Med 1976;60:39–45.

41. Simon EB, Ling J, Mendizabal RC, Midwall J. Radiation induced coronary artery disease. Am Heart J 1984;108:1032–1034.

42. Tracy GP, Brown DE, Johnson LW, Gottleib AJ. Radiation induced coronary artery disease. JAMA 1974;228:1660.

43. Iqbal SM, Hanson EL, Gensini GG. Bypass graft for coronary arterial stenosis following radiation therapy. Chest 1977;71:664–666.

44. Kirkpatrick JB. Pathogenesis of foam cell lesions in irradiated arteries. Am J Pathol 1967;50:291–309.

45. Narayan K, Cliff WJ. Morphology of irradiated microvasculature: A combined in vivo and electron microscopic study. Am J Pathol 1982;106:47–62.

46. Applefeld MM, Slawson RG, Spicer FC, et al. The long term cardiac effects ot radiotherapy in patients treated for Hodgkin's disease. Cancer Treat Rep 1982;66: 1003–1013.

47. Strender LE, Lindahl J, Larsson LE. Incidence of heart disease and functional significance of changes in the electrocardiogram 10 years after radiotherapy for breast cancer. Cancer 1986;57:929–934.

48. Artom C, Lofland HB Jr, CIarkson TB. Ionizing radiation, atherosclerosis, and lipid metabolism in pigeons. Radiat Res 1965;26:165–177.

49. Amronin GG, Gildenhorn HC, Solomon RD, et al. The synergism of x irradiation and cholesterol fat feeding on the development of coronary artery lesions. J Atheroscler Res 1964;4:325–334.

Comparison of Endovascular and External Beam Irradiation for the Prevention of Restenosis

Monique M.H. Marijianowski, PhD,
Keith Robinson, PhD, and Ian R. Crocker, MD

Introduction

Endovascular radiation has been shown effective in reducing restenosis-like arterial pathological responses to angioplasty in several animal models.[1–5] Both gamma and beta radiation inhibited neointima formation in a linear dose-response fashion, and at high doses, beta radiation suppressed constrictive arterial wall remodeling.[1,2,6]

Endovascular radiation treatment, in one study, was found to be more effective when delivered 2 days following the intervention than at the time of the intervention.[1] Limitations associated with the use of endovascular irradiation include the additional time that a catheter must remain within the coronary vessel at the time of angioplasty and the inability to optimize the treatment time in relationship to the intervention. In addition, adverse late effects of treatment are related to large dose per fraction radiotherapy; an improvement in the therapeutic ratio is usually obtained by fractionation of the dose. This could be easily accomplished with external beam irradiation but not with endovascular therapies.

Early studies of external radiation for prevention of restenosis have shown contradictory results (Table 1).[7–14] Five groups[7,10,11,13,14] have shown that external radiation treatment was beneficial in reducing arterial neointima formation following injury. In contrast, there have been three other studies that showed no benefit or an exacerbation of neointima.[8,9,12] Some of these negative studies have been criticized on the basis of either the animal model or the radiation doses.

The objective of the study described below was to evaluate the potential benefit of external beam irradiation at doses similar to those used successfully for endovascular studies on the restenosis-like response of pig coronary arteries to overstretch balloon catheter injury. Additionally, we examined the histopathological consequences of endovascular and external irradiation in this setting.

From Waksman R (ed.). *Vascular Brachytherapy, Third Edition.* Armonk, NY: Futura Publishing Co., Inc.; © 2002.

Table 1

Studies of External Irradiation in Animal Models of Restenosis

Author	Animal/Vessel	Radiation Source	Result
Abbas[7]	Rabbit/iliacs	Linac	6 Gy no benefit; 12 Gy benefit at 5 days postangioplasty
Gellman[8]	Rabbit/iliacs	Orthovoltage	Increased neointima with 3 and 9 Gy postangioplasty
Hehrlein[9]	Rabbit/iliacs	Linac	Neointima significantly worse with radiation (8–16 Gy) poststent implantation
Hirai[10]	Rabbit/femorals	Orthovoltage	2,5 Gy no benefit; 10Gy and 20 Gy reduced neointima postair drying
Sarac[11]	Rats/carotid	Tele^{192}Ir	Reduction in neointima with all dose levels (5–10–15Gy)
Schwartz[12]	Pig/coronaries	Orthovoltage	Neointima significantly worse with radiation (4–8Gy) poststent implantation
Shefer[13]	Rabbit/central arter of the ear	Tele^{90}Sr	Decreased neointima with 9 Gy; optimal at 2 days post-angioplasty
Shimatokahara[14]	Rats/carotids	Tele^{137}CS	Reduced neointima following balloon angioplasty

Materials and Methods

Experimental Protocol and Dosimetry

External Irradiation

The experimental protocol for overstretch injury has been described extensively in previous publications.[15,16] For external radiation treatment, an initial treatment plan was designed using computed tomography (CT) simulation. With use of PRISM (in-house treatment planning software), the dose distribution was calculated for equally weighted anterior-posterior–posteroanterior (AP-PA) fields using 6-mV x-rays. In this idealized plan, the 100% isodose line encompassed the heart, with a small area on the anterior surface receiving a maximum dose of 107%. There was little variation in dose from one artery to the next. For each pig, an individual treatment field was designed. The cardiac silhouette was marked on the anterior chest wall of each sedated pig under fluoroscopy. The pig was set up at 100 cm source-to-axis distance (SAD) and an initial port film was obtained based on the field previously marked. Minor modifications were made with a repeat film obtained, in most cases, prior to treatment. A dose of 14 Gy was prescribed to the midplane. Following radiotherapy and injury, the pigs were returned to routine care and tissue was harvested at 4 weeks.

Beta and Gamma Irradiation

The same model of overstretch injury was used as referenced above. One of the injured coronary arteries in each swine was randomly assigned to receive radiation treatment (3.5, 7, 14, 28, or 56 Gy) to a radial distance of 2 mm from the source center, with use of either a beta-(^{90}Sr/Y; Novoste Corp., Norcross, GA) or gamma- (^{192}Ir; Best Industries, Springfield, VA) source train. The delivery catheter, without the radioactive source, was placed in the control injured artery in the same manner as for the treated vessel. The absorbed dose distribution and dose rate around the 2.5-cm ^{90}Sr/Y line source was calculated with the use of the Monte Carlo electron transport code ITS. The dose distribution and dose rate around the 3-cm ^{192}Ir source train was calculated by use of a commercial treatment planning system (CMS Modulex). There was no self-centering of the catheter within the arterial lumen, nor was there any attempt made to account for curvature of the artery.

Histopathology and Histomorphometry

The injured segments of the left anterior descending coronary artery (LAD) and left circumflex (LCX) were located with the guidance of the coronary angiograms, and dissected free from the heart with accompanying perivascular tissues. Serial 2- to 3-mm transverse segments were processed and embedded in paraffin, such that the entire length of injury plus proximal and distal uninjured regions were contained within the same block and would be present on the same slide. Sections (5 μm) were stained with hematoxylin-eosin (H&E) and Verhoeff-van Gieson (VVG) elastin stain. Morphometric analysis was performed on those sections with evidence of medial fracture, by use of a computer-assisted planimetry after instrument calibration (Image ProPlus software, MediaCybernetics Inc.), as previously described.[2] The VVG-stained sections were magnified at 20x, digitized, and stored in the frame-grabber board. Measurements were obtained by tracing the lumen perimeter, vessel perimeter, adventitial perimeter, and neointima perimeter. The following areas were then generated via ImageProPlus: luminal area, vessel area, adventitial area, and intimal area. The maximal intimal thickness was determined by a radial line drawn from the lumen to the external lamina at the point of greatest tissue growth. The arc length of the medial fracture, traced through the neointima from one dissected medial end to the other, was obtained for use as a measure of the extent of injury. The ratio of intimal area-to-fracture length (IA/FL) was made to correct for extent of injury and changes in vessel size. Repeat measurements were made on randomly selected samples and found to vary by less than 10%, except adventitial area, which varied approximately 15%. Each specimen was evaluated for the presence of medial dissection and morphological appearances of the cells within the media, adventitia, and neointima. Sections were also evaluated for the presence of intraluminal thrombus and intramural hemorrhage.

Picrosirius Red Staining

Sirius red specifically stains all types of fibrillar collagens.[17] All sections (endovascular beta and gamma from all dose groups as well as externally irradiated specimens) were stained with sirius red F3BA dissolved in saturated picric acid (pH 2.0).

Immunohistochemistry

Approximately half of the vessels from each group were randomly selected for immunohistochemical staining. HHF-35 (Dako Corporation, CA) is a monoclonal antiactin antibody, which is raised against muscle-specific actin. It recognizes α- and γ-actin isotypes common to all muscle cells, including smooth muscle cells (SMCs). This is in contrast to CGA-7 (Enzo Diagnostics Inc., NY), which is an antibody raised against α- and γ-actin isotypes, specific for SMCs. The specificity of these antibodies has been described previously.[18–21] Factor VIII-RAg (Dako Corporation) was used to identify endothelial cells and CD3 (Dako Corporation) was used to localize T-lymphocytes.

A strepavidin-biotin complex (SABC)/horse radish peroxidase (HRP) technique was used as previously described.[22] Endogenous peroxidase activity was blocked with methanol and 0.3% H_2O_2. HRP activity was visualized with use of diaminobenzidine as a chromogen.

Results

Morphometric Analysis

External Irradiation

The luminal and vessel cross-sectional areas were significantly reduced in the irradiated animals compared to controls, whereas the amount of neointima was less in the treated vessels than in the controls (Table 2). Traditionally, the intimal area value is divided by the fracture length value (IA/FL) to normalize the intimal response for the degree of injury to the vessel. When this is done, there is no evidence that radiation reduces the amount of intima formation compared with controls. To account for possible shrinkage of the vessel with radiation treatment, we have added a second correction to this product by dividing it by the vessel size. This calculation reveals that external radiation treatment did result in significant reduction in neointima. Overall, there was no significant difference in the adventitial area of the irradiated pigs compared to the controls.

Endovascular Irradiation

With both gamma and beta irradiation the lumen area was significantly larger in the irradiated animals in comparison with controls, with a significant reduction in neointima formation (Table 2). Neither gamma nor beta irradiation had an effect on vessel area with the exception that an increase in vessel size was observed with the highest doses in the beta group.

Table 2

Results of Computer-Assisted Histomorphometric Analysis of VVG-Stained Sections from Arteries of Pigs in Control and in 14-Gy-Irradiated Endovascular and External-Treated Vessels

| | 14-Gy endovascular irradiation (2 wk) | | | 14-Gy external radiation (4 wk) | |
	Control	Beta Radiation	Gamma Radiation	Control	Radiation
Lumen area	1.91±0.85	2.46±1.20*	2.76±1.20*	1.95±0.6	1.10±0.52*
Vessel area	3.77±1.10	3.83±1.13	4.14±1.44	4.45±1.05	2.75mw*
Intimal area (IA)	1.09±0.07	0.58±0.54*	0.33±0.35*	1.36±0.61	0.793mw*
Fracture length (FL)	2.28±1.19	3.45±1.77	2.04±0.90	2.19±0.58	1.63±0.61*
Max int. thick IA/FL	0.47±0.15	0.34±0.23*	0.22±0.12*	0.66±0.17	0.55±0.16
	0.47±0.25	0.19±0.20*	0.17±0.16*	0.61±0.15	0.583±0.18

Max. int. thick. = maximal intimal thickness; Values are ±SD. *$P<0.05$ versus controls; mwrepresents data sets that violated assumptions of normal distribution in which the Mann-Whitney rank sum test was used for between-groups comparisons.

Morphology

In injured segments of both control and irradiated vessels there was a variable degree of rupture of the tunica media, resulting in a vessel wall defect. Controls showed that neointimal growth replaced the disrupted media and consisted mostly of stellate and spindle-shaped cells in a loose extracellular matrix. The neointima of endovascular irradiated arteries was markedly smaller in size than the controls, with some sections showing a virtual absence of neointima, especially at higher doses.[1,2] Neointimal tissue occasionally contained unresolved mural thrombi covered at the luminal aspect by one or more layers of spindle-shaped and stellate cells. Additionally, in rare cases unresolved intramural hemorrhages were seen within submedial dissection planes and in the perivascular space. There was no difference in the morphology between arteries irradiated using beta- and gamma-emitting isotopes.

Unresolved intramural hemorrhages were seen more frequently in the samples irradiated by use of the external beam technique. Unresolved mural thrombi within the neointima were seen with approximately the same frequency as in arteries treated with use of endovascular irradiation; this no different than controls.

Immunohistochemistry

Vessel Wall

There were no differences in staining intensity or density between beta- and gamma-irradiated vessels. The cells of the neointima have been identified as being of smooth muscle origin by showing positive staining for α-actin as described previously.[15,23–25] The SMCs in both the control and irradiated vessels showed positive staining for HHF-35 at 2 weeks after balloon injury. However, at this same time the neointima of control vessels showed a distinct staining for CGA-7, which was absent in the irradiated vessels. Even at 6 months after treatment, the control tissues stained more intensely for CGA-7 than endovascular irradiated arteries. The neointima in external beam irradiated vessels showed some CGA-7 positive cells at 4 weeks after irradiation.

In almost all samples of endovascular and externally irradiated arteries, there was a complete coverage of the luminal surface by a monolayer of endothelial-like cells showing positive staining for factor VIII antibodies. The exceptions were the 28 and 56 Gy groups at 2 weeks after endovascular irradiation; they showed occasional areas with no endothelial lining. Despite the absence of endothelium, none of these sections showed evidence of substantial fresh thrombus at the site of injury.

An inflammatory response could be seen primarily in the adventitial area in both endovascular and externally treated arteries as well as controls, as detected by an anti-CD3 antibody for T-lymphocytes compared to controls.

Picrosirius red staining showed that the fibrocellular tissue of control arteries contained collagen that surrounded the SMCs. When neointima was present in endovascular irradiated vessels, there was a dense collagen layer at the luminal surface of the vessel. The external irradiated vessels revealed a major increase in collagen in both neointimal and adventitial areas. The increase in collagen at 4 weeks after external irradiation was more pronounced than that seen in tissues harvested at 6 months after endovascular irradiation. In the neointima there was a lacunar arrangement of the SMCs within the dense collagen matrix.

Myocardium

The left ventricular myocardium adjacent to the endovascular irradiated arteries showed no interstitial fibrosis at 2 weeks or 6 months after irradiation. Perivascular fibrosis was occasionally seen in both control and endovascular irradiated vessels, but external irradiation consistently resulted in both interstitial and perivascular fibrosis. Patchy areas with myocyte necrosis, fibroblast proliferation, and inflammation were found. The results are summarized in Table 3.

Discussion

The major finding from our studies is that external radiation treatment, in comparison to endovascular brachytherapy, is ineffective in preventing restenosis-like neointima formation and constrictive remodeling. Secondarily, we have observed that external irradiation of the whole heart at this dose in a single fraction (14 Gy) is associated with myocardial damage. Both endovascular and external approaches seem to alter the healing process of the vessel wall at early time points (2 and 4 weeks) with persistence of an abnormal synthetic phenotype of SMCs at 6 months in arteries undergoing endoluminal brachytherapy.

After external radiation treatment there was a reduction in the lumen of the coronary arteries that was apparently due to shrinkage of the vessel rather than intimal hyperplasia. Other authors have shown that negative remodeling is a major cause of restenosis,[26–28] and in our study it appeared to be exacerbated by external radiation treatment of the heart. This is in contrast to the larger lumens

Table 3

Histologic Comparison for Endovascular versus
External Beam Irradiated Coronary Arteries

Tissue Region	Marker	Control		Endovascular Irradiation		External Irradiation
		2wk	6mo	2wk	6mo	4wk
Neointima	CGA-7*	±	+	−	±	±
	HHF-35Ü	+	+	+	+	+
Vessel lumen	Factor VIII-rAg	±	+	±	+	+
Entire section	T-cells	−	−	+adventitia	+adventitia	+adventitia
	Collagen	+	+	⇑ neointima	⇑ neointima	⇑⇑ neointima and ⇑ adventitia

*CGA-7 is specific for α and γ-actin of smooth muscle cells, whereas ÜHHF-35 is specific for α and γ-actin of isotypes of all muscle cells.
In the neointima of control arteries there is an arrangement of collagen surrounding smooth muscle cells;
⇑ = this is increased in the neointima of irradiated arteries;
⇑⇑ = an even more pronounced increase.

and reduced neointima formation observed almost universally by ourselves and others after endovascular treatment (either beta or gamma). There are many limitations to the use of external radiation as carried out in our study. Treatment was delivered to a very large field encompassing almost entire heart and with a large single dose of radiation. It is possible that some of the negative effects of radiation treatment in our study may have related to the techniques used, but other authors, using alternative methods, have reported similarly disappointing results.

It is widely accepted that the major cell type involved in neointimal proliferation is of vascular SMC origin. It is also known that the phenotypic expression of vascular SMCs may adapt to pathological conditions.[19,24,29–31] There are two different phenotypes of SMCs: the synthetic phenotype is present in the medial layer of the artery during fetal and postnatal periods and is mainly involved in extracellular matrix production; the contractile phenotype, on the other hand, provides both vasomotion and structural support to the vessel.[32] SMCs are capable of reversion to a synthetic phenotype during the processes of atherogenesis and intima formation after endothelial injury.[30,33,34] Electron microscopic studies of coronary arteries from patients with stable and unstable angina pectoris and postangioplasty restenosis have revealed phenotypic modulation of SMCs.[35]

In the early stages of healing after balloon injury and radiation, the cells in the neointima stained positive with HHF-35, but almost no reactivity was obtained with CGA-7. This contrasted with the control injured vessels, where there was positive staining for CGA-7 as well as HHF-35. At 6 months after injury, the control tissues still showed more intense staining for CGA-7 compared to the irradiated vessels. Since CGA-7 marks both α- and γ-actin isotypes of SMCs whereas HHF-35 stains all types of muscle cells, it appears that the SMC phenotype involved in the vascular injury response is modified by radiation therapy. In particular, expression of smooth muscle-specific filaments seems to be inhibited by irradiation given at the time of balloon injury. This is important because it has been assumed that the fibrocellular tissue response at sites of balloon angioplasty is complete at approximately 2 to 3 months.[36] Our findings show that radiation prevents or delays the reversion of neointimal SMC into a "mature" SMC (ie, transform from the postinjury synthetic SMC back into a contractile phenotype). Because these synthetic SMCs may still be involved in the production of extracellular matrix components, it seems clear that the effect of vascular radiotherapy should be examined at later timepoints (>6 months) than were undertaken in this study. The persistence of this immature phenotype may be indicative of a long-term arterial pathophysiology caused by irradiation.

This study also shows that there is a considerable amount of collagen present in the neointima of balloon-injured coronary arteries irradiated by both external and endovascular approaches (although there is little neointima formation with high-dose endovascular irradiation). The amount of collagen in the externally irradiated vessels at 4 weeks exceeds the amount present even at 6 months in endovascular irradiated specimens. There are a number of possible explanations for these observations. With the endovascular technique we targeted the doses of 7 or 14 Gy at a 2-mm radial distance from the source center. At distances closer than 2 mm, considerably higher doses of radiation are delivered. On the other hand, with external radiation treatment no part of the vessel wall or heart received more than 14 Gy. In a 3-mm-diameter vessel, a substantially higher dose of radiation was delivered to portions of the intima and media with use of the catheter-based endovascular technique for a nominal dose of 14 Gy at 2 mm. Not only was the distribution of dose different between external and endovascular irradiated vessels, but there was a major difference in the volume of tissues that received high doses of radiation. With external radiation treatment, virtually the entire heart received the prescribed dose of 14 Gy, as opposed to endovascular irradiation, where only the tissues enclosed within a 4-mm-diameter cylinder (3 cm in length) received that dose. This may explain the presence of interstitial and perivascular fibrosis in the myocardium in the externally irradiated animals that was absent in the endovascular irradiated vessels. It is therefore important that in reporting studies of vascular radiotherapy, there be clear descriptions of the dose and method of delivery.

Conclusions

Further research should be focused on mechanisms by which radiation treatment delays the arterial wound-healing response to balloon injury and on the potential of small-field, conformal external techniques in reducing restenosis.

Acknowledgments: The authors would like to acknowledge the contributions of Terry Styles, MD for carrying out most of the external interventional procedures. Dr. Ron Waksman and Gustavo Cipolla were instrumental in the initial investigation of endovascular brachytherapy. Donna Forestner was responsible for the immunohistochemical staining. None of the work could have been carried out without the support of Spencer B. King III, Director of Interventional Cardiology at Emory.

References

1. Waksman R, Robinson KA, Crocker IR, et al. Endovascular low-dose irradiation inhibits neointima formation after coronary artery balloon injury in swine: A possible role for radiation therapy in restenosis prevention. Circulation 1995;91:1533–1539.

2. Waksman R, Robinson KA, Crocker IR, et al. Intracoronary low-dose β-irradiation inhibits neointima formation after coronary artery balloon injury in the swine restenosis model. Circulation 1995;92:3025–3031.
3. Wiedermann JG, Marboe C, Amols H, et al. Intracoronary irradiation markedly reduces restenosis after balloon angioplasty in a porcine model. J Am Coll Cardiol 1994; 23:1491–1498.
4. Wiedermann JG, Marboe C, Amols H, et al. Intracoronary irradiation markedly reduces neointimal proliferation after balloon angioplasty in swine: Persistent benefit at 6-month follow-up. J Am Coll Cardiol 1995;25:1451–1456.
5. Mazur W, Ali NM, Dabaghi SF, et al. High dose rate intracoronary radiation suppresses neointimal proliferation in the stented and ballooned model of porcine restenosis [abstract]. Circulation 1994;90(suppl I):I652.
6. Waksman R, Rodrigez JA, Robinson KA, et al. Intracoronary radiation affects restenosis in the swine model by reduction of cell proliferation and favorable remodeling [abstract]. Circulation 1996;8(suppl I):I108.
7. Abbas M, Afshari N, Stadius M, et al. External beam irrdiation inhibits neointimal hyperplasia following balloon angioplasty. Int J Cardiol 1994;44:191–202.
8. Gellman J, Healey G, Qingsheng C, et al. The effect of very low dose irradiation on restenosis following balloon angioplasty. A study in the atherosclerotic rabbit. Circulation 1991;84:46A–59A.
9. Hehrlein C, Kaiser S, Kollum M, et al. External beam radiation fails to inhibit neointima formation in stented rabbit arteries [abstract]. Circulation 1996;94(suppl):1219.
10. Hirai T, Korogi Y, Harada M, Takashashi M. Intimal hyperplasia in an atherosclerotic model: Prevention with radiation therapy [abstract]. Radiology 1994;872.
11. Sarac TP, Riggs PN, Williams JP, et al. The effects of low dose radiation on neointimal hyperplasia. J Vasc Surg 1995;22(1):17–24.
12. Schwartz RS, Koval TM, Edwards WD, et al. Effect of external beam irradiation on neointimal hyperplasia after experimental coronary artery injury. J Am Coll Cardiol 1992;19:1106–1113.
13. Shefer A, Eigler NL, Whiting JS, Litvack FI. Suppression of intimal proliferation after balloon angioplasty with local beta irradiation in rabbits [abstract]. J Am Coll Cardiol 1993;21(2):185A.
14. Shimotakahara S, Mayberg MR. Gamma irradiation inhibits neointimal hyperplasia in rats after arterial injury. Stroke 1994;25:424–428.
15. Karas SP, Gravanis MB, Santoian EC, et al. Coronary intimal proliferation after balloon injury and stenting in swine: An animal model of restenosis. J Am Coll Cardiol 1992;20:467–474.
16. Schwartz RS, Murphy JG, Edwards WD, et al. Restenosis after balloon angioplasty. A practical proliferative model in porcine coronary arteries. Circulation 1990;82: 2190–2200.
17. Junqueira LC, Bignolas G, Brentani RR. Picrosirius staining plus polarization microscopy: A specific method for collagen detection in tissue sections. Histochem J 1979; 11:447–455.
18. Gown AM, Vogel AM, Gordon D, Lu PL. A smooth muscle-specific monoclonal antibody recognizes smooth muscle actin isozymes. J Cell Biol 1985;100:807–813.
19. Gown AM, Tsukada T, Ross R. Human atheroscerosis. II. Immunocytochemical analysis of the cellular composition of human atherosclerotic lesions. Am J Pathol 1986;125: 191–207.
20. Tsukada T, Tippens D, Gordon D, et al. HHF-35, A muscle-actin-specific monoclonal antibody. I. Immunocytochemical and biochemical characterization. Am J Pathol 1987;126:51–60.
21. Tsukada T, McNutt MA, Ross R, Gown AM. HHF35, a muscle actin-specific monoclonal antibody. II. Reactivity in normal, reactive and neoplastic human tissues. Am J Pathol 1987;127:389–402.
22. Coggi G, Dell'orto P, Viale G. Avidin-biotin methods. In: Polak JM, van Noorden S (eds.): Immunocytochemistry. Modern Methods and Applications, 2nd Edition. Bristol: Wright; 1986:54–70.
23. Gravanis MB, Robinson KA, Santoian EC, et al. The reparative phenomena at the site

of balloon angioplasty in humans and experimental models. Cardiovasc Pathol 1993;24:263–273.

24. Gravanis MB, Roubin GS. Histopathologic phenomena at the site of percutaneous transluminal coronary angioplasty: The problem of restenosis. Hum Pathol 1989;20: 477–485.

25. Robinson KA. Pig coronary artery model of post-angioplasty restenosis. In: Waksman R, King SB, Crocker IR, Mould RF (eds.): Vascular Brachytherapy. AX Veenendaal, The Netherlands: Nucletron BV; 1996:30–40.

26. Kakuta T, Currier JW, Haudenschild CC, et al. Differences in compensatory vessel enlargement, not intimal formation, account for restenosis after angioplasty in the hypercholesterolemic rabbit model. Circulation 1994;89:2809–2815.

27. Lafont A, Chisolm G, Whitlow P, et al. Postangioplasty restenosis in the atherosclerotic rabbit: Proliferative response or chronic constriction [abstract]? Circulation 1993;88: 521.

28. Mintz G, Kovach J, Javier S, et al. Geometric remodeling is the predominant of late lumen loss after coronary angioplasty [abstract]. Circulation 1993;88:I654.

29. Chamley-Campbell J, Campbell GR, Ross R. The smooth muscle cell in culture. Physiol Rev 1979;59:1–61.

30. Campbell JH, Kocher O, Skalli O, et al. Cytodifferentiation and expression of alpha-smooth muscle actin mRNA and protein during primary culture of aortic smooth muscle cells. Correlation with cell density and proliferative state. Arteriosclerosis 1989;9: 633–643.

31. Ueda M, Becker AE, Tsukada T, et al. Fibrocellular tissue response after percutaneous transluminal coronary angioplasty. An immunocytochemical analysis of the cellular composition. Circulation 1991;83:1327–1332.

32. Schwartz SM, Campbell GR, Campbell JH. Replication of smooth muscle cells in vascular disease. Circ Res 1986;58:427–444.

33. Campbell GR, Chamley-Campbell JH. The cellular pathobiology of atherosclerosis. Pathology 1981;13:423–440.

34. Kocher O, Gabbiani F, Gabbiani G, et al. Phenotypic features of smooth muscle cells during the evolution of experimental carotid artery intimal thickening. Biochemical and morphologic studies. Lab Invest 1991;65:459–470.

35. Chen YH, Chen YL, Lin SJ, et al. Electron microscopic studies of phenotypic modulation of smooth muscle cells in coronary arteries of patients with unstable angina pectoris and postangioplasty restenosis. Circulation 1997;95:1169–1175.

36. Serruys PW, Luijten HE, Beatt KJ, et al. Incidence of restenosis after successful coronary angioplasty: A time-related phenomenon. A quantitative angiographic study in 342 patients at 1, 2, 3, and 4 months. Circulation 1988;77:361–371.

## Chapter 23

Intracoronary Gamma Irradiation in the Swine Model of Restenosis

Ron Waksman, MD

Restenosis after successful percutaneous transluminal coronary angioplasty (PTCA) is primarily mediated by an uncontrolled proliferation and extracellular matrix synthesis by modified smooth muscle cells (SMC) that have migrated to the site of the injury.[1] The development of the neointimal component of the restenosis lesion is the endpoint of a healing process initiated by vascular injury, predominantly to the nonatheromatous aspect of the dilated artery.[2]

Ionizing radiation, even at low doses, affects renewing dividing cells, resulting in reduction of cell proliferation by damaging the nucleus, in single- or double-strand breaks of the purine and pyrimidine bases of DNA.[3–8]

Therefore, it was hypothesized that low-dose gamma radiation delivered intraluminally could reduce the extent of neointima formation after balloon injury. The balloon-injured swine restenosis model, a reliable model for testing antiproliferative therapies that was intended for interventional cardiology, was chosen to examine this hypothesis.

The gamma radiation studies in the swine model are summarized in Table 1. This chapter contains detailed description of the initial gamma radiation studies and discussion on consensus and controversy issues related to these studies that used gamma sources.

The Experimental Protocol

The model of overstretch injury has been described previously and is detailed in this book.[9–12] The following is a detailed description of the classic experimental protocol for catheter-based systems that was used in the majority of the experiments described in this book. Vascular neointimal lesions resembling human restenosis were created in the coronary arteries of normal pigs by overstretch balloon angioplasty injury with a 3.5-mm angioplasty balloon positioned in the proximal segments of the left anterior descending (LAD), left circumflex (LCX), and right coronary (RCA) arteries.

One of the injured coronary arteries in each swine was assigned randomly to receive radiation treatment. Over a flexible 0.014" wire, a 4F noncentered delivery

From Waksman R (ed.). *Vascular Brachytherapy, Third Edition.* Armonk, NY: Futura Publishing Co., Inc.; © 2002.

Table 1

Animal Studies Utilizing Gamma Radiation

Author	Animal/Vessel	Radiation Source	Result
Wiedermann[21]	Pig/coronaries	iridium 192	Vasoreactivity studies in a noninjured artery
Wiedermann[16]	Pig/coronaries	iridium 192	Decreased neointima with 20 Gy to the vessel wall
Waksman[12]	Pig/coronaries	iridium 192	Decreased neointima with 3.5–14 Gy; sustained benefit at 6 months with 7 & 14 Gy
Weinberger[19]	Pig/coronaries	iridium 192	Decreased neointima with 15–20 Gy; worse with 10 Gy; benefit at 6 months with 20 Gy
Mazur[18]	Pig/coronaries	iridium 192 HDR afterloader	Decreased neointima with 10, 15, and 25 Gy following stent and balloon angioplasty
Waksman[20]	Pig/coronaries Repeat injury	iridium 192	Decreased neointima only after the second injury; no effect on neointima from initial injury
Waksman[22]	Pigs/stented coronaries	iridium 192	Radiation prior to stenting reduced neointima formation at 30 days

HDR = high dose rate.

catheter (USCI) was introduced to the injury site of the assigned artery, the guidewire was withdrawn, and a ribbon with either placebo or ^{192}Ir radioactive seeds was inserted manually into the catheter and was positioned at the site of injury in the target vessel with use of cinefluoroscopic visualization within the delivery catheter. It was left in place for a period sufficient to deliver the assigned dose to a depth of 2 mm (8 to 38 minutes, depending both on dose and source activity).

Radiation Planning

Radiation dose was determined in a standard fashion by entering the activity and length of the ^{192}Ir ribbon into a radiation treatment planning system (CMS Modulex). The dose rate at the prescribed point was then calculated by the system by use of standard brachytherapy dose algorithms. No in vivo dosimetry was performed; the dose rate calculations, and subsequent determination of dose at a distance from the source, was the product of this treatment planning system. Since the delivery catheter was not self-centered within the lumen, there was potential variability in the dose delivered to the artery wall, ranging from 2.9 to 0.6 times the prescribed dose, depending on the catheter dimensions and whether the catheter was opposed to the ipsilateral or contralateral side, respectively.

After irradiation, the ribbon and the guiding catheters were removed and the femoral cutdown was repaired. Nitroglycerin ointment (1″) was administered topically and the animals were returned to routine care.

Tissue Analysis

The injured segments of the treated arteries were located with the guidance of the coronary angiograms, then dissected free from the heart. Serial 2- to 3-mm transverse segments were processed and embedded in paraffin. Cross sections (4 μm) were stained with hematoxylin and eosin (H&E) or Verhoeff-van Gieson elastin (VVG). The H&E-stained sections were examined by an experienced observer who was blinded to the treatment group. Each specimen was evaluated for the presence of neointima formation, luminal encroachment, medial dissection, alteration of the internal and external elastic lamina, and morphological appearance of the cells within the media, adventitia, and neointima. Sections were also evaluated for the presence of intraluminal thrombus and inflammatory cell infiltrate.

Morphometric analysis was performed on each segment with evidence of medial fracture (1 to 5 in each artery). The histopathological features were measured with use of a computerized IBM-based system (Bioscan 2, Thomas Optical Measurement System Inc., Columbus, GA). VVG-stained sections were magnified at 26 ×, digitized, and stored in a frame-grabber board. The maximal intimal thickness (MIT) was determined by a radial line, drawn from the lumen to the external lamina at the point of greatest tissue growth. The arc length of the medial fracture (FL), traced through the neointima from one dissected medial end to the other, was used as a measure of the extent of injury. Area measurements were obtained by tracing the lumen perimeter [luminal area (LA), mm^2], neointima perimeter [intimal area (IA), mm^2, defined by the borders of the internal elastic lamina, lumen, media, and external elastic lamina], and external elastic lamina [vessel area (VA), mm^2]. Calculations were performed to correct for vessel size and extent of injury: ratio of intimal area to fracture length (IA/FL).

Short-Term Study Groups

In the initial studies performed at Emory by Waksman et al, there were four treatment groups with three different doses of radiation: 3.5 Gy (10 arteries), 7 Gy (12 arteries), and 14 Gy (9 arteries), delivered immediately after injury, and one group 7 Gy (10 arteries) given 48 hours after the injury. These pigs were sacrificed 14 days after treatment. The effect of radiation dose and timing in the short-term study, on four descriptors of the vessel response to injury, is shown in Table 2. By analysis of variance (ANOVA), a significant treatment effect of irradiation on MIT (F = 48.2, $P<0.0001$), IA (F = 982.67, $P<0.0001$), IA/FL (F = 26.85, $P<0.0001$), and residual lumen (F = 9.33, $P<0.0001$) was observed (Table 2 and Fig. 1). Post hoc analysis by t test showed significant reductions comparing each treatment group to the control group for all dependent variables except MIT and IA for the 3.5 Gy group. In addition, there was a linear relationship between the dose (control, 3.5, 7, 14) and IA/FL ratio (m = -0.0028, $P<0.0001$, r = -0.75). There were also significant reductions in the indices of neointima formation in the group that had 2-day delayed irradiation at 7 Gy compared to the same dose given immediately after injury (Table 2 and Fig. 2).

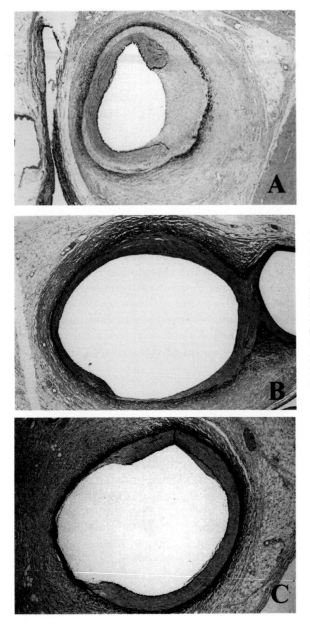

Figure 1. Representative micrographs, at 40x instrument magnification, of Verhoeff-van Gieson-stained thick sections from injured pig coronary arteries comparing healing responses at 2 weeks, from four treatment groups. In all micrographs, L = lumen; M = dissected ends of tunica media; N = neointima. Samples from: **A)** control group, **B)** 7 Gy-treated group, and **C)** 14 Gy-treated group.

Table 2

Results of Computer-Assisted Histomorphometric Analysis of VVG-Stained Thick Sections from Arteries of Pigs in Control and Radiation-Treated Groups

	Control	3.5 Gy	7 Gy	7 Delay Gy	14 Gy
# arteries analyzed	20	10	10	11	8
# Segments analyzed	43	36	32	38	30
Maximal intimal thickness (MIT, mm)	0.47±0.21	0.47±0.09	0.37±0.18*	0.27±0.1*,▲	0.22±0.12*
Intimal area (IA, mm²)	0.96±0.7	1.23±0.47	0.70±0.44*	0.48±0.25*,▲	0.33±0.35*
Fracture length (FL, mm)	1.61±0.8	3.53±1.5*	1.55±1.06	2.04±0.9	2.68±1.25*
Intimal area to fracture length ratio (IA/FL)	0.59±0.23	0.38±0.21*	0.42±0.16**	0.24±0.10*,▲	0.17±0.16*

Values are mean ±SD. *$P<0.0001$ vs. control; **$P<0.001$ vs. control; ▲ = $p<0.01$ vs. 7 Gy at time of injury. 7 Delay = dose given 2 days after arterial injury. VVG = Verhoeff-van Gieson.

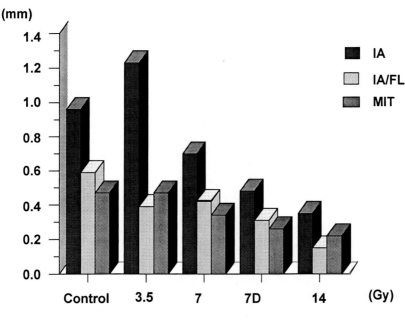

Figure 2. Effect of four doses of radiation (3.5 Gy, 7 Gy, 7 Gy delayed, and 14 Gy) on indices of neointima formation. IA = intimal area, mm²; IA/FL = intimal area to fracture length ratio; MIT = maximal intimal thickness, mm. A significant inhibitory effect of radiation treatment on MIT, IA, and particularly IA/FL was observed. In addition, delay of radiation for 2 days after balloon injury suppressed neointima formation compared to the same dose at the time of injury.

Long-Term Study Group

Seven miniature pigs with a mean weight of 23.3±4.0 kg underwent over-stretch balloon injury similar to the other treated groups, with an additional injury in the right coronary artery as an internal control, and were given 7 Gy (7 arteries) and 14 Gy (6 arteries) immediately after the injury in the LAD and LCX. Six months later the animals had a repeat angiogram of the coronary arteries and tissue was retrieved for morphometric analysis. There were no differences in artery size or extent of injury in the long-term group. Angiography prior to balloon injury revealed a mean artery size of vessel of 2.5±0.3 mm. Balloon-to-artery ratio was 1.42 There were two (10%) arteries without evidence of medial tear. There were no substantial differences in the morphological appearance of coronary arteries from animals killed 6 months as compared to 2 weeks after injury, and there was no evidence of excess fibrosis within the arterial wall, in the perivascular space, or in the adjacent myocardium compared to 2-week or control arteries. There were no differences in the morphological appearance of carotid arteries that were irradiated compared to the nonirradiated control arteries. There was a significant inhibition of intimal thickening in arteries treated by 7 and 14 Gy as demonstrated by a reduction in the intimal area, maximal intimal thickness, and IA/FL ratio (Fig. 3, Table 3).

Repeat Balloon Injury Model

Waksman[22] studied the effect of radiation in the repeat injury model in porcine coronary arteries, using ^{192}Ir to deliver 14 Gy at the time of the second in-

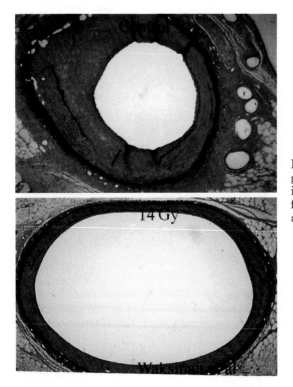

Figure 3. Low-magnification micrographs of **A)** control and **B)** 14 Gy-irradiated injured coronary arteries from miniature pigs killed 6 months after injury.

Table 3

Results of Computer-Assisted Histomorphometric Analysis of VVG-Stained
Thick Sections from Arteries of Miniswine after 6 Months in Control and
Radiation-Treated Groups

	Control	7Gy	16Gy
# arteries analyzed	6	7	6
# segments analyzed	24	26	21
Maximal intimal thickness (MIT, mm)	0.49±0.22	0.33±0.16*	0.33±0.12*
Intimal area (IA, mm²)	1.25±085	0.86±0.47*	0.62±045**
Fracture length (FL, mm)	2.58±1.42	2.63±1.21	1.98±0.96
Intimal area to fracture length ratio (IA/FL)	0.50±0.20	0.35±0.18**	0.31±0.16 ▲
Residual lumen (RL)	0.57±0.14	0.67±0.14	0.80±0.14 ▲▲

Values are mean±SD. *$P = 0.05$ vs. control; **$P<0.01$ vs. control; ▲ = $P = 0.001$ vs. control; ▲▲ = $P = 0.0008$ vs. control.

jury (1 month following the initial injury). Seven domestic pigs underwent similar balloon injury to both coronary arteries; 1 month later both arteries underwent repeat balloon injury to the same site as before, but this time one of the injured arteries was assigned to radiation treatment of 14 Gy with the same radiation details described above. One month following that, the animals were sacrificed and the arteries were studied by histologic and morphological analysis. This study demonstrated that radiation had no ablative effect on the neointima formation induced by the initial injury However, the treated arteries demonstrated the inhibitory effect on a secondary wave of proliferation in response to the repeat balloon injury (Fig. 4). The morphometric results of this study demonstrated that there is no radiation effect on the existing neointima from the initial injury (Table 4). However, intracoronary irradiation immediately after the second balloon injury attenuates new intimal hyperplasia due to that injury.

Consensus and Controversy in Animal Studies with Gamma Radiation

Several experimental protocols were conducted to examine the following questions: does low-dose gamma radiation delivered intraluminally reduce the extent of neointima formation after balloon injury? If so, how can we define the minimum effective dose, the time of maximum effective therapy, the durability of the effect over a period of 6 months, and the effect of radiation treatment in the presence of neointima formation as a result of a prior injury? Another important question which remains open is whether low doses below the minimum effective dose can stimulate proliferation in an injured vessel. The consensus is that doses from 14 to 25 Gy result in reduction of neointima formation.

More consistent evidence of the efficacy of radiotherapy came from groups using catheter-based brachytherapy techniques (Table 1). Groups led by Waksman[12] from Emory and Wiedermann[16,17] from Columbia have evaluated the potential benefit of intraluminal ^{192}Ir with doses between 14 and 20 Gy, using hand loading

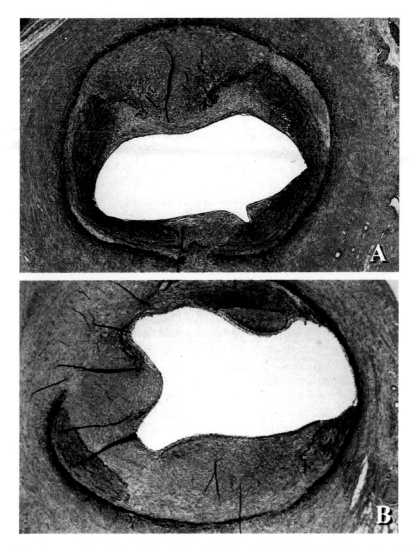

Figure 4. Low-magnification micrographs of **A)** control and **B)** 14 Gy-irradiated injured coronary arteries in a repeat injury porcine model. These specimens are at 2 months after first injury and 1 month after second injury and irradiation.

sources via a noncentered perfusion catheter with a dwelling time of 30 to 60 minutes. Mazur et al[18] from Baylor (Houston, TX) also evaluated the effect of ^{192}Ir with use of a high dose rate afterloader to deliver doses between 15 and 25 Gy within 5 to 10 minutes. All of these investigators have shown the benefits of endovascular brachytherapy in the porcine model of restenosis. Some discrepancies exist among the groups regarding dose-response relationships, but all have shown that doses in the range of 14 to 25 Gy delivered immediately following or prior to balloon angioplasty significantly diminished the amount of neointimal hyperplasia in the short-term follow-up (2 to 4 weeks). Waksman et al[12] and Wiedermann et al[17] have shown that this effect appears to be durable at 6 months without any excess of fibrosis or

Table 4

Results of Computer-Assisted Histomorphometric Analysis of VVG-Stained Thick Sections from Arteries of Swine 1 Month after Repeat Injury in Control and Radiation-Treated Groups

	Control	14Gy
# arteries analyzed	7	7
# segments analyzed	24	28
Maximal intimal thickness (MIT, mm)	0.68±0.08	0.57±0.18
Intimal area(IA, mm²)	1.38±033	0.93±035*
Fracture length (FL, mm)	1.78±1.29	1.97±0.74
Intimal area to fracture Length ratio (IA/FL)	0.78±0.13	0.48±0.11**

Values are mean ± SD, t tests using the Bonferroni correction, to analyze specific group differences. *$P = 0.008$ vs. control; **$P = 0.03$ vs. control.

other adverse effects in the treated arteries and the adjacent segments. Some controversies still exist: Raizner,[18] in contrast to the work of others, found that radiation was not effective in the RCA. The unfavorable results in the RCA were explained by anatomic differences (size and curve) of the RCA versus LAD or LCA arteries and by differences in the physiological response: for example, spasm. The lack of a centering catheter to deliver the dose in a homogenous way could be another explanation to this phenomenon. Wiedermann reported that low doses of 10 Gy can stimulate intimal hyperplasia (Fig. 5); this is in contrast to the work of Waksman et al,[12] who demonstrated partial response without stimulatory effect using lower doses, such as 3.5 and 7 Gy, after balloon injury in the same model. These questions obviously bear further studies. One common finding to all studies is the specific histologic pattern after radiation which shows nearly no neointima formation in the irradiated segments as displayed in Figure 1.

Wiedermann et al[21] demonstrated that noninjured irradiated arteries vasoconstrict in response to acetylcholine, which may imply an immediate impairment of the endothelium by the radiation, probably due to acute radiation injury. However, at 32 days the normal vasodilatatory effect of these segments in response to acetylcholine was restored. Waksman also demonstrated, by electron microscopy, complete reendothelialization at 14 days in arteries that underwent balloon injury and radiation therapy with 14 Gy. These studies confirm the hypothesis that injury of low-dose radiation is reversible in terms of reendothelialization and endothelial function. In addition, radiation was shown to be an adjunct therapy to intracoronary stenting.[22] These findings facilitated the clinical trials combining these two technologies.

Discussion

The major finding of these studies is that low-dose radiation reduced the extent of neointima formation after oversized balloon injury in the pig model of coro-

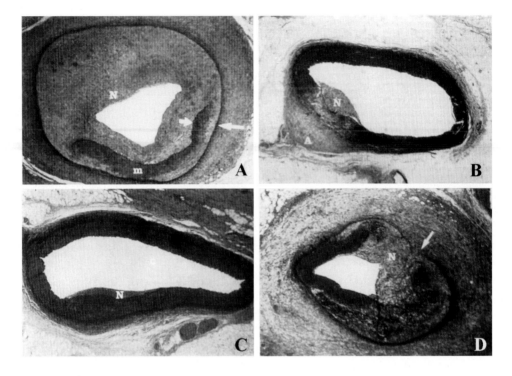

Figure 5. Representative micrographs from the gamma radiation in the porcine model at 40x instrument magnification, from injured pig coronary arteries comparing healing responses at 4 weeks from four treatment groups. In all micrographs, L = lumen; M = dissected ends of tunica media; N = neointima. Samples from **A)** control group, **B)** 15 Gy-treated group, **C)** 20 Gy-treated group, **D)** 10 Gy-treated group suggesting a stimulatory effect of low doses of 10 Gy. From the work of Weinberger et al.

nary restenosis. There is a dose response to low doses of radiation, and 14 Gy prescribed to a distance of 2 mm showed the greatest decrease in neointima formation at 2 weeks post injury. While the duration of the radiation effect is maintained at 6 months, administrating the radiation 1 month post injury does not have any ablative effect on previously formed neointima.

In all dose groups the SMC of the intact media, as well as the fibroblasts of the adventitia, did not appear different morphologically from these same cell populations in the control group, displaying no regions of substantial pyknosis or necrosis.

Previous studies with immunostaining for proliferating cell nuclear antigen (PCNA) have qualitatively demonstrated peak replicative activity at 2 to 3 days.[13,14] This finding, and the possibility of potentiating the radiation effect by exposure during peak replicative activity, led the investigators to test the efficacy of a 2-day delay in irradiation. The results of these experiments, showing that the effect of radiation on neointima formation is more pronounced when administered 48 hours after the vessel injury, suggest that radiation given near the peak of mitotic activity may more effectively suppress subsequent neointima formation.

Other models of injury have shown that dividing cells are more susceptible to the effects of radiation during the G_2/M phase of the cell cycle. [3,6,7] It is not known precisely when the arterial wall cells in this injury model enter into the proliferative phase, and it seems likely that there is considerable overlap in cycling among cell subpopulations; however, ongoing studies using specific proliferative markers with quantitative serial timepoint analysis may identify the time of maximal radiosensitivity. The data regarding lower doses are confusing due to the reports of Wiedermann that 10 Gy may be a stimulatory dose. This contradicts the findings of Waksman, who reporteded that single doses of 3.5 Gy or 7 Gy, and recently 5 Gy, did not demonstrate a stimulatory effect. The 3.5 and 7 Gy even showed some effectiveness in reducing the neointima formation compared with control. Fibrosis was reported with the use of external radiation, especially in patients who underwent radiotherapy for Hodgkin's disease.[15] To specifically address the potential for coronary fibrosis or accelerated arteriosclerosis with endovascular irradiation, Waksman et al administered the 7- and 14-Gy doses in injured coronary arteries, and 14 Gy in the uninjured carotid arteries of mature miniature pigs, and examined the arteries and adjacent tissues at 6 months post treatment. In none of the samples did they detect evidence of excess of fibrosis in the media, adventitia, or perivascular space, which differed from that observed in control injured but nonirradiated arteries. Myocardium adjacent to the irradiated arteries showed a normal appearance, without evidence of fibrosis in the interstitium or blood vessels. Furthermore, the long-term irradiated arteries , which also received balloon injury, demonstrated that the inhibitory effect of endovascular irradiation on neointima formation was maintained. A trend toward maintenance of the dose-response effect was observed, but did not attain statistical significance.

Summary

Low-dose intracoronary gamma irradiation delivered to the site of coronary arterial overstretch balloon injury in pigs inhibited subsequent intimal thickening (hyperplasia). A dose-response relationship was demonstrated, and delay of treatment for 48 hours appeared to augment the inhibitory effect. Six months' follow-up demonstrated the durability of the beneficial effect in the treated group without fibrosis or arteriosclerosis. However, intracoronary irradiation had no ablative properties in existing neointima, but it potentially can prevent recurrence of hyperplasia in the treatment of restenotic lesions. There are several remaining issues regarding gamma radiation in the porcine model; for example, the stimulatory effect of low doses and the importance of centering, especially in larger arteries such as the RCA.

Overall, the data from the experimental studies with gamma radiation on a platform of a catheter-based system suggest that intracoronary radiation therapy may be a tool in the fight to prevent clinical restenosis.

References

1. Holmes DR Jr, Vlietstra RE, Smith HC, et al. Restenosis after percutaneous transluminal coronary angioplasty (PTCA): A report from the PTCA registry of the National Heart, Lung and Blood Institute. Am J Cardiol 1984;53:77C–81C.
2. Forrester JS, Fishbein M, Helfant R, Fagin J. A paradigm for restenosis based on cell biology: Clues for the development of new preventive therapies. J Am Coll Cardiol 1991;17:758–769.

3. Hall EJ. Cell-survival curves. In: *Radiobiology for the Radiologist (3rd ed)*. Philadelphia: Lippincott; 1988:18–38.
4. Puck TT, Morkovin D, Marcus PI, et al. Action of x-rays on mammalian cells: II. Survival curves of cells from normal human tissues. J Exp Med 1957;106:485–500.
5. Sinclair WK. Cyclic x-ray response in mammalian cells in vitro. Radiat Res 1968;63:620–643.
6. Fischer-Dzoga K, Dimitrievich GS, Griem ML. Differential radiosensitivity of aortic cells in vitro. Radiat Res 1984;99:536–546.
7. Fischer-Dzoga K, Dimitrievich GS, Schaffner T. Effect of hyperlipemic serum and irradiation on wound healing in primary quiescent cultures of vascular cells. Exp Mol Pathol 1989;52:1–12.
8. Nickson JJ, Lawrence W Jr, Rachwalsky I, et al. Roentgen rays and wound healing: II. Fractionated irradiation: Experimental study. Surgery 1953;34:859–862.
9. Gravanis MB, Robinson KA, Santoian EC, et al. The reparative phenomena at the site of balloon angioplasty in humans and experimental models. Cardiovasc Pathol 1993;2(4):263–273.
10. Karas SP, Gravanis MB, Santoian EC, et al. Coronary intimal proliferation after balloon injury and stenting in swine: An animal model of restenosis. J Am Coll Cardiol 1992;20:467–474.
11. Gravanis MB, Roubin GS. Histopathologic phenomena at the site of percutaneous transluminal coronary angioplasty: The problem of restenosis. Hum Pathol 1989;20: 477–485.
12. Waksman R, Robinson KA, Crocker IR, et al. Endovascular low dose irradiation inhibits neointima formation after coronary artery balloon injury in swine: A possible role for radiation therapy in restenosis prevention. Circulation 1995;91:1553–1559
13. Clowes AW, Schwartz SM. Significance of quiescent smooth muscle migration in the injured rat carotid artery. Circ Res 1985;56:1390–1345.
14. Windsor JH, Santoian EC, Tarazona N, et al. Smooth muscle cell proliferation during neointimal development after PTCA in swine: Identification of site and sequence using proliferating cell nuclear antigen staining [abstract]. J Am Coll Cardiol 1994;235A.
15. Borvin IF. Coronary heart disease mortality after irradiation for Hodgkin's disease.
16. Wiedermann JG, Marboe C, Schwartz A, et al. Intracoronary irradiation reduces restenosis after balloon angioplasty in a porcine model. J Am Coll Cardiol 1994;23: 1491–1498.
17. Wiedermann JG, Marboe C, Amols H, et al. Intracoronary irradiation markedly reduces neointimal proliferation after balloon angioplasty in the swine: Persistent benefit at 6-month follow-up. J Am Coll Cardiol 1995;25:1451–1456
18. Mazur W, Ali MN, Dabaghi SF, et al. High dose rate intracoronary radiation suppresses neointimal proliferation in the stented and ballooned model of porcine restenosis. Int J Radiat Oncol Biol Phys 1996;36:778–788.
19. Wienberger J, Amols H, Ennis RD, et al. Intracoronary irradiation: Dose response for the prevention of restenosis in swine. Int J Radiat Oncol Biol Phys 1996;36:767–775.
20. Waksman R, Robinson KA, Crocker IR, et al. Intracoronary radiation decreases new additional intimal hyperplasia in a repeat balloon angioplasty swine model of restenosis. Int J Radiat Oncol Biol Phys 1997;376:767–777.
21. Wiedermann JG, Leavy JA, Amols H, et al. Effects of high dose intracoronary irradiation on vasomotor function and smooth muscle histopathology. Am J Physiol 1964;267: H125–H126.
22. Waksman R. Intracoronary radiation adjunct therapy to stenting. J Int Cardiol 1977; 10:2133–2136.

Endovascular Beta Radiation in the Swine Model

Ron Waksman, MD

The use of low-dose gamma radiation to inhibit neointima formation after balloon injury has been demonstrated in several animal models. Wiedermann et al,[1] Mazur et al,[2] and Waksman et al[3] have demonstrated the efficacy of endovascular low-dose gamma radiation, using ^{192}Ir to inhibit neointima formation after balloon overstretch injury in pig coronaries. With 6 months follow-up, the durability of the beneficial effect in the treated group, without evidence of excess fibrosis, was demonstrated in two studies.[3,4] In these studies, the radiation was delivered either by a high dose rate afterloader or by an ^{192}Ir ribbon delivered manually to the treatment site. Although their dosimetry is known and simple to apply for use in animal studies and peripheral arteries,[5] gamma emitters such as the ^{192}Ir isotope have serious limitations for use in human coronaries, as they are deeply penetrating and are not effectively shielded by standard lead aprons. Use of gamma emitters would require the cardiology staff to leave the proximity of the patient during treatment. In addition, the highest activity (300 mCi) commercially available (Best Medical Industry, Springfield, VA) gamma emitter that is hand-delivered requires a treatment time of approximately 20 minutes for delivering 15 Gy at a 2-mm distance, during which time the delivery catheter is continuously present in the coronary artery. The advantage of using a high dose rate afterloader is the ability to reduce the treatment time with a very high-activity (10 Ci) [192]Ir source, which is delivered under remote control to the treatment site. These high-activity sources require special shielding beyond that which is present in most cardiac catheterization suites. Although the treatment time might be reduced, the potential need to add shielding to the catheterization suite or to transfer the patient to a radiation oncology facility for treatment presents significant problems and is not practical.

Since 1993, as a result of the above concerns, several investigators have initiated the development of new treatment devices for endovascular irradiation that use pure beta emitters such as ^{90}Y, ^{90}Sr/Y, ^{32}P, [186]Re, ^{133}Xe, [62]Cu, [188]Re, and [188]W. The majority of these are pure beta emitters, although some have a weak gamma in addition to the beta source.

The beta emitters have favorable characteristics in terms of permitting delivery of dose to the required depth in tissue (2 to 3 mm) with little dose measured beyond 1 cm from the source. The treatment time for beta emitters ranges from 2 to 8 minutes, depending on the dose and the activity of the emitters.

From Waksman R (ed). *Vascular Brachytherapy, Third Edition.* Armonk, NY: Futura Publishing Co., Inc.; © 2002.

Several investigators performed a series of studies using catheter-based beta radiation. These studies are summarized in Table 1, and they addressed the following questions:

1. Does beta radiation inhibit neointima formation after balloon overstretch injury as effectively as gamma radiation such as [192]Ir?
2. What is the radiation exposure to the patient, whole-body, and to the operator from clinical use of beta-emitting sources?
3. What are the advantages and limitations in the use of beta emitters for vascular brachytherapy?

Table 1

Preclinical Studies with Beta Radiation for Vascular Brachytherapy

Author	Animal/Vessel	Radiation Source	Outcome
Waksman[6]	Pig/Coronaries	[90]Sr/Y	Benefit with 7 and 56 Gy post angioplasty inhibition of neointima formation
Verin[17]	Rabbit/Carotid +Iliac	[90]Y	Decreased neointima with 18 Gy; no benefit with 6 and 12 Gy
Raizner[24]	Pig/Coronaries	[32]P centering catheter and an afterloader	Doses 20–35 Gy demonstrated reduction of neointima formation following stenting or balloon injury
Eigler[23]	Pig/Coronaries	[188]Re liquid-filled balloon	Dose response 16–29 Gy to suppress neointima formation in stented arteries
Weinberger[24]	Pig/Coronaries	[188]Re liquid-filled balloon	13.5–30 Gy on the surface of the balloon, inhibition of neointima formation after injury
Robinson[22]	Pig/Coronaries	[186]Re liquid-filled balloon	Dose response 5–30 Gy suppress neointima formation and enhances lumen size
Waksman[21]	Pig/Coronaries	[90]Y centered balloon and an afterloader	18 Gy to a distance of 1.2mm from the surface of the balloon resulted in suppression of neointima after balloon injury and stent arteries.
Waksman[20]	Pig/Coronaries	[133]Xe gas-filled balloon	Doses 7.5–30 Gy suppress neointima formation after balloon injury
Waksman[26]	Pig/Coronaries	[188]Re coiled wire	Dose of 15 Gy to a distance of 2mm from the source showed reduction of neointima formation after balloon injury

Catheter-Based Systems for Beta Emitters

Several groups have developed brachytherapy systems based on beta emitters, and have conducted series of preclinical studies in animal models. The pure beta emitters that underwent preliminary evaluation are ^{90}Y as a wire, ^{90}Sr/Y in radioactive seeds delivered manually by hydraulic system to the treatment site, ^{32}P as a line source delivered by a high dose rate afterloader, liquid-filled balloon systems containing ^{188}Re and ^{186}Re sources, and gas-filled balloon systems containing ^{133}Xe gas.

Verin and Popowski, and colleagues,[17,18] have used a ^{90}Y emitter on a wire delivered via a centering balloon catheter, in atherosclerotic rabbit iliac and carotid arteries, to treat with doses of 6, 12, and 18 Gy to the surface of the centering catheter. At 6 weeks, the percent-area stenosis and the number of neointimal cell layers were both significantly reduced in the group of arteries exposed to 18 Gy compared to the control group. However, there was no significant reduction of the histologic indices in the 6 Gy and the 12 Gy groups. The authors concluded that 18 Gy should be sufficient for long-term inhibition of neointima formation after balloon injury, and thus they selected this dose for their clinical study. A series of studies was performed at Emory University (Atlanta, GA) and published by Waksman et al,[6,19] who used a catheter-based beta radiation system with ^{90}Sr/Y, a pure beta emitter, as the radioactive source (Novoste Corp., Norcross, GA). This isotope, like the other beta emitters, has favorable characteristics in terms of permitting delivery of the dose to the required depth in tissue (2 to 3 mm) with little dose measured beyond 1 cm from the source. It has a half-life of approximately 29 years, which does not require day-to-day activity and dwelling time calculations. The ^{90}Sr/Y isotope was delivered manually via a low-profile approximately 5F noncentered catheter, and required a short treatment time of less than 4 minutes to deliver doses of 14 Gy. The preclinical studies for this system were designed to determine the efficacy of this isotope and to determine if ^{90}Sr/Y could inhibit neointima formation after balloon overstretch injury as effectively as ^{192}Ir. Doses of 7, 14, 28, and 56 Gy were delivered following balloon angioplasty in porcine coronary arteries. Morphometric indices of maximal intimal thickness (MIT) and intimal area (IA) corrected for the extent of injury (fracture length) (IA/FL) of irradiated vessels with both beta and gamma radioisotopes were examined and compared at 14 Gy. The morphometric analysis demonstrated similar effectiveness of ^{90}Sr/Y in reduction of neointimal hyperplasia, as demonstrated previously with ^{192}Ir (Table 2). Higher doses of 28 Gy and 56 Gy showed a more consistent effect in the reduction of neointimal hyperplasia without an excess of adverse effects to the treated vessel and the surrounding area (Fig. 1).

The group from Baylor University (Houston, TX)[2,24] also examined the effectiveness of ^{32}P, a pure beta emitter, in a wire configuration by use of a centering helical catheter and an automatic afterloader technique. Consistent results of reduction of neointima formation were obtained only with doses of 32 to 35 Gy. The group also reported similarity to previous studies in the same model with the gamma source ^{192}Ir.[25] These studies demonstrated significant reduction of neointima formation when radiation was applied both after balloon angioplasty and post stenting in the porcine coronaries.

Table 2

Results of Computer-Assisted Histomorphometric Analysis of
VVG-Stained Thick Sections from Arteries of Pigs in Control and
Radiation-Treated Groups with ^{90}Sr/Y Beta Emitter

	Control	7Gy	14Gy	28Gy	56Gy
No. arteries analyzed	16	9	9	2	2
No. segments analyzed	59	45	38	10	8
Maximal intimal thickness (MIT, mm)	0.47±0.15	0.40±0.18	0.34±0.23*	0.23±0.14***	0.08±0.09ι
Vessel perimeter (mm)	7.19±1.08	7.12±1.10	7.40±1.25	9.15±0.8ι	7.79±1.39
Vessel area (mm²)	3.77±1.10	3.63±1.17	3.83±1.13	5.25±0.91***	4.34±1.46
Luminal area (mm²)	1.91±0.85	2.01±0.82	2.46±1.20*	3.85±0.77***	3.70±1.36**
Intimal area (IA, mm²)	1.09±0.70	0.81±0.49*	0.58±0.54***	0.47±0.55**	0.10±0.15ι
Fracture length (FL, mm)	2.28±1.19	2.39±0.95	3.45±1.77***	4.57±1.47***	3.62±1.38*
Intimal area to fracture length ratio (IA/FL)	0.47±0.25	0.34±0.18*	0.19±0.20**	0.08±0.09ι	0.02±0.02ι

Values are mean±SD. *$P <0.03$ vs. control; **$P <0.001$ vs. control; ***$P<0.0001$ vs. control;
ι = $P<0.00001$;ιι = $P<0.0000001$. VVG = Verhoeff van Gieson.

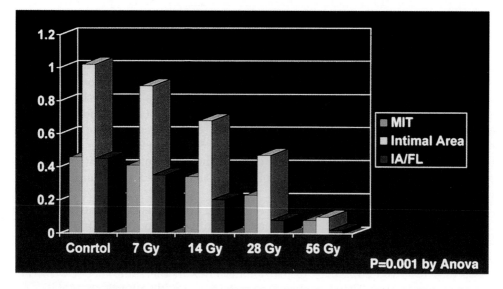

Figure 1. Dose-response effects of ^{90}Sr/Y delivered into pig coronaries following balloon
overstretch injury. MIT = maximal intimal thickness; IA = intimal area; FL = fracture
length (degree of injury).

Experimental Protocols

The swine model of restenosis, based on oversized balloon catheter inflation in the coronary arteries of normal juvenile pigs, was used to test the primary hypothesis regarding neointima formation and to determine the mechanisms by which intracoronary irradiation reduces neointima formation.

The model of overstretch injury has been described previously.[7–11] In summary, female domestic pigs were given aspirin (325 mg) 1 day before, and on the day of the procedure. Coronary overstretch injury was performed with a 3.5-mm angioplasty balloon, which was positioned in the proximal segments of the left anterior descending (LAD) and left circumflex (LCX) arteries, and inflated to 10 atm three times for 30 seconds in each artery. Inflation periods were separated by 1-minute deflation periods to restore coronary perfusion. After the completion of the third inflation the angioplasty balloon was withdrawn, and additional nitroglycerin (200 μg) was administered to limit coronary spasm. Repeat angiography was then performed to assess vessel patency and degree of injury. One of the injured coronary arteries in each swine was assigned randomly to receive radiation treatment and the contralateral artery was treated with a sham catheter. The pigs were killed 14 days after the initial injury, and the coronary vasculature was perfusion-fixed. Morphometric analysis was performed on each segment with evidence of medial fracture (2 to 6 in each artery). Intramural deposits of fibrin as well as larger organized mural thrombi were included in the area measurements of neointima. The samples were compared with one control artery in the same pig. A radial line, drawn from the lumen to the external lamina at the point of greatest tissue growth, determined the MIT. The arc length of the medial fracture (FL), traced through the neointima from one dissected medial end to the other, was used as a measure of the extent of injury. Area measurements were obtained by tracing the lumen perimeter (luminal area [LA] mm^2), neointima perimeter (intimal area [IA] mm^2, defined by the borders of the internal elastic lamina, lumen, media, and external elastic lamina), and external elastic lamina (vessel area [VA] mm^2). IA/FL was calculated to correct for the extent of injury. The MIT and the absolute IA reflected the new tissue formation after vessel injury and served as reliable indicators of the capacity for a potential therapy to inhibit neointima formation after injury. The IA/FL ratio was somewhat more precise, since it provides an adjustment for the extent of medial fracture, to which IA is directly correlated.[11]

Studies with the ^{90}Sr/Y System

With use of the porcine model described above, a delivery catheter (Novoste) was introduced over a flexible 0.014″ wire to the injury site of the assigned artery and positioned at the angioplasty site. The guidewire was then withdrawn, and a 2.5-cm length train with five seeds of ^{90}Sr/Y was positioned at the site of injury in the target vessel by use of cinefluoroscopic visualization, within the delivery catheter. It was left in place for a period sufficient to deliver the assigned dose (7, 14, 28, or 56 Gy) to a depth of 2 mm (90 to 720 sec). The delivery catheter without the radioactive source was placed in the control injured artery in the same manner as in the treated artery.

In the two arteries, the effect of beta irradiation with 14 Gy on reendothe-lialization of the luminal surface at 14 days after injury was examined by scanning electron microscopy. Control arteries and irradiated arteries with 14, 28, and 56 Gy were examined 48 to 72 hours post treatment to detect immediate vasculopathy as a result of the radiation.

Radiation Dosimetry and Exposure to ^{90}Sr/Y

The activity of each seed and the total source train was determined by the manufacturer with a National Institute of Standards and Technology (NIST) traceable standard. The absorbed dose distribution and dose rate around the 2.5-cm ^{90}Sr/Y line source was calculated by use of the Monte Carlo electron transport code ITS.[12] The beta energy spectrum of ^{90}Sr/Y was obtained from Cross et al.[13] As part of the verification of ITS, a determination of the dose distribution around the ^{192}Ir line source from our previous study was carried out and compared to the calculations done with the CMS Treatment Planning System. There was no self-centering of the catheter within the arterial lumen, nor was there any attempt made to account for curvature of the artery and the radiation line source. The radiation exposure at the bedside measured 0.009 mSv with the ^{90}Sr/Y versus 0.14 mSv with ^{192}Ir, and the total-body exposure to the pig was 0.19 versus 1000 mSv, respectively, during treatment with 14 Gy targeted to a depth of 2 mm (Table 3).

Study Results with ^{90}Sr/Y

The neointima from beta-irradiated arteries was markedly smaller in size than the controls, with some sections showing a virtual absence of neointima formation (especially 28 and 56 Gy) (Table 2). When present, the cells of the neointima were morphologically similar to those of the controls. In a moderate number of samples there were mural fibrin deposits. In the majority of the samples there was complete coverage of the luminal surface by a monolayer of endothelial-like cells. However, in the arteries treated with 28 and 56 Gy, some regions revealed no luminal cell lining; nevertheless, few of these sections showed evidence of thrombosis. Furthermore, significant necrosis or nuclear pyknosis in the media or adventitia was not observed in either the control or the radiation treatment groups. The perivascular nerve fibers, adipose tissue, and adjacent myocardium appeared normal. The overall histologic findings in arteries treated with 56 and

Table 3

Measured Exposures with ^{90}Sr/Y Source Train

	Effective Dose Rate (mSv/hr)	Total Effective Dose for 14 Gy in 4 minutes (mSv)
Surface of transfer device	15	1
Chest surface	1.4	0.09
At bedside	0.14	0.009

Total source activity of 16 mCi.

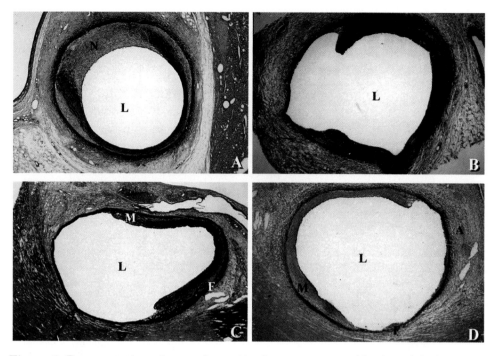

Figure 2. Representative micrographs at 40× instrument magnification of thick sections from injured pig coronary arteries, stained with Verhoeff-van Gieson elastin. Healing responses at 2 weeks in five treatment groups are compared. L = lumen; M = dissected ends of tunica media; N = neointima; F = fibrin dissection-plane hematoma. Samples from: **(A)** control group, **(B)** 14-Gy-treated group, **(C)** 28-Gy-treated group, and **(D)** 56-Gy-treated group.

28 Gy were similar. Low-magnification micrographs of Verhoeff-van Gieson (VVG)-stained sections from injured coronary arteries of porcine control and treated groups are shown in Figure 2.

Scanning Electron Microscopy

Representative low-magnification images of control and 14-Gy–irradiated, balloon-injured arteries are shown in Figure 3. Arteries from both groups displayed a largely confluent lining of endothelial-like cells showing occasional leukocyte adherence with apparent spreading and endothelial diapedesis, as well as rare small (approximately 200 to 500 μm^2) nonreendothelialized areas. No regions of significant mural thrombosis were seen in either control or irradiated vessels.

Histologic Analysis

Hematoxylin-eosin (H&E)- and VVG-stained sections of all arterial segments were examined. In injured segments of both control and beta-irradiated arteries there was a variable degree of rupture of the tunica media, resulting in a vessel wall defect. Control arteries showed replacement of the medial defect with a substantial neointima consisting mostly of stellate and spindle-shaped cells, in a loose

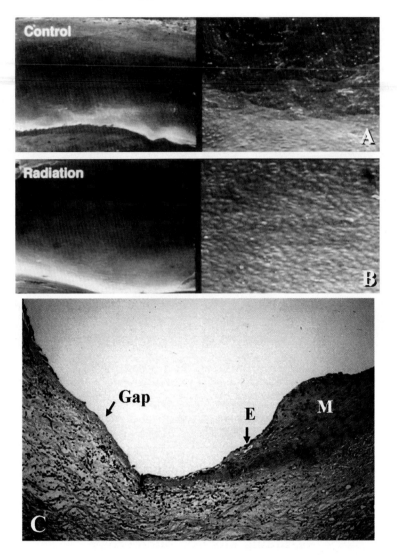

Figure 3. Representative scanning electron micrographs at 350× instrument magnification of **(A)** control, and **(B)** 14-Gy irradiated coronary artery luminal surfaces from samples harvested at 14 days after overstretch injury and radiation treatment. Rare small areas of incomplete reendothelialization (arrow) can be seen, as well as occasional adherent leukocytes (WBC); both phenomena were observed with approximately equal frequency in treated versus control arteries. G = gap; E = endothelial cells.

extracellular matrix. A moderate number of sections showed hematomas in the media-adventitia dissection planes. In most sections there was perivascular edema and mild to moderate round cell infiltration.

Radiobiological Effect

Substantial effects of irradiation were observed on all morphometric descriptors of neointima formation. The morphometric analysis detected a response similar to that in the studies with [192]Ir. These studies indicate that there is a linear dose-response effect from single doses of 7 to 28 Gy with use of the ^{90}Sr/Y source. There is virtual eradication of neointima formation at 2 weeks with 28 Gy. Consequently, there is no further inhibition of neointima formation at 56 Gy.

The absence of a necrotizing effect on the arterial tissue, and the preservation of normal morphology in perivascular tissues and adjacent myocardium in this study suggest that these tissues are not damaged, at least not acutely, by even very high doses of beta radiation. We know from our gamma studies that doses of up to 14 Gy are unlikely to cause any injury to the vessel from the radiation treatment. Our present results from scanning electron microscopic analysis demonstrate that the inhibitory effect of 14 Gy on neointima formation does not retard reendothelialization. At 28 and 56 Gy in paraffin-embedded tissue sections, there was no evidence of recent mural thrombosis, and for the most part there was recovery of a periluminal cell layer in the medial defect. Furthermore, the results in three miniature pigs at 6 months provide evidence that there is no chronic injury to the arterial wall or surrounding tissues, including adjacent myocardium, that is induced by beta radiation at doses of 7 and 14 Gy. It remains to be seen in ongoing chronic beta studies whether higher doses (28 and 56 Gy) will also be free of any adverse effect from radiation treatment.

Late Effects

One of the concerns with the use of beta emitters in the coronary porcine model is the absence of efficacy at 6 months. None of the isotopes (^{90}Sr/Y, ^{32}P, ^{90}Y) used so far reported satisfactory results. In some of the studies harmful effects were noted, such as an increase in the late thrombosis and mortality rate in pigs that were exposed to radiation therapy. The overall neointima formation in this studies showed similar indices when compared with controls. Excluding the late thrombosis phenomenon, these findings are limited to the animal model and have not been seen in humans. This discrepancy raises the question of whether the porcine model at 6 months has value to predict late clinical outcome. On a positive note, the long-term animal studies did not demonstrate perforation or late aneurysm of coronaries exposed to radiation.

90Y, Centering Catheter, and an Automatic Afterloader in the Porcine Model

In a study performed by Waksman et al[21] at the Washington Hospital Center, the effectiveness of ^{90}Y delivered into a new segmented centering balloon closed-end lumen catheter (Schneider, Bullach, Switzerland) via an automatic remote afterloader was examined. In this study, 12 pigs (16 arteries LAD, LCX, and RCA) underwent balloon injury with a 3.5-mm balloon, and 8 pigs (16 arteries) underwent 3.5-mm stent implantation. Intracoronary radiation prior to stenting was administered in 8 arteries. A 2.5- to 3.0-mm segmented balloon catheter automatically loaded with ^{90}Y was introduced into one of the injured arteries in each animal to deliver 18 Gy prescribed at 2 mm from the surface of the balloon. The dose rate varied from 11.9 to 5.6 Gy/min. Two weeks after the balloon injury and 4 weeks after stenting, the animals were killed and the arteries were analyzed. IA and IA/FL were

Table 4

Effects of ^{90}Y Delivered Intracoronary on Reduction of Neointima Formation Indices

	IA	IA/FL	Late Loss in Stented Arteries
^{90}Y (n-14)	0.25±13	0.09±0.05	0.004 (mm)
Control (n = 18)	0.99±0.19	0.55±0.08	0.60 (mm)
P value	0.008	0.0002	0.007

IA = intimal area; IA/FL = intimal area to fracture length ratio.

smaller in the irradiated versus the control arteries (Table 4). Angiograms detected less stenosis in arteries that received radiation prior to stent implantation. This study demonstrates that intracoronary delivery of ^{90}Y via a centering catheter and automatic afterloader is feasible and safe and results in consistent, homogenous inhibition of neointima formation post injury in the porcine model.

^{133}Xe-Filled Balloon System

Another novel technology is the gas-filled balloon. We tested a gas-filled balloon system using a ^{133}Xe radioactive gas (Cook, Bloomington IN). To examine the effectiveness of ^{133}Xe in the inhibition of neointima formation, balloon injury was performed in the coronaries LAD, LCX, and RCA in 10 pigs. Following the injury, 3.0- to 3.5-mm balloons of 30 mm in length were positioned to overlap the injured segment. After a vacuum was obtained in the balloon, 2.5 cc of ^{133}Xe gas with an activity of 300 mCi was injected to fill the balloon. A dose of 15 Gy was delivered to a distance of 0.25 mm from the surface of the balloon. The dwell time of the catheter was 2.0±0.2 minutes. Localization of the ^{133}Xe in the balloon was verified by a gamma camera, which acquired images during treatment and after retrieval of the gas and the catheter from the treated artery. The radiation exposure on the heart measured 100 mR/h, and at the bedside, 6 mR/h. Two weeks following the treatment, the animals were killed, the arteries were perfusion-fixed, stained, and analyzed by histomorphometric techniques. The IA and IA/FL were compared among the irradiated and control arteries. Significant reduction of neointima formation was observed in the arteries treated with the ^{133}Xe gas-filled balloon system (Table 5). This method also demonstrated feasibility and effectiveness in reduction of neointima in the porcine model and may be an attractive modality for clinical use.

Table 5

Effect Of ^{133}Xe on the Neointima Formation Following Balloon Injury in Porcine Coronary Arteries

	Control (n = 8)	^{133}Xe 15 Gy (n = 9)	P Value
IA (mm^2)	1.51±0.19	0.10±0.07	0.009
IA/FL	0.76±0.08	0.04±0.02	0.0001

IA = intimal area; IA/FL = intimal area to fracture length ratio.

^{188}Re Wire Coiled System

The effectiveness of ^{188}Re isotope (half-life 17 hours), which has both beta and gamma energies, was tested in another study. Eight pigs underwent balloon over-stretch injury to 16 coronary arteries. Following the injury, a 30-mm in length radioactive ^{188}Re coiled wire 1 mm in diameter was introduced to cover the angioplasty site in 8 of the injured arteries. The prescribed dose was 15 Gy delivered to a distance of 2 mm into the artery wall, and the dose rate varied from 9 to 2 Gy/min. Two weeks after the procedure the animals were killed and the arteries were perfusion-fixed, stained, and examined by histologic and morphometric techniques. Complete inhibition of neointima formation was demonstrated in the irradiated arteries, regardless of the difference in the dose rate. IA and IA/FL were smaller in the irradiated arteries versus control (Fig. 4). There was no excess of

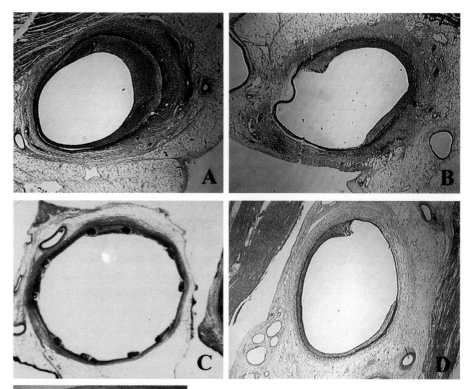

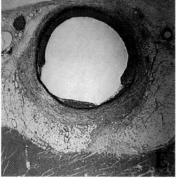

Figure 4. Representative micrographs at 40× instrument magnification of thick sections from injured pig coronary arteries, stained with Verhoeff-van Gieson elastin. Healing responses at 2 weeks in five treatment groups are compared. Samples from **(A)** control group, **(B)** ^{90}Y 18-Gy-treated group, **(C)** ^{90}Y 18-Gy-treated stented group, **(D)** ^{188}Re 15-Gy-treated balloon group, and **(E)** ^{133}Xe, 133-Gy balloon-treated group.

thrombus, fibrin, or fibrosis in the irradiated arteries compared to control. [188]Re was shown to be feasible and safe, and resulted in consistent homogenous inhibition of neointima formation in the porcine model.

[188]W Wire Coiled Wire-Based System

The effectiveness of coiled wire-based system was demonstrated in the porcine model with doses of 22 Gy at 2 mm from the center of the source. The Tungsten source has a similar design to the [186]Re source with the advantages of prolonged half-life of 70 days. The delivery system used in this study was similar to the one used in the [192]Ir (The CheckMate catheter of Cordis, and the closed end lumen of Medtronic). Complete inhibition of the neointima formation in the balloon overstretched injury and the stent model have been obtained.

[186]Re and [188]Re Liquid-Filled Balloon Systems

The concept of a liquid filled-balloon with a beta emitter was tested in the porcine model by three groups. The isotopes selected for this were either [186]Re, a pure beta emitter provided from a reactor by Mallinckrodt in St. Louis, Missouri,[22] or [188]Re milked from a generator in the hospital.[24,25]

The doses reported to show effectiveness in reduction of neointima formation ranged between 15 and 30 Gy prescribed to a distance of 0.5 mm from the balloon surface into the vessel wall (Table 6). One concern regarding the studies with the liquid-filled balloon is the edge effect that may result from underdosing at the edge of the treated lesion.

A Novel [32]P Deployable Balloon System

The RDX ^{32}P deployable balloon system uses the radioisotope ^{32}P integrated into the balloon material. The activity is less than 30 mCi, and dwell time to deliver 20 Gy at 1.0 mm into the vessel wall ranges from 6 to 10 minutes. Studies using the deployable balloon system in the porcine coronary model of restenosis demonstrated the effectiveness and safety of this system in the porcine balloon and the stent injury model. Domestic swines underwent balloon overstretch injury (BI) in 20 coronary arteries and were randomized to receive a dose of 0, 15, or 20 Gy,

Table 6

Effect of [186]Re on Neointima Formation Following Balloon Injury in Porcine Coronary Arteries

Dose	0Gy	5Gy	10Gy	15Gy	20Gy	30Gy
Lumen (mm²)	1.29	0.66*	1.1	1.2	2.14**	2.17*
Vessel (mm²)	3.17	2.4	2.81	3.02	3.35	3.44
Intima (mm²)	1.08	1.07	0.79	0.89	0.31***	0.14***

*$P<0.01$ versus control; **$P<0.001$ versus control; ***$P<0.0001$ versus control.

prescribed to 1 mm from the surface of the radioactive balloon material. The animals were killed 4 weeks following the procedure. Vessel parameters, intimal area, and thrombus area were analyzed by computer-aided histomorphometry. Neointimal formation after BI was reduced in the radiated groups as compared to control ($P<0.05$). Vessels treated with 20 Gy underwent vascular remodeling and had an increase in the total thrombus area ($P<0.05$). These studies demonstrated that the new ^{32}P deployable balloon system is feasible and safe. Radiation doses of 15 Gy were sufficient to inhibit the neointimal response in the porcine coronary balloon injury model. Long-term studies in the stent model were not favorable at 6 months.

Beta versus Gamma Catheter-Based Systems

These studies demonstrate that an endovascular beta emitter can inhibit neointima formation in porcine coronary arteries as effectively as gamma emitters. Similar to our previous study using the gamma emitter ^{192}Ir, the present findings demonstrate that both 7 and 14 Gy at a 2-mm depth had a significant effect in decreasing neointima formation compared to control at 2 weeks post injury. The histologic and histomorphometric analyses of coronary arteries treated with the same doses of beta and gamma radiation demonstrate overall similarity.[19] An interesting difference is the gradient of the radiation dose between beta and gamma. While beta radiation is usually associated with higher doses to the vessel wall, gamma has the ability to deliver higher doses at the periadventitia area. This can be of an importance if we identify clearly that the target is at the adventitia or beyond. The similarity in the preclinical results with the use of the various emitters does not seem to be influenced by this theory, or, it is possible that the therapeutic range is so wide that differences cannot be seen. It can be summarized, therefore, that the biological effect on neointima formation is dependent on the absorbed dose and not on the type of isotope or the variation in treatment times seen with the different approaches.

Conclusions

Intracoronary irradiation with a variety of beta emitters is feasible for use in a standard catheterization laboratory following coronary intervention. Radiation doses between 7 and 56 Gy have effectively inhibited neointima formation at 2 weeks after coronary balloon injury. No dose response has been seen beyond 28 Gy. These study results suggest that endovascular radiation reduces the new neointima formation by inhibiting the first wave of cell proliferation in the adventitia and the media. Histologic and histomorphometric results are similar in arteries irradiated with gamma (^{192}Ir) and beta emitters (^{32}P, ^{188}Xe, ^{188}Re, ^{188}W and ^{90}Sr/Y). However, the use of beta irradiation for this application appears to possess distinct advantages in terms of both safety and practicality for patients and health care workers.

References

1. Wiedermann JG, Marboe C, Schwartz A, et al. Intracoronary irradiation reduces restenosis after balloon angioplasty in a porcine model. J Am Coll Cardiol 1994; 23:1491–1498.

2. Mazur W, Ali MN, Dabaghi SF, et al. High dose rate intracoronary radiation suppresses neointimal proliferation in the stented and ballooned model of porcine restenosis. Int J Radiat Oncol Biol Phys 1996;36:778S-788S.

3. Waksman R, Robinson KA, Crocker IR, et al. Endovascular low dose irradiation inhibits neointima formation after coronary artery balloon injury in swine: A possible role for radiation therapy in restenosis prevention. Circulation 1995;91:1553–1559.

4. Wiedermann JG, Marboe C, Schwartz A, et al. Intracoronary irradiation markedly reduces neointimal proliferation after balloon angioplasty in swine: Persistent benefit at 6-month follow-up. J Am Coll Cardiol 1995;25:1451–1456.

5. Liermann, DD, Boettcher HD, Kollatch J, et al. Prophylactic endovascular radiotherapy to prevent intimal hyperplasia after stent implantation in femoro-popliteal arteries. Cardiovasc Intervent Radiol 1994;17:12–16.

6. Waksman R, Robinson KA, Crocker IR, et al. Intracoronary low dose β-irradiation inhibits neointima formation after coronary artery balloon injury in the swine restenosis model. Circulation 1995;92:3025–3031.

7. Karas SP, Gravanis MB, Santoian EC, et al. Coronary intimal proliferation after balloon injury and stenting in swine: An animal model of restenosis. J Am Coll Cardiol 1992;20:467–474.

8. Gravanis MB, Robinson KA, Santoian EC, et al. The reparative phenomena at the site of balloon angioplasty in humans and experimental models. Cardiovasc Pathol 1993;2:263–273.

9. Gravanis MB, Roubin GS. Histopathologic phenomena at the site of percutaneous transluminal coronary angioplasty: The problem of restenosis. Hum Pathol 1989;20:477–485.

10. Wanibuchi H, Ueda M, Dingemans KP, Becker AE. The response to percutaneous transluminal coronary angioplasty: An ultrastructural study of smooth muscle cells and endothelial cells. Cardiovasc Pathol 1992;1:295–306.

11. Waksman R, Robinson KA, Sigman SR, et al. Balloon overstretch injury correlates with neointima formation and not with vascular remodeling in the pig coronary restenosis model [abstract]. J Am Coll Cardiol 1994; Feb:138A.

12. Halbleib JA, Mehlhorn TA. ITS: The integrated TIGER series of coupled electron/photon Monte Carlo transport codes. CCC-467 Radiation Information Shielding Center, Oak Ridge National Laboratory.

13. Cross WG, Ing H, Freedman N. A short atlas of beta-ray spectra. Phys Med Biol 1983;28:1251–1260.

14. Cascade PN, Peterson LE, Wajszczuk WJ, Mantel J. Radiation exposure to patients undergoing percutaneous transluminal coronary angioplasty. Am J Cardiol 1987;59:996–997.

15. Pattee PL, Johns PC, Chambers RJ. Radiation risk to patients from percutaneous transluminal coronary angioplasty. J Am Coll Cardiol 1993;22:1044–1051.

16. Jeans SP, Faulkner K, Love HG, Bardsley RA. An investigation of the radiation dose to staff during cardiac radiological studies. Br J Radiol 1985;58:419–428.

17. Verin V, Popowski Y, Urban P, et al. Intra-arterial beta irradiation prevents neointimal hyperplasia in a hypercholesterolemic rabbit restenosis model. Circulation 1995; 92:2284–2290.

18. Popowski Y, Verin V, Papirov I, et al. High dose rate brachytherapy for prevention of restenosis after percutaneous angioplasty: Preliminary dosimetric tests of a new source presentation. Int J Radiat Oncol Biol Phys 1995;33:211–215.

19. Waksman R, Robinson KA, Crocker IA, et al. Efficacy and safety of β versus γ radioisotopes for endovascular irradiation in prevention of intimal hyperplasia after balloon angioplasty in swine coronaries [abstract]. Circulation 1995;92:I146.

20. Waksman R, Chan RC, Vodovotz Y, et al. Radioactive 133-Xenon gas-filled angioplasty balloon: A novel intracoronary radiation system to prevent restenosis. J Am Coll Cardiol 1998:31:2356A.

21. Waksman R, Saucedo JF, Chan RC, et al. Yttrium-90 delivered via a centering catheter and remote afterloader, uniformly inhibits neointima formation after balloon injury or stenting in swine coronary arteries. J Am Coll Cardiol 1998;31:2278A.

22. Robinson KA, Pipes DW, Van Bibber R, et al. Dose response evaluation in balloon-injured pig coronary arteries of beta emitting 186-Re liquid-filled balloon catheter system for endovascular brachytherapy. Advances in Cardiovascular Radiation Therapy II. 1998: abstract 7.

23. Eigler N, Whiting J, Makkar R, et al. Radiant™ liquid isotope intravascular radiation system. Advances in Cardiovascular Radiation Therapy II. 1998:234–237.
24. Gieldd KN, Amols H, Marboe CC, et al. Effectiveness of a beta emitting liquid-filled perfusion balloon to prevent restenosis [abstract]. Circulation 1997;96:I220.
25. Raizner AE, Calfee RV. The Guidant Intravascular Brachytherapy System. In: Waksman R, Serruys PW (eds.): Handbook of Vascular Brachytherapy. London: Martin Dunitz; 1998:53–58.

## Chapter 25

Local Delivery of Radionuclides to Prevent Restenosis

Ron Waksman, MD, Rosanna C. Chan, PhD, Lisa R. Karam, PhD, and Brian E. Zimmerman, PhD

Local drug delivery was introduced as an alternative to the systemic administration of a variety of agents that failed to reduce the restenosis rate.[1] The concept was an attempt to reduce restenosis by pharmacology agents with a highly concentrated dose while avoiding the side effects associated with systemic administration. The technology is based on the success of delivering sufficient concentration of the drug (much higher than the human body can tolerate by systemic administration) to, or nearby, the treated segment in the coronary tree.[2–4]

A variety of pharmacological agents and device therapies have been introduced and tested in clinical trials as means to prevent or limit restenosis. The devices used for this application deliver the drugs either passively or actively. These devices are designed to deliver the drug either intraluminally or intramurally via several techniques. Among these are porous, microporous, and double-balloon catheters, hydrogel-coated balloons, microinjectors, and iontophoretic and electrophoretic catheters.[5–12]

Antithrombotic and antimitotic drugs, as well as gene therapy etc., could use liposomes, microparticles, microspheres, and viruses to enhance the efficiency of the delivery to the vessel wall.[13,14] Another approach to improving the efficiency of the drugs is to modify the active agents and prolong their residence time or release at the site of delivery. Another technique is to use agents that, as a consequence of extremely high affinity or covalent bonding, manifest prolonged activity even following a single delivery.

Local delivery of a wide range of agents using a number of devices has been associated with limited biologic and clinical efficacy despite high local concentrations achieved at the time of the delivery. Several potential explanations for this failure have been suggested, and include the following: the limited residence time of the delivered agent to the target segment due to washout, the lack of finding an effective agent, or an additional injury caused by the device that could not be corrected by the agent selected for treatment.[15]

Ionizing radiation delivered intraluminally via catheter-based systems has been shown to reduce neointima formation in animal models. Both beta and gamma emitters have demonstrated effectiveness and safety in the porcine coronary model of restenosis. We propose a new method to deliver the radiation to the

From Waksman R (ed.). *Vascular Brachytherapy, Third Edition.* Armonk, NY: Futura Publishing Co., Inc.; © 2002.

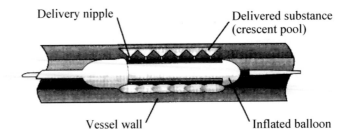

Delivery nipple

Delivered substance (crescent pool)

Vessel wall

Inflated balloon

Figure 1. The Infiltrator™ device used for delivery of [99m]Tc. Note the three rows of small nipples on its surface that are in contact with the vessel wall.

target site by directly injecting the radioisotopes into the vessel via a local delivery catheter system.[16–20]

The Delivery Device "The Irradiator"

The Infiltrator™ (Interventional Technologies, San Diego, CA), a true intramural drug depoting system, was selected as the delivery device. This is an angioplasty balloon catheter that has three rows of small nipples on its surface (Fig. 1). The nipples are in communication with small channels. During inflation of the balloon, the nipples penetrate the vessel wall. The radioisotopes can be delivered, through the channels of the nipples, into the vessel wall and into the adventitia. The device incorporates a low-pressure positioning balloon with a series of microminiaturized injector ports mounted on its surface and connected to a fluid flow channel independent of the inflation/deflation system. The balloon has been crafted such that the injector ports are recessed during maneuvering in the artery, but upon inflation these injector ports radially extend and enter the vessel wall. A multiplicity of individual ports facilitates injection of the drug over an area encompassing $360' \times 15$ mm (length). Microliter quantities of drug can therefore be delivered into the tunica media of the arterial wall in a precise fashion. Injection of the drug is accomplished in less than 10 seconds, without substantial intimal damage and with 90% plus delivery efficiency and minimal luminal washout.[21,22]

Prior studies with this device[21,22] have demonstrated that small amounts of fluid (0.4 mL) can be delivered into the vessel wall without acute or significant subacute damage to the wall and without escape of the substance. The coverage area can be increased with tandem applications. Including balloon up/down time, a single injection application is unlikely to take more than 60 seconds.

Liposome Encapsulation of Technetium 99m

The encapsulation of [99m]Tc (lipid bilayer vesicles) is hoped to improve residence time of the isotope in the coronary artery, and we have developed a method for rapid synthesis of such vesicles, suitable for use in radiopharmacy. Studies were performed using generator-produced [99m]Tc (as [99m]TcO$_4$) and commercially available liposome formulations of various chemistries and charge (positive, negative, or neutral) to determine efficacy and stability of encapsulation. Paper chromatography with detection by phosphor plate (Fuji) imaging and liquid scintillation was used to determine the amount of free technetium. Encapsulation efficiency and stability over the course of up to 6 hours (at room temperature) was determined. Since both positive membrane and neutral membrane samples were similarly efficient (and slightly more efficient than negatively charged) and the chemistry of the neutral membrane liposome is nontoxic, we decided to use the neutral formulation in subsequent animal (pig) studies in which coronary artery perfusion with both free pertechnetate and liposome-encapsulated ^{99m}Tc were done.[23]

Encapsulation efficiency of ^{99m}Tc was consistently on the order of 97% for all chemistries and there was no measurable leakage of ^{99m}Tc from the liposomes during the time course followed. Addition of blood to the prepared ^{99m}Tc liposomes, to simulate in vivo conditions, did not induce release of the ^{99m}Tc from the liposomes during a period of 4 hours However, as previous literature suggested, experiments indicate that addition of Sn^{+2} ions as a reducing agent to the liposome formulation before addition of the generator-produced ^{99m}TcO is required for complete encapsulation. Initial studies in animals demonstrated enhanced uptake of the labeled liposomes in the coronary artery relative to free ^{99m}TcO, with significant residual activity present after 2 hours. (Fig. 2). This approach demonstrates the rapidity by which ^{99m}Tc can be packaged for delivery to the perfusion site after percutaneous transluminal coronary angiography. The fact that liposome-encapsulated ^{99m}Tc resides at the perfusion site, with less washout than free ^{99m}Tc, suggests the possibility of using this same method for other isotopes.

Animal Studies and Detection of the Injected Isotope

The ability to deliver free ^{99m}Tc versus encapsulated ^{99m}Tc in liposomes directly into the arterial wall of 12 porcine coronaries was examined by injecting 0.4 mL of the isotopes (4 to 14 mCi) via the intra-aortic balloon catheter. Isotope uptake at different timepoints from injection was determined by gamma camera. Gamma camera images were detected at different timepoints following the injection of the isotope (Table 1). The isotope was delivered successfully to all treated vessels, and the animal tolerated the procedure. There was immediate washout of the free-^{99m}Tc isotope following the injection and the removal of the catheter. However, the liposome ^{99m}Tc remained in the vessel wall with up to 30% of its radioactivity at 20 minutes versus the control.

This study proves the principle that radionuclides can be delivered safely locally to the vessel wall. Liposome ^{99m}Tc resides longer in the vessel wall compared to free ^{99m}Tc. The challenge of this technology is to deliver locally into the adventitia cumulative doses of 10 to 15 Gy. These doses, based on the catheter-based systems, should be sufficient to reduce the intimal hyperplasia following balloon injury.

In another study[23] the liposome ^{99m}Tc with activities between 4 and 14 mCi was injected following balloon injury into the vessel wall. At 4 weeks following the treatment, the animals were killed and histomorphometric studies were performed. There was no evidence of reduction of neointima formation in the irradiated arteries. This can be explained by an insufficient dose to reside at the injured segment.

Another approach that does not require binding to liposomes is the use of ^{99m}Tc sestamibi. Activities of up to 80 mCi could be safe for this application, due to the short half-life of this isotope. The presence of the isotopes in other organs is still considered safe. The future of this technology depends on the ability to im-

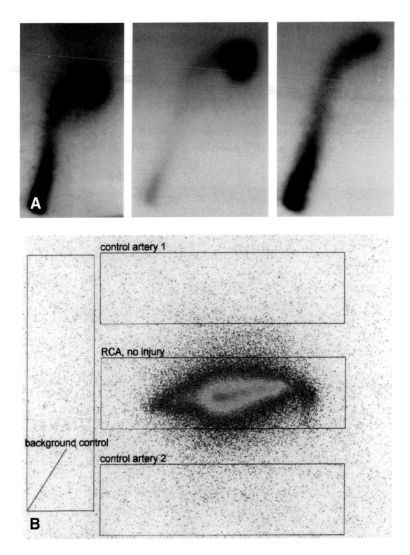

Figure 2. Detection of the ^{99m}Tc after injection intramurally to the coronary artery by phosphor plate (Fuji) imaging by paper chromatography 2 hours after injection **(A)**, and by gamma camera 20 minutes following injection **(B)**.

Table 1

Detection of Free ^{99m}Tc versus Liposome-^{99m}Tc by Gamma Camera*

Time from Injection (minutes)	0	5	10	20	40
Free ^{99m}Tc	100	20	10	5	0
Liposome-^{99m}Tc**	100	50	40	30	10

*After injection of 4 mCi of the isotope intramurally in the porcine coronary artery via the Infiltrator™.
**P value by paired t-test = 0.034.

prove the residence time, specifically in the target area, the media, the adventitia, and the residual plaque.

References

1. Wolinsky H, Taubman MD. Local delivery to the arterial wall: Pharmacologic and molecular approaches. In: Holmes DR Jr, Vlietstra RE (eds.): Coronary Balloon Angioplasty. Boston: Blackwell; 1994:156–186.
2. Riessen R, Isner JM. Prospects for site-specific delivery of pharmacologic and molecular therapies. J Am Coll Cardiol 1994;23:1234–1244.
3. Femando-Ortiz A, Meyer BJ, Mailhac A, et al. A new approach for local intravascular drug delivery: Iontophoretic balloon. Circulation 1994;89:1518–1522.
4. Rogers C, Karnovsky MJ, Edelman ER. Inhibition of experimental neointimal hyperplasia and thrombosis depends on type of vascular injury and the site of drug administration. Circulation 1993;88:1215–1221.
5. Hong MK, Wong C, Farb A, et al. Feasibility and drug delivery efficiency of a new balloon angioplasty catheter capable of performing simultaneous local drug delivery. Coron Artery Dis 1993;4:1023–1027.
6. Lambert CR, Leone JE, Rowland SM. Local drug delivery catheters: Functional comparison of porous and microporous designs. Coron Artery Dis 1993;4:469–475.
7. Plante S, Dupuis G, Mongeau CJ, Durand P. Porous balloon catheters for local delivery: Assessment of vascular damage in a rabbit iliac angioplasty model. J Am Coll Cardiol 1994;24:820–824.
8. Leung W-H, Kaplan AV, Grant GW, et al. Local delivery of antithrombin agent by an infusion balloon catheter reduces platelet deposition at the site of balloon angioplasty. Coron Artery Dis 1991;2:699–706.
9. Santoian EC, Gravanis MB, Anderberg, et al. Use of a porous infusion balloon in swine coronary arteries: Low pressure minimizes arterial damage [abstract]. Circulation 1992;86(suppl 11):591.
10. Rasheed Q, Cacchione JG, Berry J, et al. Local intramural drug delivery using an infusion balloon following angioplasty in normal and atherosclerotic vessels. Cathet Cardiovasc Diagn 1994;31:240–245.
11. Nabel EG, Yang Z, Liptay S, et al. Recombinant platelet-derived growth factor B gene expression in porcine arteries induces intimal hyperplasia in vivo. J Clin Invest 1993;91:1822–1829.
12. Wolinsky H, Thung SN. Use of a perforated balloon catheter to deliver concentrated heparin into the wall of the normal canine artery. J Am Coll Cardiol 1990;15:475–481.
13. Simons M, Edelman ER, DeKeyser J-L, et al. Anti-sense c-myb oligonucleotides inhibit intimal arterial smooth muscle cell accumulation in vivo. Nature 1992;359:67–70.
14. Shi Y, Fard A, Vemani P, Zalewski A. C-myc antisense oligomers reduce neointima formation in porcine coronary arteries [abstract]. J Am Coll Cardiol 1994;23:395A.
15. Rome JJ, Shayani V, Flugelman MY, et al. Anatomic barriers influence the distribution of in vivo gene transfer into the arterial wall. Arterioscler Thromb 1994;14:148–161.
16. Waksman R, Robinson KA, Crocker IR, et al. Endovascular low dose irradiation inhibits neointima formation after coronary artery balloon injury in swine: A possible role for radiation therapy in restenosis prevention. Circulation 1995;91:1533–1539.
17. Wiedermann JG, Marboe C, Schwartz A, et al. Intracoronary irradiation reduces restenosis after balloon angioplasty in a porcine model. J Am Coll Cardiol 1994;23:1491–1498.
18. Mazur W, Ali MN, Dabaghi SF, et al. High dose rate intracoronary radiation suppresses neointimal proliferation in the stented and ballooned model of porcine restenosis. Int J Radiat Oncol Biol Phys 1996;36:777–788.
19. Verin V, Popowski Y, Urban P, et al. Intra-arterial beta irradiation prevents neointimal hyperplasia in a hypercholesterolemic rabbit restenosis model. Circulation 1995;92:2284–2290.
20. Waksman R, Robinson KA, Crocker IR, et al. Intracoronary low dose beta irradiation inhibits neointima formation after coronary artery balloon injury in the swine restenosis model. Circulation 1995;92:3025–3031.

21. Barath P, Popov A, Dillehay GL, et al. Infiltrator angioplasty balloon catheter: A device for combined angioplasty and intramural site-specific treatment. Cathet Cardiovasc Diagn 1997;41:333–341.
22. Pavlides GS, Barath P, Maginas A, et al. Intramural drug delivery by direct injection within the arterial wall: First clinical experience with a novel intracoronary delivery-infiltrator system. Cathet Cardiovasc Diagn 1997;41:287–292.
23. Karam LR, Zimmerman BE, Chan RC, Waksman R. Liposome encapsulation of ^{99m}Tc for use in intravascular brachytherapy. Advances in Cardiovascular Radiation Therapy 1998: Syllabus 33. Abstract 29.

## Chapter 26

Intravascular Red Light Therapy:

Long-Term Results from the Human Clinical Trial

Nicholas N. Kipshidze, MD, PhD,
Ivan DeScheerder, MD, PhD, Upendra Kaul, MD,
Victor Nikolaychik, MD, PhD, Harry Sahota, MD,
Martin B. Leon, MD, Jeffrey W. Moses, MD,
and Michael H. Keelan, Jr., MD

Introduction

The first coronary balloon angioplasty, performed by Andreas R. Gruentzig in 1977, introduced a new dimension to the field of interventional cardiology. Since then, percutaneous transluminal coronary angioplasty (PTCA) has offered an alternative to surgical treatment of patients with various forms of coronary artery disease. More than 1 million patients worldwide will undergo percutaneous interventions. The frequent appearance of restenosis (20 to 50%), however, significantly limits the long-term clinical benefits of this very well established procedure.

It is believed that restenosis following coronary interventions is the result of endothelial disruption, thrombus formation, vascular remodeling, and smooth muscle cell (SMC) migration and proliferation. Coronary stents provide luminal scaffolding that virtually eliminates elastic recoil and remodeling, and have been shown to reduce the likelihood of restenosis by approximately 30%. Stents, however, do not decrease myointimal hyperplasia and in fact lead to an increase in the proliferative comportment of restenosis. We have previously demonstrated that intravascular low-power red laser light therapy (IRLT) prevents restenosis in atherosclerotic rabbit and pig stented models.[1,2] An initial feasibility and safety study in humans was recently reported.[3] The objective of the study was to investigate the feasibility and safety of IRLT after coronary stenting in humans and to evaluate the short- and long-term clinical and angiographic follow-up. The study protocol was approved by ethics and academic review boards of the University Hospitals in Leuven, Belgium and the Batra Hospital and Medical Research Center, in New Delhi, India.

From Waksman R (ed.). *Vascular Brachytherapy, Third Edition*. Armonk, NY: Futura Publishing Co., Inc.; © 2002.

Intravascular Red Light Therapy

Equipment

The illumination system used in this study consisted of a 3.5F rapid-exchange balloon catheter with a proximal and distal marker. The balloon material was polyethylene of 2.5, 3, 3.5, and 4.0 mm in diameter with lengths of 20 and 30 mm. The catheter had fiber optics within the balloon, with a diffusion tip at the distal end to provide uniform illumination. Low-power red light was transmitted from a diode laser at an energy level of 10 mW. Minimal internal diameter of the guiding catheter was 6 F. The system used a CL illuminator, and the light delivery balloon catheters were manufactured by Global Therapeutics, Bromfield, Colorado.

Procedure

Between March 1996 and May 1997, 60 patients with de novo lesions received IRLT following stent implantation. All procedures were performed with the use of a 6F, 7F, and 8F guiding catheter system and a conventional balloon angioplasty technique using a rapid-exchange balloon catheter of appropriate diameter. Following predilation, the segment was illuminated for 1 minute by use of a CL illuminator balloon of the same dimension used during PTCA. During illumination, the balloon was filled with the diluted contrast medium and was inflated at low pressures less than 4 atm, following which the standard stenting procedure with high-pressure dilatation was performed. Illumination with the CL illuminator with two 1-minute doses was performed after stenting. All patients were treated with heparin during the procedure to keep the activated clotting time above 300 seconds. Aspirin, 325 mg per day, was given to all patients indefinitely, and ticlopidine, 250 mg twice daily, was administered for 4 weeks. Oral anticoagulants were not used in this cohort of patients. Patients aged greater than 40 years undergoing angioplasty of one of the native coronary arteries because of angina were eligible for the study. The target lesion was required to have greater than 50% diameter stenosis as determined with quantitative coronary angiography (QCA), to be less than 45 mm long, and to be located in a vessel with more than 2-mm reference diameter. Patients with myocardial infarction, densely calcified lesions, or those requiring stents greater than 40 mm in length were not included in the study. Patients' baseline medical characteristics are presented in Table 1. Indications for stent placement were those currently used in many institutions, and included: (1) suboptimal angiographic results with a significant residual stenosis and (2) bail-out situations following balloon angioplasty.

Clinical and Angiographic Follow-Up

Patients or their physicians were contacted by telephone at 1, 3, and 6 months after the procedure. Clinical examination, 12-lead electrocardiogram, and exercise stress testings were performed at 3 and 6 months before the second coronary angiography at 6 months. When prompted by recurrent symptoms or signs of ischemia, the follow-up angiography was done before the 6-month follow-up. All angiograms were analyzed with the QCA analysis system. Restenosis was considered

Table 1

Clinical Characteristics

Age	62.5±8.5
Male	82%
Hyperlipidemia	49%
Diabetes mellitus	16%
Previous MI	40%
Hypertension	68%
Smoking history	42%

MI=myocardial infarction.

to have occurred if the percent-diameter stenosis was greater than 50%. The immediate luminal gain was defined as the minimal luminal diameter immediately after the procedure minus the minimal luminal diameter before the procedure. Late luminal loss was defined as the minimal luminal diameter immediately after the procedure minus the minimal luminal diameter at follow-up. The late loss index was defined as the late luminal loss divided by the immediate luminal gain.

Endpoints

A successful procedure was defined as one resulting in less than 30% residual stenosis after the procedure, and successful illumination of the arterial segments subjected to stent implantation without acute myocardial infarction, bypass surgery, or stent thrombosis within the first 25 days after the procedure. The primary endpoints were angiographic restenosis, late loss, and late loss index. Secondary endpoints were clinical restenosis, target lesion revascularization, death, or myocardial infarction.

Statistical Analysis

All data were recorded on standardized forms, entered into a computerized database, and expressed as mean ± standard deviation. Since no concurrent group of nonstented patients were included for analysis, the only comparison that was tested was the preprocedure minimal luminal diameter versus the postprocedure minimal luminal diameter and at 6 months' follow-up, for which the paired tests were used. All tests of significance were two-tailed and values of less than 0.05 were considered to indicate statistical significance.

Results

Immediate Results

Baseline angiographic characteristics of the 60 patients who participated in the study are presented in Tables 1 and 2. IRLT was delivered successfully with no patient developing ischemia, arrhythmia, coronary spasm, or any other major

Table 2

Angiographic Characteristics

Location of target lesion	
LAD	48
RCA	9
CX	6
Reference vessel	2.0–4.5 mm
Lesion length	12.6±6.5 mm
Type B and C	84%
Diffuse disease	26%

LAD = left anterior descending; RCA = coronary artery; CX = circumflex.

complication during the procedure (Table 3). In none of the cases was IRLT interrupted. The mean minimal luminal diameter after the procedure was 2.74±0.39, and the mean residual percent-diameter stenosis after the procedure was 7±22%. There was no instance of acute or subacute stent thrombosis. In-hospital events are presented in Tables 3 and 4 for both groups of patients. There were two vascular complications (hematomas); however, none of them required a transfusion or emergency surgery.

Follow-Up

All patients were clinically evaluated at 3 months. Two patients presented with symptoms suggesting restenosis, which was documented by coronary angiography done at 3 and 4 months, respectively. Both patients required angioplasty, rotational atherectomy, and balloon angioplasty. Fifty-one patients from this group underwent coronary angiography at 6 months (Table 4). Six patients developed angiographic evidence of restenosis on follow-up, 5 of whom were asymptomatic, with only 3 having a positive treadmill test. Four patients who developed restenosis had 2.5-mm-diameter stents implanted. The other two patients had long lesions and they required double or triple stent implantation. Three patients had distal diffused lesions with thrombus before the procedure. Except for

Table 3

Procedural Results

Procedural success	100%
In-hospital events	
Mortality	0
Subacute closure	0
MI	0
ER CABG	0
Vascular complications	2

MI = myocardial infarction; ER CABG = emergency coronary artery bypass graft.

Table 4

Angiographic Follow-Up in 53 Patients Following IRLT and Stenting

	All patients 2.0–4.5 mm	Arteries >3.0 mm	Arteries 2.5–3.0	Arteries <2.5
Number of patients	53	17	28	9
Reference vessel (mm)	2.81±0.76	3.10±0.59	2.86±0.61	2.49±0.41
MLD before (mm)	1.07±0.46	1.02±0.61	1.1±0.48	1.1±0.63
MLD after (mm)	2.74±0.39	2.98±0.57	2.68±0.68	2.46±0.75
MLD at 6 months (mm)	2.38±0.45	2.73±0.61	2.18±0.51	1.84±0.48
Late loss (mm)	0.46±0.68	0.25±0.31	0.50±0.53	0.62±0.35
Late loss index	0.28	0.12	0.31	0.45
Restenosis	8(15%)	0(0%)	4(14%)	4(44%)

IRLT = intravascular red light therapy; MLD = minimal luminal diameter.

one patient in whom angiography showed total occlusion of the stented segment, all the other patients' arteries remained patent, with a mean luminal diameter at the late follow-up of 2.28±0.45 and a mean residual stenosis of 28.6±19.2%. The late loss for the entire cohort was 0.46±0.68 mm, and late loss index was 0.28±0.54. There were three patients with negative late loss and eight patients with less than 10% diameter stenosis at follow-up. At 10.9±3.5 months' clinical follow-up, the survival rate free of myocardial infarction, bypass surgery, or revascularization of the target lesion was 90.5%. Five patients underwent repeat angioplasty for in-stent restenosis. None of the patients developed complications or an illness that could be related to the effects of low-power laser light therapy.

Discussion

Vascular Effect of Low-Power Laser

Interest in the interactions between light and the vascular wall dates to the beginning of the last century. In 1919, Adler[4] first demonstrated photorelaxation of the vascular SMCs. In 1955, Furchgott et al[5] showed that interaction of low-power light and smooth muscle of the vascular wall could result in a reduction of the muscular tone. With the first applications of the laser irradiation in biology and medicine, Steg et al[6] demonstrated endothelium-independent relaxation of rabbit aortic SMC following laser irradiation at 632 nm. These findings were confirmed by others.[7,8] Gal et al[9] documented that laser light induced vascular relaxation in vivo. They were able to reverse pharmacologically induced spasm of rabbit iliac arteries and document it angiographically. In 1993 Van Breugel and Bar[10] demonstrated that it is possible to photobiomodulate fibroblasts in vitro. By varying the energy levels, the authors were able to stimulate or inhibit the cell growth in vitro. Deckelbaum et al[11] documented that laser irradiation at 530 nm inhibits SMC migration in vitro. In 1985, one of the present authors and his colleagues[12] studied the interaction of low-power laser/tissue interaction, and later they demonstrated that intravascular low-power red light inhibits SMC proliferation and restenosis following balloon angioplasty in the atherosclerotic rabbit model.[1] These studies were confirmed by DeScheerder et al[2] in a pig stented model. The authors were able to prevent adverse stent-induced changes including SMC migration and proliferation documented by QCA, planimetric, and histologic data. Although the precise mechanisms by which low-power laser irradiation prevents restenosis have not been clearly identified, reduction of vascular reactivity, stimulation of endothelial repair, followed by inhibition of SMC migration are potential mechanisms.

One of the possible mechanisms of the stimulative effect of low-power laser irradiation on endothelial reproduction could be enhanced release of the different growth factors. In vitro experiments in our laboratory indicated that low-power laser irradiation of human SMCs and fibroblasts in cultured media, using a dosage similar to that used in humans, resulted in significant increase of secretion of vascular endothelial growth factor (VEGF) measured by sandwich enzyme immunoassay technique (Fig. 1). It was also demonstrated that SMC conditioned media stimulated endothelial cell growth in a dose-response manner. This may create a spatial gradient of VEGF towards denuded area following balloon injury, permitting endothelial cell migration and proliferation. The precise mechanism of increased production of the VEGF is unknown; however, it may be a response to light-induced cell hypoxia involving nitric oxide (NO) synthase pathway.

Nitric oxide is involved in promoting reendothelialization, preventing platelet and leukocyte adherence, and inhibiting cellular proliferation. A decline in NO production after PTCA induces the vascular SMC overgrowth.

Interestingly, several authors have reported elevated levels of cyclic GMP (cGMP) in blood vessels exposed to UV or blue light in vitro,[8,13–17] in which the level of cGMP correlated with the degree of vasorelaxation.[13] Chaundry et al speculated that light absorption by vascular tissue leads to either activation of guanylate cyclase or inhibition of its hydrolysis by phosphodiesterase.[8] They have also postulated that direct light absorption by the heme of guanylate cyclase is not the mechanism for the increase of cGMP level. They have investigated whether NOS might be the photoactivating enzyme for photovasorelaxation. However, two NO inhibitors, N-monomethyl-L-arginine (NMMA) and N-amino-L-arginine (NAA),

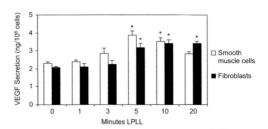

Figure 1. Vascular endothelial growth factor (VEGF) secretion in cell culture; laser treatment results in VEGF secretion. Smooth muscles and fibroblasts were subjected to low-power laser irradiation (LPLI) treatment for 1 to 20 minutes. The untreated cells were used as controls (0). The amount of VEGF secreted in the tissue culture medium was quantified using an ELISA kit from R&D Systems (Minneapolis, MN, USA). The results are expressed as ng/10^6 cells (Y-axis). Error bars show the SD from at least three experiments. A statistically significant increase at 5, 10, and 20 minutes and at 5, 10, and 20 minutes of treatment with LPLI can be seen in smooth muscle cells and fibroblasts, respectively. (*=$P<0.001$ and **=$P<0.01$).

did not alter UV-induced relaxation in vitro, indicating that NO was not activated. Similarly, Goud et al[17] showed that photorelaxation is not attenuated by inhibition of the NO-cGMP pathway.

Our recent in vivo experiments in an atherosclerotic rabbit model, however, do not correspond with these observations; these studies demonstrate significant overexpression of iNOS and an increase of vascular cGMP levels after endoluminal laser irradiation versus uninjured control.[18] This finding corresponds with previous in vitro observations.[18,19] Lovren and Triggle[19] postulated that photovasorelaxation is mediated via a NO/cGMP–dependent, and perhaps, direct light activation of potassium channels. Morimoto et al[20] demonstrated that vascular relaxation by pulsed-UV light in vitro is partially related to NO. In control uninjured arteries we observed a very low level of iNOS expression, and this was due to the atherosclerotic changes of the vessel wall. Interestingly, balloon dilatation did not induce iNOS. Steady-state levels of cGMP are the products of the rate of synthesis stimulated by NO and the rate of degradation by phosphodiesterase (PDE). This balance appears to be differentially influenced by balloon injury. Balloon + laser treatment, however, tended to restore the expression of iNOS.

Consistent with this model, endoluminal low-dose laser irradiation demonstrated enhanced reendothelialization and, subsequently, a reduction of neointimal hyperplasia in balloon-injured arteries in a rabbit model.

Comparison with Previous Stent Implantation Studies

Freedom from the major adverse events including myocardial infarction, coronary artery bypass surgery, or target vessel revascularization was seen in 90% of patients at 1 year. These results exceed the results from the BENESTENT I and II Trials,[21,22] as well as the stent group in the STRESS Trial,[23] despite the fact that the patient population in the IRLT Study contained 14 patients with 2.5-mm-diameter stents. Moreover, angiographic success was even more dramatically improved with restenosis of 0% in BENESTENT/STRESS equivalent lesions (0% versus 31%, 22%, and 13%) (Table 5). Compared to reports with the second generation of stents,[24] the restenosis and target lesion revascularization was similarly reduced by IRLT (0% versus 12%, 10%, 10%, and 12%). Also, the late luminal loss and late loss index compares favorably with the values of 0.38 and 0.12,

Table 5

Clinical and Angiographic Follow-Up in STRESS/BENESTENT Equivalent Lesions (n=21)

	IRLT=Stent	STRESS	BENESTENT I	BENESTENT II
Angiographic restenosis	0%	31.6%	22%	13%
Freedom from major adverse clinical events	100%	80.5%	82.6%	86%

IRLT = intravascular red light therapy.

respectively, reported in the treated group of the catheter-based radiation therapy study reported recently by Teirstein et al.[24] These figures are lower than the late luminal loss reported in the BENESTENT[21,22] and STRESS[23] Trials and more recent clinical studies.[25] Although this study has no control arm, the long-term follow-up angiograms in 75% of the patients demonstrate diameter stenosis less than 30%, suggesting that this mode of therapy might be useful in limiting neointimal hyperplasia following stent implantation.

Conclusion

This study reports a new treatment in humans with clinical and angiographic follow-up to 6 months. It demonstrates that intravascular illumination with the low-power red laser light using a catheter-based system is feasible and can be performed safely with no procedural complications or in-hospital adverse events. A large randomized study is under way to further evaluate the clinical efficacy of this new modality of treatment.

References

1. Kipshidze M, Sahota H, Komorowski R, et al. Photoremodeling of arterial wall reduces restenosis after balloon angioplasty in an atherosclerotic rabbit model. J Am Coll Cardiol 1998;31:1152–1157.
2. DeScheerder I, Wang K, Zhou XR, et al. Intravascular low power red laser light as an adjunct to coronary stent implantation evaluated in a porcine coronary model. J Invas Cardiol 1998;10:269–273.
3. Kipshidze NN, DeScheerder I, Arie S, et al. Intravascular red light therapy: The first human clinical experiences. Circulation 1997;96:I649.
4. Adler L. Uber Lichtwirkungen auf uberlebende glattmuskelige Organe. Arch Exp Pathol Pharmakol 1919;85:152–177.
5. Furchgott RF, Sleator W Jr, McCaman MW, et al. Relaxation of arterial strips by light, and influence of drugs on this photodynamic effect. J Pharmacol Exp Ther 1955;113:22.
6. Steg PG, Gal D, Rongione AJ, et al. Effect of argon laser irradiation on rabbit aortic smooth muscle: Evidence for endothelium-independent contraction and relaxation. Cardiovasc Res 1988;22:747–753.
7. Steg PG, Rongione AJ, Gal D, et al. Pulsed ultraviolet laser irradiation produces endothelium-independent relaxation of vascular smooth muscle. Circulation 1989;79:189–197.
8. Chaudhry M, Lynch M, Schomacker K, et al. Relaxation of vascular smooth muscle induced by low- power laser irradiation. Photochem Photobiol 1992;58:661–669.
9. Gal D, Chokshi SK, Mosseri M, et al. Percutaneous delivery of low-level laser energy versus histamine- induced spasm in an atherosclerotic Yucatan microswine. Circulation 1992;35:756–758.
10. Van Breugel HHFI, Bar PR. He-Ne laser irradiation affects proliferation of cultural rat Schwann cells in a dose dependent manner. J Neurocytol 1993;22:185–190.
11. Deckelbaum LI, Scott JJ, Stetz ML. Photoinhibition of smooth muscle cell migration: Potential therapy for restenosis. Lasers Surg Med 1993;13:4–11.
12. Petrosyan YS, Kipshidze NN, Putilin SA. Clinical experience with the use of laser radiation energy in the treatment of atherosclerosis. Cor Vasa 1989;31:118–127.
13. Karlsson JOG, Axelsson KL, Anderson RGG. Effects of ultraviolet radiation on the tension and the cyclic GMP level of bovine mesenteric arteries. Life Sci 1984;34:1555–1563.
14. Lincoln TM, Laks J, Johnson RM. Ultraviolet radiation-induced GMP decreases in tension and phosphorylase formation in rat aorta. J Cyclic Nucleotide Protein Phosphorylation Res 1985;10:525–533.
15. Furchgott RF, Jothianandau D. Endothelium dependent and independent vasodilation

involving cyclic GMP, relaxation induced by nitric oxide, carbon monoxide and light. Blood Vessels 1991;28:52–61.

16. Karlsson JOG, Axelsson K, Elwing J, Anderson RGG. Action specta of photoactivated cyclic GMP metabolism and relaxation in bovine mesenteric artery. J Cyclic Nucleotide Protein Phosphorylation Res 1986;11:155–166.

17. Goud C, Watts SW, Webb RC. Photorelaxation is not attenuated by inhibition of the nitric oxide-cGMP pathway. J Vasc Res 1996;33:299–307.

18. Kipshidze N, Keelan MH, Petersen JR, et al. Photoactivation of vascular iNOS and elevation of cGMP in vivo: Possible mechanism for photovasorelaxation. Photo Photobiol 2000;72:579–582.

19. Lovren F, Triggle CR. Involvement of nitrosothiols, nitric oxide and voltage-gated K+ channels in photorelaxation of vascular smooth muscle. Eur J Pharmacol 1998; 24:347(2–3):215–221.

20. Morimoto Y, Arai T, Matsuo H, Kikuchi M. Possible mechanisms of vascular relaxation induced by pulsed-UV laser. Photochem Photobiol 1998;68:388–393.

21. Serruys PW, de Jaegere P, Kiemeneij F, et al, for the Benestent Study Group. A comparison of balloon expandable stent implantation with balloon angioplasty in patients with coronary artery disease. N Engl J Med 1994;331:489–495.

22. Serruys PW, Emanuelsson H, van der Giessen W, et al, on behalf of the Benestent-II Study Group. Heparin-coated Palmaz-Schatz stents in human coronary arteries: Early outcome of the Benestent-II pilot study. Circulation 1996;93:412–422.

23. Fishman DL, Leon MB, Baim DS, et al, for the Stent Restenosis Investigators. A randomized comparison of coronary stent placement and balloon angioplasty in the treatment of coronary artery disease. N Engl J Med 1994;331:496–501.

24. Teirstein PS, Massullo V, Jani S, et al. Catheter based radiotherapy to inhibit restenosis after coronary stenting. N Engl J Med 1997;336:1697–1703.

25. Yokoi M, Kimura T, Mamasaki N, et al. Coronary stenting for STRESS/BENESTENT equivalent lesions: Comparison of four different types of stent. J Am Coll Cardiol 1998;31(suppl A):313.

## Chapter 27

Current Status of Photodynamic Therapy for the Prevention of Restenosis

Robert I. Grove, PhD, Ian Leitch, PhD, Steve Rychnovsky, PhD, and Jeffrey Walker, MD

Introduction

Electromagnetic energy in the form of ionizing radiation (brachytherapy) and in the use of light-activated drugs (photodynamic therapy [PDT]) has been investigated as a treatment for cancer.[1,2] Both approaches rely on the transmission of energy via the electromagnetic spectrum to generate free radicals in target cells. Free radicals are well known mediators of damage at the molecular level and cause the destruction of essential cell molecules. Ionizing radiation breaks linkages in the nucleic acids and induces a population of cells that is incapable of proliferating. PDT generates reactive oxygen species which inhibit cell proliferation by inducing apoptosis or cell suicide.[3–5] Because of this potential to inhibit cell proliferation, PDT may have a clinical benefit in the treatment of cardiovascular diseases that have a proliferative component such as restenosis.

Rat Restenosis Model Studies

The possibility that PDT could inhibit or prevent restenosis was initially investigated in the rat carotid model.[6–9] In these early studies, systemic administration of one of several different photoactive drugs was followed by carotid artery injury with a balloon denudation technique.[6–10] Visible light produced by an external light source was then used to activate the drug in the exposed carotid artery. The results demonstrated a dramatic PDT-induced prevention of intimal hyperplasia that resulted in inhibition of restenosis at 21 days.[6–9] Furthermore, PDT treatment was found to induce a profound depletion of artery wall smooth muscle cells within the first several days that correlated well with the more chronic inhibition of hyperplasia.[7,10] The data suggested that PDT inhibited restenosis by first reducing or eliminating the neointimal precursor cells from the vessel medial wall.

In addition to depleting cells in the vessel wall presumably by an apoptosis-mediated process,[5,7,10,11] further mechanistic studies indicated that PDT treat-

From Waksman R (ed.). *Vascular Brachytherapy, Third Edition.* Armonk, NY: Futura Publishing Co., Inc.; © 2002.

ment of vessel walls resulted in alterations in the collagenous extracellular matrix.[11,12] It was suggested that the alterations in extracellular matrix were due to reactive oxygen-mediated cross-linking of collagen components in the vessel wall.[12] These alterations were shown to inhibit migration of smooth muscle cells, strengthen the carotid artery as determined from burst pressure studies, facilitate reendothelialization of the vessel lumen, and promote healing of the injured vessel wall.[8,11] Six months following PDT in rats there was no evidence of side effects and PDT-treated arteries appeared normal.[7,13]

Swine Restenosis Model Studies

PDT was equally effective in inhibiting neointimal hyperplasia in swine models of restenosis. When swine femoral arteries were injured using atherectomy procedures, PDT significantly reduced intimal hyperplasia typical in that model.[14,15] Following local administration of the photosensitive drug Photofrin™ (QLT, Inc., Vancouver, BC, Canada), an optical fiber with a light-diffusing distal end was positioned endovascularly within a catheter at the atherectomy site to deliver the light dose. A saline flush was used to limit absorption by the intervening blood layer. At 21 days, PDT inhibited hyperplasia by approximately 90%.[14] In another swine model in which arteries were first subjected to angioplasty overstretch injuries, PDT using 5-aminolevulinic acid (ALA) inhibited restenosis in both iliac and coronary arteries.[16] Furthermore, a strong correlation was established in swine between induction of vessel wall acellularity at early time points and inhibition of intimal hyperplasia at 28 days.[16,17]

Clinical Studies

The dramatic results in rat and swine models suggested that PDT might be efficacious in the clinic. Since ALA was safe based on previous anticancer clinical studies,[18,19] a safety study was initiated using ALA in patients with advanced peripheral artery disease.[20] ALA was administered intravenously and after sufficient time to allow uptake into arterial tissues, a catheter device was used percutaneously to localize light to the target tissue. Eight arteries in seven elderly patients with advanced atherosclerotic lesions were treated and the results of the study suggested that PDT with ALA was safe.[20] A larger study is being planned to determine if PDT with ALA is efficacious for peripheral artery restenosis.

Miravant Preclinical Studies

Rat Carotid Model Studies

An intensive screening project was initiated at Miravant to identify new second generation photosensitive drugs with improved characteristics such as potency, rapid clearance, and low toxicity. In rat model studies using one of these new compounds (MV6401), near total depletion of carotid smooth muscle and adventitial cells was observed after external light (665 nm) administration (Fig. 1).[21] The depletion of vessel wall cells occurred as early as 1 to 3 days post-PDT treatment and was dose-dependent. At 21 days, the vessels were still largely devoid of

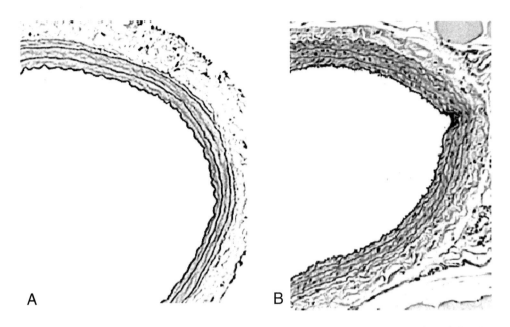

Figure 1. Transverse section (light microscopy) of a rat carotid artery at 3 days following **(A)** treatment with photodynamic therapy (PDT) (with MV6401 and light irradiation) and **(B)** light irradiation only (sham control). Note the depletion of vascular smooth muscle cells in the medial layer in the PDT section.

medial smooth muscle cells and, in addition, intimal hyperplasia was inhibited by greater than 90% (Fig. 2). The doses of MV6401and light required to induce vessel wall acellularity correlated well with doses required to inhibit restenosis. In other studies, MV6401 gave similar results when small light delivery catheters were used to administer endovascular light.

These dramatic PDT effects on rat arterial tissue did not appear to alter blood vessel function or cause deleterious effects in the animals. PDT-treated carotid arteries were patent, appeared to be in the process of reendothelializing, and the lumenal area was larger than in untreated controls (Fig. 2). These results are consistent with previous observations that depletion of the vessel wall cells did not cause side effects even after 6 months, and that reendothelialization and normalization of the treated arteries were rapid.[7,8,13]

Swine Model Studies

Initial PDT studies using endovascular light delivery catheters confirmed that MV6401 induced dose-dependent acellularity in normal swine iliac arteries.[22,23] The effects of PDT on the more acceptable swine coronary artery restenosis model were investigated in collaboration with Dr. Ron Waksman at MedStar Research Institute in Washington D.C. Requirements for interventional procedures at the coronary level are more rigorous compared with peripheral artery procedural requirements. Thus, it is important that endovascular light delivery catheters for the coronaries are guidewire-compatible and capable of delivering the required light dose in acceptably short periods of time. The Miravant en-

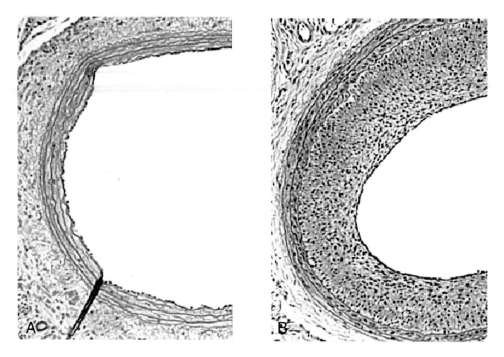

Figure 2. Carotid artery of a rat subjected to balloon deendothelialization injury followed by **(A)** treatment with PDT (MV6401 and light irradiation) and **(B)** light irradiation only (sham control). Note the absence of neointima in the PDT section at 21 days.

dovascular light delivery catheter was designed to meet these clinically relevant criteria.[23]

Acute studies with uninjured swine coronary arteries harvested at 3 days indicated that PDT using intravenous administration of MV6401 and the Miravant endovascular light delivery catheter depleted medial smooth muscle and adventitial cells (Fig. 3) with a dose-dependent mechanism. In sham control arteries irradiated with light alone, there was no evidence of depletion of intimal, medial, or adventitial cells.

In coronary arteries that were subjected to balloon overstretch injury and PDT, an overall inhibitory effect on restenosis was observed. Fourteen days after balloon injury, control arteries displayed extensive neointimal development as typically seen in this model,[24,25] while PDT with MV6401 dramatically inhibited intimal hyperplasia (Fig. 4). Administration of MV6401 in swine caused no detectable abnormalities in coronary artery patency, electrocardiography, heart rate, blood pressure, morbidity, or mortality. The light delivery catheters were also safe in that they tracked over the guidewire well[23] and did not cause heart function side effects.

Conclusions

A potential clinical role for PDT in preventing restenosis is supported by evidence from a number of preclinical studies where PDT safely decreased or prevented intimal hyperplasia. The magnitude of inhibition usually was on the order

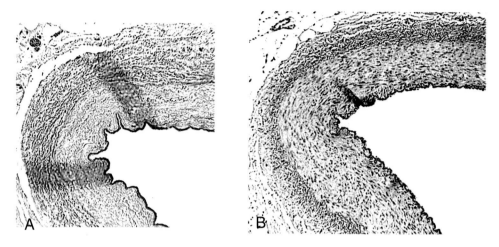

Figure 3. Transverse section of a swine coronary artery at 3 days following **(A)** treatment with PDT (MV6401 and light irradiation) and **(B)** endovascular light irradiation only (sham control). Note the depletion of vascular smooth muscle cells in the media and adventitial cells in the PDT section.

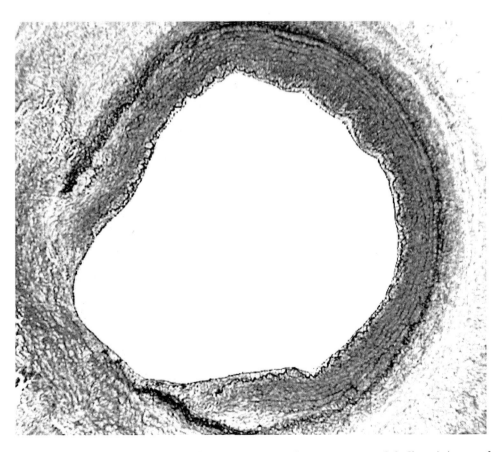

Figure 4. Coronary artery (LAD) of a swine subjected to an overstretch balloon injury and treated with the photosensitive drug MV6401 (2 mg/kg, IV) and endovascular light. Note the absence of neointima at 14 days after PDT.

of that seen in brachytherapy studies.[24–27] Furthermore, initial clinical studies in peripheral arteries suggested that PDT may be safe for cardiovascular indications.[20,28] This safety record is due in part to the use of nontoxic photosensitive compounds and a safer form of electromagnetic radiation (visible light). Thus, PDT may have advantages over brachytherapy for cardiovascular indications, including improved safety for patient and health care professionals, lack of requirements for additional personnel such as radiation safety officers and physicists, and fewer long-term side effects such as late stage thrombosis, aneurysmal formation, or tumor induction.

MV6401, a potent new photosensitive drug developed for the cardiovascular program at Miravant, effectively inhibited restenosis in rat and swine coronary models. The swine coronary PDT studies were performed using clinically relevant light delivery catheters specifically designed for the cardiovascular program. Although more work is needed, PDT with MV6401 and the Miravant light delivery catheter may have clinical utility in the prevention of post-angioplasty coronary restenosis as well as other forms of hyperproliferative vascular disease.

Acknowledgments: We would like to thank the following people for their technical contributions to this research: John Roessler, Dylan Bennett, Alistair Wilson, Van Caldwell, Heidi Nielsen, Mark Purter, Ross Heath, Edessa Diaz, Jennifer Barton, Dr. Christina Waters, Pamela Cates, Dr. Han Soo Kim, Dr. Hamid Yazdi, Rufus Seborn, and Tim Hunt.

References

1. Roberts DJH, Cairnduff F. Photodynamic therapy of primary skin cancer: A review. Br J Plastic Surg 1995;48:360–370.
2. Ackerman LV. The pathology of radiation effects on normal and neoplastic tissue. Am J Roentgenol Radium Ther Nucl Med 1972;114:447–459.
3. Weishaupt KR, Gomer CJ, Dougherty TJ. Identification of singlet oxygen as the cytotoxic agent in photoinactivation of a murine tumor. Cancer Res 1976;36:2326–2329.
4. Henderson BW, Dougherty TJ. How does photodynamic therapy work? Photochem Photobiol 1992;55:931–948.
5. Oleinick NL, Evans HH. The photobiology of photodynamic therapy: Cellular targets and mechanisms. Radiation Res 1998;150(suppl):S146-S156.
6. Ortu P, LaMuraglia GM, Roberts G, et al. Photodynamic therapy of arteries: A novel approach for treatment of experimental intimal hyperplasia. Circulation 1992; 85:1189–1196.
7. Grant WE, Speight PM, MacRobert AJ, et al. Photodynamic therapy of normal rat arteries after photosensitisation using disulphonated aluminum phthalocyanine and 5-aminolaevulinic acid. Br J Cancer 1994;70:72–78.
8. LaMuraglia GM, ChandraSekar NR, Flotte TJ, et al. Photodynamic therapy inhibition of experimental intimal hyperplasia: Acute and chronic effects. J Vasc Surg 1994; 19:321–331.
9. Nyamekye I, Anglin S, McEwan J, et al. Photodynamic therapy of normal and balloon-injured rat carotid arteries using 5-amino-levulinic acid. Circulation 1995;91:417–425.
10. Nyamekye I, Buonaccorsi G, McEwan J, et al. Inhibition of intimal hyperplasia in balloon injured arteries with adjunctive phthalocyanine sensitised photodynamic therapy. Eur J Vasc Endovasc Surg 1996;11:19–28.
11. Heckenkamp J, Leszczynski D, Schiereck J, et al. Different effects of photodynamic therapy and gamma-irradiation on vascular smooth muscle cells and matrix: Implication for inhibiting restenosis. Arterioscler Thromb Vasc Biol 1999;19:2154–2161.
12. Overhaus M, Heckenkamp J, Kossodo S, et al. Photodynamic therapy generates a matrix barrier to invasive vascular cell migration. Circ Res 2000;86:334–340.
13. Grant WE, Buonaccorsi G, Speight PM, et al. The effect of photodynamic therapy on the mechanical integrity of normal rabbit carotid arteries. Laryngoscope 1995;105:867–871.

14. Gonschior P, Gerheuser F, Fleuchaus M, et al. Local photodynamic therapy reduces tissue hyperplasia in an experimental restenosis model. Photochem Photobiol 1996;64:758–763.
15. Gonschior P, Vogel-Wiens C, Goetz AE, et al. Endovascular catheter-delivered photodynamic therapy in an experimental response to injury model. Basic Res Cardiol 1997;92:310–319.
16. Jenkins MP, Guonaccorsi GA, Mansfield R, et al. Reduction in the response to coronary and iliac artery injury with photodynamic therapy using 5-aminolaevulinic acid. Cardiovasc Res 2000;45:478–485.
17. Jenkins MP, Buonaccorsi G, MacRobert A, et al. Intra-arterial photodynamic therapy using 5-ALA in a swine model. Eur J Vasc Endovasc Surg 1998;16:284–291.
18. Regula J, MacRobert AJ, Gorchein A, et al. Photosensitisation and photodynamic therapy of oesophageal, duodenal, and colorectal tumours using 5-aminolaevulinic acid induced protoporphyrin IX: A pilot study. Gut 1995;36:67–75.
19. Webber J, Kessel D, Fromm D. Plasma levels of protoporphyrin IX in humans after oral administration of 5-aminolevulinic acid. J Photochem Photobiol B 1997;37:151–153.
20. Jenkins PM, Buonaccorsi GA, Raphael M, et al. Clinical study of adjuvant photodynamic therapy to reduce restenosis following femoral angioplasty. Br J Surg 1999;86:1258–1263.
21. Leitch IM, Nielsen H, Waters C, et al. Photodynamic therapy with the new photosensitizer drug MV6401 prevents neointima formation in balloon injured rat carotid arteries. Circulation 2000 (AHA abstracts) Circulation 2000;102(suppl II):A423.
22. Leitch IM, McElroy CA, Stephens PW, et al. Acute effects of endovascular photodynamic therapy using local intra-arterial delivery of the new photosensitizer MV6401 in balloon injured swine iliac arteries. Circulation 1999;100(suppl 1):A1697.
23. Grove RI, Rychnovsky S, Stephens P, et al. The Miravant light delivery device for photodynamic therapy. In: Waksman R, Serruys PW (eds.): Handbook of Vascular Brachytherapy, 2nd Edition. London: Martin Dunitz; 2000:176–182.
24. Waksman R. Endovascular beta radiation in the swine model. In: Waksman R (ed.): Vascular Brachytherapy, 2nd Edition. Armonk, NY: Futura Publishing Co., Inc.; 1999:273–286.
25. Waksman R. Intracoronary gamma irradiation studies in the swine model of restenosis. In: Waksman R (ed.): Vascular Brachytherapy, 2nd Edition. Armonk, NY: Futura Publishing Co., Inc., 1999:245–256.
26. Condado JA, Waksman R, Gurdiel O, et al. Long term angiographic and clinical outcome after percutaneous transluminal coronary angioplasty and intracoronary radiation therapy in humans. Circulation 1997;96:727–732.
27. Teirstein PS, Massullo V, Jani S, et al. Catheter based radiotherapy to inhibit restenosis after coronary stenting. N Engl J Med 1997;336:1697–1703.
28. Rockson SG, Lorenz DP, Cheong WF, et al. Photoangioplasty: An emerging clinical cardiovascular role for photodynamic therapy. Circulation 2000;102:591–596.

Part V

Stents and Radiation

The Calculation and Measurement of Radiation Dose Surrounding Radioactive Stents:

The Effects of Radionuclide Selection and Stent Design on Dosimetric Results

Charles W. Coffey, II, PhD, and Dennis M. Duggan, PhD

Introduction

Intravascular brachytherapy has been shown in clinical trials to be safe and effective for the treatment of restenosis of coronary arteries following percutaneous transluminal angioplasty. A variety of isotopes have been used, including high-energy photon emitters, such as ^{192}Ir, and beta emitters, such as ^{32}P, ^{90}Sr, ^{90}Y, and ^{188}Re, in a variety of forms including seed trains, wires, stents, and liquid-filled balloons. These isotopes fall into two groups: radioactive stents used as low dose rate, permanent implants, and catheter-based emitters used as high dose rate, temporary implants. Presently, all the radioactive stents used in clinical trials have contained ^{32}P, a beta emitter; to date, the catheter-based emitters have been much more successful.

Radioactive stents do have practical advantages over catheter-based emitters. First, the technique for implanting a stent is familiar to interventional cardiologists and is almost the same whether or not the stent is radioactive.[1] Second, since a radioactive stent is a permanent implant and is close to the lesion, its activity can be low and its emissions need not be very penetrating. That means that its use need not add significantly to the radiation exposure of any of the personnel in the catheterization laboratory. Third, again because it is a permanent implant, procedures for routinely removing the source, returning it to storage, and verifying safety after the treatment are not needed.

If radioactive stents are to be successful, two serious problems must be overcome. These problems have been reported in animal models and human clinical trials of radioactive stents, but they have also been observed in patients who received intravascular brachytherapy from catheter-based sources immediately after implantation of a cold stent. The first problem is edge restenosis,[2] or the "candy wrapper" effect. This restenosis 2 to 3 mm distal and proximal to a stent may be

From Waksman R (ed.). *Vascular Brachytherapy, Third Edition.* Armonk, NY: Futura Publishing Co., Inc.; © 2002.

due to the failure to deliver an adequate dose to those tissues after they have been injured by angioplasty and stent implantation. The second problem is delayed healing and thrombosis at the surface of the stent which may be partly due to excessive dose there.[3-7] Solving these problems requires evaluation and correlation of the physics parameters of the dose distribution with the suboptimal clinical results. As suggested by Carter and Fischell,[8] Surruys and Kay,[5] and Amols,[9] it also requires optimization of stent design for radiation dose delivery and evaluation of alternative radionuclides and dosing strategies.

This chapter serves as a review of the dosimetric issues involved in the calculation and measurement of radiation-absorbed dose and subsequent dose distributions surrounding radioactive stents, and as an overview of the dosimetric issues associated with the radionuclide selection and stent design which may result in improvements in radiation dose delivery. It is believed that, for radioactive stents to be clinically successful, the radionuclide and its distribution on the stent must have the following properties: the activity must be high enough everywhere on the stent to achieve the threshold dose rate necessary to prevent restenosis,[3,5,10] even at the stent margins,[2] yet the lifetime dose should be minimal[11] to prevent late injury to the vessel wall. Since neointimal hyperplasia occurs only in the first few weeks after angioplasty,[12-14] the half-life should be no more than a few weeks. The penetration of the emitted particles must be sufficient[15] to reach the target cells,[5] while depositing minimal surface dose. The emitted particles should also penetrate calcified plaque, with its higher density and effective atomic number, in the lumen well enough to reach target cells on the other side.[16] Yet the penetration beyond the target cells must also be minimal to avoid normal tissues there. Finally, to make it possible to develop a quality assurance program of the kind that is standard practice in conventional brachytherapy[17] and recommended for intravascular brachytherapy,[18] the stent should emit particles that are sufficiently penetrating so that the activity (or at least the activity relative to a standard) can be verified with conventional technologies.[19]

Background and Significance

Percutaneous transluminal coronary angioplasty (PTCA) is an interventional procedure in cardiology to open obstructed (stenotic) coronary arteries. However, restenosis[20] is a significant problem associated with balloon angioplasty procedures. It has been reported that two distinct processes are likely to contribute to restenosis following PTCA procedures: vessel constriction and excessive neointimal proliferation (hyperplasia).[12,21,22] Stents[23] have been shown to reduce the vessel constriction (remodeling) process when compared to balloon angioplasty alone, but to increase neointimal hyperplasia perhaps secondary to chronic vessel wall irritation. Recently, catheter-based endovascular radiation has been demonstrated to inhibit this proliferation after angioplasty in both animal studies[24-26] and human clinical trials[27-30] for catheter-based gamma and beta sources.

Fischell et al[31,32] have suggested that if stents could be made radioactive then perhaps both processes associated with restenosis, remodeling and neointimal hyperplasia, could be reduced. Several investigators[6,7,33-36] have reported using radioactive stents to prevent smooth muscle cell proliferation and neointimal hyperplasia in rabbit, canine, and pig models using ^{32}P, ^{90}Y, and ^{198}Au. Safety and feasibility study results with ^{32}P radioactive stents[37-39] have now been reported in human clinical trials in Europe. Albiero et al[40] have recently reported the dose dependence of the response at 6-month follow-up of 82 patients with ^{32}P radioactive stents.

Although human clinical trials continue, the exact tissue and cellular targets remain unknown[41] and radiobiological studies continue on the response of vascular smooth muscle cells and endothelial cells to radiation.[42,43] The present aim in intravascular brachytherapy remains to deliver sufficient radiation to the angioplasty site without exceeding tissue tolerance. Although these tissue tolerances are not well defined, recent studies have demonstrated that vascular radiation therapy from both high dose rate catheter-based systems[25,26] and low dose rate radioactive stents[44,45] delay the recovery of arterial luminal surface reendothelialization in animal models. Taylor et al[46,47] found delayed healing within canine coronary stents implanted with ^{32}P stents and incomplete reendothelialization in vessels with high-activity (high dose) ^{32}P stents; these data also suggested that the delay in reendothelialization is dose-dependent. Carter et al[3] also reported a dose-dependent formation of an atheromatous neointima in the porcine coronary model using ^{32}P radioactive stents. Vodovotz et al[48] recently published results from a porcine balloon-injury model which demonstrated an effect of intracoronary radiation on thrombus formation and thrombus morphology. Their findings also suggest that healing of irradiated arteries is delayed.

The potential for increased occurrence of intracoronary thrombus in patients undergoing endovascular brachytherapy[41] is critical because it can lead to acute myocardial infarction, ventricular arrhythmia, and sudden death. Two recent reports on human clinical trials[49,50] indicate a higher incidence (9.1% versus 1.2% in one trial and 6.6% versus 1.5% in the other) of sudden late thrombotic coronary occlusion after intracoronary radiotherapy versus a placebo following PTCA. In a recent editorial Waksman[51] has coined the phase "late, late thrombosis" for the higher incidence of late occlusion seen in the intravascular brachytherapy setting. Costa et al[50] suggested that the variables that might be involved include: overlapping (nonradioactive) stents, unhealed dissections, less than optimal antiplatelet therapy, and delay of the healing process by radiation. Waksman[51] lists the following as potential causes of late thrombosis after radiation: delayed reendothelialization, fibrin deposition and platelet recruitment,[52] impaired vasoreactivity and spasm, tissue erosion around a stent, and unhealed dissections. Whatever the exact causes, it is believed that higher radiation doses to the vascular tissue, especially very close to the surface of radioactive stents, exacerbate the delayed reendothelialization effect of intracoronary radiation.

Several clinics[37,39,40] have proven that use in humans of stents with 0.75 to 6 μCi of ^{32}P is both feasible and safe: for example, Albiero et al[40,53] treated 91 lesions in 82 patients with ^{32}P stents, with activities ranging from 0.75 to 12 μCi. They reported a dose-dependent decrease in intrastent restenosis. However, they also observed intralesion restenosis across all dose groups because of late lumen loss at the stent edges. They coined the term "candy-wrapper" to describe this new restenosis pattern. They attributed this edge restenosis to the combination of the rapid fall-off in the dose just beyond the ends of the stent and an overly aggressive stent implantation strategy which included the use of an overstretched balloon with an excessive length and diameter. It is presumed that this effect was also present in animal models but was never appreciated. Since the first observation of edge restenosis, others[54,55] have reported the same effect in human trials of ^{32}P stents. Furthermore, edge restenosis is not limited to patients treated with radioactive stents; it has also been reported in several human trials of catheter-based ^{192}Ir sources,[4,56,57] including a recent follow-up analysis of the patients in the SCRIPPS trial.[2] Honda et al[58] also observed edge restenosis in porcine coronary arteries treated with a balloon filled with the beta emitter [188]Re. The conclusions drawn from all these studies of edge restenosis in arteries with stents (both radioactive and nonradioactive) after treatment with gamma or beta emitters were that the effect is due to intimal hyperplasia and insufficient dose at the margins of the stent combined with suboptimal antiplatelet therapy.[4]

In a recent editorial, Serruys and Kay[5] concluded that, due to balloon oversizing, a dose adequate to inhibit neointimal proliferation must be delivered as far as 2.7 mm distal and proximal to a radioactive stent, and that ^{32}P stents with activities just high enough to inhibit neointimal proliferation within the stent deliver an insufficient dose to tissues beyond the ends of the stent. They suggested that various modifications of the system used for stent implantation and intravascular brachytherapy must be considered, including: a square-shouldered balloon, a self-expanding radioactive stent, a radioactive stent with ends colder than the middle, a radioactive stent with ends hotter than the middle, a hybrid of a radioactive stent and a catheter-based radioactive source, and a photon-emitting stent. They note that all of the last three modifications would increase the dose at the stent edges, either by increasing the activity near the ends or increasing the penetration of the radiation. This would be an example of a strategy, suggested by Lansky et al,[2] that directs radiation treatment to the stented segment while including the margins of the stent.

Waksman[51] warned that with any novel technique, like intravascular brachytherapy, unexpected complications may dampen early high expectations and result in pessimism and skepticism. He concluded that only time, experience, and complete data analysis will determine the utility of any new procedure. As investigations continue into the radiobiological and dosimetric causes of the complications associated with intravascular brachytherapy, the redesign of sources for radioactive stenting to give a better dose distribution in the arterial wall may help to alleviate the suboptimal clinical results presented to date.

Materials and Methods

Experimental Methods

At present, there have been dosimetric evaluation and subsequent animal-model experiments using ^{32}P, ^{90}Y, [198]Au, [103]Pd, and [48]V radioactive stents. Characteristics of each radionuclide suggested for use in radioactive stents are seen in Table 1. To date, only beta-emitting ^{32}P stents have been used in human clinical investigations. These radioactive stents are prepared, in general, using three methodologies; neutron activation of a target species in the stent material, the ion implantation of the radioactive species into the stent material, or coating of the radioactive species onto the stent material.

Investigators[59–63] have reported using thermoluminescent techniques, scintillation counter methods, extrapolation ionization chamber measurements, and BANG gel dosimetry to determine absorbed dose surrounding beta-emitting sources. However, because of the anticipated presence of high surface doses and large dose gradients associated with radioactive stents, other investigators[7,64,65] have chosen

Table 1

Characteristics of Radionuclides of Consideration for Use in IVB
Radioactive Stenting Procedures

Radionuclide	Decay Product of Interest	Maximum Energy (keV)	Half-life
^{32}P	Beta$^-$	1710	14.3 days
^{48}V	Beta$^+$	690	16.0 days
^{90}Y	Beta$^-$	2280	64.1 hours
^{198}Au	Beta$^-$	960	2.7 days
^{103}Pd	photon	21	17.0 days
^{125}I	photon	35	60.1 days
^{131}Cs	photon	30	9.7 days

radiochromic media because both high- and low-sensitivity, high-resolution films are commercially available. These investigators have presented methodologies for radiochromic media use for beta-emitting stent dosimetry; to date, our laboratory has performed dose measurement experiments using radiochromic media for beta-emitting stents, ^{32}P and ^{90}Y, and for low-energy photon-emitting ^{103}Pd stents.

When performing absolute dose and relative dose distribution measurements for either beta-emitting stents or low-energy photon-emitting stents, data must be measured in very precise geometries. Hence, there is a need to develop and fabricate very geometrically accurate water (tissue) equivalent phantoms. Various phantom designs and their use have been described by various investigators.[7,64,66] Figure 1 and Figure 2 show representative phantoms used in our laboratory for the assessment of absolute and relative dose surrounding radioactive stents. The phantoms shown can be used to determine absolute dose, radial dose distributions from the central axis of the stent, and longitudinal dose distributions along the long axis of the stent.

Dose Calculations

Various early investigators[67–70] have studied a calculational concept known as the dose point kernel (DPK) for determination of dose in water from beta-emitting sources. NCRP Report No. 108,[71] which explains this DPK methodology, contains equations for calculating dose to a target volume from beta-emitting point sources uniformly distributed throughout a finite right circular cylinder. Prestwich et al[72,73] have presented results of DPK calculations for the dose distributions surrounding a circular cylinder with ^{32}P point sources uniformly distributed on its surface in order to obtain information relative to the clinical use of radioactive stents. One of the present authors[65] has extended the DPK models of Berger[68] and Brookeman et al[70] to include the dose distributions radially from ^{32}P stents, modeled as ^{32}P point sources uniformly distributed throughout a thin finite-length cylindrical shell, as a function of distance along the stent long axis.

Janicki et al[74] calculated the near-field dose of a ^{32}P impregnated vascular stent using the ^{32}P point dose kernel to numerically simulate the specific wire mesh geometry of a Palmaz-Schatz stent. A later report by Janicki et al[66] introduced a point dose kernel model which allowed for the calculation of doses from

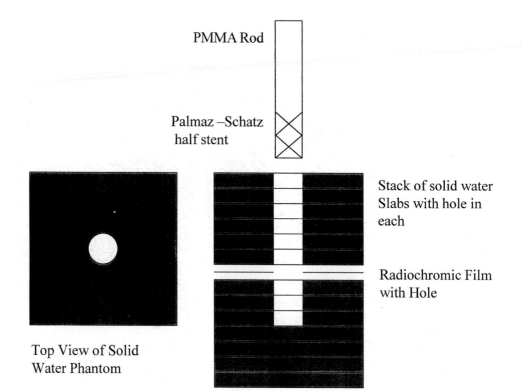

Figure 1. A diagram of the solid water phantom used for exposing radiochromic film. Radiochromic films with holes in their centers were placed in between sheets of solid water with holes in their centers. The holes were aligned and the stent placed in the hole. Note that the lumen of the stent (Palmaz-Schatz half-stent) was mounted on a nearly tissue-equivalent plastic (polymethylmethacrylate PMMA rod). Reproduced with permission from Reference 65.

[32]P stents in the presence of nonwater equivalent (heterogeneous) materials. Subsequently, Rahdert et al[75] measured the actual density and atomic composition of a large number of plaque samples from human coronary arteries. They also used this data to calculate the effects of plaque on the dose from beta-emitting stents. Janicki et al[76] has further extended this point dose kernel concept to include the photon emitters, [103]Pd and [131]Cs. For the case of a uniform and homogeneous medium, Janicki et al state that the DPK for a beta point source can be replaced by a photon source. The DPK functions for photon emitters can be derived from Berger[77] or from recent mono-energetic photon data compilation by Luxton and Jozsef.[78] For photons in a nonhomogeneous system, Janicki et al suggest that the Sievert integral can be used for the calculations. Another investigator[79] has proposed numerical integration of the source distribution radial dose function given in the AAPM TG-43 report[80] for photon emitters.

Other investigators[64,76,81–83] have used Monte Carlo dose calculation codes to theoretically predict the dose and dose distributions surrounding radioactive stents. The radionuclides studied have included: [48]V, ^{32}P, [198]Au, [103]Pd, and [131]Cs. Monte Carlo dose calculations differ with respect to the specific calculational code used, the specific energy spectrum assumed for the radioactive source, the specific architecture assumed for the stent, the specific depth of the radioactive species in

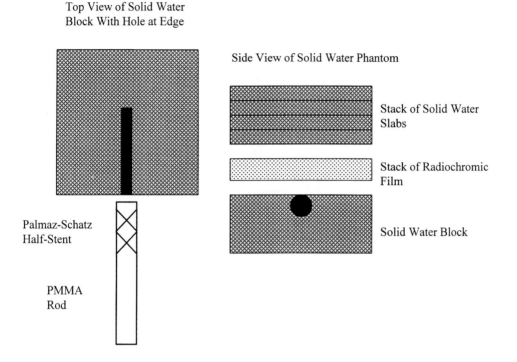

Figure 2. A diagram of a solid water phantom used for exposing radiochromic film perpendicular to the stent axis. The stent (Palmaz-Schatz half-stent), mounted on a PMMA rod, was placed in a hole in the edge of a thick block leaving a narrow strip exposed through a slit in the face of the solid water block. Radiochromic film was stacked on top of the stent and then solid water sheets were stacked on the film. Reproduced with permission from Reference 65.

or on the stent material, the inclusion or exclusion of the effects of absorption and scatter by the stent struts, and the inclusion or exclusion of the presence of non-homogeneous material(s).

Two investigators, Amols[79] and Kirisits,[84] have extended the calculations of dose from radial and longitudinal distributions to dose volume histograms. Kirisits et al[84] have used the Janicki et al[74] point dose kernel model for homogeneous medium and the intravascular ultrasound (IVUS) anatomic data to calculate the dose to surrounding tissues for 10 patients who received ^{32}P radioactive stent implantation in a European clinical trial.

Results

The architecture of coronary stents has become a very important variable in the resultant dose distributions surrounding radioactive stents. Figure 3 illustrates the architecture of a Palmaz-Schatz stent. The architectural pattern results in regions of peak and valley doses that correlate with the position of the strut lattice and resulting "holes." For correlation between theory and calculation, it is essential that phantoms are designed and constructed of tissue-like materials and of accurate geometric dimensions. Figures 1 and 2 show phantoms used

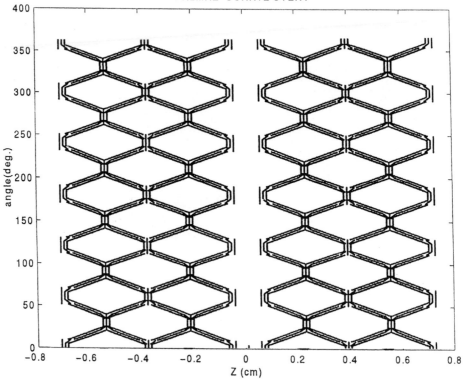

Figure 3. Schematic illustration of the geometry of a 3.5-mm diameter Palmaz-Schatz stent. The stent is made by articulation of two one-half stents, each 7.5 mm in length. The resulting architecture of the stent results in peaks and valleys in the dose distribution. Reproduced with permission from Reference 74.

by the present investigators for measuring radial and longitudinal dose distributions surrounding both beta-emitting and photon-emitting stents.

Figure 4 shows the radial dose distribution for a ^{32}P beta-emitting stent with a correlation between theory and experimental data utilizing radiochromic film and the tissue-equivalent phantom that is seen in Figure 1. Figure 5 shows similar results using the phantom in Figure 2 to assess the longitudinal dose distribution as a function of radial dose from a ^{32}P beta-emitting stent. The near-field dose distributions are very nonuniform for radial distances of up to 200 microns due to the architecture of the stent (Fig. 3), which results in peaks and valleys in dose. With radial distances greater than 200 microns, the dose distribution becomes generally uniform along the length of the stent. The agreement between the DPK model and radiochromic film is within experimental error as illustrated in Figure 6.

The DPK model has been extended by Janicki to include scaling factors that allow for areas and regions of nonhomogeneous material. Figure 7A shows the results of the DPK model taking into account the presence of the film stack illustrated in Figure 2. Additionally in Figure 7B, the DPK model is extended to include layers of a plaque-like high-density material. Again, the agreement between DPK model results using scaling factors and radiochromic film data is within ex-

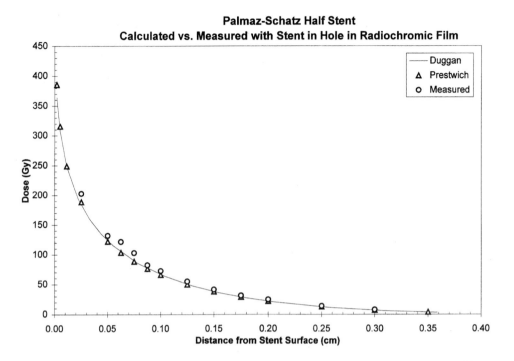

Figure 4. A plot of the radial dependence of the dose from a Palmaz-Schatz stent midway between the ends of the stent. The plot compares the values calculated with a finite cylindrical shell model to those measured with radiochromic film in a phantom of the type shown in Figure 1. Reproduced with permission from Reference 65.

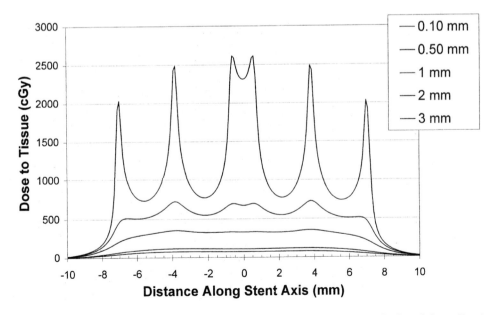

Figure 5. Near-field dose along the length of Palmaz-Schatz stent–calculated dose distribution along a 3.5-mm diameter and 15-mm length ^{32}P Palmaz-Schatz stent of 1.0 μCi activity after 14 days. One notes the peaks and valleys in the dose distribution for radial distances of less than 250 microns due to the stent architecture (Fig. 3). Reproduced with permission from Reference 74.

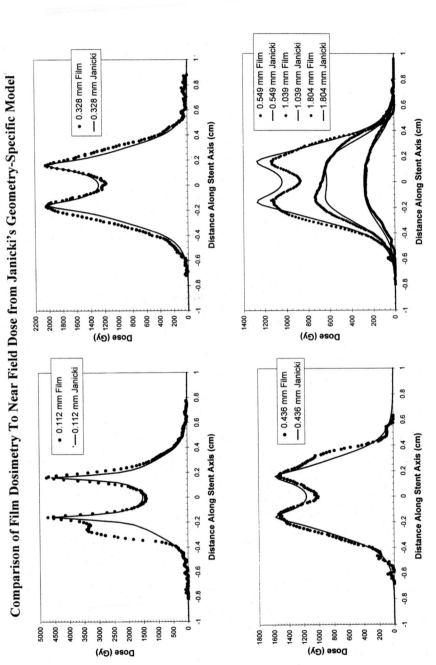

Figure 6. Measured dose profiles (dots) and the dose point kernel (DPK) model predictions (solid lines) taken along the long axis of a 3.5-mm diameter, one-half Palmaz-Schatz ^{32}P stent at radial distances of 0.112 mm, 0.328 mm, 0.436 mm, 0.549 mm, 1.039 mm, and 1.804 mm exterior to the stent surface. The agreement between the experimental dose profiles and the DPK model predictions is very satisfactory. Reproduced with permission from Reference 74.

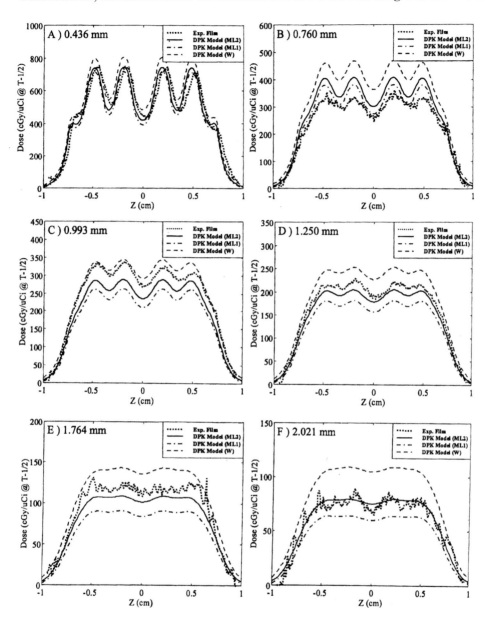

Figure 7A. Axial profiles of the radiochromic film results (dots) and the DPK multiplayer ML2 model (solid lines) at radial distances of 0.436 to 2.021 mm.

perimental error. Rahdert et al[75] have evaluated the physical density of plaque materials. Only IVUS could estimate the presence of plaque and the thickness of the plaque; plaque-corrected dose distributions will be difficult in a real-time catheterization laboratory environment.

Figures 8 and 9 illustrate the intravascular brachytherapy use of radio-nuclides for stents other than [32]P. Figure 8 shows the radial dose distribution of the betas from ^{90}Y versus the betas from ^{32}P using radiochromic film methods. The higher energy ^{90}Y betas penetrate deeper than ^{32}P betas; at 1 and 2 mm radii, [90]Y

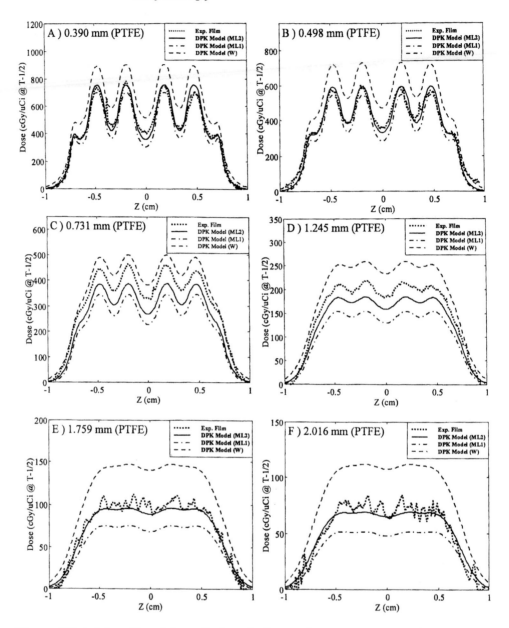

Figure 7B. Axial profiles of the radiochromic film results (dots) and the DPK multiplayer ML2 model (solid line) with the presence of 0.386 mm of polytetrafluoroethylene used to simulate the presence of high-density plaque. Reproduced with permission from Reference 66.

betas offer a 10% increase in dose per decay over ^{32}P betas. In Figure 9, percentage depth doses normalized to a 0.5 mm radius are plotted for ^{103}Pd and ^{131}Cs low-energy photons versus ^{32}P betas. There is an approximate 20% gain in percentage depth dose at radial distances of 1 and 2 mm for ^{103}Pd and ^{131}Cs photons versus ^{32}P betas. The dose calculations for Figure 9 were determined using the MCNP-4B Monte Carlo code. The simulated stent was modeled as a cylindrical steel shell, 100

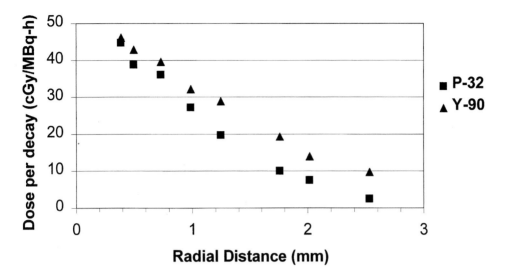

Figure 8. Radial dose distribution plots using radiochromic film from ^{32}P and ^{90}Y BX beta-emitting stents. The graphs are normalized to dose per decay. The gain in tissue penetration by the higher energy betas from ^{90}Y is illustrated.

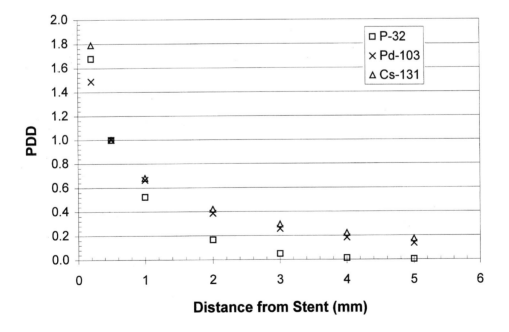

Figure 9. Percentage depth doses (PDDs) for three isotopes averaged over stent length. Monte Carlo (MCNP-4B)-calculated radial dose distribution plots from ^{32}P beta-emitting, and [103]Pd and [131]Cs photon-emitting simulated cylindrical steel shell stents. It is observed that the low-energy photons from [103]Pd and [131]Cs penetrate deeper into arterial tissues than ^{32}P betas.

microns thick, 3.5 mm in outside diameter, and 15 mm in length, with rectangular holes. A uniform coating was simulated by a large number of appropriately weighted point sources. Twenty-one percent of the total surface area was assumed to be strut material with the remainder representing the rectangular holes.

Because edge restenosis is such an important concern in the clinical use of radioactive stents, Figure 10 shows the radiation doses at the ends of simulated ^{103}Pd and ^{131}Cs photon stents versus ^{32}P beta stents. The graphs represent data within ± 2.5 mm of the stent ends plotted as the ratio of the dose at the point of interest to the dose at the middle of the stent for radial distances of 0.5 mm (Fig. 10A), 1.0 mm (Fig. 10B), and 2.0 mm (Fig. 10C) from the stent surface. A small but significant gain in relative dose for the low-energy photons of ^{103}Pd and ^{131}Cs over the betas of ^{32}P can be noted; the magnitude of this gain increases as the radial distance from the stent surface increases.

The effect of increased penetration of the low energy-photons from ^{103}Pd at the stent edge can be further enhanced by increasing the ^{103}Pd activity at the ends of the simulated stent. This enhancement, plotted as the ratio of the dose at the point of interest to the dose at the middle of the stent, is illustrated in Figures 11A, 11B, and 11C for radial distances of 0.5, 1.0, and 2.0 mm, respectively. The simulated stent in this illustration was 15 mm in length; each 3-mm end segment contained three times the activity as the central 9-mm segment. The dose enhancements at the stent ends resulting from the nonuniform activity distribution and the low-energy photons of ^{103}Pd versus ^{32}P betas are presented in Table 2. The Monte Carlo dose data presented in Figures 10 and 11 were calculated using the same simulated model stent characteristics described previously.

Figure 12 presents the longitudinal dose distributions surrounding ^{32}P and ^{198}Au radioactive stents using the Monte Carlo EGS4 dose code. Individual Monte Carlo dose evaluations are dependent on the stent architecture assumed, depth of the radioactive species from the stent surface, and the stent strut absorption assumptions. Again, one notes the nonuniform dose distributions seen within 250 microns of the stent surface. The radial isodose distribution from a simulated ^{103}Pd stent using Monte Carlo EGS4 dose calculations is presented in Figure 13.

Figure 14A shows a representative transverse cut from an IVUS study for a patient undergoing a ^{32}P radioactive stent implantation procedure. Using IVUS-generated anatomic data radially from the stent surface as a function of the longitudinal distance along the stent and the Janicki DPK model[76] (without inhomogeneity corrections), Kirisits et al[84] calculated dose volume histograms (DVH). Figure 14B shows the cumulative DVH for two patients with the data analyzed only over the total length (intrastent) of the ^{32}P stent. Figure 14C shows the cumulative DVH for the same 2 patients with the data analyzed over the total length of the stent and including the 2.5 mm both proximal and distal (peristent) to the stent. It can be seen that the volume containing 90% of the normalized dose (DV$_{90}$) is significantly reduced when including the dose evaluated in the peristent volumes versus the dose evaluated in the intrastent volumes only. This DVH analysis by Kirisits is the first clinical attempt to present dose data for the adjacent tissues involved in a radioactive stent implantation procedure.

In Figure 15 are seen the peristent cumulative DVH data for the same patient data as presented in Figure 14, however, the dose evaluations were made using Monte Carlo calculations for ^{103}Pd photons instead of the Janicki DPK model for ^{32}P betas. It is seen that for both patient simulated calculations, an analysis

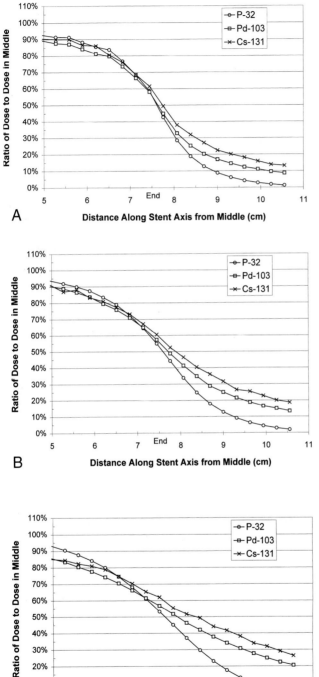

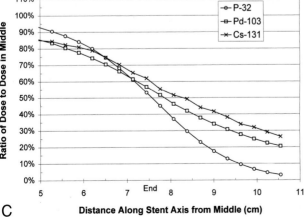

Figure 10. Monte Carlo (MCNP-4B)-calculated radial dose distribution plots (as a function of radial distance from the stent surface) near the stent ends for ^{32}P beta-emitting, and ^{103}Pd and ^{131}Cs photon-emitting simulated stents. Figures 10A, 10B, and 10C represent radial distances from the stent surface of 0.5 mm, 1.0 mm, and 2.0 mm, respectively. It is hoped that the increased penetration at the ends of the stents using ^{103}Pd and ^{131}Cs compared to ^{32}P will help to prevent the edge stenosis ("candy wrapper") effect.

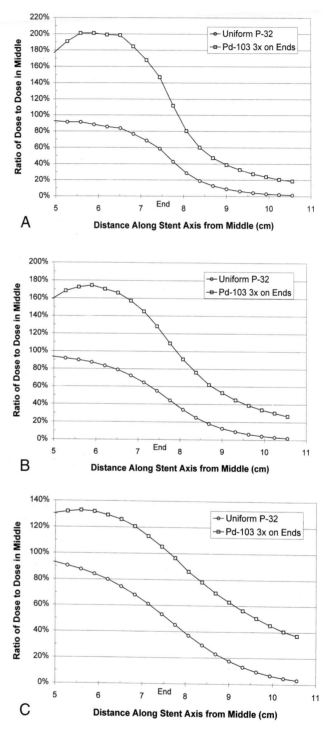

Figure 11. Monte Carlo (MCNP-4B)-calculated dose distribution plot from a ^{103}Pd photon-emitting simulated stent with higher activity ^{103}Pd deposited at the stent ends. The simulated stent was 15 mm in overall length; each 3-mm end segment contained three times the activity as the central 9-mm segement. Figures 11A, 11B, and 11C represent radial distances from the stent surface of 0.5 mm, 1.0 mm, and 2.0 mm, respectively. The higher penetration of ^{103}Pd photons combined with higher activity at the stent ends may assist in the prevention of edge restenosis.

Table 2

Monte Carlo (MCNP-4B) Dose Calculations* for Simulated
(Cylindrical Steel Shell Model) ^{32}P and ^{103}Pd Stents

Radial Distance from Stent Surface	Stent	Position Along Stent Axis			
		Stent Center	Stent End	1 mm Distal	2 mm Distal
0.5 mm	^{32}P	2000 cGy	1150 cGy	350 cGy	100 cGy
	$1 \times {}^{103}$Pd	2000 cGy	1150 cGy	470 cGy	270 cGy
	$3 \times {}^{103}$Pd	2180 cGy	3190 cGy	1220 cGy	640 cGy
1.0 mm	^{32}P	1060 cGy	580 cGy	240 cGy	80 cGy
	$1 \times {}^{103}$Pd	1340 cGy	770 cGy	440 cGy	270 cGy
	$3 \times {}^{103}$Pd	1550 cGy	1890 cGy	1050 cGy	600 cGy
2.0 mm	^{32}P	320 cGy	170 cGy	90 cGy	40 cGy
	$1 \times {}^{103}$Pd	780 cGy	450 cGy	320 cGy	230 cGy
	$3 \times {}^{103}$Pd	990 cGy	900 cGy	640 cGy	450 cGy

*Assuming 20 Gy prescribed at 0.5 mm radial from stent surface at stent center.
$1 \times {}^{103}$Pd indicates uniform activity along stent length.
$3 \times {}^{103}$Pd indicates nonuniform activity (three times the activity at the stent ends).

of the peristent volumes result in an increased DV_{90} for the low-energy photons of ^{103}Pd versus ^{32}P betas.

Discussion and Conclusions

Dosimetry and Quality Assurance

The theoretical approaches to radioactive stent dosimetry (DPK and Monte Carlo) have proven, in general, to be in agreement with the best dosimetry data (radiochromic film) for homogeneous conditions. Improved iterations of these models are providing corrections for inhomogeneous medium conditions including the presence of assumed finite dimensions of plaque-like materials. When attempting to correlate DPK and Monte Carlo calculations with experimental results, one must be careful to accurately define the geometry and boundary conditions and the presence of both homogeneous and inhomogeneous materials in the theoretical dose calculation parameters. Additionally, for both the DPK and Monte Carlo methods, it is important to investigate the effects of specific stent architecture, the effects of ion implantation and specialty coating processes on the depth of the radioactive atoms relative to the stent surface, and the effects of scatter and absorption of the radiation by the stent strut architecture itself. Also for Monte Carlo calculations, the important variable of specific source energy spectra must be considered.

Of course, to rely on the theoretical DPK and Monte Carlo calculations, it is assumed that the apparent activity of the radioactive stent is known. These activity values, as specified by the manufacturers,[7,85] are often determined via a relative activity measurement technique by comparison to standard sources. As intravascular brachytherapy, with both radioactive stents and catheter-based

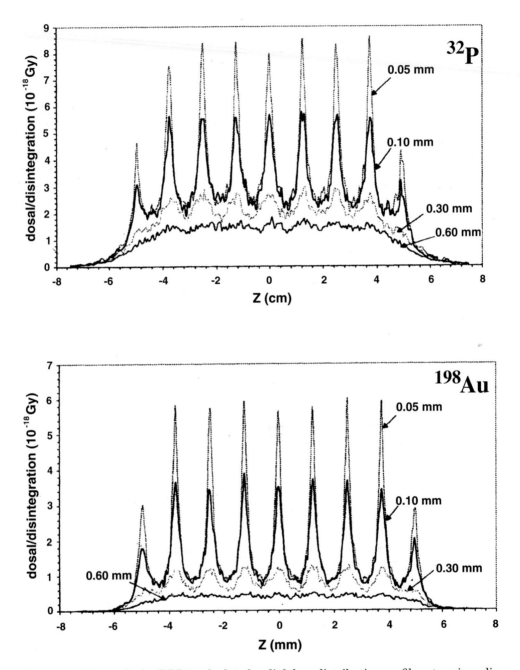

Figure 12. Monte Carlo (EGS4)-calculated radial dose distribution profiles at various distances from two simulated ACS-Multi Link radioactive stents, ^{32}P and ^{198}Au. The effect of the peak and valley doses becomes negligible at distances greater than 300 microns from the stent surfaces for both radionuclides. Reproduced with permission from Reference 82.

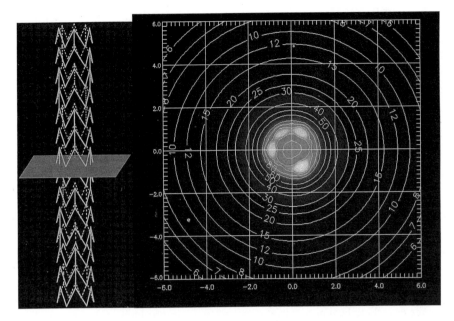

Figure 13. Monte Carlo (EGS4)-generated radial dose distribution profiles from a mathematically simulated ^{103}Pd radioactive stent. The isodose curves represent total dose (Gy) delivered over the lifetime of a 1 mCi stent. Reproduced, with permission of the author, from Reference 83.

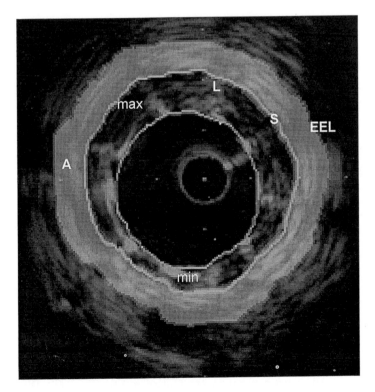

Figure 14A. Intravascular ultrasound cross-section of a stented artery. The inner contour indicates the vessel lumen (L) along the stent struts (S). The outer contour delineates the external elastic lamina (EEL). The highlighted area marks the adventitia (A), arbitrarily defined as a layer of 0.5-mm thickness.

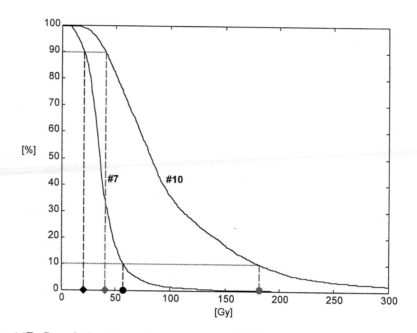

Figure 14B. Cumulative dose volume histogram (DVH) for two patients, #7 and #10, analyzing the dose distribution within the adventitia along the body of the stent (intrastent). The DVH for patient #7 shows that the adventitia received predominantly low doses with a small high dose region. The DVH for patient #10 indicates a dose distribution that is more heterogeneous over much of the dose range. Diamonds (◆) correspond to the DV_{90} values, 19.6 Gy and 39.4 Gy, for patients #7 and #10. DV_{10} values marked by (●) are 56.3 Gy and 180.6 Gy for patients #7 and #10.

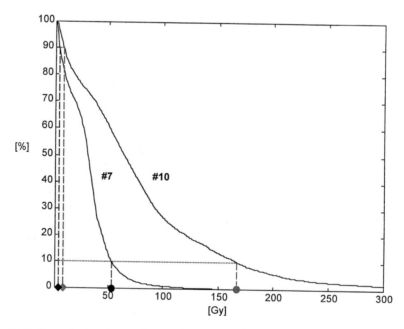

Figure 14C. Cumulative dose volume histogram for the same two patients as in Figure 14B, analyzing the dose distribution within the adventitia along the center of the stent including the tissues 2.5 mm proximal and 2.5 mm distal to the stent (peristent). The shape of the curves above 50 Gy are as for the intrastent adventitia (Fig. 14B). DV_{10} for patients #7 and #10, marked by (●), is 52.2 Gy and 165.8 Gy, respectively. At lower doses the DVH curves are markedly affected by the dose distribution within the peristent volume. The indented shape in this dose range results in a decrease of DV_{90} (◆) to 3.4 Gy (patient #7) and 7.3 Gy (patient #10). Reproduced with permission from Reference 84.

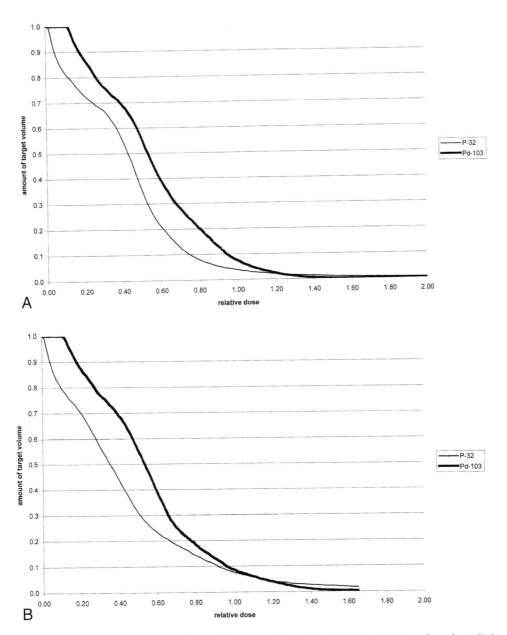

Figure 15. Cumulative dose volume histogram for patient #7 (Fig. 15A) and patient #10 (Fig. 15B) (both patients are the same as in Fig. 14C) analyzing the dose distribution to the adventitia within the peristent volume, assuming the stents were coated with ^{103}Pd. Monte Carlo (MCNP-4B) dose calculations were performed for ^{103}Pd photons in comparison to the DPK dose calculations for ^{32}P betas. One observes the predicted increase in DV_{90} for patient #7 in Figure 15A and for patient #10 in Figure 15B with ^{103}Pd photons over the DV_{90} values in both patients (Fig. 14C) for ^{32}P betas. Reproduced, with permission of the author, from Reference 103.

systems, moves toward widespread clinical applications, there is a need for "in-house" determination or secondary verification of manufacturers' stated activities. The AAPM Task Group-60 report[18] suggests that measured activity of radioactive stents should be traceable to national standards and that the method used to determine the activity should be an appropriate transfer technique.

For low-energy, low-activity photon-emitting stents, relative activity can be assessed via secondary standard photon sources and a well-ionization or reentrant chamber. For low-activity beta-emitting stents, relative activity may be determined via secondary standard beta sources and the use of very sensitive well-ionization counters or scintillation detectors. A more difficult problem is encountered when the sterile beta-emitting stent packaging may not allow for the techniques above. The present authors[19] presented a relative counting technique for sterile packaged beta-emitting stents using a sodium iodide (NaI) scintillator bremsstrahlung counting method. Whether low-energy, low-activity photon-emitting, or low-activity beta-emitting stents, there is a need for standardization of stent size (diameter and length), stent holder device, and positioning within the well-counter to allow for counting accuracies within the limits of clinical use. These very practical secondary well-ionization counter techniques mentioned above are exceedingly useful for relative measurements, but it should be cautioned that primary[86,87] and secondary standards[88] are needed to first calibrate the instrument(s). We suggest that relative activity analysis should be done at the receipt of the radioactive stent for labeling identification and inventory recording; stent activity should be checked again prior to the initiation of the patient treatment procedure.

Radiation Dosing Strategies

Human clinical trial results using ^{32}P radioactive stents have repeatedly shown the "candy wrapper" effect. Many animal and human clinical trials show pristine results inside the radioactive stent center; however, there is often neo-intimal hyperplasia near and beyond the ends of the stent, which frequently results in luminal narrowing and restenosis. As previously mentioned,[5,79] it is suspected that the increased hyperplasia at the ends of the stent is due to dose inhomogeneities resulting in underdosing of the tissues in that region and/or balloon injury at the stent edges. In a clinical trial using ^{32}P, the radiation dose at the stent ends was increased by raising the total activity along the entire length of the stent. This trial, first reported by Alberio et al,[53] combined the effects of increased total stent activity and a nonaggressive ballooning technique, which limited the balloon injury outside the stent. In a later report, Alberio et al[89] concluded that increased ^{32}P stent activity did reduce intrastent neointimal hyperplasia compared to stents of lesser activity; however, it did not solve the problem of edge restenosis even if a nonaggressive stent implantation strategy was used. Alberio further concluded that the edge restenosis in this clinical model was thought to be due to remodeling effects.

Albiero et al[89] have reported that two different modifications of existing ^{32}P radioactive BX stents are currently under investigation in Europe: (1) the hot-ends stent and (2) the cold-ends stent. It is hoped that the hot-ends stent, which has a higher activity level at its proximal and distal ends, will diminish the problem of edge restenosis related to tissue growth and/or remodeling by extending the area of irradiation beyond the balloon-injured area outside the stent. The rationale for the cold-ends stent is that lengthening the stent with a nonradioactive section on each end of the stent might minimize the edge effect related to negative remodeling. From this rationale, a patent[90] has recently been issued for a radioactive stent that has radioactivity along the center of the stent, but no radioactivity for a limited length, at each end section of the stent. To date, results from these clinical trials are incomplete.

Other Radionuclides

Theoretical dose distributions from DPK and Monte Carlo dose models have prompted investigators in the search for a solution to the restenosis problem to consider the potential clinical results of substituting other beta-emitting species for ^{32}P. Of note are three radionuclides, ^{48}V, ^{198}Au, and ^{90}Y, which have been suggested for radioactive stenting. Although it is acknowledged that both ^{48}V and ^{198}Au are not pure beta-emitting species, the dose given to the tissues immediately surrounding the target area does come primarily from the dose deposited locally as a result of emitted beta particles. Conclusions from initial animal investigations[7,81] show an increased neointimal formation for the ^{198}Au studies and a significantly reduced lumen narrowing in moderately injured coronary porcine vessels using ^{48}V. The higher energy associated with ^{90}Y betas results in an increased range when compared to ^{32}P betas (Fig. 8). The radial dose distribution normalized to dose per decay suggests that ^{90}Y betas should result in increased radiation dose (approximately 5 to 10%) at distances of 1.0 to 2.5 mm from the stent surface, and thus perhaps offer a clinical advantage of ^{90}Y over ^{32}P betas. However, any advantage in increased range was overshadowed by the adverse results of increased neointimal area, frequent total occlusions, and incomplete neointimal healing at 90 days for activities of 16 to 32 μCi as reported by Taylor et al.[6] Carter et al[85] reported mixed porcine results assayed at 28 days with neointimal inhibition for 0.5 to 2μCi ^{90}Y stents and adverse radiation effects for animals with stents of 16 to 32 μCi. For similar cumulative doses comparing ^{32}P and ^{90}Y response in the porcine model, Carter et al have concluded that dose rate rather than cumulative dose may be the more significant contributing factor to arterial tissue(s) response. Thus, the modest range advantage afforded by the higher energy ^{90}Y betas may be overshadowed by the dose rate kinetics inherent in the ^{90}Y half-life of 3.8 days versus the 14-day half-life of ^{32}P.

With the apparent shortcomings of ^{32}P and other beta-emitting species to solve restenosis and overcome the edge effects, use of low-energy photon-emitting stents has been suggested.[5,16,75,79] With half-lives and time-dose kinetics similar to that of ^{32}P, the low-energy photon emitters, ^{103}Pd and ^{131}Cs, have been suggested as potential substitutes for ^{32}P betas. DPK and Monte Carlo dose models predict that the dose to the tissues surrounding the proximal and distal ends of radioactive stents is enhanced with the substitution of ^{103}Pd or ^{131}Cs photons versus ^{32}P betas (Fig. 10). Experiments in our laboratory using radiochromic film are presently underway to measure the dose distributions surrounding ^{103}P stents and compare them with the distribution using Monte Carlo methods. Although ^{125}I has been suggested as a radionuclide for vascular brachytherapy,[91] its time-dose kinetics (60-day half-life) is not within the favorable range thought to be optimal.

Two animal experiments using ^{103}Pd radioactive stents are under way, the first in a rabbit iliac model,[92] the second in a porcine coronary model,[93] with no published results to date. The experiment with the rabbit iliac model[92] has yielded preliminary results similar to that reported for ^{32}P stents; neointimal hyperplasia within the central portion of the stent decreases with increasing stent activity (1 to 4 mCi of ^{103}Pd). However, to date, the hoped-for result of reduced edge effects with the more penetrating photons from ^{103}Pd was not realized in the early investigational analysis.

Stent Design

Another porcine study is under way investigating the effects of a novel stent design[94] in which the central body of the stent contains ^{32}P, with the addition of ^{103}Pd at each of the stent ends. No results from this study have been reported to date. Although this stent design has assumed clinical advantages, the stent would probably be expensive to manufacture and the design would make it difficult to quantitate activity with "in-house" measurement techniques. From the early results of the ^{103}Pd animal study above,[92] and the results shown in Figure 11 and Table 2, it could be that a ^{103}Pd stent manufactured with increased ^{103}Pd activity at the stent ends would be a stent fabrication design worthy of a follow-up animal study.

A subtle effect not considered by the early theoretical models for ^{103}Pd and ^{131}Cs is the emission of low-energy auger and conversion electrons[95] from the decay schemes encountered with ^{103}Pd and ^{131}Cs. These low-energy electrons are of sufficient energy to escape the outer surface layer of the stent and deposit their energy within the first few microns of the arterial wall surface. These electrons will contribute undesired radiation dose in addition to the desired dose from the emitted low-energy photons; the combined dose from electrons and photons could lead to excessive fibrosis and delayed healing to tissues closely adjacent to the stent wires. The present authors[96] and Janicki et al[76] believe that these low-energy electrons can be attenuated and absorbed by the addition of a coating material overlaying the ^{103}Pd material. Janicki has shown that a 4 micron coating of stable palladium can reduce these low-energy electrons by three orders of magnitude while only reducing the low-energy photons by 10%. It is of note, however, that some metallic coating materials and methods have been shown to have deleterious effects on arterial tissues in human trials after extended observation times.[97] Additionally, physicists and manufacturers must be aware that with the use of metallic coating materials, there is an increased incidence of bremsstrahlung production from low-energy electrons interacting with high-Z material atoms. Hence, the low-energy electrons that are attenuated and absorbed in the metallic coatings can result in the production of low-energy bremsstrahlung x-rays which again deposit their energy locally at the adjacent arterial wall surface. To reduce this potential effect, the coating materials could be made from low-Z materials. There is an animal experiment in progress[93] in which stable palladium is used to coat a radioactive ^{103}Pd stent; at present no data is available from this investigation.

The increased hyperplasia and delayed healing seen in radioactive stent trials and the late, late thrombosis reported in both radioactive stent and catheter-based trials may be attributed in part to the very high dose gradients that exist at the stent- or catheter-arterial wall surface. This high dose gradient effect is a result of the inverse square law associated with radioactive emitters and the very short distances involved in intravasular brachytherapy. This high dose gradient effect for radioactive stents is exacerbated by the stent architecture (Fig. 3). At the strut intersections, the radiation dose is higher relative to the holes in the stent architecture; this is referred to as areas of peak and valley doses. This effect of peak and valley doses can be overcome by a relative reduction in the peak to valley ratio; however, the optimum design of solid stent walls would not be tolerated clinically. Hence, perhaps the only solution for creating dose homogeneity from radioactive stents is the coating of stents with 100 to 200 microns of a low-Z material that would allow for the absorption of those high dose gradients within the coating material. The use of coating materials to decrease surface dose inhomogeneities combined with the prolonged use of antiplatelet therapies[51] may further reduce the incidence of late, late thrombosis.

Two manufacturers[98] have recently entered into a joint agreement to develop a biocompatible porous polymer-coated vascular stent. This polymer-coated stent is envisioned to reduce restenosis by providing a means for either local radiation delivery, drug delivery, or gene therapy within the polymer. An immediate application of this polymer-coated stent would be in improved dose homogeneity afforded by the attenuation of auger and conversion electrons, the reduction and subsequent attenuation of any bremsstrahlung radiation, and the absorption of the peak and valley doses associated with the stent struts and holes. A second application is the use of the coating medium for application in targeted radioimmunotherapy applications as proposed by Mosseri et al.[99] They have reported that specially prepared bovine serum albumin (BSA)-coated stainless steel wires, when incubated with ^{125}I-labeled anti-BSA, have shown a specific binding of the anti-BSA to the BSA-coated wire which results in an enhanced uptake of ^{125}I radioactivity over the ^{125}I uptake on control wires. This concept could potentially allow for in vivo targeted immunotherapy by injecting radioactive labeled compounds intravenously and binding the radioacative label onto the surface of previously implanted, specially coated stents. Of course, the success of this immunotherapy technique process would be highly dependent on the specificity and percentage uptake of the labeled anti-BSA compound by the BSA present on the stent coating.

Future Directions

An issue addressed by theoretical calculations and, as of yet, untested in animal and human models, is the effect of absorption and attenuation of radiation by higher density plaque materials. Janicki et al,[66] Rahdert et al,[75] Stabin et al,[100] and Li et al[101] have shown these effects to be extensive in theoretical models. It can only be assumed that in vivo plaque present at the time of implantation in human trials has affected the resulting dose distribution and, subsequently, the clinical results. Plaque models and theoretical calculations have shown that betas are attenuated more by plaque materials than are low- energy photons. Additionally, it is known that ^{131}Cs 30 keV photons have less attenuation in calcified plaque than do the photons of ^{103}Pd, due to the decreased attenuation coefficient of the higher energy ^{131}Cs photons in calcium compared to the 20 keV photons emitted by ^{103}Pd.[102] With its low-energy photons and time-dose kinetics similar to ^{103}Pd, and its decreased photon dose absorption by calcium, ^{131}Cs has been suggested as the next radionuclide for evaluation.

A significant publication by Kirisits et al[84] has evaluated 10 patients who received ^{32}P stents using IVUS to determine anatomic regions and distances from the stent surfaces. Using the Janicki DPK model for ^{32}P betas, DVHs have been determined along the stent axis for distances radially 1 to 2 mm from the stent surface. These three-dimensional dose distributions have given more physics and biological dose data than has ever been reported previously. A thorough and continuing follow-up analysis of these patients may show correlations of clinical response (both good and poor) versus absorbed dose. These data may for the first time allow the analysis of a true dose-response study; results from these patients can be used as hypotheses for further clinical trials. At present, theoretical calculations[103] using ^{103}Pd in conjunction with the IVUS patient data show that ^{103}Pd low-energy photons improves the DV_{90} values surrounding ^{103}Pd radioactive stents compared to ^{32}P betas (Fig. 15).

In conclusion, we need to pursue radioactive stenting issues on three fronts: physics and dosimetry, animal and biological models, and human trials. For physics and dosimetry, there is a need to find the optimal radionuclide, to use dose calculation methods to predict resulting dose and dose distributions from novel stent designs, and to perfect the measurement of apparent activity in a clinical environment to ensure the best correlation between theoretical and actual dose given. On the animal and biological front, there is a need to continue to study the effects that are presently predicted by theoretical models, in terms of: photons versus betas, nonuniform activity loadings, coated versus noncoated stents, and ^{131}Cs versus ^{103}Pd photons. And finally, on the clinical trials front, there is a need to continue investigating the long-term effects of radioactive stenting and to correlate these clinical effects with dosimetry and anatomic data. It is imperative to continue IVUS studies and correlate three-dimensional dose distributions and clinical endpoints, as was demonstrated by the Kirisits study. Last, following successful animal studies, clinical investigators must be willing to proceed to clinical trials in the quest to find the optimal radionuclide and the best stent design strategy to achieve a radiation dose distribution that prevents restenosis and leads to clinical solutions for the "candy wrapper" and late thrombosis effects.

References

1. Fischell TA, Carter AJ, Fischell DR, et al. Radioisotope stents. In: Waksman RW, Serruys P (eds.): Handbook of Vascular Brachytherapy. London: Martin Dunitz, Ltd.; 1998:59–67.
2. Lansky AJ, Popma JJ, Massullo V, et al. Quantitative angiographic analysis of stent restenosis in the scripps coronary radiation trial to inhibit intimal proliferation post stenting (SCRIPPS) trial. Am J Cardiol 1999;84:410–414.
3. Carter AJ, Scott D, Bailey L, et al. Dose-response effects of ^{32}P radioactive stents in an atherosclerotic porcine coronary model. Circulation 1999;100:1548–1554.
4. Waksman R, Mehran R, Bhargava B, et al. Recurrent restenosis after "failed" intracoronary radiation therapy: Angiographic patterns and predictors [abstract]. Circulation 1999;100:222.
5. Serruys PW, Kay IP. I like the candy, I hate the wrapper: The ^{32}P radioactive stent. Circulation 2000;101:3–7.
6. Taylor AJ, Gorman PD, Hudak C, et al. The 90-day coronary vascular response to 90Y β particle-emitting stents in the canine model. Int J Radiat Oncol Biol Phys 2000;46:1019–1024.
7. Schulz C, Nidereer MS, Andres C, et al. Endovascular irradiation from β-particle-emitting gold stents results in increased neointima formation in a porcine restenosis model. Circulation 2000;101:1970–1975.
8. Carter AJ, Fischell TA. Current status of radioactive stents for the prevention of in-stent restenosis. Int J Radiat Oncol Biol Phys 1998;41:127–133.

9. Amols HI. Designing the ideal radioactive stent [abstract]. Cardiovascular Radiation Therapy IV Symposium. February 16–18, 2000.

10. Carter AJ, Jenkins JS, Bailey LR, et al. Dose rate and cumulative dose effects of P-32 radioactive stents [abstract]. J Am Coll Cardiol 1999;33:20.

11. Teirstein PS. Vascular radiation therapy: The devil is in the dose. J Am Coll Cardiol 1999;34:567–569.

12. Clowes AW, Reidy MA, Clowes MM. Mechanisms of stenosis after arterial injury. Lab Invest 1983;49:208–215.

13. Geary RL, Williams JK, Golden D, et al. Time course of cellular proliferation, intimal hyperplasia, and remodeling following angioplasty in monkeys with established atherosclerosis: A nonhuman primate model of restenosis. Arterioscler Thromb Vasc Biol 1996;16:34–43.

14. Labinaz M, Pels K, Hoffert C, et al. Time course and importance of neoadventitial formation in arterial remodeling following balloon angioplasty of porcine coronary arteries. Cardiovasc Res 1999;41:255–266.

15. Hausleiter J, Li A, Makkar R, et al. Localization of target tissue and the minimum effective dose in intracoronary radiation therapy [abstract]. J Am Coll Cardiol 1999;33:44.

16. Sioshansi P, Bricault RJ. Low energy 103Pd gamma (X-Ray) source for vascular brachytherapy. Radiat Med 1999;1:278–287.

17. American College of Radiology Standards 1997. Reston, VA: American College of Radiology; 1997.

18. Nath R, Amols HI, Coffey C, et al. Intravascular brachytherapy physics: Report of the AAPM Radiation Therapy Committee Task Group No. 60. Med Phys 1999;26:119–152.

19. Coffey CW, Duggan DM, Reddick RC. Dosimetric considerations and dose measurement analysis of phosphorus 32 beta-emitting stents: A review. In: Waksman R (ed.): Vascular Brachytherapy, 2nd Edition. Armonk, NY: Futura Publishing Company; 1999:313–332.

20. Holmes DR, Vlietstra RE, Smith HC, et al. Restenosis after percutaneous transluminal coronary angioplasty (PTCA): A report from the PTCA registry of the National Heart, Lung, and Blood Institute. Am J Cardiol 1984;53:77C–81C.

21. Schwartz RS, Murphy JG, Edwards WD, et al. Restenosis after balloon angioplasty: A practical proliferative model in porcine coronary arteries. Circulation 1990;82:2190–2200.

22. Karas SP, Gravanis MB, Santoian EC, et al. Coronary intimal proliferation after balloon injury and stenting in swine: An animal model of restenosis. J Am Coll Cardiol 1992;20:467–474.

23. Haude M, Erbel R, Issa H, et al. Quantitative analysis of elastic recoil after balloon angioplasty and after intracoronary implantation of balloon-expandable Palmaz-Schatz stents. J Am Coll Cardiol 1993;21:26–34.

24. Waksman R, Robinson KA, Crocker IR, et al. Endovascular low-dose irradiation inhibits neointima formation after coronary artery balloon injury in swine: A possible role for radiation therapy in restenosis prevention. Circulation 1995;91:1533–1539.

25. Waksman R, Robinson KA, Crocker IR, et al. Intracoronary radiation before stent implantation inhibits neointima formation in stented porcine coronary arteries. Circulation 1995;92:1383–1386.

26. Wiedermann JG, Marboe C, Amols H, et al. Intracoronary irradiation markedly reduces neointimal proliferation after balloon angioplasty in swine: Persistent benefit at 6-month follow-up. J Am Coll Cardiol 1995;25:1451–1456.

27. Teirstein PS, Massullo V, Jani S, et al. Catheter-based radiotherapy to inhibit restenosis after coronary stenting. N Engl J Med 1997;336:1697–1703.

28. Waksman R, White LR, Chan RC, et al. Intracoronary radiation therapy for patients with in-stent restenosis: 6 month followup of a randomized clinical study [abstract]. Circulation 1998;98:651.

29. King SB, Williams DO, Chougule P, et al. Endovascular beta-radiation to reduce restenosis after coronary balloon angioplasty: Results of the beta energy restenosis trial (BERT). Circulation 1998;97:2025–2030.

30. Teirstein PS, Massullo V, Jani S, et al. Two-year follow-up after catheter-based radiotherapy to inhibit coronary restenosis. Circulation 1999;99:243–247.

31. Fischell RE, Fischell TA. Intra-arterial stent with capability to inhibit internal hyperplasia. US Patent No. 5,059,166. October 22, 1991.

32. Fischell TA, Kharma BK, Fischell DR, et al. Low-dose, beta-particle emission from 'stent' wire results in complete, localized inhibition of smooth muscle cell proliferation. Circulation 1994;90:2956–2963.
33. Hehrlein C, Gollan C, Donges K, et al. Low dose radioactive endovascular stents prevent smooth muscle cell proliferation and neointimal hyperplasia in rabbits. Circulation 1995;92:1570–1575.
34. Laird JR, Carter AJ, Kufs WM, et al. Inhibition of neointimal proliferation with low-dose irradiation from a beta-particle-emitting stent. Circulation 1996;93:529–536.
35. Carter AJ, Laird JR, Bailey LR, et al. Effects of endovascular radiation from a beta-particle-emitting stent in a porcine coronary restenosis model: A dose-response study. Circulation 1996;94:2364–2368.
36. Waksman R, Kim WH, Chan R, et al. Effectiveness of a beta-emitting radioactive stent for the treatment of in-stent restenosis in porcine arteries [abstract]. Circulation 1998;99:779.
37. Hehrlein C, Brachmann J, Hardt S, et al. P-32 stents for prevention of restenosis: Results of the Heidelberg safety trial using the Palmaz-Schatz stent design at moderate activity levels in patients with restenosis after PTCA [abstract]. Circulation 1998;99:780.
38. Albiero R, DiMario C, DeGregorio J, et al. Intravascular ultrasound (IVUS) analysis of beta-particle emitting radioactive stent implantation in human coronary arteries: Preliminary, immediate, and intermediate results of the MILAN study [abstract]. Circulation 1998;99:780.
39. Wardeh AJ, Kay IP, Sabate M, et al. Beta-particle-emitting radioactive stent implantation: A safety and feasibility study. Circulation 1999;100:1684–1689.
40. Albiero R, Adamian M, Kobayashi, et al. A short- and intermediate-term results of ^{32}P radioactive beta-emitting stent implantation in patients with coronary artery disease: The Milan dose-response study. Circulation 2000;101:18–26.
41. Salame MY, Verheye CS, Robinson KA. The paradox of vascular radiation therapy: Restenosis inhibition but delayed arterial healing with increased thrombogenicity. Vasc Radiother Mon 1999;2:35–45.
42. Farb A, Fischell DR, Fischell RE, et al. Effects of endovascular radiation from a beta-particle-emitting stent in a porcine coronary restenosis model. Circulation 1996; 96:2364–2368.
43. Fareh J, Martel R, Kermani P, et al. Cellular effects of beta-particle delivery on vascular smooth muscle cells and endothelial cells: A dose-response study. Circulation 1999;99:1477–1484.
44. Farb A, Tang A, Virmani R. The neointima is reduced but endothelialization is incomplete 3 months after P-32 beta-emitting stent placement [abstract]. Circulation 1998;98:779.
45. Shroff SS, Farb A, Sweet WL, et al. Sustained neointimal inhibition with delayed healing 6 months after placement of 32P β-emitting stents [abstract]. Circulation 1999;100:155.
46. Taylor AJ, Gorman PD, Farb A, et al. Differential effect of 32P beta particle-emitting stent on the intima and adventitia in the dog model [abstract]. Circulation 1998;98:779.
47. Taylor AJ, Gorman PD, Farb A, et al. Long-term coronary vascular response to (32)P beta-particle-emitting stents in a canine model. Circulation 1999;100:2366–2372.
48. Vodovotz Y, Waksman R, Kim WH, et al. Effects of intracoronary radiation on thrombosis after balloon overstretch injury in the porcine model. Circulation 1999;100:2527–2533.
49. Waksman R, Bhargava B, Chan RC, et al. Late total occlusions following intracoronary radiation therapy for patients with in-stent restenosis [abstract]. Circulation 1999;100:222.
50. Costa MA, Sabat M, van der Giessen W J, et al. Late coronary occlusion after intracoronary brachytherapy. Circulation 1999;100:789–792.
51. Waksman R. Late thrombosis after radiation: Sitting on a time bomb. Circulation 1999;100:780–782.
52. Salame M, Lampkin J, Mulkey P, et al. Effects of endovascular irradiation on platelet recruitment at site of balloon angioplasty in pig coronary arteries [abstract]. J Am Coll Cardiol 1999;33:44.
53. Albiero R, Adamian MG, Amato A, et al. Radioactive 32P beta emitting stents in patients with CAD: Do higher initial activity levels combined with a nonaggressive implantation strategy "unwrap the candy"? [abstract] Circulation 1999;100:221.
54. Adamian MG, Albiero R, Nishida T, et al. Restenosis following implantation of ra-

dioactive P-32 stents: Long-term clinical followup after treatment [abstract]. Circulation 1999;100:221.

55. Hansen A, Hehrlein C, Hardt S, et al. Is the "candy-wrapper" effect of beta-particle emitting stents due to remodeling or neointimal hyperplasia? [abstract] Circulation 1999;100:155.

56. Ahmed J, Mintz GS, Harrington D, et al. Mechanism of in-stent restenosis: a serial intravascular ultrasound study [abstract]. Circulation 1999;100:222.

57. Lansky AJ, Weissman NJ, Desai KJ, et al. Predictors and mechanisms of in-stent and stent edge restenosis in patients treated with iridium192 brachytherapy: Results from the GAMMA I trial [abstract]. Circulation 1999;100:221.

58. Honda H, Makkar R, Li A, et al. Experimental stent edge stenosis after intravascular radiation therapy [abstract]. Circulation 1999;100:223.

59. Popowski Y, Verin V, Papirov I, et al. High dose rate brachytherapy for prevention of restenosis after percutaneous transluminal coronary angioplasty: Preliminary dosimetric tests of a new source presentation. Int J Radiat Oncol Biol Phys 1995;33:211–215.

60. Xu Z, Almond PR, Deasy J. The dose distribution produced by a ^{32}P source for endovascular irradiation. Int J Radiat Oncol Biol Phys 1996;36:933–939.

61. Bambynek M, Fluhs D, Quast U, et al. A high-precision, high-resolution and fast dosimetry system for beta sources applied in cardiovascular brachytherapy. Med Phys 2000;27:662–667.

62. Soares C, Halpern P, Wang CK. Calibration and characterization of beta-particle sources for intravascular brachytherapy. Med Phys 1998;25:339–346.

63. Hafeli U, Roberts W, Meier D, et al. Dosimetry of a W-188/Re-188 beta line source for endovascular brachytherapy. Med Phys 2000;27:668–675.

64. Li A, Eigler N, Litvack F, et al. Characterization of a positron emitting V48 nitinol stent for intracoronary brachytherapy. Med Phys 1998;25:20–27.

65. Duggan D, Coffey C, Levit S. Dose distribution for a ^{32}P impregnated coronary stent: Comparison of theoretical calculations and measurements with radiochromic film. Int J Radiat Oncol Biol Phys 1998;40:713–720.

66. Janicki C, Duggan D, Gonzalez A, et al. Dose model for a beta-emitting stent in a realistic artery consisting of soft tissue and plaque. Med Phys 1999;26:2451–2460.

67. Loevinger R, Berman MA. Formalism for calculation of absorbed dose from seven radionuclides. Phys Med Biol 1968;13:205–217.

68. Berger MJ. Beta ray dosimetry calculations with the use of point kernels. In: Cloutier RJ, Edwards CS, Synder WS (eds.): Medical Radionuclides: Radiation Dose and Effect. U.S. Atomic Energy Commission Report CONF-691212. Springfield, VA: National Technical Center; 1970:63–68.

69. Simpkin DJ Mackie TR. EGS4 Monte Carlo determination of the beta dose kernel in water. Med Phys 1990;17:179–186.

70. Brookeman VA, Fitzgerald LT, Morin RL. Electron dose reduction coefficients for seven radionuclides and cylindrical geometries. Phys Med Biol 1978;23:852–864.

71. National Council on Radiation Protection and Measurements. Conceptual Basis for Calculations of Absorbed Dose Distributions. NCRP Report No. 108. Bethesda, MD, 1991.

72. Prestwich WV, Kennet TJ, Fus FW. The dose distribution produced by a ^{32}P coated stent. Med Phys 1995;22:313–320.

73. Prestwich WV. Analytic representation of the dose from a ^{32}P coated stent. Med Phys 1996;23:9–13.

74. Janicki C, Duggan D, Coffey C, et al. Radiation dose from a phosphorous-32 impregnated wire mesh vascular stent. Med Phys 1997;24:437–445.

75. Rahdert DA, Sweet WL, Tio FO, et al. Measurement of density and calcium in human atherosclerotic plaque and implications for arterial brachytherapy. Cardiovas Radiat Med 1999;1:358–367.

76. Janicki C, Duggan D, Rahdert D. A dose point kernel (DPK) model for a low energy gamma emitting stent in a heterogeneous medium. Submitted to Med Phys.

77. Berger MJ. Energy depostion in water by photons from point isotropic sources (MIRD Pamphlet No. 2) J Nucl Med 1969;1(suppl):17–25.

78. Luxton G, Jozsef G. Radial dose distribution, dose to water and dose rate constant for monoenergetic photon point sources from 10 keV to 2 MeV: EGS4 Monte Carlo model calculation. Med Phys 1999;26:2531–2538.

79. Amols HI. Methods to improve dose uniformity for radioactive stents in endovascular brachytherapy. Cardiovas Radiat Med 1999;1:270–277.

80. Nath R, Anderson L, Luxton G, et al. Dosimetry of interstitial brachytherapy sources: Recommendations of the AAPM Radiation Therapy Committee Task Group No. 43. Med Phys 1995;22:209–234.

81. Eigler N, Whiting J, Li A, et al. Effects of a positron-emitting Vanadium-48 nitinol stent on experimental restenosis in porcine arteries. Cardiovas Radiat Med 1999; 1:239–251.

82. Reynaert N, Verhaegen F, Taeymans Y, et al. Monte Carlo calculations of dose distributions around ^{32}P and ^{198}Au stents for intravascular brachytherapy. Med Phys 1999;26:1484–1491.

83. McLemore L. Dosimetric characterization of a palladium-103 implanted stent for intravascular brachytherapy. MS thesis. The University of Texas, Health Science Center at Houston, Graduate School of Biomedical Sciences, Houston, Texas. August, 2000, p 80.

84. Kirisits C, Wexberg P, Gottsauner-Wolf M, et al. Dose volume histograms based on serial intravascular ultrasound: A calculation model for radioactive stents. Radiotherapy Oncol 2001;59:329–337.

85. Carter AJ, Jenkins S, Sweet W, et al. Dose and dose rate effects of beta particle emitting radioactive stents in a porcine model of restenosis. Cardiovasc Radiat Med 1999;1:327–335.

86. Seltzer SM, Lamperti PJ. Status of NIST primary standards for I-125 and Pd-103 therapy seeds based on the wide-angle-free-air chamber (WAFAC). In: CIRMS Workshop on Measurements and Standards for Prostate Seed Therapy. Gathersburg, MD, 1994.

87. Coursey BM, Colle R. Activity measurements of beta-particle emitting radionuclides for use in intravascular brachytherapy [abstract]. Med Phys 1997;24:994.

88. Words MJ, Munster AS, Stephton JP, et al. Calibrations of the NPL secondary standard radionuclide calibrator for ^{32}P, ^{90}Sr, and ^{90}Y. Nucl Instrum Methods Phys Res 1996;369:698–702.

89. Albiero R, Nishida T, Adamian M, et al. Edge restenosis after implantation of high activity P-32 radioactive beta-emitting stents. Circulation 2000;101:2454–2459.

90. Columbo A, Fischell RE. Radioisotope stent with non-radioactive end sections. US Patent No. 6,099,455. August 3, 2000.

91. Amols HI. Review of endovascular brachytherapy physics for prevention of restenosis. Cardiovas Radiat Med 1999;1:64–71.

92. Bradley Strauss (personal communication) 2000.

93. Anthony Armini (personal communication) 2000.

94. Anthony Armini (personal communication) 2000.

95. Johns HE, Cunningham JR. The Physics of Radiology, 4th Edition. Springfield, IL: Charles C. Thomas Publishing Co.; 1983:84–90.

96. Duggan DM, Coffey CW. Pd-103 Coated Stents for Arterial Restenosis. Presented at Cardiovascular Radiation Therapy IV, Washington, D.C., 2000.

97. Kastrati A, Schomig A, Dirschinger J, et al. Increased risk of restenosis after placement of gold-coated stents. Circulation 2000;101:2478–2486.

98. Anthony Armini (personal communication) 2000.

99. Mosseri M, Vodovotz Y, Symon Z, et al. A novel gamma emitting radioactive stent constructed by targeted radioimmunotherapy [abstract]. J Am Coll Cardiol 2000;35:83.

100. Stabin MG, Konijnberg M, Knapp FF, et al. Monte Carlo modeling of radiation dose distributions in intravascular radiation therapy. Med Phys 2000;27:1086–1092.

101. Li XA, Wang R, Yu C, et al. Beta versus gamma for catheter-based intravascular brachytherapy: Dosimetric perspectives in the presence of metallic stents and calcified plaques. Int J Radiat Oncol Biol Phys 2000;46:1043–1049.

102. Johns HE, Cunningham JR. The Physics of Radiology, 4th Edition. Springfield, IL: Charles C. Thomas Publishing Co.; 1983:733.

103. Christian Kirisits (personal communication) 2000.

## Chapter 29

Radioactive Stents:

The Milan Experience

Remo Albiero, MD, and Antonio Colombo, MD

Introduction

Although stent placement in selected lesions has demonstrated a 30% relative reduction in restenosis rate compared with balloon angioplasty,[1,2] it has not solved the problem of restenosis, mainly due to intimal hyperplasia.[3] Intracoronary radiation therapy delivered by catheter-based systems has been shown to reduce restenosis in patients with coronary artery disease.[4,5] In the animal model,[6,7] low dose beta radiation delivered by a stent was effective in preventing restenosis by inhibition of subsequent intrastent neointimal cell proliferation. The first implantation of a ^{32}P radioactive beta-emitting Palmaz-Schatz (PS 153) stent into human coronary arteries was performed in the fall of 1996.[8] The radioisotope ^{32}P, a pure beta-particle emitter, was used because of its short half-life of 14.3 days and because it has a low degree of tissue penetration: the maximum penetration depth is 8.3 mm, and at 2 to 3 mm from the stent surface, the activity is almost negligible due to a significant drop-off. This physical characteristic can be considered an advantage in terms of minimum exposure of the surrounding tissue as well as of the catheterization staff, and also with regard to ease of shielding ^{32}P by plastic material, but it is a disadvantage in terms of dose distribution to the target vessel wall.

The safety, feasibility, and efficacy of ^{32}P radioactive beta-particle emitting stent implantation in patients with symptomatic de novo or restenotic native coronary lesions has been evaluated in the pilot Isostent for Restonosis Intervention Study (IRIS). Fifty-seven patients were enrolled: 32 patients in the low dose IRIS 1A (0.5 to 1.0 µCi),[9] and 25 patients in the IRIS 1B (0.75 to 1.5 µCi).[10] This pilot clinical trial found that ^{32}P radioactive Palmaz-Schatz stents can be safely implanted. However, coronary angiography, performed in 52 of 57 patients (92.9%) at 6-month follow-up, showed a binary intralesion (both within the stent and at the edges) restenosis in 21 of 52 patients (40.4%),[11] a result that is not different from that with currently available nonradioactive stents.

Clinical study with ^{32}P radioactive stents started in Europe (Heidelberg, Rotterdam, and Milan) in 1997. The Heidelberg[12] and the early Rotterdam experiences[13] with ^{32}P radioactive Palmaz-Schatz or BX stents at low-to-intermediate

From Waksman R (ed.). *Vascular Brachytherapy, Third Edition*. Armonk, NY: Futura Publishing Co., Inc.; © 2002.

activity have been reported. In the Heidelberg study,[12] 11 [32]P Palmaz-Schatz coronary stents with activities of 1.5 to 3 μCi were implanted in 11 patients with restenosis after previous percutaneous transluminal coronary angioplasty (PTCA). At 6-month follow-up, the restenosis rate was 54% (6/11), found mainly at the articulation of the stents; it was observed at a lower rate at the proximal and distal edges.[14] In the Rotterdam study,[13] a total of 31 radioactive stents with activities of 0.75 to 1.5 μCi were implanted in 26 patients. At 6-month follow-up, the restenosis rate was 17% and no restenosis was observed at the stent edges.

The Milan Experience

A clinical dose-finding study with ^{32}P radioactive stents began in October 1997, at Centro Cuore Columbus, in Milan, Italy. Inclusion criteria for enrollment were the presence of a de novo or restenotic lesion of a major, native coronary artery with a reference artery size visually estimated to be appropriate for the available stent diameters (3.0 to 3.5 mm).

Two types of radioactive stents (Isostent, Inc., Belmont, CA) were implanted: initially the Palmaz-Schatz PS 153 with activities of 0.75 to 3.0 μCi and, later, the BX stent with activities up to 21 μCi. The stent was mounted on a compliant balloon covered with an integral sheat (delivery system), and with a lucite radiation shield attached to the distal end of the stent delivery system to prevent operator exposure to the radiation.

The BX stent, designed by a computed-aided technique, was selected to provide flexibility and to have a more favorable effect on dose distribution along the length of the stent, as it does not have a central articulation. The BX stent has been demonstrated to favorably influence the vascular response in normal porcine coronary arteries compared to the Palmaz-Schatz stent.[15]

Medical Regimen and Stenting Procedure

Patients received aspirin 325 mg daily, continued long-term, and ticlopidine 250 mg twice daily for 3 months post procedure. The technique used for implantation of a radioactive stent is nearly identical to that required for an optimal intravascular ultrasound (IVUS)-guided placement of a nonradioactive stent. After lesion predilatation, mostly using a 20-mm long balloon, the delivery system was advanced to the target lesion site and the 15-mm long stent delivered at the recommended pressure of 8 to 10 atm. The stent was premounted on a 20-mm long compliant balloon so that 2.5 mm of the length of the delivery balloon emerged beyond each stent edge. Further stent expansion using a larger and usually shorter balloon at higher pressure was used to achieve an optimal angiographic result. After high-pressure inflation, IVUS was performed. Further expansion was indicated if the stent was not fully apposed to the vessel wall or if the cross-sectional area was not appropriately large compared to the adjacent reference segments.

Low-to-Intermediate Activity Stents (0.75 to 3 μCi)

The experience with radioactive stents in Milan started in October 1997 using low-to-intermediate activity stents. Twenty-seven lesions (93% de novo) in 25 patients were treated by implantation of 31 [32]P Palmaz-Schatz PS 153 stents with an initial activity ranging from 0.75 to 3 μCi (mean 1.55 μCi).[16]

After 4 to 6 months, intralesion binary restenosis (defined as ≥50% luminal reduction occurring inside the stent or at the proximal and distal reference segments) occurred in 10 of 19 lesions (52%) of patients who underwent angiographic follow-up. The analysis of the pattern of restenosis showed that in 5 lesions (26%) restenosis occurred only in the reference segments (at the edges of the stent), in one lesion (5%) at the edges and in the first 1 to 3 mm inside the stent, and in one lesion (5%) the stent was occluded (this late occlusion was not associated with a clinical event). Finally, a pure intrastent restenosis (defined as ≥50% luminal reduction occurring only inside the stent with absence of restenosis in the proximal and distal reference segments) occurred in 3 lesions (16%). In this group of patients, the incidence and the pattern of restenosis were similar to that which was observed in the group of 11 patients enrolled in the Heidelberg study, in whom the rate of restenosis was observed to be 54% at the articulation of the stents, with a lower rate at the proximal and distal edges.[14] In addition, the incidence of pure intrastent restenosis was similar to that observed in the group of 26 patients enrolled in Rotterdam,[13] treated by radioactive stents with activities of 0.75 to 1.5 μCi, in whom restenosis was 17% (no restenosis was observed at the stent edges).

High-Activity Stents (3 to 12 μCi)

From December 1997 through October 1998, 32 lesions (91% de novo) in 29 patients were treated by implantation of 39 ^{32}P BX stents with an initial activity of 3 to 6 μCi (mean 4.25 μCi), and 32 lesions (100% de novo) in 30 patients were treated by implantation of 53 ^{32}P BX stents with an initial activity of 6 to 12 μCi (mean 9.30 μCi).[16]

After 4 to 6 months, in the patients who underwent angiographic follow-up (>80%), the intralesion restenosis rate was 41% in the 3 to 6 μCi group, and 50% in the 6 to 12 μCi group. This intralesion restenosis rate was similar to, or perhaps higher than, that of currently available nonradioactive stents. However, the analysis of the pattern of restenosis showed that pure intrastent restenosis occurred in only 1 patient (3%) in the 3 to 6 μCi group, and in no patients (0%) in the 6 to 12 μCi group, even though in 3 patients of this latter group the stent was occluded at follow-up (only one occlusion was associated with a clinical syndrome of stent thrombosis 1 week after the patient stopped both aspirin and ticlopidine 3 months after stenting). Thus, restenosis occurred mostly in the reference segments at the stent edges. We summarized the presence of a good intrastent result combined with an "edge effect," coining the term "candy wrapper" (Fig. 1).[16,17] The precise mechanism by which the "edge effect" occurs remains poorly understood. It could be the result of a low dose of radiation at the stent edges, due to a sharp decline of dose rate within millimeters from the stent margins,[18] in combination with the balloon injury in the segments adjacent to the stent. The injury at the stent margins has been advocated as one of the mechanisms of restenosis at these sites after nonradioactive stent implantation.[19,20]

To clarify the mechanism of the "edge effect," we compared the lesions with and without edge restenosis. By univariate analysis, we found that the ratio of the maximum diameter of the longest balloon (used to predilate, deploy, or postdilate the stent) to the reference vessel diameter was significantly higher in the lesions

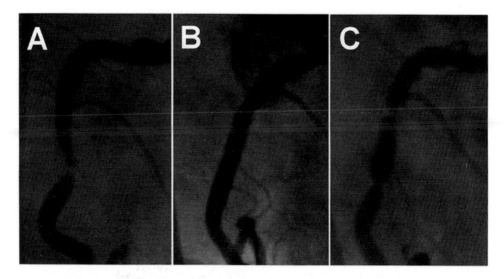

Figure 1. Representative lesion with the "candy wrapper" pattern of restenosis 6 months after implantation of a ^{32}P radioactive 15-mm long BX stents with an initial activity of 17.3 μCi. **(A)** Baseline angiogram showing a significant stenosis in the mid right coronary artery. **(B)** Post-stenting angiogram. **(C)** Six-month follow-up angiogram, showing no late lumen loss inside the stent, but a focal significant stenosis at both of the stent edges.

with edge restenosis compared with the lesions without edge restenosis. In addition, the lesions with edge restenosis had a significant smaller reference lumen diameter and a smaller final minimum lumen diameter by angiography than the group without restenosis. Finally, serial IVUS analysis of the 13 lesions treated by a single radioactive stent and with restenosis at follow-up, showed that the late lumen loss in the first 1 to 3 mm outside the stent (at the sites of balloon injury) was mainly due to neointimal hyperplasia.

The results of the Milan dose-finding study in radioactive stents of 6 to 12 μCi are consistent with the results of the Rotterdam group in radioactive stents with the same range of activity. While there were no cases of edge restenosis in ^{32}P radioactive stents of 0.75 to 1.5 μCi,[13] a restenosis rate of 43% was reported, occurring only at the stent edges, in an additional group of lesions treated by ^{32}P radioactive stents with a higher activity of 6 to 12 μCi.[21]

High-Activity Stents (12 to 21 μCi)

Despite the fact that the restenosis rate in the 3 to 12 μCi radioactive stents was not lower, and was perhaps even higher, than that of currently available nonradioactive stents, we continued the Milan dose-finding study, supported by animal safety data testing activities up to 24 μCi.[22] Our purpose was to evaluate whether stents with a higher initial activity combined with a nonaggressive stent implantation strategy could solve the problem of edge restenosis. The stent implantation technique was more conservative, selecting nonoversized balloons to predilate the lesion and deploy the stent, and postdilating the stent at high pressure using a shorter balloon to avoid mechanically damaging the reference segments.

From October 1998 through April 1999, 54 lesions were treated by single ^{32}P radioactive BX stents of 12 to 21 μCi, using a nonaggressive approach. The results of these lesions were compared with the results of 42 lesions treated by single ^{32}P radioactive BX stents with a lower initial activity of 3 to 12 μCi.[23] This study demonstrated that single ^{32}P radioactive beta-emitting stents with an initial activity greater than 12 μCi, implanted using a nonaggressive approach, significantly reduced intrastent neointimal hyperplasia compared with the lower dose group; this did not solve the problem of edge restenosis, however, which still occurred in 30% of the lesions, mostly at the edges (26%). A representative example of the "candy wrapper" appearance with restenosis at both edges after implantation of a 17.3 μCi stent is shown in Figure 1. The mechanism of the "edge effect" which occurred in this latter group of 12 to 21 μCi stents was elucidated by IVUS. Serial IVUS analysis (after stenting and at follow-up) showed that the late lumen loss in the first 1 to 3 mm from the stent margins was mainly due to remodeling (shrinkage of the vessel),[23] as opposed to our prior observation in 3 to 12 μCi stents (implanted aggressively), which was mainly due to tissue growth (intimal hyperplasia).[16] In addition, in-stent intimal hyperplasia was lower in the central 5 mm compared with the proximal and distal 5 mm of the stent. Therefore, by increasing the stent activity and limiting the balloon-induced injury outside the stent, we reduced the component of edge restenosis that was related to plaque growth, but not the component related to negative remodeling.

To reduce the vascular changes that affect edge restenosis of the stent, we evaluated two of the proposed[17] modifications to existing radioactive stent morphology: the "cold-ends" and the "hot-ends" stent.

The "Cold Ends" Stent

The rationale for using a "cold ends" stent was the prevention of negative remodeling at the stent edges. This concept was supported by the results of our study on 12 to 21 μCi stents implanted using a nonaggressive strategy,[23] which demonstrated a reduction of edge restenosis related to plaque growth but not of that related to negative remodeling.

The "cold ends" [32]P stent consists of a 25-mm BX stent with a radiated center segment of 15.9 mm in length, which has an activity level between 6 and 24 μCi, and nonradioactive end segments of 5.7 mm in length. From June until July 1999, we treated 10 de novo lesions in native coronary arteries by implantation of 10 "cold ends" [32]P stents.

Some procedural and angiographic results are shown in Table 1. All 10 patients (100%) underwent the 6-month angiographic follow-up. Restenosis occurred in 4 patients (40%) only in the nonradioactive part of the stent. One patient had also a symptomatic late (after 3.5 months) occlusion after discontinuation of any antiplatelet therapy.

The "Hot Ends" Stent

The rationale for using radioactive stents with higher activity at the proximal and distal ends of the stent ("hot ends") was the chance to diminish the problem of edge restenosis by extending the area of irradiation beyond the balloon-injured area.

Table 1

Results of the "Cold Ends" Stents

Lesions, n	10
Radioactivity, μCi	10.67±2.67
Vessel	
LAD, n (%)	8 (80)
LCx, n (%)	1 (10)
RCA, n (%)	8 (10)
Reference diameter, mm	2.96±0.53
Lesion length, mm	14.1±5.3
Balloon-to-artery ratio	1.15±0.23
MLD, preintervention, mm	0.99±0.46
MLD, post stenting, mm	2.78±0.43
Restenosis rate (DS >50%), n (%)	4/10 (40%)

LAD = left anterior descending coronary artery; LCx = left circumflex artery; RCA = right coronary artery; MLD = minimum lumen diameter.

The "hot ends" ^{32}P radioactive stent has a length of ~18 mm. The initial maximal activity is 2.6 μCi/mm in the proximal and distal 2 mm of the stent, and 0.57 μCi/mm in the central 14 mm of the stent. Thus, the initial maximal total activity of the stent is ~18.5 μCi (10.4 μCi at the ends plus 7.98 μCi in the middle of the stent). From July until November 1999, we treated 36 patients with 39 de novo lesions in native coronary arteries by implantation of 39 "hot ends" stents. Table 2 shows the acute results. The 6-month follow-up results are pending, but cases of edge restenosis have been observed in the patients who have had an angiographic follow-up.

Table 3 summarizes the complete Milan experience with radioactive stents.

Late Stent Occlusions

Due to the significant incidence (up to 15%) of late occlusions (>30 days) after intracoronary radiation therapy using catheter-based systems, we analyzed the incidence of this event after ^{32}P radioactive stent implantation.[24] In Milan,

Table 2

Results of the "Hot Ends" Stents

Patients, n	36
Lesions, n	39
Radioactivity, μCi	14.1±2.4
Reference diameter, mm	2.92±.64
Lesion length, mm	13.1±.62
Max pressure, atm	14.0±2.9
Balloon-to-artery ratio	1.19±.17
MLD, preintervention, mm	.90±.53
MLD, post stenting, mm	2.92±.62

MLD = minimum lumen diameter.

Table 3

Summary of the Complete Milan Experience with Radioactive Stents

Type of Radioactive Stent	Period	Lesions (n)	Intralesion Restenosis (%)
Low-mid Activity (0.75–3 μCi)	Oct–Dec '97	27	52%
Mid-high Activity (3–6 μCi)	Dec '97 until	32	41%
High-activity (6–12 μCi)	Oct '98	32	50%
Highest activity (12–21 μCi)	Oct '98–Apr '99	83	43%
"Cold ends"	Apr–July '99	10	40%
"Hot ends"	July–Nov '99	39	?
Total		223	45%

from September 1997 until October 1999, 260 ^{32}P radioactive stents were implanted in 223 lesions in 192 patients. After stenting, all patients received aspirin plus either ticlopidine 250 mg BID or clopidogrel 75 mg QD for ≤3 months. A 6-month angiographic follow-up study was performed in 163 patients (85%) with 190 lesions (86%).

A late occlusion occurred in 10 lesions (5.3%) in 10 patients (6.1%): (a) 6 occlusions (3.2%) were asymptomatic and documented between 76 and 315 days (mean 168 days) after stenting; (b) 4 occlusions (2.1%) were symptomatic for acute myocardial infarction which occurred between 102 and 147 days after stenting in patients who discontinued ticlopidine (2 of the 4 patients discontinued both ticlopidine and aspirin). Only 2 of the 4 symptomatic occlusions were documented at the time of acute myocardial infarction, while in the other 2 patients the vessel was patent at the time of the lately performed coronary angiogram. One of these 4 patients died 15 days after the documented stent thrombosis due to left ventricular failure. In the 4 patients with symptomatic late occlusion, the initial stent activity was between 9.8 and 20 μCi. In the 6 patients with asymptomatic late occlusion, mean lesion length before stenting was 31.6 mm, the mean number of stents per lesion was 2.67, mean reference vessel diameter was 2.44 mm, and mean initial stent activity level was 9.28 μCi.

In conclusion, in the whole Milan experience with ^{32}P radioactive stents, a late occlusion occurred in 5.3% of the lesions. The late occlusions were mostly asymptomatic (3.2%). These asymptomatic late occlusions occurred in long lesions in small vessel treated with multiple stents. A late occlusion symptomatic for acute myocardial infarction occurred in 4 patients (2.1%) who discontinued ticlopidine or any antiplatelet therapy between 3 and 6 months after stenting. Thus, a prolonged antiplatelet therapy with ticlopidine/clopidogrel for 6 to 12 months after radioactive stent implantation is recommended.

Long-Term Follow-Up

We analyzed the outcome of a repeat percutaneous coronary intervention (PCI) for the occurrence of restenosis after radioactive stent implantation. Restenosis at 6 months after stent implantation occurred in 90 lesions (in 31 lesions ≥2 radioactive stents were implanted) of 75 patients, with the following pattern: at the proximal edge in 37%, at the distal edge in 18%, at both edges in 20%, and inside the stent in 24% of the lesions. The mean length of the restenotic lesion was 11±6 mm. A repeat PCI was performed in all the lesions with angiographic restenosis even if the patients were asymptomatic and had no objective evidence of ischemia. New stents were implanted in 34%, traditional balloon angioplasty was performed in 39%, Cutting Balloon™ angioplasty in 26%, and directional atherectomy in 6% of the lesions. Angiographic success was achieved in all the lesions and the clinical success rate was 96%. A non-Q-wave myocardial infarction occurred in 4% of the patients and no other major adverse cardiac events occurred during the hospitalization. Clinical follow-up was obtained in all eligible (≥3months) patients (n=72) after 8.4±5 months (the results are presented in Table 4), and the outcome appears favorable.

Mechanism of Edge Restenosis

Edge restenosis could be simply explained by the basic physics of a radioactive stent, which delivers a lower dose of radiation at the ends compared with the central part of the stent. In other words, edge restenosis could be the result of the shorter length of the prescription isodose compared with the length of the radioactive stent.

In some circumstances radioactive stents can stimulate rather than inhibit intimal hyperplasia, as reported by Carter at al[7] in the porcine model of restenosis. They demonstrated that 1.0 μCi stents had a significant greater neointimal formation and luminal narrowing than the control nonradioactive stents. Other animal studies[26,27] have analyzed the effect of radiation delivery by a stent on the extracellular matrix deposition. Hehrlein et al,[26] in the rabbit model, demonstrated by immunocytochemical analysis an increase in the expression of collagen type I after radioactive stent implantation, whereas collagen type III and IV production was unchanged. We do not have data regarding the composition of the plaque at the edges of the stent in the lesions with edge restenosis. However, we observed that these plaques had a low echodensity by IVUS and were easily treated with balloon inflations at low pressure, suggesting that these plaques probably consisted mostly of extracellular matrix. Finally, a study of Carter et al[28] in cholesterol-fed pigs demonstrated stimulation of intimal hyperplasia when radioactive stents were implanted 1 month after angioplasty.

Table 4

Long-Term (>6 months) Clinical Follow-Up Results After Repeat Percutaneous Transluminal Coronary Angioplasty

Patients, n	72
Death	1 (1%)
CABG	2 (3%)
MI	1 (1%)
Second repeat TLR	16 (22%)
Second repeat TVR	17 (24%)

CABG = coronary artery bypass graft; MI = myocardial infarction; TLR = Target lesion revascularization; TVR = Target vessel revascularization.

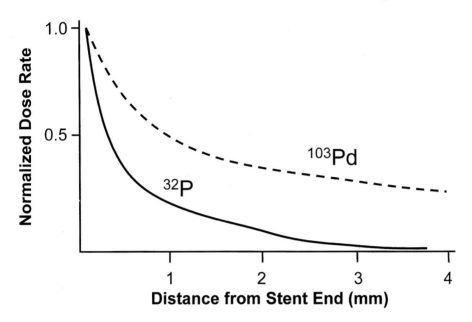

Figure 2. Normalized dose rate versus distance from the stent end (mm) of a ^{32}P and a [103]Pd radioactive stent. Note the lower dose fall-off of [103]Pd compared to ^{32}P, that may allow delivery of a higher dose of radiation in the first 2 to 3 mm beyond the [103]Pd stent edge.

Conclusions and Future Directions

Radioactive ^{32}P beta-emitting stents with an initial activity of 3 to 21 μCi are effective in inhibiting intrastent neointimal hyperplasia and in reducing intrastent restenosis to less than 4%. However, a high intralesion restenosis rate (~30 to 50%) due to an "edge effect" has been observed. We summarized these two findings, coining the term "candy wrapper." The "edge effect" is possibly the result of a low dose of radiation at the edges of the stent in combination with the systematic vessel wall injury induced by balloon inflation outside the stent margins. The "cold ends" and the "hot ends" stent are two of the approaches proposed to solve the problem of edge restenosis. In the Milan experience, after implantation of [32]P "cold ends" stent, restenosis occurred in the nonradioactive ends, while the results of the "hot ends" stent are pending. Finally, there is a rationale for using a gamma-emitting (Palladium, [103]Pd) stent. This isotope ([103]Pd) has a lower dose fall-off than [32]P (Fig. 2), and may allow delivery of a higher dose of radiation in the first 2 to 3 mm beyond the stent edge.

References

1. Fischman DL, Leon MB, Baim DS, et al. A randomized comparison of coronary-stent placement and balloon angioplasty in the treatment of coronary artery disease. Stent Restenosis Study Investigators. N Engl J Med 1994;331:496–501.
2. Serruys PW, de Jaegere P, Kiemeneij F, et al. A comparison of balloon-expandable-stent implantation with balloon angioplasty in patients with coronary artery disease. Benestent Study Group. N Engl J Med 1994;331:489–495.
3. Hoffmann R, Mintz GS, Dussaillant GR, et al. Patterns and mechanism of in-stent restenosis: A serial intravascular ultrasound study. Circulation 1996;94:1247–1254.

4. Teirstein PS, Massullo V, Jani S, et al. Catheter-based radiotherapy to inhibit restenosis after coronary stenting. N Engl J Med 1997;336:1697–1703.

5. King SB III, Williams DO, Chougule P, et al. Endovascular beta-radiation to reduce restenosis after coronary balloon angioplasty: Results of the beta energy restenosis trial (BERT). Circulation 1998;97:2025–2030.

6. Hehrlein C, Stintz M, Kinscherf R, et al. Pure beta-particle-emitting stents inhibit neointima formation in rabbits. Circulation 1996;93:641–645.

7. Carter AJ, Laird JR, Bailey LR, et al. Effects of endovascular radiation from a beta-particle-emitting stent in a porcine coronary restenosis model: A dose-response study. Circulation 1996;94:2364–2368.

8. Fischell TA, Hehrlein C, Fischell RE, et al. The impact of stent design and delivery upon the long-term efficacy of radioisotope stents. J Invasive Cardiol 2000;12:162–167.

9. Fischell TA, Carter A, Foster M, et al. Lessons from the feasibility radioactive (IRIS) stent trials. In: Waksman R (ed.): Vascular Brachytherapy, 2nd Edition. Armonk, NY: Futura Publishing Co., Inc.; 1999:475–481.

10. Moses J, Ellis S, Bailey S, et al. Short-term (1 month) results of the dose response IRIS feasibility study of a beta-particle emitting radioisotope stent [abstract]. J Am Coll Cardiol 1998;31:350A.

11. Moses J. U.S. IRIS trials low-activity 32P stent: Advances in Cardiovascular Radiation Therapy III [abstract]. Washington, DC, 1999:387–388.

12. Hehrlein C, Brachmann J, Hardt S, et al. P-32 stents for prevention of restenosis: Results of the Heidelberg safety trial using the Palmaz-Schatz stent design at moderate activity levels in patients with restenosis after PTCA [abstract]. Circulation 1998;98:I-780.

13. Wardeh AJ, Kay IP, Sabate M, et al. Beta-particle-emitting radioactive stent implantation: A safety and feasibility study. Circulation 1999;100:1684–1689.

14. Hansen A, Hehrlein C, Hardt S, et al. Is the "candy-wrapper" effect of beta-particle emitting stents due to remodeling or neointimal hyperplasia? [abstract] Circulation 1999;1000:I-155.

15. Carter AJ, Scott D, Rahdert D, et al. Stent design favourably influences the vascular response in normal porcine coronary arteries. J Invasive Cardiol 1999;11:127–134.

16. Albiero R, Adamian M, Kobayashi N, et al. Short- and intermediate-term results of (32)P radioactive beta-emitting stent implantation in patients with coronary artery disease: The Milan Dose-Response Study. Circulation 2000;101:18–26.

17. Serruys PW, Kay IP. I like the candy, I hate the wrapper: The (32)P radioactive stent. Circulation 2000;101:3–7.

18. Janicki C, Duggan DM, Coffey CW, et al. Radiation dose from a phosphorous-32 impregnated wire mesh vascular stent. Med Phys 1997;24:437–445.

19. Dussaillant GR, Mintz GS, Pichard AD, et al. Small stent size and intimal hyperplasia contribute to restenosis: A volumetric intravascular ultrasound analysis. J Am Coll Cardiol 1995;26:720–724.

20. Ikari Y, Hara K, Tamura T, et al. Luminal loss and site of restenosis after Palmaz-Schatz coronary stent implantation. Am J Cardiol 1995;76:117–120.

21. Wardeh AJ, Knook AHM, Kay IP, et al. The European P-32 Dose Response Trial: The Rotterdam contribution [abstract]. Am J Cardiol 1999;84:84P.

22. Carter AJ, Scott D, Bailey L, et al. Dose-response effects of 32P radioactive stents in an atherosclerotic porcine coronary model. Circulation 1999;100:1548–1554.

23. Albiero R, Nishida T, Adamian M, et al. Edge restenosis after implantation of high activity (32)P radioactive beta-emitting stents. Circulation 2000;101:2454–2457.

24. Albiero R, Nishida T, Amato A, et al. Late total occlusions following 32P radioactive β-particle-emitting stent implantation in patients with CAD [abstract]. Eur Heart J 2000;21(suppl):399.

25. Fischell TA, Carter AJ, Laird JR. The beta-particle-emitting radioisotope stent (isostent): Animal studies and planned clinical trials. Am J Cardiol 1996;78:45–50.

26. Hehrlein C. Radioactive stents: The European Experience. In: Waksman R (ed.): Vascular Brachytherapy, 2nd Edition. Armonk, NY: Futura Publishing Company; 1999:333–342.

27. Carter AJ, Jenkins JS, Bailey LR, et al. Dose rate and cumulative dose effects of P-32 radioactive stents [abstract]. J Am Coll Cardiol 1999;33:20A.

28. Carter AJ, Scott D, Bailey LR, et al. High activity 32P stents promote development of atherosclerosis at six months in a porcine model [abstract]. Circulation 1997;96:I-607.

## Chapter 30

New Concepts for Radioactive Stents

Christoph Hehrlein, MD, and Tim A. Fischell, MD

Introduction

Early clinical results worldwide with more than 400 implants of balloon-expandable [32]P Palmaz-Schatz and BX radioisotope stents have demonstrated safety of the technology with excellent procedural and 6-month event-free survival. According to the early trials, thrombotic occlusion of the coronary artery after stent-based coronary irradiation is a rare event (rate <2%). The clinical trials indicate that restenosis rates are decreased in a dose-dependent fashion within the bodies of radioisotope stents. However, the major problem with these radioactive implants is restenosis at the stent edges, leading to revascularization rates similar to conventional stenting. The typical angiographic appearance of restenosis after implantation of radioactive stents is narrowing at the proximal and distal stent edges, which was called a "candy-wrapper." This problem occured exclusively with the balloon-expandable radioactive stent delivery system. The biological reasons for restenosis occurring exclusively at stent edges are mostly unknown, and the mechanisms are complex. Radiation dose in the fall-off zone, for instance, interacts with variable degrees of vascular injury (barotrauma) at the stent ends depending on the means of stent delivery and pre- and post-dilatation procedures. It may be possible to overcome the edge restenosis problem with improvement in balloon-expandable stent delivery systems by minimization of barotrauma at the stent ends, application of sufficient radiation doses to counteract dose fall-off, and evaluation of new isotopes or local radiosensitizers. Future directions for this technology may also include alternative radiation delivery platforms such as self-expanding radioactive stents, which may improve results by favorable arterial remodeling combined with the inhibition of neointimal hyperplasia.

Background

Despite the benefits of stenting to treat coronary artery disease, in-stent restenosis remains a significant problem after intracoronary stenting, particularly in long lesions and smaller diameter vessels.[1] Experimental and clinical data have demonstrated that in-stent restenosis is principally caused by neointimal formation.[2] Radiation therapy is known to be effective in reducing benign dermatosis, keloid formation, or heterotopic bone formation.[3] Studies that systematically evaluated the effects of radiation on atherosclerotic arteries began in 1965.[4]

From Waksman R (ed.). *Vascular Brachytherapy, Third Edition.* Armonk, NY: Futura Publishing Co., Inc.; © 2002.

Later, cell culture studies showed that both migration and proliferation of vascular cells are inhibited by the application of ionizing radiation.[5-7] Despite an obvious therapeutic benefit, many studies also showed that ionizing radiation can induce damage to the skin and nearby vascular structures.[8] The late effect of high-volume external beam irradiation, for instance, is fibrosis, which can cause severe carotid or coronary artery stenosis.[9,10] Recently, however, the approach to endovascular irradiation has been shown to be a highly effective method to reduce neointimal formation and thus, prevent restenosis.[11,12]

Intravascular radiation using an ^{192}Ir and a ^{90}Sr/^{90}Y source has been effective in reducing neointimal formation after balloon injury in a porcine restenosis model and in subsequent clinical studies.[13,14] An alternative, and perhaps simpler approach to temporary intravascular radiation is the use of a stent as the platform for local radiation delivery as a means to prevent restenosis. Experimental studies have demonstrated that stents ion-implanted with ^{32}P reduce neointimal formation at activities as low as 0.5 μCi.[15-17]

Processes of Stent Activation

There are at least three methods for the fabrication of a radioisotope stent. These include, but are not limited to: (1) bombardment of metallic stents with charged particles (ie, deuterons or protons); (2) direct ion implantation of stents with radioisotopes; and (3) chemical methods for radioisotope incorporation into the metallic stents or stent coatings.

Stents can be placed in a cyclotron and bombarded with charged particles.[18] Furthermore, it is technically possible to selectively implant a single type of radioisotope, ie, ^{32}P or ^{103}Pd, into the stent surface. ^{32}P is a "pure" beta-particle emitter with a half-life of 14.3 days and maximum energy of 1.71 MeV. The portion of bremsstrahlung produced by a stent incorporating ^{32}P decays into the stable isotope ^{32}S. After 5 months, the radiation has essentially disappeared. The maximum penetration depth of the radiation from ^{32}P in tissue is 8.3 mm. In tissue, the dose decrease is very steep. ^{103}Pd is a weak gamma-emitter with a longer radial and transversial penetration depth, a maximum energy of 21 KeV, and a half-life of 17 days.

Finally, chemical methods using radioactive polymer films coated onto the stent surface (electrochemical deposition) provide alternative, and possibly more cost-effective, means for fabrication of radioisotope stents using ^{32}P or ^{103}Pd, or other potentially valuable isotopes.

Dosimetry

Despite very low activities compared to catheter-based irradiation devices and the low dose rates, the near-field cumulative dose can be quite high with stents in the higher activity ranges. The dosimetry of a ^{32}P stent has previously been described in detail. Janicki et al characterized the near-field dose of a 1.0 μCi 15-mm length Palmaz-Schatz (Cordis, a Johnson and Johnson Co., Warren, NJ) using a modification of the dose point kernel method.[19] Modification of the dose distribution around a uniform cylinder of ^{32}P to account for the geometry of a tubular-slotted Palmaz-Schatz stent with mathematical modeling allowed construction of three-dimensional dose maps. The nonuniformity of dosing reflective of the stent geometry decreases at distances of 1 to 2 mm from the surface. However, it may be important to optimize uniformity of dosing in the near-field of radioactive stents. The dosimetry predicted by the dose calculations correlated well with the measured dose using radiochromic film. While these data provide an in vitro analysis of dosing from a radioactive stent, the actual dose distribution will be affected by variations in atherosclerotic plaque morphology and symmetry of stent expansion. Because the cumalative radiation doses to the subendothelium are quite high, ie, several 100 Gy for 6 to 48 µCi ^{32}P stents, radioisotope stents impregnated with radiosensitizers may reduce radiotoxicity and improve long-term results. Stent design appears to be an important denominator of dose pertubations of vascular irradiation. If stents are irradiated by beta particles from endovascular radiation sources, thicker struts with high atomic numbers induce cold spots in the dose distribution adjacent to the wires.[20]

Biology of Stent-Based Vessel Irradiation

Stent-based vessel irradiation causes localized inibition of smooth muscle cell migration and proliferation.[7] In addition, radiation-induced apoptosis appears to play a role by maintaining hypocellularity of the newly formed neointimal layer after stent implantation.[21] Interestingly, both in rabbit and porcine restenosis models, neointima lesion formation after stent-based vessel irradiation consists predominantly of excessive extracellular matrix formation.[15,22] Excessive matrix formation after stent implantation and vessel irradiation appears to occur dose-dependently to a greater extent at high radiation doses.[23] Largely unexplained is the occurrence of a certain type of restenosis, ie, the so-called "black hole," a process of lumen narrowing difficult to detect by conventional intravascular ultrasound (IVUS) techniques.

Clinical Pilot Trials with Radioisotope Stents

American Studies

The initial clinical experience with beta-particle–emitting stents occurred in the U.S. beginning in October 1996. The phase 1 Isostent for Restenosis Intervention Study (IRIS IA and B) were nonrandomized trials designed to evaluate the safety of implanting very low-activity (0.5 to 1.5 µCi) ^{32}P 15-mm length Palmaz-Schatz coronary stents in patients with symptomatic de novo or restenosis native coronary lesions.[24,25]

Stent placement was successful in all patients. The mean stent activity at the time of implant in the IRIS trials was 0.7 µCi. There were no cases of acute or subacute stent thrombosis, target lesion revascularization, death, or other major cardiac events within the first 30 days (primary safety endpoint), thus demonstrating acceptable early event-free survival. At 6-month follow-up there was a binary restenosis rate of 31% (10/32) and a clinically driven target vessel revascularization (TVR) rate of 21%. Interestingly, there was only 1 restenosis (proximal to stent) out of the 10 patients treated for restenosis lesions (10%) and only 18% for patients receiving stents greater than 0.75 µCi. There were no further TVR events between 6 months and 12 months. By IVUS there was a significant amount of diffuse disease as noted by a mean of 41% cross-sectional area stenosis in the reference vessel at the time of stent implantation. Optimal stent implantation, by IVUS, was achieved in only 56% of cases, due mainly to high plaque burden preventing an optimal ratio of stent to reference vessel cross-sectional area. Quantitative angiographic follow-up at 6 months demonstrated a lesional late loss of 0.94 mm for the group as a whole and 0.70 mm for the restenosis subgroup.[24]

European Studies

A small pilot feasibility trial using 1.5 to 3 μCi 15-mm length [32]P Palmaz-Schatz stents started in June 1997 in Heidelberg, Germany. Eleven stents were implanted successfully in patients with coronary artery restenosis. The main inclusion criteria were age, 50–75 years, restenosis after conventional PTCA, and stabile angina pectoris. The main exclusion criteria were acute myocardial infarction, unstable angina, not eligible for bypass surgery, and allergies to aspirin and ticlopidine. Exclusion criteria related to the coronary artery disease were reference diameters greater than 3.5 mm and less than 3.0 mm, tortuosity of artery (>45° bend), in-stent restenosis, bypass graft lesions, and multivessel disease. Optimal stent deployment was controlled by IVUS guidance. The patients received ticlopidine for a period of 2 months after stent implantation. There were no major adverse cardiac events (death, myocardial infarction, coronary artery bypass graft) noted at the 30-day safety endpoint and after 6 months. However, the study was terminated early because angiographic restenosis rates were high (54%) due to the edge effects occuring in particular at the bridging strut of the Palmaz Schatz stent.[26] After this trial, only radioactive stents without an articulation (BX stents) were used in further studies.

The vast majority of patients receiving radioisotope stents were enrolled in trials conducted at the Thoraxcenter in Rotterdam and at the Columbus Hospital in Milan.

Experience at the Thoraxcenter, Rotterdam

Twenty-six patients with coronary ^{32}P stents at activity levels of 0.75 to 1.5 μCi were studied in a nonrandomized fashion. The clinical results were different from the IRIS trials. In contrast to American studies with coronary ^{32}P stents of the same activity range, restenosis rates were low, ie, in-stent restenosis occurred in 17% of the patients and 13% had repeat vascularization. No restenosis was observed at the stent edges. However, the angiographic late loss of 0.99±0.59 and loss index of 0.53±0.35 were comparable to data from the IRIS trials and known results of conventional stent implantation.[27] In a series of 42 patients receiving 6 to12 μCi ^{32}P stents, two uneventful vessel closures occurred in the follow-up period. All other vessels remained patent after 6 months and had no in-stent restenosis; however, the rate of edge restenosis was 44%. In this study, one non-Q-wave acute myocardial infarction was noted due to transient thrombotic closure of the coronary artery. The group in Rotterdam is currently studying a series of patients, in which radioisotope stents with "hot"- and "cold-ends" have been implanted into the coronary arteries. The Rotterdam group first described a peculiar finding by IVUS within ^{32}P radioactive stents, which was called the" black hole."

The morphology of the "black hole" corresponds most likely with a specific array of glycoproteins assembled in a newly formed bulk of extracellular matrix.

Experience at the Colombus Hospital in Milan

Albiero et al[28] recently reported on a cohort of 122 patients studied after implantation of three groups of ^{32}P coronary stents in the activity range from 0.75 to 12 μCi. At 6-month follow-up, no deaths had occurred, and only 1 patient had stent thrombosis. The intrastent restenosis rate was 16% for stents with activities of 0.75 to 3 μCi (group 1), 3% for stents with activties of 3 to 6 μCi (group 2), and 0% for stents with activities of 6 to 12 μCi (group 3). The intralesion restenosis rate, however, was 52% in group 1, 41% in group 2, and 50% in group 3 due to restenosis at the stent edges. The authors concluded that an "aggressive approach" to stenting in combination with a dose fall-off at the stent end below therapeutic levels was responsible for the results of this procedure. In a subsequent study of only moderate- to high-activity stents (3 to 12 μCi), the authors reported a rate of edge restenosis (peristent-intrastent restenosis) of 24 to 38%.[29] The edge restenosis process appears to occur independently of the activity levels used in the study. These findings were made despite a "gentle" implantation technique using stent deployment pressures of only 8 to 10 atm, and despite a post-dilatation technique using a shorter balloon inside the stent to avoid mechanical damage (barotrauma) at the stent ends.[29]

New Concepts

The unsolved problem of edge restenosis after radioisotope stenting initiated the intense search for better stent-based radiation sources. Because the dose falls off by 50% at the ends of a homogenously coated ^{32}P stent, stents were manufactured with increasing activity levels at the edges ("hot-ends") to prevent edge restenosis. Higher activities at the stent ends could counteract a "stimulatory effect" of low-dose radiation for smooth muscle cell proliferation. The concept of "cold-end" radioactive stents is based on the assumption that hyperproliferative neointimal smooth muscle cells piling up at the stent ends are allowed to migrate into the stent ends to "smoothen out edge restenosis." In theory, migration of smooth muscle cells occurs from the stent ends into the stent until it is stopped by the radioactive portion of the stent body (electron fence hypothesis). Another hypothesis related to the "candy wrapper" problem is the following: the radioactivity at the stent ends induces constrictive vascular remodeling. The solution here could also be a nonradioactive stent end. These two concepts ("hot" and "cold" end) are currently being tested clinically.

Two other concepts are in a pre-clinical testing phase: (1) self-expanding radioisotope stents, which potentially eliminate balloon barotrauma beyond the stent edges because they lack a balloon delivery system, and (2) gamma-emitting stents, ie, using the isotope ^{103}Pd, which provide higher longitudinal penetration depth than beta radiation. Apart from these four concepts, there are multiple new design strategies for stent delivery balloons to reduce edge effects ranging from minimal balloon overhang and square-shouldered balloons to hybrid stent/catheter-based systems.[30]

Animal studies using pig and rabbit restenosis models with the ^{32}P self-expanding stent and the ^{103}Pd balloon-expandable stent have been conducted in the U.S., and the histomorphometric data from these studies are currently being evaluated. First results of the ^{103}Pd balloon-expandable stents indicate that occurrence of edge restenosis correlates with the extent of vessel injury at the stent ends, ie, it is more pronounced at distal stent end if the vessel tapers. These early animal findings suggest that even the "direct-stenting technique" may not improve clinical results.

In Japan, a novel gamma stent using the isotope ^{133}Xe has been sucessfully tested in a pre-clinical study, however, the edge problem has not been addressed.[31] Whether alternative radioisotopes impregnated to a balloon-expandable stent platform could prevent edge restenosis in patients is the subject of further trials.

Conclusion

It is now known from many clinical trials studying catheter-based radiation, that vascular brachytherapy can potently inhibit restenosis. It is clear that the clinical event of a subacute coronary thrombosis is rare after stent-based irradiation in coronary arteries, even if a rather brief period of combined antithrombotic therapy for 3 months was applied. However, the edge restenosis after radioactive stenting is a serious problem, which is now addressed in several ongoing studies. The major issues in solving this problem are related to dose-tissue interactions in the radiation fall-off zone at the stent ends, and to the impact of geographical miss due to pre- and post dilatation of the lesion. By improving stent delivery systems, minimizing or eliminating balloon barotrauma at the stent ends, and applying sufficient radiation doses to inhibit excessive proliferation, it may be possible to overcome the edge problem of radioactive stents.

References

1. Serruys PW, de Jaegere P, Kiemeneij F, et al. A comparison of balloon-expandable-stent implantation with balloon angioplasty in patients with coronary artery disease. N Engl J Med 1994;331:489–495.
2. Schwartz RS, Edwards WD, Bailey KR, et al. Differential neointimal response to coronary artery injury in pigs and dogs: Implications for restenosis models. Arterioscler Thromb 1994;14:395–400.
3. Escarmant P, Zimmermann S, Amar A, et al. The treatment of 783 keloid scars by iridium 192 interstitial irradiation after surgical excision. Int J Radiat Oncol Biol Phys 1993;26:245–251.
4. Friedman M, Byers SO. Effects of iridium 192 radiation on thromboatherosclerotic plaque in the rabbit aorta. Arch Path 1965;80:285–291.
5. Ootsuyama A, Tanooka H. Threshold-like dose of local beta irradiation repeated throughout the life span of mice for induction of skin and bone tumors. Radiat Res 1991;125:98–101.
6. Maity A, McKenna WG, Muschel RJ. The molecular basis for cell cycle delays following ionizing radiation: A review. Radiother Oncol 1994;31:1–13.
7. Fischell TA, Kharma BK, Fischell DR, et al. Low-dose, beta-particle emission from "stent" wire results in complete, localized inhibition of smooth muscle cell proliferation. Circulation 1994;90:2956–2963.
8. Hopewell JW, Sieber VK, Heryet JC, et al. Dose- and source-size-related changes in the late response of pig skin to irradiation with single doses of beta radiation from sources of differing energy. Radiat Res 1993;133:303–311.

9. Silverberg GD, Britt RH, Goffinet DR. Radiation-induced carotid artery disease. Cancer 1978;41:130–137.
10. Brosius FC, Waller BF, Roberts WC. Radiation heart disease: Analysis of 16 young (aged 15 to 33 years) necropsy patients who received over 3,500 rads to the heart. Am J Med 1981;70:519–530.
11. Tierstein PS, Massullo V, Popma JJ, et al. Catheter-based radiotherapy to inhibit restenosis after coronary stenting. N Engl J Med 1997;336:1697–1703.
12. Condado JA, Waksman R, Gurdiel O et al. Long-term angiographic and clinical outcome after percutaneous transluminal coronary angioplasty and intracoronary radiation therapy in humans. Circulation 1997;96:727–732.
13. Wiedermann JG, Marboe C, Amols H, et al. Intracoronary irradiation markedly reduces restenosis after balloon angioplasty in a porcine model. J Am Coll Cardiol 1994;23:1491–1498.
14. Waksman R, Robinson KA, Crocker IR, et al. Intracoronary low-dose beta-irradiation inhibits neointima formation after coronary artery balloon injury in the swine restenosis model. Circulation 1995;92:3025–3031.
15. Hehrlein C, Gollan C, Dönges K, et al. Low-dose radioactive endovascular stents prevent smooth muscle cell proliferation and neointimal hyperplasia in rabbits. Circulation 1995;92:1570–1575.
16. Hehrlein C, Stintz M, Kinscherf R, et al. Pure beta-particle-emitting stents inhibit neointima formation in rabbits. Circulation 1996;93:641–645.
17. Carter AJ, Laird JR, Bailey LR, et al. Effects of endovascular radiation from a beta-particle-emitting stent in a porcine coronary restenosis model: A dose-response study. Circulation 1996;94:2364–2368.
18. Fehsenfeld P, Golombeck M, Kleinrahm A, et al. On the production of radioactive stents. Sem Interv Cardiol 1998;3:157–161.
19. Janicki C, Duggan DM, Coffey CW, et al. Radiation dose from a phosphorus-32 impregnated wire mesh vascular stent. Med Phys 1997;24:437–445.
20. Amols HI, Trichter F, Weinberger J. Intracoronary radiation for prevention of restenosis: Dose pertubations caused by stents. Circulation 2000;98:2024–2029.
21. Hehrlein C, Kollum M, Arab A, et al. Increased apoptotic cell death in the neointima after stent-based vascular irradiation: Role of radiation-induced apoptosis for restenosis reduction. J Intervent Cardiol 1999;12:299–305.
22. Carter AJ, Douglas S, Bailey L, et al. Dose-response effects of 32P radioactive stents in an atherosclerotic porcine coronary model. Circulation 1999;100:1548–1554.
23. Hehrlein C, Kaiser S, Riessen R, et al. External beam radiation increases neointimal hyperplasia by augmenting smooth muscle cell proliferation and extracellular matrix accumulation. J Am Coll Cardiol 1999;34:561–566.
24. Fischell TA, Hehrlein C. The radioisotope stent for the prevention of restenosis. Herz 1998;23:373–379.
25. Hehrlein C, Fischell TA. History of the radioisotope stent. Vasc Radiother Mon 1999;1:66–69.
26. Hehrlein C, Hardt S, Brachmann J, et al. P32 stents for the prevention of restenosis: Results from the Heidelberg safety trial using the Palmaz-Schatz stent design at moderate activity levels in patients with restenosis after PTCA [abstract]. Circulation 1998;98(suppl 1):I-780.
27. Wardeh AJ, Kay IP, Sabate M, et al. Beta-particle emitting radioactive stent implantation: A safety and feasibilty study. Circulation 1999;100:1684–1689.
28. Albiero R, Adamian M, Kobayashi N, et al. Short-and intermediate-term results of ^{32}P radioactive β-emitting stent implantation in patients with coronary artery disease. Circulation 2000;101:18–26.
29. Albiero R, Nishida T, Adamian M, et al. Edge restenosis after implantation of high activity ^{32}P radioactive β-emitting stents. Circulation 2000;101:2454–2460.
30. Serruys PW, Kay IP. I like the candy, I hate the wrapper: The ^{32}P radioactive stent. Circulation 2000;101:3–7.
31. Watanabe S, Osa A, Sekine T, et al. Production of radioactive endovascular stents by implantation of ^{133}Xe ions. Appl Radiat Isot 1999;51:197–202.

## Chapter 31

Long-Term Effects of ^{32}P Radioactive Stents in Experimental Models

Andrew J. Carter DO, and Joerg Lehmann, PhD

Radioactive stents have been proposed as a means to reduce in-stent restenosis by inhibiting neointimal formation.[1-5] Fischell et al proposed that continuous low dose rate irradiation delivered by a radioactive stent would be sufficient to impair the ability of smooth muscle cells (SMCs) to proliferate following vascular injury after stent placement.[1] Experimental studies have demonstrated that stents ion-implanted with activities as low as 0.14 µCi of ^{32}P reduce neointimal formation at 28 days in porcine iliac arteries.[3] Hehrlein et al, however, reported a reduction in neointima after 12 weeks in rabbit iliac arteries only after placement of radioactive stents with 13 µCi ^{32}P.[5] Stents with 4 µCi of ^{32}P were histologically similar to nonradioactive stents. In the porcine coronary restenosis model, we observed an unusual biphasic biological response to low (0.5 µCi)-, intermediate (1.0 µCi)-, and high (>3.0 µCi)-activity 7-mm length ^{32}P Palmaz-Schatz stents at 28 days.[4] The low-activity ^{32}P radioactive stents reduced neointimal formation to a similar degree as reported in the porcine iliac model with 0.14 µCi ^{32}P radioactive stents. The intermediate-activity stents, however, promoted the formation of a matrix proteoglycan-rich neointima while the high-activity stents reduced neointimal formation, but with histologic evidence of delayed vascular repair. Thus, the data suggest important dose-, time-, species-, and model-dependent variations in the vascular response to ^{32}P radioactive stents. The purpose of this chapter is to review the long-term experimental results of radioactive stents.

Long-Term Experimental Studies in the Porcine Model

We evaluated the long-term (6 months) dose-response effects of radioactive stents ion-implanted with activities of 0 to 12.0 µCi of ^{32}P in a porcine atherosclerotic coronary model.[6] Fibrocellular coronary arterial lesions were created by overstretch balloon injury and cholesterol feeding.[7] The methods used to manufacture a radioactive stent have been described previously.[2-5] In brief, commercially available 15-mm length tubular-slotted balloon-expandable stainless steel stents were rendered radioactive using ion implantation of ^{32}P into the stent. Janicki et al characterized the near-field dose of a 1.0 µCi 15-mm length Palmaz-Schatz (Cordis, a Johnson and Johnson Co., Warren, NJ) using a modification of

From Waksman R (ed.). *Vascular Brachytherapy, Third Edition.* Armonk, NY: Futura Publishing Co., Inc.; © 2002.

the dose point kernel method.[8] For a 1.0 μCi 15-mm length ^{32}P stent, at a distance of 0.1-mm, dose values of ≈2500 cGy are delivered at the strut wires (peaks) and ≈800 cGy between the wires (valleys) over one half-life (14.3 days). Sixty 3.0- to 4.0-mm diameter, 15-mm length, balloon-expandable stainless steel tubular-slotted stents (19 control and 41 radioactive) were implanted (mean stent to artery ratio 1.00±0.08) in the coronary arteries of 31 miniature swine at 28 days after balloon injury. The animals were treated with ticlopidine, 250 mg daily for 28 days, and aspirin, 325 mg daily for 6 months, post implant. Angiography and histology were performed at 6 months.

Subacute Stent Thrombosis

Three of 29 animals (10.3%) with successful stent placement had sudden death secondary to subacute thrombosis of a stent. Subacute stent thrombosis occurred in 3 of 39 radioactive stents (7.7%) and none of the nonradioactive stents ($P=0.54$). Stent thrombosis occurred on day 4, day 27, and day 28 after implant. The radioactive stents with subacute thrombosis were in the 6.0 μCi ^{32}P activity group at the time of implant.

Histology of the coronary arteries from the animal with sudden death on day 4 revealed an occlusive thrombus distal to a 6.0 μCi ^{32}P stent implanted in the left anterior descending artery. Focal compression of the plaque and media was present without deep vessel wall injury within the stent. Analysis of the proximal and distal reference sections failed to identify a cause for stent thrombosis such as a medial dissection. The nonradioactive stent in left circumflex coronary artery was patent with a thin neointima consisting of an organized fibrin-thrombus with inflammatory cells and SMCs. Focal necrosis of the plaque and media underneath the struts was more prominent for the radioactive than the nonradioactive stent.

The histology of the stents from the animals with sudden death on days 27 and 28 revealed a large organizing thrombus in one case and mural thrombus associated with neointimal proliferation in the other case. In the animal with sudden death on day 27, a 6.0 μCi ^{32}P stent implanted in the left anterior descending coronary artery had a fibrin-rich thrombus with 80% luminal narrowing. The animal with sudden death on day 28 had abundant neointimal formation in a 6.0 μCi ^{32}P radioactive stent implanted in the right coronary artery. The neointima consisted of a proteoglycan-rich matrix with occasional SMC and fibrin adjacent to the struts resulting in greater than 75% luminal narrowing. A mural thrombus was present in this case but without evidence of complete occlusion of the lumen. A nonradioactive stent implanted in the left anterior descending coronary artery was patent with mild neointimal thickening and evidence of surface endothelialization on light microscopy.

Dose-Response Effects on Arterial Morphology

The results of vessel morphometry are summarized in Table 1. The area of the plaque + media was similar for the control (1.88±0.52 mm^2) and radioactive stents (1.73±0.53, $P= 0.12$). The mean neointimal area (mm^2) for the stents with ≈3.0 μCi ^{32}P (3.57±1.21) was significantly greater than the nonradioactive stents (1.78±0.68, $P< 0.0001$), resulting in greater in-stent stenosis (53±14 versus

Table 1

Summary of Vessel Morphometry 6 Months After ^{32}P Radioactive Stent Placement in Atherosclerotic Porcine Coronary Arteries and Comparison to Control Stent Vessels

Stent Activity	Adventitia	Stent/IEL	Neointima	Lumen	%Stenosis	Injury Score
Control (n = 16)	1.43 ± 0.54	6.40 ± 1.27	1.78 ± 0.68	4.62 ± 1.07	28 ± 9	0.57 ± 0.54
0.5–1.0 μCi (n = 8)	1.33 ± 0.43	6.52 ± 1.17	2.23 ± 0.66	4.30 ± 1.04	34 ± 10	0.94 ± 0.89*
3.0 μCi (n = 9)	1.56 ± 0.56	6.58 ± 1.08	3.39 ± 1.10†	3.24 ± 1.02‡	51 ± 14§	0.83 ± 0.36
6.0 μCi (n = 8)	2.02 ± 1.06‖	6.12 ± 1.08	3.37 ± 1.02†	2.85 ± 0.92‡	53 ± 16§	0.94 ± 0.46
12.0 μCi (n = 10)	2.52 ± 1.09‖	7.14 ± 1.04	3.94 ± 1.21†	3.23 ± 0.82‡	54 ± 13§	0.81 ± 0.41

Data expressed as mean area (mm^2) ± SD.

*P=0.045 for 0.5–1.0 μCi versus control.

†P<0.006 for 3.0, 6.0, and 12.0 μCi versus control and = 1.0 μCi.

‡P<0.002 for 3.0, 6.0, and 12.0 μCi versus control and = 1.0 μCi.

§P<0.0001 for 3.0, 6.0, and 12.0 μCi versus control and = 1.0 μCi.

‖P=0.03 for 6.0 and 12.0 μCi versus control and = 1.0 μCi.

28±9, $P <$ 0.0001). The mean neointimal area and the percent in-stent stenosis positively correlated with increasing stent activity (r=0.64, $P <$ 0.001). The neointimal area correlated with the injury score for the control stents (r=0.33, P=0.009), but not the radioactive stents (r=0.02, P=0.86).

The neointima of the nonradioactive stents consisted of well-organized SMCs within a collagen matrix. Neovascularization was present adjacent to the strut wires. The adventitia contained collagen, fibroblasts, and neovascular capillaries. The neointima of the radioactive stents with ≈1.0 μCi of ^{32}P appeared similar to the nonradioactive stents. Occasional regions of cholesterol-rich macrophages were identified adjacent to the stent struts. Neovascularization of the neointima and adventitia was also similar to the nonradioactive stents.

The morphology of the high-activity stents was somewhat variable. The neointima contained areas of SMCs in a proteoglycan-collagenous matrix mostly localized in the region of the struts with other areas rich in macrophages, necrotic debris, cholesterol clefts, and giant cells (Fig. 1). Calcification was observed in some cases. Neovascularization was more prominent in the neointima as compared with the control and 1.0 μCi ^{32}P stents. The media was compressed underneath the stent struts, and, in other locations, the media was of normal thickness

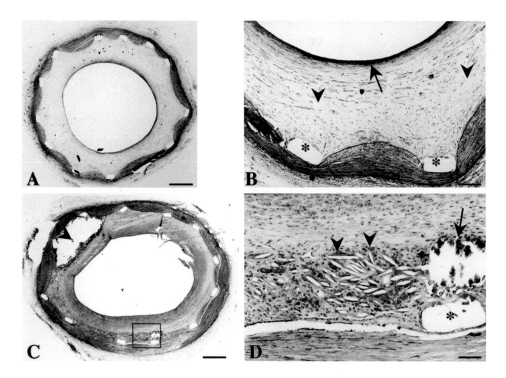

Figure 1. Low- and high-power photomicrographs of coronary arteries at 6 months after placement of 6.0 μCi ^{32}P radioactive stents in separate animals. **(A)** shows a markedly thickened neointimal layer with scant smooth muscle cells (SMCs) in a proteoglycan-rich matrix. A high-power view **(B)** of the same section illustrates the low SMC content within the neointima near the struts (*). In **(C)** a section from another 6.0 μCi ^{32}P stent shows eccentric neointimal thickening with focal areas of cholesterol clefts, macrophage infiltration (**D**, arrow) near the struts (*), and calcium deposits in a necrotic region of the neointima (**E**, arrows). Measurement bars are 500 μm in A and C, 100 μm in B and D, and 50 μm in E.

and appearance. Only rare areas of severe medial disruption were observed. At other sites near the stent struts, the neointima was markedly hypocellular and consisted of a loose proteoglycan matrix with occasional SMCs and some condensation of SMCs near the lumen. The adventitia was significantly thickened without any inflammatory infiltrate in the stents with ≈6.0 μCi of ^{32}P.

Late Effects of Continuous Low Dose Rate Endovascular Irradiation

The 6-month data, unlike previous 28-day studies in the porcine coronary model of restenosis, failed to demonstrate a significant reduction in neointimal formation for low-activity (0.5 to 1.0 μCi ^{32}P) radioactive stents at 6 months in atherosclerotic pig coronary arteries.[3,4,6]The lack of efficacy at 6 months in this model for the low-activity ^{32}P stents suggests inadequate cumulative radiation dose, dose rate, or delayed neointimal growth after 28 days. The higher injury score observed in the 0.5 to 1.0 μCi ^{32}P group, however, suggests that stent-induced arterial trauma may have contributed to the failure at this activity. Importantly, a dose-dependent increase in neointimal formation was observed with increasing the activity of ^{32}P on the stent at the time of implant.

The histologic features of the 3.0 to 12.0 μCi ^{32}P radioactive stents observed in the porcine model are consistent with radiation-induced arteriopathy.[9–12] Experimental studies in canine and rabbit models indicate external beam irradiation of the aorta or vascular grafts causes intimal hyperplasia and accelerated atherosclerosis after 6 months with single doses greater than 30 Gy.[9–12] Hoopes et al reported that large single intraoperative radiation doses (60 Gy) delivered to the canine aorta resulted in decreased or delayed intimal proliferation and lumen narrowing when compared to lower fractionated doses.[12] Our data suggest that the cumulative dose delivered by a ≈3.0 μCi ^{32}P radioactive stent exceeds vascular tissue tolerance in the atherosclerotic porcine coronary model. The estimated lifetime cumulative tissue dose at a distance of 0.5 mm from the surface of a 3.0 to 12.0 μCi radioactive stent is ≈20 to 125 Gy. Importantly, the lifetime cumulative near-field (0.1 mm from the stent surface) dose for a 3.0 μCi ^{32}P stent is greater than 125 Gy. Therefore, the arterial tissue immediately adjacent to the struts of a permanently implanted 3.0 μCi ^{32}P stent receives a lifetime cumulative dose nearly fivefold greater than a single dose of irradiation known to induce an arteriopathy.

Several experimental and initial clinical trials have demonstrated efficacy in preventing restenosis after stenting by treatment with 8- to 30-Gy irradiation given in a single dose via a high dose rate (1200 to 5000 cGy/h) ^{192}Ir catheter-based system.[13–16] In the atherosclerotic porcine coronary model, the 28-day cumulative dose (10 Gy) or initial dose rate (3 cGy/h at implant) delivered by a 1.0 μCi ^{32}P radioactive stent at a distance of 0.1 mm was insufficient to reduce neointimal formation and in-stent stenosis at 6 months. The arterial morphology of the 1.0 μCi ^{32}P radioactive stents did not exhibit the pathological features identified in the 3.0 to 12.0 μCi ^{32}P radioactive stents consistent with a radiation-induced arteriopathy. Together, these data suggest that dose rate may be a critical factor in predicting efficacy for the prevention of restenosis with endovascular irradiation, while the cumulative dose predicts toxic radiation-induced late tissue responses.

Hehrlein et al also reported a series of experiments with similar activities of ^{32}P stents in rabbit iliac arteries.[5] In contrast to the porcine experiments, these authors reported a dose-dependent reduction in neointimal formation with the maximal effect evident at 3 months after placement of a 13.0 µCi 7-mm length stent. The contrasting results with the doses of continuous beta-particle irradiation used in these experimental studies suggest a species- or model-dependent response to endovascular irradiation delivered via a stent. Others have demonstrated species differences in response to nonradioactive stent implantation that may be related to endothelial cell regeneration or the intrinsic fibrinolytic capacity of the animal.[17,18] A study by Taylor et al in a canine coronary model, however, failed to demonstrate species differences in the response to stent-based irradiation.[19]

Farb et al reported data in the rabbit iliac model that confirmed the earlier observations of Hehrlien et al.[20] At 3 months, there was a significant dose-dependent inhibition of neointimal growth with 6 and 24 µCi ^{32}P radioactive stents. However, the authors reported that nonhealing of the intimal surface was evident, consisting of a hypocellular, fibrin-rich matrix. Inflammatory cells were more numerous in the radioactive stent groups, and inflammation post stenting has been associated with increased neointimal growth.[21] Importantly, only one third of the stent surface of the 6 µCi stents was endothelialized, and increased intimal cellular proliferation was evident in the radioactive stent groups. In view of the incomplete healing, the authors recommended longer term studies to determine whether the inhibition of intimal growth seen at 3 months will be maintained at 6 months, 1 year, or longer.

Comparison with Clinical Studies of Radioactive Stents

The phase 1 Isostent Restenosis Intervention Study (IRIS) was designed to evaluate the safety of implantation of 0.5 to 1.0 µCi ^{32}P radioactive Palmaz-Schatz stents in patients with focal de novo or restenotic coronary arterial lesions. Thirty-two patients underwent successful placement of 32 radioactive stents with a mean activity of 0.72 µCi ^{32}P without a major adverse clinical event (death, myocardial infarction, coronary artery bypass graft). There were no cases of subacute stent thrombosis during the 6-month follow-up interval. Target lesion revascularization was completed in 10 of 32 patients (31%) for recurrent ischemic symptoms or at the time of 6-month angiographic restudies.[22]

The IRIS trial demonstrated the feasibility and safety of low-activity ^{32}P radioactive stents for use in native focal coronary arterial obstructions. Unfortunately, late restenosis was similar to that expected for a nonradioactive Palmaz-Schatz stent. This suggests that the dose prescribed by a 0.5 to 1.0 µCi ^{32}P stent was insufficient to inhibit neointimal formation in atherosclerotic human coronary arteries. As a result, an expanded phase 1 IRIS trial and the Milan dose-response study were designed to evaluate the safety and dose response effects of radioactive stents with 0.75 to 24.0 µCi of ^{32}P.[23–25]

Albiero et al recently reported a dose-dependent reduction in intrastent neointimal hyperplasia with a treatment threshold of 3 to 6 µCi ^{32}P activity using a 15-mm long Palmaz-Schatz or BX stent in the Milan study.[24,25] Unfortunately, restenosis was common at the margins for the high-activity radioactive stents (≈40%) and has since been termed the "candy-wrapper" phenomena by the authors of the study. Subsequent intravascular ultrasound data suggests, as noted in the porcine model, a stimulatory effect of irradiation with the lower doses delivered by high-activity ^{32}P radioactive stents at the proximal and distal margins.[3,26] Several alternative approaches have been proposed in order to address problems with dosimetry to the vessel wall at the margins of the radioactive stent, including the application of other isotopes, hybrid or dual isotope radioactive stents, and stents with "hot" or "cold" ends.

Novel Strategies for Radioactive Stents

We, and others, have proposed the use of a gamma-emitting isotope for radioactive stents.[2,27] In theory, gamma-emitting isotopes have a potential advantage over beta-emitting isotopes because of the longer range of photons compared to electrons. The dose fall-off for gamma emitters is therefore shallower, as has been documented by others, and may enhance radial dose distribution as well as the dose distribution along the vessel axis.

In the radial direction from the stent surface, a shallower dose fall-off leads to a potentially more homogenous coverage of the target region. The near-field dose on the surface of the stent is comparably lower while a therapeutic dose can be delivered to the target tissue at a greater radial distance from the source (Fig. 2). In the longitudinal direction, parallel to the stent axis, the longer range of the

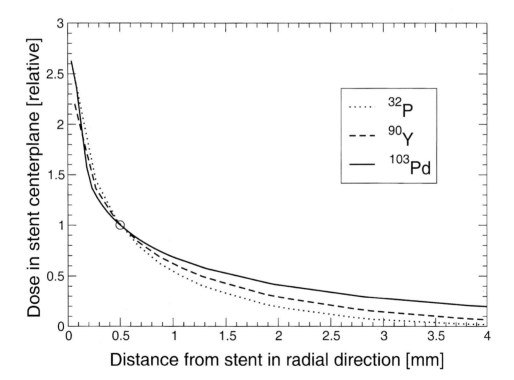

Figure 2. Radial dose distribution in the center plane of an expanded 16-mm long stent (diameter 3.5 mm) for the beta emitters, ^{32}P and ^{90}Y, and the gamma-emitting ^{103}Pd. The dose is displayed as a function of the radial distance from the stent surface and has been normalized to 0.5 mm, the AAPM-recommended prescription point. The fall-off for the ^{103}Pd is shallower, resulting in a lower near-field dose with the potential to deliver the therapeutic dose to greater radial distances.

gamma radiation can potentially reduce a dose-dependent "edge" effect. This is especially important since, with radioactive stents, in contrast to catheter-based endovascular irradiation, the isotope can only be placed in the treated region. Also, the half-life of the gamma-emitting radioisotope ^{103}Pd is similar to ^{32}P, the beta-particle-emitting isotope currently used in stents. Therefore, an activity of ^{103}Pd with a similar dose rate at implant can be selected to deposit the same long-term cumulative dose as with ^{32}P.

The dose distribution of ^{103}Pd versus ^{32}P is shown in Figure 3. This figure demonstrates that the dose is more homogenous over the length of the stent for the beta-particle emitter while the gamma emitter delivers a higher tissue dose in the body of the stent due to the longer range of photons. Therefore, a beta-emitting isotope appears ideal for homogenous dose delivery to the target tissue in the body of the stent while a gamma emitter is optimal at the stent ends to enhance the tissue dose in the axial dimensions. Such a hybrid radioisotope stent design with ^{32}P on the stent body and a spike of ^{103}Pd activity at each end (Implant Sciences Co., Wakefield, MA) is currently under investigation.

Although recent clinical data suggest that nonmeasurable device injury may cause restenosis at the edges of the treatment field for catheter-based radiation,

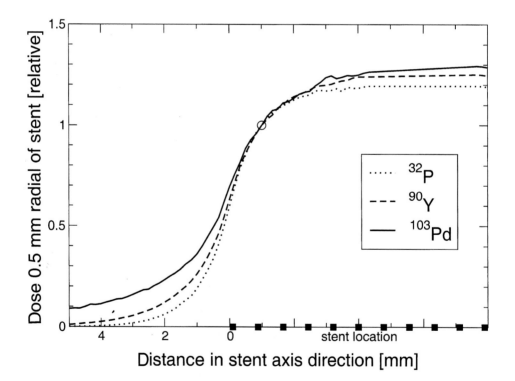

Figure 3. Dose distribution parallel to the stent axis at a 0.5-mm radial distance from an expanded 16-mm long stent (diameter 3.5 mm) for ^{32}P, ^{90}Y, and ^{103}Pd. The dose has been normalized to the values at 1 mm from the end of the stent for each isotope for comparison of the dose distribution characteristics. The dose from the gamma-emitting ^{103}Pd extends further beyond the margins of the stent, potentially preventing the dose-dependent "edge" effect. The dose penetration of ^{103}Pd is also deeper over the body of the stent than with ^{32}P. The beta-particle-emitting radioistope ^{32}P shows a more homogeneous dose distribution over the center part of the stent and a sharper fall-off at the ends.

it appears that certain doses of radiation delivered by radioactive stents may stimulate intimal proliferation.[26,28] Thus, low-energy, and short-range, isotopes that only act in the immediate vicinity of the stent strut, such as [35]S (β-, half-life 87.5 days, 0.17 MeV) and [185]W (β-, half-life 75.1 days, 0.43 MeV), may be potential candidates for radioisotope stents.

Conclusions

The experimental and clinical data with radioactive stents demonstrates time-, species-, and model-dependent variations in the dose-response effects of ^{32}P stents. The human clinical intrastent dose-response effects of ^{32}P radioactive stents correlate best with the 3-month data from the rabbit iliac model.[2,24,25,27] The human clinical trials with ^{32}P radioactive stents, however, have long-term follow-up data only at 4 to 6 months after stent implantation.[24,25] This intermediate term of clinical follow-up is insufficient to allow comparison with 6-month data in the porcine model. In addition, there are several important limitations to experimental models utilized for testing novel device and restenosis therapies such as a radioactive stent.

The atherosclerotic pig coronary lesions created by balloon injury and high cholesterol diet differ from the complex atherosclerotic lesions in humans in which focal plaque rupture, and necrosis and calcification are often observed. The diet- and injury-induced lesions in the porcine atherosclerotic coronary model consist primarily of SMCs. The extent of atherosclerotic plaque is substantially less in this model than that encountered when stenting diseased human coronary arteries. These factors will have significant effects on radiation dose distribution to the vessel wall due to variations in tissue density and plaque mass as well as uniformity of stent expansion. The long-term porcine data, however, defines the late tissue responses to continuous low dose rate irradiation delivered by a 0.5 to 12 μCi ^{32}P radioactive stent in an experimental model of restenosis. Therefore, these data may be useful for predicting dose-dependent long-term effects of ^{32}P radioactive stents with a similar dose delivered to the adventitia in human coronary arteries.

References

1. Fischell TA, Kharma BK, Fischell DR, et al. Low-dose, β-particle emission from stent wire results in complete, localized inhibition of smooth muscle cell proliferation, Circulation 1994;90:2956–2963.
2. Hehrlein C, Gollan C, Donges K, et al. Low-dose radioactive endovascular stents prevent smooth muscle cell proliferation and neointimal hyperplasia in rabbits. Circulation 1995;92:1570–1575.
3. Laird JR, Carter AJ, Kufs W, et al. Inhibition of neointimal proliferation with a beta particle emitting stent. Circulation 1996;93:529–536.
4. Carter AJ, Laird JR, Bailey LR, et al. The effects of endovascular radiation from a β-particle emitting stent in a porcine restenosis model: A dose response study. Circulation 1996;94:2364–2368.
5. Hehrlein C, Stintz M, Kinscherf R, Schlosser K, et al. Pure β-particle emitting stents inhibit neointima formation in rabbits. Circulation 1996;93:641–645.
6. Carter AJ, Laird JR, Kufs W, et al. Changes in arterial geometry after placement of a novel balloon expandable stent in atherosclerotic porcine coronary arteries. J Am Coll Cardiol 1996;27:1270–1277.

7. Carter AJ, Scott D, Bailey LR, et al. High activity ^{32}P radioactive stents promote the formation of an "atheromatous" neointima in porcine coronary arteries. Circulation 1999;100:1548–1554.
8. Janicki C, Duggan DM, Coffey CW, et al. Radiation dose from a phosphorous-32 impregnated wire mesh vascular stent. Med Phys 1997;24:437–445.
9. Fajardo LF, Stewart JR. Experimental radiation induced heart disease. Am J Pathol 1970;59:299–315.
10. Gillette EL, Powers BE, McChesney SL, et al. Response of aorta and branch arteries to experimental intraoperative irradiation. Int J Radiat Oncol Biol Phys 1987;17:1247–1255.
11. Johnstone PA, Sprague M, DeLuca AM, et al. Effects of intraoperative radiotherapy on vascular grafts in a canine model. Int J Radiat Oncol Biol Phys 1994;29:1015–1025.
12. Hoopes PJ, Gillette EL, Withrow SJ. Intraoperative irradiation of the canine abdominal aorta and vena cava. Int J Radiat Oncol Biol Phys 1987;13:715–722.
13. Waksman R, Robinson KA, Crocker IR, et al. Intracoronary radiation before stent implantation inhibits neointima formation in stented porcine coronary arteries. Circulation 1995;92:1383–1386.
14. Teirstein PS, Massullo V, Jani S, et al. Catheter-based radiotherapy to inhibit restenosis after coronary stenting. N Engl J Med 1997;336:1697–1703.
15. Condado JA, Waksman R, Gurdiel O, et al. Long-term angiographic and clinical outcome after percutaneous transluminal coronary angioplasty and intracoronary radiation therapy in humans. Circulation 1997;96:727–732.
16. King SB, III, Williams DO, Chougule P, et al. Endovascular beta-radiation to reduce restenosis after coronary balloon angioplasty: Results of the beta energy restenosis trial (BERT). Circulation 1998;97:2025–2030.
17. Muller DWM, Ellis SG, Topol EJ. Experimental models of coronary restenosis. J Am Coll Cardiol 1992;19:418–432.
18. Schwartz RS, Edwards WD, Bailey KR, et al. Differential neointimal response to coronary artery injury in pigs and dogs: Implications for restenosis models. Arterioscler Thromb 1994;14:395–400.
19. Taylor AJ, Gorman PD, Farb A, et al. Long-term coronary vascular response to [32]P β-particle–emitting stents in a canine model. Circulation 1999;100:2366–2372.
20. Farb A, Tang AL, Shroff S, et al. Neointimal responses 3 months after [32]P β-emitting stent placement. Int J Radiat Oncol Biol Phys 2000;48:889–898.
21. Rogers C, Welt FG, Karnovsky MJ, Edelman ER. Monocyte recruitment and neointimal hyperplasia in rabbits: Coupled inhibitory effects of heparin. Arterioscler Thromb Vasc Biol 1996;16:1312–1318.
22. Baim DS, Fischell T, Weissman NJ, et al. Short-term results of the IRIS feasibility study of a beta-particle emitting radioisotope stent. Circulation 1997;96:I-218.
23. Wardeh AJ, Kay IP, Sabaté M, et al. β-particle–emitting radioactive stent implantation: A safety and feasibility study. Circulation 1999;100:1684–1689.
24. Albiero R, Nishida T, Adamian M, et al. Edge restenosis after implantation of high activity ^{32}P radioactive β-emitting stents. Circulation 2000;101:2454–2457.
25. Albiero R, Adamian M, Kobayashi N, et al. Short and intermediate term results of ^{32}P radioactive β-emitting stent implantation in patients with coronary artery disease. Circulation 2000;101:18–26.
26. Kay IP, Sabate M, Costa MA, et al. Positive geometric vascular remodeling is seen after catheter based radiation followed by conventional stent placement but not after radioactive stent implantation. Circulation 2000;102:1434–1439.
27. van der Geissen W, Serruys P. Radioactive stents radiate enthusiasm in search for effective prevention of restenosis. Circulation 1996;94:2358–2360.
28. Kozuma K, Costa MA, Sabate M, et al. Three-dimensional intravascular ultrasound assessment of noninjured edges of β-irradiated coronary segments. Circulation 2000; 102:1484–1489.

Pathology of Radioactive Stents

Renu Virmani, MD, Andrew Farb, MD,
Michael John, BA, and Allen J. Taylor, MD

Introduction

The advent of balloon angioplasty in 1978 resulted in the ability of the interventional cardiologist to treat coronary artery atherosclerosis percutaneously; however, the procedure has been limited by a high rate of arterial restenosis (30 to 40% of cases).[1] Although coronary stents have resulted in a significant reduction in restenosis rates to 25 to 30% when they have been deployed in ideal lesions, in-stent restenosis remains an important clinical problem.[2] Additionally, as stenting is performed more frequently (>70% of purcutaneous coronary interventions), and in less than ideal lesions, the incidence of restenosis is likely to increase.[3,4] Currently, over 1 million percutaneous coronary procedures are performed annually, worldwide, and if conservative estimates are used, at least 300,000 individuals will require another procedure for restenosis; of these, more than half will have persistent restenosis.[5,6] Despite the availability of a large number of different stent designs, the rate of in-stent restenosis has not changed. Therefore, the field of interventional cardiology requires novel procedures to prevent and treat restenosis.

At the present time, attention is focused on brachytherapy, the "most promising" new anti-restenosis technology.[7,8] Gamma radiation and beta radiation have been delivered to atherosclerotic human coronary arteries via catheter- and stent-based delivery systems. In a case-controlled study performed at Scripps Clinic (La Jolla, CA) by Teirstein et al,[8] the rate of recurrent restenosis following intravascular gamma radiation was 33% in the radiated arm compared to 64% in patients treated with balloon angioplasty alone. However, it should be noted that the control group had 8 more high-risk patients than the brachytherapy group. Recently, both gamma- and beta-delivered brachytherapy have been shown to reduce restenosis following treatment for in-stent restenosis.[9,10] With respect to radioactive stents, in the recently reported Milan Dose-Response Study of ^{32}P beta-emitting stents, there was a dose-dependent reduction in pure intrastent restenosis rates at 6-month follow-up.[11]

However, multiple concerns have been raised regarding the long-term efficacy and safety of coronary brachytherapy. In the Scripps Study, angiography at 3 years showed a trend toward increased diameter stenosis from 6 months to 3 years

The opinions and assertions contained herein are the private views of the authors and are not to be construed as official or reflecting the views of the Department of the Army or the Department of Defense.
From Waksman R (ed.). *Vascular Brachytherapy, Third Edition.* Armonk, NY: Futura Publishing Co., Inc.; © 2002.

in the radiated arm (14 to 26%, *P*=0.15), but remained unchanged in nonradiated arteries (21 to 23%).[8] Because of the small number of patients (17 in the brachytherapy group and 10 in the control group), no significant difference was observed. Radioactive stents have been associated with the development of adverse edge effects, resulting in an increased frequency of nontarget lesion revascularization (see below).[11,12] Also, patients treated with intravascular gamma and beta brachytherapy have been reported to have an unacceptably high rate of subacute arterial thrombosis (6.6 to 9.1%) at 2 to 15 months.[13–15]

This chapter will discuss the effects of ^{32}P beta-emitting stents on arterial responses following varying intervals after implantation. Experimental animal data will be reviewed first, followed by a comparison to human clinical studies.

Radioactive Stents

In 1994, Fischell et al showed that a ^{32}P-impregnated titanium stent wire inhibited smooth muscle cell proliferation preferentially as compared to endothelial cells.[16] This led to the manufacturing of radioactive ^{32}P beta-emitting stents, which could be implanted in animal coronary and peripheral arteries.[17] Most of the early animal work was carried out by Hehrlein, who showed that radioactive stents containing a mixture of isotopes (^{56}Co, ^{51}Cr, ^{52}Mn, ^{57}Ni, and ^{55}Fe) within the metal emitting beta, gamma, and x-radiation (with half-lives between 17.5 hours [^{56}Co] and 2.7 years [^{55}Fe]) could prevent neointimal formation.[18] Laird et al showed that neointimal inhibition could be accomplished following implantation of low dose (0.14 µCi) beta-emitting radioactive stents in pig iliac arteries with complete endothelialization at 28 days.[19]

Hehrlein et al reported a few-long term studies following implantation of ^{32}P beta-particle-emitting stents, with activities ranging from 3.9 to 35 µCi, in the rabbit iliac artery model with analysis at 4, 12, and 52 weeks.[18] The lowest stent activity failed to show any difference between radiated and nonradiated arteries at 4 weeks; however, at higher activities, there was a dose-related reduction in the neointimal area at 4, 12, and 52 weeks. Published photomicrographs illustrate healed lesions with neointimal smooth muscle cells and endothelialization at 4 weeks following deployment of high-activity stents.[18] Subsequent to the above report, ^{32}P-impregnated Palmaz-Schatz stents with 4 and 13 µCi activity suppressed neointimal formation in rabbit iliac arteries at 3 months.[20] The number of smooth muscle cells in the neointima was less than controls and was least in the high-activity group. Also, endothelial cells were identified but were reported to be less dense than conventional stents.[20] However, no quantitative data was reported, and no immunohistochemical stains for factor VIII were illustrated. From the illustrations and text descriptions, it was implied that the healing was complete at 4 and 12 weeks following radioactive stent implantation.

Our first study of 6 and 24 µCi ^{32}P beta-emitting stents was completed in rabbit iliac arteries with histologic analysis 3 months post-stent placement.[21] We noted a significant decrease in neointima formation (Fig. 1) and incomplete healing consisting of persistent neointimal fibrin deposition, fewer smooth muscle cells, and increased inflammatory cells with poor endothelialization compared to nonradioactive stents (which showed complete healing consisting of smooth muscle cells within a collagen/proteoglycan matrix) (Fig. 2). Endothelial function was assessed by methylene blue dye injection prior to euthanasia to determine endo-

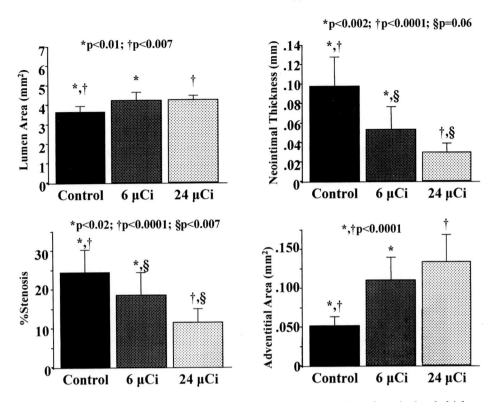

Figure 1. Increased lumen area and adventitial area with reduced neointimal thickness and arterial stenosis 3 months after deployment of ^{32}P beta-emitting stents in rabbit iliac arteries (mean±SD).

thelial permeability. Radioactive stents showed extensive blue staining over most of the luminal surface, indicative of impaired endothelial integrity, whereas control arteries showed no blue staining of the arterial wall. This finding was further confirmed by scanning electron microscopy, which showed incomplete endo-thelialization and adherence of platelets and inflammatory cells in the radio-

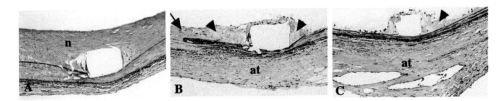

Figure 2. Rabbit iliac artery morphology 3 months after ^{32}P beta-emitting stent placement. A nonradioactive control stent (**A**) demonstrates a mature neointima (n) consisting of numerous smooth muscle cells in a proteoglycan/collagen matrix. In a 6 μCi stent (**B**), the neointima is significantly smaller versus the control stent. A hypocellular proteoglycan/collagen matrix (arrow) is present that is partially endothelialized. Stent struts are surrounded by fibrin-containing trapped erythrocytes (arrowheads). Minimal intima is present only adjacent to 24 μCi stent struts (**C**) consisting of fibrin (arrowhead). A layer of inflammatory cells lines the arterial lumen surface. There is no proteoglycan/collagen extracellular matrix within the stent. Adventitial thickening (at) is present in both 6 and 24 μCi stents.

active stents, and complete endothelialization of control nonradioactive stents. In this 3-month study, we did not observe "edge effects" in the adjoining non-stented artery segments.

We then posed the question of whether there would be a persistent decrease in neointimal formation with complete healing and endothelialization at 6 months.[22] In this study, we noted no significant difference in neointimal area and thickness between 6 μCi stents and control stents, but there was significant neointima inhibition with 24 and 48 μCi stents versus nonradioactive controls (Fig. 3). However, there was persistent incomplete healing with fibrin deposition and inflammatory cell infiltration, with incomplete endothelialization in 24 and 48 μCi stents. We also observed definite "edge effects" in the 24 and 48 μCi stents, especially at the arterial edge distal to the stents consisting of increased neointimal and adventitial thickness. The area within the arterial internal elastic lamina was significantly smaller in the distal non-stented edge sections in the high dose stent groups (24 and 48 μCi) compared to nonradioactive control arteries, consistent with negative arterial remodeling.

We have extended our observations to 1 year following deployment of 6, 24, and 48 μCi ^{32}P beta-emitting stents in rabbit iliac arteries.[22] The neointima at 1 year was significantly reduced in the 24 and 48 μCi stent groups compared to control nonradioactive and 6 μCi stents (Fig. 4). However, there was greater inflammation with 24 and 48 μCi stents, and focal atherosclerotic change was observed in 30 to 50% of animals, respectively. The inflammatory infiltrate was predomi-

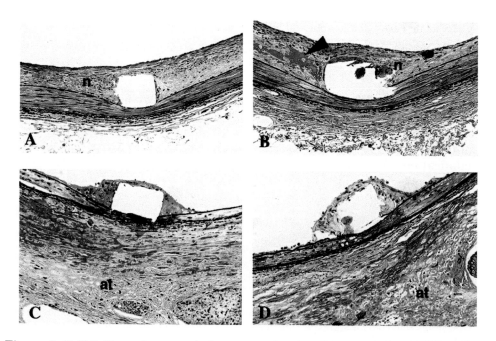

Figure 3. Rabbit iliac artery morphology 6 months after ^{32}P beta-emitting stent placement. A nonradioactive control stent is shown in **A**. In contrast to neointimal inhibition seen at 3 months with 6 μCi stents, neointimal thickness was similar to controls at 6 months (**B**). The intima is relatively hypocellular and contains trapped fibrin (arrowhead). There was reduced in-stent neointimal growth within the 24 μCi (**C**) and 48 μCi stents (**D**). Both high-activity stents were associated with marked adventitial thickening (at).

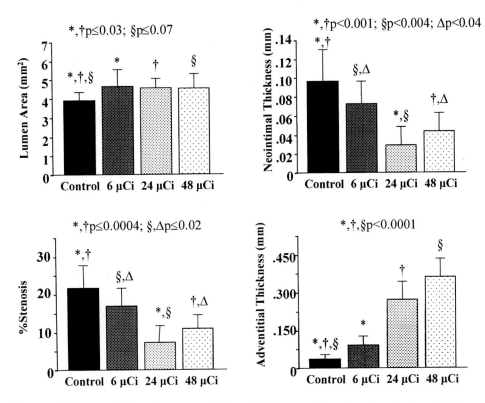

Figure 4. Increased lumen area and adventitial area with reduced neointimal thickness and arterial stenosis 12 months after deployment of ^{32}P beta-emitting stents in rabbit iliac arteries (mean±SD).

nantly limited to the neointima and mostly consisted of macrophages, giant cells, and lymphocytes; further, neutrophil infiltration was occasionally observed. We also observed a significant increase in cellular proliferation (BrdU-labeling) in the high dose stented arteries versus nonradioactive control stents.

Beta-Emitting Stents in Normal Canine Coronary Arteries

Balloon angioplasty studies of normal canine and porcine coronary artery show divergent results; the pig uniformly demonstrates arterial restenosis with negative remodeling, and the dog shows neither restenosis nor negative remodeling. The porcine coronary model has been thought to be a superior model of human coronary artery disease compared with the dog. Therefore, our initial studies of radioactive stents were performed in the pig. Since studies of ^{32}P beta-emitting stents in pig coronary arteries (discussed elsewhere in the text) showed greater neointimal area and arterial stenosis at 3 and 6 months compared to control stents, we wanted to determine if this response was unique to the pig or common to other large animal coronary arteries.[23–25] Therefore, we implanted beta-emitting ^{32}P stents in dog coronary arteries using doses similar to those employed in the pig (3.5 to 14.4 μCi stents).[24,25] Histologic analysis at 15 weeks showed a greater percent arterial stenosis and increased neointimal fibrin area in the high-activity group (6.5 to 14.4 µCi) compared to nonradioactive stents (Figs. 5 and 6). The adventitial/neointimal area ratio was significantly reduced in the radioactive stents. No edge effects were observed. These findings clearly indicate that stent-based beta radiation is associated with incomplete arterial healing and no reduction in neointimal growth in the canine coronary model.

Evidence from large animal studies indicates that one of the major limitations with ^{32}P as an isotope for radioactive stents is both its failure to prevent neointimal growth and its inhibition of complete neointimal healing (requiring 3 to 6 months to resolve, using doses <15 µCi.) In contrast, in the rabbit model at 6 and 12 months, high-activity stents (24 and 48 µCi) result in reduced in-stent neointimal growth, but there is also delayed healing characterized by persistent fibrin, greater inflammation, and poor endothelialization. A potential contributor to these healing effects is the relatively long half-life (14.3 days) and low dose rate of ^{32}P. To clarify this issue, we implanted a shorter half-life, higher dose rate ^{90}Y stent in canine coronary arteries. ^{90}Y has a half-life of 2.7 days, and a ^{90}Y 16 µCi stent has a dose rate of 18 cGy/h (compared to a ^{32}P 12 µCi stent). The cumulative dose was much less for ^{90}Y (1500 cGy for a 16 µCi stent) compared with ^{32}P (4000 cGy for a 12 µCi stent) stents. In this study, ^{90}Y stents, varying in activities from 4.5 to 32 µCi, were implanted in dog coronary arteries for 3 months. The neointimal area and luminal stenosis were similar in low-

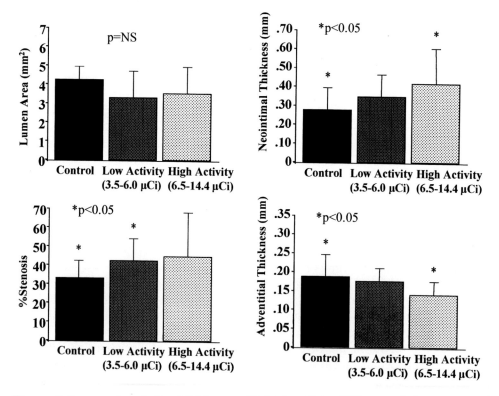

Figure 5. Increased neointimal thickness with high activity ^{32}P beta-emitting stents and increased arterial stenosis with low-activity stents 15 weeks after deployment in normal canine coronary arteries (mean±SD).

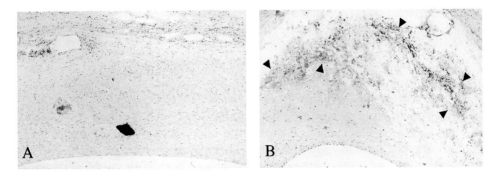

Figure 6. Fibrin II immunostaining of canine coronary arteries 15 weeks after placement of a control stent (**A**) and a high-activity (6.5 to 14.4 µCi) ^{32}P beta-emitting stent (**B**). There is marked intimal fibrin deposition (arrowheads) within the thick neointima of the radioactive stent. Reproduced from Reference 24, with permission from the American Heart Association.

activity (4.5 and 8 µCi) stents and control stents. Higher activity (16 and 32 µCi) stents were associated with total occlusions in 5 of 18 stents, 28%; P=0.008. Further, there was a 40% increase in neointimal area (P=0.024 versus controls) in the 16 µCi stent group. Incomplete neointimal healing and a trend toward reduced neointimal cell density were observed in 16 and 32 µCi groups. Therefore changing characteristics of the beta-emitting stent did not result in significant benefit.[25]

Clinical Trials with Radioactive Stents

In a preliminary study, implantation of 0.75 to 1.5 µCi beta-emitting ^{32}P stents in coronary arteries at 6 months showed a 17% restenosis rate, and 13% of patients required revascularization.[26] Stent edge restenosis was not observed. However, these results were not substantially different than those seen in the BENESTENT Trials, in which the restenosis rate in similar lesions and vessel sizes was 12%.[27,28]

Colombo and colleagues implanted low dose ^{32}P beta-emitting radioactive stents (0.75 to 12 µCi) in human coronary arteries and performed angiographic follow-up studies at 4 to 6 months.[11] The patients were divided into three groups based on stent activity: group I, 0.75 to 3.0 µCi; group II, 3.0 to 6.0 µCi; and group III, 6.0 to 12.0 µCi. At 6 months, no deaths had occurred, and only 1 patient had stent thrombosis. In-stent restenosis was observed in 16% in group I, 3% in group II, and 0% in group III. However, intralesional restenosis (defined as >50% luminal reduction occurring inside the stent or at the proximal or distal reference segments) was high in all three groups (50% in group I, 41% in group II, and 50% in group III).[11] Therefore, studies in humans were quite similar to those observed at 6 and 12 months in our rabbit arteries utilizing 24 and 48 µCi stents. These higher activity stents in the rabbit showed minimal in-stent intimal thickening, but adverse edge effects were present, especially at the distal edges. In a subsequent study of beta-emitting stents in humans coronary arteries, results at 6 months of higher activity stents (12 to 21 µCi) were compared to lower activity stents (3 to 12 µCi).[12] Rates of intrastent restenosis (4% and 5%) and intralesional restenosis (30% and 38%), including total occlusions, was similar in the two groups of stent activities. However, intravascular ultrasound measurement of intrastent plaque volume was significantly less in the higher activity stents (4.4 ± 5.6 mm^3) than in the low-activity stents (15.1 ± 14.1 mm^3, $P<0.01$).[12]

Summary

Experimental pig and rabbit studies uniformly show a decrease in neointimal area and percent stenosis at all activities at 3 months. Both ^{32}P and ^{90}Y beta-emitting stents in the dog coronary arteries at 3 months do not reduce neointimal growth compared to control nonradioactive stents. Thus, shortening the half-life and increasing dose rate of the beta-emitting stents does not improve outcome. However, high-activity stents ^{32}P beta-emitting stents (24 and 48 µCi) in the rabbit model show a decrease in in-stent neointimal growth at 6 and 12 months, but edge effects become apparent, similar to observations in human clinical trials.

References

1. Popma JJ, Califf RM, Topol EJ. Clinical trials of restenosis after coronary angioplasty. Circulation 1991;84:1426–1436.
2. Serruys PW, de Jaegere P, Kiemeneij F, et al. A comparison of balloon expandable stent implantation with balloon angioplasty in patients with coronary artery disease. N Eng J Med 1994;331:489–495.
3. Edelman ER, Rogers C. Hoop dreams: Stents without restenosis. Circulation 1996;94:1199–1202.
4. Peterson ED, Lansky AJ, Anstrom KJ. Evolving trends in interventional device use and outcomes: Results from the National Cardiovascular Network Database. Am Heart J 2000;139:198–207.
5. Linnemeier TJ. In-stent restenosis: Is the "stent-wich" the answer? Cath Cardiovasc Interv 2000;49:382–383.
6. Mach F. Toward new therapeutic strategies against neointimal formation in restenosis. Arterioscl Thromb Vasc Biol 2000;20:1699–1700.
7. Serruys PW, Kay IP. I like the candy, I hate the wrapper: The (32)P radioactive stent. Circulation 2000;101:3–7.
8. Teirstein PS, Massullo V, Jani S, et al. Three-year clinical and angiographic follow-up after intracoronary radiation: Results of a randomized clinical trial. Circulation 2000;101:360–365.
9. Waksman R, White RL, Chan RC, et al. Intracoronary gamma-radiation therapy after angioplasty inhibits recurrence in patients with in-stent restenosis. Circulation 2000;101:2165–2171.
10. Waksman R, Bhargava B, White L, et al. Intracoronary beta-radiation therapy inhibits recurrence of in-stent restenosis. Circulation 2000;101:1895–1898.
11. Albiero R, Adamian M, Kobayashi N, et al. Short- and intermediate-term results of (32)P radioactive beta-emitting stent implantation in patients with coronary artery disease: The Milan Dose-Response Study. Circulation 2000;101:18–26.
12. Albiero R, Nishida T, Adamian M, et al. Edge restenosis after implantation of high activity (32)P radioactive beta-emitting stents. Circulation 2000;101:2454–2457.
13. Costa MA, Sabate M, van der Giessen WJ, et al. Late coronary occlusion after intracoronary brachytherapy. Circulation 1999;100:789–792.
14. Waksman R, Bhargava B, Leon MB. Late thrombosis following intracoronary brachytherapy. Catheter Cardiovasc Interv 2000;49:344–347.
15. Waksman R, Bhargava B, Mintz GS, et al. Late total occlusion after intracoronary brachytherapy for patients with in-stent restenosis. J Am Coll Cardiol 2000;36:65–68.
16. Fischell TA, Kharma BK, Fischell DR, et al. Low-dose, β-particle emission from 'stent' wire results in complete, localized inhibition of smooth muscle cell proliferation. Circulation 1994;90:2956–2963.

17. Fischell TA, Carter AJ, Laird JR. The beta-particle-emitting radioisotope stent (isostent): Animal studies and planned clinical trials. Am J Cardiol 1996;78:45–50.
18. Hehrlein C, Gollan C, Donges K, et al. Low-dose radioactive endovascular stents prevent smooth muscle cell proliferation and neointimal hyperplasia in rabbits. Circulation 1995;92:1570–1575.
19. Laird JR, Carter AJ, Kufs WM, et al. Inhibition of neointimal proliferation with low-dose irradiation from a beta-particle-emitting stent. Circulation 1996;93:529–536.
20. Hehrlein C, Stintz M, Kinscherf R, et al. Pure beta-particle-emitting stents inhibit neointima formation in rabbits. Circulation 1996;93:641–645.
21. Farb A, Tang AL, Shroff S, et al. Neointimal responses 3 months after ^{32}P β-emitting stent placement. Int J Radiat Oncol Biol Phys 2000;48:889–898.
22. Farb A, Shroff S, John M, et al. Late arterial responses (6 and 12 months) after 32P β-emitting stent placement: sustained intimal suppression with incomplete healing. Circulation 2001;103:1912–1919.
23. Carter AJ, Scott D, Bailey LR, et al. High activity 32P stents promote development of atherosclerosis at six months in a porcine model. Circulation 1997;96:I-607.
24. Taylor AJ, Gorman PD, Farb A, et al. Long-term coronary vascular response to (32)P beta-particle-emitting stents in a canine model. Circulation 1999;100:2366–2372.
25. Taylor AJ, Gorman PD, Hudak C, et al. The 90-day coronary vascular response to (90)Y-beta particle-emitting stents in the canine model. Int J Radiat Oncol Biol Phys 2000;46:1019–1024.
26. Wardeh AJ, Kay IP, Sabate M, et al. Beta-particle-emitting radioactive stent implantation: A safety and feasibility study. Circulation 1999;100:1684–1689.
27. de Feyter PJ, Kay P, Disco C, Serruys PW. Reference chart derived from post-stent implantation intravascular ultrasound predictors of 6-month expected restenosis on quantitative coronary angiography. Circulation 1999;1999:1777–1783.
28. Serruys PW, Emanuelsson H, van der Giessen W, et al. Heparin-coated Palmaz-Schatz stents in human coronary arteries: Early outcome from the Benestent-II pilot study. Circulation 1996;93:412–422.

## Chapter 33

Targeted Immunotherapy and Radioactive Stents

*Morris Mosseri, MD, Zvi Symon, MD,
and Ron Waksman, MD*

Introduction

Restenosis of coronary arteries following percutaneous transluminal angioplasty may result from vessel wall recoil, arterial remodeling, and/or neointimal formation.[1-6] Stent implantation abolishes recoil completely, but does not prevent neointimal hyperplasia. Brachytherapeutic intravascular radioactive modalities have proved to prevent neointimal hyperplasia and in-stent restenosis in animal experiments and clinical trials.[7,8] Most of these modalities prolong the invasive treatment in the catheterization laboratory and share logistical problems related to supply, handling, and disposal of radioactive material with a specific half-life, and to providing the appropriate level of radiation to the patient. Radioactive stents as a platform are easy and practical to use compared with other intravascular radioactive modalities. The benefit of recently tried beta-emitting stents is hampered by excess of neointimal hyperplasia at the stent edges due to the low radiation dose at these segments. Theoretically, a gamma-emitting stent may prevent this "candy wrapper" effect. Gamma radiation has several drawbacks, including the need to shield and monitor staff and equipment in the catheterization laboratory, and the presence of radiation personnel to support the procedure. In this chapter, we present a novel concept for producing a gamma-emitting radioactive stent to overcome these problems.

Current Brachytherapy Modalities

Current brachytherapy techniques are used in the angiography suite immediately following angioplasty and do not subject the patient to further procedures. These modalities, however, prolong the procedure and have several biological and logistical disadvantages with regard to their application in cardiac angioplasty.

Limitations on Radiation Timing and Fractionation

All radioactive modalities end in a common pathway – the generation of free radicals which are lethal to cells during vulnerable mitotic phases. Neointimal

From Waksman R (ed.). *Vascular Brachytherapy, Third Edition.* Armonk, NY: Futura Publishing Co., Inc.; © 2002.

hyperplasia following angioplasty occurs secondary to release of cytokines and growth factors from damaged endothelial cells and accumulating platelets at the traumatized luminal surface. Several studies have shown that mRNAs associated with cell proliferation appear 48 hours after angioplasty, and that the optimal time for a single treatment of vascular brachytherapy is 1 to 2 days after angioplasty.[9–11] Ideally, radiation therapy should be administered at this time. Immediate vascular radiotherapy is premature as cellular elements are not optimally vulnerable at this time. Delayed irradiation is not possible to accomplish unless another invasive procedure is performed.

The hallmark of modern day radiotherapy is fractionation. This is a process whereby a large single dose of radiation is divided into many smaller doses that are given over a longer period of time. Fractionation offers several significant therapeutic advantages. It traps a greater percentage of proliferating cells in their vulnerable mitotic phases, allowing for a more complete therapeutic effect, and it limits the toxicity of nonproliferating cells in the surrounding tissue by permitting them more time to recover.[12] Because fractionation would require repeated invasive procedures, its application is impractical for most brachytherapy vascular procedures.

Logistical Considerations

Many radioactive sources used in brachytherapy have short half-lives and shelf lives, which require local means of producing or means for periodic replacing. A full-time radiation oncologist and radiation physicist must be present during each procedure to introduce, monitor, and withdraw the radiation device. In order to ensure for a radioactive dwell time of 20 minutes, the procedure of vascular brachytherapy may require more than 40 minutes. Increased procedure time is costly, it exposes the patient to increased risk of acute cardiovascular complications such as arrhythmias and bleeding, and it may induce more ischemia in the diseased heart. Finally, setting up a catheter laboratory capable of performing brachytherapy requires a program of staff education and training to ensure both worker and patient safety, as well as appropriate shielding and radioactive monitoring for gamma sources.

Dosing Inhomogeneity

A major problem in brachytherapy relates to nonhomogeneous dose distribution in the vessel wall. Atheromatous plaques in diseased coronary arteries are located along the vessel walls, very frequently creating an eccentric lumen. Even after balloon angioplasty, the resultant lumen is frequently nonspherical with heterogeneous wall thickness. In this setting, placement of a brachytherapeutic device into the diseased artery may create very uneven radiation fields. With a gamma (photon) source such as ^{192}Ir, the delivered dose to the vessel wall may range between 0.6 to 2.9 times the prescribed dose depending on the eccentricity of positioning.[9,13] The risk of radiation nonhomogeneity to the vessel wall is even more crucial and disturbing with beta (electron)-emitting sources which have a rapid dose fall-off.[14,15] Small to moderate doses reported by beta brachytherapy investigators were generally calculated for tissues at some distance (eg, 2 mm) from the source, whereas actual doses attained at closer distances are much higher and reach 50 Gy and more. Such high levels of localized radiation may ultimately lead to undesirable local and late toxicity. Centering balloon catheters partially overcomes arterial asymmetric configuration, but not the problem of radiation fall-off.

Radioactive stent implantation may overcome many of the above limitations; a low activity applied continuously over several weeks or months serves as the ultimate fractionation and includes all mitotic phases during this period of time, and the stent's proximity to the vessel wall may overcome part of the inhomogeneity problem related to wall asymmetry. However, the results of beta-emitting stents used in recent clinical trials were disappointing with neointimal hyperplasia at the stent edges, possibly due to fall-off in radiation dose at the stent edges.[16,17] It has been suggested that gamma-emitting stents may result in a substantially higher radial penetration depth than beta-particle radiation, and thus may allow for enhanced dosing to injured vascular tissue beyond the stent margins.[18]

A Novel Gamma-Emitting Stent Constructed by Targeted Radioimmunotherapy

Introduction to Radioimmunotherapy

Radioimmunotherapy (RIT) is a promising experimental treatment, which uses antibodies, peptides, or other constructs to target radiation to tumors. The targeting ligands are conjugated to a radionuclide, and when injected systemically or regionally, can bind specifically to tumor-associated antigens or receptors uniquely expressed or overexpressed on tumor cells or tumor vasculature. The capability of systemically targeted therapy to treat disease in multiple scattered locations and to target microscopic subclinical disease provides the rationale for the investigation of RIT in clinical trials for the treatment of disseminated cancer, such as advanced non-Hodgkin and Hodgkin's lymphomas, leukemia, and solid tumors.[19–22] RIT has been most successful for the treatment of B cell lymphomas. Most studies have use intact IgG antibodies labeled with ^{131}I or [90]Y. Treatment of relapsed B cell lymphoma patients with high dose ^{131}I-anti-CD20 monoclonal antibody and autologous stem cell rescue has resulted in a complete response rate of 79% and an overall response rate of 86%.[23] However, the treatment of other solid tumors has been less successful.[19]

One of the main limitations of systemic RIT has been the low uptake of radioactivity (generally <0.001% injected dose/g) in tumors, which is affected by many factors such as tumor vascularity, antibody size, affinity and avidity, density of cell surface tumor associated antigens, and interstitial pressure in tumors.[24] After more than 20 years of studies in animals and in human subjects, it is evident that optimization of carrier-delivered radionuclide therapy is highly dependent on matching and maximizing a number of biological and physical parameters. The introduction of genetically engineered antibody fragments, bispecific antibodies that can bind both tumors and metal chelates, linker chelators that bind a variety of isotopes, and different pre-targeting strategies that amplify the receptor density on the target have considerably improved tumor to normal tissue uptake.[24] The optimization of RIT with these technologies has somewhat reduced the exposure of the bone marrow to radiation, thus attenuating myelosuppression, which has been the major dose-limiting toxicity of RIT. Other approaches to improve the therapeutic ratio have been the use of cytokines and hyperthermia to increase tumor uptake of radiolabeled antibody and radiosensitizers such as cisplatin, which enhance the effect of radiation.[19]

Notwithstanding the progress made in optimizing RIT, considerable challenges remain. These include immunogenicity of some of the constructs, physiological barriers to tumor uptake, and inefficient clearance of radiolabeled chelates from the body. The doses calculated for RIT are much less accurate than for external beam radiotherapy because of limited dose input data and inhomogeneous dose distributions. The fundamental data are acquired by sequential imaging using planar scintillation cameras or single-photon emission tomography (SPECT). A mathematical model known as Medical Internal Radiation Dose (MIRD) is then applied to estimate the dose to the target and critical normal structures.[25]

The theoretical advantage of RIT compared with external beam radiotherapy in irradiating neoplasms is the potential for increased dose to the target with little effect on the surrounding normal tissue. The advent of conformal three-dimensional treatment planning in external beam radiotherapy has achieved favorable therapeutic ratios with target to nontarget ratios of 10:1. However, external beam radiotherapy does not differentiate between tumor and normal tissue in the irradiation field. By selectively targeting neoplastic tissues on the macroscopic and cellular levels, carrier-delivered radionuclide therapy may present an attractive alternative form of radiotherapy.

The Rationale for the Investigation of Radioimmunotherapy for the Prevention of In-Stent Restenosis

Based on the principles of RIT, we recently devised a method and device to utilize carrier-delivered radionuclide therapy for the in vivo production of a radioactive stent. The idea that an implantable device such as a stent can be densely coated with an antigen in vitro, be inserted into an artery and then later, outside the catheterization laboratory, be targeted with a systemic venous injection of a radiolabeled antibody to render the stent radioactive at a time that coincides with the peak of neo-endothelial proliferation is appealing (Fig.1). This technology if successful, would permit the delivery of subsequent fractions without repeat catheterization. While technically challenging, the additional degree of freedom gained by being able to coat the stent in vitro allows full control of the nature, specificity, density, and uniformity on the target. This and the lower dose required to prevent restenosis suggest that in-stent restenosis may indeed be an ideal model to investigate targeted RIT.

Methods and Results

Proof of Concept

1. Six aluminum strings coated with avidin and six aluminum control strings were incubated in biotinylated horseradish peroxidase and then immersed shortly in 3,3'-diaminobenzidine solution with cobalt chloride enhancer. Avidin strings were stained dark brown compared to no stain in controls.

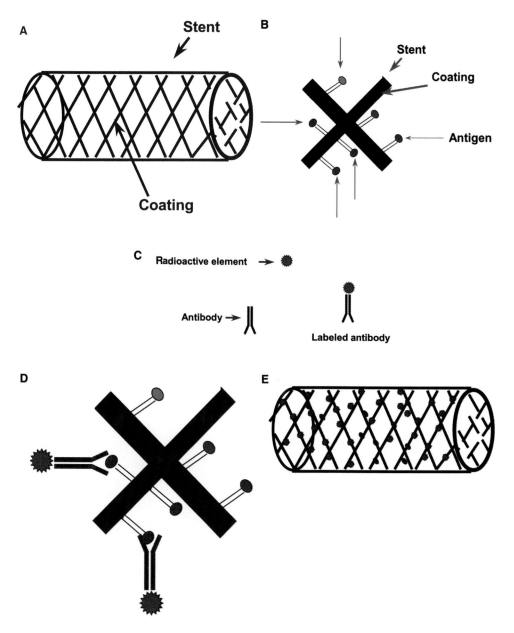

Figure 1. Rendering a nonradioactive stent into radioactive in vivo. **A.** An implantable stent is coated in vitro. **B.** An antigen is embedded into the stent coating. Different antigens (illustrated by different colors) are embedded into the stent coating. The stent is implanted in the patient's vessel at the catheterization laboratory. **C.** Antibodies specific to the antigens in (B) are labeled with a radioactive element. **D.** Labeled antibodies are injected intravenously outside of the catheterization laboratory and targeted to the antigen. **E.** The stent becomes radioactive.

2. Stainless steel coupons coated with bovine-serum-albumin (BSA) and stainless steel uncoated control coupons (Guidant, Santa Clara, CA) were treated with a 0.02 μg/mL solution of mouse monoclonal anti-BSA antibodies (Sigma). The coupons were then incubated with biotinylated secondary antibody coupled to alkaline phosphatase and subjected to colorimetric analysis. BSA-coated coupons showed specific binding of the anti-BSA manifested by stable red staining of the coupons. Control coupons, in contrast, had no staining.

3. Stainless steel BSA-coated coupons and stainless steel uncoated control coupons were treated with mouse monoclonal anti-BSA antibodies. All coupons were incubated with biotinylated antibody horseradish peroxidase, subjected to enhanced enzyme chemiluminescence analysis, and put instantly on standard x-ray films in a dark room for 1 to15 minutes. Developed x-ray films showed dark imaging of BSA-coated coupons but not of controls (Fig. 2).

Construction of a Radioactive Stent

4. Five BSA-coated and five control-coated ACS Multilink stents (Guidant) were incubated with a 0.02 μg/ml solution of 0.1 μCi/mL 125-iodinated mouse monoclonal anti-BSA antibodies (Sigma) for 4 hours. The BSA-

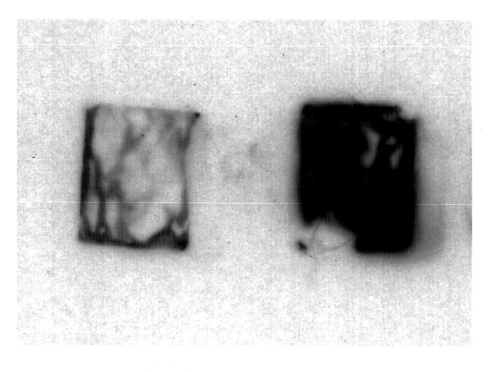

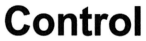

Figure 2. Enhanced chemiluminescence experiment (see text).

Table 1

Stent type	Activity μCi	n
Control-coated	0.017 ± 0.009	5
BSA-coated	0.23 ± 0.06 *	5

$P < 0.001$.
BSA = bovine-serum-albumin.

coated stents exhibited a 13-fold greater radioactivity as compared to controls, with activities in the range of 0.16 to 0.31 μCi (Table 1 and Fig. 3). The radioactivity of the BSA-coated stents was stable when incubated in porcine blood for 3 hours and then started leaching (Fig. 4).

Discussion

Radioactive stents may overcome many of the disadvantages of other intravascular brachytherapy modalities. Radioactive stents used in clinical trials were produced by bombarding stainless steel stents with ^{32}P atoms, or by embedding ^{31}P atoms onto stents and rendering them radioactive in a linear accelerator. Both methods require expensive equipment and facilities, and the results of clinical trials with such beta-emitting stents have been disappointing due to in-

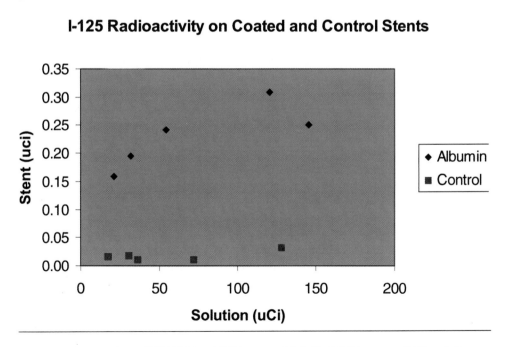

I-125 Radioactivity on Coated and Control Stents

Figure 3. Preparation of ^{125}I BSA/anti-BSA stents. Multilink BSA-stents ("Albumin") were incubated for 3 hours with solutions containing ^{125}I-anti-BSA antibody, and produced labeling up to 0.31 μCi.

Retained I-125 Activity during Leaching

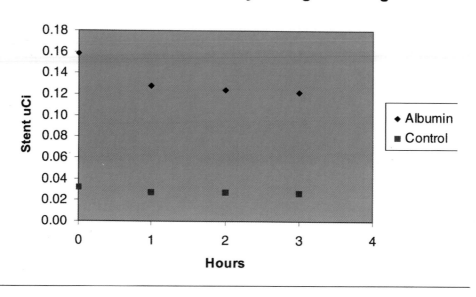

Figure 4. Leaching rate studies of ¹²⁵I BSA/anti-BSA ("Albumin") stents performed at room temperature in porcine blood.

creased restenosis at the stent edges, the "candy-wrapper effect." It is believed that gamma-emitting stents may overcome this side effect. Furthermore, current radioactive stents are not devoid of logistical drawbacks. As soon as a radioactive isotope is attached to the stent, it must be handled according to the strict regulations for all radioactive material. Shipping such radioactive stents is far more complicated than shipping the corresponding nonradioactive stent.

The results presented above demonstrate the feasibility of producing ¹²⁵I stents using the antigen/antibody methodology. The embodiment we envision is of a non-radioactive-coated stent which will be implanted into the diseased vessel. The stent will then be rendered into a radioactive stent outside of the catheterization laboratory by intravenous injection of a radioactive antigen targeted to its specific antibody which will be embedded in the stent coating. This implement has benefits related to the elimination of the radioactive procedure from the catheterization laboratory, as well as important logistical and biological advantages. It will avoid the need for expensive shielding of the catheterization laboratory from radioactive radiation, and the presence of radiation personnel in the catheterization laboratory will not be required. It will also shorten expensive procedural time at the catheterization laboratory. Delaying the initiation of the radioactive treatment for hours or days will coincide with the advent of smooth muscle cell proliferation, and possibly fractionate or boost the treatment with additional doses. It may be used with various radioactive sources (beta or gamma) with a possibly higher and more beneficial dose rate than the currently studied ³²P stents. The results presented here, however, suggest that further optimization is needed, in order to increase the radioactivity of these stents as well as to minimize leaching rate. Future research directions will include investigation of a more densely coated stent, other stable and high affinity RIT reagents, and various radioactive sources. It is also prudent to exploit techniques used in RIT to increase targeting while minimizing sequestration in normal tissues.

The concept presented is, in a broader sense, a method for targeted treatment of a tissue with an effector by a "lock and key" system. The "lock and key" system includes a "lock" attached to a biomedical device, which is inserted into a subject as part of a regular insertion procedure. The "key" is attached to an effector. The effector/key combination is then injected into the subject, or is otherwise introduced into the subject, at a site that may be at any suitable distance from the point of insertion of the biomedical device. The key enables the effector/key combination to be localized to the biomedical device, by interaction of the key and the lock on the biomedical device. Thus, the effector is specifically targeted to the tissue surrounding the biomedical device. The term "effector" includes any molecule, combination of molecules, or even a complete cell, which has a therapeutic effect. For example, the effector could be a radioactive isotope, drug, hormone, growth factor, cytokine, T cell, endothelial cell, or toxin. The effector could be selected in order to inhibit tissue growth, eg, to treat or prevent restenosis. Examples of suitable combinations of lock and key systems include an antibody and antigen combination, nonimmunological proteins such as avidin and biotin, and nonprotein macromolecules such as complex carbohydrate ligands and receptors.

The same concept applied ex vivo would comprise a more convenient method of manufacturing radioactive stents compared with the current process. In addition, this would allow separate shipping of the stent and the radioactive isotope, which then may be combined shortly before the stent is inserted into the patient at the end user facility, or alternatively, by the manufacturer according to the logistics of the delivery.

Conclusions

Labeled compounds may be targeted to coated stents to render them radioactive in vitro. This concept should allow for numerous variations in dose as well as isotope, and may be extended to in vivo targeted RIT by injecting labeled compounds intravenously. This approach has biological and logistical advantages and eliminates the handling of radioactive sources in the catheterization laboratory.

References

1. Goldberg JD, Stemerman MB, Schnipper LE, et al. Vascular smooth muscle cell kinetics: A new assay for studying patterns of cellular proliferation *in-vivo*. Science 1979;205:920–922.
2. O'Connel TX, Mowbray JF. Effect of humoral transplantation antibody on the arterial intima in normal rabbits. Circ Res 1973;29:478–487.
3. Moore S. Responses of the arterial wall to injury. Diabetes 1975;2(suppl):8–13.
4. Gajdusek KM, Shwartz SM. Ability of endothelial cells to condition culture medium. J Cell Physiol 1982;110:35–44.
5. Smith EB, Staples EM, Dietz HZ. Role of endothelium in sequestration of lipoprotein and fibrinogen in aortic lesions, thrombi and graft pseudo-intimas. Lancet 1979:712–816.
6. Dejana E, Cazenave JP, Hatton MWC, et al. The effect of thrombi and platelet accumulation on the vessel wall—influence of heparin and aspirin. Thromb Haemostasis 1983;50:567–571.

7. Tierstein P, Massullo VM, Jani SK, et al. Catheter-based radiotherapy to inhibit restenosis after coronary stenting. N Engl J Med 1997;336:1697–1703.
8. Waksman R, White RL, Chan RC, et al, for the Washington Radiation for In-Stent Restenosis Trial (WRIST) Investigators. Intracoronary gamma-radiation therapy after angioplasty inhibits recurrence in patients with in-stent restenosis. Circulation 2000;101:2165–2169.
9. Waksman R, Robinson KA, Crocker IR, et al. Endovascular low-dose irradiation inhibits neointima formation after coronary artery balloon injury in swine: A possible role for radiation therapy in restenosis prevention. Circulation 1995;91:1533–1539.
10. Mayberg MR, Luo Z, London S, et al. Radiation inhibition of intimal hyperplasia after arterial injury. Radiat Res 1995;142:212–220.
11. Shimotakahara S, Mayberg MR. Gamma irradiation inhibits neointimal hyperplasia in rats after arterial injury. Stroke 1994;25:424–428.
12. Koh WJ, Mayberg MR, Chambers J, et al. The potential role of external beam radiation in preventing restenosis after coronary angioplasty. Int J Radiat Oncol Biol Phys 1996;36:829–834.
13. Teirstein P, Massullo V, Jani S, et al. Catheter-based radiotherapy to inhibit restenosis after coronary stenting. N Engl J Med 1997;336:1697–1703.
14. Popowski Y, Verin V, Papirov I, et al. Intra-arterial ^{90}Y brachytherapy: Preliminary dosimetric study using a specially modified angioplasty balloon. Int J Radiat Oncol Biol Phys 1995;33:713–717.
15. Waksman R, Robinson KA, Crocker IR, et al. Intracoronary low dose beta radiation inhibits neointimal formation after coronary artery balloon injury in the swine restenosis model [abstract]. Circulation 1995;92:3205–3231.
16. Albiero R, Adamian M, Kobayashi N, et al. Short- and intermediate-term results of (32)P radioactive beta-emitting stent implantation in patients with coronary artery disease: The Milan Dose-Response Study. Circulation 2000;101:18–26.
17. Albiero R, Nishida T, Adamian M, et al. Edge restenosis after implantation of high activity (32)P radioactive beta-emitting stents. Circulation 2000;101:2454–2457.
18. Fishell T. Gamma emitting radioactive stents. The 4th Cardiovascular Radiation Therapy Meeting. Washington, DC, February 16–18, 2000.
19. Knox SJ, Meredith RF. Clinical Radioimmunotherapy. Semin Radiat Oncol 2000;10:73–93.
20. Wilder RB, DeNardo GL, DeNardo SJ. Radioimmunotherapy: Recent results and future directions. J Clin Oncol 1996;14:1383–1400.
21. Kaminski MS, Estis M, Regan J. Frontline treatment of advanced B-cell low-grade lymphoma with radiolabeled anti-B1 antibody: Initial experience [abstract]. J Clin Oncol 1997;16:15a.
22. Jurcic JG, Caron PC, Nikula TK, et al. Radiolabeled anti-CD33 monoclonal antibody M195 for myeloid leukemias. Cancer Res 1995;55(suppl):5908S-5910S.
23. Liu SY, Eary JF, Petersdorf SH, et al. Follow-up of relapsed B-Cell lymphoma patients treated with iodine 131-labeled anti-CD20 antibody and autologous stem cell rescue. J Clin Oncol 1998;16:3270–3278.
24. Wessels BW, Meares CF. Physical and chemical properties of radionuclide therapy. Semin Radiat Oncol 2000;10:115–122.
25. Fisher DR. Internal dosimetry for systemic radiation therapy. Semin Radiat Oncol 2000;10:123–132.

## Chapter 34

Intravascular Ultrasound
Observations from the
Radioactive Stent Trials

Remo Albiero, MD

Introduction

Brachytherapy by implantation of a radioactive stent is an alternative approach to catheter-based systems to reduce restenosis. In the pilot clinical trial currently in progress, it has been demonstrated that the use of ^{32}P radioactive beta-emitting stents with activities up to 24 μCi has resulted in a reduction in intrastent restenosis at 6 months in a dose-related manner.[1-6] However, binary intralesion (both within the stent and at the edges) restenosis was not different (17%,[4] 40.4%,[6] 52%,[1] and 54%[5]), and was perhaps higher than that of currently available nonradioactive stents, due to restenosis at the stent edges ("edge effect"). We tried to summarize these two findings (the "good" intrastent result and the "bad" effect at the edges) coining the term "candy wrapper." Serial intravascular ultrasound (IVUS) imaging (after stenting and at follow-up) and dosimetric analysis was used to help elucidate the mechanism of the "candy wrapper" pattern.

Methodology

The Radioactive [32]P Beta-Particle-Emitting Stent

The radioisotope ^{32}P, a pure beta-particle emitter, is currently being used in the pilot clinical trial because of its short half-life (14.3 days) and limited range of tissue penetration. Two types of radioactive 15-mm long stents have been used: initially the Palmaz-Schatz (PS 153) with an initial activity up to 3 μCi, and later, the BX stent with an initial higher activity between 3 and 24 μCi. To make the stent radioactive, the radioisotope ^{32}P was embedded beneath the surface of the stent using an ion implantation technique (Isostent, Inc., Belmont, CA).

Dosimetry

For radioactive stent dosimetry it is recommended[7] that the doses be specified in gray (Gy) delivered over a time period of 28 days at a 0.5-mm radial distance from the stent surface. However, we preferred to specify the dose as the min-

From Waksman R (ed.). *Vascular Brachytherapy, Third Edition.* Armonk, NY: Futura Publishing Co., Inc.; © 2002.

imum dose rate (the speed at which the radiation dose was delivered) at the adventitia (the target tissue) in centigray per hour (cGy/h) at the time of stent implantation, calculated according to the model of Janicki et al[8] as illustrated in Figures 1 and 2. The dose rate was calculated by using IVUS to measure the maximum radial distance between the stent struts and the external elastic membrane (EEM) a shown in Figure 3. The calculated average minimum dose rate at the adventitia in the central part (5 mm) of the stent was correlated with the tissue growth at follow-up in the same segment, to evaluate the effect of the dose delivered in inhibiting subsequent neointimal tissue growth. The radiation dose delivered by a stent is not homogeneous; however, this nonuniformity of dosing, which depends on the stent geometry, decreases at distances greater than 0.5 to 1 mm from the stent surface, as shown in Figures 1 and 2. Designed by computer-aided technique to provide flexibility without a central articulation, the BX Isostent has a more homogeneous dosimetry along the length of the stent, and has been demonstrated to favorably influence the vascular response in normal porcine coronary arteries compared with the Palmaz-Schatz stent.[9]

IVUS Imaging and Analysis

IVUS imaging was done after stenting and at 4- to 6-month follow-up using the Cardiovascular Imaging System (CVIS, Sunnyvale, CA) and a motorized trans-

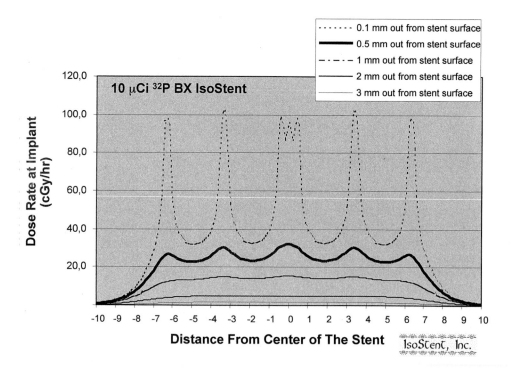

Figure 1. Calculated dose rate (cGy/hr) distribution at radial distances of 0.1, 0.5, 1, 2, and 3 mm along a 3.0-mm diameter and 15-mm long ^{32}P BX Isostent of 10 μCi. The dose rates were calculated using the model of Janicki et al[8] (source, Isostent, Inc.). Note the nonuniformity of the dose distribution, which depends on the stent geometry and decreases at radial distances greater than 0.5 to 1 mm from the stent surface.

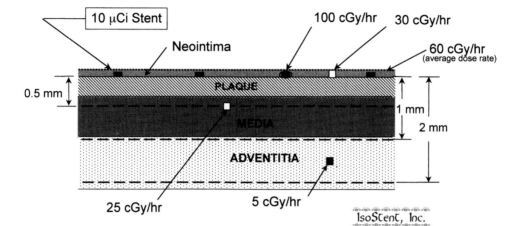

Figure 2. Calculated dose rates for a 10 μCi ^{32}P 15-mm long BX Isostent based on the model of Janicki et al[8] (source, Isostent, Inc.).

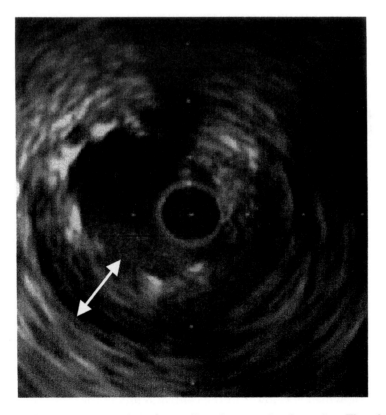

Figure 3. IVUS image cross section after radioactive stent implantation. The white arrow indicates the maximum distance between the stent struts and the external elastic membrane. This distance was used to calculate the minimum dose rate at the adventitia based on the model of Janicki et al.[8]

ducer pullback at a speed of 0.5 mm/s. Quantitative IVUS analysis was performed offline measuring stent/EEM cross-sectional area (CSA), lumen CSA , and plaque CSA in 15 segments inside the stent and, when feasible, in 10 reference segments proximal and distal to the stent. The image cross sections analyzed were 1 mm apart. In-stent plaque volume was calculated at follow-up based on Simpson's rule and was, therefore, the product of the 15 plaque CSAs and the distance of 1 mm separating them. For each of the 15 segments inside the stent and for the reference segments, the following calculations were made: remodeling = post-intervention (PI) stent or EEM CSA – follow-up (FU) stent or EEM CSA; late lumen loss = PI lumen CSA – FU lumen CSA; tissue growth = FU plaque CSA – PI plaque CSA.

The Milan Experience

Radioactive ^{32}P Stents with Initial Activities of 0.75 to 12 μCi

In the early Milan experience from October 1997 to October 1998, a total of 122 ^{32}P radioactive beta-emitting stents (initially the Palmaz-Schatz and later the BX Isostent) with initial activities of 0.75 to 3 μCi (group1), 3 to 6 μCi (group 2), and 6 to12 μCi (group 3) were implanted in 91 lesions in 82 patients. At 6-month follow-up, pure intrastent binary angiographic restenosis was reduced in a dose-related manner (16% in group 1, 3% in group 2, and 0% in group 3). However, in the 3 groups we observed a high intralesion restenosis (52% in group 1, 41% in group 2, and 50% in group 3) due to an "edge effect."[1] Figures 4 and 5 show two representative patients with the "candy wrapper" pattern of restenosis in the mid left anterior descending coronary artery, which occurred approximately 4 months after implantation of a single ^{32}P BX Isostent with an initial activity of approximately 8 μCi. IVUS images in Figure 4 show a low amount of plaque burden in the contiguous proximal and distal reference segments after stenting. At 4-month follow-up: (1) there is no intimal hyperplasia inside the stent, and (2) the reduction of the lumen CSA outside the stent is due to "tissue growth," without vessel shrinkage (negative remodeling). The plot in the upper part of Figure 5 shows that the late lumen loss at the edges was entirely due to "tissue growth" without remodeling. In this lesion, the maximum increase of the neointimal tissue occurred in the first millimeter outside the stent, but there was also a large amount of neointima in the adjacent 3 to 4 mm inside and outside the stent margins. Figure 6 summarizes the results of 13 lesions with restenosis in which a single BX Isostent with an initial activity of 3 to12 μCi was implanted during the early Milan experience. Late lumen loss in the proximal and distal reference segments outside the stent was higher than inside the stent and was mainly due to tissue growth (intimal hyperplasia) in the first 1 to 3 mm and to negative remodeling (shrinkage of the vessel) in the last 4 to10 mm from the stent edges. Inside the stent, no remodeling was observed and late lumen loss was only due to tissue growth, which was lower in the central 5 mm of the stent compared with the proximal and distal 5 mm. This edge effect was possibly the result of a low-activity level of radiation at the stent margins[8] combined with systematic balloon injury at these sites.

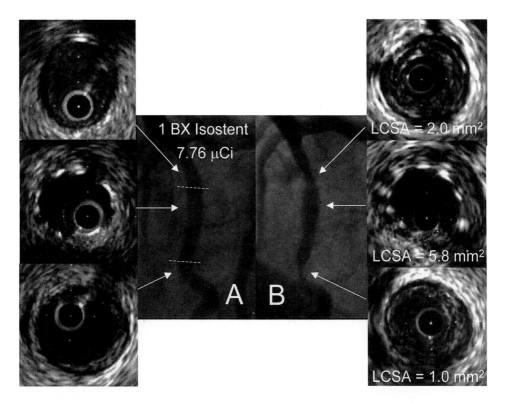

Figure 4. Representative lesion with the "candy wrapper" pattern of restenosis approximately 4 months after implantation of a ^{32}P radioactive 15-mm long BX Isostent with an initial activity of 7.76 μCi. **(A)** Angiogram after stent implantation in the mid LAD. **(B)** Four-month follow-up angiogram, showing the persistence of a good result inside the stent, but a significant stenosis at both of the stent edges. IVUS images after stenting (left side of the figure) show very little plaque burden of the contiguous proximal and distal reference segments (left upper and lower panels). IVUS images at 4-month follow-up (right side of the figure) show that there is no intimal hyperplasia inside the stent (right middle panel), and that the reduction of the lumen CSA in the proximal and distal reference segments outside the stent (right upper and lower panels) is due to "tissue growth," without vessel shrinkage (negative remodeling).

Radioactive [32]P Stents with Initial Activities of 12 to 21 μCi

From October 1998 to April 1999, we evaluated whether ^{32}P radioactive BX Isostents with higher activity levels (12 to 21 μCi) combined with a nonaggressive approach to stenting could solve the problem of edge restenosis.[2] A very low (<4%) intrastent binary restenosis was observed. However, the intralesion (intrastent plus peri-stent) restenosis rate was still greater than 30%.

Figure 7 summarizes the results of lesions with edge restenosis (proximal edge, n=8; distal edge, n=5) treated by a single ^{32}P BX Isostent of 12 to 21 μCi during the late Milan experience: late lumen loss in the first 1 to 3 mm from the stent margins was mainly due to remodeling (shrinkage of the vessel),[2] as opposed to our prior observations in 3 to 12 μCi stents, in which late lumen loss was mainly

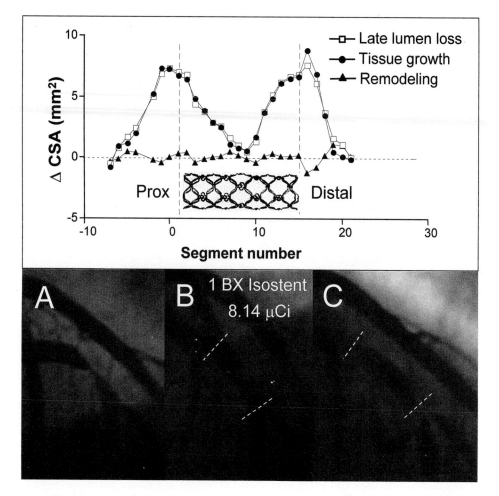

Figure 5. Impressive example of the "candy wrapper" pattern of restenosis approximately 4 months after implantation of a ^{32}P radioactive 15-mm long BX stent with an initial activity of 8.14 μCi. **(A)** Baseline angiogram showing a stenosis in the mid LAD. **(B)** Post-stenting angiogram. **(C)** Four-month follow-up angiogram, showing a "freezed" result in the mid part of the stent at the site of the original lesion, but a tight stenosis at both the stent edges. The upper part of the figure is a plot of the late lumen loss, tissue growth, and remodeling (in mm^2). Point represents differences in CSA measured in slices 1 mm apart inside the stent and in proximal and distal reference segments. CSA indicates the cross-sectional area. The plot shows that the late lumen loss at the edges was entirely due to "tissue growth" without remodeling. In addition, the maximum increase of the neointimal tissue occurred in the first millimeter outside the stent, but there was also a large amount of neointima in the adjacent 3 to 4 mm inside and outside the stent margins.

due to tissue growth (intimal hyperplasia).[1] In addition, IVUS imaging confirmed the dramatic reduction of neointimal tissue inside the stent.

Edge Restenosis

Although there are no data regarding the composition of the neointima at the edges of radioactive stents, we observed by IVUS that this tissue was soft with a

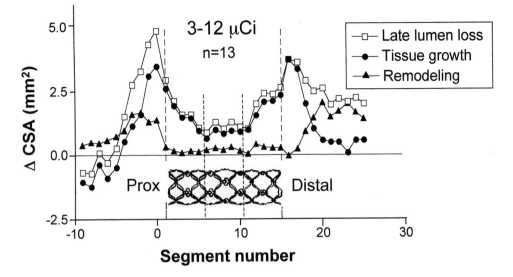

Figure 6. Plot of mean of late lumen loss, tissue growth, and remodeling (in mm²) in 13 lesions with restenosis treated with a single BX Isostent of 3 to12 μCi. Point represents differences in CSA measured in slices 1 mm apart inside the stent and in the proximal and distal reference segments. CSA indicates the cross-sectional area.

very low echodensity, and often difficult to distinguish. In addition, the easiness of retreatment by balloon inflations at low pressure suggests that this soft tissue was probably mostly constituted by extracellular matrix. This deduction is also consistent with the results reported in the rabbit model by Hehrlein,[10] who analyzed the effect of radiation delivery by a stent on the extracellular matrix deposition, and demonstrated by immunocytochemical analysis an increase in the expression of collagen type I.

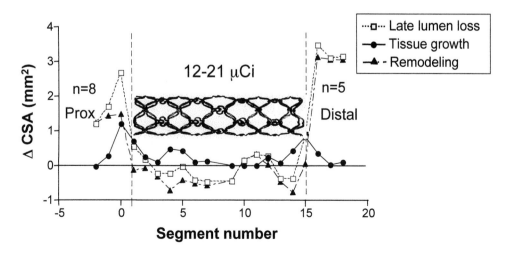

Figure 7. Plot of mean of late lumen loss, tissue growth, and remodeling (in mm²) in lesions with edge restenosis (proximal edge, n=8; distal edge, n=5) treated with 12 to 21 μCi BX stents. CSA indicates the cross-sectional area.

Inhibition of In-Stent Neointima Hyperplasia

IVUS Intrastent Plaque Measurement

Serial IVUS imaging and quantitative analysis was performed in 69 of the 119 lesions treated in Milan by single 15-mm long ^{32}P radioactive stents. As shown in Figure 8, intrastent neointimal hyperplasia measured as plaque volume at 4- to 6-month follow-up was inversely related to the initial stent activity, with a significantly lower amount of neointima in lesions treated by 12 to 21 μCi stents (n=32) than in lesions treated by 3 to 12 μCi (n=33) and 0.75 to 3 μCi stents (n=4). In Figure 9, the same data are shown as a line graph that illustrates the distribution of plaque along the long axis of the stent. Note a dose-dependent reduction of the neointima inside the BX stent and its increase at the central articulation of the Palmaz-Schatz stent and toward the stent edges.

Dosimetric Analysis

Dosimetric analysis might help to clarify the mechanism by which radioactive stents prevent intrastent neointimal hyperplasia. The 6-month results of radioactive stents with activities up to 12 μCi are consistent with the hypothesis, proposed by Fishell et al,[11] that inhibition of intrastent neointimal hyperplasia is the result of the inhibition of the migration of smooth muscle cells and myofibroblasts from the tunica media and adventitia into the neointima, as these cells

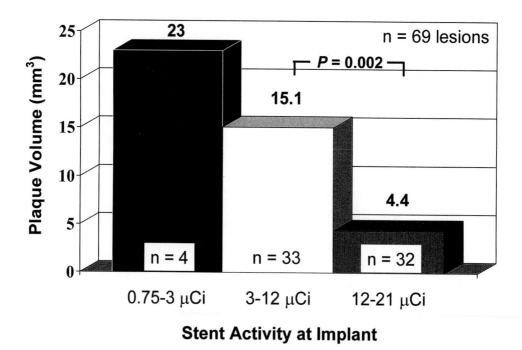

Stent Activity at Implant

Figure 8. Plaque volume measured at 4 to 6 months after implantation of a single ^{32}P radioactive BX Isostent. Plaque volume decreased with increasing radiation activity.

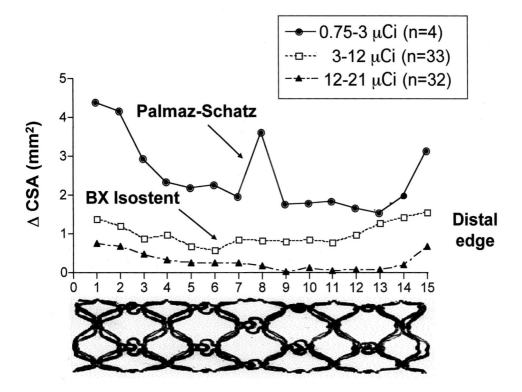

Figure 9. Line graph showing the distribution of the plaque (measured as plaque CSA in mm²) along the long axis of single ^{32}P radioactive stents with activities ranging from 0.75 to 21 μCi. There is a dose-dependent reduction of intrastent neointimal tissue. Note the increase of neointima at the central articulation of the Palmaz-Schatz stent and toward the stent edges.

pass through the "electron fence" at the plane of the stent wires. However, this theory cannot explain the significantly lower amount of neointima found inside ^{32}P radioactive stents with a higher activity of greater than 12 μCi compared with 3 to 12 μCi stents. This latter finding could be explained in two ways: (1) as the result of the longer time the stent remains effective as "a fence" before it decays below the (unknown) minimum activity level required to inhibit cell migration into the neointima (eg, the efficacy duration as "a fence" of a ^{32}P 16 μCi stent with a half-life of 14.3 days is approximately 1 month longer than a 4 μCi stent); and/or (2) the result of a deeper effect on the media and adventitia similar to that seen with catheter-based radiation therapies, in which the cells are disabled (killed) before their attempt to migrate into the neointima. To verify the second hypothesis, we calculated the mean minimum dose rate in centigray/hour at the adventitia at the time of stent implantation in the central 5 mm of the stent (this target segment was selected based on our prior observation of greater inhibition of neointimal proliferation in the central part of radioactive stents; see Fig. 6). This dose rate was correlated with the mean tissue growth (plaque volume, mm³) at follow-up in the same segment, as shown in the plot of Figure 10. By regression analysis, there was a significant nonlinear logarithmic inverse correlation between the minimum dose rate delivered at the adventitia at stent implant and intrastent

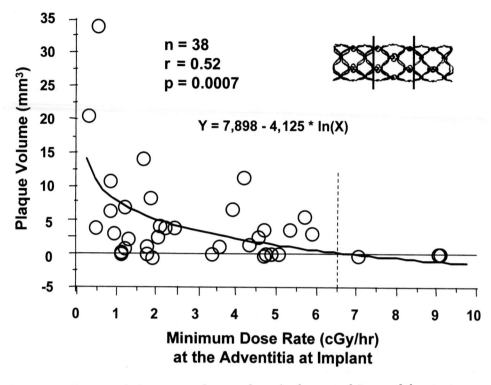

Figure 10. Decrease in intrastent plaque volume in the central 5 mm of the stent correlated with increase in minimum dose rate (cGy/h) at the adventitia at the time of stent implantation in the same segment in 38 lesions in which a single 15-mm ^{32}P radioactive stent was implanted. By regression analysis, this nonlinear logarithmic inverse correlation was statistically significant (*P*=0.0007).

plaque volume at 6-month follow-up.[12] Note that when the minimum dose rate at the adventitia at stent implant was greater than 6 to 7 cGy/h (a dose rate commonly achieved by ^{32}P radioactive stents with an initial activity greater than 5 to 6 μCi), the intrastent plaque volume was nearly zero. This observation is concordant with an in vitro study on human smooth muscle cells by Williams et al (Johns Hopkins University, personal communication), in which 80 to 90% of the cells were killed by dose rates of 3 to 6 cGy/h.

"Black Holes"

"Black holes" have been called the dark spots occasionally observed by IVUS behind and between the struts of radioactive stents 4 to 6 months after stenting. Figure 11 shows an illustrative case of "black holes" observed 6 months after implantation of a ^{32}P radioactive "hot ends" stent. Note that, by angiography, the vessel appears slightly larger at follow-up (panel B) than after stenting (panel A). The dark spots ("black holes," indicated by arrows in the right of the figure) behind and between the stent struts, were not visible at the same sites immediately after stenting (left side of the figure). The significance of this observation is unknown. If we exclude stent malapposition, this finding might be the consequence of a sort

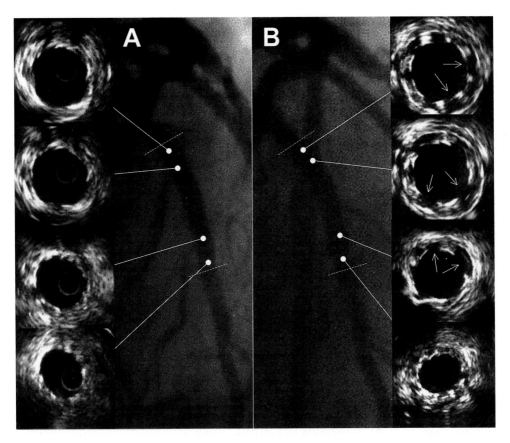

Figure 11. Illustrative case of "black holes" observed 6 months after implantation of a ^{32}P radioactive "hot ends" stent of 18.5 μCi in the mid LAD. The "hot ends" stent has a length of 18 mm. The initial activity in the proximal and distal 2 mm of the stent is 2.6 μCi/mm, while in the central 14 mm, it is 0.57 μCi/mm. The initial maximum total stent activity is therefore 18.5 μCi (10.5 μCi at the ends plus approximately 8 μCi in the middle). By angiography, the vessel appears slightly larger at follow-up (**B**) than after stenting (**A**). The IVUS images on the right show the presence of dark spots ("black holes," indicated by arrows) behind and between the stent struts, which were not visible at the same sites immediately after stent implantation (left side of the figure).

of plaque melting/erosion outside the stent. We think that if this phenomenon occurs, it is probably followed by deposition of new soft, poorly echogenic tissue similar to that observed at the sites of edges restenosis. The clinical relevance (tendency to late stent thrombosis) of the "black holes" is unknown.

The Rotterdam Experience

The Rotterdam group did not observe cases of edge restenosis in ^{32}P radioactive stents of 0.75 to 1.5 μCi.[4] However, they reported a restenosis rate of 43%, occurring only at the stent edges, in an additional group of lesions treated by ^{32}P radioactive stents of 6 to 12 μCi.[3]

They compared the serial IVUS results (performed after stenting and at 6-month follow-up) of a group of 18 patients treated by conventional stents (Multilink n=8, NIR n=10) with those of 12 patients treated by high-activity (6 to 12 μCi) BX radioactive stents.[13] The changes in lumen volume and total vessel volume were assessed at the stent edge (up to 5 mm proximal and distal to the stent) and inside the stent, by measuring stent volume, intrastent neointimal hyperplasia, and plaque volume behind the stent. Stent edge renarrowing occurred after both conventional and high-activity radioactive stent implantation, without a statistically significant difference between the 2 groups. However, the decrease in lumen volume observed at the edges of radioactive stents was higher than that of nonradioactive stents (-11.24 versus -9.1 mm^3), and was due to a higher increase in plaque volume ($+3.3$ versus $+1.47$ mm^3) with a similar decrease in the total vessel volume (-8.68 versus -8.46 mm^3). In addition, they demonstrated that intrastent neointimal hyperplasia was significantly reduced after implantation of high-activity radioactive stents compared with nonradioactive stents (8.90 versus 20.18 mm^3, $P<0.05$) with no change in total vessel volume or plaque volume behind the stent between the two groups.

The Vienna Experience

The Vienna group experience with radioactive stents began in January 1999.[14] These investigators reported the results of 36 patients treated by ^{32}P radioactive BX stents of 5.36 to 20.77 μCi (mean±SD, 12.77±4.69 μCi).[15] At 6-month clinical follow-up, 15 patients (42.9%) required target vessel revascularization (TVR) mostly due to edge restenosis (n=13, 87.7%). Using IVUS and dosimetric analysis, the relationship between the dose delivered and the inhibition of neointimal hyperplasia was studied. The absorbed dose in a defined artery volume (dose volume histograms [DVH]) was calculated by an original model and correlated with the 6-month IVUS results. This model was applied in 11 patients who had serial (after stenting and at follow-up) IVUS documentation. Based on post-implantation IVUS measurements at seven defined segments (five within the stent, one at 2 mm proximal and distal to the stent, respectively), the doses delivered to 10 and 90% (DV10, DV90), and the mean target dose within the assumed target volume, ie, the adventitia (defined as 0.5-mm thickness outside the external elastic lamina), were calculated by an elaborate computer algorithm. Plaque volume was calculated by multiplying each segments plaque area by the segment length both for the stent body and the peri-stent segments, and its changes after 6 months were evaluated. In all patients, there was a clear trend towards lower neointima growth at higher doses within the stent body. This inverse correlation reached significance for DV10 (r=0.72, $P=0.006$) and a borderline significance for DV90 (r=0.52, $P=0.051$). The same trend was observed in the peri-stent segments for DV90 (r=0.44, $P=0.018$). The initial activity at implantation did not correlate with plaque growth. This analysis of DVH confirms our findings[12] of a dose-dependent reduction of intrastent neointima formation after ^{32}P radioactive coronary stenting.

Conclusions

IVUS analysis has contributed to the identification of the mechanism by which the "candy wrapper" pattern occurs. Radioactive ^{32}P stents with activities of 3 to 21 μCi reduce intrastent neointimal hyperplasia in a dose-related manner. The high edge restenosis rate observed after implantation of 3 to 12 μCi stents was mainly due to tissue growth in the first 1 to 3 mm from the stent edges and negative remodeling in the last 4 to 10 mm from the stent margins. By increasing the initial stent activity (12 to 21 μCi) and limiting the balloon-induced injury outside the stent, edge restenosis did not disappear: there was a reduction of the component of edge restenosis due to plaque growth, but not of that due to negative remodeling. Finally, the significance and the clinical relevance (potential tendency of late stent thrombosis) of the so-called "black holes" is unknown.

References

1. Albiero R, Adamian M, Kobayashi N, et al. Short- and intermediate-term results of (32)P radioactive beta-emitting stent implantation in patients with coronary artery disease: The Milan Dose-Response Study. Circulation 2000;101:18–26.
2. Albiero R, Nishida T, Adamian M, et al. Edge restenosis after implantation of high activity (32)P radioactive beta-emitting stents. Circulation 2000;101:2454–2457.
3. Wardeh AJ, Knook AHM, Kay IP, et al. The European P-32 Dose Response Trial: The Rotterdam contribution [abstract]. Am J Cardiol 1999;84(suppl):84P.
4. Wardeh AJ, Kay IP, Sabate M, et al. Beta-particle-emitting radioactive stent implantation: A safety and feasibility study. Circulation 1999;100:1684–1689.
5. Hansen A, Hehrlein C, Hardt S, et al. Is the "candy-wrapper" effect of beta-particle emitting stents due to remodeling or neointimal hyperplasia? [abstract] Circulation 1999;1000:I-155.
6. Moses J. U.S. IRIS trials low-activity 32P stent [abstract]. Advances in Cardiovasc Radiation Therapy III. Washington, DC, 1999:387–388.
7. Nath R, Amols H, Coffey C, et al. Intravascular brachytherapy physics: Report of the AAPM Radiation Therapy Committee Task Group No. 60. American Association of Physicists in Medicine. Med Phys 1999;26:119–152.
8. Janicki C, Duggan DM, Coffey CW, et al. Radiation dose from a phosphorous-32 impregnated wire mesh vascular stent. Med Phys 1997;24:437–445.
9. Carter AJ, Scott D, Rahdert D, et al. Stent design favourably influences the vascular response in normal porcine coronary arteries. J Invas Cardiol 1999;11:127–134.
10. Hehrlein C. Radioactive stents: The European experience. In: Waksman R (ed.): Vascular Brachytherapy, 3rd Edition. Armonk, NY: Futura Publishing Company; 1999:333–342.
11. Fischell TA, Carter AJ, Laird JR. The beta-particle-emitting radioisotope stent (isostent): Animal studies and planned clinical trials. Am J Cardiol 1996;78:45–50.
12. Albiero R, Nishida T, Amato A, et al. IVUS and dosimetric analysis of 32P radioactive β-particle-emitting stents [abstract]. Eur Heart J 2000;21(suppl):399.
13. Kay IP, Sabaté M, Costa MA, et al. Stent and stent-edge remodeling after conventional and radioactive stent implantation [abstract]. J Am Coll Cardiol 2000;35(suppl A):22.
14. Wexberg P, Beran G, Sperker W, et al. Six month follow-up of radioactive BX stents with an initial activity of up to 24 μCi: The Vienna P-32 Dose Response Study [abstract]. Eur Heart J 2000;21(suppl):622.
15. Wexberg P, Kirisits C, Gottsauner-Wolf M, et al. Radioactive stents decrease neointima growth during six months in a dose-dependent manner: Dose volume histograms based on serial IVUS measurement [abstract]. Eur Heart J 2000;21(suppl):399.

## Chapter 35

Lessons from the Feasibility Radioactive (IRIS) Stent Trials

Tim A. Fischell, MD, Andrew Carter, DO,
Malcolm Foster, MD, Robert E. Fischell, ScD,
and David R. Fischell, PhD

Despite improvements in long-term outcomes following intracoronary stent placement, restenosis remains a significant problem, particularly in long lesions and smaller diameter vessels.[1,2] Experimental and clinical data have demonstrated that in-stent restenosis is principally caused by neointimal formation.[3–6] Endovascular radiation has been proposed as a method to reduce neointimal formation and, thus, prevent restenosis.[7–17]

Intravascular radiation using an ^{192}Ir source has been effective in reducing neointimal formation after balloon injury in a porcine model.[15] Additional studies have also demonstrated the efficacy of a strontium/yttrium source in a porcine model.[16] A centered ^{32}P wire-based radiation system was also shown to reduce neointimal hyperplasia with doses of 2500 to 4500 cGy targeted 0.5 mm deep to the intimal surface.

Teirstein et al[12] recently reported approximately 75% reduction in late lumen loss and restenosis in a randomized, placebo-controlled clinical trial using 8- to 25-Gy irradiation delivered via an endovascular ^{192}Ir source, combined with stenting, in patients with restenosis lesions. While this landmark study established the clinical efficacy of endovascular irradiation in the prevention of restenosis, the impracticalities and safety issues related to the use of a gamma source may limit the acceptance of this therapy. An alternative approach using a beta-emitting source has proven feasible and possibly effective.[17]

Another alternative, and perhaps a simpler approach to intravascular radiation, is the use of a stent as the platform for local radiation delivery as a means to prevent restenosis. Low-dose beta particle irradiation inhibits smooth muscle proliferation and migration in vitro.[13] Experimental studies have demonstrated that stents ion-implanted with ^{32}P reduce neointimal formation at activities as low as 0.14 μCi.[7,8,10,14] The purpose of this chapter is to review the current status of radioactive stents from the recent clinical phase 1 feasibility trials.

The dosimetry of a ^{32}P stent has previously been described in detail. Janicki et al[18] characterized the near-field dose of a 1.0-μCi, 15-mm-length Palmaz-Schatz (Cordis, a Johnson and Johnson Co., Warren, NJ) using a modification of the dose point kernel method. Modification of the dose distribution around a uniform cylin-

From Waksman R (ed.). *Vascular Brachytherapy, Third Edition.* Armonk, NY: Futura Publishing Co., Inc.; © 2002.

der of ^{32}P to account for the geometry of a tubular slotted Palmaz-Schatz stent with mathematical modeling allowed construction of three-dimensional dose maps. For a 1.0-µCi, 15-mm-length ^{32}P stent, at a distance of 0.1 mm, dose values of ≈ 2500 cGy were delivered at the strut wires (peaks) and ≈ 800 cGy were delivered between the wires (valleys) over one half-life (14.3 days). The dosimetry for a 1.0-µCi, 15-mm-length ^{32}P Palmaz-Schatz stent is shown in Figure 1. The nonuniformity of dosing reflective of the stent geometry decreased at distances of 1 to 2 mm from the surface. The dosimetry predicted by the dose calculations correlated well with measured dose with use of radiochromic film. While these data provide an in vitro analysis of dosing from a radioactive stent, the actual dose distribution is affected by variations in atherosclerotic plaque morphology and the symmetry of stent expansion.

Hehrlein et al[10] also reported a series of experiments with varying activities of ^{32}P stents in rabbit iliac arteries. In contrast to the porcine experiments, these authors reported a substantial dose-dependent reduction in neointimal formation with the maximal effect evident at 3 months after placement of a 13.0-µCi, 7-mm-length stent. The contrasting results with the doses of continuous beta particle irradiation used in these experimental studies suggests a species- or model-dependent response to endovascular irradiation delivered via a stent. Others have demonstrated species differences in response to nonradioactive stent implantation that may be related to endothelial cell regeneration or the intrinsic fibrinolytic capacity of the animal.[19-21] Studies are under way to examine species differences in the response to stent-based irradiation which may have important implications for the selection of animal models used to evaluate radioactive stents. Ultimately, the safety and efficacy of this approach to inhibit restenosis in humans with atherosclerotic coronary artery disease requires carefully planned clinical trials.

The initial clinical experience with beta-particle–emitting stents occurred at three FDA approved investigation centers in the United States beginning in October 1996. The phase 1 Isostent for Restenosis Intervention Study (IRIS) was a nonrandomized trial designed to evaluate the safety of implanting very low activity (0.5 to 1.0 µCi) ^{32}P, 15-mm-length Palmaz-Schatz coronary stents in patients with symptomatic de novo or restenosis native coronary lesions. The enrollment for this trial was completed on January 14, 1997, with 32 patients receiving a beta-particle–emitting stent.

Stent placement was successful in all patients. The mean stent activity at the time of implant in the IRIS trial was 0.7 µCi. There were no cases of subacute stent thrombosis, target lesion revascularization, death, or other major cardiac events within the first 30 days (primary safety endpoint), thus, demonstrating acceptable early event-free survival. At 6-month follow-up there was a binary restenosis rate of 31% (10/32) and a clinically driven target vessel revascularization (TVR) rate of 21%. Interestingly, there was only 1 restenosis (proximal to stent) out of the 10 patients treated for restenosis lesions (10%) and only 18% for patients receiving stents greater than 0.75 µCi. There were no further TVR events between 6 months and 12 months. Of note, in the de novo subgroup the mean reference vessel diameter was 2.85 mm, and 7 of 22 reference vessels in this subgroup were less than 2.50 mm. One stent was implanted in a vessel with a reference vessel size of 1.95 mm.

By intravascular ultrasound (IVUS) there was a significant amount of diffuse disease as noted by a mean of 41% cross-sectional area stenosis in the reference vessel at the time of stent implantation. Optimal stent implantation, by IVUS,

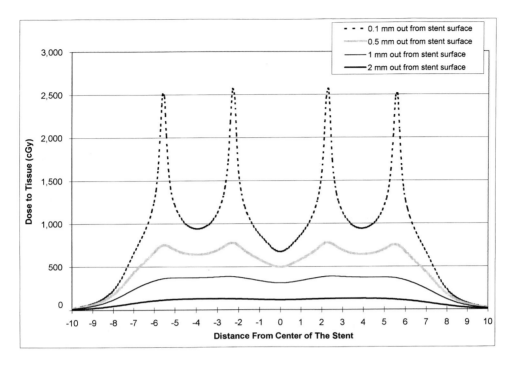

Figure 1. Two-dimensional plot of cumulative 2-week dose from a radioactive ^{32}P Isostent, implanted in a 2.5-mm vessel with an activity of 1.0 µCi at the time of stent implantation. Longitudinal dose distribution is shown for a Palmaz-Schatz stent. Note the marked fall-off of near-field radiation dose at the edges and at the articulation of the Palmaz-Schatz stent.

was achieved in only 56% of cases, due mainly to high plaque burden preventing an optimal ratio of stent to reference vessel cross-sectional area. Quantitative angiographic follow-up at 6 months demonstrated a lesional late loss of 0.94 mm for the group as a whole and 0.70 mm for the restenosis subgroup. These data are similar to late loss data from contemporary stent trials with nonradioactive stents. It should be emphasized that this was a small feasibility trial that was not intended to detect differences in restenosis with these very low activity stents. Two examples of the 6-month angiographic and IVUS follow-up studies are shown in Figures 2 and 3. In both of these cases the radioactive stent was used to treat a restenosis lesion. In both cases there is minimal neointima observed by angiography and IVUS at 6 months.

Based on human smooth muscle cell experiments looking at effects of continuous low dose rate beta irradiation, we currently estimate the effective stent activity for de novo lesions to be in the 4.0- to 12.0-µCi range (IRIS 1A mean activity was 0.7 µCi). It should be noted that in some animal models the effective activity was as high as 26 µCi. It is possible that a lower stent activity can be effective in restenosis lesions if the proliferating target tissue derives from the recently formed neointima rather than the adventitia, as is likely for de novo lesions.

The Phase 1 IRIS trial (1B) was recently expanded to test the safety of higher activity (0.75 to 1.5 mCi) stents at five additional medical centers in the United States (The University of Texas, San Antonio; Lenox Hill Hospital; Fairfax Hos-

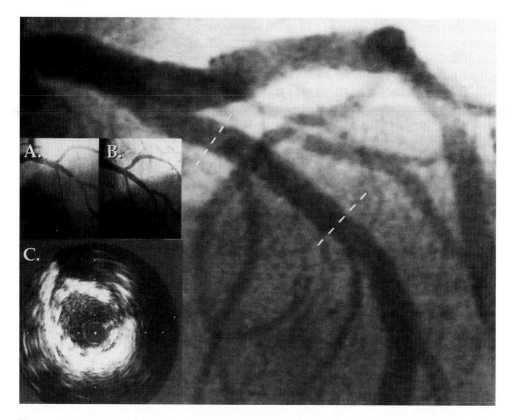

Figure 2. Six-month follow-up after treatment of left anterior descending (LAD) restenosis lesion with 0.65-μCi ^{32}P Isostent. Dotted lines on angiogram demarcate location of stent. **A.** Restenosis lesion prior to stenting. **B.** Acute result after Palmaz-Schatz Isostent implantation. **C.** Intravascular ultrasound (IVUS) image showing 6-month follow-up IVUS image at site of initial lesion, with minimal neointimal hyperplasia.

pital; The Cleveland Clinic; and Scripps Clinic). Twenty-five patients have been enrolled in this extension of the phase 1 trial, with a mean stent activity of 1.14 μCi at the time of implantation. All 25 cases were performed successfully, without reported adverse events at 1-month safety follow-ups. A small safety trial with 3.0-μCi, 15-mm-length ^{32}P stents has started in Heidelberg, Germany. To date, nine stents have been implanted successfully. There were no adverse events noted in this group at the 30-day safety endpoint. Follow-up data from these cohorts demonstrated a high rate of restenosis especially at the edges.

Future Directions

Stent restenosis often occurs in the mid stent at the site of the central articulation of the 15-mm-length Palmaz-Schatz stent.[3] The central articulation is a 1-mm single metal filament connecting two 7-mm hemistents. The articulation provides longitudinal flexibility to enable the stent to be placed in coronary arteries. Several second generation stents have been developed by use of computer-assisted modeling that have sufficient compressive resistance and longitudinal

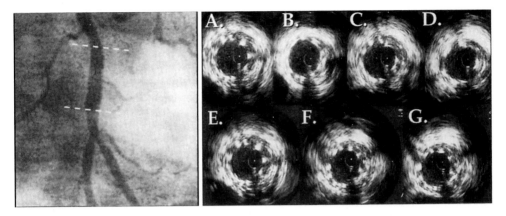

Figure 3. Six-month angiographic and intravascular ultrasound (IVUS) follow-up after treatment of left circumflex restenosis lesion with 0.8-μCi ^{32}P Isostent. Dotted lines on angiogram demarcate location of stent. IVUS is shown from proximal edge of the stent (**A**) moving through to the mid stent (**D**) and to the distal edge of the stent (**G**). Note the lack of neointimal hyperplasia.

flexibility with a continuous or nonarticulated geometry. The BX™ (IsoStent Inc., San Carlos, CA) is a novel stainless steel balloon expandable stent designed without a central articulation. The BX has honeycomb-shaped cells linked by alternating articulation geometries that provide longitudinal flexibility while maintaining the radial strength of the stent. The uniform geometry of the BX appears to have a favorable effect on the dose distribution for a ^{32}P stent. The difference between maximal and minimal near-field tissue dose of irradiation is less for the BX than for the Palmaz-Schatz design. In theory, this would provide a more uniform dose distribution to the arterial wall and minimize areas of insufficient or potentially toxic doses of irradiation. European trials are now under way in Milan and in Rotterdam with approximately 50 radioactive ^{32}P BX stent implants at stent activities ranging from 0.75 to 6.0 μCi. The results from these implants are reported in Chapter 29 of this book.

The clinical results with catheter-based brachytherapy techniques for the prevention of restenosis have been encouraging. Teirstein et al[12] reported $\approx$ 75% reduction in late lumen loss and angiographic restenosis in a randomized, placebo-controlled clinical trial with 8- to 25-Gy irradiation delivered via an endovascular ^{192}Ir source in patients with refractory restenosis. Similar 6-month results were reported with the beta emitter ^{90}Y/Sr in the Beta Particle Radiation Restenosis Trial.[17] These investigators prescribed a dose of radiation that was similar to the cumulative dose provided by a 1.0-μCi ^{32}P radioactive at a distance of 0.1 mm from the stent surface, but less than 20% of the catheter-delivered dose in the deeper vessel wall. The catheter-based approach gives the radiation at a much greater dose rate, which may be as important as the cumulative dose in preventing neointimal formation. A short-acting radioisotope with a higher energy than ^{32}P would allow higher dose rates to be achieved via a radioactive stent. One such candidate isotope is ^{90}Y, with a 64-hour half-life and a maximal energy of 2.28 MeV ($\approx$ 25% greater than ^{32}P). A 15-mm-length BX stent implanted with approximately 8 to 16 mCi of ^{90}Y would provide a dose rate of 40 to 100 cGy/h at a distance of 0.5 mm from the stent surface. The cumulative dose prescribed by an 8-

to 16-mCi ^{90}Y stent would approximate 30 to 70 Gy over the lifetime of the isotope at a distance of 0.5 mm from the surface. It is possible that ^{90}Y will prove to be an effective alternative radioisotope.

Conclusions

Clinical data support the idea that radiation therapy may be effective in the prevention of restenosis. The early clinical results with more than 120 implants of low-activity ^{32}P Palmaz-Schatz and BX radioactive stents have demonstrated excellent procedural and 30-day, event-free survival. Further dose finding safety trials are anticipated in 1998. Implementation of a large-scale randomized clinical trial will commence if and when early safety and efficacy data suggest a therapeutic effect from this technology. Thus, future studies will focus on optimal stent design and will evaluate alternative isotopes and dosing strategies.

References

1. Serruys PW, De Jaegere P, Kiemeneij F, et al, for the Benestent Study Group. A comparison of balloon-expandable-stent implantation with balloon angioplasty in patients with coronary artery disease. N Engl J Med 1994;331:489–495.
2. Fischman DL, Leon MB, Baim DS, et al, for the Stent Restenosis Study Investigators. A randomized comparison of coronary-stent placement and balloon angioplasty in the treatment of coronary artery disease. N Engl J Med 1994;331:496–501.
3. Painter JA, Mintz GS, Wong SC, et al. Serial intravascular ultrasound studies fail to show evidence of chronic Palmaz-Schatz stent recoil. Am J Cardiol 1995;75:398–400.
4. Hoffmann R, Mintz G, Dussaillant G, et al. Patterns and mechanisms of in-stent restenosis: A serial intravascular ultrasound study. Circulation 1996;94:1247–1254.
5. Edelman ER, Rogers C. Hoop dreams: Stents without restenosis. Circulation 1996;94: 1199–1202.
6. Serruys PW, Kutryk JB. The state of the stent: Current practices, controversies, and future trends. Am J Cardiol 1996;78(suppl 3A):4–7.
7. Laird JR, Carter AJ, Kufs W, et al. Inhibition of neointimal proliferation with a Beta particle emitting stent. Circulation 1996;93:529–536.
8. Carter AJ, Laird JR, Bailey LR, et al. The effects of endovascular radiation from a b-particle emitting stent in a porcine restenosis model: A dose response study. Circulation 1996;94:2364–2368.
9. Hehrlein C, Gollan C, Dönges K, et al. Low-dose radioactive endovascular stents prevent smooth muscle cell proliferation and neointimal hyperplasia in rabbits. Circulation 1995;92:1570–1575.
10. Hehrlein C, Stintz M, Kinscherf R, et al. Pure b-particle emitting stents inhibit neointima formation in rabbits. Circulation 1996;93:641–645.
11. Waksman R, Robinson KA, Crocker IR, et al. Intracoronary radiation before stent implantation inhibits neointima formation in stented canine coronary arteries. Circulation 1995;92:1383–1386.
12. Teirstein PS, Massullo V, Jani S, et al. Radiotherapy reduces coronary restenosis: Late follow-up. J Am Coll Cardiol 1997;29:397A.
13. Fischell TA, Kharma BK, Fischell DR, et al. Low-dose, b-particle emission from stent wire results in complete, localized inhibition of smooth muscle cell proliferation. Circulation 1994;90:2956–2963.
14. Rivard A, Leclerc G, Bouchard M, et al. Low-dose B-emitting radioactive stents inhibit neointimal hyperplasia in porcine coronary arteries: An histological assessment. J Am Coll Cardiol 1997;29:238A.
15. Waksman R, Robinson KA, Crocker IA, et al. Intracoronary low-dose B-irradiation inhibits neointima formation after coronary artery balloon injury in the swine restenosis model. Circulation 1995;92:3025–3031.

16. Waksman R, Robinson KA, Crocker IA, et al. Endovascular low-dose irradiation inhibits neointima formation after coronary artery balloon injury in swine: A possible role for radiation therapy in restenosis prevention. Circulation 1995;91:1553–1559.
17. King SB, Williams DO, Chougule P, et al. Intracoronary beta irradiation inhibits late lumen loss following balloon angioplasty: Results of the BERT-1 Trial. Circulation 1997;96:1211–1219.
18. Janicki C, Duggan DM, Coffey CW, et al. Radiation dose from a phosphorous-32 impregnated wire mesh vascular stent. Med Phys 1997;24:437–445.
19. Schwartz RS, Murphy JG, Edwards WD, et al. Restenosis after balloon angioplasty: A practical proliferative model in porcine coronary arteries. Circulation 1990;82: 2190–2200.
20. Muller DWM, Ellis SG, Topol EJ. Experimental models of coronary restenosis. J Am Coll Cardiol 1992;19:418–432.
21. Schwartz RS, Edwards WD, Bailey KR, et al. Differential neointimal response to coronary artery injury in pigs and dogs: Implications for restenosis models. Arterioscler Thromb 1994;14:395–400.

Part VI

Vascular Radiation and Peripheral Vascular Disease

Peripheral Vascular Radiation Therapy:

Problems Related to Technical Applications

Louis G. Martin, MD

Introduction

Restenosis following percutaneous angioplasty is not a problem limited to the coronary circulation. It is a problem that has vexed interventional angiographers for more than 30 years. To date, it has not been significantly affected by the numerous attempts to alter its course. These attempts have included: laser, directional, and rotational atherectomy; metallic stents; and pharmacological measures (Fig. 1). We and others have been encouraged by the results of radiation therapy in laboratory animals for the purpose of reducing restenosis due to myointimal hyperplasia (MIH),[1-4] and its early clinical success in the coronary circulation.[5,6] Although the mechanism responsible for the restenosis is the same in the coronary and noncoronary circulations, the lesions, vessels, and organs are not similar and the clinical situations in the peripheral circulation are more diverse.

In 1994, with the approval of our Investigational Review Board, we began the investigation of irradiation to reduce restenosis following angioplasty and stenting in patients who failed initial conventional efforts at revascularization. These patients included those with long or multifocal stenoses in the femeropopliteal artery, stenoses of dialysis graft anastomoses and brachiocephalic veins, and recurrent stenosis following stent placement. Sixteen patients were studied prior to Food and Drug Administration notification that an Investigational Device Exemption (IDE) must be obtained prior to continuation of investigation. Our early investigation was very helpful in defining the technical aspects of radiation delivery, vessel characteristics, patient transportation, and handling considerations that were instrumental in obtaining an IDE for the Peripheral Artery Radiation Investigation Study (PARIS) Trial, which is discussed in this chapter.

Delivery of the Radiation Source

Delivery issues include: when, in relation to the angioplasty, the radiation should be delivered; whether a gamma or beta radiation source should be used;

From Waksman R (ed.). *Vascular Brachytherapy, Third Edition.* Armonk, NY: Futura Publishing Co., Inc.; © 2002.

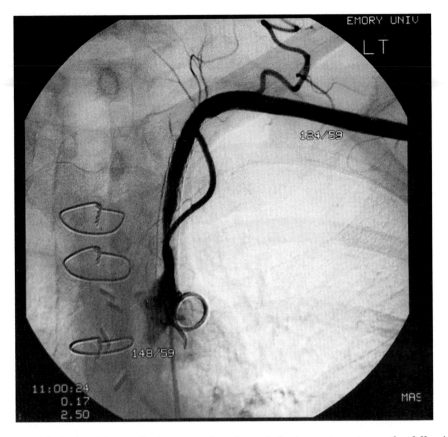

Figure 1. Neointimal hyperplasia narrowing the subclavian artery 4 months following stent placement.

and whether the treatment should be administered in the interventional suite or in the radiation oncology department. Animal studies suggest that it does not make any difference whether the irradiation treatment is delivered several days prior to or after the angioplasty. The limits of the effective time range are unknown. Present evidence in our animal laboratory[1] suggests that up to 7 days before or after angioplasty may be reasonable; however, except in unusual circumstances, most treatments are performed immediately before or after vessel dilatation.

Unlike in the coronary circulation, most of the peripheral vessels treated are greater than 3 mm in diameter; in fact many are 7 to 10 mm in diameter and some may be as large as 20 mm. It is therefore necessary to use a gamma radiation source because it would be difficult to irradiate the subintimal tissue with a beta source centered in a large vessel. Hand delivery of a gamma source would expose the operator to excessive amounts of radiation. Although it would be possible to bring the high dose rate afterloader (HDRA) to the cardiovascular suite to deliver the radiation, room modifications necessary to meet radiation safety requirements make this impractical. It therefore is evident that the treatment must be delivered by an HDRA in the radiation oncology department.

The radiation source wire contained within the HDRA is reused. It is therefore important that it does not come into contact with the patient's blood or any body tissue. In order to prevent contamination, a coaxial system has been constructed. It includes: (1) a dummy source wire (DSW), which is used for planning radiation therapy. During treatment this will be replaced by the radioactive wire that is delivered by the HDRA; (2) a source guiding catheter (SGC) into which the DSW can be introduced while remaining external to patient contact. This is analogous to a surgeon's gloved hand remaining external to an operative field; and (3) a vascular sheath or angiographic guiding catheter into which the SGC is introduced and which protects the recently treated vessel wall (Fig. 2). The SGC we have used is 5F in diameter, 100 cm long, and rather rigid. It was not designed for intravascular use. SGCs are being designed that will be more compliant and less likely to cause intimal damage, permitting them to be introduced without the vascular sheath. Following angioplasty or stenting, it is now necessary to introduce a vascular sheath or angiographic guiding catheter that extends from the percutaneous puncture site to a point beyond the lesion to be treated. The lumen must be large enough to accommodate the 5F SGC. Once this catheter has been introduced, a DSW is placed through it and radiographs are obtained for treatment planning (Fig. 3, panel C).

Vessel Characteristics

Restenosis following peripheral angioplasty is a problem in the arterial and venous systems as well as in bypass graft anastomoses and arteriovenous dialysis grafts (AVGs). The vessels to be treated vary considerably in size, wall thickness, curvature, and orientation. The lesions requiring treatment vary in length and number and they may be concentric or eccentric within the vessel wall. Although these issues are discussed in previous chapters and are not repeated here, several examples may serve to illustrate the scope of the problem of restenosis in the peripheral vascular system.

The angiograms in Figure 3 are those of a 35-year-old woman who had a femero-tibial vein bypass graft in the right lower extremity. The proximal end of the graft required revision. The graft required percutaneous transluminal angioplasty (PTA) of the distal suture line of the revised segment because of early restenosis detected by screening ultrasound. Following thrombolysis and re-angioplasty for graft occlusion on two occasions, a metallic stent was used to treat the area of restenosis. Four months later rethrombosis because of MIH at the stent margin was treated with thrombolysis PTA and intravascular radiation

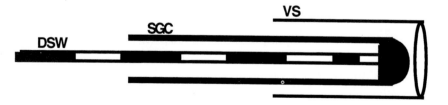

Figure 2. Intravascular components of the brachytherapy planning system: vascular sheath (VS), source guiding catheter (SGC), and dummy source wire (DSW).

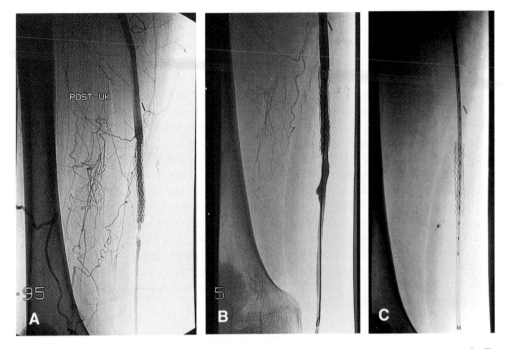

Figure 3. A. Angiogram following thrombolysis of a femeropopliteal vein bypass graft. **B.** Angiogram following percutaneous transluminal angioplasty of the stent and proximal graft margins. **C.** The coaxial system used for radiation treatment planning that is illustrated in Figure 2.

therapy. The patient has remained asymptomatic for the 8 months prior to this writing.

Atheromatous plaque that lines the aorta often causes stenosis of the renal artery. Balloon angioplasty is often unsuccessful in treating these lesions because the plaque falls like a curtain over the vessel ostium shortly after the balloon is deflated (Fig. 4). Stenting can prevent this type of early restenosis, however MIH limits long-term patency in 27% to 40% of stented renal arteries.[7] The angiograms in Figure 5 demonstrate restenosis in a left renal artery 9 months after initially successful bilateral stenting of ostial renal artery stenoses in a 66-year-old woman. Treatment of this renal artery with irradiation would be complicated by the acute angulation of its origin. This may be lessened in some circumstances by introducing the catheters from the axillary rather than the femoral artery. This acutely angled origin also increases the potential for trauma to the vessel because of the stiff coaxial system now in use.

Transjugular intrahepatic porto-systemic shunting is a very effective treatment for portal hypertension, however a restenosis rate of 31% significantly limits its efficacy.[8] This is most commonly due to MIH, which narrows the hepatic side of the stented shunt between the portal and hepatic veins. This problem is demonstrated angiographically in Figure 6. This is an ideal lesion to treat now that the problem of centering in large vessels has been solved by the development of centering balloons.

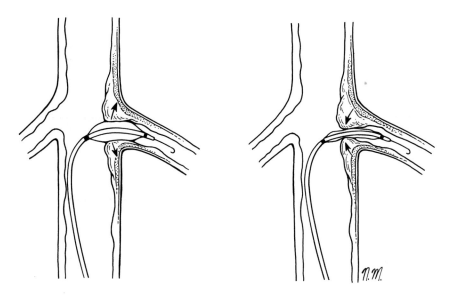

Figure 4. In the illustration on the left, a curtain of aortic plaque is displaced by the expanded angioplasty balloon. When the balloon is deflated, the ostium of the artery narrows.

The angiograms in Figure 7 demonstrate right subclavian vein stenosis occurring in the ipsilateral arm of a patient in chronic renal failure receiving dialysis through an AVG. The stenosis is caused by both MIH occurring within the vessel and perivascular fibrotic reaction secondary to insertion of catheters used for temporary dialysis during the course of this patient's treatment. Although initial angioplasty and stenting may be successful, these stenoses almost always recur due to MIH.[9,10] Successful treatment with radiation in these central veins would depend on the ability to center the source in vessels that are 15 to 20 mm in diameter. Eccentric placement of the radiation source in a large vessel could result in very high radiation exposure to the wall and adjacent tissues. It is readily evident that centering would be a major problem in the cases illustrated in Figures 5, 6, and 7 if the radiation source wire followed the course of the angiographic guidewire. In these cases, the treatment would be unevenly distributed to the vessel walls. As illustrated in Figure 8, this can also be a problem in a relatively straight vessel such as the superficial femoral artery (SFA), where vascular calcification in the wall of the vessel or the rigid nature or the SGC may cause uneven delivery of the radiation to the vessel wall.

Patient Handling and Transport

The choice of the percutaneous puncture site, anticoagulation, transportation, and observation during treatment must be considered for each patient. It is important to administer the treatment in a straight line because angulation of the SGC

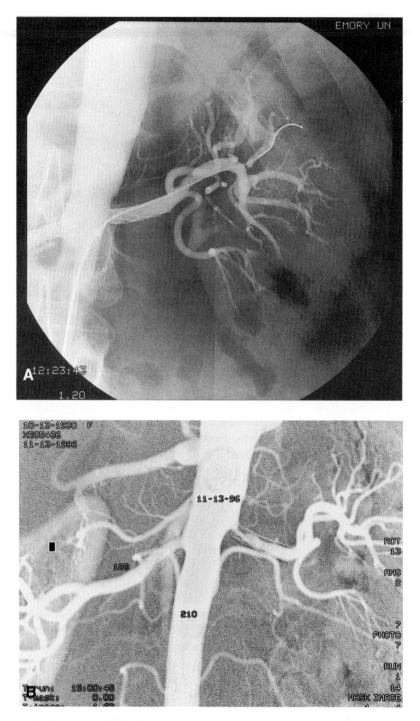

Figure 5. A. Aortogram following placement of bilateral renal artery stents. **B.** Eight-month follow-up showing intimal hyperplasia narrowing the left stent.

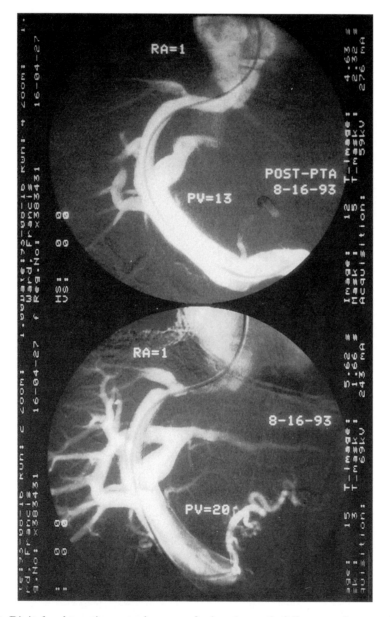

Figure 6. Digital subtraction arteriograms during 9-month follow-up of a transjugular intrahepatic porto-systemic shunting procedure. Bottom: stenosis at superior margin of the stent and in the hepatic vein. Top: angiogram following treatment with balloon angioplasty. RA = right atrium; HV = hepatic vein; PV = portal vein. Numerals indicate intravascular pressures in mm Hg.

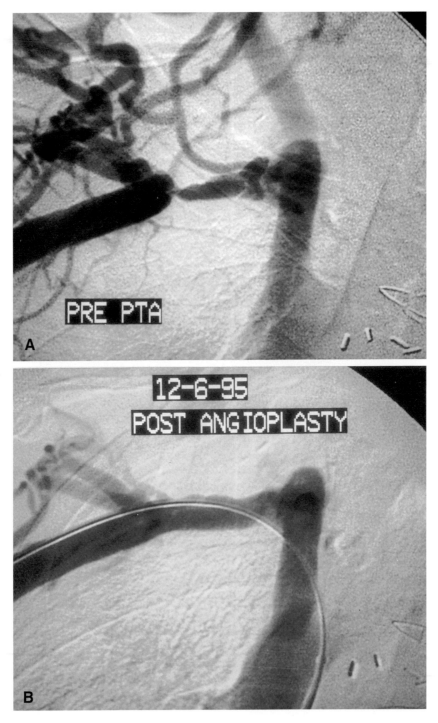

Figure 7. Digital subtraction angiograms before (**A**) and after (**B**) percutaneous transluminal angioplasty of a right subclavian vein stenosis. Note the eccentric location of the guidewire in the vessel.

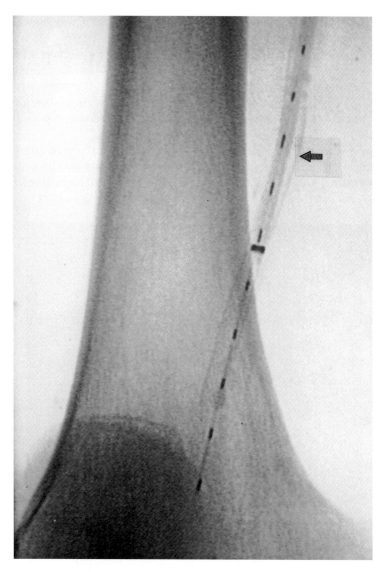

Figure 8. Superficial femoral artery treated by irradiation following PTA and stenting. Eccentric calcification (arrow) displaces the vascular sheath and dummy source wire laterally.

will cause resistance to passage of the radiation source wire. This usually is easily accomplished by use of an antegrade arterial puncture for treatment of the lower extremities, but occasionally previous surgery, physical deformity, or obesity may make the path more acutely angled or necessitate introduction of the radiation by a contralateral (retrograde) approach. This may result in increased resistance within the delivery catheter, which is not a serious problem when the source is being delivered by hand because the operator can easily recognize the situation and push the wire more forcefully; however, the HDRA is unable to make this adjustment and will either abort the treatment or deliver the treatment to the wrong area. The problem of delivering irradiation over an acutely angled iliac bifurcation is illustrated in Figure 9. Multiple previous surgeries precluded treating the restenosis via an antegrade right common femoral artery puncture. It was necessary to substitute a more rigid guiding catheter for the vascular sheath that was initially used. A similar problem may occur when the treatment is being delivered to the iliac or femoral vessels from a left axillary or brachial puncture site because of the acute angle that frequently exists between the aorta and the left subclavian artery. The distance from the puncture site to the lesion requiring treatment may also be a problem. The length of the source wire and its catheter is too short to permit treatment of the popliteal artery from an axillary approach.

The necessity to transport the patient to a remote site for irradiation will necessitate anticoagulation, the degree of which will depend on the time necessary for transportation, treatment, and observation prior to catheter removal. It is im-

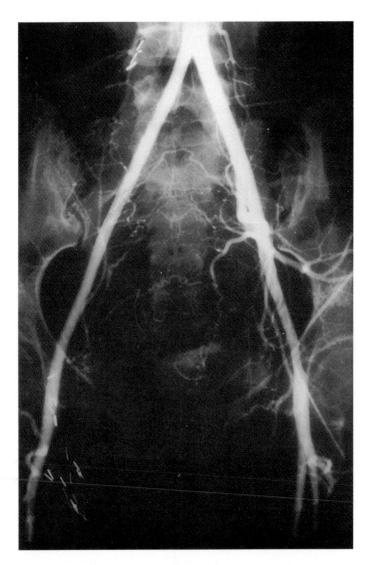

Figure 9. A pelvic arteriogram on the patient treated in Figure 3. The acute angle of the iliac arteries makes delivery of the radiation source from the contralateral side difficult.

portant that the SGC does not move during transportation. We exercise great care in securing the catheter to the patient and transferring the patient onto the gurney. Since radiation treatment can be performed on the same gurney, this patient movement should only have to be performed one time, even if it is necessary to take the patient by ambulance to a remote site to complete the treatment. Needless to say, it is important that the patient is under continuous observation during his or her transportation and treatment.

Summary

It is important to recognize that, although intravascular irradiation is a promising treatment to inhibit restenosis, it is not being proposed as a cure for a technically poor angioplasty. First the angioplasty must be optimized, and only then is radiation a therapeutic consideration. The technical aspects of radiation for peripheral applications are rather straightforward. Issues of patient care and transportation are easily solved. Centering the radiation source in the vessel is of critical importance.

In order to successfully treat the lesion and prevent complications, the radiation dose must be evenly and reliably administered to the subintimal cells. Attention is now being directed toward developing centering catheters and devices that can direct treatment to the larger peripheral vasculature and to branch vessels which may arise at an acute angle.

References

1. Waksman R, Robinson KA, Crocker IR, et al. Endovascular low-dose irradiation inhibits neointima formation after coronary artery balloon injury in swine. A possible role for radiation therapy in restenosis prevention. Circulation 1995;91:1533–1539.
2. Waksman R, Robinson KA, Crocker IR, et al. Intracoronary radiation decreases the second phase of intimal hyperplasia in a repeat balloon angioplasty model of restenosis. Int J Radiat Oncol Biol Phys 1997;39:475–480.
3. Wiedermann JG, Marboe C, Amols H, et al. Intracoronary irradiation markedly reduces restenosis after balloon angioplasty in a porcine model. J Am Coll Cardiol 1994;23:1491–1498.
4. Weinberger J, Amols H, Ennis RD, et al. Intracoronary irradiation: Dose response for the prevention of restenosis in swine. Int J Radiat Oncol Biol Phys 1996;36:767–775.
5. Teirstein PS, Massullo V, Jani S, et al. Catheter-based radiotherapy to inhibit restenosis after coronary stenting. N Engl J Med 1997;336:1697–1703.
6. Condado JA, Waksman R, Gurdiel O, et al. Long-term angiographic and clinical outcome after percutaneous transluminal coronary angioplasty and intracoronary radiation therapy in humans [see comments]. Circulation 1997;96:727–732.
7. Rees CR, Palmaz JC, Becker GJ, et al. Palmaz stent in atheroselerotic stenoses involving the ostia of the renal arteries: Preliminary report of a multicenter study. Radiology 1991;181: 507–514.
8. Rossle M, Haag K, Ochs A, et al. The transjugular intrahepatic portosystemic stent-shunt procedure for variceal bleeding [see comments]. N Engl J Med 1994;330: 165–171.
9. Quinn SF, Schuman ES, Hall L, et al. Venous stenoses in patients who undergo hemodialysis: Treatment with self-expandable endovascular stents. Radiology 1992;183: 499–504.
10. Criado E, Marston WA, Jaques PF, et al. Proximal venous outflow obstruction in patients with upper extremity arteriovenous dialysis access. Ann Vasc Surg 1994;8: 530–535.

Restenosis in Peripheral Vascular Disease

Alan B. Lumsden,MD, M. Julia MacDonald, RN, and Changyi Chen, MD, PhD

Background

Intimal hyperplasia is the usual response to vascular injury and complicates all types of vascular intervention. It is the primary cause of restenosis in the first year after vascular bypass and is responsible for stenosis rates of up to 50% after percutaneous transluminal angioplasty of the infrainguinal vessels. The median patency of arteriovenous grafts (AVGs), the most frequently implanted graft in vascular surgery, is only 15 months, and 90% of the stenoses are due to an accelerated form of intimal hyperplasia at the venous anastomosis.

In a prospective ultrasound study of surgical carotid endarterectomy, a 21% restenosis rate (>50%) was noted at 1-year follow-up. Restenosis in peripheral vascular surgery is therefore common, morbid, and expensive. It has, furthermore, markedly limited the application of endovascular procedures in the infrainguinal vasculature.

This chapter focuses on two specific types of common vascular surgical procedure (AV access grafts and infrainguinal bypass), reviewing the incidence of neointimal hyperplasia, its pathophysiology in each location, and why these sites were selected for evaluation of endoluminal radiation therapy.

Arteriovenous Grafts

Repetitive angioaccess for chronic hemodialysis is most commonly provided by ePTFE AV vascular grafts. Unfortunately, these grafts fail on average 15 months after placement, with a reported primary occlusion rate of 15% to 50% at 1 year. Development of venous anastomotic intimal hyperplasia is particularly rapid (Fig. 1) and may be promoted by several factors: turbulence, compliance mismatch, peritissue vibration, and platelet deposition. Although the majority of initial occluding events may be temporarily salvaged by thrombectomy and patch angioplasty, the secondary patency rates remain a meager 3 months. These grafts, therefore, have a high frequency of outcome events. Patients can be closely followed, providing accurate patency rates, and their superficial nature provides ease of imaging by duplex ultrasound.

From Waksman R (ed.). *Vascular Brachytherapy, Third Edition.* Armonk, NY: Futura Publishing Co., Inc.; © 2002.

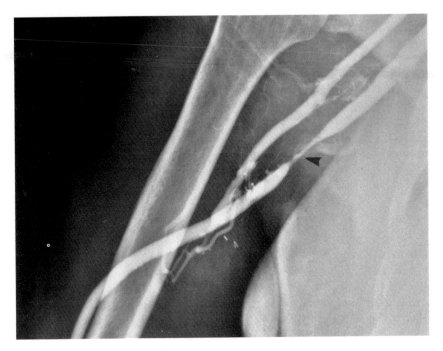

Figure 1. Arteriogram of venous anastomotic lesion.

Thrombogenicity

We studied several markers of thrombosis in patients with PTFE bridge grafts: (1) platelet activation was evaluated via serum concentrations of platelet factor 4 (PF4) and B-thromboglobulin (BTG) for 15 patients; (2) stimulation of individual platelets was determined by expression of ligand-induced binding sites (LIBS) on the Gp IIb/IIIa receptor; and (3) thrombin generation was measured by assay of serum fibrinopeptide-A (FPA) and thrombin-antithrombin complexes (TAT). Platelet deposition on chronic grafts was quantitated by measurement of ^{111}In platelet deposition for five cases. A serum level of PF4 was 21.9+35.2 I c/mL; mean (+SD) BTG was 155.1+36.81/mL; FPA was 13.5+12.9 nM; and TAT peptide was 8.0+4.1 ng/mL, all of which were higher than values in normal adults ($P<0.05$).

LIBS expression was also increased, with 7444+4809 epitopes per platelet versus 2569+1328 in controls ($P<0.01$). Platelet deposition on the grafts at 2 hours was 10.94+1.76×109 (Fig. 2). The graft-to-blood ratio of radioactivity remained significantly ($P>0.05$) elevated at 24 and 36 hours, with ratios of 33.0 and 49.6, respectively.

We conclude: (1) platelet activation occurs in patients with ePTFE grafts, as demonstrated by increased circulating platelet markers and expression of LIBS; and (2) significant platelet deposition continues to occur in chronically implanted grafts.

Composition of the Restenotic Lesion

We studied the venous anastomoses of 12 chronically implanted human AV PTFE grafts removed at the time of fistula revision. Immunoperoxidase technique

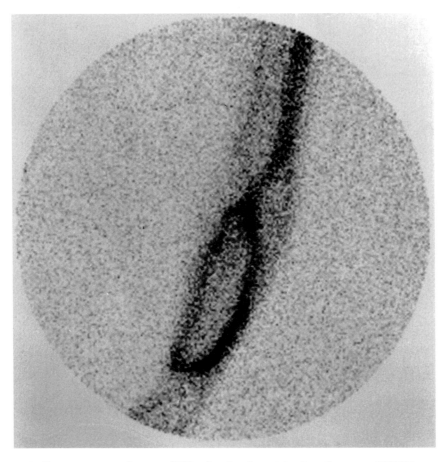

Figure 2. Gamma camera image of [111]Ir platelet deposition in a forearm ePTFE loop graft.

was used to determine the present of proliferating cell nuclear antigen (PCNA) as an index of cell proliferation (Fig. 3). Relative cellularity, extracellular matrix (ECM) composition, and distribution of a newly described ECM protein (tenascin) were described.

The venous anastomotic neointimal hyperplastic lesion was analyzed in three layers, each one third of the thickness. PCNA indices (percentage of cells that were PCNA-positive (mean ± SD) were: luminal layer 29±11%, middle layer 9±5%, deep layer near the graft 9±7%, and microvessel-containing intimal fields 67±4%. The cell proliferation rate in the luminal layer was significantly higher than those in the middle and deep layers of neointima ($P<0.05$). The PCNA index in micro-vessel containing intimal fields was three to eight times that of avascular fields ($P<0.001$).

We further measured the cellular and ECM volumes which made up the venous anastomotic neointima. The luminal layer consisted of 34±13% cells and 66±13% ECM volume. The middle layer contained 14±3% cells and 86±3% ECM in volume. The deep layer near the grafts comprised 21+14% cells and 79±14% ECM in volume. Statistical analysis showed that the ECM volume percentage in the luminal layer of neointima was significantly lower than that in the middle and deep layers

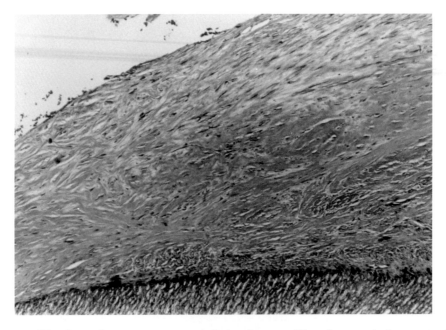

Figure 3. Histology of venous anastomotic lesion from an AV graft stenosis demonstrating large numbers of smooth muscle cells overlaying the PTFE graft.

of neointima ($P<0.05$). However, there was no significant difference between the ECM volume percentages in the middle and deep layers of neointima ($P>0.05$).

Tenascin (TN) was distributed in the neointima as follows: (1) in the luminal layer, all lesions were intensely stained; (2) in the middle layer, 9 of 12 (75%) lesions had moderate reactivity, and 3 of 12 (25%) lesions were strongly stained, 5 of 12 (42%) had moderate reactivity, and 4 of 12 (33%) had weak positive staining; and (3) $90\pm6\%$ of microvessels within the neointima showed intense periendothelial staining.

This study quantitatively demonstrates that ECM comprises the bulk of occlusive human neointimal hyperplastic lesions in AVGs and that the deep two-thirds layer of neointima has more ECM component than the luminal layer. TN is distributed in a pattern similar to cell proliferation in human neointimal hyperplastic lesions. The results suggest that inhibition of ECM production might be an effective treatment strategy for preventing graft occlusion, without the need to inhibit smooth muscle cell (SMC) migration or proliferation. TN expression may be an important mechanism of neovascularization and cell proliferation in human AV PTFE graft failure.

Experimental Approach to Control of Venous Anastomotic Neointimal Hyperplasia

PTFE-based local infusion devices were implanted bilaterally as femoral AV conduits in six dogs (Table 1). The venous anastomoses were the sites of continuous delivery of fibroblast growth factor-saporin, a plant mitotoxin (FGF-Sap) (2.7 mg/kg/day) to one side and vehicle (4.6 mL/kg/day) as control to the contralateral

Table 1

Neointimal Hyperplasia in Treated and Untreated Animals

Venous Anastomosis	Treated	Control	Reduction	P value
Intimal thickness (mm)	0.27±0.12	0.40±0.11	32±30%	0.047
Intimal area (mm²)	0.26±0.17	0.46±0.23	40±25%	0.044
BrdU index (%)	4.95±2.33	8.48±4.86	33±22%	0.036

side for 14 days. Morphometric measurements and cell proliferation by BrdU index analysis were performed at both arterial and venous anastomoses.

There were no significant differences in intimal hyperplasia and intimal cell proliferation at the arterial anastomoses between the treated grafts and the control grafts. By contrast, rFGF2-SAP significantly reduced intimal thickness by 32%, intimal area by 40%, and cell proliferation index by 33% at the treated venous anastomoses as compared with the control venous anastomoses.

These data demonstrate that continuous local infusion of rFGF2-SAP significantly reduces venous anastomotic intimal hyperplasia and cell proliferation.

Restenosis in Infrainguinal Bypass Procedures

The most commonly performed lower extremity bypass procedure is femoral popliteal grafting with reversed saphenous vein (80% 5-year patency) and polytetrafluoroethylene grafts (60% 5-year patency). Bypass grafting can be successively applied to both long segment and short segment occlusive disease. Vein grafts fail due to development of perianastomotic and intrinsic stenoses. Indeed, the incidence of stenosis development is up to 30% within the first 24 months.

The etiology of these stenoses is uncertain and probably multifactorial, including neointimal hyperplasia, valve stenoses, and clamp injury. The incidence is so high, however, and the salvage rates for failed grafts so low, that most surgeons practice duplex surveillance to permit prophylactic intervention for developing stenoses. Salvage procedures usually consist of patch angioplasty or segmental graft replacement since lesions are often resistant to balloon angioplasty and recurrences are common.

Bypass grafting has remained the procedure of choice for infrainguinal occlusive disease because of the lack of durability of endovascular procedures. Angioplasty, stenting, atherectomy, and stent grafting have all had limited application in treatment of infrainguinal occlusive disease. They are most efficacious for stenoses rather than occlusions and for short segment (<4 cm) disease. Initial technical success rates are high, development of restenosis being the single major factor that has limited widespread application of these techniques. Effective control of this lesion would drastically alter the treatment selection for infrainguinal occlusive disease.

Animal Models of Bypass & Endarterectomy

Since bypass grafting and endarterectomy are among the most commonly performed peripheral vascular procedures, we have developed clinically relevant,

Table 2

Time Course of Intimal Development

Time Course (week)	Intimal Thickness (μm)	Intimal Area (mm²)	Stenosis Level (%)	Nuclear Density ($\times 10^3$/mm²)	ECM Volume (%)	BrdU Index (%)
1	78.79±19.09	0.45±0.13	13.34±4.15	6.91±0.70	29.26±7.19	19.40±4.12
2	131.73±35.33	0.85±0.19	23.17±7.81	5.73±0.51	40.26±5.33	6.70±0.72
12	160.50±69.21	1.09±0.56	37.05±14.16	5.64±0.91	42.20±9.21	2.55±0.71

quantitative, reproducible animal models: eversion carotid and femoral endarterectomy and interposition ePTFE aortoiliac, carotid, and femoral grafts. These models all have a similar healing pattern, with initial injury being followed by a short-term burst of SMC proliferation (peak proliferation at 3 to 5 days), SMC migration into the intima, and subsequent elaboration of extracellular matrix.

The pattern of smooth muscle cell proliferation in these models is very different from that which occurs in AV grafts. In the latter it is likely that ongoing injury results from the high flow, turbulence, and compliance mismatch which occurs at the venous anastomosis. Ongoing platelet activation due to the graft itself and repeated dialysis may further contribute to the accelerated neointima formation. We would anticipate that this is likely to result in reduced efficacy from single pulse interventions.

Carotid Endarterectomy Model

Seventeen dogs underwent surgical endarterectomies of the carotid and femoral arteries. Eleven, 10, and 9 patent arteries were subjected to morphological and histologic analyses at 1, 2 and 12 weeks post operation, respectively. The results (mean ± SD) of morphological and histologic analyses are given in Table 2.

These data demonstrate that the intimal hyperplastic lesion and ECM volume increase throughout the duration of this study and the SMC proliferation is most active at 1 week and does not subside to baseline at 12 weeks following the injury. This model is a reproducible, quantitative approach for testing strategies designed to reduce neointimal hyperplasia.

References

1. Bell, DD & Rosenthall JJ, Arteriovenous graft life in chronic hemodialysis, Arch Surg 1988;123:1169–1172.
2. Bernstein EF, Harker LA, Gent M, Scala TE, Koziol J, The San Diego Restenosis Group: Preoperative asprin and dipyridamole in the prevention of carotid artery reatenosis: a controlled trial, in: Current Critical Problems in Vascular Surgery. Veith FJ (ed), 1992;3:416–419, Quality Medical Publishing: St. Louis.
3. Capek P, Mclean GK, Berkowitz HD, Femoropopliteal angioplasty: factors influencing long term success, Circulation 1992;83(Suppl I):70–80.
4. Chen C, Hanson SR & Lumsden AB, Boundary layer infusion of heparin prevents

thrombosis and reduces neointimal hyperplasia in venous PTFE grafts without systemic anticoagulation, J Vas Surg 1995;22:237–247.

5. Chen C, Mattar SG, Hughes JD, Pierce GF, Cook, JE, Ku DN, Hanson SR & Lumsden AB, Recombinant mitotoxin, basic fibroblast growth factor-saporin, reduces venous anastomotic hyperplasia in the arteriovenous graft, Circulation 1995;94:1989–1995.

6. Chen C, Suwyn CR, Matter SG, Coyle KA, Ku DN & Lumsden AB, Distribution of tenascin in human neointimal hyperplastic lesions, Surg Forum 1994;15:382–385.

7. Clowes AW, Gown,AM, Hanson SR & Reidy MA, Mechanism of arterial graft failure. Role of cellular proliferation in early healing of PTFE prostheses, Am J Pathol 1985;118:43–54.

8. Clowes AW & Kohler T, Graft endothelialization: the role of angoigenic mechanisms, J Vasc Surg 1991;13:734–736.

9. Clowes AW, Reidy MA & Clowes MM, Kinetics of cellular proliferation after arterial injury. I. Smooth muscle growth in the absence of endothelium, Lab Inves 1983;49:327–333.

10. Etheredge EE, Haid SD, Maeser MN et al., Salvage operations for malfunctioning PTFE hemodialysis access grafts, Surgery 1983;94:464–470.

11. Etheredge EE, Haid SD, Maeser MN, Sicard GA & Anderson CB, Salvage operations for malfunctioning PTFE hemodialysis access grafts, Surgery 1983;94:64–47.

12. Hobson RW, O'Donnel JA, Jamil Z & Mehta K, Below-knee bypass for limb salvage: Comparison of autogenous saphenous vein, polytetrafluoroethylene and composite dacron-autogenous vein grafts, Arch Surg 1980;115:833–837.

13. Johnston KW, Femoral and popliteal arteries: reanalysis of results of balloon angioplasty, Radiology 1992;183:767–771.

14. Lumsden AB, Chen C & Ku DN, Neovascularization in the venous neointimal hyperplastic lesions of arteriovenous grafts, JASN 1994;5:421.

15. Matsi PJ, Manninen HI, Suhonen MT, Prinen AE & Soimakallia S, Chronic critical lower limb ischemia: prospective trail of angioplasty with 1–36 months follow-up, Radiology 1993;188:382–387.

16. Palder SR, Kirkman RL, Whittemore AD et al, Vascular access for hemodialysis. Patency rates and results of revision, Ann Surg 1985;202:235–239.

17. Palder SR, Kirkman RL, Whittemore AD, Hakim RM, Lazarus JM & Tilney NL, Vascular access for hemodialysis. Patency rates and results of revision, Ann Surg 1985; 202, 235–239.

18. Schwab SJ, Raymond JR, Saeed M et al, Prevention of hemodialysis fistula thrombosis. Early detection of venous stenoses, Kidney Int 1989;36:707–711.

19. Schwab, SJ, Raymond JR, Saeed M, Newman GE, Dennis PA & Bollinger RR, Prevention of hemodialysis fistula thrombosis. Early detection of venous stenoses, Kidney Int 1989;36:707–711.

20. Weiner SN, Complications of vascular access devices for hemodialysis, Angiology 1985; 202:275–284.

## Chapter 38

Intravascular Irradiation Therapy

Dieter D. Liermann, MD, R. Bauernsachs, MD,
Bernhard Schopohl, MD, and H.D. Böttcher, MD

Introduction

Treatment for the restenosis in stented vascular segments causes injuries to the vascular wall, almost always resulting in intimal hyperplasia.[1–16] Some authors presume that because of this, the use of stents alone does not appreciably improve patency rates compared to percutaneous transluminal angioplasty (PTA).[17–22] One possible alternative is to combine the methods available for treating intimal hyperplasia.

The good results obtained in treating keloids by means of irradiation therapy[23–34] was the basis for our therapeutic concept for the prophylactic irradiation of hyperproliferative vascular wall reactions. The development of small caliber probes for afterloading therapy in the biliary tract[35] allowed us to use these for therapy in the vascular system.

Together with the initiator of these afterloading methods, H.D. Böttcher, our considerations were converted into a clinical trial. Before proceeding further, all risks and problems, together with ethical reservations in the context of using afterloading methods for treating arterial occlusive disease in the peripheral vascular system, were discussed in detail and taken into consideration when planning the procedure. In addition to interventional management, significance was also accorded to stipulation of the individual dose, the follow-up regimen, and adequate patient information.

Materials & Methods

The entire treatment was carried out under heparin therapy: 100 IU/kg body weight. On conclusion of recanalization and PTA of restenosed, stented vascular segment, a 9F recanalization catheter was inserted through the positioned 9F sheath via guidewire, and positioned so that its tip was just below the affected vascular segment. The inner diameter of this catheter permitted insertion of a special catheter having a diameter of 5 French. The pointed tip of the catheter means that the measuring rod and special catheter can only be pushed forward to just before the tip of the recanalization catheter, without being able to pass through the catheter opening. This particular feature allows for exact measure-

From Waksman R (ed.). *Vascular Brachytherapy, Third Edition.* Armonk, NY: Futura Publishing Co., Inc.; © 2002.

ment and calculation of the length of the stented vascular segment and of the insertion length of the afterloading probe under stable, reproducible conditions.

After stipulation of the distal point of the catheter, the sheath and recanalization catheter were fixed on the skin to avoid any displacement. The measuring rod, whose distal segment marks the lower end of the irradiation field and protrudes 1 cm distally beyond the actual irradiation field, was then exchanged with the 5F special catheter. This catheter was inserted through the 9F catheter as far as possible with its independently sealed tip, and was again firmly fixed (Fig. 1).

It later accommodated the ^{192}Ir source of 1.1 mm diameter. This was inserted during the afterloading procedure, after the proximal end of the special catheter had been connected to the outlet valve of the 10 Ci ^{192}Ir high dose rate (HDR) source. We used a microSelectron-HDR™ planning system version 10.10 for exact calculation, monitoring, and control of the afterloading procedure. The reference dose was 1200 cGy.

After calculating the exact irradiation dose for the afterloading method, the program controls and monitors the insertion and removal of the ^{192}Ir source from the afterloader into the special catheter through to the tip, and then monitors the irradiation duration. The exposure time depends on the activity of the source and was around 200 seconds. During this time, a surface dose of 12 Gy was applied to the vascular wall in one session in the affected region.

Subsequently, the catheter material was removed and pressure was carefully applied by hand to the puncture point for 10 to 20 minutes. An elastic pressure

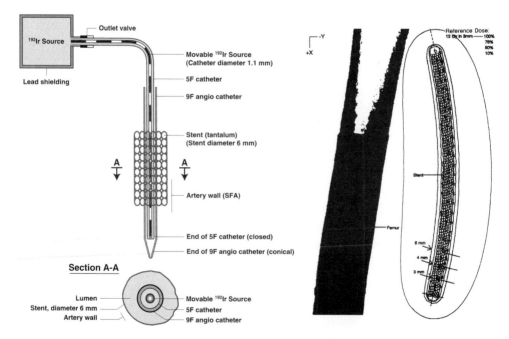

Figure 1. [192]Ir afterloading irradiation technique within the stent of the superficial femoral artery. Diagram showing the catheter and loading system for endovascular irradiation and the isodose distribution for endovascular irradiation in the region of the stented superficial femoral artery.

bandage was then applied for 24 hours and the patient was treated for 72 hours with a dose of heparin 1000 IU/hour via a perfusor. A 6-month course of Marcumar therapy was then initiated.

Follow-Up

Follow-up examinations were carried out at precisely defined intervals, consisted of routine ankle-arm indices (AAI) before and during the intervention, after 3 and 6 months, and then at six month intervals, together with a study of the case history and examination of the patient. Additionally, magnetic resonance imaging (MRI) examinations were carried out before and after treatment and at six month intervals.

The examinations were performed in a FLASH gradient, spin echo sequence with a flip angle of 30°, in vertical and coronary sections (1.0 Tesla unit in a cervical coil [300]). An intravenous digital subtraction angiography (DSA) was also carried out after 6 months or upon MRI evidence of stenotic lesions. The clinical parameters were stipulated according to the Fontaine classification.

Indications

Indications for endovascular afterloading therapy were restricted to clinically relevant stenoses or recurrent occlusions in the stented vascular segment occurring within less than 8 months after repeated PTA treatment. All patients must have had a long history of arterial occlusive disease, with recurrent vascular occlusions following PTA treatment in a vascular segment of the superficial femoral artery prior to stent implantation.

In the event of restenosis or occlusion in the stented vascular segment, at least one successful treatment of the recurrence must have been carried out by conventional PTA or by using the Nd-YAG laser with matted sapphire tip. Prior to repetition of the PTA in the stented segment with subsequent irradiation therapy, angiogram control must have been performed, together with diagnostic atherectomy by means of the Simpson catheter to obtain histologic material.

In order to minimize the somatic tumor risk as a consequence of the radiation therapy, only patients in their seventh decade of life or older were admitted for such treatment. Contraindications to heparin and Marcumar therapy were not to be present following stent implantation and radiation therapy.

Patient Data

To date a total of 30 patients (10 women and 20 men) have been treated with endovascular afterloading. All patients suffered from clinically relevant reocclusions or restenoses in stented vascular segments of the superficial artery following successful laser or PTA treatment, within 6 to 8 months after last therapy.

The patients were aged from 54 to 84 years with a mean of 68.4 years. All patients had generalized arterial occlusive disease. Fifteen patients had concurrent diabetes mellitus, 21 had high blood pressure, and 22 nicotine abuse over a period of more than 20 years. According to the Fontaine classification, before the repeated PTA treatment (28 cases) or laser therapy (2 cases), 10 of the patients were clinical stage IIb and 20 patients were stage III. The histologic analysis indicted intimal hyperplasia as the cause for restenosis in all 30 patients.

The case histories for all patients revealed PTAs as a treatment for reocclusion in the superficial femoral artery prior to implantation of one or more stents. The length of stented vascular segments ranged from 4.5 cm to 14 cm with a mean of 6.7 cm, with the stent diameter ranging from 6 mm to 7 mm.

Results

In all 30 patients it was possible to perform re-PTA treatment without remaining residual stenoses in the stented region. Subsequent irradiation therapy with the ^{192}Ir HDR afterloading method was successfully performed. In all cases, the dose was 12 Gy in the plane of the vascular; the exposure time was approximately 200 seconds. The additional time required in comparison to a sole PTA procedure was approximately 45 minutes, with most of this time consisting of transport between the treatment room and afterloading room. After conclusion of the treatment, there was no bleeding from the puncture sites. The follow-up period for the 30 patients had a range from 4 to 68 months.

According to the Fontaine classification, it was possible to improve the clinical stage for 11 patients from stage IIb to stage I, and for 12 patients stage III to stage I. It was only possible to improve two patients from stage IIb to stage IIa, and four patients from stage III to stage IIa. In these cases, contralateral occlusion was present as a limiting factor. In the fourth case, it was possible to improve the clinical stage from III to IIa, but after approximately 2 years this patient suffered from an occlusion which became manifest in the exit of the superior femoral artery, resulting in a bypass.

During the follow-up examinations, there was no deterioration of the clinical stage and no recurrent stenosis for 22 patients. One patient suffered from an acute thrombosis approximately 3 months after stent implantation, without a cause being found. Histologic examination using the atherectomy catheter revealed fresh thrombotic material, as expected. Following local lysis therapy, the thrombosis was entirely eliminated. We suspect that the thrombosis was due to an underdose of Marcumar in an otherwise physically active patient.

One other patient had a stenosis 3 cm above the stented vascular segment 12 months after irradiation treatment. During treatment to eliminate the severe stenosis, angioscopic and angiogram controls revealed no evidence of constrictions or intimal hyperplasia in the stented and irradiated region. The restenosis above the stent was successfully eliminated.

In a third case, approximately 10 months after the combined therapy restenosis occurred in a vascular segment approximately 8 cm long that had not been included in the irradiation treatment. It occurred between two treated sections in the superficial femoral artery, and was successfully removed by PTA treatment. In this case also, there was no intimal restenosis in the vascular segment previously treated by stent implantation, PTA, and irradiation. In three cases we had a reocclusion in the long-term follow-up.

Follow-up examinations have revealed no evidence of nerve lesions following irradiation therapy. The tissue surrounding the artery showed no recordable change following irradiation therapy, either in the CT, color-coded Doppler, endo-vascular ultrasonic scanning, or MRI.

No complaints of discomfort were reported during or after irradiation. With the exception of the changes described above, and the one acute thrombosis likely caused by an underdose of Marcumar, there was no evidence of any complications (Figs. 2 and 3).

Late Clinical Follow-Up

From May 1990 to May 1997, 30 patients with 31 lesions were treated with PTA for in-stent restenosis at the superficial femoral artery followed by endovas-cular brachytherapy. Follow-up time ranged from 7 to 84 months (median of 32.9 months). The findings of 28 patients from this cohort are as follows: 3 patients de-veloped stenosis within the treated segment (target lesion revascularization); 2

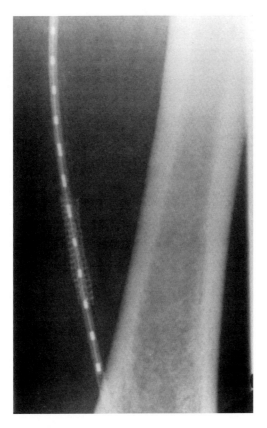

Figure 2. The measuring chain with standardized intervals of 1 cm between each mark-ing for precise measurement of the dose. The insert and removal length, together with the length of the vascular segment, has been positioned in the stent region. It can be seen that according to the real conditions after introduction of the ^{192}Ir source, the probe protrudes 2 cm beyond the distal end of the stent. The stop of the 5F guide catheter which is visibly closed at the distal end accommodating the afterloading probe, is defined by the conical tip of the open ended 9F catheter.

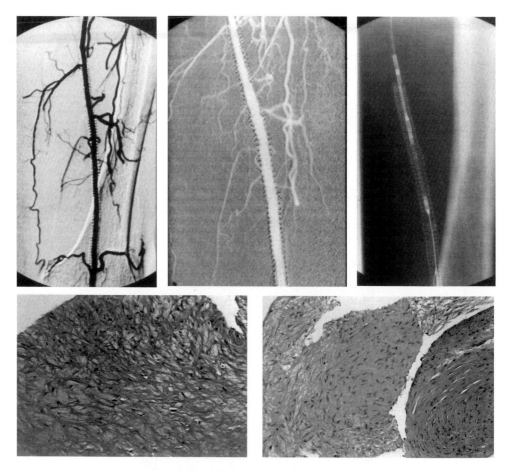

Figure 3. The case shown in this set of pictures is an example of the use of endovascular irradiation, histologic monitoring, and interpretation in the case of occlusion of the left superficial in an 80-year-old female patient.

(a) The angiogram shows free passage following re-PTA and irradiation treatment.

(b) The control examination 1 year after revision and radiation therapy shows occlusion of a segment of the superficial femoral artery above the radiated, stented region.

(c) Tissue material is sampled from various sectors of the vascular wall in the stented region and the vascular lumen not exposed to irradiation by means of the Simpson atherectomy catheter in order to proceed with histological analysis.

(d) The HE coloring of a section with material from the vascular segment not exposed to irradiation, showing expansive, myoxide degeneration of the basic substance, with irregular distribution of the smooth muscle cells and myofibroblasts, as in highly active, florid atherosclerosis.

(e) HE coloring of a section with material from the stented region shows a more compact arrangement of the smooth muscle cells and myofibroblasts, indicating lesser florid intimal lesion possibly the result of the mitosis inhibiting effect of irradiation.

patients developed stenosis at 41 and 48 months in the same vessel but not at the treated site; 2 patients presented with closure of the vessel due to acute thrombosis at 16 and 37 months; 1 patient underwent surgery at the target lesion due to a crushed stent at the treated segment; and 1 patient died 18 months post treatment not related to the radiation treatment.

Discussion

Afterloading irradiation is a therapeutic concept for treating recurrent intimal hyperplasia in stented vascular segments that must be applied under extremely strict provisos. From an ethical point of view, the methods should be compared with radiation therapy nonmalignant disorder[23,30,31,34] and it is essential to make a strict distinction between this kind of radiation therapy and irradiation of malignant growths where a far higher dose is required and there is a greater risk of induction of malignant secondary disorders. The afterloading technique allows for drastic reductions in the radiation dose to the tissues surrounding the affected organ, which in turn reduces somatic risk.

The dose distribution for ^{192}Ir gives a surface dose of 1200 cGy at a depth of 3 mm, 877 cGy at a depth of 4 mm, 551 cGy at a depth of 6 mm, 396 cGy at a depth of 8 mm, and 303 cGy at a depth of 10 mm. The risk to the nearby nerves can be considered as slight. In the medical literature, the tolerance for a maximum single dose is 15 Gy.[36,37]

For ethical reasons, this pilot study was restricted to older patients. In addition, the case histories of prospective patients had to reveal multiple restenoses with short recurrence intervals for the vascular segment concerned, together with a clinical stage of IIb to IV. Our therapeutic approach was discussed in detail with the patients, together with other possible alternatives.

Interarterial afterloading therapy became possible because the diameter of the ^{192}Ir afterloading source had been considerably reduced during development of treatment for malignant growths in the biliary tract.[35]

In contrast to percutaneous irradiation, which has to be applied in a fractionated form to avoid severe side effects to the surrounding tissue, the endovascular afterloading method achieves the same effect in the vascular wall with only a single application lasting 200 seconds with a steep dose fall-off for the surrounding tissue.

Based on experience with antihyperproliferative treatment of keloids,[23–34] we thought it possible that irradiation would have a suppressive effect on hyperproliferative reactions following stent implantation. The initial small number of patients, however, does not allow us to make any definitive statements, but our follow-up results are sufficiently encouraging to prompt us to proceed with further development of afterloading irradiation as an antihyperproliferative therapy following stent implantation. With the exception of the somatic risk during irradiation therapy described above, we saw no other relevant short-term or long-term complications.

Potential short-term effects include an increased thrombosis risk following an edema or inflammatory reaction to irradiation, although such effects were not detected.[38,39] Cicatrization with corresponding lumen constriction of the iliac artery is a feared long-term effect of high-dose radiation therapy.[40–44] Various analyses about the effect of irradiation show that cicatrization in the vascular system only occurs following high doses with complete tissue necrosis. Cicatrization is not anticipated following endovascular application of low doses of 12 Gy.

The dose we have used in our therapy causes a significant reduction of mitosis only in the most exposed cells with only isolated cell necrosis.[39,43,45-53] This effect, combined with reduction in myofibroblast migration velocity, is possibly responsible for the lack of restenoses in our patient population.[54]

It should be noted that recurrences have also been observed in our patients. Zeitler and colleagues, who also use our procedure, have indicated a higher recurrence rate than our group using a single dose of 10 Gy applied to the vascular wall. Our application of 12 Gy also gives rise to doubts whether the dose is always homogeneously distributed in the vascular wall, achieving the same antiproliferative effect all over, or whether certain adjacent areas may be differentially exposed resulting from the decentral position of the probe.

In order to minimize this effect, I have developed a catheter that can accommodate the probe system with an inner lumen of just 6 French, but which has an outer diameter of approximately 8 French with balloons for centering the catheter in the lumen during dose application. Preliminary experimental test have already been successfully completed here.

In comparison to alternative methods for treatment of intimal hyperplasia, endovascular afterloading irradiation is the only method which is used locally in the stented region with success under clinical conditions. Some models use heparin, Marcumar, aspirin, low molecular weight heparin, corticoid, or other substances to influence intimal hyperplasia, but therapeutically effective doses all have systematic side effects.[55-70]

Knowledge about the mediators responsible for prolific growth after any kind of damage to the vascular wall led to the development of substances aimed at interrupting or reducing this process. Unfortunately, such processes are always only aimed at one or two growth factors, while leaving others largely unaffected.[19,56,59,69,71,72]

Another model favors the genetic influence on the vascular wall.[73-76] A few animal experiments have been carried out with rather discouraging results following implantation of so-called "coated stents." Hyperproliferation has been observed at the transition zones between stent end and vascular wall.[77,78] There are also a few initial models in which the stent is prepared with heparin or other chemotherapeutic substances to reduce intimal hyperproliferation following implantation.[58,78]

Finally it is worth mentioning the development of so-called biocompatible stents which have been tested in animal experiments.[79,80] Most of these models are still only in the experimental stage, so it is necessary to wait for further developments. When all is said and done, it is only the use of a functioning antihyperproliferative therapy, of whatever type, that makes it possible to proceed with routine use of stents for the treatment of arterial occlusive disease in the peripheral vascular system.

References

1. Clowes AW, Karnovsky MJ. Suppression by heparin of smooth muscle cells proliferation in injured arteries. Nature 1977;265:625–626.
2. Clowes AW, Reidy MA, Clowes MM. Kinetics of cellular proliferation after arterial injury. Lab Invest 1983;49:327–334.
3. Cox JL, Gottlieb AL. Restenosis following percutaneous transluminal angioplasty: Clinical, physiological and pathological features. Can Med Assoc J 1986;136:1129–1132.

4. Essed CE, Van Den Brand M, Becker AE. Transluminal coronary angioplasty and early restenosis: Fibrocellular occlusion after wall laceration. Br Heart J 1983;49:393–396.

5. Faxon DP, Sanborn TA, Weber VJ. Restenosis following transluminal angioplasty in experimental atherosclerosis. Arteriosclerosis 1984;4:189–195.

6. Faxon DP, Sanborn TA, Hauenschild. Mechanism of angioplasty and its relation to restenosis. Am J Cardiol 1987;60:5B-9B.

7. Friedman JR, Burns R. Role of platelets in the proliferative response of the injured artery. Prog Hemost Thromb 1978;4:249–278.

8. Garth EA, Ratliff NB, Hollman J, et al. Intimal proliferation of smooth cells as an explanation for recurrent coronary artery stenosis after percutaneous transluminal coronary angioplasty. J Am Coll Cardiol 1985;62:372.

9. Hashizume M, Yang Y, Galt S. Intimal response of saphenous vein to intraluminal trauma by simulated angioscopic insertion. J Vasc Surg 1987;75:862–868.

10. Imparato AM, Bracco A, Kim GE, Zeff R. Intimal and neointimal fibrous proliferation causing failure of arterial reconstructions. Surgery 1972;172:1007–1017.

11. Ip JH, Fuster V, Badimon L, et al. Syndromes of acceleration atherosclerosis: Role of vascular injury and smooth muscle cell proliferation. J Am Coll Cardiol 1990;15:1667–1687.

12. Laerum BF, Vlodaver Z, Castaneda-Zuniga WR, et al. The mechanism of angioplasty. Fortschr Röntgenstr 1982;136:573–576.

13. Nobuyoshi M, Kimura T, Ohishi H, Horiuchi H. Restenosis after percutaneous transluminal coronary angioplasty: Pathologic observations in 20 patients. J Am Coll Cardiol 1991;176:433–439.

14. Spaet TH, Stemermann MB, Veith FJ, Lejnieks I, Intimal injury and regrowth in the rabbit aorta. Medial Smooth muscle cells as a source of neotima. Circ Res 1975;36:58–70.

15. Ueda M, Becker AE, Fujimoto T. Pathological changes induced by repeated percutaneous transluminal coronary angioplasty. Br Heart J 1987;58:635–643.

16. Zollikofer CL, Cragg AH, Hunter DW, et al. Mechanism of transluminal angioplasty. In: Castaneda-Zuniga WR, Tadavarthy SM (eds.): Interventional Radiology. Baltimore: Williams and Wilkins; 1992:249–298.

17. Leung DYM, Glagov S, Matthews MB. Cyclic stretching stimulates synthesis of matrix components by arterial smooth muscle cells in vitro. Science 1976;191:475–477.

18. Liermann D, Bötcher HD, Kollath J, et al. Intimal hyperplasia after stent implantation in peripheral arteries: Treatment by endovascular afterloading. J Cardiovasc Intervent Radiol 1994;17:12–16.

19. Liu MW, Roubin GS, King SB. Restenosis after coronary angioplasty: Potential biologic determinants and role of intimal hyperplasia. Circulation 1989;79:1374–1387.

20. Palmaz JC, Windeler SA, Garcia F. Atherosclerotic rabbit aortas: Expandable intraluminal grafting. Radiology 1986;160:723–726.

21. Rollins N, Wright KC, Charnsangavej C, Gianturco C. Self-expanding metallic stents: Preliminary evaluation in an atherosclerotic model. Radiology 1987;163:739–742.

22. Rousseau H, Joffre F, Raillat C, et al, Self-expanding endovascular stent experimental atherosclerosis. Radiology 1989;170:773–778.

23. Baensch W. Über die Strahlenbehandlung der Keloide. Strahlentherapie 1937;60:204–209.

24. Craig RDP, Person D. Early post-operative irradiation in the treatment of keloid scars. Br J Past Surg 1965;18:369–375.

25. Crocett DJ. Regional keloid susceptibility. Br J Plas Surg 1964;17:245–253.

26. Dalicho W. Zur therapie der keloide mit besoderer berückshrigung der Radiumbestrahlubg. Strahlentherapie 1949;78.

27. Enhamre A, Hammar H. Treatment of keloids with excision and postoperative x-ray irradiation. Dermatologica 1983;167:90–93.

28. Graul EH. Zur klinik des keloids. Strahlentherapie 1955;98:119–132.

29. Kovalic JJ, Perez CA. Radiation therapy following keloidektomie: A 20 year experience. Radiat Oncol Biol Phys 1989;17:77–80.

30. Krüger A. Über keloide und ihre Behandlung unter besonderer Berücksinchtigung der Strahlentherapie. Strahlentherapie 1945;93:426–433.

31. Levy DS, Salter MM, Roth RE. Postoperative irradiation in the prevention of keloids. Am J Roentgenol 1981;127:509–510.

32. Ollstein RN, Siegel HW, Gilloley JF, Barsa JMM. Treatment of keloids by combined sur-

gical excision and immediate postoperative x-ray therapy. Ann Plast Surg 1981;7: 281–284.

33. Scherer E. Kontaktbestrahlung mit radioaktiven Stoffen. in: Hdb Med Radiol, Bd XVI/2. Springer, 1970:136–146.
34. Wagner W, Schopohl B, Böttcher HD, Scheppner E. Ergebnisse der Narbenkeloidpro-phylaze durch Kontaktbestrahlung mit Strintium 90. Rôntgenpraxis 1989;42:248–252.
35. Brambs HJ, Freund U, Bruggmoser G, Wannenmacher M. Kombrte intraduktale perkutane Radiotherapie bei malignen Gallengangonstruktionen mit anschliessender prothetischer Versorgung. Onkologie 1987;10:84–89.
36. Kinsella TJ, Sindelar EF, De Luca AM. Threshold dose to peripheral nerve injury fol-lowing intraoperative radiotherapy (IORT) in a large animal model. Int J Radiat On-col Biol Phys 1988;16:205.
37. Le Couteur RA, Gilette EL, Powers BE, et al. Peripheral neuropathies following ex-perimental intraoperative radiation therapy (IORT). Int J Radiat Oncol Biol Phys 1989;17:583–590.
38. Rosen EM, Vinter DW, Golberg ID. Hypertrophy of cultured bovine aortic endothelium following irradiation. Radiat Res 1989;117:395–408.
39. Schartwz RS, Koval TM, Edwards WD, et al. Effect of external beam irradiation on neointimal hyperplasia after experimental coronary artery injury. J Am Coll Cardiol 1992;19:1106–1113.
40. Drescher W, Bache ST, Schumann E. Arterielle Spätkomplikationene nach strahlen-therapie. Strahlentherapie 1984;160:505–507.
41. Johnson AG. Large artery damage after x-radiation. Br J Radiol 1969;42:937–938.
42. Kolar J. Strahlenfolgen am Herz und grossen Gefässen. Med Klin 1971;66:661–668.
43. Scherer E, Streffer C, Trott KR (eds.): Radiopathology of Organs and Tissues. Berlin: Springer; 1991.
44. Schwartz RS, Murphy JG, Edwards WD, et al. Restenosis occurs with internal elastic lamina laceration and it's proportional to severity of vessel injury in a porcine coronary artery model. Circulation 1990;82:656.
45. Amronin GG, Gildenhorn HC, Solomon RD, et al. The synergism of x irradiation and cholesterol fat feeding on the development of coronary artery lesions. J Atheroscler Res 1964;4:325–334.
46. Artom C, Lofland HB, Clarkson TB. Ionizing radiation, atherosclerosis, and lipid me-tabolism in pigeons. Radiat Res 1965;26:165–177.
47. Battegay EJ, Raines EW, Seifert RA, et al. TGF-B induces bimodal proliferation of con-nective tissue cells via complex control of an autocrine PGDF loop. Cell 1990;63: 515–524.
48. Fischer JJ. Proliferation of rat aortic endothelial cells following x irradiation. Radiat Res 1982;92:405–410.
49. Hirst DG, Denekamp J, Hobson B. Proliferation studies of the endothelial and smooth muscle cells of the mouse mesentery after irradiation. Cell Tissue Kinet 1980;193:91–104.
50. Kirkpatrick JB. Pathogenesis of foam cell lesions in irradiated arteries. Am J Pathol 1967;50:291–309.
51. Liermann D, Schopohl B, Hermann G, Kollath HD. Endovaskuläres afterloading als therapiekonzept zur prohylaxe der intimalen hyperplasia in peripheren gefässen nach stentimplantation. in: Kollath J, Liermann D (eds.): Stents. Konstanz: Schnetztor Ver-lag; 1992:80–92.
52. Narayan K, Cliff WF. Morphology of irradiated microvasculature: A combined in vivo and electron microscopic study. Am J Pathol 1982;106:47–62.
53. Sholley MM, Gimbrone MA, Coltran RS. The effect of leukocyte depletion on corneal neovascularization. Lab Invest 1978;38:32–40.
54. Sholley MM, Gimbrone MA, Cotran RS. Cellular migration and replication in endo-thelial regeneration: A study using radiated endothelial cultures. Lab Invest 1977;36:18.
55. Betz E, Hämmerle H, Strohscheider T. Vergleich von wirkungen einzelner pharmaka auf die proliteration von gefäaamuskelzellen in vivo und in vitro. In: Fischer H, Betz E (eds.): Gefasswandelemente In Vivo und Vivo. Wiss Verlagsgesellschaft: Stuttgart; 1984:43–57.
56. Betz E, Hämmerle H, Strohschneider T. Inhibition of smooth muscle cell proliferation

and endothelial permeability with fluranizine in vifro and in experimental atheromas. Res Exp Med 1985;325–340.

57. Courier JW, Power TK, Haudenschild CC, et al. Low molecular weight heparin (eno-aparin) reduces restenosis after iliac angioplasty in the hypercholesterolemic rabbit. J Am Coll Cardiol 1991;17:118–125.

58. Cwikiel W, Stridbeck H, Stenram U. Electrolytic stents to inhibit tumor growth: An experimental study in vitro and in rats. Acta Radiologica 1993;34:1–5.

59. Dartsch PC, Betz E, Ischinger T. Wirkung von Dihatoporphyrin-Deraten aut kultivierte glatte muskelzellen des menschen aus normalen und atherosklertosch veränderten Gefässegmenten. Übersicht er bisherige ergebnisse und impliktationen für einr photodynamische therapie. Z Kardio 1991;80:6–14.

60. Eilis SG, Roubin GS, Wilentz J. Results of a randomized trial of heparin and aspirin vs aspirin alone for prevention of acute closure and restenosis after angioplasty (PTCA). Circulation 1987;76:213.

61. Guyton J, Rosenburg R, Ciowes A, Karnowsky M. Inhibition of rat arterial smooth muscle cell proliferation heparin: zin vivo studies with anticoagulant and nonanticoagulant heparin. Circ Res 1980;46:625–634.

62. Hagen B. Einflüsse der medikamentösen Nachbehandlung auf die mittelfristigen Ergebnisse von stent-implanmtationen der a femoropolitea. J Card Vasc Interv Radiol 1994;17:65.

63. Heras M, Chesebro JH, Penny WJ, et al. Effects of thrombin inhibition on the development of acute platelet thrombus deposition during angioplasty in pigs. Heparin versus recombinant hirudin, a specific thrombin inhibitor. Circulation 1989;79:657–665.

64. Hoepp LM, Elbadawi M, Cohn M, et al. Steroids and immunosuppresion effect on anastomotic intim hyperplasia femoral arterial dacron grafts. Arch Surg 1979;114:273–276.

65. Hoover R, Rosenburg R, Hearing W, Karnovsky M. Inhibition of rat arterial smooth cell proliferation by heparin: II in vitro studies. Circ Res 1980;47:578–583.

66. Kramsch DM, Aspen AJ, Rozler LJ. Suppresion of experimental atherosclerosis by the Ca++ antagonist lanthanum. J Clin Invest 1980;65:967–981.

67. Liu MW, Roubin GS, Robinson KA. Trapidil in preventing restenosis after balloon angioplasty in the atherosclerotic rabbit. Circulation 1990;81:1089–1093.

68. Pepine CJ, Hirschfeld JW, MacDonald RG. A controlled trial of corticosteroids to prevent restenosis after coronary angioplasty. Circulation 1990;81:1753–1761.

69. Powell JS, Clozel JP, Müller KM. Inhibitors angiotensin-converting enzyme prevent myointimal proliferation after vascular injury. Science 1989;245:186–188.

70. Reis GJ, Boucher TM, Sipperly ME. Randomized trial of fish oil for prevention of restenosis after coronary angioplasty. Lancet 1989;2:1753–1761.

71. Castellot JJ Jr., Addonizio ML, Rosenberg R, Kamovsky MJ. Cultured endothelial cells produce a heparin like inhibitor of smooth muscle cell growth. J Cell Biol 1990;373–379.

72. Nilsson J, Sjölund M, Palmberg L, et al. Arterial smooth muscle cells in primary culture produce a platelet-derived growth factor like protein. Cell Biol 1985;82:4418–4422.

73. Dichek DA, Neville RF, Zwiebel JA, et al. Seeding of intravascular stents wrth genetically engineered endothelial cells. Circulation 1989;80:1347–1353.

74. Leclerc G, Isner JM, Kearny M, et al. Evidence implicatrng nonmuscle myosin in restenosis: Use of in situ hybridization to analyze human vascular lesions obtained by directional atherectomy. Circulation 1992;85:1–11.

75. Nabel EG, Plautz G, Nabel GJ. Site specific expression in vivo by direct into arterial wall. Science 1990;249:1285–1288.

76. Wilcox JN. Analysis of local gene expression in human atherosclerotic plaques by in situ hybridization. Trends Cardiol Med 1991;1:17–24.

77. Roeren T, Palmaz JC, Garcia O, et al. Percutaneous vascular grafting with a coated stent. Radiology 1990;177:202.

78. Strecket EP, Hagen B, Liermann D, Kuhn FP. Komplikationen bei der implantation arterieller Tantastent und deren Behandlung. Zentralblatt der Radiologie. Radiology 1993;147:799.

79. Murphy JG, Schwartz RS, Kennedy K, et al. A new biocompatible polymeric coronary stent: Designs and early results in the pig model. J Am Coll Cardiol 1990;1:10.

80. Slepian MJ, Schindler A. Polymeric endoluminal paving/sealing: A biodegradable alternative to intracoronary stenting. Circulation 1988;78:409.

## Chapter 39

Peripheral Vascular Brachytherapy in the United States

Ron Waksman, MD

Introduction

As the manifestation of coronary atherosclerosis and peripheral artery disease is primarily evident in older patient populations, and with the generation of baby boomers nearing their 60's, the full impact of peripheral and coronary atherosclerosis in the U.S. is becoming evident. Vascular medicine is the fastest growing field of medicine today. It is estimated that in 1999, there were 270,000 peripheral endovascular procedures performed, and by the end of the year 2000, this rate is expected to increase to more than 550,000. Whereas coronary vascular procedures increase at a rate of 8% per year, there is greater growth in the frequency of peripheral procedures, estimated at 19% per year. Despite new advances such as stents, atherectomy devices, thrombectomy, and endoluminal grafts, the restenosis rate after peripheral artery intervention continues to peak and compromise the overall success of these procedures.

Vascular brachytherapy is a promising technology with the potential to reduce restenosis rates. Clinical trials to evaluate the effectiveness and safety of this technology are still ongoing with nearly 5000 patients enrolled in trials. Three-year follow-up of clinical and angiographic data collection on patients treated with intracoronary radiation for the prevention of restenosis has recently been released. These studies demonstrate different levels of efficacy and raise further questions regarding proper dosimetry, the incidence of edge effect, the late thrombosis phenomenon, and late restenosis. While the majority of vascular brachytherapy trials have focused on the use of radiation therapy for the prevention of coronary in-stent restenosis, more data is still needed to determine the effectiveness of beta and gamma sources, and the use of centering delivery systems.

Currently, the clinical experience with vascular brachytherapy for the peripheral system is limited and planned trials are designed to evaluate the restenosis rates of several vascular sites with the use of endovascular radiation therapy following vascular intervention (ie, balloon angioplasty, stent placement, atherectomy, or laser ablative techniques). Target sites and/or patients for such preventive therapy have been identified as: saphenous femoral artery lesions, renal artery stenosis, and patients who are undergoing hemodialysis with the arteriovenous graft stenosis, a subclavian or brachiocephalic vein, and following trans-

From Waksman R (ed.). *Vascular Brachytherapy, Third Edition.* Armonk, NY: Futura Publishing Co., Inc.; © 2002.

jugular intrahepatic portosystemic shunt (TIPS) procedures for patients with portal hypertension.

Mechanisms of Restenosis

The use of percutaneous transluminal angioplasty (PTA) has improved considerably the revascularization rates of many patients. Unfortunately, the long-term efficacy of PTA is limited by its high 6- to 12-month rate of restenosis.[1] Restenosis following PTA occurs in response to the healing process associated with overinflation of the balloon during angioplasty and subsequent overstretching of the vessel. The main mechanisms of restenosis are acute recoil, intimal hyperplasia, and late vascular constriction (negative remodeling).[2–5]

In the peripheral system, restenosis following PTA is mainly seen in small and medium peripheral arteries, such as the saphenous femoral-popliteal arteries (SFA) and renal arteries. Although not as common, and found to have less of an effect on patency, lower rates of restenosis have also been reported in larger arteries, such as the aorto-iliac and carotid arteries, following intervention.[6–12] Other sites affected by restenosis include bypass graft anastomosis, arteriovenous dialysis grafts, and following the placement of TIPS.[13] Factors that affect long-term vessel patency following PTA include the length of the lesion, the degree of the stenosis, the plaque burden, vessel size, and proximal and distal flow. For peripheral short focal lesions, short-term (6-month) patency rates as high as 75% have been reported. In contrast, more complex and longer areas of stenosis, those with poor distal runoff and those performed for limb salvage, may have a 6-month patency rate as low as 25%, and a 5-year patency rate of only 16%.[14]

Many attempts have been made to reduce restenosis by adding adjunct pharmacological therapy to PTA, or by the use of mechanical devices, including atherectomy, laser angioplasty, and intravascular stenting. It appears that instrumentation of these vessels by the balloon or the devices is responsible for inducing restenosis, as none of these alternative approaches significantly retard the neointimal hyperplasia or improve and preserve long-term vascular patency.[15–18] Indeed, the hyperplastic response post revascularization remains an outstanding issue for all vascular interventional modalities.

Intraluminal delivery of radiation following vascular intervention is viewed as a viable solution to inhibit restenosis.[19–29] Exposing the vessels to low dose radiation following angioplasty modifies wound healing by inhibiting the excessive neointima formation. Intravascular radiation in the peripheral system, however, requires special considerations when selecting the isotope and the delivery system to deliver the radiation to the target site.

Radiation Physics and Dosimetric Considerations

Different isotopes on various platforms and systems have been developed for the use of endovascular brachytherapy. The main platforms for radiation delivery are catheter-based systems and radioactive stents. Catheter-based systems contain a solid form such as line source wires, radioactive seeds or radioactive balloons, or nonsolid sources such as radioactive gas and liquid-filled balloons.

As there are several different gamma and beta isotopes available, selecting the most appropriate one depends on the anatomy of the vessel, the properties of the treated lesion, and the proper identification of the target tissue that needs treatment. Anatomically important parameters which also need consideration include the diameter and the curvature of the vessel, the eccentricity of the plaque, the lesion length, the composition of the plaque, the amount of calcium, and the presence or absence of a stent in the treated segment. These factors influence which source to use, as different sources have varying properties that warrant using one over another.

Requirements for choosing the ideal radiation system for vascular brachytherapy should include dose distribution of a few millimeters from the source with a minimal dose gradient, low dose levels to surrounding tissues, and a dwell time less than 15 minutes. Other considerations for source selection include source energy, half-life for multiple applications, available activity, penetration, dose distribution, radiation exposure to the patient and the operator, shielding requirement, availability, and cost. An example of dose distribution of ^{192}Ir is shown in Figure 1.

In order to determine an accurate dosimetry, it is essential to identify the target tissue, the right dose, and the treatment margins. It has been argued that the adventitia is the target, but when considering the success of previous trials, it is difficult to deny the fact that high dose exposure to the vessel wall and residual plaque may be essential to obtain efficacy.[30,31] The doses prescribed today in clinical studies are empirical; they are based on doses used in animal studies and the limited experience gained from treating other benign diseases. Since a wide range of doses has been demonstrated to be effective in pre-clinical studies, a therapeutic window must exist that allows some flexibility in selecting the isotope for this application.

Understanding Gamma Radiation

Gamma rays are photons originating from the center of the nucleus and differ from x-rays, which originate from the orbital outside of the nucleus. Gamma

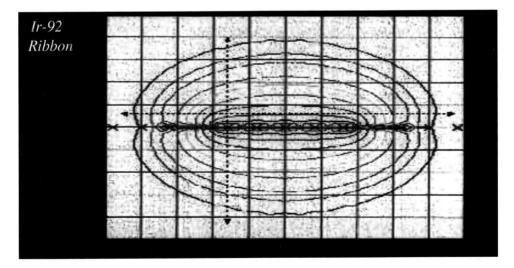

Figure 1. Example of dose distribution along an ^{192}Ir 5-seed ribbon.

rays have deep penetrating energies between 20 keV and 20 MeV which require an excess of shielding, as compared to beta and x-ray emitters. The only gamma ray isotope currently in use is ^{192}Ir. There are isotopes that emit both gamma and x-rays, such as ^{125}I and ^{103}Pd. These isotopes have lower energies, however, and require higher activity levels in order to deliver a prescribed dose in the acceptable dwell time (<15 min). Using these isotopes for vascular brachytherapy is difficult, as they are either not available in high-activity levels or they are too expensive for this application. The dosimetry of ^{192}Ir is well understood and is associated with an acceptable dose gradient, as ^{192}Ir has a lesser fall-off in dose than beta emitters. ^{192}Ir is available in activities of up to 10 Ci, but due to high penetration, patients need to be transferred to the radiation oncology shielded room, as the average shielding of a catheterization lab will not be enough to handle more than 500 mCi source in activity. Focal stenosis in smaller diameter arteries can be treated with lower activities of ^{192}Ir in the catheterization lab and will require an average of 20 minutes of dwell time for doses above 15 Gy when prescribed at a 2-mm radial distance from the source.

Understanding Beta Radiation

Beta rays are high-energy electrons emitted by nuclei and contain too many or too few neutrons. These negatively charged particles have a wide variety of energies, including transition energies, particularly between parent-daughter cells and a diverse range of half-lives from several minutes (^{62}Cu) up to 30 years (^{90}Sr/Y). Beta emitters are associated with a higher gradient to the near wall, as they lose their energy rapidly to surrounding tissue and their range is within 1 cm of tissue. Vascular brachytherapy using beta emitters appears promising, as safety levels are high when radiation exposure to nontargeted areas is low. In order to use beta emitters for the peripheral application, they must be in proximity with the vessel wall and should be used with as high an activity level as possible.

Radiation Systems for the Peripheral Vascular System

Several radiation systems for peripheral endovascular brachytherapy have been suggested and are currently under development. These systems are discussed in the following sections.

External Radiation

External beam radiation is a viable option for the treatment of peripheral vessels. It allows a homogenous dose distribution with the possibility of fractionation. To date, an attempt to treat SFA lesions and arteriovenous dialysis grafts with external radiation to reduce the restenosis rate, was reported as without success. Using stereotactic techniques to localize the radiation to the target area may improve the results of this approach.

Radioactive Stents

The radioactive stent is an attractive device because it requires minimum shielding and is easy to use. The dosimetry of radioactive stents is even more complicated and depends on the geometry of the stent, which varies across stent designs. Current tested radioactive stents lack dose homogeneity across the entire length of the stent. This could affect the biological response to radiation, especially at the stent edges. The lack of an even dose distribution may also result in an improper delivery to specific injured sites, causing additional growth. This problem, known as the edge effect, and identified as the major limitation of radioactive stents in coronary trials, may result from a stimulatory response from the vessel. Low-activity radioactive stents may be associated with an ineffective low dose rate. While radioactive stents with high activities may deliver toxic doses to the stented area that delay reendothelialization, higher radiation doses might promote stent thrombosis and tissue necrosis to the area surrounding the stent. New studies are under way which will evaluate whether higher activities will minimize the edge effect phenomenon. Other approaches to improving the results with radioactive stents include changes to the geometry of the stent, and altering the isotope or the activity level at the stent's edges. A new approach, using radioactive nitinol self-expanding stents with gamma emitters, is currently under investigation as a potential therapy for primary SFA lesions.

Catheter-Based Systems

Several catheter-based systems are available for the peripheral vascular system. However, the only system used in clinical trials is the microSelectron-HDR (Nucletron-Odelft, The Netherlands). This system uses a high dose rate afterloader that consists of a computerized system which delivers a 3-mm stepping 10 Ci in activity of ^{192}Ir source into a centered closed-end lumen segmented balloon radiation catheter. There are many advantages to using a remote afterloading system for vascular brachytherapy. Namely, the remote afterloading system drives the radiation source quickly to the treatment site, avoiding radiation exposure to nontreated arteries. In addition, radiation exposure to clinical personnel is eliminated by remotely programming the automatic advancement of the radiation source from a shielded safe to the treatment site. The radiation dose can be controlled and shaped using the computerized afterloader device to accurately adjust the source position and treatment time. By using an afterloader, it continually monitors the radiation dose and automatically retracts the source into the shielded safe after treatment. Treatment time is automatically adapted for the radioactive decay of the source, and the afterloader can handle a very high-activity source (10 Ci) which results in shorter dwell times. The afterloader used in the microSelectron-HDR system is pictured in Figure 2.

The Peripheral Brachytherapy Centering Catheter (PARIS™ catheter; Guidant, Santa Clara, CA) is currently being used in the multicenter Peripheral Artery Radiation Investigational Study (PARIS). This catheter is a double-lumen catheter with multiple centering balloons near its distal tip. One lumen is for inflation of the centering balloon; the second lumen is for the guidewire and for the closed-end lumen sheath which, after the catheter is in position, is introduced fol-

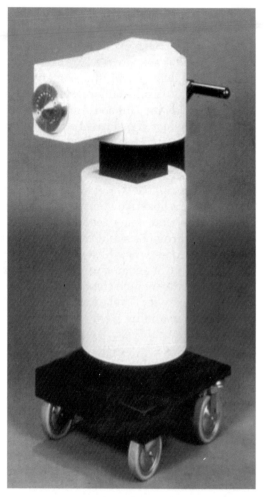

Figure 2. The microSelectron-HDR afterloader (Nucletron-Odelft, The Netherlands).

lowing removal of the guidewire. The inflated balloons engage the walls of the vessel and allow centering. The shaft diameter is a 7 F closed-end lumen catheter (Fig. 3) and it comes with balloons of 4 to 8 mm in diameter and 10 to 20 cm in length, enabling the catheter to be in the center of the lumen of large peripheral vessels during inflation. Other designs of catheters, such as the helical balloon, will overcome the centering problem and provide flow and perfusion during centering.

Another catheter-based system available for use in the catheterization lab includes the use of a ^{192}Ir radioactive wire that is delivered manually or by hand into a closed-end lumen catheter. The activity of the source is limited to 500 mCi and the system is only practical to use for short lesions in small vessels (diameters of <4.0 mm) that require a dwell time of 20 minutes. Similar to this gamma system, the eventual use of a catheter-based system using high-activity beta sources may also be an option for intermediate-sized vessels.

The angioplasty balloon is another platform that can be used to deliver radiation for the peripheral system. These balloons can be filled with either a liquid isotope such as ^{188}Re or ^{186}Re, or radioactive ^{133}Xe gas. The advantage of using these systems is the uniform dosimetry and proximity of the beta emitter to the

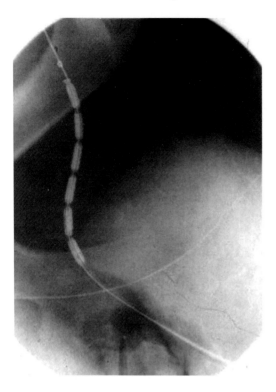

Figure 3. PARIS™ Centering Catheter (Guidant Corporation, Santa Clara, CA).

vessel wall. Special care, however, is required when using the liquid-filled balloon to prevent spilling of the isotope outside of the balloon. The radioactive balloon catheter is particularly attractive for peripheral applications since it is associated with apposition of a solid beta ^{32}P source attached to the inner balloon surface. With inflation of the balloon, the source is attached to the lumen surface. The system is limited to lesions less than 30 mm in length with one step, but it can accommodate longer lesions with manual stepping. To date, there is no clinical data to support the use of this technology.

An alternative and attractive approach would be the use of low x-ray energy delivered intraluminally via a catheter. The emitter would be between 5 to 7 mm in length and 1.25 to 2.0 mm in diameter. It could be administered distally to the lesion and pulled back to cover the entire lesion length. If effective, it would alleviate the need for the use of radioisotopes in the catheterization laboratory. Miniaturizing the emitter is a technical challenge and there is no pre-clinical data yet to support this theory.

Limitations to Brachytherapy

Although clinical trials using vascular brachytherapy for both coronary and peripheral applications have demonstrated positive results in reducing restenosis rates, these trials have also identified two major serious complications related to the technology: late thrombosis and edge stenosis effects seen at the edges of radiation treatment segments. Late thrombosis is probably due to the delay in healing associated with radiation. It has been estimated that late thrombosis can be remedied through the prolonged administration of antiplatelet therapy following intervention.

Identified as a major limitation to radioactive stents and explained above, the edge effect phenomenon is not only exclusive to stented lesions. The incidence of edge effect has also been known to occur with catheter-based systems utilizing both beta and gamma emitters, especially when the treated area is not covered with wide enough margins. The main explanation for the incidence of the edge effect is a combination of low dose at the edges of the radiation source and an injury created by the device for intervention that is not covered by the radiation source. It is hypothesized that wider radiation margins of radiation treatment to the intervening segment may eliminate or significantly reduce the edge effect seen thus far in all radiation trials.

Clinical Trials

The first application of vascular brachytherapy for the prevention of restenosis was performed in the peripheral arteries and was initiated by Liermann and Schopohl (Frankfurt, Germany). Known as the "Frankfurt Experience," the first pilot study of endovascular radiation was conducted in 30 patients with in-stent restenosis in their superficial femoral arteries (SFA).[32] The patients underwent atherectomy and PTA followed by endovascular radiation using the microSelectron-HDR afterloader and a noncentering catheter. The gamma source ^{192}Ir was used to deliver a dose of 12 Gy, 3 mm into the vessel wall. The actual dose, however, varied from 8 to 28 Gy. No adverse effects from the radiation treatment were reported up to a follow-up period of 7 years. The 5-year patency rate of the target vessel was 82% with only 3 of 28 (11%) stenosis within the treated segment reported. Late total occlusion developed in 2 of 28 patients (7%) after 16 and 37 months, respectively.

The Emory Experience

A subsequent pilot study was conducted at Emory University (Atlanta, GA) in 1994, which studied the effects of endovascular radiation in the superficial femoral arteries of 4 patients following PTA and stenting. Of the 4 patients, 1 patient with a Palmaz stent needed subsequent surgery 1-year post-radiation therapy because of a crushed stent. The histology of the irradiated stent segment in this patient demonstrated minimal intimal hyperplasia surrounding the stent struts, thus indicating the inhibitory effect of radiation therapy in stented SFAs.

The Vienna Experience

The effectiveness of the Nucletron HDR system was tested in a randomized placebo-controlled trial in Vienna using ^{192}Ir, a noncentering close-end lumen catheter, and a prescribed dose of 12 Gy in 100 patients following PTA to the SFA and the popliteal arteries. This study demonstrated a 50% reduction in the clinical restenosis rate in the irradiated group versus control.[33] The group from Vienna continued to investigate a series of patients with higher dose 18 Gy, and also a series of patients who were treated with primary stenting of the SFA followed by radiation therapy. The group receiving higher dosages experienced a late thrombosis rate of 10%. Prolonged antiplatelet therapy was initiated to further prevent this complication.

The PARIS Trial

The PARIS Trial is the first FDA approved multicenter randomized double-blind control study involving 300 patients following PTA to SFA stenosis using gamma radiation ^{192}Ir source. Utilizing the microSelectron-HDR afterloader, the treatment dose is 14 Gy delivered via a centered segmented end lumen balloon catheter. The primary objectives of this study are to determine angiographic evidence of patency and a reduction of greater than 30% of the treated lesion's restenosis rate at 6 months. A secondary endpoint is to determine the clinical patency at 6 and 12 months by treadmill exercise and by the ankle-brachial index (ABI). The clinical endpoints are improvements in treadmill exercise time of greater than 90 seconds, improvement of ABI 0.10 compared to pre PTA values, and an absence of repeat interventions to the treated vessel. This study was designed based on recently published recommendations and general principles of the evaluation of new interventional devices and technologies.[34,35] The data from this study should ultimately determine whether endovascular radiation therapy has a role in prevention of restenosis in patients following PTA for SFA lesions.

In the feasibility phase of PARIS, 41 patients with claudication were enrolled in the study and underwent PTA to SFA. Only 35 patients, however, were treated with radiation therapy. Mean lesion length was 9.8±3.0 cm and mean reference vessel diameter was 5.2±3.1 mm. Following successful PTA, a segmented centering balloon catheter was positioned to cover the PTA site. The patients were transported to the radiation oncology suite and treated with a high dose rate microSelectron-HDR afterloader using a ^{192}Ir source with a prescribed dose of 14 Gy, 2 mm into the vessel wall. ABI was evaluated at 1, 6, and 12 months and angiographic follow-up was conducted at 6 months.

Radiation was delivered successfully to 35 of 40 patients. There were no procedural complications. Exercise and rest ABI were higher at 1 year (0.74±0.26; 0.89±0.18) compared to the baseline prior to PTA (0.55±0.28; 0.67±0.19) ($P<0.03$). Maximum walking time on treadmill increased from 3.56±2.7 to 4.62±2.7 minutes at 30 days and was 4.04±2.8 minutes at 12 months, $P=0.01$. Angiographic binary restenosis at 6 months was 17.2% and the clinical restenosis at 12 months was 13.3%. There were no angiographic or clinical adverse events related to the radiation.

Arteriovenous Dialysis Studies

A pilot study was initiated at Emory in 1994 to determine whether intravascular low dose radiation retards neointimal hyperplasia in patients who had failed PTA at the distal venous anastomosis of arteriovenous dialysis grafts.[34]

Patients who failed prior PTAs to their arteriovenous graft and had less than 50% luminal stenosis were enrolled in the study and underwent balloon dilatation at the narrowed segment. Following PTA, a sheath was placed across the lesion and a closed-end lumen 5 F noncentered radiation delivery catheter was positioned at the angioplasty site. The catheter position was verified by radio-opaque marker bands on a dummy source wire that was placed into the catheter. The sheath and the catheter were fixed to the skin and the patients were transported to the radiation oncology suite. The patients were treated with a high-activity ^{192}Ir source delivered to the treatment site by a microSelectron-HDR afterloader. The treatment dose was 14 Gy delivered to a depth of 2 mm into the arterial wall. After the radiation treatment, the sheath and the catheter were retrieved and the patients were sent home on the same day. Bimonthly clinical follow-up including color-flow Doppler evaluation was performed, and the majority of the patients underwent angiographic follow-up at 6 months. Eleven patients with 18 lesions were treated. A 40% patency rate at 44 weeks was reported.

Although the procedure was successful in all patients, the long-term results of this study were similar to the practice reported so far by stand-alone PTA without radiation. In summary, this study demonstrated only the feasibility and safety of intravascular radiation therapy post PTA using the microSelectron-HDR afterloader for patients with arteriovenous dialysis graft stenosis.

This feasibility study had several limitations: the study population was small and heterogeneous, many patients had several PTA failures prior to the procedure, and there was heterogenicity on the type of the treated grafted shunts. Several patients in this study had thrombotic events within 3 months following the procedure and underwent thrombectomy or lytic therapy. Although the prescribed dose was 14 Gy, the actual calculated dose given to the patients ranged between 7 and 90 Gy. This occurred because a centering catheter was not utilized in a large conduit. The effectiveness of intravascular radiation therapy in the arteriovenous dialysis grafts, however, is unclear. Utilizing a centered catheter to deliver radiation to large vessels will be essential to control the uniformity of the dose given to the vessel wall in such large conduits. Larger randomized studies are required to determine the value of this new technology for patients with arteriovenous dialysis graft failure.

A pilot study utilizing external radiation in a fractionated method for arteriovenous dialysis in 12 patients failed to maintain any of these grafts within the first year. New studies for this application are currently under way, using low dose external radiation to reduce restenosis of vascular access for arteriovenous grafts of hemodialysis patients. Other studies using a centering device to deliver an accurate homogenous dose of radiation following PTA are currently under design.

Recently, a new study was initiated at Scripps Clinic (San Diego, CA) utilizing endovascular radiation therapy for the prevention of restenosis following TIPS for patients with portal hypertension. Overall, the restenosis rate due to intimal hyperplasia of TIPS at 6 months has been reported as high as 70%. Complete thrombosis as early as 2 weeks after the procedure has also been reported.[35] However, in the long term, brachytherapy may be the best means of preventing occlusion for these patients.

Other potential targets for vascular brachytherapy include renal arteries and subclavian vein stenosis.

Conclusion

Despite the new technologies and devices, restenosis remains the major limitation of intervention in the peripheral vascular system. The results from preliminary studies demonstrate that radiation has the potential to alter the rate of restenosis following intervention. With the further progression of these studies and their promising results, the use of vascular brachytherapy will dramatically change the practice of peripheral intervention, resulting in an improved long-term patency for patients.

References

1. Tripuraneni P. Catheter-based radiotherapy for peripheral vascular restenosis. Vascular Radiotherapy Monitor 1999;1:70–77.
2. Haude M, Erbel R, Issa H, Meyer J. Quantitative analysis of elastic recoil after balloon angioplasty and after intracoronary implantation of balloon-expandable Palmaz-Schatz stents. J Am Coll Cardiol 1993;21:2634.
3. Consigny PM, Bilder GE. Expression and release of smooth muscle cell mitogens in arterial wall after balloon angioplasty. J Vasc Med Biol 1993;4:1–8.
4. Mintz GS, Popma JJ, Pichard AD, et al. Arterial remodeling after coronary angioplasty: A serial intravascular ultrasound study. Circulation 1996;94:35–43.
5. Isner JM. Vascular remodeling: Honey, I think I shrunk the artery. Circulation 1994;89:2937–2941.
6. Murray RR Jr, Hewews RC, White RI Jr, et al. Long-segment femoro-popliteal stenoses: Is angioplasty a boon or a bust? Radiology 1987;162:473–476.
7. Johnston KW. Femoral and popliteal arteries: Re-analyses of results of balloon angioplasty. Radiology 1992;183:767–771.
8. Vroegindeweij D, Kemper FJ, Teilbeek AV, et al. Recurrence of stenosis following balloon angioplasty and Simpson atherectomy of the femoropopliteal segment: A randomized comparative 1 year follow-up study using color flow duplex. Eur J Vasc Surg 1992;6:164–171.
9. Rees CR, Palmaz JC, Becker GJ, et al. Palmaz stent in atherosclerotic stenosis involving the ostia of the renal arteries: Preliminary report of a multicenter study. Radiology 1991;181:507–514.
10. Hunink MFM, Magruder CD, Meyerovitz MF, et al. Risks and benefits of femoropopliteal percutaneous balloon angioplasty. J Vasc Surg 1993;17:183–194.
11. White GF, Liew SC, Waugh RC, et al. Early outcome of intermediate follow-up of vascular stents in the femoral and popliteal arteries without long term anticoagulation. J Vasc Surg 1995;21:279–281.
12. Kotb MM, Kadir S, Bennett JD, Beam CA. Aortoiliac angioplasty: Is there a need for other types of percutaneous intervention. J Vasc Int Radiol 1992;3:67–71.
13. Dolmath BL, Gray RJ, Horton KM, et al. Treatment of anastomotic bypass graft stenosis with directional atherectomy: Short term and intermediate-term results. J Vasc Int Radiol 1995;6:105–113.
14. Johnston KW. Femoral and popliteal arteries: Reanalysis of results of angioplasty. Radiology 1987;162:473–476.
15. Robinson KA. Arterial biologic response to ionizing radiation. In: Waksman R, Bonan R (eds.): Vascular Brachytherapy: State of the Art. London: Remedica Publishing; 1999:15–24.
16. Hillegass WB, Ohman EM, Califf RM. Restenosis: The clinical issues. In: Topol EJ (ed.): Textbook of Interventional Cardiology, 2nd Edition. Vol. 1. Philadelphia: WB Saunders, Inc.; 1994:415–435.
17. Pickering JG, Weir L, Jekanowski J, et al. Proliferative activity in peripheral and coronary atherosclerotic plaques among patients undergoing percutaneous revascularization. J Clin Invest 1993;91:1469–1480.
18. Strandness DE, Barnes RW, Katzen B, Ring EJ. Indiscriminate use of laser angioplasty. Radiology 1989;172:945–946.
19. Waksman R, Robinson KA, Crocker IR, et al. Long term efficacy and safety of endovascular low dose irradiation in a swine model of restenosis after angioplasty. Circulation 1995;91:1533–1539.
20. Weidermann JG, Marboe C, Amols H, et al. Intracoronary irradiation markedly re-

duces restenosis after balloon angioplasty in a porcine model. J Am Coll Cardiol 1994;23:1491–1498.

21. Weiderman JG, Marboe C, Amols H, et al. Intracoronary irradiation markedly reduces neointimal proliferation after balloon angioplasty in swine: Persistent benefit at 6-month follow-up. J Am Coll Cardiol 1995;25:1456–1461.

22. Mazur W, Ali MN, Dabhagi SF, Criscard C, et al. High dose rate intracoronary radiation suppresses neointimal proliferation in the stented and balloon model of porcine restenosis. Int J Radiat Oncol Biol Phys 1996;36:777–788.

23. Borok TL, Bray M, Sinclair I, et al. Role of ionizing irradiation for keloids. Int J Radiat Oncol Biol Phys 1988;15:865–870.

24. Van den Brenk HAS, Minty CCJ. Radiation in the management of keloids and hypertorphic scar. Br J Surg 1959/1960;47:595–605.

25. Nickson JJ, Lawrence W, Rachwalsky I, et al. Roentgen rays and wound healing: Fractionated irradiation. Experimental study. Surgery 1953;34:859–868.

26. Insalsingh CHA. An experience in treating 501 patients with keloids. Johns Hopkins Med J 1974;134:284–290.

27. Grillo HC, Potsaid MS. Studies in wound healing. Ann Surg 1961;154:741.

28. MacLennon I, Keys HM, Evarts CM, Rubgin P. Usefulness of post-operative hip irradiation in the prevention of heterotrophic bone formation in a high risk group of patients. Int J Radiat Oncol Biol Phys 1984;10:49–53.

29. Van den Brenk HAS. Results of prophylactice post-operative irradiation in 1300 cases of pterygium. AJR 1968;103:723.

30. Mintz GS, Pichard AD, Kent KM, et al. Endovascular stents reduce restenosis by eliminating geometric arterial remodeling: A serial intravascular ultrasound study. J Am Coll Cardiol 1995;35A:701–705.

31. Waksman R, Rodriquez JC, Robinson KA, et al. Effect of intravascular irradiation on cell proliferation, apoptosis and vascular remodeling after balloon overstretch injury of porcine coronary arteries. Circulation 1996;96:1944–1952.

32. Liermann DD, Bottcher HD, Kollath J, et al. Prophylactic endovascular radiotherapy to prevent intimal hyperplasia after stent implantation in femoropopliteal arteries. Cardiovasc Intervent Radiol 1994;17:12–16.

33. Minar E. SFA brachytherapy: The Vienna Experience [abstract]. Cardiovascular Radiation Therapy III Syllabus 1999;431.

34. Waksman R, Crocker IA, Kikeri D, et al. Long term results of endovascular radiation therapy for prevention of restenosis in the peripheral vascular system. Circulation 1996;94I-300:1745.

35. Raat H, Stockx L, Ranschaert E, et al. Percutaneous hydrodynamic thrombectomy of acute thrombosis in transjugular intrahepatic portosystemic shunt (TIPS): A feasibility study in five patients. Cardiovasc Intervent Radiol 1997;20:180–183.

## Chapter 40

Peripheral Vascular Brachytherapy in Europe

Erich Minar, MD, Boris Pokrajac, MD, Roswitha Wolfram, MD, and Richard Pötter, MD

Introduction

Peripheral vascular disease from the aortic bifurcation to the runoff vessels is common, and the efficacy of percutaneous transluminal angioplasty (PTA) has been well documented in numerous trials. The advantages of PTA include low morbidity and mortality, and a shorter hospital stay. However, restenosis has remained until now a major limitation of the clinical usefulness of PTA, especially in the femoropopliteal and crural region. A poor long-term patency rate after PTA of longer femoropopliteal lesions was repeatedly reported, and complex and longer areas of stenosis may have a 6-month patency rate as low as 23%.[1] Therefore, angioplasty is not generally accepted for treatment of longer (>10 cm) femoropopliteal lesions by many interventional radiologists, and especially by vascular surgeons, despite the increasing primary success rates due to experience and technical improvements. Angioplasty for recurrence after previous PTA has a further reduced long-term success rate.[2] A 1-year patency rate of 41% and a 3-year patency rate of only 11% was reported after PTA of recurrent femoropopliteal lesions with lesion lengths of 1 to 5 cm. The use of newer interventional devices such as stents has not improved these long-term results.[3] While stents can reduce the constricting effect of vascular remodeling, the major drawback of stent implantation is the enhanced occurrence of neointimal proliferation within the stent, and therefore, currently available metallic stents have not significantly improved the outcome of femoropopliteal PTA.[3]

Since pharmacological adjuncts have been tried without success after peripheral angioplasty with/without stent implantation, there is urgent need for new approaches to deal with the problem of restenosis. Increasing knowledge about the pathophysiology of the process leading to restenosis has given the rationale to investigate the potential role of radiation in the prevention of restenosis. Compared to the rapidly increasing experience in the coronary circulation, there is until now only a very limited number of studies with clinical data concerning the use of brachytherapy (BT) in the peripheral circulation. Most of the studies in the peripheral system have been done in the femoropopliteal region, and this chapter deals with the experience with peripheral vascular BT in Europe.

From Waksman R (ed.). *Vascular Brachytherapy, Third Edition.* Armonk, NY: Futura Publishing Co., Inc.; © 2002.

External Percutaneous Radiation Therapy

External beam radiotherapy has some advantages from biological, physical, logistic, and patient-related points.[4] However, due to some technical problems, this approach has been investigated in the femoropopliteal region only in one small German study. Steidle[5] applied percutaneous radiation therapy on 5 consecutive days with a single dose of 2.5 Gy–thus resulting in a total dose of 12.5 Gy–in 11 patients after femoropopliteal PTA and stent implantation (Strecker stent). During a 7-month follow-up, only 2 of 11 patients suffered from occlusion (compared with 5 of 13 patients treated with stent implantation without further irradiation).

Endovascular Radiation Therapy

Frankfurt Trial

The first clinical trial using endovascular BT after femoropopliteal angioplasty was initiated in the early 1990s by the Frankfurt group. Böttcher et al.[6] were the first to present data showing that endovascular irradiation is both feasible and safe in humans. Between 1990 and 1997, 30 patients were treated with PTA followed by endovascular BT for in-stent restenosis in the superficial femoral artery. The length of the stented vascular segments ranged from 4.5 to 14 cm, with a mean of 6.7 cm. A dose of 12 Gy–prescribed at a radial distance of 3 mm corresponding to the vessel surface–was administered by a microSelectron-HDR remote afterloader (Nucletron-Odelft, The Netherlands) using an ^{192}Ir source via a noncentering 5 F closed-end lumen catheter. Because of the eccentric position of the catheter in the vessel (due to noncentering and eccentric plaques), the calculated dose to various sectors of the vessel wall varied from 8 to 28 Gy. This group used a dose of 12 Gy because of the long experience and positive results with this dose in the prevention of keloids and hypertrophic scars. The optimistic primary results have been confirmed recently by long-term results, with a range of follow-up of 7 to 84 months (median 33 months). In the 28 patients available for follow-up, the 5-year patency rate (determined clinically and by ultrasound) was 82%. Three patients developed restenosis within the treated segment, while 2 patients presented with acute thrombotic occlusion after 16 and 37 months, respectively.[7] Furthermore, these investigators observed (by magnetic resonance imaging) no evidence of side effects to the vessels, nerves, or soft tissue surrounding the femoral artery.

Switzerland Trial

A Swiss group in Bern began a three-phase trial in 1997 investigating the role of endovascular BT in femoropopliteal lesions.[8] In the first phase, the feasibility of BT was examined using a dose of 12 Gy prescribed at a radial distance of 3 mm. In the second phase, a randomized trial with and without BT, the same dose is prescribed at a larger radial distance of 5 mm. Phase III is a four-arm trial randomizing patients to: (a) PTA + aspirin; (b) PTA + aspirin + BT; (c) PTA + aspirin + probucol; or (d) PTA + aspirin + probucol + BT. The radiation dose in this phase III trial (inclusion of 80 patients is planned in each arm) is 14 Gy prescribed at the reference radius plus 2 mm. Neither centering devices nor stents are used in this study. Results of these trials are not yet available.

Rotterdam Trial

The Vascular Radiation (VARA) Trial is currently being performed in Rotterdam addressing the effect of endovascular BT after femoropopliteal PTA without stenting.[9] The design is like the Peripheral Artery Radiation Investigational Study (PARIS) with the use of a centering device.

The Vienna Experience

In May 1996, a group in Vienna began to investigate the feasibility and efficacy of endovascular BT after femoropopliteal angioplasty.

In all trials, an ^{192}Ir source with a diameter of 1.1 mm was delivered by using a high dose rate remote afterloader (microSelectron).

Vienna 01 Trial

In this pilot study, 10 patients with long-segment (mean length, 16 cm; range, 9 to 22 cm) restenosis after former PTA underwent angioplasty followed by endovascular irradiation.[10] A dose of 12 Gy was targeted to the inner intimal layer of the vessel. Follow-up examinations included measurement of ankle-brachial index (ABI) and color duplex sonography with calculation of the peak velocity ratio (PVR); intra-arterial angiography was performed when a recurrence was suspected. Endovascular BT was technically feasible in all patients without complications. In 6 patients, the dilated and irradiated segment remained widely patent on color duplex sonography, with corresponding excellent hemodynamic and clinical results after 12 months. In 4 patients, arteriography demonstrated 60 to 90% diameter restenosis. Considering the negative selection of patients with a high risk of restenosis, the results of this pilot study were promising concerning the possibility of reduction of restenosis by means of endovascular BT after long-segment femoropopliteal PTA without stent implantation.

Vienna 02 Trial

From November 1996 to August 1998, 113 patients (63 males, 50 females; mean age 71 years) with de novo ($\geq$5 cm) or recurrent (any length) femoropopliteal lesions were included in this randomized trial comparing the angiographically verified restenosis rate after PTA plus BT (N=57) versus PTA (N=56) without stent implantation.[11] The mean treated length of the artery was 16.7 cm (PTA + BT) versus 14.8 cm (PTA), respectively. In patients randomized to PTA + BT, a reference dose of 12 Gy was prescribed in 3 mm distance from the source axis using the high dose rate remote afterloader with an ^{192}Ir source. The length of the artery to be irradiated corresponded to the total length of the angioplastic site with an additional 1 cm at each end, which has been chosen as a safety margin. The mean irradiation time was approximately 4 minutes. Transportation to the

BT unit, and the irradiation protocol, prolonged the PTA procedure by about 30 minutes.

Treatment with 100 mg of aspirin per day was initiated at least 2 weeks before the intervention and was prescribed as long-term treatment. During the intervention, 5000 IU of standard heparin were administered; further administration in a dosage of 1000 IU/h was started before transportation to the BT unit and was continued until the next morning.

Follow-up examinations were performed the day after PTA and after 1, 3, 6, 12, 18, and 24 months after PTA. Follow-up examinations were assessment of symptoms, clinical examination, and noninvasive laboratory testing including ankle-brachial arterial pressure measurement with Doppler ultrasound to calculate the ABI, and color duplex sonography of the femoropopliteal segment. The maximum peak systolic velocity (PSV) in the dilated region was determined and compared to the PSV in the preceeding normal arterial segment. A PVR of greater than or equal to 2.4 was considered indicative of a stenosis of greater than 50% at that site. If recurrent stenosis was suspected on the basis of clinical or laboratory findings, intra-arterial angiography was performed with eventual further PTA. According to the high sensitivity of color duplex sonography for detection of greater than 50% stenosis, control angiography was not mandatory in case of normal hemodynamic results.

The primary endpoint of the study was patency of the recanalized segment after 6 months. Restenosis was defined as an angiographically verified stenosis of greater than 50% narrowing of the luminal diameter within the recanalized segment compared with the diameters of normal segments of the vessel on the follow-up angiograms. Clinical success of the procedure was defined by immediate improvement by at least one clinical category according to the criteria defined by Rutherford and Becker.[12] Patients with tissue damage had to move up at least two categories and reach the level of claudication to be considered improved. Clinical patency was defined by sustained improvement without further intervention.

The irradiation procedure was technically feasible in all patients without complications. The follow-up period was 12±6 months. Control angiography was performed in 69 patients (64%), 37 in the PTA group and 32 in the PTA + BT group.

In 107 patients, information concerning patency could be obtained after 6 months. The overall angiographically verified recurrence rate was 15 of 53 (28.3%) in the PTA + BT group versus 29 of 54 (53.7%) in the PTA group (chi-square test, $P<0.05$). The cumulative patency rates at 12-month follow-up were 63.6% in the PTA + BT group and 35.3% in the PTA group (log rank test, $P<0.005$).

The cumulative clinical patency rates at 12-month follow-up were 51.9% in the PTA group and 73.6% in the PTA + BT group, respectively (log rank test, $P<0.05$).

The angiographic appearance of restenosis after BT was quite different compared to the well known kind of restenosis after long-segment angioplasty without BT. While, in these patients, the typical pattern of long-segment recurrence with a high degree of stenosis covering mostly the total length of the former dilated segment was observed (Fig. 1), the morphological pattern in the case of restenosis after BT was characterized by only circumscript stenosis with segments of normal lumen width between (Fig. 2). These findings suggest a detectable radiation effect also in patients with recurrence.

There was no observation of an edge effect as reported in studies using BT after stent implantation or in studies with radioactive stents. This may be due to

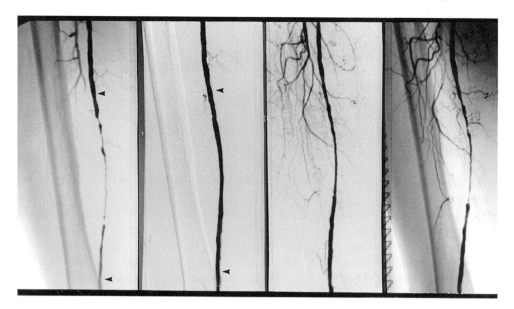

Figure 1. Left: Long-distance recurrence after former percutaneous transluminal angioplasty (PTA). **Mid left:** Angiogram after PTA. **Mid right:** Angiogram after 3 months with moderate restenosis. **Right:** Angiogram after 6 months with the typical pattern of long-segment recurrence within the dilated segment.

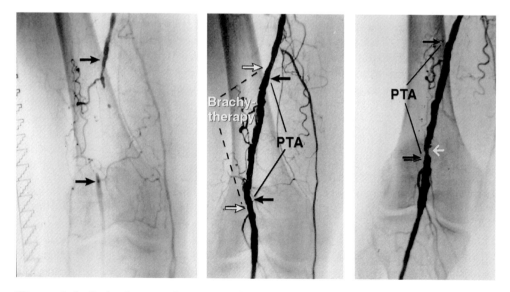

Figure 2. Left: Angiogram of a 60-year-old male with occlusion of the proximal popliteal artery. **Middle:** Angiogram immediately after angioplasty (the dilated segment is between the black arrows; the irradiated segment is between the white arrows). **Right:** Control angiogram obtained 6 months later (the formerly dilated segment is between the black arrows) demonstrates moderate circumscript restenosis (white arrow) after angioplasty followed by brachytherapy.

the use of a safety margin of 1 cm of irradiation surpassing the angioplasty length at each end.

Late thrombotic occlusion was not a problem in this study since, in cases of recurrence, all patients in the BT group presented with restenosis, and no patient had thrombotic reocclusion.

Despite the significant reduction of recurrence in this randomized trial, the investigators could not prevent restenosis in about one third of the patients. The nominal dose used in this trial was lower than the dose given in most intracoronary trials using gamma sources.[13] This may not be adequate for complete inhibition of neointimal hyperplasia. Another important factor that can account for the observed restenoses in this study may be the dose inhomogeneity due to an eccentric catheter position. With long treatment lengths, a noncentered catheter can often be eccentrically located at various points along the vessel length. An eccentric plaque can further accentuate this noncentering, resulting in significant dose inhomogeneity to the target volume. In our experience, decentering of the source with the technique applied was not uncommon although some centering may be achieved by the 5 F radiation delivery catheter and the 6 F sheath. Otherwise, source centering for gamma emitters such as ^{192}Ir is not as critical as it is for beta emitters.[14] New catheters with centering capabilities have been designed and are being used in ongoing clinical trials. The reduction in "hot spots" along the intimal surface by a source centering system may also improve the overall therapeutic ratio, by reducing restenosis rates without a corresponding increase in toxicity. However, even if the source is perfectly centered, dose asymmetries will continue to result from eccentrically located plaques, or where the target length incorporates a significant angulation or curvature.

In summary, this was the first randomized study to demonstrate the efficacy of endovascular BT for prophylaxis of restenosis after femoropopliteal PTA. However, the results of this trial need to be confirmed by a double-blind, randomized multi-institutional study using an adequate centering device before the use of endovascular BT can be generally recommended for prophylaxis of restenosis after femoropopliteal PTA.

Vienna 03 Trial

In November 1998, enrollment began in an Austrian multicenter trial using a new catheter with source centering capabilities similar to the one utilized in the PARIS Trial. This trial was also designed as a randomized, double-blinded study comparing the restenosis rate after PTA + BT versus the rate after PTA alone. However, in contrast to the PARIS protocol, patients with longer lesions (total occlusions >5 cm) are eligible and the prescribed dose is 18 Gy delivered to the adventitia of the artery. The primary endpoint is angiographically demonstrable restenosis after 12 months.

Vienna 04 Trial

To evaluate the interaction of endovascular BT and peripheral arterial stenting, a pilot study was completed in patients with long-segment femoropopliteal angioplasty + stent implantation. Thirty-three patients were enrolled between October 1998 and June 1999. The mean treated length was 17 cm (range 5 to 30 cm), and a dose of 14 Gy was prescribed at 2 mm beyond the average luminal radius using the PARIS™ centering catheter. All patients received clopidogrel (75 mg/day) for 1 month (following a loading dose of 300 mg in the catheter laboratory immediately after stent implantation) and were maintained on long-term aspirin (100 mg/day). The 6-month angiographic results demonstrated recurrence in 10 of 33 patients (30%). Three patients presented with stenosis, and 7 patients with sudden late thrombotic occlusion of the stented segment, occurring between 3.5 and 6 months after the intervention. Such late thrombotic events have also been reported in patients receiving intracoronary BT in conjunction with stenting, and are believed to be due to delayed reendothelialization of the newly implanted stents in the irradiated vessels.[15] Therefore, the protocol has changed and all patients now continue on clopidogrel for at least 6 months. The other patients showed an excellent angiographic result without any luminal narrowing within the stent, or at the stent edges (Figs. 3A and 3B). Intravascular ultrasound demonstrated no, or only minimal (<0.5 mm) intimal hyperplasia in these patients.

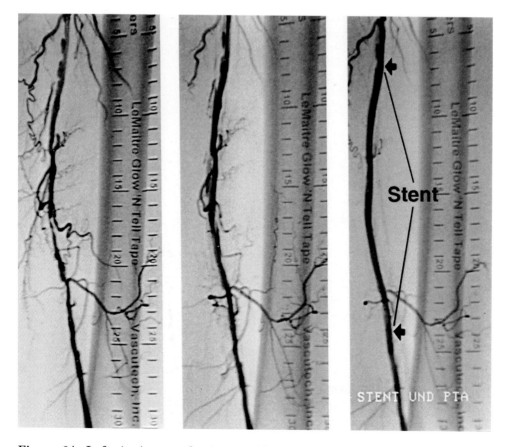

Figure 3A. Left: Angiogram of a 64-year-old male with long-segment femoropopliteal stenosis. **Middle:** Angiogram immediately after angioplasty demonstrates dissection and residual stenosis. **Right:** Angiogram immediately after long-segment stent implantation.

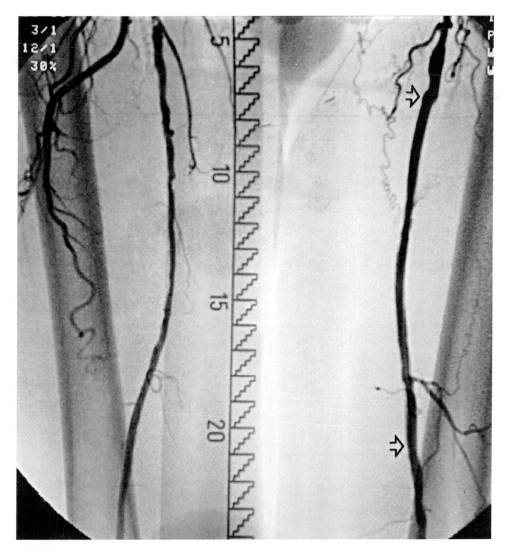

Figure 3B. Control angiogram obtained 6 months after stent implantation followed by brachytherapy (the stented segment is between the arrows).

Vienna 05 Trial

Based on the results from the Vienna 04 Study, a double-blind, randomized trial was initiated comparing the angiographically verified recurrence rate after femoropopliteal stenting and BT versus stenting alone. The primary endpoint of this study is the angiographically verified patency rate after 6 months. The study began in June 1999; study design and dose prescription are identical to the Vienna 04 Trial, except that all patients will receive clopidogrel for at least 1 year. Eighty patients have been enrolled by April 2001 in this ongoing trial.

Discussion

The results available until now from the described European trials are very promising concerning the possibility of significant and clinically relevant reduction of restenosis after femoropopliteal angioplasty.

One of the major problems with the currently used approach is that it cannot be performed in the normal interventional radiology suite due to the special shielding requirements for such high-activity sources. However, compared to coronary interventions, transportation of patients to the BT unit can be performed without problems after peripheral interventions.

The rather high incidence of late thrombotic occlusion after long-segment femoropopliteal stenting and endovascular BT requires optimization of the antithrombotic regimen.

In the interests of standardizing the prescription, and to allow meaningful interinstitutional comparisons, a task group of the American Association of Physicists in Medicine (AAPM) has recently published recommendations.[16] For peripheral BT, the AAPM now recommends prescribing the dose at 2 mm beyond the average luminal radius (average vessel radius + 2 mm = prescription point).

References

1. Murray RR Jr, Hewes RC, White RI Jr, et al. Long-segment femoropopliteal stenoses: Is angioplasty a boon or a bust? Radiology 1987;162:473–476.
2. Treiman GS, Ichikawa L, Treiman RL, et al. Treatment of recurrent femoral and popliteal artery stenosis after percutaneous transluminal angioplasty. J Vasc Surg 1994;20:577–587.
3. Vroegindeweij D, Vos LD, Tielbeek AV, et al. Balloon angioplasty combined with primary stenting versus balloon angioplasty alone in femoropopliteal obstructions: A comparative randomized study. Cardiovasc Intervent Radiol 1197;20:420–425.
4. Nori D. Principles of external radiation for vascular applications. Cardiovascular Radiation Therapy IV, Syllabus 2000:204.
5. Steidle B. Preventive percutaneous radiation therapy to avoid hyperplasia of the intima after angioplasty combined with stent-implantation. Strahlenther Onkol 1994;170:151–154.
6. Böttcher HD, Schopohl B, Liermann D, et al. Endovascular irradiation: A new method to avoid recurrent stenosis after stent implantation in peripheral arteries—technique and preliminary results. Int J Radiat Oncol Biol Phys 1994;29:183–186.
7. Liermann DD, Bauernsachs R, Schopohl B, et al. Intravascular irradiation therapy. In: Waksman R (ed.): Vascular Brachytherapy, 2nd Edition. Armonk, NY: Futura Publishing Company; 1999:395–405.
8. Greiner RH, Do DD, Mahler F, et al. Peripheral endovascular radiation for restenosis prevention after percutaneous transluminal angioplasty. Endovascular Brachytherapy Workshop 10/5/98; Napoli, Italy;Syllabus:49–50a.
9. Gescher FM, Coen VMLA, van Tongeren RBM, et al. Endovascular brachytherapy preventing restenosis after percutaneous transluminal angioplasty. Endovascular Brachytherapy Workshop 10/5/98; Napoli, Italy;Syllabus:43–46a.
10. Minar E, Pokrajac B, Ahmadi R, et al. Brachytherapy for prophylaxis of restenosis after long-segment femoropopliteal angioplasty: Pilot study. Radiology 1998;208:173–179.
11. Minar E, Pokrajac B, Maca TH, et al. Endovascular brachytherapy for prophylaxis of restenosis after femoropopliteal angioplasty: Results of a prospective, randomized study. Circulation 2000;102:2694–2699.
12. Rutherford RB, Becker GJ. Standards for evaluating and reporting the results of surgical and percutaneous therapy for peripheral arterial disease. Radiology 1991; 181:277–281.

13. Waksman R. Intracoronary radiation therapy for restenosis prevention: Status of the clinical trials. Cardiovasc Radiat Med 1999;1:20–29.
14. Jani SK. Gamma vs. beta irradiation: Which is superior? Cardiovasc Radiat Med 1999;1:102–106.
15. Costa MA, Sabaté M, van der Giessen WJ, et al. Late coronary occlusion after intra-coronary brachytherapy. Circulation 1999;100:789–792.
16. Nath R, Amols H, Coffey C, et al. Intravascular brachytherapy physics: Report of the AAPM Radiation Therapy Committee Task Group No. 60. Med Phys 1999;26:119–152.

## Chapter 41

External Radiation Therapy for Patients with Arteriovenous Dialysis Shunts

Suhrid Parikh, MBBS, MS, MCh and Dattatreyudu Nori, MD

Background

For a long time, the full potential of hemodialysis was limited by the lack of a means for repeated access to the vascular system. At the outset, repeated cutdowns were made on the artery and the vein for each dialysis, after which the vessels were ligated. The duration of a course of dialysis was obviously limited to the treatment of acute renal failure. Successful, long-term hemodialysis requires a vascular access that is readily available, and sustains an intradialytic blood flow of at least 200 mL/min without thrombosis.[1] Such an access is usually achieved today by the surgical creation of an arteriovenous (AV) fistula.

Physiology of Arteriovenous Fistulas

A fistula may be formed directly between an adjacent artery and vein or, if these vessels are separated, by connecting them with a conduit limb of variable diameter and length. The direction of flow in both the proximal artery and vein is normal in all fistulas. Fistulas for therapeutic purposes are usually large (fistula "orifice" diameter >75% of the arterial lumen) and the blood flow in the distal artery and vein is usually reversed.

When a fistula is first created, there is a fall in the peripheral resistance that leads to an increase in cardiac output. The proximal arterial flow is increased, and accompanying this there is an increase in the proximal venous outflow. The highest pressure in the distal artery is usually only two thirds of systemic pressure, which is still higher than the pressure at the fistula opening, leading to a retrograde flow in the distal artery. Blood in the distal fistula vein flows retrograde until at some point the valves are able to withstand the pressure. The blood in the distal vein is carried cardiad by venous collaterals which open off the vein. With time, there is significant increase in the number of collateral vessels formed between the proximal and distal arteries and the proximal and distal veins. With time, there is a lengthening and dilatation of the proximal and distal veins and the proximal artery

From Waksman R (ed.). *Vascular Brachytherapy, Third Edition.* Armonk, NY: Futura Publishing Co., Inc.; © 2002.

in addition to the vascular collaterals. The proximal artery develops smooth muscle hypertrophy in addition to dilatation, and then elongates. Later the muscle atrophies and the vessel becomes tortuous and aneurysmal. The veins continue to dilate for up to 8 months, and gradually become arterialized and tortuous.

Types of Access

External Arteriovenous Shunt

The development of the external AV shunt in 1960 provided the first successful method for long-term hemodialysis. Quinton et al[2] described their technique, which basically consists of a loop of Silastic tubing lying on the volar aspect of the forearm, connecting Teflon cannulae in the radial artery and nearby wrist vein. Although it was quickly and widely adopted as a practical means of providing access in chronic renal failure, several disadvantages soon became apparent: (1) a high rate of infection due to bacterial contamination at the entry sites in the skin; (2) frequent thrombosis of the shunt due to the small size of the conduits; (3) restriction of the patient's daily activities; and (4) use of vessels and vascular sites potentially available for more permanent vascular access.[3] Consequently, these are rarely used today.

Autogenous, Subcutaneous Arteriovenous Fistula

First described in 1966 by Brescia et al,[4] the autogenous, subcutaneous AV fistula is currently the procedure of choice. The fistula is most commonly constructed by a direct anastomosis between the radial artery and the cephalic vein at the wrist of the nondominant hand, although several variants have been described. At surgery, under local anesthesia, the radial artery and cephalic vein are mobilized and anastomosed in one of several different configurations (Fig. 1). This fistula is associated with the longest useful patency and lowest rates of infection, and is the least likely to thrombose. The fistula is unobtrusive and does not interfere with patient activities. It does, however, require an artery large enough to support a high rate of blood flow, and veins that will arterialize and dilate. It also takes about 3 to 5 weeks from the time of fistula construction for maturation of the veins into large, thick-walled vessels that can be repeatedly and reliably punctured. During this period, dialysis may be maintained with use of a Scribner shunt, central venous cannulation, or by peritoneal dialysis.

The Cimino fistula may function for a long time. Eventually, though, it fails due to sclerosis of the veins as a result of repeated venipunctures or following renal transplant, when biochemical changes restore coagulation to normal.

Vascular Grafts (Bridge Fistulas)

Vascular substitutes are used in access surgery when suitable arteries or veins are not available for the construction of a standard peripheral AV fistula. There can be several reasons for this: (1) the peripheral vessels have already been used for

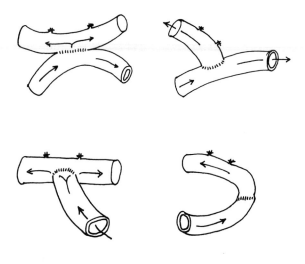

Figure 1. Various configurations for a Brescia-Cimino fistula between the radial artery and the basilic vein at the wrist.

previous access procedures; (2) the peripheral veins have been rendered unusable by drug abuse or intravenous therapy; (3) severe peripheral vascular disease exists, especially in diabetics; and (4) obesity with inadequate superficial veins.

These fistulas take on various configurations. If the vein and artery are close to each other, the bridge material may run in a loop or lie in a U configuration. If the artery and vein are some distance apart, the bridge graft lies in a straight or curved line (Fig. 2). Bridge fistulas can be placed between almost any suitably sized superficial artery and vein in the body. After implantation, these easily palpable conduits can be readily punctured by needles for dialysis (thus, they do not require suitable veins for arterialization, and are more widely applicable). Location of the fistula in the arm is almost always the first choice (traditionally between the radial artery and cephalic or basilic vein, or between the brachial artery and cephalic or basilic vein), because there is a lower risk of infection and distal limb ischemia.

Expanded polytetrafluoroethylene (PTFE) is the most commonly used material today for bridge fistulas.[5] These grafts do not require preclotting. They are widely available, easily inserted, easily thrombectomized or recanalized (with reasonable patency), and they have a moderate resistance to infection and a low incidence of aneurysm formation.[6,7] The usual graft diameter is 6 to 8 mm, although tapered grafts are often preferred in order to minimize graft-vessel mismatch.

Complications

Complications associated with AV access are the most common cause of hospitalization for patients on long-term hemodialysis.[8,9] Preservation of access sites is of paramount importance as patients are being carried on hemodialysis for longer periods (almost 50% at 5 years).[5] Understandably, vascular access has been referred to as the "Achilles' heel of the hemodialysis patient."[10] The most common complication is partial or complete obstruction of the access blood flow due to thrombosis or vascular stenosis; these account for over 80% of all complications (Fig. 3).[5] Less common complications include, aneurysm and pseudoaneurysm formation, steal syndrome, distal extremity edema, high-output congestive heart failure, and infection.

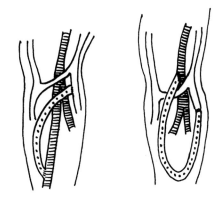

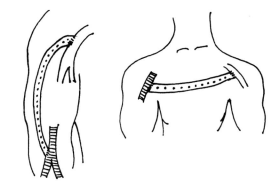

Figure 2. Examples of configurations for bridge fistulas using polytetrafluoroethylene (PTFE) or other graft materials.

While the conventional approach to stenotic accesses is an interventional radiology procedure of some sort, usually a percutaneous transluminal balloon angioplasty, the results are seldom durable (Fig. 4)[5,11–13] Post-percutaneous transluminal angioplasty (PTA) adjuncts have also had very little impact on the dismal natural history of this process. With over 200,000 patients on hemodialysis in the United States alone, there is an acute need for more effective therapy. There is a growing recognition that the post-PTA process is essentially a growth disorder (with a striking resemblance to a neoplastic process, especially when one considers the biology at a molecular level [Fig. 5]), and this new paradigm forms the basis for the use of ionizing radiation in this setting.[14,15]

Following the reported success of Liermann et al using high dose rate endovascular brachytherapy in the femoral arteries, attempts were made to duplicate their results in the U.S. One of the first endovascular experiences was reported by Waksman et al from Emory University (Atlanta, GA). Their pilot study included a number of patients with compromised dialysis accesses. After a successful intervention, a high dose rate remote afterloader was used to deliver 14 Gy, prescribed to the "adventitia." Eighteen lesions, including some subclavian stenoses, were treated. At a mean of 44-weeks follow-up, 61% of the lesions were still patent. One subclavian lesion showed a suggestion of a pseudoaneurysm formation, probably as a result of an eccentric catheter lie resulting in inadvertent overdosing of the inner wall of the vein. This data has been reported only in ab-

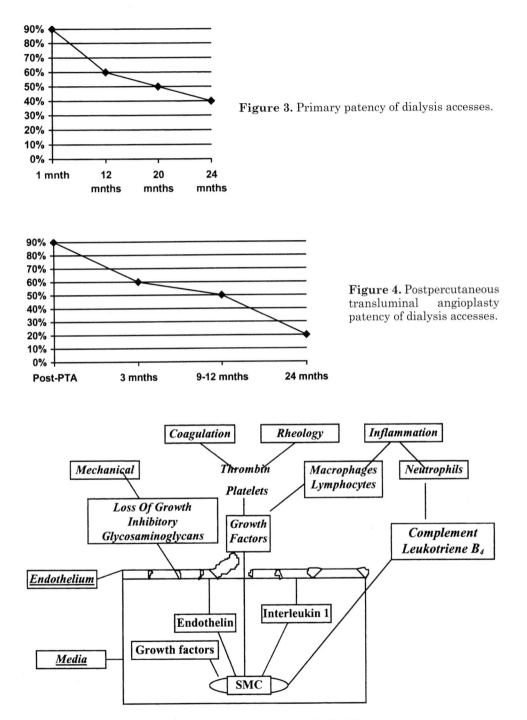

Figure 3. Primary patency of dialysis accesses.

Figure 4. Postpercutaneous transluminal angioplasty patency of dialysis accesses.

Figure 5. Stimuli to the medial smooth muscle cell (SMC) following percutaneous transluminal angioplasty (PTA).

stract form[16]; details about the exact dose prescription (how was the "adventitial" dose prescription point determined?), post-procedure dosimetry, adequacy of margins, etc., are rather sketchy. Also, there have been no further reports on this patient cohort regarding any possible late complications from the therapy. Another report describes a similar endovascular approach for the sequential treatment of two separate lesions in the subclavian vein of a single patient–a durable response was observed up to 15 months.[17] One of the potential problems in vascular radiotherapy is the danger of using a "one size fits all"approach. Thus, while the basic pathophysiological mechanism of restenosis may be similar in the coronary arteries, the peripheral arteries, and the dialysis accesses, there are several features that are specific to each site.

Pathophysiology of Access Failure

There is surprisingly little literature available on the actual pathology and pathogenesis of access failures. Most of the information has been extrapolated from the examination of failed vein grafts in the coronary or peripheral arterial circulation.[15,18] There are some basic conceptual problems with this approach; significant anatomic and physiological differences exist between arteries and veins (Tables 1 and 2), and a vein segment that has been harvested to use as a vascular graft at a distant site may behave quite differently from a vein that is left in situ without significant alteration in its blood supply (as is the case with the dialysis accesses). Also, while it is true that the basic underlying process is probably one of fibrointimal hyperplasia (FIH), the access lesions differ from the arterial lesions in terms of the initiating stimuli and the composition of the lesion. Restenosis in the arterial tree is triggered by the angioplasty "injury." It is this "trauma" that is believed to be responsible for the initiation of a series of events that culminate in the activation of the medial smooth muscle cell (SMC), which then proliferates and migrates to form the neointimal lesion of restenosis.[18] Thus, in the arterial system there is no ongoing stimulus to the SMC, apart from the PTA injury, and any therapeutic modality that inhibits the SMC activation/proliferation in the immediate

Table 1		
Anatomic Differences between Arteries and Veins		
	Vein	Artery
Endothelial cells	Larger, thinner, less firmly anchored to subendothelium	Smaller, thicker, more firmly anchored to the subendothelium
Tunica intima	More permeable	Less permeable
Internal elastic lamina	Poorly defined	Well defined
Media	Thin	Thick
Elastic lamellae	Absent	Present
Medial smooth muscle cells	Few, circular and longitudinal in arrangement, widely separated by collagen	Circular arrangement, orderly array with collagen, elastic fibers and matrix
Vasa vasorum	More anastomoses	Fewer anastomoses
Valves	Present	Absent

Table 2

Physiologic Differences between Arteries and Veins

	Vein	Artery
Elasticity	Relatively inelastic at arterial pressures	Elastic at arterial pressures
Role of collagen	Inconsequential	Important
Lipolysis	Slower	More rapid
Lipid uptake	Rapid	Slower
Lipid synthesis	More active	Less active
Prostacyclin production	Less	More
Endothelium	Stimulatory to smooth muscle cell contraction	Inhibitory to smooth muscle cell contraction
Vasoconstrictors	More sensitive	Less sensitive
Vasodilators	Less sensitive	More sensitive

postangioplasty period is likely to result in durable inhibition of restenosis. The situation in compromised accesses is quite different.[15] Altered local hemodynamics, with the resultant stresses on the vein wall, play a major role in access compromise. Turbulent blood flow, increased intraluminal pressures, and cyclical stretching of the vein wall in association with the arterial pulse, shear stresses, and mismatched compliances are all very important in the pathogenesis of access compromise.[19-27] Even more important is the fact that all of these factors continue to act at the anastomosis distinct from the angioplasty injury, and thus constitute a continuous, ongoing stimulus to FIH. This fits in well with the recent observation by Lumsden et al,[28] who studied the pathophysiology of access compromise in PTFE grafts. They found convincing evidence of chronic platelet activation in these patients, as evidenced by elevation of serum platelet factor 4 and β-thromboglobulin. They also found overexpression of the ligand-induced binding sites on the Gp IIb/IIIa receptor (indicative of stimulation of individual platelets) and increased thrombin generation, as measured by serum fibrinopeptide-A and thrombin/antithrombin complexes. They concluded that " . . . *significant platelet deposition continues to occur in chronically implanted PTFE grafts.*"[28] Apart from the platelet interaction with the PTFE graft, the extracorporeal circulation through the dialysis circuit is another important mechanism of chronic platelet activation in these patients.

The access lesions may also differ in composition. While the SMC forms the bulk of the postangioplasty restenotic lesion, extracellular matrix (ECM) forms a significant component of the occlusive neointimal hyperplastic lesions in the PTFE grafts. Further indications of the importance of the ECM come from the demonstration of tenascin in the neointima, especially in the luminal layer.[29] The tenascins are a family of large multimeric ECM proteins consisting of repeated structural modules including heptad repeats, epidermal growth factor (EGF)-like repeats, fibronectin type III repeats, and a globular domain shared with the fibrinogens.[30] Of the three tenascins, tenascin-C, -R, and -X, tenascin-C is prominent during tissue remodeling and is linked to cell migration, proliferation, and apoptosis. There is also evidence that the induction of tenascin may be critical to growth factor-dependent SMC proliferation. Thus, strategies aimed at inhibiting the ECM formation and/or tenascin expression may play an important role in preserving the dialysis accesses.

Postangioplasty Adjuvants

As in the coronaries and in other parts of the arterial tree, pharmacological adjuvants have had little, if any, impact on the natural history of post-PTA hemodialysis accesses. However, unlike in the arterial circulation, where stents have had a positive impact,[31] stents have not been proven beneficial to these post-PTA patients.[32] Thus, while stents may help the interventional radiologist by improving the immediate post-PTA patency rates in difficult venous lesions (resistant and/or residual stenoses, long segments, central venous stenosis, etc), they have had little impact on long-term patency in this setting.[33] There may be several reasons for this. One of the main mechanisms by which stents help in the arterial system is by acting as an "internal scaffolding" and preventing negative remodeling (this is the late lumen loss as a result of "circumferential constriction" of the arterial wall, quite akin to the phenomenon of wound contracture). It is not clear if this negative remodeling plays a significant role in the setting of the dialysis accesses, due to anatomic/structural differences between a muscular coronary artery and the vein/PTFE graft of the access. On the other hand, it is well known that stents do cause an increase in the neointimal proliferation as a result of the "chronic" injury to the vessel wall by the stent struts.[34] Thus, while the advantage of preventing negative remodeling outweighs the increase in neointima in the coronaries (resulting in an absolute reduction in the post-PTA restenosis rate by approximately 15%), in the dialysis accesses the problem of increased neointimal proliferation outweighs any possible short-term gains, such that long-term patency rates with stents are less than 20% at 2 years.[33] Differences in the structure of the vein wall—especially after it has been subjected chronically to turbulent, high-pressure flows and to relatively low flow states (which further increase the neointima formation)—may further contribute to the dismal results that are seen with venous stenting. This distinction is of more than mere academic importance. There is some evidence to suggest that post-PTA external beam radiotherapy may actually worsen the negative remodeling while still inhibiting the neointimal hyperplasia in the arteries.[35] However, if negative remodeling is not an important pathophysiological mechanism in access restenosis, external beam radiotherapy may be a simple and valid therapeutic option in this setting.

Potential Problems with Endovascular Brachytherapy in Arteriovenous Fistulas

Lesion Topography

In the coronary arteries, post-PTA restenosis develops on a background of atherosclerotic disease. These lesions are almost always eccentric and have a substantial intramural component; as a result, the arterial wall thickness varies widely along the circumference of the vessel.[36,37] These lesions are also short, usually less than 3 to 4 cm in length (although longer lesions and diffuse disease can be seen, especially in diabetics). As compared to this, the venous limb of the dialysis access is inherently normal and is subjected to high (but uniformly high) circumferential, pulsatile pressures. The venous stenosis is therefore more often concentric, with little, if any, intramural plaque. As a result of this, one would expect a more uniform thickness around the circumference of the "diseased" vein. The venous lesions can also be quite long (several centimeters), and tandem, and multiple lesions are not uncommon.[38]

Need for Source Centering

Most of the early studies in the peripheral arteries and the coronaries did not use any special mechanism to ensure that the source was centered in the vessel lumen. The coronary arteries have an average diameter of 3 to 3.5 mm. Also, as discussed above, the plaque is quite eccentric; thus, even if the source is centered with respect to the lumen, the actual target (ie, the vessel wall) would be at varying distances from the source. Last, the source is constantly being subjected to a pulsatile blood flow, a feature that has been claimed to minimize the effects of an eccentric lie. Despite these theoretical issues, eccentric plaques can result in very high doses to small areas of the intima that actually come in contact with the catheter.

The issue of centering becomes very important when endovascular brachytherapy is used in the dialysis accesses—and even more so when it is used post-PTA in the central veins. The average diameter of the vein/graft junction, or the outflow vein, is approximately 6 to 8 mm (the subclavian vein can measure 12 mm or even more). Given the absence of an intraluminal or intramural plaque, the centering catheter would truly be able to center the source, not only in relation to the lumen but also with respect to the target layer of the vessel. Also, as discussed above, the lesions can be several centimeters long and the blood flow through the vein is slower and nonlaminar when compared to that through a comparable sized artery. In the absence of a centering system, these factors greatly increase the likelihood of non-homogeneous dose distribution, both along the long axis and in the radial direction along the circumference of the vein (Fig. 6).

Choice of Isotope

There is an ongoing discussion about the ideal isotope for endovascular brachytherapy. Radiation protection issues and the ability to perform the procedure in an unmodified catheterization laboratory make the beta isotopes a very attractive choice: the Beta-Cath Study, which evaluates the ^{90}Sr source in a double-blinded, randomized fashion, will provide an answer to the therapeutic efficacy of the beta source in the intracoronary setting. In the larger vessels, including the femoropopliteal arteries, in the dialysis accesses, and especially in the larger central veins, gamma emitters such as ^{192}Ir are probably preferable. The main reason for this is the less rapid fall-off of dose with distance from the source. While this allows us to prescribe the dose at a greater distance from the source, the radial dose fall-off is also less, thus providing a safety margin in case the source is not perfectly centered in the lumen. If we assume a 6-mm-diameter vessel (the average diameter of the access graft or the femoral artery), have a centered source, and prescribe 14 Gy to a depth of 2 mm within the vessel wall, the dose at the luminal surface

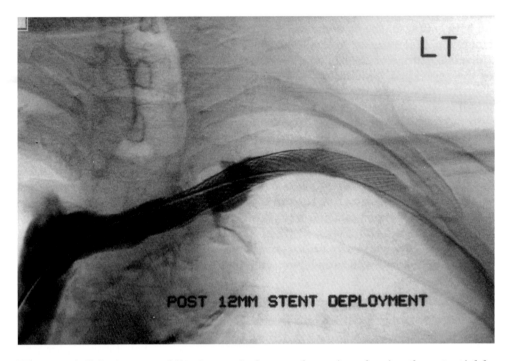

Figure 6. A dialysis access, following angioplasty and stenting, showing the potential for dose inhomogeneity if an endovascular radiation approach is used without a centering device.

and at a depth of 1 mm would be 24.15 Gy and 17.77 Gy, respectively, with use of an ^{192}Ir high-dose–rate afterloader. With use of a ^{90}Sr source, doses at the same depths would be as high as 30 Gy and 65 Gy, respectively; in this setting, the dose with ^{90}Sr at a distance of 2 mm from the source would be as high as 140 Gy–this could be a real issue with even the least bit of off-center catheter positioning (Fig. 7)! Of course, external beam radiotherapy would give the most uniform longitudinal, circumferential, and radial dose with a very precise dosimetry.

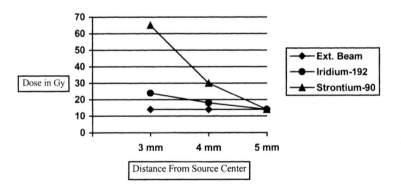

Figure 7. Radial dose variation with different approaches to irradiation of a 6-mm-diameter access. (Centered source employed; dose of 14 Gy prescribed at 5 mm from source center.)

Expectations from Vascular
Radiotherapy in the Dialysis Accesses

With a better understanding of the chronic proliferative stimuli to which the vein/PTFE graft is subjected, it may be unrealistic to expect a pulsed intervention like post-PTA radiotherapy to cure the patient of the restenosis problem. Borrowing some of the oncological terminology, a more reasonable expectation from post-PTA radiotherapy for these "malignant" restenosis may be a significant prolongation of the "disease-free interval," ie, a significant prolongation of the time to the next episode of access compromise. Given that over 40,000 patients undergo at least one access revision each year, and that these patients undergo up to 15 days of hospitalization per year for access-related complications, this would still be a very substantial achievement.

This concept, however, leads to the very important issues of re-treatment and radiation tolerance. If the main goal of radiation therapy is to delay the onset of restenosis, we must consider the possibility of re-treating these patients at a subsequent episode of access compromise. It is important to consider this issue while designing any clinical trial, especially when most laboratory and clinical trials either have a dose escalation protocol or employ a dose that is supposedly the highest possible "safe" dose. Basic radiation therapy principles, as well as the need for safe re-treatment, make it essential for us to determine the lowest possible dose that is compatible with durable freedom from restenosis.[39] Endovascular brachytherapy is again at a disadvantage in this setting; even if the prescribed dose is "low," an ^{192}Ir-based system will deliver almost twice as much to the intima, while a beta emitter like ^{90}Sr will give close to four times the prescribed dose to the intima. Radiation tolerance, or late tissue complication probability, also raises the issue of dose fractionation, since, if it were delivered in multiple fractions, a much higher total dose could be delivered with the same late side effects. Again, it is difficult to conceive of an endovascular approach that would allow us to do this. All of these issues can be very easily and effectively addressed by an external beam radiotherapy program.[40]

External Beam Radiotherapy for
Arteriovenous Fistulas

New York Hospital Medical Center of Queens Pilot Study

Ten patients were treated in a Phase I study with fractionated external beam radiotherapy as described below. Entry to the study was limited to patients aged 55 years or older who had a currently compromised access, as evidenced by angiography or a thrombosed access site. All the patients had an adequate angioplasty with/without prior thrombolysis, prior to the institution of the radiotherapy. History of prior radiation to the area to be treated or a history of collagen vascular disorders were absolute exclusion criteria.

Five of the 10 patients had at least one prior access, which had ceased to function. Five of the 10 patients had one or more recanalization procedures performed on the current access. The interval from the last intervention ranged from 2 1/2 to 14 months. The length of the stenosis ranged from 2 to 9 cm, with a median of

5 cm. All patients had a successful angioplasty; 3 patients required placement of a stent to optimize the angioplasty results.

Following angioplasty, the interventional radiologist marked the proximal and distal extents of the dilated segment on the skin for radiation therapy planning. Estimate of the depth of the access from the skin was made by clinical palpation (since most of these are subcutaneous) and by taking an orthogonal film with a graduated radio-opaque marker on the skin. After all the interventional hardware was withdrawn and hemostasis was achieved, the patient was discharged to the Department of Radiation Oncology. The radiation therapy target volume was defined as the angiographic target lesion plus a 1-cm margin, in keeping with standard radiation therapy principles. An appropriate electron energy was selected by a computerized treatment planning system such that the 90% isodose covered the target volume in all dimensions. Seven patients were treated with 9 MeV electrons, while the other 3 were treated with 12 MeV electrons because of a concern that the proximal portion of the target volume (near the axilla) was a little deeper.

As per the U.S. Food and Drug Administration (FDA) mandates, the first 5 patients were treated with 8 Gy. The second group of 5 patients received 12 Gy since that was the nominal dose used in the German arterial study without any complications. Based on in vitro and animal data, the radiation dose was delivered in two equal fractions with the first fraction being delivered immediately post angioplasty and the second fraction after 48 hours, ie, on day 2. Follow-up included evaluation of the efficacy of dialysis by recirculation and venous pressure measurements, as well as an anatomic evaluation of the fistula by fistulograms, at 3-, 6-, and 12-month intervals. The patients also have a long-term follow-up in the Department of Radiation Oncology to monitor any possible late side effects from the radiation therapy. The implementation of the protocol was easy and there were no procedure-related complications. At a median follow-up of 6 months, 4 patients developed restenosis, 3 at the site of the original target lesion and 1 at the edge of an implanted stent. In keeping with the natural history of this process, new lesions developed in 5 patients. Unfortunately, with a longer follow-up, all patients had restenosed by 18 months.[41,42] This lack of durability is probably a reflection of the patient population as well as the fairly low dose that was used.

Taiwan Study

Kuan et al[43] reported on 20 patients with at least two previous episodes of access compromise. These were randomized to PTA alone or PTA followed by external beam radiotherapy to a dose to 1500 cGy in three daily fractions. The radiated group showed a 2-month prolongation in mean access patency time, a difference that was marginally statistically significant even with the small number of patients.

Temple University Study

Cohen et al[44] reported on the efficacy of low-dose external beam irradiation in 31 patients with 41 lesions in their dialysis shunts. Seven had native arteriovenous fistulas, and 24 had PTFE grafts. The stenoses were either venous outflow stenoses (68%) or central stenoses (32%). The patients were randomized to PTA and/or stent placement alone (n=15), or to the same intervention followed by external beam irradiation (n=16 patients; 21 lesions). A cobalt 60 unit was used to deliver 14 Gy in two 7 Gy fractions; the first fraction was delivered within 24 hours of the intervention, and the second fraction within the next 24 hours. The restenosis rate at 6 months was 45% in the irradiated group and 67% in the control group. However, the patient population was very heterogenous and the patients were not stratified by risk factors (patients with peripheral venous and subclavian stenoses were not separated; similarly, there was no distinction made between the patients who required stenting and those who did not). There are also several issues regarding adequacy of margins, as well as the actual implementation of the radiation therapy (since the patients were planned with the arm in a different position from what it was during the actual treatment). There was no failure analysis to define the contribution of these treatment-related factors to the incidence of target lesion failures.[45] Further studies in a larger and more homogenous population are needed to really assess the benefit of external beam irradiation in this setting.

Why Did These Early Studies "Fail"?

Whether radiation therapy is delivered in one fraction, or as a fractionated regimen, the biologically effective dose (BED) is expressed as:

$$BED = D\left(1 + \frac{d}{\alpha/\beta}\right)$$

When one considers the BEDs as outlined in the Table 3, it is not surprising that Parikh et al[42] did not observe any significant benefit from the low doses of 4 Gy × 2 and 6 Gy × 2, and the Taiwan study observed only marginally positive results with 5 Gy × 3, while Cohen et al observed marginally positive results with

Table 3

Examples of Biologically Effective Doses (BED)
Used in Vascular Radiotherapy Studies

	BED (Acute–"Efficacy")	BED (Late–"Side Effects")
20 Gy × 1 (START) β radiation	60	153.33
18 Gy × 1 (BetaCath) β radiation	50.4	126
16 Gy × 1 (START) β radiation	41.6	101.33
15 Gy × 1 (WRIST) γ radiation	37.5	90
14 Gy × 1 (BetaCath) β radiation	33.6	80
7 Gy × 3 (RENAL Study)	35.7	70
8 Gy × 2 (RENAL Study)	28.8	58.6
7 Gy × 2 (Cohen et al)	23.8	46.6
5 Gy × 3 (Kwan et al)	22.5	40
6 Gy × 2 (Parikh, Nori et al)	19.2	36
4 Gy × 2 (Parikh, Nori et al)	11.2	18.6

BED = biologically effective doses.

7 Gy × 2. The consistently positive results in the coronary/peripheral arterial studies have all been obtained with doses in the range of 12 to 14 Gy. These are prescribed doses, delivered at a depth in the vessel wall, with the inner layers of the vessel wall actually getting even higher doses. Based on the BED analysis, doses of 8 Gy × 2 daily fractions and 7 Gy × 3 daily fractions may be equivalent to these brachytherapy doses (Table 3). These doses have a BED (acute) equivalent to brachytherapy doses of 12 to 14 Gy, while the BED (late) is actually less than that with the brachytherapy doses (ie, these doses should result in less late tissue changes when compared to brachytherapy).[46] Based on this, we have obtained FDA approval to initiate the RENAL (Radiation to ExteNd Access Life) Study. This will incorporate an initial dose-escalation phase in which 20 patients will be treated to a dose of 8 Gy × 2, and the next 20 patients will receive 7 Gy × 3. This will be followed by a randomized, multi-institutional study.

There are several other ongoing studies in this area evaluating the efficacy of external beam radiotherapy in prolonging access patency. Thus, New York-Presbyterian Hospital (New York, NY) has an ongoing Phase I study on patients with de novo AV grafts. Two weeks post surgery, patients have a baseline venogram and 4 weeks post surgery the patients are treated to either a single dose of 8 Gy, or two fractions of 8 Gy each (on consecutive days), using electrons. Twenty patients will be enrolled in this study. Duke University (Durham, NC) has a similar dose-finding Phase I study testing a single fraction of 8 or 10 Gy in the de novo setting with the radiation scheduled to be delivered 1 to 3 days post surgery. Levendag et al (personal communication) are conducting a double-blinded, randomized study using two daily fractions of 9 Gy each versus no further treatment. The study is still under accrual.

Summary and Conclusions

There are several unique issues involved in radiation therapy to dialysis accesses. Given the uncertainties of the dose prescription point, the need for centering an endovascular source, and the smaller margin of safety with the beta sources, it is likely that any endovascular approach would have to be based on a gamma-emitting isotope such as ^{192}Ir. This approach has its own logistical problems. Radiation safety would be an issue if the procedure were to be done in the interventional suite; furthermore, this would preclude the use of a remote high dose rate afterloader. On the other hand, if the radiation was to be delivered in the radiation oncology suite, there would be important issues related to patient transportation with intravascular catheters in place, infection potential, etc. Also, endovascular approaches would have the inherent problem of a radial dose gradient across the vessel wall, and it is difficult to conceive of an endovascular approach that would allow us to vary the timing of the radiation therapy (in relation to the PTA) or allow for fractionation of the radiation dose.

External beam radiation therapy with electrons offers an easy answer to most of these problems. It is simple, noninvasive, and universally applicable in the community. The dosimetry is very well established and a precise, uniform dose can be delivered to any segment of the vein or graft without any worry about axial, radial, or longitudinal dose inhomogeneity. The timing of the radiation can be varied in relation to the angioplasty in keeping with available information on post-PTA cell kinetics. Similarly, dose fractionation is easy and may allow us to deliver a higher dose (if required) for a given level of late side effects. The question of integral dose has often been raised as a problem with external beam therapy. Among the different vascular sites being treated with post-PTA radiation, the dialysis accesses are uniquely suited for external beam therapy because of their very superficial location, usually just beneath the skin. This allows us to use a low electron energy (9 MeV in most cases). Even if the integral dose is slightly higher, the advantages listed above, including the absence of a radial dose gradient (with consequent "overdosing" of the intima), make this a very attractive approach for access compromise. The only disadvantage is the inability to treat central venous stenosis—endovascular approaches using a gamma emitter and centering catheters would be required for adequate treatment at these sites.

Acknowledgments: The authors gratefully acknowledge the assistance of Adrian Osian, MS, Huili Wang, PhD, and Albert Sabbas, PhD (Radiation Physics, New York Hospital Medical Center of Queens, and New York Hospital-Cornell Medical Center) in helping with the dosimetry data.

References

1. Kumpe DA, Cohen MAH. Angioplasty/thrombolytic treatment of failing/failed hemodialysis access sites: Comparison with surgical treatment. Prog Cardiovasc Dis 1992;34(4):263–278.
2. Quinton WE, Dillard D, Scribner BH. Cannulation of blood vessels for prolonged hemodialysis. Trans Am Soc Artif Intern Organs 1960;6:104–113.
3. Chazan JA, London MR, Pono LM, et al. Long-term survival of vascular access in a chronic hemodialysis population. Nephron 1995;69:228–233.
4. Brescia MJ, Cimino J, Appel K, et al. Chronic hemodialysis using venipuncture and a surgically created arteriovenous fistula. N Engl J Med 1966;275:1089–1092.
5. Kherlakian GM, Rodersheimer LR, Arbaugh JJ, et al. Comparison of autogenous fistula versus expanded polytetrafluoroethylene graft fistula for angioaccess in hemodialysis. Am J Surg 1986;152:238–243.
6. Haimov M, Burrows L, Shanzer H. Experience with arterial substitutes in the construction of vascular access for hemodialysis. J Cardiovasc Surg 1980;21:149.
7. Valji K, Bookstein JJ, Roberts AC. Pharmacomechanical thrombolysis and angioplasty in the management of clotted hemodialysis grafts: Early and late clinical results. Radiology 1991;178:243–247.
8. Wilson SE. Complications of vascular access procedures. In: Wilson SE, Owens ML (eds.): Vascular Access Surgery. Chicago, IL: Yearbook Medical; 1980:185–207.
9. Swedberg SH, Brown BG, Sigley R. Intimal fibromuscular hyperplasia at the venous anastomosis of PTFE grafts in hemodialysis patients. Circulation 1989;80:1726–1736.
10. Kjellstrand C. The Achilles' heel of the dialysis patient. Arch Intern Med 1978;138:1063.
11. Munda R, First RF, Alexander JW. PTFE graft survival in hemodialysis. JAMA 1983;249(2):219–222.
12. Tordoir JHM, Herman JMMPH, Kwan TS. Long term followup of PTFE prosthesis as an arteriovenous fistula for hemodialysis. Eur J Vasc Surg 1987;2:3–7.
13. Jenkins AM, Buist TAS, Glover SD, et al. Medium term followup of forty autogenous and forty PTFE grafts for vascular access. Surgery 1980;88(5):667–672.
14. Nori D, Parikh S, Moni J. Management of peripheral vascular disease: Innovative approaches using radiation therapy. Int J Radiat Oncol Biol Phys 1996;36(4):847–856.
15. Parikh S, Nori D. Endovascular brachytherapy: Current status and future trends. J Brachytherapy International 1997;13:167.
16. Waksman R, Crocker IR, Lumsden AB, et al. Long term results of endovascular radiation therapy for prevention of restenosis in the peripheral vascular system. Circulation 1996;94(suppl):I–300.
17. Wong F, Kwok P, Ngan R, et al. Prevention of restenosis of central venous stricture after percutaneous transluminal angioplasty and endovascular stenting by brachytherapy. Kidney Int 1999;55:724–732.
18. Cox JL, Chiasson DA, Gotlieb AL. Stranger in a strange land: The pathogenesis of

saphenous vein graft stenosis with emphasis on structural and functional differences between veins and arteries. Prog Cardiovasc Dis 1991;34:45–59.

19. Rittgers SE, Karayannacos PE, Guy JF. Velocity distribution and intimal proliferation in autologous vein grafts in dogs. Circ Res 1978;42:792–801.

20. Leung DY, Glasgov S, Mathews MB. Cyclic stretching stimulates synthesis of matrix components by arterial smooth muscle cells in vitro. Science 1976;191:475–477.

21. Boerboom LE, Olinger GE, Tie-Zhu L. Histologic, morphologic and biochemical evolution of vein bypass grafts in nonhuman primate model. III Long term changes and their modification with platelet inhibition by aspirin and dipyridamole. J Thorac Cardiovasc Surg 1990;99:426–432.

22. Dobrin P, Canfield T, Moran J. The physiological basis for differences in flow with internal mammary artery and saphenous vein grafts. J Thorac Cardiovasc Surg 1977;74:445–453.

23. Fujiwara T, Kajiya F, Kanazawa S. Comparison of blood-flow velocity waveforms in different coronary artery bypass grafts. Sequential saphenous vein grafts and internal mammary grafts. Circulation 1988;78:1210–1221.

24. LoGerfo FW, Soncrent T, Tell T. Boundary layer separation in models of side-to-end arterial anastomoses. Arch Surg 1979;114:1369–1373.

25. Ross R. The pathogenesis of atherosclerosis–An update. N Engl J Med 1986;314:488–500.

26. Clark RE, Apostoulou S, Kardos JL. Mismatch of mechanical properties as a cause of arterial prosthesis thrombosis. Surg Forum 1976;27:208–210.

27. Myhre HO, Halvorsen T. Intimal hyperplasia and secondary changes in vein grafts. Acta Chir Scand 1985;529(suppl):63–67.

28. Lumsden AB, MacDonald MJ, Chen C. Restenosis in peripheral vascular disease. In: Waksman R, King SB, Crocker IR, Mould RF (eds.): Vascular Brachytherapy. The Netherlands: Nucletron B.V.; 1996:258–265.

29. Chen C, Ku DN, Kikeri D, Lumsden AB. Tenascin: A potential role in human arteriovenous PTFE graft failure. J Surg Res 1996;60(2):409–416.

30. Chiquet-Ehrismann R. Tenascins, a growing family of extracellular matrix proteins. Experientia 1995;51(9–10):853–862.

31. Mintz G, Pichard A, Kent K, et al. Endovascular stents reduce restenosis by eliminating geometric arterial remodeling: A serial intravascular ultrasound study. J Am Coll Cardiol 1995;26:701–705.

32. Beathard GA. Gianturco self-expanding stent in the treatment of stenosis in dialysis access grafts. Kidney Int 1993;43:872–877.

33. Rogers D. Venous interventions in dialysis patients. Proceedings of The International Seminar On The Current Status Of Radiotherapy In The World: Brachytherapy In The Next Millennium. New York, NY: April 17–19, 1997.

34. Kimura T, Kaburagi S, Tashima Y, et al. Geometric remodeling and intimal regrowth as mechanisms of restenosis: Observations from the Serial Ultrasound Analysis of Restenosis (SURE) Trial. Circulation 1995;(92):I76.

35. Styles TJ, Marijianowski MMH, Robinson KA, et al. Effects of external irradiation of the heart on the coronary artery response to balloon angioplasty injury in pigs. Proceedings of The Advances In Cardiovascular Radiation Therapy Conference. Washington, DC: February 20–21, 1997.

36. Waller BF, Pinkerton CA, Orr CM, et al. Morphological observations late after clinically successful coronary balloon angioplasty. Circulation 1991;83:28–41.

37. Nobuyoshi M, Kimura T, Ohishi H, et al. Restenosis after percutaneous transluminal coronary angioplasty. Pathologic observations in 20 patients. J Am Coll Cardiol 1991;17:433–439.

38. Parikh S, Nori D. Prolonging the utility of dialysis accesses. Presented at: The International Seminar On The Current Status Of Radiotherapy In The World: Brachytherapy In The Next Millennium; April 17–19, 1997; New York, NY.

39. Rubin P. Personal communication.

40. Parikh S, Nori D. Radiation therapy to prevent stenosis of AV dialysis accesses. Semin Radiat Oncol 1999;9:144–154.

41. Parikh S, Nori D, Rogers D, et al. External beam radiation therapy to prevent postangioplasty dialysis access restenosis: A feasibility study. Cardiovasc Radiat Med 1999;1:36–41.

42. Nori D, Parikh S, et al. External beam radiotherapy to prevent post-angioplasty restenosis of compromised arterio-venous dialysis accesses: A Phase I Study. Int J Radiat Oncol Biol Phys 1998;42(suppl 1):347.

43. Kuan P, Chiang S, Liou J, et al. Effect of vascular access external beam radiation on prevention of restenosis. Proceedings of Cardiovascular Radiation Therapy III, Washington, DC, 1999.

44. Cohen GS, Freeman H, Ringold MA. External beam irradiation as an adjunctive treatment in failing dialysis shunts. JVIR 2000;11:321–326.

45. Parikh S, Nori D. Re: Cohen et al: External beam irradiation as an adjunctive treatment in failing dialysis shunts (Letter to the Editor). JVIR 2000;11:1364.

46. Nori D, Parikh S. Do we really need to invade foreign territories? Proceedings of The 5th Annual Conference on Vascular Brachytherapy, "Winning The Fight Against Restenosis," New York, NY, June 9, 2000.

Part VII

Imaging and Analysis

## Chapter 42

Quantitative Coronary Angiography Methodology in Vascular Brachytherapy I

Evelyn Regar, MD, Ken Kozuma, MD,
George Sianos, MD, Stephane G. Carlier, MD,
and Patrick W. Serruys, MD, PhD

Introduction

The application of intracoronary radioactivity represents a relatively new therapeutic tool for the cardiologist. Radioactivity is administered by various techniques, eg, intracoronary afterloading,[1–5] radioactive stents,[6–10] or radioactive balloons[11–13] using gamma- or beta-emitting sources. The particular physics, application modalities, and mechanisms of action of this new treatment modality force us to adapt the procedural practice and the methodological approach of angiographic outcome assessment.[14,15]

Recently, a number of phenomenons associated with intracoronary brachytherapy, such as positive remodeling,[16] relocation of the minimal lumen diameter (MLD),[17] geographic miss,[18] and edge effect[19] have been described. These entities have been recognized in the past; however, their incidence and their impact on clinical outcome has reached new and so far unknown dimensions. While, after standard balloon angioplasty, neointimal hyperplasia and vessel shrinkage at the site of injury is the usual response,[20,21] in balloon angioplasty followed by irradiation, an increase in the MLD at the treated segment is predominantly seen[16] as a result of positive remodeling and neointimal inhibition.[22] This systematic change in vessel response after brachytherapy prompts us to adapt new angiographic approaches, taking into account the relocation of MLD at follow-up from its pre-interventional location. Similarly, the growing knowledge of the deleterious effects of geographic miss and the awareness of possible edge effects underline the need for standardized and detailed angiographic assessment.

This chapter will review standard quantitative coronary analysis and describe the current approach for vascular brachytherapy.

Classical Quantitatitve Coronary Angiography Analysis

Quantitative coronary angiography (QCA) is the well-established gold standard for the assessment of coronary angiograms.[23] In classical QCA analysis, the

From Waksman R (ed.). *Vascular Brachytherapy, Third Edition.* Armonk, NY: Futura Publishing Co., Inc.; © 2002.

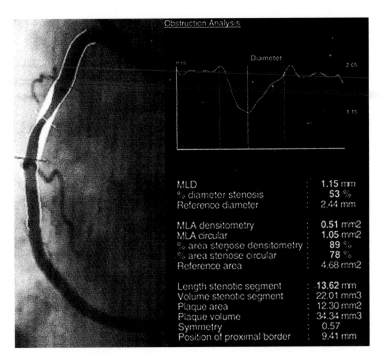

Figure 1. Classical quantitative coronary angiography (QCA) analysis. The analyst defines the vessel segment of interest bordered by major proximal and distal side branches. Minimal lumen diameter (MLD) and interpolated reference diameter (RD) at the site of MLD is calculated.

analyst defines the vessel segment of interest. Sophisticated edge detection algorithms define automatically the obstructed target segment. Within the target segment, MLD, interpolated reference diameter (RD), and diameter stenosis (DS) are calculated (Fig. 1).[24–28] Pre-interventional, post-interventional, and follow-up measurements are compared to analyze treatment efficacy in such terms as residual DS, acute lumen gain, late lumen loss, or dichotomous restenosis rate.[29–37]

Limitations of Classical Quantitative Coronary Angiography Analysis

Classical QCA analysis is comprehensive from a clinical perspective, as it detects reliably whether or not relevant lumen changes occurred in a previously treated vessel segment. From a scientific perspective, however, this method is of limited value: it fails to describe precisely the anatomic location of lumen changes, as it does not provide information on the topography of the MLD within the target vessel segment at the time of repetitive measurement. Recent studies after balloon angioplasty have demonstrated that changes in RD and in the anatomic position of the MLD occur during follow-up, invalidating direct comparison of quantitative parameters over time.[38] This "relocation" makes the direct comparison of MLD questionable.[39] The dynamic lumen changes have various causes such as plaque progression, unmasking of new lesions, or remodeling, and might be triggered intentionally by intervention or nonintentionally by periprocedural vessel injury. To overcome these problems, our group, over the last 15 years, has applied a strategy of analyzing a treated "vessel segment," rather than a focal spot representing the site of pre-interventional MLD. The treated "vessel segment" encompasses the culprit lesion and is defined in length by the most proximal and distal side branch. These side branches serve as reproducible landmarks for the follow-up analysis.[40] Similarly, the TOSCA group introduced the concept of "target lesion work length," defined as the length of contiguous target segment exposed to balloon inflation.[41] Thus, not only is the segment of the original angiographic lesion analyzed, but also the vessel segment over the entire treated length.

New Concepts of Angiographic Assessment on Brachytherapy

Principle of Dose-Based Segmental Assessment

Intracoronary radiation has complex and dose-dependent effects on arterial tissue.[42–50] It is usually used as an adjunctive therapeutic tool to other debulking and/or angioplasty devices. Thus, angiographic assessment must include radiation dose, proximal and distal vascular injury, and possible interactions of both (determinants of the edge effect), rather than the isolated target lesion. Based on these considerations, quantitative assessment of irradiated vessels should include different vessel segments, which are defined below (Fig. 2).

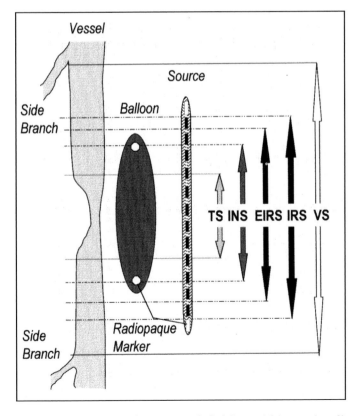

Figure 2. Schematic of dose-based segment definition within an irradiated coronary artery. TS = target segment; INS = injured segment; EIRS = effective irradiated segment; IRS = irradiated segment; VS = vessel segment.

Target Segment

The target segment is defined by the proximal and distal margin of the obstructed segment.

Injured Segment

The macroscopic injured segment is defined as the segment encompassed by the most proximal and most distal position of the angioplasty device (eg, rotablator burr) or marker of the angioplasty balloon as assessed by fluoroscopy.

Effective Irradiated Segment

The effective irradiated segment is the vessel segment receiving the full prescribed therapeutic radiation dose (>90% isodose rate). In catheter-based line sources, the length of this full radiation dose segment is slightly shorter than the distance between the radiopaque markers as a result of the dose fall-off caused by the limited size of the source train (Fig. 3). The dose-fall characteristics vary in different isotopes.

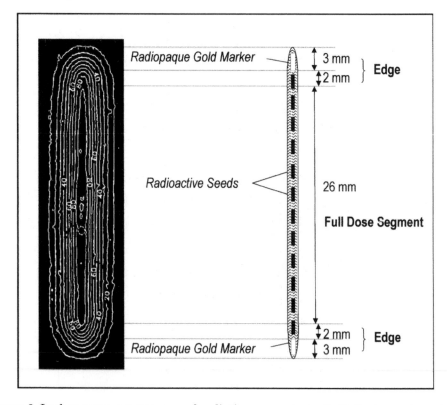

Figure 3. Isodose rate contour map and radiation source train. **Left:** Isodose rate contour map measured at a depth of 1.89 mm (contour intervals: 10 mGy/s) as described by the National Institute of Standards and Technology. The depth (1.89 mm) illustrates an isodose model to resemble the radius of a coronary artery. Longitudinal dose fall-off may be extrapolated from this graphic. **Right:** Radiation source train (Beta-Cath, Novoste Corp.). The central part receives an approximately full radiation dose.

Similarly, the effective irradiated segment is slightly shorter than the stent length in radioactive stents, because of the dose fall-off at the extremities of the stent, involving the most proximal and the most distal stent struts. The length of the fall-off zone varies as it is dependent on isotope and stent design. Furthermore, the dose profile is not homogeneous, but peaks behind every individual strut. This effect varies depending on the distance and the angle of observation.

Irradiated Segment

In practice, the exact delineation of the effective irradiated segment is complicated, as it requires the knowledge of the individual dose profiles for each isotope and source design. Correction for the dose fall-off at the extremities of the irradiated segment is a matter of a few millimeters. Exact length measurement, however, is often hampered by the anatomy of the artery and foreshortening.

For these practical reasons, quantitative analysis is performed on an *irradiated segment,* which is defined as the segment encompassed by the inner edge of the radiopaque markers of the source train or the length of the radioactive stent.

Edge Segments

Edge segments are the vessel segments at the extremities of the radiation source (catheter-based source, radioactive stent, or balloon), which do not receive the full therapeutic radiation dose. The lengths of the edge segments are dependent on the isodose profile of the individual source.

Geographic Miss Segment

In coronary brachytherapy, this is defined as a mismatch between injured and irradiated segment: geographic miss is present when the entire length of the injured segment is not completely covered by the irradiated segment.

Vessel Segment

The vessel segment is the coronary segment bordered by angiographically visible side branches which encompass the original lesion, all angioplasty devices, and the radiation source.

Image Acquisition and Procedural Implications

In order to allow for such detailed analysis, image acquisition and angiographic documentation need to be performed in an accurate and standardized fashion. Angiography should be done in biplane views at a frame rate of 25 frames per second. The electrocardiogram (ECG) tracing must be visible on screen. Before each angiogram, nitrates should be administered by intracoronary infusion. Each angiogram should be performed at mid-inspiration. The empty (guiding) catheter[51] should be documented for calibration, preferably near the center of the screen. At the start of the procedure, two projections should be selected with more than 30 degrees celsius difference in rotation and avoiding foreshortening and side branch overlapping. The entire procedure should be filmed in identical projections. Any instrumentation (eg, balloons or stents) should be filmed at the site of treatment surrounded by contrast medium in identical projections. The radioactive source should be filmed in place with contrast medium repeating the same projections. Follow-up angiography must performed using the same imaging projections, same contrast medium at 37°C, and documentation of the unfilled catheter. Again, intracoronary nitrates should be administered before each angiogram.

The meticulous documentation of all angioplasty devices and the radiation source using the same projections is essential. Inadequate angiographic documentation of the procedure, hampering proper angiographic assessment of geographic miss, is seen in up to 50% of the cases enrolled in brachytherapy trials.

Angiographic Analysis of Brachytherapy

Qualitative Assessment

The introduction the concept of "geographic miss," originating from radiation oncology,[52] into the scenario of intracoronary brachytherapy stressed the importance of assessment of the injured segment in relation to the radiation source.

To assess whether geographic miss is present or not, multiple angiographic loops and ECG-matched still frames should be displayed simultaneously, side by side, on the screen (eg, Rubo Medical Imaging, Uithoorn, The Netherlands). This approach allows definition of the location of the various subsegments (irradiated segment, injured segment, edges) in relation to side branches, and the correct matching of the angiograms. By identifying the relationship between the irradiated segment and its edges relative to the injured segment, the occurrence of geographic miss can be determined (Fig. 4). Using this method, the agreement rate of two independent cardiologists is as high as 90%.

The procedure should be considered as not interpretable in the following cases: (a) lack of correct filming with the radiation source and the balloons deflated with contrast injection, so as to allow the location of the irradiated segment, injured segment, and the edges in relation to anatomic landmarks; (b) more than 10 degrees difference in the angiographic projections, not allowing for correct matching; (c) interventions reported in the technician's worksheet, but not filmed.

Quantitative Coronary Analysis

Dedicated analysis software (CAAS II System; Pie Medical, Maastricht, The Netherlands) allows for simultaneous assessment of the different segments. By displaying an angiographic sequence showing the lesion pre-intervention, positions of angioplasty devices, and radiation source simultaneously on a screen, the analyst indicates the different analysis segments according to the location of the angioplasty devices and radiation source relative to the original lesion (Fig. 5). The proximal (or distal) side branch within the vessel segment can be used as an index anatomic landmark to assess additionally the distances (measured on the

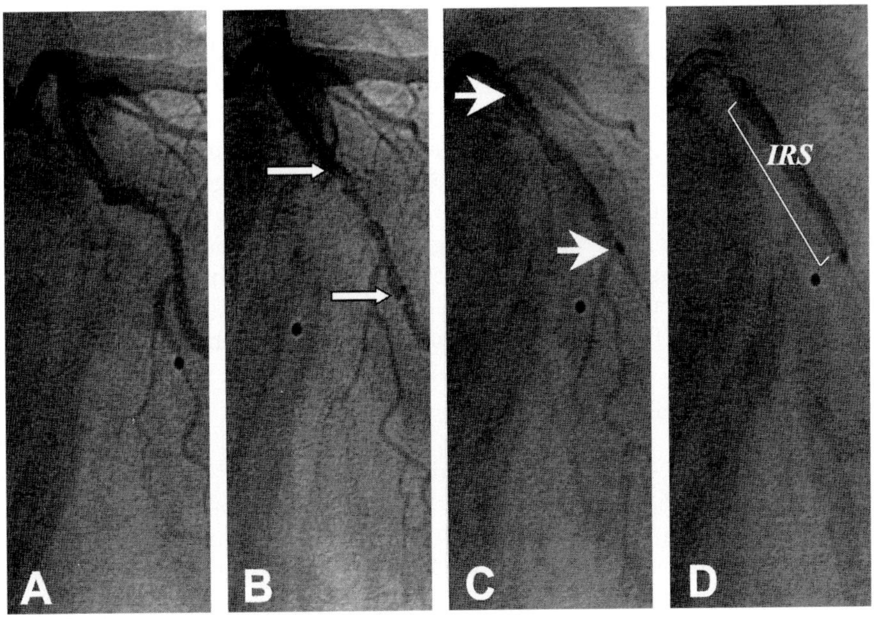

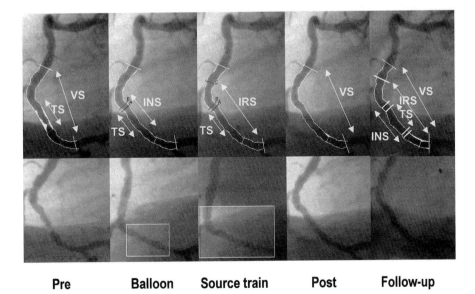

Figure 4. Qualitative assessment of geographic miss. Pre-intervention lesion **(A)**, balloon **(B)** and radiation source **(C)** (Radiance RDX radiation balloon, Radiance Corp.) have been filmed in the same imaging plane, allowing for accurate assessment of the injured and the irradiated segments. The injured segment is distally not completely covered by the irradiation source, resulting in distal geographic miss.

Figure 5. Dose-based definition of vessel segments within an irradiated coronary artery. **Lower panels:** The pre-intervention lesion, any instrumentation (balloon and source train), the post-interventional result, and follow-up have been filmed in identical projections and are displayed simultaneously on a screen. **Upper panels:** The vessel segment (VS) is defined by the analyst; the target segment (TS) is automatically defined by the quantitative coronary angiography system; the injured segment (IS) is defined as the segment encompassed by the most proximal and most distal radiopaque marker of the angioplasty balloon; the irradiated segment (IRS) has been defined between the radiopaque markers of the source.

center line) to: (1) the inner part of the proximal radiopaque marker of the radiation source; (2) the proximal marker of the angioplasty balloon; (3) the proximal margin of the obstruction segment; (4) the distal margin of the obstruction segment; (5) the distal marker of the angioplasty balloon; and, (6) the inner part of the distal radiopaque marker. All regions of interest are superimposed on the pre- and post-procedural angiograms. Thus, the occurrence of geographic miss can be directly assessed and quantified (Fig. 6). The accuracy of such quantification of geographic miss in the direction of the longitudinal vessel axis, however, is strongly dependent on an imaging projection without foreshortening. In all analysis segments, the MLD is determined by edge detection and the RD is automatically calculated. The percent DS is calculated from the MLD and the RD (Fig. 7).

Analysis of Restenosis: Regional Restenosis

As in classical QCA analysis, dichotomous restenosis is defined as greater than 50% DS. As long-term radiation effects on the coronary vessel wall have shown to be dependent on dose and injury, possibly resulting in the "candy wrapper" or "edge effect," it is important to describe late outcome with respect to the dose-based subsegments.

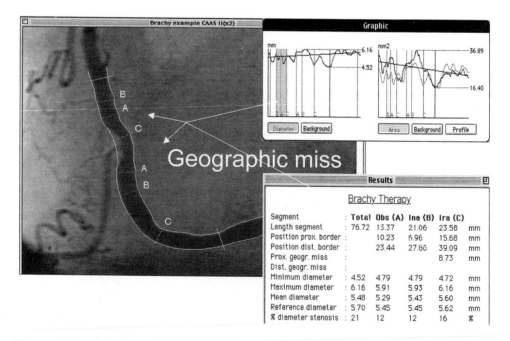

Figure 6. Quantitative assessment of geographic miss. Using the quantitative analysis software, the target segment **(A)**, injured segment **(B)**, and irradiated segment **(C)** have been defined. Ideally, the borders of the irradiated segment are most proximally and most distally situated, encompassing both, the target segment and the injured segment. Automated comparison of the position of the proximal and distal borders of each individual segment detects any deviation from this ideal pattern, indicating geographic miss. In the example, the proximal border of the irradiated segment is located more distal than the proximal border of the injured segment, indicating proximal geographic miss. The length of the geographic miss segment is 8.73 mm.

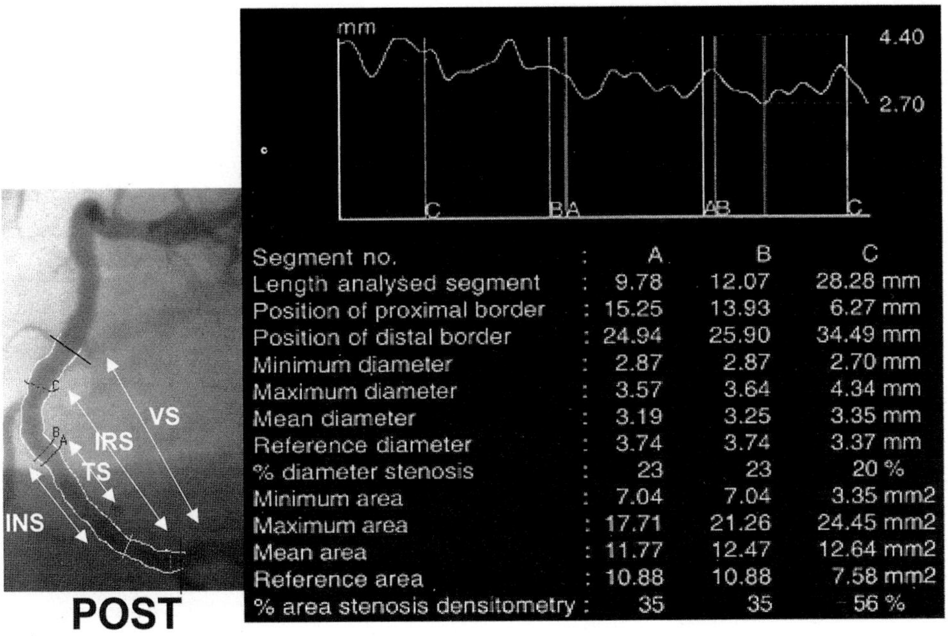

Segment no.	:	A	B	C
Length analysed segment	:	9.78	12.07	28.28 mm
Position of proximal border	:	15.25	13.93	6.27 mm
Position of distal border	:	24.94	25.90	34.49 mm
Minimum diameter	:	2.87	2.87	2.70 mm
Maximum diameter	:	3.57	3.64	4.34 mm
Mean diameter	:	3.19	3.25	3.35 mm
Reference diameter	:	3.74	3.74	3.37 mm
% diameter stenosis	:	23	23	20 %
Minimum area	:	7.04	7.04	3.35 mm2
Maximum area	:	17.71	21.26	24.45 mm2
Mean area	:	11.77	12.47	12.64 mm2
Reference area	:	10.88	10.88	7.58 mm2
% area stenosis densitometry	:	35	35	56 %

Figure 7. Quantitative coronary analysis of dose-based segments. Within the vessel segment (VS) quantitative parameters such as segment length, minimal lumen diameter, or reference diameter, are calculated for each segment individually. **(A)** represents the analysis for the target segment (TS); **(B)** represents the analysis for the injured segment (INS); **(C)** represents the analysis for the irradiated segment (IRS).

The pre-, post-intervention, and follow-up angiograms with the dose-based subsegments are superimposed and compared in two orthogonal projections. Thus, the location of the segment with restenosis can be assessed in relation to the dose-based segments. Regional restenosis is classified as restenosis in the irradiated segment, edge restenosis (proximal and/or distal), and restenosis outside the injured segment. The criterion for binary restenosis might be fulfilled in more than one subsegment in the same vessel segment.

Subsegmental QCA Analysis: Relocation

Using current analysis software, subsegmental analysis can be performed within the vessel segment. The vessel segment is automatically divided into subsegments of equidistant length (on average, 5 mm). In each subsegment MLD, RD, and percentage DS is automatically calculated.

Relocation For relocation analysis, the subsegment containing the MLD at baseline is taken as the index segment. Relocation is defined whenever the MLD in subsequent analysis is located in a subsegment other than the index segment. Sequential analysis may refer to pre-interventional to post-interventional MLD, or post-interventional (Fig. 8) to follow-up MLD (Fig. 9).

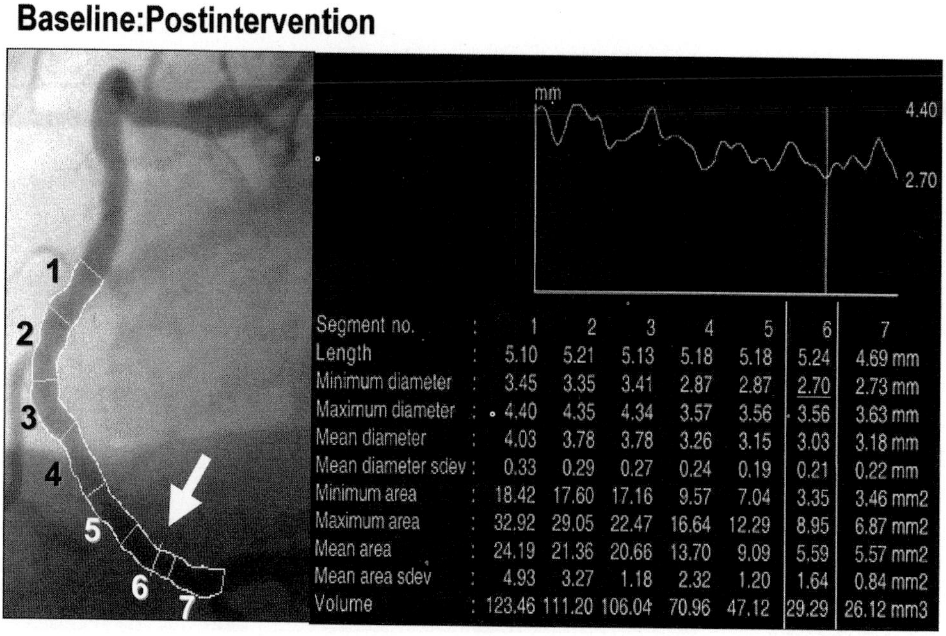

Baseline:Postintervention

Segment no.	:	1	2	3	4	5	6	7
Length	:	5.10	5.21	5.13	5.18	5.18	5.24	4.69 mm
Minimum diameter	:	3.45	3.35	3.41	2.87	2.87	2.70	2.73 mm
Maximum diameter	:	4.40	4.35	4.34	3.57	3.56	3.56	3.63 mm
Mean diameter	:	4.03	3.78	3.78	3.26	3.15	3.03	3.18 mm
Mean diameter sdev	:	0.33	0.29	0.27	0.24	0.19	0.21	0.22 mm
Minimum area	:	18.42	17.60	17.16	9.57	7.04	3.35	3.46 mm2
Maximum area	:	32.92	29.05	22.47	16.64	12.29	8.95	6.87 mm2
Mean area	:	24.19	21.36	20.66	13.70	9.09	5.59	5.57 mm2
Mean area sdev	:	4.93	3.27	1.18	2.32	1.20	1.64	0.84 mm2
Volume	:	123.46	111.20	106.04	70.96	47.12	29.29	26.12 mm3

Figure 8. Subsegmental analyis. The vessel segment is automatically divided into subsegments of equidistant length (on average 5 mm). In each subsegment minimal lumen diameter (MLD), reference diameter (RD), and percentage diameter stenosis is automatically calculated.

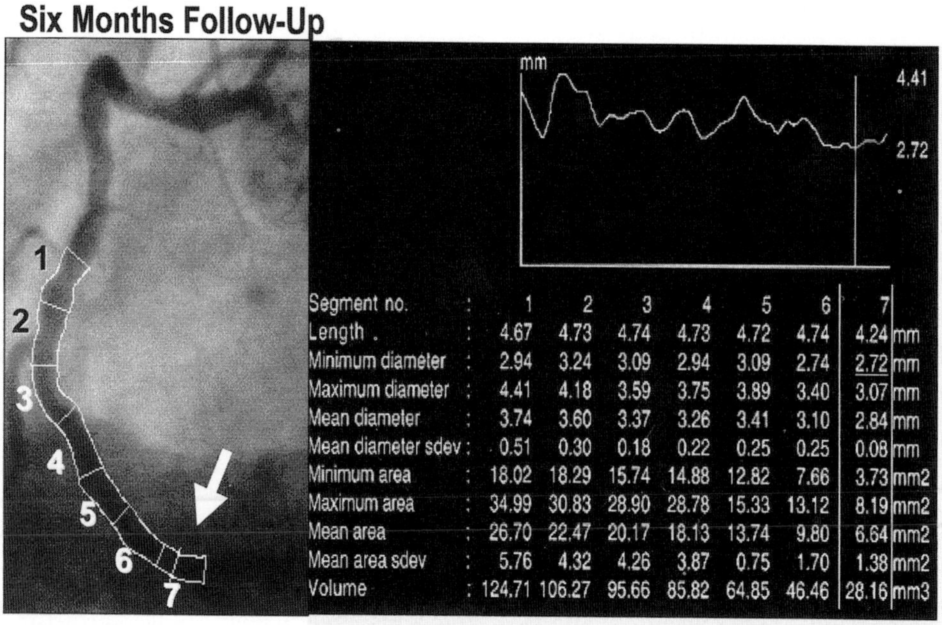

Six Months Follow-Up

Segment no.	:	1	2	3	4	5	6	7
Length	:	4.67	4.73	4.74	4.73	4.72	4.74	4.24 mm
Minimum diameter	:	2.94	3.24	3.09	2.94	3.09	2.74	2.72 mm
Maximum diameter	:	4.41	4.18	3.59	3.75	3.89	3.40	3.07 mm
Mean diameter	:	3.74	3.60	3.37	3.26	3.41	3.10	2.84 mm
Mean diameter sdev	:	0.51	0.30	0.18	0.22	0.25	0.25	0.08 mm
Minimum area	:	18.02	18.29	15.74	14.88	12.82	7.66	3.73 mm2
Maximum area	:	34.99	30.83	28.90	28.78	15.33	13.12	8.19 mm2
Mean area	:	26.70	22.47	20.17	18.13	13.74	9.80	6.64 mm2
Mean area sdev	:	5.76	4.32	4.26	3.87	0.75	1.70	1.38 mm2
Volume	:	124.71	106.27	95.66	85.82	64.85	46.46	28.16 mm3

Figure 9. Subsegmental analysis–relocation of minimal lumen diameter (MLD). This figure shows the same coronary artery as Figure 8 at 6-month follow-up. At post intervention (Fig. 8), the MLD is located in subsegment no. 6. At subsequent follow-up analysis (Fig. 9), the MLD is located in subsegment no. 7.

Definition of Reference Diameter

Methods of Reference Diameter Calculation In the early years of quantitative angiographic assessment, the RD was "user-defined." The analyst set proximal and distal calipers at "normal" reference sites (Fig. 10). This method, however, was strongly user-dependent and showed high variability in measurements. To circumvent this limitation, the concept of the "interpolated reference diameter" was introduced in 1982. The interpolated RD is calculated at the site of the MLD and represents the diameter of the artery when the obstruction would not be present. This method is completely automated and user-independent, once the margins of the vessel segments are given (Fig. 11).

These concepts of RD definition are based on the assumption that a non-treated reference segment preserves its stable dimensions over time. Following intracoronary radiation, however, therapy-associated changes in vessel dimensions have been consistently observed due to edge effect, relocation of the MLD, and positive remodeling. Under these circumstances, the interpolated RD became less reliable. To overcome these problems, "computer-constructed reference diameter analysis" has been developed. The method is not influenced by development of a new (edge) stenosis close to the original treatment site as the RD is calculated apart from the treatment side. In the first step, proximal and distal boundaries for diameter construction are automatically set at 5% and 95% of the vessel length under study. This reference position is averaged over a width of 3 mm to suppress the influence of noise on the local diameter. In the second step, the computer-constructed RD is then reconstructed at the position of the MLD, based on a line fitted through the proximal and distal boundaries by linear interpolation. Thus, this approach gives more reliable reference dimensions over serial measurements;

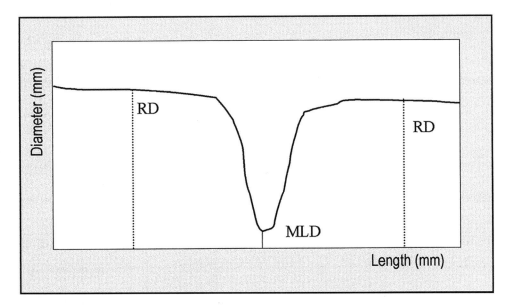

Figure 10. User-defined reference diameter. Diameter profile of a stenotic coronary artery segment. The analyst set proximal and distal markers at "normal" reference sites. MLD = minimal lumen diameter; RD = reference diameter.

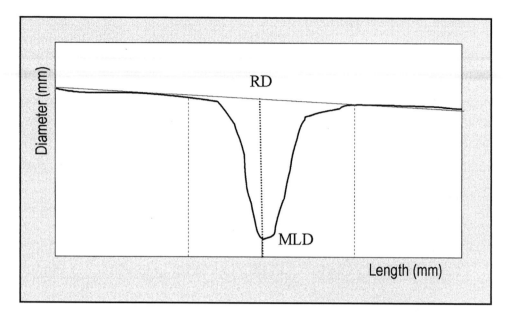

Figure 11. Interpolated reference diameter (RD). Diameter profile of a stenotic coronary artery segment. The "interpolated reference diameter" is automatically calculated at the site of the minimal lumen diameter (MLD) and represents the diameter of the artery when the obstruction is not present.

however, it does not cure the principal problem of relocation of the MLD. In consequence, the RD might be calculated at different positions within a vessel segment at baseline and follow-up measurement (Fig. 12).

Selection of Reference Diameter   Analysis of dose-based segments and subsegmental analysis gives an MLD and an RD for each individual segment. This might be helpful in the analysis of specific mechanistic questions. For the analysis of treatment efficacy and side effects, however, all measurements should de referred to one single "reference diameter." The RD calculated for the vessel segment is considered to best represent the "true" vessel dimensions, and thus, should be used for standardized reporting.

Clinical Implications

Intracoronary radiation has shown an effective inhibition of neointimal proliferation. The local mechanisms of action are poorly understood. Recent intravascular ultrasound studies demonstrated that mechanic vessel injury in combination with radioactivity can cause both beneficial and deleterious effects. Irradiation may prevent shrinkage after balloon angioplasty[53] and even promote positive remodeling at the irradiated site.[54] In contrast, edge segments show an increase in plaque volume without adaptive remodeling.[10,22,55] These findings have indicated a need to differentiate between the reporting of angiographic outcomes.

Dose-based segmental analysis allows for an accurate description of local lumen changes in different portions of the irradiated vessel. This is a prerequisite to study both the therapeutic and the side effects. Based on this methodology, angiographic analysis could demonstrate, that geographic miss plays a key role in

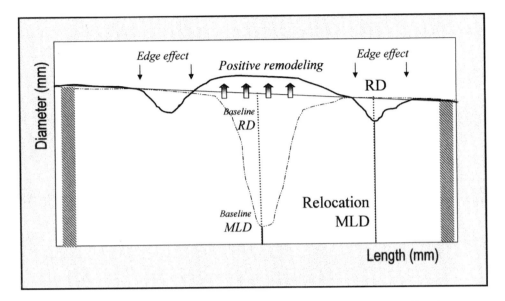

Figure 12. Computer constructed reference diameter (RD). Diameter profile of a stenotic coronary artery segment. At the proximal and the distal end of the vessel segment, boundaries (shaded area) for diameter calculation are automatically set. The "computer constructed reference diameter" is reconstructed at the position of the minimal lumen diameter (MLD), based on a line fitted through the proximal and distal boundaries by linear interpolation. In this example there is relocation of the MLD due to the edge effect. Thus, the RD is calculated at different positions within a vessel segment at baseline (gray lines) and follow-up (black line).

restenosis after (beta) brachytherapy,[18,56] emphasizing the need for complete coverage of the injured segment.

It could also been shown that late lumen loss differs considerably according to the selected segment. In consequence, the dichotomous restenosis rate varied from 3.1% in the "target segment" to 13.8% when analysis was extended to the "vessel segment" (Table 1).[17] Consistently, others found variation within a similar range (14.2% to 28.8%).[57] This has important impact on the reporting, interpretation, and comparison of study results.

Detailed analysis of computer-defined subsegments is of great help to gain insights in pathophysiological effects, and might be highly recommended for in vitro and/or "mechanistic" studies. Such detailed angiographic analysis could demonstrate that within the target segment, positive remodeling is a major effect of irradiation therapy, whereas relocation of the MLD within the injured segment has a substantially higher incidence after brachytherapy compared to conventional angioplasty.[17] Possible mechanisms of relocation include: tapering of the vessel; development of new coronary lesions in any of the dose-based subsegments; "unmasking " of pre-existing plaque (stenosis) outside the irradiated segment, which becomes angiographically apparent over follow-up time; progression of disease inside (treatment failure, edge effect?) or outside the irradiated area; and geographical miss. Further studies are needed to understand the complex interactions and mechanisms of action of radiation, dose, and normal and atherosclerotic arterial tissue. Analysis of the "target segment" may demonstrate the effect of brachytherapy in optimal conditions (maximum injury fully covered by radiation),

Table 1

Quantitative Coronary Angioplasty Data for Dose-Based Coronary Vessel Segments*

	TS	INS	IRS	VS
MLD pre-intervention (mm)	1.06±0.2	1.06±0.2	1.06±0.2	1.06±0.2
MLD post-intervention (mm)	2.17±0.5	1.99±0.4	2.00±0.4	1.91±0.4
MLD follow-up (mm)	2.36±0.5	1.97±0.5	1.97±0.5	1.84±0.5
DS follow-up (%)	20.3±11	33.2±11	33.4±11	37.9±10
Acute gain (mm)	1.12±0.4	0.93±0.4	0.94±0.4	0.85±0.4
Late loss (mm)	−0.18±0.4	0.01±0.4	0.03±0.4	0.07±0.3
Restenosis rate (%)	2 (3.1)	5 (7.7)	6 (9.2)	9 (13.8)
Segment length (mm)	5.0±0.3	18.7±4.2	22.9±3.5	36.9±8.4

*From Reference 17.

MLD = minimal lumen diameter; DS = diameter stenosis; TS = target segment; INS = injured segment; IRS = irradiated segment; VS = vessel segment.

while analysis of the injured segment and the edge segments may be helpful to identify potential causes of failure (ie, geographic miss, non injury-related edge effect, etc.).

In clinical trials, however, treatment effectiveness is the major endpoint. Angiographic outcome measurements should therefore be referred to the clinically relevant "vessel segment." This represents the targeted region used in most of the historical trials, under the assumption that the patients symptoms and need for re-intervention are driven by flow-limiting lesions within the treated vessel, irrespective of the precise anatomic position. A restrictive definition of the "target segment" with follow-up analysis of the site of the initial MLD pre-treatment would be misleading and would make any comparison to previous nonradiation studies inaccurate.

References

1. Verin V, Urban P, Popowski Y, et al. Feasibility of intracoronary beta-irradiation to reduce restenosis after balloon angioplasty: A clinical pilot study. Circulation 1997;95:1138–1144.
2. Teirstein PS, Massullo V, Jani S, et al. Catheter-based radiotherapy to inhibit restenosis after coronary stenting. N Engl J Med 1997;336:1697–1703.
3. King SB III, Williams DO, Chougule P, et al. Endovascular beta-radiation to reduce restenosis after coronary balloon angioplasty: Results of the beta energy restenosis trial (BERT). Circulation 1998;97:2025–2030.
4. Waksman R, White RL, Chan RC, et al. Intracoronary gamma-radiation therapy after angioplasty inhibits recurrence in patients with in-stent restenosis. Circulation 2000;101:2165–2171.
5. Waksman R, Bhargava B, White L, et al. Intracoronary beta-radiation therapy inhibits recurrence of in-stent restenosis. Circulation 2000;101:1895–1898.
6. Fischell TA, Hehrlein C. The radioisotope stent for the prevention of restenosis. Herz 1998;23:373–379.
7. Wardeh AJ, Kay IP, Sabate M, et al. Beta-particle-emitting radioactive stent implantation: A safety and feasibility study. Circulation 1999;100:1684–1689.

8. Albiero R, Adamian M, Kobayashi N, et al. Short- and intermediate-term results of (32)P radioactive beta-emitting stent implantation in patients with coronary artery disease: The Milan Dose-Response Study. Circulation 2000;101:18–26.

9. Serruys PW, Kay IP. I like the candy, I hate the wrapper: The (32)P radioactive stent. Circulation 2000;101:3–7.

10. Kay IP, Sabate M, Costa MA, et al. Positive geometric vascular remodeling is seen after catheter-based radiation followed by conventional stent implantation but not after radioactive stent implantation. Circulation 2000;102:1434–1439.

11. Amols HI, Reinstein LE, Weinberger J. Dosimetry of a radioactive coronary balloon dilatation catheter for treatment of neointimal hyperplasia. Med Phys 1996;23:1783–1788.

12. Weinberger J. Intracoronary radiation using radioisotope solution-filled balloons. Herz 1998;23:366–372.

13. Hoeher M, Woehrle J, Wohlform M, et al. Intracoronary beta-irradiation with liquid rhenium-188 to prevent restenosis following coronary angioplasty: Interim results from the randomized ECRIS-trial. Eur Heart J 2000;21:622.

14. Quast U, Fluhs D, Bambynek M. Endovascular brachytherapy: Treatment planning and radiation protection. Herz 1998;23:337–346.

15. Waksman R. Intracoronary brachytherapy in the cath lab. Physics dosimetry, technology and safety considerations. Herz 1998;23:401–406.

16. Condado JA, Waksman R, Gurdiel O, et al. Long-term angiographic and clinical outcome after percutaneous transluminal coronary angioplasty and intracoronary radiation therapy in humans. Circulation 1997;96:727–732.

17. Sabate M, Costa MA, Kozuma K, et al. Methodological and clinical implications of the relocation of the minimal lumen diameter after intracoronary radiation therapy. J Am Coll Cardiol 2000;101:2467–2471.

18. Sabate M, Costa MA, Kozuma K, et al. Geographic miss: A cause of treatment failure in radio-oncology applied to intracoronary radiation therapy. Circulation 2000;101:2467–2471.

19. Albiero R, Nishida T, Adamian M, et al. Edge restenosis after implantation of high activity (32)P radioactive beta-emitting stents. Circulation 2000;101:2454–2457.

20. Mintz GS, Popma JJ, Pichard et al. Arterial remodeling after coronary angioplasty: A serial intravascular ultrasound study. Circulation 1996;94:35–43.

21. Di Mario C, Gil R, Camenzind E, et al. Quantitative assessment with intracoronary ultrasound of the mechanisms of restenosis after percutaneous transluminal coronary angioplasty and directional coronary atherectomy. Am J Cardiol 1995;75:772–777.

22. Sabate M, Serruys PW, van der Giessen WJ, et al. Geometric vascular remodeling after balloon angioplasty and beta- radiation therapy: A three-dimensional intravascular ultrasound study. Circulation 1999;100:1182–1188.

23. Foley DP, Escaned J, Strauss BH, et al. Quantitative coronary angiography (QCA) in interventional cardiology: Clinical application of QCA measurements. Prog Cardiovasc Dis 1994;36:363–384.

24. Zijlstra F, van Ommeren J, Reiber JH, Serruys PW. Does the quantitative assessment of coronary artery dimensions predict the physiologic significance of a coronary stenosis? Circulation 1987;75:1154–1161.

25. Reiber JH, van der Zwet PM, Koning G, et al. Accuracy and precision of quantitative digital coronary arteriography: Observer-, short-, and medium-term variabilities. Cathet Cardiovasc Diagn 1993;28:187–198.

26. Haase J, Escaned J, van Swijndregt EM, et al. Experimental validation of geometric and densitometric coronary measurements on the new generation Cardiovascular Angiography Analysis System (CAAS II). Cathet Cardiovasc Diagn 1993;30:104–114.

27. Haase J, van der Linden MM, Di Mario C, et al. Can the same edge-detection algorithm be applied to on-line and off-line analysis systems? Validation of a new cinefilm-based geometric coronary measurement software. Am Heart J 1993;126:312–321.

28. Keane D, Haase J, Slager CJ, et al. Comparative validation of quantitative coronary angiography systems: Results and implications from a multicenter study using a standardized approach. Circulation 1995;91:2174–2183.

29. Rensing BJ, Hermans WR, Deckers JW, et al. Lumen narrowing after percutaneous transluminal coronary balloon angioplasty follows a near gaussian distribution: A

quantitative angiographic study in 1,445 successfully dilated lesions. J Am Coll Cardiol 1992;19:939–945.

30. Beatt KJ, Serruys PW, Luijten HE, et al. Restenosis after coronary angioplasty: The paradox of increased lumen diameter and restenosis. J Am Coll Cardiol 1992; 19:258–266.

31. Kuntz RE, Gibson CM, Nobuyoshi M, Baim DS. Generalized model of restenosis after conventional balloon angioplasty, stenting and directional atherectomy. J Am Coll Cardiol 1993;21:15–25.

32. Serruys PW, Rutsch W, Heyndrickx GR, et al. Prevention of restenosis after percutaneous transluminal coronary angioplasty with thromboxane A2-receptor blockade: A randomized, double- blind, placebo-controlled trial. Coronary Artery Restenosis Prevention on Repeated Thromboxane-Antagonism Study (CARPORT). Circulation 1991;84:1568–1580.

33. Multicenter European Research Trial with Cilazapril after Angioplasty to Prevent Transluminal Coronary Obstruction and Restenosis (MERCATOR) Study Group. Does the new angiotensin converting enzyme inhibitor cilazapril prevent restenosis after percutaneous transluminal coronary angioplasty? Results of the MERCATOR study: A multicenter, randomized, double-blind placebo-controlled trial. Circulation 1992;86:100–110.

34. Serruys PW, Klein W, Tijssen JP, et al. Evaluation of ketanserin in the prevention of restenosis after percutaneous transluminal coronary angioplasty: A multicenter randomized double-blind placebo-controlled trial. Circulation 1993;88:1588–1601.

35. Serruys PW, de Jaegere P, Kiemeneij F, et al. A comparison of balloon-expandable-stent implantation with balloon angioplasty in patients with coronary artery disease. Benestent Study Group. N Engl J Med 1994;331:489–495.

36. Serruys PW, van Der Giessen W, Garcia E, et al. Clinical and angiographic results with the multi-link stent implanted under intravascular ultrasound guidance (West-2 Study). J Invas Cardiol 1998;10(suppl B):20B–27B.

37. Serruys PW, Foley DP, Jackson G, et al. A randomized placebo-controlled trial of fluvastatin for prevention of restenosis after successful coronary balloon angioplasty; final results of the fluvastatin angiographic restenosis (FLARE) trial. Eur Heart J 1999;20:58–69.

38. Beatt KJ, Luijten HE, de Feyter PJ, et al. Change in diameter of coronary artery segments adjacent to stenosis after percutaneous transluminal coronary angioplasty: Failure of percent diameter stenosis measurement to reflect morphologic changes induced by balloon dilation. J Am Coll Cardiol 1988;12:315–323.

39. Hermans WR, Foley DP, Rensing BJ, Serruys PW. Morphologic changes during follow-up after successful percutaneous transluminal coronary balloon angioplasty: Quantitative angiographic analysis in 778 lesions: Further evidence for the restenosis paradox. MERCATOR Study Group. Am Heart J 1994;127:483–494.

40. Serruys P, Foley D, de Feyter P. Quantitative Coronary Angiography in Clinical Practise. Dordrecht: Kluwer Academic Publishers; 1994.

41. Buller CE, Dzavik V, Carere RG, et al. Primary stenting versus balloon angioplasty in occluded coronary arteries: The Total Occlusion Study of Canada (TOSCA). Circulation 1999;100:236–242.

42. Kanaar R, Hoeijmakers JH, van Gent DC. Molecular mechanisms of DNA double strand break repair. Trends Cell Biol 1998;8:483–489.

43. Wiedermann JG, Marboe C, Amols H, et al. Intracoronary irradiation markedly reduces restenosis after balloon angioplasty in a porcine model. J Am Coll Cardiol 1994;23:1491–1498.

44. Mazur W, Ali MN, Khan MM, et al. High dose rate intracoronary radiation for inhibition of neointimal formation in the stented and balloon-injured porcine models of restenosis: Angiographic, morphometric, and histopathologic analyses. Int J Radiat Oncol Biol Phys 1996;36:777–788.

45. Weinberger J, Amols H, Ennis RD,et al. Intracoronary irradiation: Dose response for the prevention of restenosis in swine. Int J Radiat Oncol Biol Phys 1996;36:767–775.

46. Waksman R. Response to radiation therapy in animal restenosis models. Semin Interv Cardiol 1997;2:95–101.

47. Rubin P, Williams JP, Riggs PN, et al. Cellular and molecular mechanisms of radiation

inhibition of restenosis. Part I: Role of the macrophage and platelet-derived growth factor. Int J Radiat Oncol Biol Phys 1998;40:929–941.

48. Nath R, Amols H, Coffey C, et al. Intravascular brachytherapy physics: Report of the AAPM Radiation Therapy Committee Task Group no. 60. American Association of Physicists in Medicine. Med Phys 1999;26:119–152.

49. Fareh J, Martel R, Kermani P, Leclerc G. Cellular effects of beta-particle delivery on vascular smooth muscle cells and endothelial cells: A dose-response study. Circulation 1999;99:1477–1484.

50. Sabate M, Marijnissen JP, Carlier SG, et al. Residual plaque burden, delivered dose, and tissue composition predict 6-month outcome after balloon angioplasty and beta-radiation therapy. Circulation 2000;101:2472–2477.

51. Di Mario C, Hermans WR, Rensing BJ, Serruys PW. Calibration using angiographic catheters as scaling devices: Importance of filming the catheters not filled with contrast medium. Am J Cardiol 1992;69:1377–1378.

52. Paterson R. The Treatment of Malignant Diseases by Radiotherapy. London: Edward Arnold, LTD; 1963.

53. Meerkin D, Tardif JC, Crocker IR, et al. Effects of intracoronary beta-radiation therapy after coronary angioplasty: An intravascular ultrasound study. Circulation 1999;99:1660–1665.

54. Costa MA, Sabate M, Serrano P, et al. The effect of 32P beta-radiotherapy on both vessel remodeling and neointimal hyperplasia after coronary balloon angioplasty and stenting: A three-dimensional intravascular ultrasound investigation. J Invas Cardiol 2000;12:113–120.

55. Kozuma K, Costa MA, Sabate M, et al. Three-dimensional intravascular ultrasound analysis of non-injured edges of beta-irradiated coronary segments. Circulation. In press.

56. Sabate M, Kay IP, Gijzel AL, et al. Compassionate use of intracoronary beta-irradiation for treatment of recurrent in-stent restenosis. J Invas Cardiol 1999;11:582–588.

57. Popma J, Heuser R, Suntharalingam M, et al. Late clinical and angiographic outcomes after use of 90Sr/90Y beta radiation for the treatment of in-stent restenosis: Results from the stents and radiation therapy (START) trial. ACCIS 2000 presentation. 2000.

Quantitative Coronary Angiography Methodology in Vascular Brachytherapy II

Alexandra J. Lansky, MD, Kartik J. Desai, MD,
Raoul Bonon, MD, Gerhard Koning, MSc,
Joan Tuinenburg, MSc, and Johan H.C. Reiber, PhD

The recent U.S. Food and Drug Administration (FDA) approval of Gamma (Cordis Corporation, A Johnson and Johnson Company, Miami Lakes, FL) and of Beta (Novoste Corporation, Norcross, GA) coronary brachytherapy devices is based on the undeniable efficacy of adjunctive radiation therapy demonstrated in a patient population typically refractory to conventional interventional therapies, specifically, patients with in-stent restenosis. Although FDA approval has been granted for beta and gamma therapies, long-term surveillance will be essential in ultimately defining their long-term safety and efficacy. In the short-run, further reductions in restenosis with optimization of radiation delivery techniques will depend, in part, on insights gained from the systematic angiographic assessment of precise radiation delivery and the relative location of disease recurrence. In this regard, the angiographic analysis of vascular brachytherapy trials has become increasingly complex as a means of explaining the peculiarities of this novel therapy. An entire lexicon of terms has emerged particular to the field of vascular brachytherapy such as "edge effect," "geographic miss," and "geographic hit," among others; however, these concepts were without precise definition at inception, and have been confused among practicing interventionalists who convincingly discourse on cause and effect, thereby effectively perpetuating misunderstanding. This has challenged the central angiographic laboratories to elucidate these new concepts by first providing precise definitions for the new lexicon, and then developing and validating methodology for the now expanded applications of conventional quantitative coronary angiography (QCA), in an attempt to prove or disprove the current observation-based theories. Although QCA can be performed with a high degree of accuracy and precision in conventional applications, the limitations of this technique must be kept in mind.[1,2] This is particularly true in cases of increasing demands in the interpretation of multidimensional measures as now expected of vascular brachytherapy applications. Newer algorithms have been developed and are currently undergoing validation that will permit all-inclusive multidimensional analyses while minimizing the excessive and burdensome user interfaces that are necessary with current generations of QCA algorithms. This chapter will review the methodology, results, and limitations of vas-

From Waksman R (ed.). *Vascular Brachytherapy, Third Edition.* Armonk, NY: Futura Publishing Co., Inc.; © 2002.

cular brachytherapy analyses performed using currently available conventional QCA algorithms, and will also present the newer generation algorithms that are currently under development.

Angiographic Methods Used in the Analysis of the Gamma Trials: The SCRIPPS, WRIST, and GAMMA I Trials

Quantitative methods used to assess serial arterial lumen changes after conventional percutaneous transluminal coronary angiography (PTCA) typically identified proximal and distal reference landmarks and a discrete point of maximal lumen narrowing (ie, the minimal lumen diameter [MLD]).[3,4] Sequential angiographic measurements are made using side branches and other anatomic structures to consistently localize the segment of analysis over time.[8,9] Using these methods, serial angiographic measurements of the reference vessel and MLD can be made with high accuracy (<0.05 mm) and precision (<0.21 mm).[5,8] The angiographic analysis of the initial Gamma Radiation Trials was more complex due to the extensive length of the segments of analysis and the multiple associated landmarks.

The SCRIPPS Trial was the first brachytherapy trial analyzed by our Angiographic Core Laboratory, and was performed using a similar methodology as that used in the analysis of the stent versus stent trials.[9,10] The quantitative angiographic analysis was performed using a validated QCA system (QCA-CMS®, including GFT, MEDIS, The Netherlands)[2] guided by the analyst's drawing of the arterial segment and its side branches, in order to demonstrate the precise location of the baseline stenosis, the stent, and the radiation delivery ribbon (Fig. 1).[9] The analysis of the SCRIPPS Trial included an analysis of the stent and a second analysis of the "stent + margin" defined by a 5-mm extension to the proximal and distal stent edge borders, enabling the identification of disease recurrence isolated to the stent edge. In the SCRIPPS Trial the Iridium 192 (^{192}Ir) seed length was

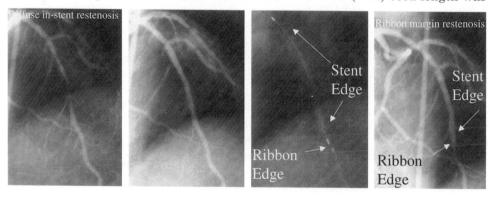

Baseline Final Result Ribbon Follow-up

Figure 1. Serial cineangiograms of the left anterior descending demonstrating the baseline stenosis (pre intervention), the position of the ribbon, and the final results (post intervention) identifying the location of the stent. The follow-up cineangiogram demonstrates restenosis at the distal margin of the stent.

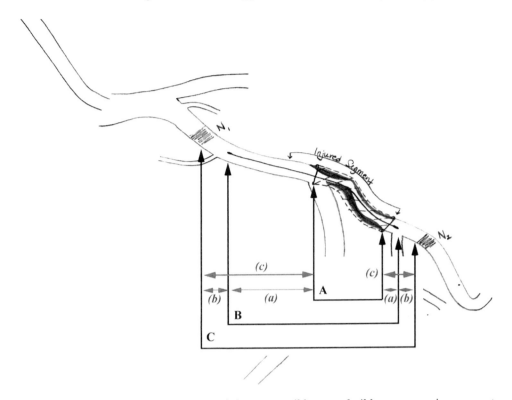

Figure 2. Schematic representation of the stent, ribbon, and ribbon + margin segment analysis. **A** (arrows) represents the axial length of the stent analysis after the procedure; **B** (arrows) represents the ribbon analysis; **C** (arrows) represents the ribbon + margin analysis including approximately 5 mm of margins beyond the ribbon (includes any injury. Five-millimeter segments of proximal and distal reference diameters are averaged to estimate the reference vessel diameter.

closely matched to the borders of the stent, thus the "stent + margin" analysis included the source train. For the purpose of the WRIST and GAMMA I Trials, the final and follow-up analyses were composed of three separate segments of analysis including the stent, the radiation source, and the source + margin, each defined by specific physical landmarks of the stent, the radiation source, and a 5-mm extension on either end (Fig. 2). This methodology was designed to detect focal restenosis isolated to the edge of each of the physical landmarks. The *stent segment* of analysis identified the MLD confined by any existing stent (in-stent restenosis) or any additional stents deployed during the procedure. The *radiated or "source segment"* of analysis identified the MLD confined by the proximal and distal border of the radiation delivery catheter. The *"source + margin"* segment of analysis extended 5 mm proximal and distal to the radiated or injured landmark. For each segment the MLD was obtained to derive the percent diameter stenosis (%DS), and restenosis was defined by a follow-up lesion %DS greater than 50%.

In an attempt to define recurrence of disease at the edge of the radiation delivery catheter due to a potential subtherapeutic proliferative radiation effect, the so-called "edge effect," this methodology was used to assess the frequency of restenosis isolated to the edges of each landmark. Stent edge restenosis was calculated as "source + margin" restenosis minus stent restenosis; restenosis at edge

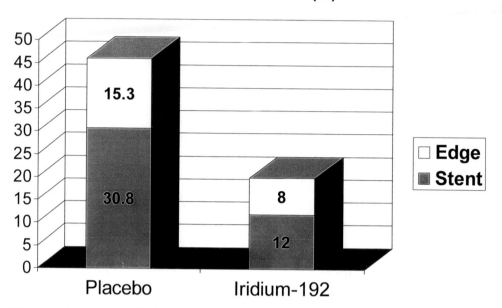

Figure 3. In the SCRIPPS Trial, treatment with ^{192}Ir reduced restenosis primarily within the stent rather than the margin. Reproduced with permission from Reference 10.

of radiated segment as "source + margin" restenosis minus source restenosis; and restenosis of non-stented but radiated segment as stent edge restenosis minus restenosis at edge of radiated segment.

Results of The SCRIPPS Trial

In the SCRIPPS trial, 55 patients were randomly assigned to receive ^{192}Ir or placebo sources after successful intervention. Procedural and 6-month follow-up cineangiograms were quantitatively reviewed in 51 patients. Treatment with ^{192}Ir reduced restenosis within the stent (12% versus 30.8%, $P=0.103$) and within the stent + margin (20.0% versus 46.1%, $P=0.048$), while the reduction in restenosis at the margin only (8.0% versus 15.3%) was not significant (Fig. 3).[9]

Results of the WRIST Trial

In the WRIST Trial, 130 patients were randomized to receive ^{192}Ir therapy or placebo after successful treatment of in-stent restenosis.[11] Baseline and follow-up angiograms technically suitable for quantitative angiographic analysis were available in 128 and in 115 of 130 patients, respectively. Compared with placebo patients, ^{192}Ir-treated patients had lower stent restenosis rates (20.3% versus 57.1%, $P<0.001$), source restenosis (22.4% versus 60.0%, $P<0.001$) and source + margin restenosis rates (23.7% versus 60.5%, $P<0.001$). Isolated stent edge restenosis occurred in only 3.4% of cases and isolated source margin restenosis occurred in 1.7% of treated lesions (Fig. 4). There was no significant increase or reduction in the

WRIST Restenosis Rates (%)

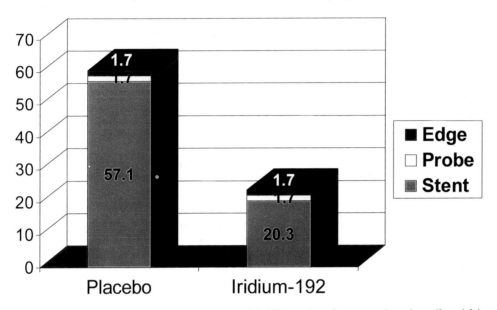

Figure 4. In the WRIST Trial, treatment with ^{192}Ir reduced restenosis primarily within the stent. Stent margin and radiation ribbon margin restenosis were minimal in both placebo and ^{192}Ir groups.

restenosis rate at the stent margin (3.4% versus 3.4% in placebo-treated patients, P=0.503) or at the source margin (1.7% versus 1.7% in placebo-treated patients) with ^{192}Ir therapy.

Source or stent margin restenosis was unrelated to the extent of coverage of the stent margins with Iridium seeds. A total of 4 patients in the Iridium group had inadequate coverage of both the proximal (mean of 2 seeds) and the distal edge (mean of 3 seeds) of the stent with active seeds. Restenosis did not occur in any of these patients. In the 2 patients with stent margin restenosis including the patient with restenosis at the edge of the radiation delivery catheter, there was extensive coverage of the proximal and distal edge areas by 6 and 10 seeds, respectively.

The distribution plot of follow-up MLDs demonstrates a near bimodal distribution with systematically larger MLDs associated with Iridium therapy when confining the analysis to the stented segment alone. When extending the analysis to include the source and its margins, the distribution of follow-up MLDs, although demonstrating more overlap, still had systematically larger MLDs with Iridium therapy compared to placebo (Fig. 5). This pattern lends further credibility to the absence of a significant "edge effect" in the WRIST trial, as the follow-up MLDs were systematically larger with Iridium therapy compared to placebo. These findings provide consistent evidence for the effectiveness of Iridium therapy in reducing restenosis within the target stented segment, and provide no evidence for a proliferative effect ("edge effect") resulting from the dose fall-off at the edge of the Iridium delivery source. The mean seed to lesion length ratio in WRIST was 1.82±0.87. The longer length of radiation delivery seeds used to cover the stent margins in this study had no apparent detrimental effects on the adjacent non-stented arterial segments at 6 months.

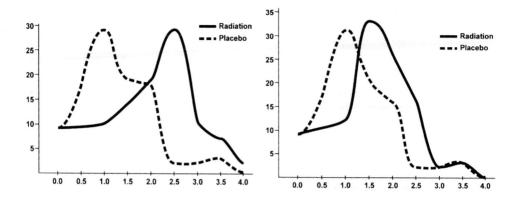

Stent Segment   Analysis Segment

Figure 5. Frequency of the minimal lumen diameters (MLDs) at follow-up demonstrating a bimodal distribution of the iridium and placebo groups using the stent MLD compared to a near normal distribution of the iridium and placebo groups using the ribbon + margin MLD.

Results of the GAMMA I Trial

In the GAMMA I trial, the first multicenter gamma trial, 252 patients were randomized to ^{192}Ir therapy or placebo after successful treatment of in-stent restenosis.[12] Complete follow-up quantitative angiographic analysis was available in 214 consecutive patients (111 ^{192}Ir and 103 placebo). [192]Ir therapy reduced the "source + margin" restenosis (55.3% versus 32.4%, $P<0.01$), and the stent restenosis rate (51.0% versus 21.6%, $P<0.001$) compared to placebo.

Restenosis at the margin of the stent was 10.8% for ^{192}Ir-treated patients and 3.8% for placebo patients. This difference was not significant. At the margin of the radiation source, there was no difference in restenosis rate between the two groups (3.8% versus 3.3% with ^{192}Ir) (Fig. 6). Among the 131 patients randomized to ^{192}Ir therapy, the univariate predictors of stent edge restenosis included a smaller reference vessel diameter (OR 7.19, $P=0.042$) and a smaller final minimal lumen dimension (OR 2.52, $P=0.203$). The only independent predictor of edge restenosis was the smaller reference vessel dimension.[13]

The results of the three gamma trials demonstrated consistency in efficacy with consistent reductions in the overall restenosis rates, ranging from 60% in the WRIST Trial to 45% in the GAMMA I Trial. Perhaps one contributing factor to the lower relative efficacy demonstrated in the GAMMA I Trial may be the higher (nonsignificant) restenosis located at the margin of the stent. The differences in stent margin restenosis among the three trials are likely multifactorial. In the SCRIPPS Trial, an attempt was made to achieve "optimal" angiographic results after intervention and before radiation therapy (final MLD, final DS). Every effort was made to precisely match the radiation delivery source wire to the confines of the stent, minimizing excessive overlap. In SCRIPPS, stent edge restenosis was reduced (14% placebo to 8% [192]Ir, $P=$NS) although the

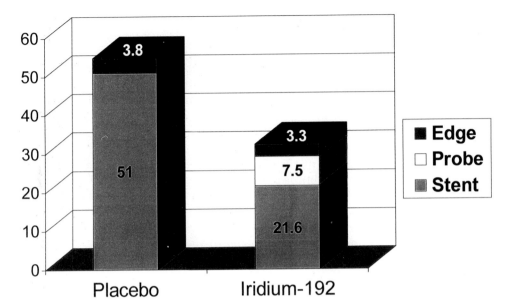

Figure 6. In the GAMMA I Trial, treatment with ^{192}Ir reduced restenosis primarily within the stent. Stent margin restenosis occurred in 10.8% with Iridium-192 versus 3.8% with placebo (*P*=NS). Small reference vessel size was the only independent predictor of stent edge restenosis among Iridium-192 treated patients.[13]

Table 1

Baseline Lesion Morphology in the WRIST Trial

	SCRIPPS Trial			WRIST Trial		
	Iridium 192 N(%)	Placebo N(%)	*P* Value	Iridium 192 N(%)	Placebo N(%)	*P* Value
Vessel location						
RCA	8 (33.3)	7 (25.0)	0.508	14 (21.5)	17 (26.2)	0.537
LAD	7 (29.2)	11 (39.3)	0.444	18 (27.7)	16 (24.6)	0.690
LM	—	—		3 (4.6)	2 (3.1)	1.000
LCx	3 (12.5)	3 (10.7)	1.00	15 (23.1)	15 (23.1)	1.000
SVG	6 (25.0)	7 (25.0)	1.00	15 (23.1)	15 (23.1)	1.000
Ostial location	3 (12.5)	6 (21.4)	0.396	15 (23.1)	18 (27.7)	0.545
Length (mm)	13.1+7.2	11.7+6.9	0.488	19.90+9.38	21.06+11.58	0.5397
Length >10 mm	14 (58.3)	12 (42.9)	0.266	47 (73.4)	46 (75.4)	0.8010
Length >20 mm	4 (16.7)	4 (14.3)	0.812	34 (53.1)	31 (50.8)	0.7970
Total occlusion	0	1.(3.6)	0.350	4 (6.2)	5 (7.9)	0.7420
ACC/AHA B2/C	13 (54.1)	13 (46.4)	0.578	41 (63.0)	41 (63.0)	
Type A	5 (20.8)	6 (21.4)	—	9 (13.8)	9 (14.3)	0.9430
Type B$_1$	6 (25.0)	9 (32.1)	—	15 (23.1)	13 (20.6)	0.7380
Type B$_2$	8 (33.3)	5 (17.9)	—	6 (9.2)	5 (7.9)	0.7940
Type C	5 (20.8)	8 (28.6)	—	35 (53.8)	36 (57.1)	0.7080

RCA = right coronary artery; LAD = left anterior descending; LM = left main; LCx = left circumflex; SVG = saphenous vein graft.

change was not significant. In the WRIST Trial, stent edge (3.4%) and probe edge (1.7%) restenosis were trivial in both the placebo and the ^{192}Ir-treated patients. The WRIST Trial also optimized acute angiographic results; however, liberalized source lengths (source to lesion length ratio 1.82±0.87) were allowed to provide more extensive source coverage of the stent margins. In the GAMMA I Trial, the overall stent edge restenosis rate was 10.8% for ^{192}Ir-treated patients and 3.8% for placebo patients, P=NS. Stent edge restenosis, in those patients randomized to ^{192}Ir therapy in GAMMA I, was predicted by a smaller reference vessel size and a smaller final MLD.

Despite different findings at the stent margins, the three gamma radiation trials demonstrated striking concordance in efficacy even with the inclusion of dose fall-off margins. Slight differences in lesion characteristics and interventional techniques including radiation delivery may contribute to the observed differences at the stent margins. Tables 1–3 compare the angiographic parameters of the three trials. Lesion length was significantly more diffuse in the WRIST and GAMMA I Trials compared to the SCRIPPS Trial.

Table 2

Quantitative Angiographic Results

	SCRIPPS Trial			WRIST Trial		
	Iridium 192	Placebo	P Value	Iridium 192	Placebo	P Value
Number of patients	24	28		49	49	
Reference, mm						
Baseline	2.93±0.57	2.77±0.47	0.266	2.71±0.53	2.72±0.56	0.9082
Final	3.17±0.77	3.00±0.51	0.364	2.79±0.50	2.85±0.50	0.5437
Follow-up	3.08±0.75	2.94±0.49	0.427	2.90±0.52	2.87±0.58	0.7960
MLD, mm						
Baseline	1.14±0.45	1.05±0.46	0.445	0.94±0.42	0.81±0.42	0.0735
Final						
Stent	2.81±0.63	2.88±0.84	0.748	2.23±0.52	2.25±0.50	0.8453
Source				2.00±0.68	2.10±0.51	0.3359
Source+margin	2.39±0.62	2.47±0.74	0.663	2.05±0.49	2.07±0.43	0.8032
Follow-up						
Stent	2.43±0.78	1.85±0.89	0.016	2.03±0.93	1.24±0.77	<0.0001
Source				1.72±0.95	1.14±0.86	0.0008
Source+margin	1.85±0.62	1.61±0.73	0.203	1.73±0.78	1.24±0.75	0.0008
% Stenosis						
Baseline	60±14	62±18	0.798	65.2±14.3	70.4±14.6	0.0471
Final						
Stent	9±22	4±23	0.452	19.4±15.4	20.4±14.9	0.6903
Source				28.4±22.9	26.2±12.0	0.5120
Source+margin	25±8	18±18	0.109	26.5±13.1	26.7±12.2	0.9366
Follow-up						
Stent	17±30	37±26	0.010	30.1±29.7	57.2±21.5	0.0001
Source				41.5±30.5	60.7±24.6	0.0003
Source+margin	38±19	45±23	0.247	40.8±23.4	57.3±20.1	0.0001

MLD = minimal lumen diameter.

Table 3

Serial Changes in Lumen Dimensions in the WRIST Trial

	SCRIPPS Trial			WRIST Trial		
	Iridium %(N/D)	Placebo %(N/D)	*P* Value	Iridium %(N/D)	Placebo %(N/D)	*P* Value
Acute gain, mm						
Stent	1.67±0.67	1.83±0.96	0.484	1.29±0.53	1.44±0.53	0.1072
Source				1.06±1.75	1.29±0.50	0.0396
Source+ margin	1.25±0.65	1.43±0.85	0.399	1.12±0.52	1.26±0.48	0.1200
Late loss, mm						
Stent	0.38±1.06	1.03±0.97	0.025	0.22±0.84	1.00±0.69	<0.0001
Source				0.28±0.73	0.88±0.64	<0.0001
Source+ margin	0.54±0.85	0.86±0.96	0.200	0.36±0.74	0.82±0.71	0.0012
Loss index						
Stent	0.12±0.63	0.60±0.43	0.002	0.22±0.08	0.65±0.15	0.0021
Source				0.26±0.12	0.58±0.15	0.0001
Source+ margin	0.30±0.72	0.60±0.49	0.082	0.36±0.08	0.67±0.06	0.0021
Restenosis rate, %						
Stent	2 (8)	11 (39)	0.010	11 (19.0)	33 (57.9)	0.0010
Source				13 (22.4)	34 (59.6)	0.0010
Source+ margin	4 (17)	15 (54)	0.010	13 (22.4)	34 (59.6)	0.0010
Stent margin	2 (8)	4 (14)	0.503	2 (3.4)	1 (1.7)	

Shifting of the Minimal Lumen Diameter with Vascular Brachytherapy

With gamma sources now ranging from 19 to 55 mm in length, the effective treatment segments have lengthened, and the residual stenosis can occur at any location spanning the radiation delivery catheter or beyond. In contrast to conventional PTCA or stenting, the follow-up MLD after brachytherapy rarely occurs at the original stenosis location.[14] In WRIST, the follow-up MLD was 0.31 mm smaller within the ribbon + margin segment than within the stent in the ^{192}Ir-treated patients (compared to 0.10 mm smaller in the placebo patients). The apparent shift in follow-up MLD away from the original lesion site with brachytherapy may occur as a result of: (1) the effectiveness of brachytherapy in reducing neointima formation within the target segment relative to adjacent no or low radiation dose margins, or (2) as a result of the location of the final MLD (proximal or distal to the stent margin in the irradiated segment or beyond), a known independent predictor of disease recurrence at follow-up.[15] Neointimal proliferation at the treatment margins has not been convincingly proven to be the cause of the shift the MLD in any of the gamma trials.

Surrogate Endpoints in Vascular Brachytherapy Trials

The angiographic binary restenosis rate has been used as a surrogate of clinical target vessel revascularization (TVR) in assessing the effectiveness of new devices or stenting in interventional cardiology.[15] Because of the apparent MLD shifting observed in vascular brachytherapy trials, the extent of the segment of analysis most relevant in the angiographic reporting of vascular brachytherapy trials must be redefined. To better understand the relationship between clinical restenosis and the relative angiographic location of restenosis, we further reviewed the angiographic methodology of WRIST. Based on the three-vessel segments individually analyzed by QCA: (1) the "stent," (2) the "radiation source," and (3) the "source + margin" segment (including 5 mm on either end of the injured or radiation ribbon segment), receiver operator curves (ROC) were used to assess the value of the follow-up percent diameter stenosis for each of the three segments in predicting TVR. The follow-up diameter stenosis obtained from the three angiographic analyses including the stent, the ribbon and the ribbon + margin segments provided reliable indexes for identifying

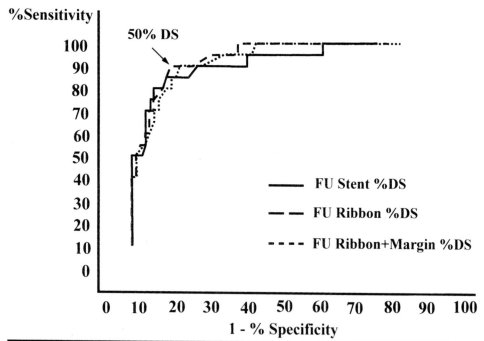

	Sensitivity	Specificity	Area ± SD	p-Value
Follow-up Stent % DS >50%	64.29%	89.19%	0.774 ± 0.121	<0.001
Follow-up Ribbon % DS >50%	66.07%	87.84%	0.804 ± 0.130	<0.001
Follow-up Ribbon+Margin % DS >50%	67.86%	86.49%	0.806 ± 0.130	<0.001

Figure 7. Receiver operator curves of the follow-up (FU) percent diameter stenosis (DS) for the stent, ribbon. and ribbon + margin analyses to determine the best surrogate of target vessel revascularization. A follow-up 50% DS obtained from the ribbon or the ribbon + margin analyses had the highest combined sensitivity and specificity for target lesion revascularization.

clinically driven target lesion revascularization (Fig. 7). The best angiographic surrogates, with the highest combined sensitivity and specificity for predicting clinically driven TVR was the binary restenosis rate (>50% DS) obtained from the ribbon + margin analysis segment (ROC area=0.806, $P<0.001$) and the ribbon analysis segment (ROC area=0.804 ± 0.130, $P<0.001$) rather than the stent analysis segment (ROC area=0.774 ± 0.121, $P<0.001$). Despite the low frequency of edge restenosis in WRIST, the restenosis rate obtained from the vessel segment inclusive of any injury and the dose fall-off zones was the best correlate of TVR. Selecting an adequate length of analysis in the angiographic assessment of vascular brachytherapy trials is particularly relevant the greater the concern or frequency of edge restenosis. These findings, although intuitive, underscore the importance of systematically including the angiographic outcome of the radiation ribbon, its dose fall-off margins as well as any zone of injury in the angiographic analysis of brachytherapy trials, and should become a standard and consistent analysis site for reporting the primary results of future vascular brachytherapy trials.

Limitations of Current QCA Versions in Assessing Vascular Brachytherapy Trials

The first and foremost limitation in the quantitative angiographic analysis of vascular brachytherapy trials is that of the acquisition. For such thorough angiographic analyses to be accurate, it is required that each step of the intervention be recorded on film, specifically in an attempt to understand the relationship between vascular injury, radiation dose fall-off, and lumen loss. Without compulsive acquisition techniques by the operator, with frequent contrast injections to precisely situate devices relative to visible side branches, such an analysis is flawed and potentially misleading. Furthermore, despite using side branches and other anatomic landmarks, the relative radiolucency of some stents makes precise localization of the stent within the artery somewhat problematic both for the angiographic analyst, and for the operator.

Current standard QCA algorithms are quickly becoming obsolete for the extensive analyses required of vascular brachytherapy trials. Each arterial segment of interest requires individual analysis with extensive editing to achieve the precise segment lengths; the trade-off is reproducibility. To better understand the interaction of arterial injury and vascular brachytherapy on disease recurrence, the addition of an injury segment of analysis has now become an integral component of any vascular brachytherapy trial analysis. Finally, although in the early gamma trials, stent margin restenosis was used as a surrogate measure of the so-called edge effect, a systematic analysis of the dose fall-off zones in all patients to assess lumen gain and loss in this region would more precisely quantify the "edge effect." The angiographic methodology of subsequent brachytherapy trials has incorporated many of these limitations including the zone of injury and the systematic isolated analysis of the dose fall-off zones. Newer, dedicated quantitative algorithms specifically designed for the analysis of brachytherapy trials are currently under development that will not only facilitate the analysis but also improve the accuracy and reproducibility of the angiographic measures.

Standardized QCA Methodology for Assessing Brachytherapy Trials

The angiographic evaluation of brachytherapy trials has become more challenging due to the extent of the segment receiving therapy (up to 60 mm in length) and the multiple associated landmarks (lesion, balloon injury, stent, and radiation delivery). Conventional QCA algorithms are limited in this regard due to the extensive editing and reanalyses required to execute these multiple segmental analyses.

Based on a consensus of experts consisting of interventional cardiologists, cardiovascular pathologists, radiation oncologists, and physicists (Ravello, Italy, March 2000), new terminology has been defined for vascular brachytherapy QCA application based on markers or physical landmarks obtained during the vascular intervention, in an attempt to achieve global consistency in the angiographic analysis and reporting of vascular brachytherapy trial results. This new terminology has been incorporated in the Brachy-option in the latest version of QCA software (MEDIS, Leiden, The Netherlands).

The main advantage of this software version is the reduced interface required by the QCA analyst in obtaining all segmental results. Guided by a detailed drawing demonstrating the precise location of each one of the landmarks, the QCA analyst will perform a single QCA analysis (at baseline, after final intervention, and at follow-up) of the entire coronary segment of analysis, by marking with pairs of flags, the positions of the procedural landmarks in the vessel or corresponding diameter function. From a practical standpoint, all parameters can be derived from this same diameter function, which results in higher consistency, while simplifying and minimizing user interface.

Definition of Terms

The *coronary segment of analysis* is the full extent of the target vessel that is used for QCA analysis. Within a coronary segment of analysis, there are four different segments that can be identified based on markers or physical landmarks and one segment that is derived from the four others (see Fig. 8):

1. The *obstructed* segment is the lesion proper (from which lesion length is derived) of the coronary segment of analysis demonstrating the stenosed area intended for conventional interventional treatment.
2. The *stented* segment is the part of the coronary segment of analysis that extends from the most proximal to the most distal stent edge or marker, when one or more new stents have been deployed or already exist as for in-stent restenosis. The unique pathophysiology of intimal hyperplasia within stented segments is the rational for distinguishing this segment from adjacent non-stented vessel segments where combined hyperplasia and negative remodeling contribute to late lumen loss. The effect of vascular brachytherapy within stented versus non-stented arterial segments can thereby be differentiated.
3. The *injured* segment is the part of the coronary segment of analysis that extends from the most proximal to the most distal marker or landmark of any physical vessel injury caused by one or multiple balloon inflations during PTCA, stent placement, or by the use of atherectomy devices. Analysis of the zones of injury may provide insight into the interaction between ves-

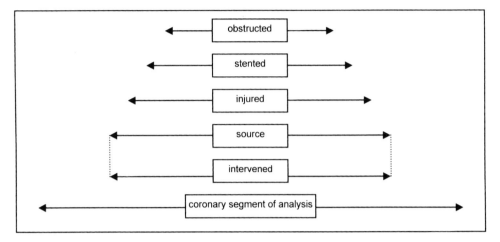

Figure 8. Ideal case with perfect line-up with definition of segments based on markers or physical landmarks.

sel injury and radiation exposure, with the caveat that this parameter is entirely dependent on operator's compulsive recording of all components of the intervention on film or CD.

4. The *source* segment is the part of the coronary segment of analysis extending from the most proximal to the most distal marker of the radiation source wire or delivery system. The specific landmark selection for the source segment analysis varies with the delivery system used and should represent over 90% of the prescribed dose at the target site.

5. The *intervened* segment is the part of the coronary segment of analysis including any marker or physical landmark of any device to which the vessel has been exposed to during the intervention (ie, the stent, balloon, source, atherectomy device, etc.). In practice, this means that the two outermost boundaries of any of the three different segments (ie, stented, injured, or source segments) define the intervened segment.

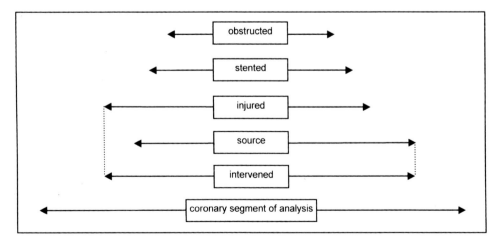

Figure 9. Mismatched case with definition of segments based on markers or physical landmarks.

In the ideal situation, each segment described is included in its successor; ie, the obstructed segment is included in the stented segment, which is included in the injured segment, which is included in the source/intervened segment, which in turn is included in the coronary segment of analysis (see Fig. 8). However, in practice, this may not be the case and segment mismatches (ie, where an individual segment is not included in its successor) may occur. In that case, the intervened segment will extend from the most proximal boundary (eg, of the injured segment) to the most distal boundary (eg, of the source segment) (see Fig. 9).

Definition and Assessment of the Segments Based on Biologically Relevant Landmarks

Within a coronary segment of analysis, there are three different biologically relevant segments that can be derived from the source segment providing pathophysiologically plausible zones of treatment. These segments are defined by the extent of radiation treatment exposure (see Fig. 10):

1. The *dose fall-off zone* segments are segments positioned around the proximal and distal boundaries of the source segment, representing the area of 90% to 10% dose fall-off. These areas straddle the proximal and the distal ends of the source and therefore are derived from the source segment. The length of the dose fall-off zone is device- and isotope-dependent; for instance, the dose fall-off length of a gamma source can be up to 10 mm, whereas that of a beta source is more focal within 5 mm (Fig. 11). Newer QCA algorithms (MEDIS) have been designed to have a prespecified default dose fall-off zone of 10 mm (5 mm on either side of the source markers, both proximally and distally), which can be changed by the analyst according to the specifications of the specific isotope and device. The biological correlate of the dose fall-off zone is the so-called "edge-effect," a proliferative effect postulated to result from a subtherapeutic radiation dose in the presence or absence of vessel injury.

2. The *prescribed dose* segment (prescribed dose segment length [PDL]) rep-

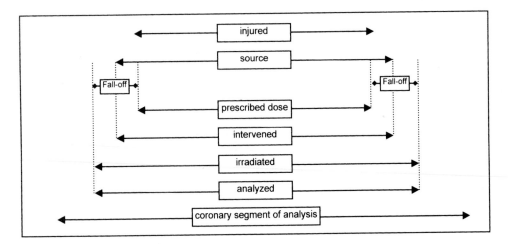

Figure 10. Segment definitions based on biologically relevant landmarks (ideal case).

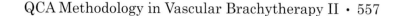

Percentage of Dose Along Source Train @ 2 mm for Sr-Y-90 and Ir-192

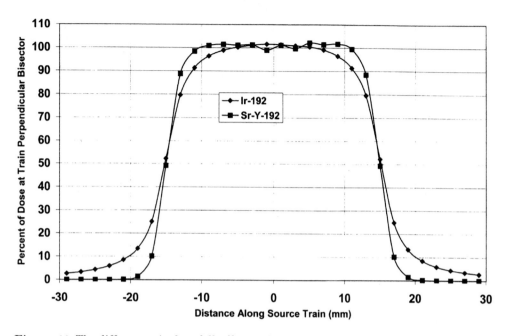

Figure 11. The differences in dose fall-off zones based on the two isotopes (Iridium-192 and Sr-Y-90) are shown. The length of the dose fall-off zone will vary based on the isotope being studied with a minimum default of 10 mm.

resents the source segment *excluding* the proximal and distal dose fall-off zones. The prescribed dose segment is the zone of radiation treatment exposed to greater than 90% of the radiation dose at the prescribed depth. The PDL is a frequently used parameter abbreviation. As for radiation oncology, vascular radiation therapy is considered successful when 90% of the prescribed dose has been delivered to the target area.

3. The *irradiated* segment (irradiated segment length [IRL]) is the source segment *including* the proximal and distal dose fall-off zones. The irradiated segment represents the full extent of the artery exposed to any radiation dose (by definition, the source segment, which includes the prescribed dose segment and its proximal and distal dose fall-off zones).

4. The *analyzed* segment is the intervened segment, *including* the proximal and distal dose fall-off zones. In practice, this means that the two outermost boundaries of any of the segments including the proximal and distal dose fall-off zones define the analyzed segment (see Fig. 10). Although the analyzed segment would be identical to the irradiated segment in an ideal situation, this is not always the case due to radiation treatment and injury mismatches.

In practice, a theoretically ideal situation may not be the case and segments mismatches (ie, where an individual segment is not included in its successor) may occur. In that case, the analyzed segment will extend from the most proximal boundary (eg, of the irradiated segment) to the most distal boundary (eg, of the injured segment) (see Fig. 12).

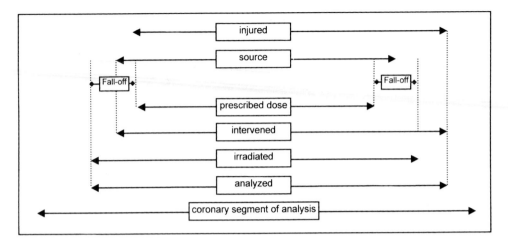

Figure 12. Segment definitions based on biologically relevant landmarks (mismatched case).

Definition and Assessment of the "Normal" Reference Vessel Segments

The *proximal and distal normal reference* segments are segments of 5 mm length both proximal and distal to the analyzed segment that represent the most normal reference vessel segment. These normal segments represent the normal "nondiseased" vessel (ie, showing normal progression/regression of the vessel), which have not been touched at all by any of the devices (see Fig. 13). The position and length of the normal segments must be user-defined based on the appearance of the coronary artery. Because of the extensive length of the coronary segment of analysis, the average of the mean diameter of the proximal and distal normal segments may be used as a measure of the average reference vessel size. Although this average value also takes any vessel tapering also into account, theoretically its value is only correct for the center position along the vessel. On the other hand, the well-known interpolated reference diameter approach, which provides a reference diameter value for each position along the vessel thereby corrected for any possible vessel tapering at each individual position, is the first choice for the correct percent stenosis measurements.

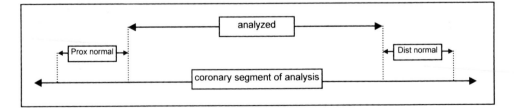

Figure 13. Defining the normal reference segments proximal and distal to the zones of treatment.

Definition and Assessment of the Radiation-Related Parts

To further describe the interrelation of radiation delivery to the extent of injury, three additional zones have been defined.[16]

1. The *geographic hit* (GH) refers to that portion of the coronary segment of analysis that has been subjected to injury *and* has been radiated with the prescribed dose. In practice, this means that the inner boundary of the dose fall-off zone (the boundary of the prescribed dose segment) and the boundary of the injured segment define the GH (see Fig. 14). In an ideal situation, GH is identical to the prescribed dose segment.

2. The *geographic extension* (GE) represent the proximal and distal parts of the coronary segment of analysis that have *not* been subjected to injury, but have been exposed to *any* radiation (including dose fall-off). In practice, the boundary of the injured segment and the outer boundary of the dose fall-off zone (the boundary of the irradiated segment) define the GE (see Fig. 14).

3. The *geographic miss* (GM) is the part of the coronary segment of analysis that has been subjected to injury, but has *not* been radiated with the prescribed dose. In practice, this means that the boundary of the injured segment and the inner boundary of the dose fall-off zone (= the boundary of the prescribed dose segment) define the GM (see Fig. 14). Only when the injured segment is completely included in the prescribed dose segment, is GM nonexistent.

The GM can be subdivided into different parts (see Fig. 15):

a) The *GM within the dose fall-off zone* (GM-fo) represents the part of GM that is within the dose fall-off zone segment. In practice, this means that the inner boundary of the dose fall-off zone (or the boundary of the prescribed dose segment) and the boundary of the injured segment, which falls *within* the outer boundary of the dose fall-off zone (or the boundary of the irradiated

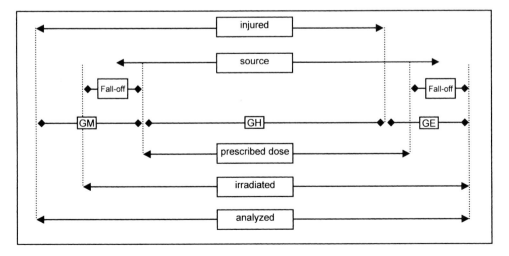

Figure 14. Definitions of the geographic hit (GH), geographic extention (GE), and geographic miss (GM).

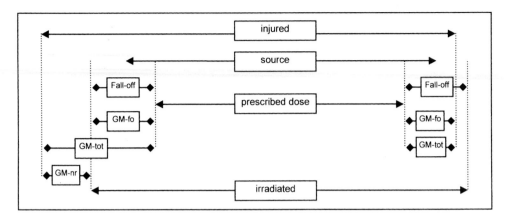

Figure 15. Definitions of the different zones of geographic miss (GM).

segment), define the GM-fo. This is the zone that is postulated to result in the proliferative "edge effect" (see right side of Fig. 15). The maximal extent of GM-fo is identical to the dose fall-off zone (see left side of Fig. 15).

b) The *GM with no radiation* (GM-nr) is the part of the GM that has *not* been exposed to any radiation. In practice, this means that the boundary of the injured segment and the outer boundary of the dose fall-off zone (= the boundary of the irradiated segment) define the GM-nr (see left side of Fig. 15).

c) The *total GM* (GM-tot) is the GM within the dose fall-off zone *plus* the GM with no radiation. In practice, this means that the boundary of the injured segment and the inner boundary of the dose fall-off zone (or the boundary of the prescribed dose segment) define the GM-tot.

Data Collection and Reporting for Vascular Brachytherapy Trials

For each of the defined segments, the following seven parameters should be reported:

Table 4

Overview Reports

Primary Report	Secondary Report	Tertiary Report
Obstructed segment	Prescribed dose segment	Subsegment analysis (Fig. 8)
Stented segment	Irradiated segment	
Injured segment	Geographic miss (proximal & distal)	
Source segment	1. GM total	
Intervened segment	2. GM dose fall-off	
Analyzed segment	3. GM no radiation	
Dose fall-off zone	Geographic extension (proximal & distal)	
(proximal & distal)	Geographic hit	
Reference segment		
(proximal & distal)		

GM = geographic miss.

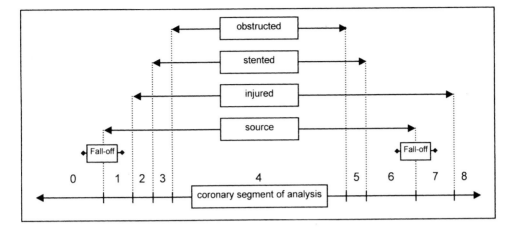

Figure 16. Definition of subsegments in a theoretically ideal (left) and not ideal (right) situation.

(1) the MLD; (2) the position of the MLD relative to the start-position of the coronary segment of analysis; (3) the mean diameter; (4) the interpolated reference diameter corresponding to a particular MLD (ie, the reference diameter measurements will be based on the interpolated reference diameter approach, which includes all the diameters over the entire coronary segment of analysis except for ectatic or aneurysmatic regions excluded by the flagging technique); (5) the percent diameter stenosis derived from the MLD and the interpolated reference diameter at the site of MLD within each segment; (6) the individual segment length; and (7) the position of the proximal and distal boundaries of an individual segment related to the start-position of the coronary segment of analysis. From all these data the detailed parameters as described in the Primary and Secondary Reports will be derived and presented automatically by the analytical software package (Table 4).

Tertiary Reporting

When traveling along the coronary segment from proximal to distal, the segment can be divided into subsegments, located between any two adjacent markers. This parameter set will be calculated and a constructed label will reflect whether the subsegment is either inside or outside a specific segment of interest (see Fig. 16) (eg, radiated/non-injured/non-stented/non-obstructed represents subsegment #1).

Conclusion

The complexity of the angiographic analysis of vascular brachytherapy trials necessary for our understanding of the mechanisms of treatment failure and for optimizing vascular brachytherapy delivery techniques has exceeded the scope of conventional QCA algorithms. Newer QCA versions, specifically designed for these purposes, have been developed based on the recommendations of a panel of experts in the field of vascular brachytherapy and are currently undergoing validation.

References

1. Lansky AJ, Popma J. Qualitative and quantitative angiography. In: Topol E (ed.): Interventional Cardiology, 3rd Edition. Philadelphia PA: WB Saunders; 1999:725–747.
2. Van der Zwet P, Reiber J. A new approach for the quantification of complex lesion morphology: The gradient field transform; basic principles and validation results. J Am Coll Cardiol 1994;24:216–224.
3. Strauss BH, Escaned J, Foley DP, et al. Technologic considerations and practical limitations in the use of quantitative angiography during percutaneous coronary recanalization. Prog Cardiovasc Dis 1994;36:343–362.
4. Foley DP, Escaned J, Strauss BH, et al. Quantitative coronary angiography (QCA) in interventional cardiology: Clinical application of QCA measurements. Prog Cardiovasc Dis 1994;36:363–384.
5. Lesperance J, Bourassa M, Schwartz L, et al. Definition and measurement of restenosis after successful coronary angioplasty: Implications for clinical trials. Am Heart J 1993;125:1394–1408.
6. Reiber J, Serruys P, Kooijman C, et al. Assessment of short-, medium-, and long-term variations in arterial dimensions from computer-assisted quantitation of coronary cineangiograms. Circulation 1985;71:280–288.
7. Popma J, Leon M, Keller M, et al. Reliability of the quantitative angiographic measurements in the New Approaches to Coronary Intervention (NACI) Registry: A comparison of clinical site and angiographic core laboratory readings. Am J Cardiol 1997; 80:19K-25K.
8. Umans V, Hermans W, Herrman J, J P, Serruys PW. Experiences of a quantitative coronary angiographic laboratory in restenosis prevention trials. In: Serruys PW, Foley D, de Feyter P (eds.): Quantitative Coronary Angiography in Clinical Practice. Dordrecht, The Netherlands: Kluwer Academic Publishers, 1994:121–135.
9. Teirstein PS, Massullo V, Jani S, et al. Catheter-based radiotherapy to inhibit restenosis after coronary stenting. N Engl J Med 1997;336:1697–1703.
10. Lansky AJ, Popma JJ, Massullo V, et al. Quantiative angiographic analysis of stent restenosis in the Scripps Coronary Radiation to inhibit intimal proliferation post stenting (SCRIPPS) trial. Am J Cardiol 1999;84:410–414.
11. Waksman R, White W, Chan RC, et al. Intracoronary gamma radiation therapy after angioplasty inhibits recurrence in patients with in-stent restenosis. Circulation 2000; 101:2165–2172.
12. Leon MB, Moses JW, Lansky AJ, et al. Intracoronary gamma radiation for the prevention of recurrent in-stent restenosis: Final results of the GAMMA I trial. Circulation 1999;100:I-75.
13. Lansky AJ, Weissman NJ, Desai KJ, et al. Predictors and mechanisms of in-stent edge restenosis in patients treated with iridium 192 brachytherapy: Results from the Gamma I trial. Circulation 1999;100(suppl I):I-221.
14. Ikari Y, Hara K, Tamura T, et al. Luminal loss and site of restenosis after Palmaz-Schatz coronary stent implantation. Am J Cardiol 1995;76:117–120.
15. Kuntz RE, Gibson CM, Nobuyoshi M, et al. Generalized model of restenosis after conventional balloon angioplasty, stenting, and directional atherectomy. J Am Coll Cardiol 1993;21:15–25.
16. Bonan R, Meerkin D, Bertrand O. Geographic miss: What is it? J Invas Cardiol 1999;11: 749–756.

## Chapter 44

Intravascular Ultrasound Assessment of the Mechanisms and Results of Brachytherapy

Gary S. Mintz, MD, and Neil J. Weissman, MD

Serial intravascular ultrasound (IVUS) studies have shown that restenosis in non-stented lesions (and late lumen loss in reference segments contiguous with edges of stents) is a balance between arterial remodeling and neointimal hyperplasia, while restenosis within stented lesions is primarily neointimal hyperplasia.[1,2] These findings are an important "backdrop" to this chapter and are discussed in detail elsewhere in this volume. The focus of this chapter will be on the mechanisms and results of brachytherapy as assessed by IVUS.

Methodological Considerations

Most brachytherapy studies have included IVUS analyses. In some cases, eg, the various Washington Radiation for In-Stent Restenosis Trials (WRIST), serial (post irradiation and follow-up) IVUS studies were performed in as many patients as possible. In other cases, IVUS was a substudy, usually site-specific, in a much smaller number of patients. These studies are noted in Table 1. It is important to note that these trials only assess the short-term (typically 6- to 9-month) effects of brachytherapy. It is also important to note that some of these substudies involved very few patients. While the in-lesion or in-stent IVUS analysis has enough statistical power to be significant with only a small number of patients, the edge analysis requires larger numbers to arrive at reasonable conclusions. This is because the dose fall-off at the edges, coupled with geographical miss, can result in a wider range of responses (eg, with both positive and negative remodeling) than is typically seen within the lesion.

In general (and unless mentioned specifically), the IVUS studies were all performed using motorized transducer pullback, and either volumetric or mean cross-sectional area (CSA), analysis. Because the lengths of segments analyzed in the many studies varied significantly, mean planar analysis may be a preferable way to compare the results of different data sets; this is especially true when comparing different in-stent restenosis studies.

Lesion site analysis, particularly in-stent neointimal hyperplasia, has become routine. The analysis of edge effects is more problematic. First, it was not

From Waksman R (ed.). *Vascular Brachytherapy, Third Edition.* Armonk, NY: Futura Publishing Co., Inc.; © 2002.

Table 1

IVUS Analyses in Various Brachytherapy Trials

Trial	No. of Patients in IVUS Study		Isotope	IVUS Analysis	
	Irradiated	Placebo		Lesion	Edge
Gamma					
SCRIPPS	18	18	^{192}Ir	X	
WRIST	47	50	^{192}Ir	X	X
Long WRIST	30	34	^{192}Ir	X	
High Dose Long WRIST	25		^{192}Ir	X	
Gamma-1	37	33	^{192}Ir	X	X
Beta					
BERT-PTCA lesions	21		^{90}Sr/^{90}Y	X	X
BERT-stented lesions	17		^{90}Sr/^{90}Y	X	X
PREVENT			^{32}P	X	X
Beta WRIST	25		^{90}Y	X	
START	24	16	^{90}Sr/^{90}Y	X	X
Beta-emitting stents					
"Standard" isostent	157		^{32}P	X	X
"Cold ends" isostent	43		^{32}P	X	X
"Hot ends" isostent	59		^{32}P	X	X

performed in all studies (Table 1). Some studies analyzed 5-mm long edge segments and reported volumetric (or mean planar) analysis of the entire edge segment; other studies report CSA analysis millimeter by millimeter over the length of the segment. Some combine proximal and distal edges and analyze them as a unit; others analyze proximal versus distal edges separately. Because edge effects can be very focal, and because the response of the edges and of the contiguous reference segments can vary over short distances beginning at the edge of the lesion (or stent), it is preferable to report edge effects as CSA analysis millimeter by millimeter over the length of the segment. This requires very careful "registration" of post-irradiation and follow-up images. Another problem with edge analyses is that on the IVUS studies, it is not possible to determine the edge of the source relative to the injured segment or to the IVUS image slices being measured. Angiography can be used as a guide. This works if the edge effect is close to the edge of the stent (within 5 mm). But this approach also has limitations. First, it requires meticulous comparison of IVUS and angiographic studies, which are usually done in different core laboratories. Second, stent edges that are intensely echorelfective are often radiolucent. Thus, most of the studies made one or more arbitrary assumptions, such as analyzing 5 mm of segment contiguous to the edge of the stent. However, this arbitrary approach also had limitations. The edge effect may be more than 5 mm from the edge of the stent, and in fact, may have no relationship to the edge of the stent. From a practical point, it is not common to image long segments of artery proximal, and especially distal, to a lesion. To properly understand edge effects, protocols must be specifically designed to image the entire length of *irradiated* (not just stented) vessel *plus* at least 5 to 10 mm of additional vessel *proximal and distal* to the irradiated segment.

Irradiation in Non-Stented Lesions

There have been no IVUS studies of gamma radiation in non-stented lesions. The data on beta irradiation of non-stented lesions is limited to extensive and detailed analysis of a small number of patients from BERT (Beta Energy Restenosis Trial). Serial (post-irradiation versus follow-up) volumetric IVUS analysis of 21 patients enrolled in BERT included a 30-mm long lesion segment and contiguous 5-mm long edges.[3] At the *lesion site* there was a significant increase in external elastic membrane (EEM) volume (451 ± 128 mm³ to 491 ± 159 mm³, $P=0.01$) which was parallel to the increase in plaque volume (201 ± 59 mm³ to 242 ± 74 mm³, $P=0.001$). As a result, lumen volume remained unchanged (251 ± 91 mm³ versus 249 ± 102 mm³, $P=NS$; Fig. 1). Changes in EEM volume showed a significant and positive correlation with changes in plaque volume ($r=0.66$, $P=0.001$; Fig. 2). Changes in lumen volume correlated significantly with changes in EEM volume ($r=0.69$, $P=0.005$), but not with changes in plaque volumes ($r=0.07$, $P=NS$). However, these "beneficial" effects on remodeling did not extend to the edges (Fig. 1). At the edges, there was an increase in plaque volume (27 ± 12 mm³ to 33 ± 10 mm³, $P=0.0001$), but no change in EEM volume (71 ± 24 mm³ to 71 ± 24 mm³, $P=NS$). As a result, there was a significant decrease in edge lumen volume (45 ± 16 mm³ to 38 ± 16 mm³, $P=0.01$).[1] At the edges, changes in lumen volume correlated significantly with changes in both EEM and plaque volume ($r=0.87$, $P<0.0001$ and $r=-0.51$, $P=0.03$); conversely, unlike at the lesion site, changes in EEM volume did not correlated with changes in plaque volume ($r=-0.03$). Thus, beta irradiation caused positive remodeling at the lesion site to prevent late lumen loss despite a significant amount of neointimal hyperplasia, but this positive remodeling did not extend to the edges.

In a secondary report, the irradiated segment (but not the edges) of 18 of these lesions were analyzed in 2-mm long subsegments (for a total of 270 subsegments).[4]

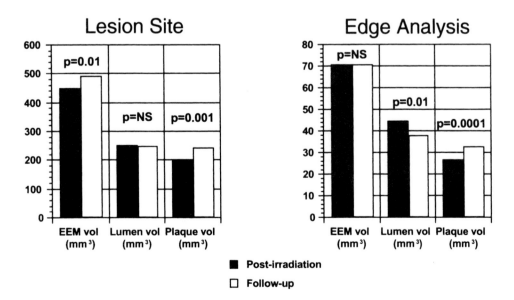

Figure 1. Lesion site and edge volumetric IVUS analysis after beta irradiation (^{90}Sr/^{90}Y) following balloon angioplasty (BERT).

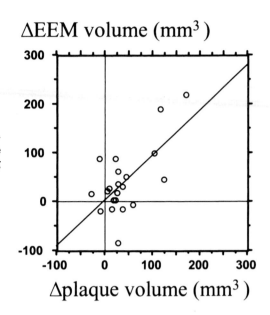

Figure 2. The correlation of ΔEEM (external elastic membrane) versus Δplaque after beta irradiation ($^{90}Sr/^{90}Y$) following balloon angioplasty (BERT).

There were three independent predictors of the absolute plaque volume at follow-up: plaque volume post-irradiation, D_{v90} at the adventitia, and the type of plaque (hard versus soft). This analysis showed that there was a wide range in the actual dose delivered to the adventitia; 26.2% of the subsegments received less than 4 Gy, 32.5% received 4.0 to 5.9 Gy, 22.8% received 6.0 to 7.9 Gy, 13.6% received 8.0 to 9.9 Gy, and 4.9% received greater than or equal to 10 Gy. The minimum effective dose delivered to 90% of the adventitia (D_{v90}) was found to be 4 Gy because subsegments receiving more than this dose demonstrated a significantly smaller increase in plaque volume versus those receiving less than 4 Gy ($P<0.01$).[4] This was also true for Δlumen volume; however, the impact on ΔEEM volume (ie, remodeling) was more variable. At lower doses, the relationship between Δlumen, Δplaque, and ΔEEM appeared to be similar to the edge analysis noted above. At higher doses, there was consistently more positive remodeling, less plaque volume growth, and greater late lumen increase (Fig. 3); in fact, above 6.0 Gy, ΔEEM was significantly greater than Δplaque to result in a late increase in lumen volume.

One of the problems with the dosimetric analysis is the unproven (and probably incorrect) assumption that adjacent subsegments behave independently. Nevertheless, in addition to being important for understanding the relationship between percutaneous transluminal coronary angioplasty (PTCA) and brachytherapy, the findings from BERT are also an important framework for understanding the IVUS findings after stenting+brachytherapy or treatment of in-stent restenosis+brachytherapy.

Beta Irradiation Followed by Stenting

Data on the use of beta irradiation prior to stenting comes from two sources. In the BERT Trial, cross-over to stent implantation was permitted for predefined endpoints (clinically significant dissection or residual stenosis >30%, n=17).[5] Within the stented segment, there was a decrease in lumen volume (129±41 mm³

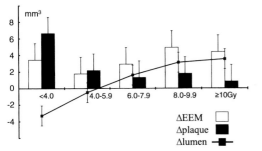

Figure 3. The impact of dose on ΔEEM (P=NS), Δplaque (P<0.0001), and Δlumen (P<0.0001) are shown (BERT). Reprinted from Reference 4 by permission of the American Heart Association.

to 122±42 mm³, P<0.05) as a result of an intimal hyperplasia (IH) volume of 7±7 mm³; there was an increase in EEM volume (259±74 mm³ to 278±90 mm³, P<0.05) as a result of an increase in peri-stent plaque volume (130±34 mm³ to 149±50 mm³, P<0.05). When proximal and distal 5-mm long edges were analyzed (and summed to make a total of 10 mm of stent edge), there was a decrease in lumen volume (73±28 mm³ to 61±26 mm³, P<0.05) as a result of a significant increase in plaque volume (61±26 mm³ to 78±29 mm³, P<0.05) without a significant change in EEM volume (133±49 mm³ to 139±47 mm³).

The Proliferation Reduction with Vascular Energy Trial (PREVENT) was a 105 patient trial of intracoronary radiation with ^{32}P, a beta-emitting source, in patients with in-stent restenosis (n=25), restenosis after PTCA (n=7), and de novo lesions in whom treatment with stents (n=64) or balloon angioplasty was allowed. As such, it represented a trial of beta-emitting radiotherapy in a broad spectrum of patients undergoing percutaneous coronary interventions.[6–8] Patients were randomized to placebo (n=25) or one of three doses. The IVUS analysis was primarily limited to the patients who received stents. Within the stented segment, there was an increase in IH volume in the irradiated patients, but this was less than in the placebo patients. An analysis of 40 stent edges in 23 patients has been presented. At the edges, there was a decrease in EEM (but no change in plaque) resulting in a decrease in lumen dimensions. ΔLumen correlated with ΔEEM (r=0.58, P=0.0001), but not with Δplaque (r=0.007). There was geographical miss in 30 of 40 edges; in these 30 edges, there was important negative remodeling in 77%. Conversely, in the 10 edges with adequate radiation coverage, there was negative remodeling in only 20%.

The SCRIPPS Trial

The first report on brachytherapy for preventing or treating in-stent restenosis was the Scripps Coronary Radiation to Inhibit Proliferation Post-Stenting (SCRIPPS) Trial.[9] The IVUS findings of this and other brachytherapy in-stent restenosis trials are summarized in Table 1. There was complete IVUS analysis in 18 treated and 18 placebo patients. Most of the lesions (62.5%) were in-stent restenosis lesions; the rest were restenotic lesions which were newly stented before being radiated.

In this study, IVUS was used to calculate dosimetry. The distance between the center of the ultrasonographic catheter (equivalent to the position of the radiation source) and the leading edge of the tunica media (the target) was measured at 1-mm intervals along the stented segment of the artery. Maximal and minimal source-to-target distances over the length of the lesion were determined. The radiation oncologist and the physicist combined this information with the specific activity of the radioactive sources to determine the time required to deliver 800 cGy to the target farthest from the radiation source, with no more than 3000 cGy delivered to the target closest to the source.

The in-stent restenosis length measured 23 ± 7 mm in the irradiated patients and 22 ± 8 mm in the placebo patients. At follow-up the increases in mean IH CSA (0.7 ± 0.9 mm^2) and volume (45 ± 39 mm^3) in the ^{192}Ir patients were less than in the placebo-treated patients (2.2 ± 1.8 mm^2 and 16 ± 23 mm^3, $P=0.01$ for both comparisons). The follow-up minimum lumen CSA measured 5.8 ± 1.4 mm^2 in the irradiated patients and 4.6 ± 2.5 mm^2 in the placebo patients ($P=0.073$).

The SCRIPPS Trial established the sensitivity of IVUS as an endpoint for brachytherapy as well as the effectiveness of this therapy. However, because edge effects were an underappreciated problem, IVUS imaging of the proximal and distal reference segments was not performed consistently.

All subsequent studies have supported the beneficial effect of brachytherapy in stented lesions. Table 2 summarizes the in-stent analysis of most of these studies.

Gamma Irradiation Treatment of In-Stent Restenosis

All gamma irradiation/in-stent restenosis studies used the same source: [192]Ir seeds delivered through 5F closed-end, noncentering catheters. The WRIST Trial was the first one specifically to address the issue of treatment of in-stent restenosis.[10] After successful intervention, 130 patients (100 native arteries and 30 vein grafts) were randomized to receive either [192]Ir (15 Gy at 2 mm) or placebo. Eighteen patients in the placebo group who developed recurrent in-stent restonosis

Table 2

Summary of IVUS "In-Stent" Findings after Brachytherapy*

Trial	Length (mm)	ΔIH CSA (mm²)			F/U Min. Lumen CSA (mm²)		
		Gamma	Placebo	P	Gamma	Placebo	P
SCRIPPS	22±8	0.7±0.9	2.2±1.8	0.01	5.8±1.4	4.6±2.5	0.073
WRIST	29±13	0.7±1.7	3.3±2.2	<0.0001	4.6±2.0	2.5±1.8	<0.0001
Long WRIST	55±15	0.6±1.1	2.3±1.5	<0.0001	2.9±1.0	1.9±1.1	0.0003
High Dose Long WRIST	67±17	0.6±1.5		4.0±1.4			
Gamma-1	32±13	0.6±1.0	1.6±1.2	0.0065	3.2±1.8	2.0±1.2	0.0035
		Beta	Placebo	P	Beta	Placebo	P
Beta WRIST	26±8	0.7±1.2			4.5±2.2		
START	21±8	−0.2±0.9	1.2±1.1	0.0003	4.0±1.6	2.8±1.5	0.027

*In an attempt to compare the various studies (whose differing lengths would, by definition, impact on volumetric findings), mean CSA findings are reported. Studies that reported only volumes are not included in this table.

IH = intimal hyperplasia; CSA = cross-sectional area; F/U = follow-up.

were crossed over to ^{192}Ir radiation and were also included in the IVUS analysis. Overall, 65 patients in the ^{192}Ir group (including 18 cross-over patients) and 50 in the placebo group had complete volumetric IVUS analysis. The length of in-stent restenosis segment analyzed measured 26±11mm in the irradiated patients versus 28±12 mm in the control group (P=NS).

At follow-up, the minimal lumen CSA was larger in the ^{192}Ir group compared to placebo (4.6±2.0 mm^2 versus 2.5±1.8 mm^2, P<0.0001). There was significantly less of an increase in IH volume (4±33 mm^3 versus 65±65 mm^3, P<0.0001) and mean IH CSA (0.7±1.7 mm^2 versus 3.3±2.2 mm^2, P<0.0001) in the ^{192}Ir group compared to placebo. As shown in Table 2, all subsequent brachytherapy studies have demonstrated an ability to reduce in-stent IH.

At the edges, there was no significant differences in ΔEEM CSA or ΔEEM volume in the ^{192}Ir group versus placebo (−0.0±2.1 mm^2 versus −0.5±1.7 mm^2, P=0.09; and −1±8 mm^3 versus −2±9 mm^3, P=0.17, respectively). The decrease in the mean lumen CSA and volume were also similar in the ^{192}Ir versus placebo groups (−0.5±1.8 mm^2 versus −0.9±1.6 mm^2, P=0.08; and −3±9 mm^3 versus −5±8 mm^3, P=0.13; respectively). The CSA and volume of tissue growth was similar (0.3±1.5 mm^2 versus 0.5±1.3 mm^2, P=0.62; and 2±8 mm^3 versus 2±7 mm^3, P=0.76; respectively). Thus, *compared to placebo,* there did not appear to be an edge effect after gamma irradiation treatment of in-stent restenosis.

However, while unusual and not different from the placebo group or previous reports of newly stented lesions, edge recurrence in gamma-irradiated patients occurred at the distal edge in eight patients. These patients were studied in more detail and compared to 21 patients with no recurrence. When compared to nonrestenotic lesions, lesions with *distal edge recurrence* had: (1) a greater decrease in distal lumen CSA (mean Δlumen CSA=−3.0±1.2 mm^2 versus −0.7±1.0 mm^2, P=0.0002); (2) no change in mean distal EEM CSA (−0.2±0.5 mm^2) versus an increase in mean distal EEM CSA of 1.0±0.9 mm^2 in nonrestenotic lesions (P=0.0047); and (3) a greater increase in mean distal plaque and media (P&M) CSA (2.9±1.2 mm^2 versus 1.7±0.6 mm^2, P=0.0103, Fig. 3).[11] These findings are similar to the edge effects of beta irradiation observed after balloon angioplasty in BERT.

Within the stented segment, the nonrestenotic lesions had no decrease in mean lumen CSA and no increase in mean IH CSA. Conversely, lesions with distal edge recurrence had a significant decrease in *mean intrastent* lumen CSA (−1.7±1.7 mm^2) and a significant increase in *mean intrastent* IH CSA (1.6±1.6 mm^2). The stented segment was then divided into four 10-mm long sections (Fig. 4). The decrease in lumen CSA and the increase in IH CSA were more pronounced closer to the distal edge of the stent. However, in the edge recurrence lesions, there was a decrease in lumen CSA and an increase in IH CSA in all four intrastent sections: within 10 mm of the distal edge, 11 to 20 mm from the distal edge, 21 to 30 mm from the distal edge, and 31 to 40 mm from the distal edge. When compared to nonrestenotic lesions, lesions with *distal edge recurrence* had a greater decrease in mean proximal lumen CSA (Δlumen CSA=−1.7±1.3 mm^2 versus −0.3±0.8 mm^2, P=0.0213). There was also a trend toward a greater increase in mean *proximal* P&M CSA (2.3±2.0 mm^2 versus 1.4±0.8 mm^2, P=0.14). These findings suggest that edge recurrence after gamma irradiation is part of diffuse treatment failure, extending even into the proximal reference.[11]

In 6 of 8 distal edge recurrence lesions there was evidence of geographical miss (versus 4/21 nonrecurring lesions, P=0.0046).[12] The lesions with geographi-

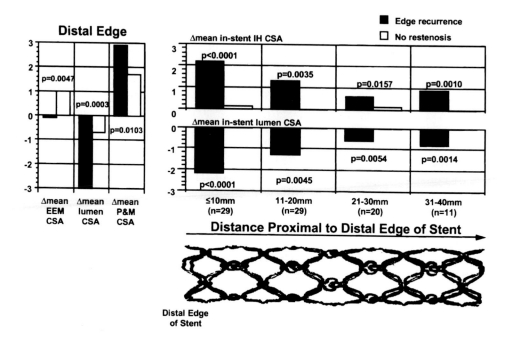

Figure 4. Edge effect in WRIST. In lesions with distal edge recurrence, there was evidence of a diffuse increase in intimal hyperplasia (IH) that was greatest in the 10-mm long segment adjacent to the distal edge, but extended into the proximal stent.

cal miss had no change in mean distal EEM CSA (0.0 ± 0.5 mm²). Conversely, the lesions with adequate radiation coverage had an increase in mean distal EEM CSA (0.8 ± 1.0 mm², $P=0.085$). Mean lumen CSA tended to decrease more in lesions with geographical miss (Δlumen$=-2.3\pm1.3$ mm² versus -1.3 ± 1.7 mm², $P=0.18$). There was no difference in mean ΔP&M CSA (2.3 ± 1.3 mm² versus 2.1 ± 1.0 mm², $P=0.6$).

One proposed solution to edge effects is to radiate longer segments. Therefore, to determine the short-term safety of this approach, we analyzed the effect of brachytherapy on irradiated, but uninjured reference segments–those segments in the artery that were more than 5 mm proximal or distal to the stent edge (Fig. 5).[13] In the proximal reference, there was a similar increase in plaque CSA in both the [192]Ir ($+0.7\pm1.1$ mm²) and placebo patients ($+0.6\pm0.9$ mm²). However, in the ^{192}Ir group, there was an increase in EEM CSA ($+0.5\pm0.6$mm²), while in the placebo group there was a decrease in EEM CSA (-0.6 ± 0.7 mm², $p<0.0001$ versus ^{192}Ir). Thus, there was no change in lumen area in the ^{192}Ir group (-0.2 ± 1.4 mm²), while in the placebo group there was a significant decrease in lumen area (-1.2 ± 1.1 mm², $P=0.0002$ versus ^{192}Ir). In the distal reference, there was a similar increase in plaque CSA in both the [192]Ir ($+1.0\pm1.0$ mm²) and placebo groups ($+0.9\pm0.9$ mm²). However, in the ^{192}Ir group there was an increase in EEM CSA ($+1.0\pm1.1$ mm²) while in the placebo group there was a slight decrease in EEM CSA (-0.4 ± 1.1 mm², $p<0.0001$ versus ^{192}Ir). As a result, in the ^{192}Ir group, there was no change in lumen CSA (0 ± 1.3 mm²), while in the placebo group there was a decrease in lumen area (-1.2 ± 1.1 mm², $P<0.0001$ versus ^{192}Ir). These changes did not vary along the length of reference segment analyzed.

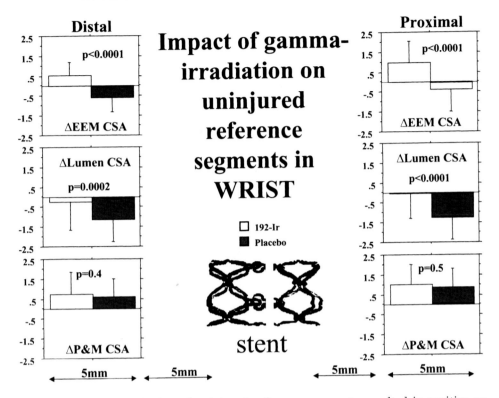

Figure 5. Gamma irradiation of uninjured reference segments resulted in positive remodeling (increase in external elastic membrane [EEM] cross-sectional area [CSA]) that prevented lumen loss (Gamma-1).

The WRIST Trial: (1) established the efficacy of gamma irradiation to prevent recurrent in-stent restenosis; (2) showed that edge effects after gamma irradiation were the result of negative remodeling and geographical miss, and were part of diffuse treatment failure; and (3) indicated that gamma irradiation promoted positive remodeling of uninjured reference segments.

Impact of Lesion Length on Gamma Radiation Treatment of In-Stent Restenosis

Long WRIST was a double-blind, placebo-controlled trial of intracoronary gamma irradiation in 120 patients with diffuse native artery in-stent restenosis lesions (length, 36 to 80 mm). The dose prescription was identical to WRIST.

Measured in-stent restenosis length was 56 ± 14 mm in the ^{192}Ir patients and 54 ± 15 mm in the placebo patients. During the follow-up period there was a decrease in lumen volume in both the [192]Ir (323 ± 134 mm^3 to 293 ± 130 mm^3, $P=0.0153$) and placebo groups (342 ± 129 mm^3 to 217 ± 114 mm^3, $P<0.0001$). This was the result of an increase in IH volume in both groups (97 ± 98 mm^3 to 132 ± 127 mm^3, $P=0.0175$; and 86 ± 52 mm^3 to 207 ± 100 mm^3, $P<0.0001$; respectively). However, in the placebo patients the increases in mean IH CSA (2.3 ± 1.5 mm^2) and volume (120 ± 81 mm^3) were significantly greater than in the irradiated patients

(0.6±1.1 mm^2 and 35±76 mm^3, $P<0.0001$ for both comparisons). At follow-up, the minimum lumen CSA measured 2.9±1.0 mm^2 in the ^{192}Ir group versus 1.9±1.1 mm^2 in the controls ($P=0.0003$).[14]

In an attempt to understand the impact of lesion length on the treatment of in-stent restenosis, native artery Long WRIST lesions were compared to WRIST lesions.[15] Post-intervention stent areas were larger in WRIST (8.9±2.5 mm^2) and smaller in Long WRIST (7.6±2.5 mm^2, $P=0.0274$) patients. In particular, minimum stent CSA in Long WRIST measured only 5.2±1.0 mm^2. This was consistent with the trend for EEM CSA to be larger in WRIST lesions versus Long WRIST lesions: 15.0±3.7 mm^2 versus 13.6±2.7 mm^2, $P=0.078$. At follow-up, there was a significant decrease in *mean* lumen areas in Long WRIST, but not in WRIST patients. There was also a greater increase in mean IH CSA in Long WRIST, but not in WRIST. Of note, the increase in maximum IH CSA was much greater in Long WRIST than in WRIST resulting in a ratio of maximum to minimum follow-up IH CSA of 7.7±13.6 mm^2 in Long WRIST versus 2.9±1.3 mm^2 in WRIST. This indicated a greater heterogeneity in neointimal recurrence over the length of the in-stent restenosis lesion in Long WRIST. As a result there was a smaller follow-up *minimum* lumen area in Long WRIST (2.9±1.0 mm^2) compared to WRIST lesions (4.2±2.0 mm^2, $P=0.0015$).

To analyze the impact of lesion geometry on the response to radiation, the maximum and minimum distances from the IVUS catheter to the EEM were measured as an index of the source-target distance. The maximum source-to-target distance was greater in Long WRIST than in WRIST (4.0±0.7 mm versus 2.8±0.4 mm, $P<0.0001$); the maximum source-to-target distance correlated directly with in-stent restenosis length ($r=0.547$, $P<0.0001$). When IVUS results were compared to the source-to-target distances, $\Delta minimum$ lumen CSA and $\Delta maximum$ IH CSA correlated with the maximum source-to-target distance ($r=0.352$, $P=0.0038$ and $r=0.523$, $P<0.0001$, respectively). The variability in neointimal reaccumulation (maximum/minimum follow-up IH CSA) also correlated with the maximum source-to-target distance ($r=0.378$, $P<0.0001$). This indicated that the greater heterogeneity in the neointimal response present in Long WRIST lesions was related to a greater variability in lesion geometry and source eccentricity.

These findings suggested that adjusting the dose would improve the effectiveness of brachytherapy in these very long lesions. A group of 25 patients were treated with an increased dose of 18 Gy at 2 mm from the source. The length of in-stent restenosis in the higher dose group was 66±17 mm. At follow-up, while the increase in mean IH CSA was similar in the High Dose Long WRIST compared to the Long WRIST patients (0.6±1.5 mm^2 versus 0.6±1.1 mm^2), the follow-up minimum lumen CSA was larger in the high dose group (4.0±1.4 mm^2 versus 2.9±1.0 mm^2, $P=0.0009$) indicating that the increased dose prescription evened out the actual dose delivered to the adventitia.

The Gamma-1 Trial

The Gamma-1 Trial was a multicenter study of gamma irradiation treatment of in-stent restenosis. The dose prescription was similar to the SCRIPPS Trial. The IVUS substudy was performed in four centers. The length of in-stent restenosis analyzed was 32±13 mm in the treated and 33±14 mm in the placebo patients. At

Table 3

IVUS Findings in Gamma-1

	192Ir	Placebo	P
N	37	33	
Proximal reference segment			
Δ mean EEM CSA (mm²)	−0.6±2.0	−1.2±2.2	0.4
Δ mean lumen CSA (mm²)	−0.9±1.8	−0.8±1.5	1.0
Δ mean P&M CSA (mm²)	0.3±1.8	−0.3±2.0	0.3
Stented segment			
Length (mm)	32±13	33±14	0.9
Δ stent volume (mm³)	3±37	2±24	0.9
Δ lumen volume (mm³)	−25±34	−48±42	0.0225
Δ IH volume (mm³)	28±37	50±40	0.0352
Distal reference segment			
Δ mean EEM CSA (mm²)	−0.5±2.0	0±2.0	0.3
Δ mean lumen CSA (mm²)	−0.8±1.9	−0.6±2.2	0.7
Δ mean P&M CSA (mm²)	0.3±1.7	0.6±2.3	0.5
Index minimum lumen area (mm²)	4.2±1.7	4.2±1.4	1.0
Follow-up minimum lumen area (mm²)	3.2±1.8	2.0±1.2	0.0035
Index area stenosis (%)	25±25	24±26	1.0
Follow-up area stenosis (%)	31±32	55±38	0.0124

EEM = external elastic membrane; CSA = cross-sectional area; P&M = plaque and media; IH = initmal hyperplasia.

follow-up, the increase in IH volume (28±37 mm³ versus 50±40 mm³, $P=0.0352$) and the increase in mean IH CSA (0.8±1.0 mm² versus 1.6±1.2 mm², $P=0.0065$) were less in the 192Ir versus placebo patients. Follow-up minimum lumen area was larger and the area stenosis (33±32% versus 55±38%, $P=0.0124$) smaller in the 192Ir compared to placebo patients. The lack of an edge effect (when the 192Ir patients were compared to placebo) that was observed in WRIST was substantiated in Gamma-1.[16] These findings are shown in Table 3 and Figure 6.

Beta Irradiation Treatment of In-Stent Restenosis

There have been two trials specifically designed to assess the efficacy of beta irradiation in treating in-stent restenosis: Beta WRIST and START (Stents and Radiation Therapy). Beta WRIST was a registry. The source was a 90Y wire that was inserted automatically by the BETAMED Intracoronary Radiation System (Boston Scientific Corporation, Nattick, MA) afterloader into a segmented centering balloon delivery catheter positioned at the treatment site. The prescribed dose was 20.6 Gy at 1 mm from the surface of the balloon. While the results were compared to the placebo group in WRIST, there was no control group. Length of in-stent restenosis was 26±8 mm. There was a decrease in IH volume from 102±53 mm³ to 118±61 mm³ which reduced lumen volume from 189±83 mm³ to 165±105 mm³.[17] There was no edge analysis in Beta WRIST.

START[18] was a randomized trial comparing the same brachytherapy system used in BERT (hydraulic delivery of 90Sr/90Y seeds) versus placebo in the treat-

Irradiated Patients in Gamma-1

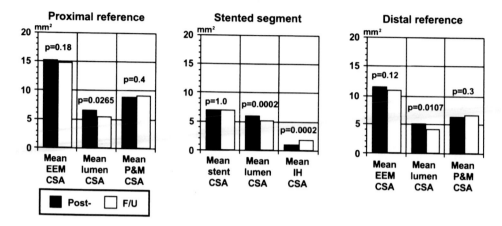

Figure 6. Intravascular ultrasound (IVUS) findings in the irradiated patients in Gamma-1.

ment of in-stent restenosis. The findings were similar to the gamma-emitter studies with no change in the neointimal hyperplasia in the treated group and a significant increase in the neointimal hyperlasia in the placebo group.

INHIBIT was also a randomized placebo-controlled trial in the treatment on in-stent restenosis. It used a beta emitter (^{32}P) delivered via a source-centering catheter. Results are pending.

Radiation-Emitting Stents

A number of analyses have looked at the efficacy of ^{32}P beta-emitting stents.[5,19–23] The dose findings of the Milan group and the core lab analysis of the global isostent experience are shown in Figures 7 and 8. The analysis from the Thoraxcenter showed an IH volume of 21 ± 12 mm^3 in the low activity group (0.75 to 1.5 µCi) and an IH volume of 9 ± 9 mm^3 in the high activity group (6.0 to 12.0 µCi). Thus, all three reached the same conclusion that increasing activity decreased in-stent neointimal hyperplasia. Of interest, in contradistinction to catheter-based beta irradiation (using ^{90}Sr/^{90}Y) followed by stent implantation, there was no evidence of positive remodeling within the length of the ^{32}P beta-emitting stent in either the low- or high activity groups.[5]

The main limitation of ^{32}P beta-emitting stents is the edge effect, the so-called "candy wrapper."[22] Both angiographically and by IVUS there is a profound, focal, and sharply demarcated lumen loss at the edge of the beta-emitting stent. When these edges were analyzed millimeter by millimeter, it was apparent that this focal edge lumen loss was the result of a focal increase in neointimal tissue which peaks approximately 1 mm outside the edge of the stent (Figs. 9 and 10).[19,20] (Whether remodeling contributes to this "candy wrapper" edge effect is the subject of some debate; however, neither of these analyses shows that remodeling contributes *importantly*.) The IsoStent experience illustrates the importance of the analysis plan in understanding the mechanism of edge effects. For example, when 5-mm long seg-

Milan IsoStent Experience

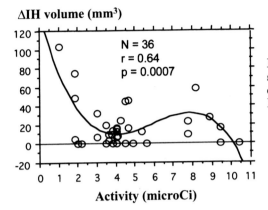

N = 36
r = 0.64
p = 0.0007

Figure 7. The Milan IsoStent dose response analysis. Reprinted from Reference 19 by permission of the American Heart Association.

Global IsoStent Experience

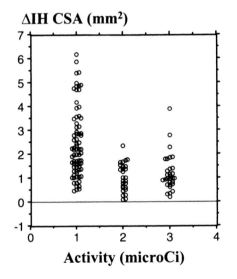

Figure 8. The core IVUS laboratory global IsoStent dose-response experience.

Milan IsoStent Experience

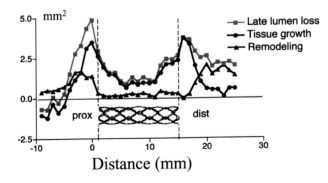

Figure 9. The Milan IVUS analysis of edge effects after beta-emitting stents. Reprinted from Reference 19 by permission of the American Heart Association.

Global IsoStent Experience

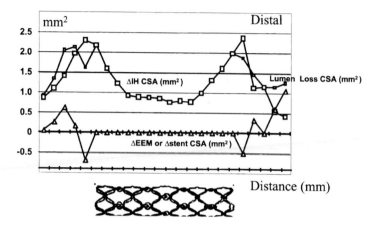

Figure 10. The core IVUS laboratory analysis of edge effects after beta-emitting stents.

ments proximal and distal to the stent edges were analyzed *as a volume,* the conclusion was quite different.[5] There was a decrease in lumen volume (from 75 ± 39 mm^3 to 67 ± 34 mm^3 in the low activity group, $P<0.05$, and from 75 ± 23 mm^3 to 63 ± 24 mm^3 in the high activity group, $P<0.05$). This was the result of a decrease in EEM volume in both groups (127 ± 58 mm^3 to 116 ± 49 mm^3 in the low activity group, $P<0.05$, and 126 ± 45 mm^3 to 118 ± 46 mm^3 in the high activity group, $P<0.05$) with *no* siginficant change in plaque volumes (51 ± 25 mm^3 to 49 ± 21 mm^3 in the low activity group and 51 ± 16 mm^3 to 55 ± 16 mm^3 in the high activity group).

Two modifications in the pattern of beta energy emission were tried. Cold ends merely broadened the peak of the "edge" IH and shifted this peak within the body of the stents (Fig. 11). In addition, there was more in-stent neointima (Fig.

"Cold" Ends IsoStent Experience

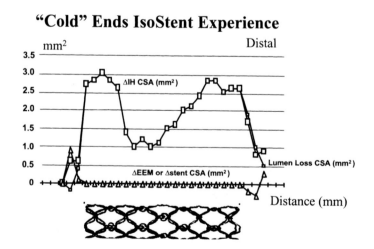

Figure 11. The core IVUS laboratory analysis of edge effects after "cold ends" beta-emitting stents.

"Hot" Ends IsoStent Experience

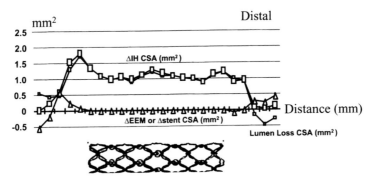

Figure 12. The core IVUS laboratory analysis of edge effects after "hot ends" beta-emitting stents.

11).[23] Conversely, hot ends appeared to attenuate the edge effect (Fig. 12); however, this was accompanied by isolated cases of marked late malapposition.

"Complications" of Brachytherapy

There are a number of IVUS observations that have been called complications of brachytherapy.

The impact of brachytherapy on the healing of post-angioplasty dissections was reported in the BERT Trial. In one study IVUS dissections were seen in 16 of 22 patients (73%) after intervention. At 6-month follow-up, 8 patients had persisting dissections; 6 had no evidence of healing and 2 had partial healing. IVUS healed dissection received a mean prescribed dose of 14 Gy and nonhealed dissection received 13.8 Gy (P=NS).[24] This finding of nonhealing of dissections after beta irradiation following balloon angioplasty was substantiated in a report by Meerkin et al.[25] Immediate post-angioplasty and 6-month follow-up IVUS studies of 94 patients in the IVUS substudy of the MultiVitamins and Probucol (MVP) trial and 26 non-stented patients in BERT were analyzed for the presence or absence of dissection. Of the 28 patients with post-angioplasty dissections in MVP, all but one had healed at 6 months. Conversely, of the 16 patients with post-angioplasty dissections in BERT, 7 had not healed (P<0.0002).

A second potential complication of brachytherapy is late stent-vessel wall malapposition. In Gamma-1, for example, late malapposition was seen in only patient; that patient was in the placebo group.[26,27] In START, there was one documented case of late malapposition in the beta-irradiated group and none in the placebo group.

A third potential complication is the "black hole" phenomenon—echolucent neointimal tissue.[28,29] It has been seen after both gamma and beta emitters and beta-emitting stents and in patients with and without stents and with and without in-stent restenosis. Directional atherectomy has been performed in 4 patients; specimens showed large myxoid areas with interspersed smooth muscle cells that were scattered in the extracellular matrix that contained proteoglycan.

It should be emphasized that none of these "complications" are unique to brachytherapy; however, they occur with marked increased frequency after radiation. Despite the suggestion that these "complications" may contribute to late thrombosis, none of the patients with these IVUS "complications" developed late thrombosis, and no patient with late thrombosis had IVUS imaging. Thus, the clinical relevance of these finding is currently unknown.

Of note, chronic stent recoil was not observed in any brachytherapy/in-stent restenosis study.

What Have We Learned?

Methodology is important to understanding mechanisms of brachytherapy, especially as they apply to edge effects. Small patient number IVUS substudies have the power to show significant treatment effects, especially as they apply to the in-lesion or in-stent analysis. The treatment effects of brachytherapy in PTCA, stenting, and treatment of in-stent restenosis seem to be similar. In PTCA, de novo stenting, and treatment of in-stent restenosis, radiation decreases neointimal hyperplasia, promotes positive remodeling in PTCA-treated lesions, and either has no effect or promotes positive remodeling along *adequately* irradiated edges and reference segments. These effects are dose-related. At the edges, where the dose is less, and especially in the presence of geographical miss, there is a combination of increased neointimal hyperplasia and either absence of positive remodeling or frank negative remodeling.

The findings in beta-emitting stents are idiosyncratic and different from beta or gamma irradiation after PTCA, de novo stenting, and treatment of in-stent restenosis. There is a dose-related decrease in intrastent neointima. Edge effects are primarily a focal exaggeration in neointimal hyperplasia which also appears to be dose-related.

References

1. Mintz GS, Popma JJ, Pichard AD, et al. Arterial remodeling after coronary angioplasty: A serial intrascular ultrasound study. Circulation 1996;94:35–43.
2. Hoffmann R, Mintz GS, Dussaillant GR, et al. Patterns and mechanisms of instent restenosis: A serial intravascular ultrasound study. Circulation 1996;94:1247–1254.
3. Sabate M, Serruys PW, van der Giessen WJ, et al. Geometric vascular remodeling after balloon angioplasty and beta-radiation therapy: A three-dimensional intravascular ultrasound study. Circulation 1999;100:1182–1188.
4. Sabate M, Marijnissen JP, Carlier SG, et al. Residual plaque burden, delivered dose, and tissue composition predict 6-month outcome after balloon angioplasty and beta-radiation therapy. Circulation 2000;101:2472–2477.
5. Kay IP, Sabate M, Costa MA, et al. Positive geometric vascular remodeling is seen after catheter-based radiation followed by conventional stent implantation but not after radioactive stent implantation. Circulation 2000;102:1434–1439.
6. Raizner AE, Oesterle SN, Waksman R, et al. Inhibition of restenosis with beta-emitting radiotherapy: Report of the Proliferation Reduction with Vascular Energy Trial (PREVENT). Circulation 2000;102:951–958.
7. Okura H, Lee DP, Handen CE, et al. Contribution of vessel remodeling to "edge effect" following intracoronary β-irradiation: A serial volumetric intravascular ultrasound study. Circulation 1999;100:I-511.
8. Lee DP, Okura H, Handen CE, et al. Reference segment and target lesion effects of ^{32}P radiation: Intravascular ultrasound results of the PREVENT Trial. Circulation 1999;100:I-517.

9. Teirstein PS, Massullo V, Jani S, et al. Catheter-based radiotherapy to inhibit restenosis after coronary stenting. N Engl J Med 1997;336:1697–1703.
10. Waksman R, White RL, Chan RC, et al. Intracoronary gamma radiation therapy after angioplasty inhibits recurrence in patients with in-stent restenosis. Circulation 2000;101:2165–2171.
11. Ahmed J, Mintz GS, Harrington D, et al. Mechanism of edge recurrence following brachytherapy treatment of in-stent restenosis: A serial intravascular ultrasound study. Circulation 1999;100:I-222.
12. Ahmed JM, Mintz GS, Kim H-S, et al. Intravascular ultrasound findings in patients with geographical miss following vascular brachytherapy treatment of in-stent restenosis. Circulation 2000;102:II-634.
13. Ahmed JA, Mintz GS, Waksman R, et al. Safety of intracoronary gamma radiation on uninjured reference segments during the first six months after treatment of in-stent restenosis: A serial intravascular ultrasound study. Circulation 2000;101:2227–2230.
14. Ahmed JM, Mintz GS, Leiboff B, et al. A serial intravascular ultrasound study to assess the efficacy of intracoronary γ-irradiation in preventing recurrent diffuse in-stent restenosis in long lesions. Circulation 2000;102:II-692.
15. Ahmed JM, Mintz GS, Waksman R, et al. Serial intravascular ultrasound analysis of the impact of lesion length on the efficacy of intracoronary gamma irradiation for preventing recurrent in-stent restenosis. Circulation 2001;103:188–191.
16. Mintz GS, Weissman NJ, Teirstein PS, et al. Effect of intracoronary gamma-radiation therapy on in-stent restenosis: An intravascular ultrasound analysis from the Gamma-1 Study. Circulation 2000;102:2915–2918.
17. Bhargava B, Mintz GS, Mehran R, et al. Serial volumetric intravascular ultrasound analysis of the efficacy of beta irradiation in preventing recurrent in-stent restenosis. Am J Cardiol 2000;85:651–653.
18. Tagaki A, Morino Y, Fox T, et al. Efficacy of intracoronary β-irradiation for the treatment on in-stent restenosis: Volumetric analysis by intravascular ultrasound. Circulation 2000;102:II-422.
19. Albiero R, Adamian M, Kobayashi N, et al. Short- and intermediate-term results of (32)P radioactive beta-emitting stent implantation in patients with coronary artery disease: The Milan Dose-Response Study. Circulation 2000;101:18–26.
20. Weissman NHJ, Titana A, Canos DA, et al. Comparison of IVUS findings of the β-emitting IsoStent versus a non-radiation control group from the HIPS trial. Circulation 2000;102:II-691.
21. Weissman NJ, Albiero R, Dimario C, et al. Final IVUS results from the IsoStent BXI multicenter dose response study. Circulation 2000;102:II-567.
22. Albiero R, Nishida T, Adamian M, et al. Edge restenosis after implantation of high activity (32)P radioactive beta-emitting stents. Circulation 2000;101:2454–2457.
23. Weissman NJ, Albiero R, De Bruyne B, et al. Final IVUS results from the multicenter "cold ends" IsoStent Study. Circulation 2000;102:II-568.
24. Kay IP, Sabate M, Van Langenhove G, et al. Outcome from balloon induced coronary artery dissection after intracoronary beta radiation. Heart 2000;83:332–337.
25. Meerkin D, Tardif JC, Bertrand OF, et al. The effects of intracoronary brachytherapy on the natural history of postangioplasty dissections. J Am Coll Cardiol 2000;36:59–64.
26. Kozuma K, Costa MA, Sabate M, et al. Late stent malapposition occurring after intracoronary beta-irradiation detected by intravascular ultrasound. J Invas Cardiol 1999;11:651–655.
27. Mintz GS, Weissman NJ, Pappas C, Waksman R. Positive remodeling, regression of in-stent neointimal hyperplasia, and late stent malapposition in the absence of brachytherapy. Circulation 2000;102:E11.
28. Castagna MT, Mintz GS, Weissman NJ, et al. "Black hole": Echolucent restenosis tissue following brachytherapy. Circulation 2001;103:778.
29. Kay IP, Ligthart JM, Virmani R, et al. The black hole: A new IVUS observation after intracoronary radiation. Circulation 2000;102:II-568.

## Chapter 45

Intravascular Ultrasound Observations for Stented and Non-Stented Procedures

Seung-Ho Hur, MD, Yasuhiro Honda, MD,
Heidi N. Bonneau, RN, MS, Paul G. Yock, MD,
and Peter J. Fitzgerald, MD, PhD

Introduction

For several decades, coronary angiography has been the primary diagnostic technique for the assessment of atherosclerotic coronary artery disease. Although it provides the location of atherosclerotic narrowings and plaque morphology, it has several significant limitations in assessing disease mechanism, plaque composition, and complications after coronary intervention. In contrast, intravascular ultrasound (IVUS) provides accurate quantitation and morphology of the plaque as well as vessel morphology. In the late 1980s, IVUS was developed mainly as a research tool, yet it now offers detailed diagnostic information as well as insight into optimizing interventional strategies. Currently, several therapeutic strategies exist for the treatment of atherosclerotic coronary artery disease, such as stents, balloons, and atheroablative devices. These devices have been implemented in the hope of reducing the incidence of restenosis, which still remains as the potential limitation after coronary intervention. In an effort to better understand the mechanisms of restenosis, numerous clinical studies that incorporate IVUS have been introduced. This chapter will review the specific research findings and current role of IVUS in the treatment and/or prevention of restenosis during stented and non-stented procedures.

IVUS During Stent Procedures

Vessel Size

Several studies have reported that stenting small vessels is associated with poor clinical outcomes. George et al[1] reported that patients receiving 2.0- or 2.5-mm Gianturco-Roubin stents had higher stent thrombosis rates than those who received larger stents for acute or threatened vessel closure after angioplasty (34% versus 19%). Similar results were supported by Agrawal et al.[2] In lesions

From Waksman R (ed.). *Vascular Brachytherapy, Third Edition.* Armonk, NY: Futura Publishing Co., Inc.; © 2002.

with stent restenosis, stent volume was smaller than nonrestenotic stents regardless of the pattern and location of in-stent restenosis.[3] Chronic stent recoil, initial stent underexpansion, and small intrinsic vessel size are believed to contribute to these results. A study by Sutton et al[4] reported that using small stent diameter, defined as a ratio less than 1.0 (stent-to-lesion diameter ratio) was highly correlated with recurrent ischemic events. However, Huang et al[5] reported a study of 40 patients with 2.5-mm Gianturco-Roubin stent implantation in small coronary arteries (<2.5 mm) utilizing high-pressure deployment techniques. In this study, no acute complications were observed and symptom-free or patent target site on repeat coronary angiography was 76%. The availability of newer generation stents and effective additional antiplatelet therapy may offer more favorable outcomes when stenting small coronary arteries. IVUS estimation of vessel size after successful balloon angioplasty has shown poor correlation with angiography.[6–8] These differences reflect the limitations of angiography in quantifying the complex, irregular lumen, which is typical following balloon angioplasty. In contrast, IVUS has shown excellent correlation with histology in measurement lumen and plaque morphology.[9] Nakamura et al[10] demonstrated that deep injury to the plaque, defined as the presence of a plaque fracture that reached the media, contributes to the discrepancy between IVUS and angiographic measurements. The most important aspect of stenting in small vessels is to identify whether these vessel subsets are actually small; often, what appears small in the angiogram is much larger when measuring the "true" vessel diameter by IVUS. Thus, investigators can decide their possible therapeutic options.

Stent Expansion/Apposition

Stent underexpansion is a frequently detected IVUS morphological finding after stent implantation. It has been reported as an increased risk for subacute thrombosis.[11] Previous studies utilizing IVUS after stent implantation have demonstrated a significant degree of underexpansion (Fig. 1) despite the initial appearance of an angiographically successful deployment.[11–17] Therefore, repeat inflations with high-pressure and/or larger balloons were performed to optimize stent deployment.[14,18–20] Colombo et al[11] demonstrated that despite aggressive high-pressure balloon strategy, 40% of the stents with an acceptable angiographic result still showed stent underexpansion. Similar findings were also supported by Carrozza et al,[20] showing only 64% of MultiLink stents achieved a lumen/reference area ratio greater than or equal to 70% following high-pressure balloon inflation. Incomplete stent apposition (stent struts separated from the vessel wall) is another IVUS detected morphological finding after stent implantation. (Fig. 1) Early stent trials showed that both optimal stent apposition to the vessel wall and adjunctive antiplatelet therapy are necessary to prevent stent thrombosis.[15,16] In the Multicenter Ultrasound Stenting in Coronaries (MUSIC) Study,[21] an aggressive IVUS-guided stent deployment protocol demonstrated a very low restenosis rate (9.7%), target vessel revascularization (TVR) rate (4.5%), and a low stent thrombosis rate (1.3%) at 6-month follow-up. However, in the era of second generation stents and/or current antiplatelet regimen, a direct association between incomplete stent apposition and subacute thrombosis is unclear. A study by Maehara et al[22] reported the relationship between incomplete stent apposition by IVUS and stent thrombosis. A total of 1081 patients were enrolled and the rate of incomplete stent apposition was 9.7%. They found that the incomplete stent apposition group had significantly

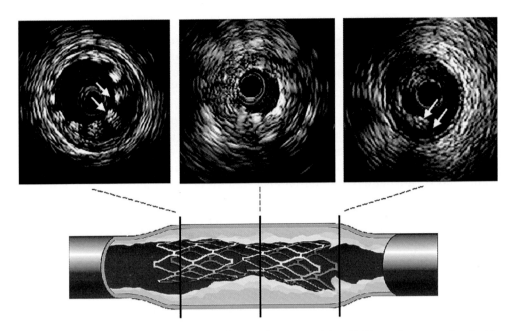

Figure 1. Ultrasound images of stent incomplete apposition (left), underexpansion (middle), edge dissection (right). The left panel shows that some portion of stent struts separated from the vessel wall (white arrows). The middle panel shows stent underexpansion relative to the vessel size. The right panel shows edge dissection (white arrows) adjacent the stent margin.

larger lumen dimensions determined by both IVUS and angiography and less plaque burden determined by IVUS, resulting in no relation between incomplete stent apposition and stent thrombosis or target lesion revascularization (TLR) at 6-month follow-up. Another study by Choi et al[17] demonstrated that although post-stent high-pressure (≥12 atm) balloon inflations resulted in an optimal angiographic result, IVUS still identified a need for additional improvement in stent apposition. Additionally, IVUS guidance was associated with low TVR and major adverse cardiac events (MACE) at 6-month follow-up.

The incidence of stent underexpansion has been reported to be 20 to 40% of cases following stent implantation,[20,23,24] whereas incomplete stent apposition has been observed in 8 to 30% of cases.[17,18,22] While the stent underexpansion is strongly associated with a higher restenosis rate, the clinical significance of incomplete stent apposition is still controversial. However, this issue may be of current interest particularly in cases using drug-coated stents where incomplete apposition may prevent effective drug delivery to tissue, and by virtue of retarding endothelialization, may increase the risk of strut thrombosis.

Minimal Stent Area /Plaque Burden and Clinical Outcomes

Minimal stent area (MSA) has been reported as the single most powerful predictor of late clinical outcomes.[25–27] With the optimization of stent deployment by IVUS, MSA or intrastent lumen cross-sectional area (CSA) was shown to increase by 11 to 80%.[14,16,25] Hoffmann et al,[25] in the IVUS analysis of 476 Palmaz-Schatz stents, demonstrated MSA, pre-interventional plaque burden, and ostial lesion location to be the most consistent predictors of angiographic in-stent restenosis. Furthermore, the inverse relation between MSA and angiographic restenosis has been reported. Moussa et al[27] demonstrated that achieving an MSA greater than or equal to 9 mm^2 in large vessels ($\geq$3 mm), and an MSA greater than or equal to 55% of average reference vessel CSA, was associated with a low restenosis rate (11% and 17%, respectively). Similar findings were reported by de Feyter et al,[26] showing two IVUS variables, MSA and stent length, as being associated with a low restenosis rate at 6-month follow-up.

The RESIST (REStenosis after Ivus-guided STenting) Study,[24] a randomized, multicenter trial, demonstrated that although there was a nonsignificant 6.3% absolute reduction in the 6-month restenosis rate and a nonsignificant difference in minimal lumen diameter (MLD) by angiography, MSA in the IVUS-guided group was 20% larger than the angiographic-guided group at 6-month follow-up (5.36±2.81 mm^{2}versus 4.47±2.59 mm^2, P=0.03). By multivariate analysis, MSA was shown to be the only independent predictior of 6-month restenosis. Another multicenter, randomized trial to determine the effect of IVUS-directed stent placement was AVID (Angiography Versus Intravascular Ultrasound-Directed stent placement).[23] This study showed a larger MSA for the IVUS-guided group than the angiographic-guided group (7.54±2.86 mm^2 versus 6.94±2.46 mm^2, P<0.001) without increased complications and reported a lower 12-month follow-up TVR for vessels less than or equal to 3.25 mm by angiography and for vein grafts (7.9% versus 14.6%, P=0.04). Recently, the CRUISE (Can Routine Ultrasound Influence Stent Expansion) Study, a substudy of the STARS (Stent Anti-thrombotic Regimen Study), showed the effectiveness of IVUS-guided stent implantation.[28] A total of 543 lesions in 499 patients were included in this study. Like AVID, the IVUS-guided group (290 lesions) had a larger MSA than the angiographic-guided group (253 lesions) (7.78±1.72 mm^2 versus 7.06±2.13 mm^2, P<0.001), a larger MLD (2.96±0.55 mm^2 versus 2.59±0.43 mm^2, P<0.001), and a lower 9-month follow-up TVR (8.5% versus 15.3%, P<0.05; relative reduction of 44%) (Fig. 2). Whether

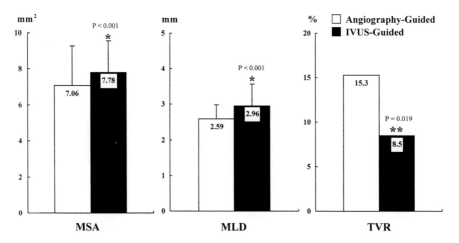

Figure 2. Final results of the CRUISE Study. Compared to the angiographic-guided group, the IVUS-guided group shows significantly larger minimal stent area (MSA) and minimal luminal diameter (MLD) after stent implantation, resulting in lower target vessel revascularization (TVR) rate at 9-month follow-up.

IVUS-guided stent deployment would offset initial catheter costs by a reduction in restenosis remains to be seen.

Edge Dissection

"Edge dissection" by IVUS (Fig. 1) is defined as a freely mobile tissue arm extending into the lumen, within 5 mm from the stent border, with clear blood speckle between this tissue structure and the vessel wall. It has been reported to occur in 11% to 20% of cases following stent implantation[29–32] and can be detected more accurately by IVUS. The transition between the stent edge and adjacent plaque interface may cause a shearing force, resulting in intimal disruption or edge tear at the stent borders. Theoretically, edge dissection may increase the risk of subacute thrombosis because it can cause flow limitations near the stented area. However, favorable acute outcomes of these lesions have been reported.[30] Recently, long-term outcomes of edge dissection were reported by Sheris et al.[32] Edge dissection lesions (11%) showed similar vessel, lumen, and plaque area in both the proximal and distal reference segments compared to nondissection lesions at 6-month follow-up. Similarly, Hong et al[31] reported long-term results of 67 minor edge dissections (19%) of 348 lesions. Late angiographic restenosis rates did not differ significantly in lesions with edge dissections compared to those without edge dissections (29.9% versus 25.3%, $P=0.540$). These observations suggest that edge dissection detected by IVUS immediately after stent implantation may not play a major role in the development of late angiographic in-stent restenosis. However, the natural history of edge dissections following drug-eluting stent implantation or intravascular brachytherapy may be different. The influences of these strategies on vascular biological components, namely inhibition of neointimal formation and/or by inhibition of the cell cycle, are similar. Intracoronary radiation has been known to prevent normal healing processes after balloon injury, resulting in unhealed dissection. As a result, edge dissection following drug-eluting stent implantation may have a different natural course compared to conventional stent-induced edge dissection.

Future Stenting and IVUS

The IVUS/Stent Delivery System device (Fig. 3), which consists of diagnostic ultrasound imaging combined with a stent delivery system, is currently being tested. This device will be able to provide interactive measurement of lumen and vessel size as well as on-line interrogation of vascular plaque components, offering immediate assessment of, and response to, stenting procedures.

From intravascular brachytherapy, we have learned that radiation-induced vascular behaviors, such as enhancement of positive remodeling and inadequate stent strut endothelialization, may result in late stent malapposition and late stent thrombosis. Drug-eluting stents have been reported to reduce vascular cell proliferation and migration in vivo and in vitro.[33–35] Following drug-eluting stent implantation, however, incomplete stent apposition or branch jail could increase the risk of acute and late stent thrombosis. To avoid these complications, IVUS may play a critical role during drug-eluting stent implantation as we en-

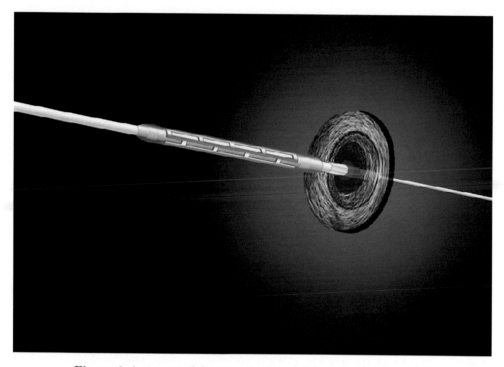

Figure 3. A concept of the combined IVUS/Stent Delivery System.

ter a new era of providing both a mechanical and a biological solution directly to coronary target segments.

IVUS During Non-Stent Procedures

Vessel Size

Vessel size has been reported to be an important predictor of acute and long-term outcome after percutaneous transluminal coronary angioplasty (PTCA) or coronary stenting. The therapeutic strategy for small-sized artery intervention is still controversial. Several studies have reported that elective stenting provides an improved clinical outcome and restenosis rate,[36,37] whereas other studies have shown an increased restenosis rate after stenting compared to conventional angioplasty.[38–40] An IVUS study by Mintz et al[41] reported that decreasing angiographic reference lumen size correlated with increasing lesion calcium, particularly in vessels less than 2.0 mm. Thus, increased calcium in small arteries can impact restenosis rate.

Modifications of therapeutic strategy, based on IVUS, have resulted in varying balloon size, balloon inflation pressure, and device selection during coronary intervention. CLOUT (Clinical Outcomes with Ultrasound Trial)[42] was a nonrandomized, single center study designed to evaluate the impact of using upsized balloon diameter, based on the mean diameter of the lumen and vessel at the reference segment, on long-term outcome. This strategy showed a significant decrease in the mean angiographic percent diameter stenosis, with a corresponding increase in MLD and a marked increase in mean lumen area without an increase in acute complication rates. Similarly, Abizaid et al[43] reported a large lumen gain and low TLR after IVUS-guided oversized balloon PTCA. The OCBAS (Optimal Coronary Balloon Angioplasty with Provisional Stenting versus Primary Stent) Trial[44] demonstrated a similar restenosis rate (19.2% versus 16.4%, P=NS) and TLR rate (17.5% versus 13.5%, P=NS) in optimal PTCA with the provisional stenting group compared to the primary stenting group. Appropriate sizing of the balloon to the arterial segment using IVUS resulted in a larger MLD, thus contributing to improved acute and late favorable outcome after PTCA.

Lesion Length

Long lesions have been associated with worse acute and late outcomes following coronary intervention.[45–48] To treat long lesions appropriately, device selection based on lesion length is seen to be an important determinant. Actual lesion length is often underestimated following angiography due to a "normal looking" reference vessel. Mintz et al[49] demonstrated that only 60 (6.8%) of 884 angiographically "normal" reference segments were normal by IVUS. In addition, reference segment disease was seen to parallel the severity of target lesion disease. Recently, Bersin et al,[50] in a follow-up study of patients treated with rotational atherectomy, reported that lesion length, not the post-procedural MLD, was the strongest predictor of subsequent TLR. Current IVUS systems, using the motorized pullback device and three-dimensional reconstruction, provide spatial orientation of the vasculature, allowing lesion length quantification with the ability to "truly" match a single stent length with the extent of disease.

Plaque Types

Compared to angiography, IVUS can provide insights into the morphology and distribution of atherosclerotic lesions in vivo.[51] Moreover, matched IVUS and histologic investigations have established an acceptance of plaque morphology.[52]

Calcified Plaque

Diagnostic Impact. Coronary calcification (Fig. 4) is a strong predictor for the presence of atherosclerotic plaque. The extent of coronary calcification is related to coronary plaque burden[53,54] as well as the potential for cardiovascular events in the future.[55,56] In heavily calcified lesions, it is difficult to gauge correctly by angiography due to distortion of the lumen geometry and contrast shadowing; thus it is often represented as angiographically ambiguous lesions. This can be particularly true at proximal branch-point in the coronary tree (eg, left main coronary artery [LMCA]). Ge et al[57] demonstrated IVUS findings of angiographically normal coronary arteries or ambiguous lesions of the LMCA. In this study, atherosclerotic plaques in the LMCA were observed in 31 of 92 (34%); eccentric plaques were in 83%, and 17% contained calcium deposits. Coronary angiography has been reported to possess several limitations to accurate detection and assessment of target lesion calcium.[58] The sensitivity and specificity of angiography were 40

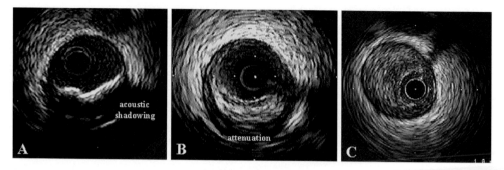

Figure 4. Ultrasound images of three different plaque types. **A:** Superficial calcification (between 3 and 7 o'clock) was located at the lumen surface. **B:** Fibrous plaque shows a strong echo reflectance (equal to adventitia) with attenuation. **C:** Fatty plaque shows echolucent homogenous echoes (more echolucent than adventitia).

to 48% and 82 to 89%, respectively.[59,60] Mintz et al[59] also reported that IVUS-detected calcium is significantly higher than angiographically detected calcium in 1155 coronary lesions (73% versus 38%, $P<0.0001$) with the sensitivity of angiography highest (85%) in lesions with four-quadrant calcium. In another study, Mintz et al[61] showed that coronary calcification is strongly related to atherosclerotic plaque burden, but not with angiographic coronary diameter stenosis. By multivariate analysis, plaque burden of target lesion and reference segment, patient age, and stable angina were the predictors of the arc of target lesion calcium.

Since calcification can strongly influence the size of dissection during balloon angioplasty, detecting the extent and location by IVUS can help triage lesions to appropriate initial therapy. The alternative therapeutic strategy for calcified plaques is high-speed rotational atherectomy (HSRA), which is designed to pulverize plaque and polish the internal lumen of the artery (Fig. 5). It has been used for the treatment of saphenous vein grafts, in-stent restenosis and ostial stenosis, and calcified, complex, and restenosic lesions in non-stented vessels.[62–67] Kovach et al[68] found that, after adjunctive PTCA, the residual plaque burden did not change from that after HSRA, and dissections in the target lesion occurred more often (77% versus 26%, $P=0.0004$) than after HSRA. This study suggested that selective atheroablation, especially for calcium, with little tissue disruption plays a role in lumen enlargement resulting from HSRA. On the other hand, a combination of HSRA and arterial dissection/expansion plays a role in lumen enlargement resulting from adjunctive PTCA. The Rotational Atherectomy Multicenter Registry,[63] an analysis of 874 lesions in 709 patients, reported a success rate of rotational atherectomy alone or with adjunctive PTCA to be 94.7% with a 6-month angiographic restenosis rate of 37.7%. In addition, previously treated lesions had significantly higher success rates than de novo lesions. Other studies have also shown favorable procedural success rates with relatively high restenosis rates.[63,69–71] Hoffmann et al[72] demonstrated the treatment strategy for calcified lesions in large (≥3.0 mm) coronary arteries. In this study, HSRA followed by adjunct stent implantation, had favorable acute and late outcomes, including infrequent complication, better acute angiographic results, and higher event-free survival at 9-month follow-up. Recently, Kobayashi et al[73] evaluated the acute and late outcomes of stenting after aggressive HSRA (final burr size ≥2.25 mm and/or final burr/vessel ratio ≥0.8) compared with stenting after less aggressive HSRA.

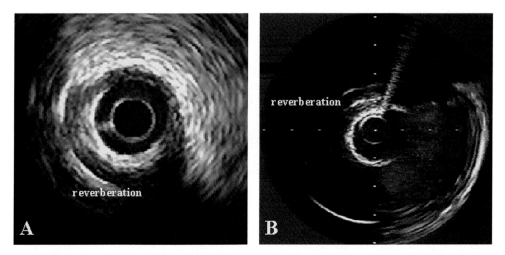

Figure 5. Ultrasound images from two cases of high-speed rotational atherectomy (HSRA). **A:** A smooth, round calcium surface with reverberations is seen following rotational atherectomy. **B:** The rotablator has created a smooth channel in a calcific lesion. This is the so-called "snowman" or "keyhole."

Although there was no significant difference in acute lumen gain after the procedure, the restenosis rate was lower in the aggressive HSRA group than in the less aggressive HSRA group (30.9% versus 50.0%, $P<0.05$). In addition, diffuse restenotic pattern, defined as lesion length of greater than 10 mm, was less frequent in the aggressive HSRA group than in the less aggressive HSRA group (9.5% versus 25.0%, $P<0.05$). These studies suggest that aggressive HSRA prior to stenting is a favorable strategy to reduce the angiographic restenosis rate in calcified lesions.

Fatty Plaque and Vessel Remodeling

Fatty plaque (Fig. 4) is relatively echolucent by IVUS and often illustrates significant segmental wall remodeling. This plaque usually consists of large lipid core, thin fibrous cap, and coronary amorphous plaque material interspersed with inflammatory component.[74–77] Recently, the association between vulnerable plaque and excessive vessel remodeling has been generated as a new concept in this important biological process. From a clinical standpoint, plaque and vascular remodeling are highly associated with clinical presentation. Gyongyosi et al[78] demonstrated that positive remodeling was associated with a larger plaque CSA. Smits et al[79] also reported that patients with unstable angina or post-myocardial infarction angina showed a larger plaque area and larger percentage remodeling compared to those with stable angina (14.8 ± 4.8 mm^2 versus 11.6 ± 4.9 mm^2, $P=0.009$ and $112\pm31\%$ versus $95\pm17\%$, $P=0.005$, respectively). More recently, the relation between the extent of remodeling and clinical presentation was studied by Schoenhagen et al.[80] This study demonstrated that positive remodeling was more common in patients with unstable syndromes (52%), whereas negative remodeling was common in those with stable syndromes (57%), thus suggesting that positive remodeling and larger plaques are related with unstable clinical presentations. Nissen et al[81] demonstrated that vulnerable plaque, as seen by IVUS, revealed a thin intimal leading edge and large intimal echolucent zones within the plaque. Other investigators[82] reported that large eccentric plaques with an echolucent zone represented vulnerable plaque, although the lumen was still preserved. The mechanism and clinical impact of vessel remodeling will be discussed in a later section *(Vascular Remodeling: Clinical Impact)*.

Minimal Lumen Diameter/Plaque Burden

The presence of a large plaque burden may limit optimal luminal dimension with percutaneous coronary intervention. Especially with stenting, debulking the plaque prior to stent deployment may provide the best anatomic conditions for stent expansion with minimal vessel injury. Several single center studies have reported that plaque burden by IVUS is highly associated with late clinical outcome. Mintz et al[83] demonstrated that the post-interventional residual cross-sectional narrowing (plaque burden) was the strongest predictor of late angiographic restenosis. This study suggested that IVUS parameters are more powerful predictors of angiographic restenosis than clinical or angiographic risk factors. The amount of plaque burden is also related to clinical presentation. From recent studies, large plaques were likely to be more vulnerable compared to small plaques, and thus were associated with unstable clinical presentations.[79,80]

The Post-IntraCoronary Treatment Ultrasound Result Evaluation (PICTURE) Trial,[84] a prospective randomized trial to evaluate IVUS parameters for the prediction of restenosis following PTCA, demonstrated that the restenosis group had larger residual plaque burden than the nonrestenosis group, although there was no statistical significance ($P=0.38$) possibly due to a relatively small sample size. Another study that evaluated the acute and late outcomes following IVUS-guided aggressive PTCA with provisional stenting was Doppler and Ultrasound Guided Balloon Therapeutics for Coronary LESionS (DOUBTLESS).[85] In this study, the authors implanted the Gianturco-Roubin II or Palmaz-Schatz stent only when post-PTCA IVUS showed a suboptimal result (minimum lumen CSA less than 65% of the average of the proximal and distal reference lumen CSA, minimum lumen CSA less than 6.0 mm^2, or major dissections). This study showed that 12-month TLR was lower in the PTCA group than in the stent group (8% versus 16%, $P=0.016$) and 50% of the patients with IVUS-guided aggressive PTCA could avoid stent implantation. Therefore, the authors concluded that IVUS-guided aggressive PTCA is an alternative strategy to avoid routine elective stenting.

Since its approval by the United States Food and Drug Administration (FDA) in 1990, directional coronary atherectomy (DCA) has been widely used for treatment of atheromatous coronary plaque lesions. This device is primarily used for treating eccentric, discrete, noncalcified lesions in proximal, nontortuous, and large vessels as well as restenotic lesions by debulking atheromatous tissue (Fig. 6).

The Guidance by Ultrasound for Decision Endpoints (GUIDE) Trial was a multicenter randomized study to evaluate angiographic and IVUS predictors of restenosis following PTCA or DCA (Fig. 7). A total of 518 lesions in 518 enrolled patients and three late endpoints were evaluated by multivariate analysis. Preliminary data from the GUIDE Trial showed that, for angiographic restenosis, only two parameters, the plaque burden or percent of plaque area by IVUS and

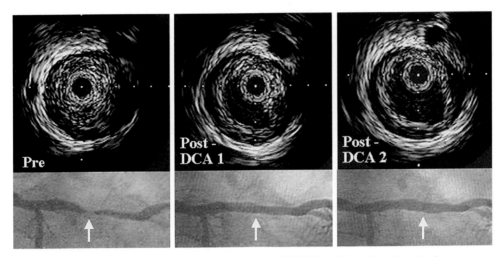

Figure 6. Ultrasound and angiographic images of IVUS-guided directional atherectomy. The large plaque burden in the culprit lesion is significantly decreased following directional atherectomy.

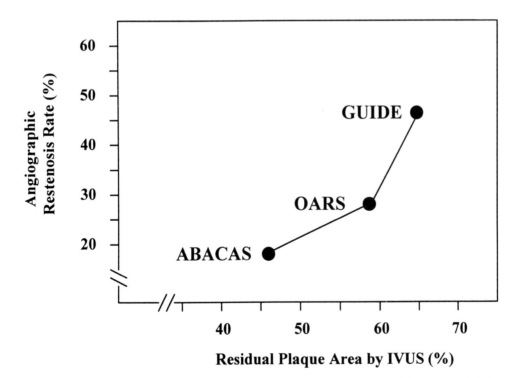

Figure 7. Relationship of residual plaque area by IVUS and angiographic restenosis. The data from the Adjunctive Balloon Angioplasty following Coronary Atherectomy Study (ABACAS), Optimal Atherectomy Restenosis Study (OARS), and Guidance by Ultrasound for Decision Endpoints (GUIDE) are superimposed.

the pre-interventional diameter stenosis by angiography, were significant predictors. For clinical restenosis, plaque burden by IVUS was the only significant predictor. For major clinical events, MLD by IVUS was the only significant predictor. In addition, the receiver operator characteristic for the percent plaque area and MLD by IVUS showed that when percent area is greater than 64.5% and the MLD is less than 1.96 mm, the restenosis rate was increased (43.7% versus 18.2%).

The Optimal Atherectomy Restenosis Study (OARS),[86] a prospective four center registry, evaluated the effect of optimal DCA in the treatment of de novo or restenotic lesions. OARS demonstrated that mean diameter stenosis was reduced from 63.5% to 7% with a reduction in plaque burden from 89 to 58%, as a result of an aggressive plaque removal and adjunct post-procedure PTCA. Moreover, the 6-month angiographic restenosis and 12-month TLR rates were lower than prior non-IVUS-guiding debulking trials (28.9% versus 50.0%, 17.8% versus 33.7%, respectively).[87]

Another prospective, randomized, multicenter trial to evaluate the effect of balloon dilatation after optimal DCA was the Adjunctive Balloon Angioplasty after Coronary Atherectomy Study (ABACAS).[88] ABACAS showed that while the average residual plaque burden was low in both groups, it was significantly lower in the DCA/PTCA group (42.6% versus 45.6%). However, the late restenosis rate and TLR were not different. These data suggest that less residual plaque after DCA results in more effective late clinical and angiographic outcome.

Recently, DCA prior to stent implantation was reported as a promising strategy for reducing stent restenosis in high-risk lesion subsets. Stenting After Optimal Lesion Debulking (SOLD),[89] a prospective single center registry, demonstrated larger acute and late post-procedural angiographic MLD in the DCA/stent group compared to the stent alone group (3.48±0.60 mm versus 3.15±0.43 mm, $P=0.0002$, and 2.57±0.87 mm versus 2.14±0.80 mm, $P=0.002$, respectively). Additionally, the DCA/stent group had a lower restenosis rate (11% versus 21%, $P=0.07$) and a lower TLR rate (7% versus 19%, $P=0.03$) than the stent alone group.

Similar results have been reported from a preliminary analysis of a single site randomized trial, the Atherectomy before Multilink Improves Lumen Gain and Clinical Outcomes (AMIGO), demonstrating a larger acute and late post-procedure angiographic MLD in the DCA/stent group compared to the stent alone group (3.34 mm versus 3.06 mm, $P=0.004$ and 2.21 mm versus 1.87 mm, $P=0.046$, respectively). DCA/stent group had a lower restenosis rate (14% versus 32%, $P=0.07$) and a lower TLR rate (8% versus 25%, $P=0.053$) than the stent alone group.

In addition, the preliminary analysis of the Debulking and Stenting in Restenosis Elimination (DESIRE) Trial[90] has demonstrated that the DCA/stent group had larger acute lumen gain compared to the stent alone group (7.2±2.1 mm² versus 5.7±1.5 mm², $P=0.02$), with a corresponding increase in minimal lumen area (8.6±2.3 mm² versus 7.2±2.6 mm², $P=0.03$).

Vascular Remodeling: Clinical Impact

In 1987, adaptive arterial remodeling (positive remodeling) (Fig. 8) in human atherosclerotic coronary arteries was first described by Glagov, who observed vessel enlargement at plaque lesion site in response to progressive accumulation of

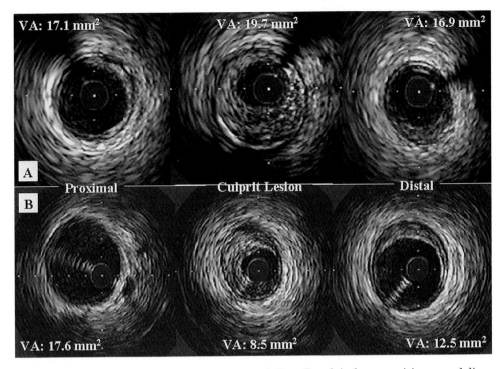

Figure 8. Ultrasound images of vascular remodeling. Panel **A** shows positive remodeling. The lesion site vessel area (VA) (19.7 mm²) was larger than at the proximal and distal reference sites (17.1 mm², 16.9 mm², respectively). Panel **B** shows negative remodeling. The lesion VA (8.5mm²) was smaller than at the proximal and distal reference sites (17.6 mm², 12.5 mm², respectively).

plaque in LMCA autopsy specimens.[91] Ensuing IVUS studies,[92,93] histopathologic studies,[94] and epicardial ultrasound studies[95] have shown that vessel enlargement occurs as a compensatory mechanism for plaque formation while the lumen area is preserved until the progressive plaque expansion exceeds the vessel remodeling. Even though most atherosclerotic plaque segments had compensatory arterial enlargement, some segments showed a decrease of vessel lumen or paradoxical shrinkage at the lesion site (negative remodeling) (Fig. 8). Nishioka et al[96] found that failure of positive remodeling was observed in 16 (46%) of 35 lesions: 26% of patients had negative remodeling and 20% had intermediate remodeling. Another study reported that arterial wall shrinkage (negative remodeling) as well as plaque increase may contribute to severe luminal narrowing in human femoral artery.[97] Shiran et al[98] reported the IVUS findings in de novo, nontreated LMCAs in 31 patients. Both positive remodeling and negative remodeling were observed in this study. In moderately diseased LMCAs (plaque burden of <50%), adaptive arterial remodeling, not plaque change, primarily contributed to luminal changes. These findings, positive remodeling and negative remodeling, have also been observed in transplant coronary artery disease[99] as well as vasospastic angina.[100] Adaptive arterial remodeling is another important mechanism of restenosis following coronary intervention. In the animal model, Kakuta et al[101] and Post et al[102] confirmed that vascular remodeling after PTCA is more correlated with angiographic late loss than intimal hyperplasia. Mintz et al[103] reported acute and follow-up IVUS findings in 212 lesions after coronary intervention. This study showed that the decrease in external elastic membrane (EEM) CSA (Δ EEM CSA) and lumen CSA (Δ lumen CSA) was significantly greater in restenotic lesions than nonrestenotic lesions (3.1 ± 3.0 mm^2 versus 0.8 ± 2.9 mm^2, 4.1 ± 2.1 mm^2 versus 1.2 ± 2.8 mm^2, respectively, both $P<0.0001$). An increase in plaque plus media CSA (Δ P+M CSA) tended to be higher in restenotic lesions than in nonrestenotic lesions (1.0 ± 2.3 mm^2 versus 0.4 ± 2.0 mm^2, $P=0.0784$). Therefore, the change in lumen CSA was more highly related with the change in EEM CSA ($r=0.751$, $P<0.0001$) than with the change in plaque plus media CSA ($r=0.284$, $P<0.0001$). The mechanisms of adaptive arterial enlargement (positive remodeling) are thought to depend on: (1) local increase in wall shear stress caused by increased blood flow velocity in a stenosis which may stimulate endothelium-dependent arterial dilatation. Nitric oxide, the gelatinase matrix metalloproteinases (MMPs), MMP-2 and MMP-4, play a role in this process, and/or (2) the development of plaque may lead to degradation of the media and adventitia, resulting in passive bulging of the plaque.[104–107] In contrast, arterial shrinkage (negative remodeling) is thought to be caused by increasing smooth muscle cell proliferation and collagen deposition in low blood flow states. The expression of mitogenic factors, such as platelet-derived growth factor and inhibition of nitric oxide, play a role in this process.[108,109]

From a clinical standpoint, unstable angina is strongly associated with positive remodeling lesions, whereas stable angina is associated with negative remodeling lesions. As stated previously, Gyongyosi et al[78] found positive remodeling in 37% of the patients with unstable angina. In other study,[110] inadequate remodeling was observed in at least 15% of chronic, focal, new coronary arterial stenoses of patients with stable angina. The process of positive remodeling is associated with plaque rupture. A post-mortem study by Pasterkamp et al[111] showed that positive remodeling with large plaque area was associated with plaque vulnerability. By histology, these investigators observed substantial macrophages and T-lymphocytes, and lack of smooth muscle cells and collagen in those lesions, suggesting that positive remodeling might enhance the risk of plaque rupture. Dangas et al[112] evaluated the influence of pre-interventional arterial remodeling on late clinical outcome. A total of 777 lesions in 715 patients treated with non-stent intervention were enrolled. The positive remodeling group had a TLR rate of 31.2% compared with 20.2% in the negative/intermediate remodeling group ($P=0.0001$). By multivariate analysis, diabetes and left anterior descending artery location were independent predictors of TLR. Clinically, stenoses due to negative remodeling may require mechanical expansion by a stent to prevent acute and/or chronic vessel recoil. For stenoses with larger plaque burdens and positive remodeling, atherectomy or other plaque removal catheters might be preferable as an initial therapeutic approach. In the future, these biologically active lesions may be ideally targeted for the combination of a local drug with a stent and a drug-eluting stent, providing both a biological and a mechanical solution.

Other Trials to Treat or Prevent Restenosis

Subsequent IVUS studies have demonstrated that the pathophysiology of in-stent restenosis is different from that of restenosis in non-stented vessels. After stent implantation, neointimal formation plays a major role in late lumen loss and restenosis.[113,114] This vascular response results from stent-derived prolonged radial strain, stent strut-induced vascular injury, and the permanent presence of foreign material in the human body.[115] In contrast, inadequate vascular remodeling is a significant contributor to late lumen loss after non-stent coronary intervention.[103,116–118] Recently, new therapeutic modalities for coronary restenosis were introduced in the field of catheter-based coronary intervention. In this section, the current knowledge of intravascular sonotherapy and cutting balloon angioplasty will be reviewed, focusing on specific findings and role of IVUS.

Therapeutic Catheter-Based Ultrasound

Ultrasound imaging is based on the release of a burst of sound waves from the ultrasound transducer and receipt of the reflected or backscattered signals. When the ultrasound signal travels the regions of impedance mismatch, the signal is more attenuated. Signal attenuation is generally more prominent with catheter-based imaging than in transcutaneous imaging because of power constraints and the use of higher frequencies for IVUS imaging (20 to 30 MHz). Recently, an over-the-wire catheter system (5F, URX™, PharmaSonics, Inc.) was developed for intracoronary sonotherapy treatment, which incorporates an ultrasonic transducer 8 mm in length, exposing an average peak ultrasonic intensity of 100 W/cm^2 at a center frequency of 700 kHz (Fig. 9). This ultrasound technology has been recently introduced into the therapeutic phase. Lawrie et al[119] demonstrated that adjunctive ultrasound exposure (1 MHz for 60 sec) can inhibit vascular smooth muscle cell proliferation in vitro, suggesting ultrasound-assisted gene therapy to prevent restenosis. Another study by Fitzgerald et al[120] evaluated the effect of intravascular sonotherapy (600 MHz for 300 sec) on intimal hyperplasia in a swine stent model. Histologic study revealed that smooth muscle cell proliferation was significantly reduced in the sonotherapy group compared to the sham group at 7 days ($24.1\pm7.0\%$ versus $31.2\pm3.0\%$, $P<0.05$), and area stenosis was significantly lower in the sonotherapy group compared to the sham group at

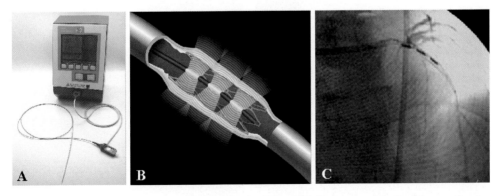

Figure 9. A: Photograph of the PharmaSonics URx IST Catheter with the PharmaSonics URx Sonotherapy Instrument. **B:** A diagram of the PharmaSonics URx IST Catheter. The over-the-wire designed 5 F catheter with three ultrasound transducers provides high radial acoustic emissions. **C:** The PharmaSonics URx IST Catheter has been placed in the left anterior descending artery.

28 days (36±24% versus 44±27%, *P*<0.05). More recently, Post et al[121] reported the effect and long-term safety of intravascular sonotherapy in stent intimal hyperplasia in the swine model. Histologic study findings at 180 days showed complete reendothelialization, reduced intimal thickness, and no edge effect. These studies suggest that intravascular sonotherapy may be an effective treatment for in-stent restenosis.

Cutting Balloon Angioplasty

The cutting balloon (Interventional Technologies, Inc., San Diego, CA) was designed as a balloon catheter, equipped with three or four microtome-sharp atherotomes (microsurgical blades), mounted on the surface of the balloon.[122] When the cutting balloon is inflated, the atherotomes-induced longitudinal incisions are directed radially into the media. The mechanism of cutting balloon has been reported as plaque compression (significant decrease of plaque area) with less vessel expansion, thus achieving luminal enlargement with less injury to the media or adventitia (Fig. 10)[123,124] and extrusion of neointimal plaque outside the stent struts.[125] Clinical trials comparing cutting balloon angioplasty with conventional angioplasty were performed in multicenter trials[126,127] as well as in single center studies.[128,129] Both the Cutting Balloon versus Angioplasty (CUBA) Trial[126] and the Restenosis Reduction by Cutting Balloon Evaluation (REDUCE) Study[127] demonstrated that cutting balloon angioplasty produced larger MLD, less coronary dissection, and more favorable late outcome compared to conventional balloon angioplasty. Recently, cutting balloon angioplasty has also been introduced as a treatment of in-stent restenosis. Several studies for the treatment of in-stent restenosis reported that late angiographic restenosis was 22% to 27% in patients with cutting balloon angioplasty compared to 47% in those with conventional angioplasty.[125,130] A nonrandomized, single center study by Lauer et

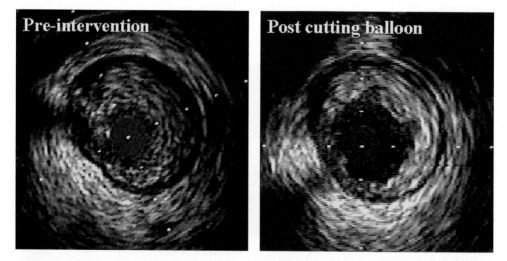

Figure 10. Ultrasound images of cutting balloon angioplasty. The **left** panel shows significant lumen narrowing with an extensive amount of fibrofatty plaque. The **right** panel shows increased lumen area with multiple small dissection following cutting balloon angioplasty.

al[131] reported long-term results of cutting balloon angioplasty for the treatment of in-stent restenosis. A total of 519 lesions with in-stent restenosis were treated with cutting balloon (200 lesions) or conventional angioplasty (319 lesions). In this study, the cutting balloon group showed greater MLD, less late lumen loss, greater net lumen gain, and a reduced TLR rate compared to conventional angioplasty. Ongoing prospective multicenter trials of REDUCE II and Restenosis Cutting Balloon Evaluation (RESCUT) may address the superiority of cutting balloon angioplasty over conventional angioplasty for the treatment of in-stent restenosis.

Conclusion

Since its emergence as a diagnostic tool for the coronary artery, the clinical utility of IVUS has increased significantly in keeping with current clinical challenges. A number of IVUS trials have contributed to our understanding of the pathology involved in coronary restenosis. IVUS can offer direct cross-sectional images as well as longitudinal images of coronary vasculature. Additionally, IVUS has provided new insight into plaque composition and vessel response to therapeutic intervention, such as coronary stenting, balloon angioplasty, directional atherectomy, rotational atherectomy, brachytherapy, and sonotherapy, thus affecting clinical decision making in the cardiac catheterization laboratory. Recently, catheter-based ultrasound has been introduced into the therapeutic interventional field, beyond its diagnostic usefulness, which may be a promising new strategy for restenosis. In the near future, new drug-eluting stents will be evaluated for their effectiveness in biologically active lesions, such as large plaque burden with compensatory vessel enlargement.

References

1. George BS, Voorhees WD, Roubin GS, et al. Multicenter investigation of coronary stenting to treat acute or threatened closure after percutaneous transluminal coronary angioplasty: Clinical and angiographic outcomes. J Am Coll Cardiol 1993;22:135–143.
2. Agrawal SK, Ho DS, Liu MW, et al. Predictors of thrombotic complications after placement of the flexible coil stent. Am J Cardiol 1994;73:1216–1219.
3. Dussaillant GR, Mintz GS, Pichard AD, et al. Small stent size and intimal hyperplasia contribute to restenosis: A volumetric intravascular ultrasound analysis. J Am Coll Cardiol 1995;26:720–724.
4. Sutton JM, Ellis SG, Roubin GS, et al. Major clinical events after coronary stenting: The multicenter registry of acute and elective Gianturco-Roubin stent placement. The Gianturco-Roubin Intracoronary Stent Investigator Group. Circulation 1994;89:1126–1137.
5. Huang P, Levin T, Kabour A, Feldman T. Acute and late outcome after use of 2.5-mm intracoronary stents in small (<2.5 mm) coronary arteries. Catheter Cardiovasc Interv 2000;49:121–126.
6. Nissen SE, Gurley JC, Grines CL, et al. Intravascular ultrasound assessment of lumen size and wall morphology in normal subjects and patients with coronary artery disease. Circulation 1991;84:1087–1099.
7. Tobis JM, Mallery J, Mahon D, et al. Intravascular ultrasound imaging of human coronary arteries in vivo: Analysis of tissue characterizations with comparison to in vitro histological specimens. Circulation 1991;83:913–926.
8. Hodgson JM, Reddy KG, Suneja R, et al. Intracoronary ultrasound imaging: Correlation of plaque morphology with angiography, clinical syndrome and procedural results in patients undergoing coronary angioplasty. J Am Coll Cardiol 1993;21:35–44.

9. Tobis JM, Mahon DJ, Moriuchi M, et al. Intravascular ultrasound imaging following balloon angioplasty. Int J Card Imaging 1991;6:191–205.
10. Nakamura S, Mahon DJ, Maheswaran B, et al. An explanation for discrepancy between angiographic and intravascular ultrasound measurements after percutaneous transluminal coronary angioplasty. J Am Coll Cardiol 1995;25:633–639.
11. Colombo A, Hall P, Nakamura S, et al. Intracoronary stenting without anticoagulation accomplished with intravascular ultrasound guidance. Circulation 1995;91:1676–1688.
12. Keren G, Pichard AD, Kent KM, et al. Failure or success of complex catheter-based interventional procedures assessed by intravascular ultrasound. Am Heart J 1992;123:200–208.
13. Deaner AN, Cubukcu AA, Rees MR. Assessment of coronary stent by intravascular ultrasound. Int J Cardiol 1992;36:124–126.
14. Goldberg SL, Colombo A, Nakamura S, et al. Benefit of intracoronary ultrasound in the deployment of Palmaz-Schatz stents. J Am Coll Cardiol 1994;24:996–1003.
15. Mudra H, Klauss V, Blasini R, et al. Ultrasound guidance of Palmaz-Schatz intracoronary stenting with a combined intravascular ultrasound balloon catheter. Circulation 1994;90:1252–1261.
16. Nakamura S, Colombo A, Gaglione A, et al. Intracoronary ultrasound observations during stent implantation. Circulation 1994;89:2026–2034.
17. Choi JW, Vardi GM, Meyers SN, et al. Role of intracoronary ultrasound after high-pressure stent implantation. Am Heart J 2000;139:643–648.
18. Gorge G, Haude M, Ge J, et al. Intravascular ultrasound after low and high inflation pressure coronary artery stent implantation. J Am Coll Cardiol 1995;26:725–730.
19. Kalmar G, Porner T, Weigand C, et al. Optimal expansion of the multi-link stent: An in vitro study with high resolution roentgen technique. Z Kardiol 1998;87:344–352.
20. Carrozza JP Jr, Hermiller JB Jr, Linnemeier TJ, et al. Quantitative coronary angiographic and intravascular ultrasound assessment of a new nonarticulated stent: Report from the Advanced Cardiovascular Systems MultiLink stent pilot study. J Am Coll Cardiol 1998;31:50–56.
21. de Jaegere P, Mudra H, Figulla H, et al. Intravascular ultrasound-guided optimized stent deployment: Immediate and 6 months clinical and angiographic results from the Multicenter Ultrasound Stenting in Coronaries Study (MUSIC Study). Eur Heart J 1998;19:1214–1223.
22. Maehara A, Apostol JC, Attubato MJ, et al. Incomplete stent apposition as determined by post-procedure intravascular ultrasound does not effect clinical outcome after elective coronary stent placement: A report from AVID and CRUISE [abstract]. J Am Coll Cardiol 2000;35(suppl A):45A.
23. Russo RJ, Attubato MJ, Davidson CJ, et al. Angiography versus intravascular ultrasound-directed stent placement: Final results from AVID [abstract]. Circulation 1999;100(suppl I):I–234.
24. Schiele F, Meneveau N, Vuillemenot A, et al. Impact of intravascular ultrasound guidance in stent deployment on 6-month restenosis rate: A multicenter, randomized study comparing two strategies—with and without intravascular ultrasound guidance. RESIST Study Group. REStenosis after IVUS-guided STenting. J Am Coll Cardiol 1998;32:320–328.
25. Hoffmann R, Mintz GS, Mehran R, et al. Intravascular ultrasound predictors of angiographic restenosis in lesions treated with Palmaz-Schatz stents. J Am Coll Cardiol 1998;31:43–49.
26. de Feyter PJ, Kay P, Disco C, Serruys PW. Reference chart derived from post-stent-implantation intravascular ultrasound predictors of 6-month expected restenosis on quantitative coronary angiography. Circulation 1999;100:1777–1783.
27. Moussa I, Moses J, Di Mario C, et al. Does the specific intravascular ultrasound criterion used to optimize stent expansion have an impact on the probability of stent restenosis? Am J Cardiol 1999;83:1012–1017.
28. Fitzgerald PJ, Oshima A, Hayase M, et al. Final results of the Can Routine Ultrasound Influence Stent Expansion (CRUISE) study. Circulation 2000;102:523–530.
29. Metz J, Mooney M, Walter P, et al. Significance of edge tears in coronary stenting: Initial observations from the STRUT registry [abstract]. Circulation 1995;92(suppl I):I-546.

30. Schwarzacher SP, Metz JA, Yock PG, Fitzgerald PJ. Vessel tearing at the edge of intracoronary stents detected with intravascular ultrasound imaging. Cathet Cardiovasc Diagn 1997;40:152–155.

31. Hong MK, Park SW, Lee NH, et al. Long-term outcomes of minor dissection at the edge of stents detected with intravascular ultrasound. Am J Cardiol 2000;86:791–795, A9.

32. Sheris SJ, Canos MR, Weissman NJ. Natural history of intravascular ultrasound-detected edge dissections from coronary stent deployment. Am Heart J 2000;139:59–63.

33. Axel DI, Kunert W, Goggelmann C, et al. Paclitaxel inhibits arterial smooth muscle cell proliferation and migration in vitro and in vivo using local drug delivery. Circulation 1997;96:636–645.

34. Sollott SJ, Cheng L, Pauly RR, et al. Taxol inhibits neointimal smooth muscle cell accumulation after angioplasty in the rat. J Clin Invest 1995;95:1869–1876.

35. Sauro MD, Camporesi DA, Sudakow RL. The anti-tumor agent, taxol, attenuates contractile activity in rat aortic smooth muscle. Life Sci 1995;56:L157–L161.

36. Savage MP, Fischman DL, Rake R, et al. Efficacy of coronary stenting versus balloon angioplasty in small coronary arteries. Stent Restenosis Study (STRESS) Investigators. J Am Coll Cardiol 1998;31:307–311.

37. Morice MC, Bradai R, Lefevre T, et al. Stenting small coronary arteries. J Invas Cardiol 1999;11:337–340.

38. Elezi S, Kastrati A, Neumann FJ, et al. Vessel size and long-term outcome after coronary stent placement. Circulation 1998;98:1875–1880.

39. Briguori C, Nishida T, Adamian M, et al. Coronary stenting versus balloon angioplasty in small coronary artery with complex lesions. Cathet Cardiovasc Intervent 2000; 50:390–397.

40. Park S, Lee CW, Hong M, et al. Randomized comparison of coronary stenting with optimal balloon angioplasty for treatment of lesions in small coronary arteries. Eur Heart J 2000;21:1785–1789.

41. Mintz GS, Pichard AD, Kent KM, et al. Interrelation of coronary angiographic reference lumen size and intravascular ultrasound target lesion calcium. Am J Cardiol 1998; 81:387–391.

42. Stone GW, Hodgson JM, St. Goar FG, et al. Improved procedural results of coronary angioplasty with intravascular ultrasound-guided balloon sizing: The CLOUT Pilot Trial. Clinical Outcomes With Ultrasound Trial (CLOUT) Investigators. Circulation 1997;95:2044–2052.

43. Abizaid A, Mehran R, Pichard AD, et al. Results of high presure ultrasound-guided "over-sized" balloon PTCA to achieve "stent-like" results [abstract]. J Am Coll Cardiol 1997;29(suppl A):280A.

44. Rodriguez A, Ayala F, Bernardi V, et al. Optimal coronary balloon angioplasty with provisional stenting versus primary stent (OCBAS): Immediate and long-term follow-up results. J Am Coll Cardiol 1998;32:1351–1357.

45. Ellis SG, Roubin GS, King SB III, et al. Angiographic and clinical predictors of acute closure after native vessel coronary angioplasty. Circulation 1988;77:372–379.

46. Hirshfeld JW Jr, Schwartz JS, Jugo R, et al. Restenosis after coronary angioplasty: A multivariate statistical model to relate lesion and procedure variables to restenosis. The M-HEART Investigators. J Am Coll Cardiol 1991;18:647–656.

47. Saucedo JF, Kennard ED, Brahimi AK, et al. Lesion length is an important independent predictor of long term clinical events in native coronary arteries [abstract]. Circulation 1997;96(suppl I):I–694.

48. Bauters C, Hubert E, Prat A, et al. Predictors of restenosis after coronary stent implantation. J Am Coll Cardiol 1998;31:1291–1298.

49. Mintz GS, Painter JA, Pichard AD, et al. Atherosclerosis in angiographically "normal" coronary artery reference segments: An intravascular ultrasound study with clinical correlations. J Am Coll Cardiol 1995;25:1479–1485.

50. Bersin RM, Cedarholm JC, Kowalchuk GJ, Fitzgerald PJ. Long-term clinical follow-up of patients treated with the coronary rotablator: A single-center experience. Cathet Cardiovasc Intervent 1999;46:399–405.

51. Yock PG, Linker DT, Angelsen BA. Two-dimensional intravascular ultrasound: Technical development and initial clinical experience. J Am Soc Echocardiogr 1989;2:296–304.

52. Rasheed Q, Dhawale PJ, Anderson J, Hodgson JM. Intracoronary ultrasound-defined plaque composition: Computer-aided plaque characterization and correlation with his-

tologic samples obtained during directional coronary atherectomy. Am Heart J 1995; 129:631–637.

53. Rumberger JA, Sheedy PF III, Breen JF, Schwartz RS. Coronary calcium, as determined by electron beam computed tomography, and coronary disease on arteriogram: Effect of patient's sex on diagnosis. Circulation 1995;91:1363–1367.

54. Sangiorgi G, Rumberger JA, Severson A, et al. Arterial calcification and not lumen stenosis is highly correlated with atherosclerotic plaque burden in humans: A histologic study of 723 coronary artery segments using nondecalcifying methodology. J Am Coll Cardiol 1998;31:126–133.

55. Detrano RC, Wong ND, Doherty TM, et al. Coronary calcium does not accurately predict near-term future coronary events in high-risk adults. Circulation 1999;99:2633–2638.

56. Taylor AJ, Burke AP, O'Malley PG, et al. A comparison of the Framingham risk index, coronary artery calcification, and culprit plaque morphology in sudden cardiac death. Circulation 2000;101:1243–1248.

57. Ge J, Liu F, Gorge G, et al. Angiographically 'silent' plaque in the left main coronary artery detected by intravascular ultrasound. Coron Artery Dis 1995;6:805–810.

58. Mintz GS, Douek P, Pichard AD, et al. Target lesion calcification in coronary artery disease: An intravascular ultrasound study. J Am Coll Cardiol 1992;20:1149–1155.

59. Mintz GS, Popma JJ, Pichard AD, et al. Patterns of calcification in coronary artery disease: A statistical analysis of intravascular ultrasound and coronary angiography in 1155 lesions. Circulation 1995;91:1959–1965.

60. Tuzcu EM, Berkalp B, De Franco AC, et al. The dilemma of diagnosing coronary calcification: Angiography versus intravascular ultrasound. J Am Coll Cardiol 1996;27:832–838.

61. Mintz GS, Pichard AD, Popma JJ, et al. Determinants and correlates of target lesion calcium in coronary artery disease: A clinical, angiographic and intravascular ultrasound study. J Am Coll Cardiol 1997;29:268–274.

62. Reisman M, Buchbinder M. Rotational ablation: The Rotablator catheter. Cardiol Clin 1994;12:595–610.

63. Warth DC, Leon MB, O'Neill W, et al. Rotational atherectomy multicenter registry: Acute results, complications and 6-month angiographic follow-up in 709 patients. J Am Coll Cardiol 1994;24:641–648.

64. MacIsaac AI, Bass TA, Buchbinder M, et al. High speed rotational atherectomy: Outcome in calcified and noncalcified coronary artery lesions. J Am Coll Cardiol 1995;26:731–736.

65. Bottner RK, Hardigan KR. High-speed rotational ablation for in-stent restenosis. Cathet Cardiovasc Diagn 1997;40:144–149.

66. Kini A, Marmur JD, Dangas G, et al. Angiographic patterns of in-stent restenosis and implications on subsequent revascularization. Cathet Cardiovasc Intervent 2000;49:23–29.

67. Thomas WJ, Cowley MJ, Vetrovec GW, et al. Effectiveness of rotational atherectomy in aortocoronary saphenous vein grafts. Am J Cardiol 2000;86:88–91.

68. Kovach JA, Mintz GS, Pichard AD, et al. Sequential intravascular ultrasound characterization of the mechanisms of rotational atherectomy and adjunct balloon angioplasty. J Am Coll Cardiol 1993;22:1024–1032.

69. Safian RD, Niazi KA, Strzelecki M, et al. Detailed angiographic analysis of high-speed mechanical rotational atherectomy in human coronary arteries. Circulation 1993;88:961–968.

70. Stertzer SH, Rosenblum J, Shaw RE, et al. Coronary rotational ablation: Initial experience in 302 procedures. J Am Coll Cardiol 1993;21:287–295.

71. Moussa I, Di Mario C, Moses J, et al. Coronary stenting after rotational atherectomy in calcified and complex lesions: Angiographic and clinical follow-up results. Circulation 1997;96:128–136.

72. Hoffmann R, Mintz GS, Kent KM, et al. Comparative early and nine-month results of rotational atherectomy, stents, and the combination of both for calcified lesions in large coronary arteries. Am J Cardiol 1998;81:552–557.

73. Kobayashi Y, Moussa I, Akiyama T, et al. Low restenosis rate in lesions of the left anterior descending coronary artery with stenting following directional coronary atherectomy. Cathet Cardiovasc Diagn 1998;45:131–138.

74. Richardson PD, Davies MJ, Born GV. Influence of plaque configuration and stress distribution on fissuring of coronary atherosclerotic plaques. Lancet 1989;2:941–944.
75. Fuster V, Badimon L, Badimon JJ, Chesebro JH. The pathogenesis of coronary artery disease and the acute coronary syndromes. N Engl J Med 1992;326:242–250.
76. Davies MJ, Richardson PD, Woolf N, et al. Risk of thrombosis in human atherosclerotic plaques: Role of extracellular lipid, macrophage, and smooth muscle cell content. Br Heart J 1993;69:377–381.
77. Pasterkamp G, Falk E, Woutman H, Borst C. Techniques characterizing the coronary atherosclerotic plaque: Influence on clinical decision making? J Am Coll Cardiol 2000;36:13–21.
78. Gyongyosi M, Yang P, Hassan A, et al. Arterial remodelling of native human coronary arteries in patients with unstable angina pectoris: A prospective intravascular ultrasound study. Heart 1999;82:68–74.
79. Smits PC, Pasterkamp G, Quarles van Ufford MA, et al. Coronary artery disease: Arterial remodelling and clinical presentation. Heart 1999;82:461–464.
80. Schoenhagen P, Ziada KM, Kapadia SR, et al. Extent and direction of arterial remodeling in stable versus unstable coronary syndromes: An intravascular ultrasound study. Circulation 2000;101:598–603.
81. Nissen SE, De Franco AC, Tuzcu EM, Moliterno DJ. Coronary intravascular ultrasound: Diagnostic and interventional applications. Coron Artery Dis 1995;6:355–367.
82. Yamagishi M, Terashima M, Awano K, et al. Morphology of vulnerable coronary plaque: Insights from follow-up of patients examined by intravascular ultrasound before an acute coronary syndrome. J Am Coll Cardiol 2000;35:106–111.
83. Mintz GS, Popma JJ, Pichard AD, et al. Intravascular ultrasound predictors of restenosis after percutaneous transcatheter coronary revascularization. J Am Coll Cardiol 1996;27:1678–1687.
84. Peters RJ, Kok WE, Di Mario C, et al. Prediction of restenosis after coronary balloon angioplasty. Results of PICTURE (Post-IntraCoronary Treatment Ultrasound Result Evaluation), a prospective multicenter intracoronary ultrasound imaging study. Circulation 1997;95:2254–2261.
85. Abizaid A, Pichard AD, Mintz GS, et al. Acute and long-term results of an intravascular ultrasound-guided percutaneous transluminal coronary angioplasty/provisional stent implantation strategy. Am J Cardiol 1999;84:1298–1303.
86. Simonton CA, Leon MB, Baim DS, et al. 'Optimal' directional coronary atherectomy: Final results of the Optimal Atherectomy Restenosis Study (OARS). Circulation 1998;97:332–339.
87. Topol EJ, Leya F, Pinkerton CA, et al. A comparison of directional atherectomy with coronary angioplasty in patients with coronary artery disease. The CAVEAT Study Group [see comments]. N Engl J Med 1993;329:221–227.
88. Suzuki T, Hosokawa H, Katoh O, et al. Effects of adjunctive balloon angioplasty after intravascular ultrasound-guided optimal directional coronary atherectomy: The result of Adjunctive Balloon Angioplasty After Coronary Atherectomy Study (ABACAS). J Am Coll Cardiol 1999;34:1028–1035.
89. Moussa I, Moses J, Di Mario C, et al. Stenting after optimal lesion debulking (SOLD) registry. Angiographic and clinical outcome. Circulation 1998;98:1604–1609.
90. Hibi K, Aizaqa T, Honda Y, et al. Impact of coronary debulking prior to stenting versus conventional stenting on early outcome: Initial IVUS findings [abstract]. J Am Coll Cardiol 2000;35(suppl A):94A.
91. Glagov S, Weisenberg E, Zarins CK, et al. Compensatory enlargement of human atherosclerotic coronary arteries. N Engl J Med 1987;316:1371–1375.
92. Hermiller JB, Tenaglia AN, Kisslo KB, et al. In vivo validation of compensatory enlargement of atherosclerotic coronary arteries. Am J Cardiol 1993;71:665–668.
93. Gerber TC, Erbel R, Gorge G, et al. Extent of atherosclerosis and remodeling of the left main coronary artery determined by intravascular ultrasound. Am J Cardiol 1994;73:666–671.
94. Clarkson TB, Prichard RW, Morgan TM, et al. Remodeling of coronary arteries in human and nonhuman primates. JAMA 1994;271:289–294.
95. McPherson DD, Sirna SJ, Hiratzka LF, et al. Coronary arterial remodeling studied by high-frequency epicardial echocardiography: An early compensatory mechanism

in patients with obstructive coronary atherosclerosis. J Am Coll Cardiol 1991;17:79–86.

96. Nishioka T, Luo H, Eigler NL, et al. Contribution of inadequate compensatory enlargement to development of human coronary artery stenosis: An in vivo intravascular ultrasound study. J Am Coll Cardiol 1996;27:1571–1576.

97. Pasterkamp G, Wensing PJ, Post MJ, et al. Paradoxical arterial wall shrinkage may contribute to luminal narrowing of human atherosclerotic femoral arteries. Circulation 1995;91:1444–1449.

98. Shiran A, Mintz GS, Leiboff B, et al. Serial volumetric intravascular ultrasound assessment of arterial remodeling in left main coronary artery disease. Am J Cardiol 1999;83:1427–1432.

99. Lim TT, Liang DH, Botas J, et al. Role of compensatory enlargement and shrinkage in transplant coronary artery disease. Serial intravascular ultrasound study. Circulation 1997;95:855–859.

100. Hong MK, Park SW, Lee CW, et al. Intravascular ultrasound findings of negative arterial remodeling at sites of focal coronary spasm in patients with vasospastic angina. Am Heart J 2000;140:395–401.

101. Kakuta T, Currier JW, Haudenschild CC, et al. Differences in compensatory vessel enlargement, not intimal formation, account for restenosis after angioplasty in the hypercholesterolemic rabbit model. Circulation 1994;89:2809–2815.

102. Post MJ, Borst C, Kuntz RE. The relative importance of arterial remodeling compared with intimal hyperplasia in lumen renarrowing after balloon angioplasty. A study in the normal rabbit and the hypercholesterolemic Yucatan micropig. Circulation 1994;89:2816–2821.

103. Mintz GS, Popma JJ, Pichard AD, et al. Arterial remodeling after coronary angioplasty: A serial intravascular ultrasound study. Circulation 1996;94:35–43.

104. Zarins CK, Weisenberg E, Kolettis G, et al. Differential enlargement of artery segments in response to enlarging atherosclerotic plaques. J Vasc Surg 1988;7:386–394.

105. Vita JA, Treasure CB, Ganz P, et al. Control of shear stress in the epicardial coronary arteries of humans: Impairment by atherosclerosis. J Am Coll Cardiol 1989;14:1193–1199.

106. Abbruzzese TA, Guzman RJ, Martin RL, et al. Matrix metalloproteinase inhibition limits arterial enlargements in a rodent arteriovenous fistula model. Surgery 1998;124:328–334.

107. Pasterkamp G, Schoneveld AH, Hijnen DJ, et al. Atherosclerotic arterial remodeling and the localization of macrophages and matrix metalloproteases 1, 2 and 9 in the human coronary artery. Atherosclerosis 2000;150:245–253.

108. Miller VM, Vanhoutte PM. Enhanced release of endothelium-derived factor(s) by chronic increases in blood flow. Am J Physiol 1988;255:H446-H451.

109. Mondy JS, Lindner V, Miyashiro JK, et al. Platelet-derived growth factor ligand and receptor expression in response to altered blood flow in vivo. Circ Res 1997;81:320–327.

110. Mintz GS, Kent KM, Pichard AD, et al. Contribution of inadequate arterial remodeling to the development of focal coronary artery stenoses. An intravascular ultrasound study. Circulation 1997;95:1791–1798.

111. Pasterkamp G, Schoneveld AH, van der Wal AC, et al. Relation of arterial geometry to luminal narrowing and histologic markers for plaque vulnerability: The remodeling paradox. J Am Coll Cardiol 1998;32:655–662.

112. Dangas G, Mintz GS, Mehran R, et al. Preintervention arterial remodeling as an independent predictor of target-lesion revascularization after nonstent coronary intervention: An analysis of 777 lesions with intravascular ultrasound imaging. Circulation 1999;99:3149–3154.

113. Hoffmann R, Mintz GS, Dussaillant GR, et al. Patterns and mechanisms of in-stent restenosis. A serial intravascular ultrasound study. Circulation 1996;94:1247–1254.

114. Mudra H, Regar E, Klauss V, et al. Serial follow-up after optimized ultrasound-guided deployment of Palmaz-Schatz stents. In-stent neointimal proliferation without significant reference segment response. Circulation 1997;95:363–370.

115. Rogers C, Edelman ER. Endovascular stent design dictates experimental restenosis and thrombosis. Circulation 1995;91:2995–3001.

116. Lafont A, Guzman LA, Whitlow PL, et al. Restenosis after experimental angioplasty. Intimal, medial, and adventitial changes associated with constrictive remodeling. Circ Res 1995;76:996–1002.
117. Di Mario C, Gil R, Camenzind E, et al. Quantitative assessment with intracoronary ultrasound of the mechanisms of restenosis after percutaneous transluminal coronary angioplasty and directional coronary atherectomy. Am J Cardiol 1995;75:772–777.
118. Kimura T, Kaburagi S, Tamura T, et al. Remodeling of human coronary arteries undergoing coronary angioplasty or atherectomy. Circulation 1997;96:475–483.
119. Lawrie A, Brisken AF, Francis SE, et al. Ultrasound enhances reporter gene expression after transfection of vascular cells in vitro. Circulation 1999;99:2617–2620.
120. Fitzgerald PJ, Moore P, Hayasse M, et al. Intravascular sonotherapy impacts neointimal hyperplasia following stent implantation in swine femoral arteries [abstract]. J Am Coll Cardiol 2000;35(suppl A):28A.
121. Post MJ, Moore P, Menahem N, et al. Intravascular sonotherapy prevents intimal hyperplasia in a coronary stent pig model without long term adverse effects [abstract]. Circulation 2000;102(suppl II):II–733.
122. Barath P, Fishbein MC, Vari S, Forrester JS. Cutting balloon: A novel approach to percutaneous angioplasty. Am J Cardiol 1991;68:1249–1252.
123. Goicolea J, Martinez D, Alfonso F. Intravascular ultrasound findings after cutting balloon angioplasty [abstract]. Circulation 1996;1996:I–635.
124. Yamaguchi T, Nakamura M, Nishida T, et al. Update on cutting balloon angioplasty. J Interven Cardiol 1998;11:S114–S119.
125. Stankovic G, Albiero R, Di Mario C, et al. Cutting balloon angioplasty for in-stent restenosis [abstract]. Am J Cardiol 2000;86(suppl 8A):24i.
126. Moris C, Bethencourt M, Gomez-Recio M, et al. Angiographic follow-up of cutting balloon vs conventional balloon angioplasty. Results of the CUBA Study [abstract]. J Am Coll Cardiol 1998;31(suppl A):223A.
127. Hosokawa H, Yamaguchi T, Kobayashi T, et al. Acute results of the Restenosis Reduction by Cutting Balloon Evaluation Study [abstract]. J Am Coll Cardiol 1998; 31(suppl A):315A.
128. Izumi M, Ysuchikane E, Otsuji S, et al. Cutting Balloon Angioplasty vs. Plain Old Balloon Angioplasty Randomized Study in Type B/C Lesions (CAPAS) [abstract]. J Am Coll Cardiol 1998;31(suppl A):315A.
129. Mori M, Kurogane H, Kajiya T, et al. Long-term angiographic and clinical outcome after "stand-alone" cutting balloon angioplasty in patients with non-complex coronary artery disease [abstract]. J Am Coll Cardiol 1998;31(suppl A):315A.
130. Ergene O, Seyithanoglu BY, Tastan A, et al. Comparison of angiographic and clinical outcome after cutting balloon and conventional balloon angioplasty in vessels smaller than 3 mm in diameter: A randomized trial. J Invas Cardiol 1998;10:70–75.
131. Lauer B, Stellbring S, Ambrosch H, et al. Cutting balloon angioplasty for treatment of in-stent restenosis [abstract]. Circulation 2000;102(suppl II):II–365.

Intravascular Ultrasound-Based Dosimetry

Stephane G. Carlier, MD, PhD, Tim Fox, PhD,
Ian R. Crocker, MD, PhD,
Peter C. Levendag, MD, PhD, Patrick W. Serruys, MD, PhD

Introduction

Since the first balloon angioplasty performed by Gruntzig et al in 1977,[1] there has been continued evolution of various mechanical approaches to percutaneously revascularize the major coronary arteries. This is essentially a remote approach that requires optimal image guidance. Interventional devices are designed to remodel, remove, or otherwise ameliorate the arterial obstruction and they involve cracking, breaking, stretching, scraping, shaving, or burning of the atherosclerotic plaque, with radiation recently being added to the interventionalist's arsenal.[2] Imaging is the major feedback mechanism and a key factor for decision making during intravascular procedures.

Despite widespread use of coronary x-ray contrast angiography over the last four decades, angiograms that are difficult to interpret are frequently encountered (ostial lesions, tortuous vessel segments, vessel overlap, intermediate lesions, dissections, and thrombus). Although the value of angiography remains unquestioned, radiographic imaging depicts a two-dimensional silhouette of the arterial lumen. This "luminogram" is a relatively poor representation of coronary anatomy and a limited standard on which to base therapeutic decisions.[3] Only lumen narrowing is well demonstrated by angiography, which is inherently limited in defining the distribution and extent of wall disease and in accurately measuring irregular lumina. Furthermore, angiography is insensitive to early atheromatous thickening of the arterial wall, partly due to vascular remodeling that allows plaque to grow to occupy an average of 40% of the vessel's cross section before luminal encroachment occurs.[4] Plaque burden in reference segments that are considered angiographically normal can reach on average 35 to 40%.[5] These shortcomings, among others, have led to the rapid growth of interest in intravascular ultrasound (IVUS) imaging.

In the late 1980s, IVUS emerged as a promising new imaging modality to assess vascular disease.[6] IVUS provides real-time tomographic images of vessel cross sections, elucidating the true morphology of the lumen and transmural components of atherosclerotic arteries. The field of IVUS imaging has led to improvements in the understanding of atherosclerotic disease and its response to various

From Waksman R (ed.). *Vascular Brachytherapy, Third Edition.* Armonk, NY: Futura Publishing Co., Inc.; © 2002.

therapeutic interventions. IVUS has been very useful in understanding the mechanisms involved in the restenosis process: elastic recoil of the artery, local thrombus formation, vascular remodeling with shrinkage of the vessel, or an exuberant healing process with neointimal cellular proliferation and matrix synthesis.[7-9] Stent implantation minimizes elastic recoil and remodeling of vessels, but exacerbates the normal proliferative reaction in response to the intervention.[10,11] Depending on the type of lesions treated, restenosis rates of 15 to 50% remain the major drawback of stent therapy.

Since radiotherapy has proven to be effective in treating the exuberant fibroblastic activity of keloid scar formation and other nonmalignant benign processes such as ocular pterygia,[12,13] it has been assumed that adjunctive radiation treatment could inhibit restenosis. Various clinical coronary applications of brachytherapy are under way and are extensively reviewed in other chapters of this book.[14-20] Reports of these groups have provided compelling experimental evidence of the efficacy of brachytherapy in the prevention of restenosis. In these studies, the short- and long-term results were evaluated by histomorphometry, measuring the amount of neointima formation after balloon overstretch injury or stent implantation.

The objective of this chapter is to emphasize the potential of IVUS imaging to guide dose prescription, to assess the results of brachytherapy in clinical trials, and to review and compare the different modalities that have been implemented so far.

Intravascular Ultrasound

Imaging Catheters

Ultrasound imaging from within the artery is achieved by placing a transducer at the tip of a catheter. These catheters are highly flexible and can be advanced on a guidewire in the epicardial coronary arteries. For coronary imaging, IVUS catheters average 3 F (1-mm diameter). While even smaller ones are being developed, others are currently combined with an angioplasty balloon or stent delivery system as depicted on Figure 1.[21] IVUS imaging has been shown to be safe, with a very low complication rate.[22]

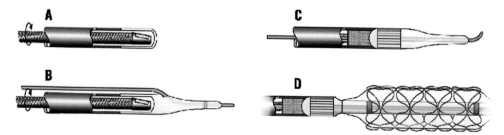

Figure 1. Schematic drawings of present intravascular echo catheters. **(A)** and **(B)** demonstrate the flex-shaft mechanically rotated single element devices, with or without the use of a guidewire, **(C)** and **(D)** are the electronically steered phased array systems, with or without the combination of a stent delivery system.

Ultrasound imaging of arteries is performed at much higher frequency than conventional diagnostic ultrasound imaging, typically 20 to 40 MHz for the coronaries, but as low as 10 MHz for large vessels. At these frequencies, shorter acoustic wavelengths result in micrometric image resolution. Typical axial and lateral resolutions for imaging catheters are of the order of 80 to 150 μm and 200 to 400 μm, respectively. High acoustic attenuation at higher frequencies is compensated by the need for interrogation of relatively short distances (5 to 15 mm). Imaging is achieved at frame rates of 20 to 30 frames per second.

Both, mechanical and solid-state imaging catheters have been developed, each with their intrinsic advantages and disadvantages. The image quality delivered by both types of imaging catheters has undergone continuous improvement. Presently, mechanical devices operate at higher frequencies (up to 47 MHz) and have been miniaturized further since they involve a single transducer element. However, the single-element transducer has a limited depth of focus and nonuniform rotation results in image artifacts.[23] Since the transducer is inside a catheter, acoustic coupling must be provided initially and maintained by flushing saline. Solid-state imaging catheters consist of arrays of transducer elements (currently 64) arranged on a flexible catheter. These elements transmit and receive ultrasound pulses that are later combined in synthetic aperture mode of operation. Electronically phasing the element responses allows dynamic focusing of the ultrasound beam at all depths.[24] Solid-state IVUS catheters are uninvolved with saline flushes and are well suited for imaging/therapy combination devices due to the lack of moving parts. Recently developed devices have combined IVUS with a stent delivery system or directional brachytherapy.

Intravascular Ultrasound Imaging

The IVUS catheters are advanced on wire before an intervention, or after the placement of a stent, and the interpretation is based on the successive cross sections obtained inside the coronary tree. A natural extension to cross-sectional ultrasound imaging is three-dimensional (3-D) imaging. To obtain a 3-D survey of the vessel, ultrasound images can be acquired during a "pullback." In this maneuver, the imaging catheter is first advanced distal to the lesion of interest and subsequently pulled back during image acquisition. Typical velocity of the pullback ranges from 0.5 to 1 mm/s. The sequence of images contains 3-D information that can be presented in various ways. A common form of presentation is the longitudinal or sagittal view that shows one of the image planes perpendicular to the set of cross-sectional images. Since during the pullback there is motion due to the pulsation of the heart, longitudinal scans may have a jagged appearance. Although this artifact does not impede the understanding of the vessel structure, the use of ECG-triggered pullbacks is also available.[25] Recently, the fusion of biplane angiography and IVUS images has been described for true 3-D reconstruction of coronary segments.[26,27]

In our patients treated with coronary brachytherapy, we have tried to systematically perform IVUS prior to the insertion of the radiation delivery catheter. Intracoronary nitrates were administered before the coronary segments were examined. The ClearView™ (CardioVascular Imaging System, CVIS, Sunnyvale, CA) was used with an IVUS catheter incorporating a 30-MHz single-element rotating transducer in a 2.9 F sheath (~1 mm). The ECG-gated image digitization system (EchoScan, TomTec, Munich, Germany) received the video signal input from the IVUS console, and the ECG signal from the patient. This system steered the ECG-gated stepping pullback device by steps of 0.2 mm. Images were acquired at end-diastole for heart cycles falling within a predetermined range (0.125 sec) around the heart rate of the patient. Premature beats and RR intervals outside this range were excluded and the IVUS catheter remained stationary. By experience, we have noticed that with these settings, on average 10 to 15% of the RR intervals are rejected, and, for a heart rate of 60 beats/min, the average pullback speed is 1 cm/min. This system assures segment-to-segment independence by not imaging during the axial movement of the IVUS catheter that occurs during the cardiac cycle.[28]

Image Analysis System

Numerous packages are presently available to perform measurements on IVUS pullbacks and standard methods have been reported elsewhere.[29,30] We use a contour detection program developed in our laboratory[31] for the automated 3-D analysis of the IVUS images corresponding to the irradiated segment. The contours of the lumen-intima and the media-adventitia boundaries are identified on two longitudinal views using a minimum-cost-based analysis algorithm. These contours are used to guide automated contour detection in every planar cross-sectional image. Scrolling through the entire data set is possible, with this Windows™-based program, for manual corrections of the contours. From these tracings, the total vessel area (encompassing the media-adventitia border) and the lumen area are determined for each cross section. The area encompassed by the lumen-intima and media-adventitia boundaries defines the luminal and the total vessel volumes, respectively. The difference between total vessel and luminal volumes defines the plaque volume. Because media thickness cannot be measured accurately, we assume that the plaque volume includes the atherosclerotic plaque and the media.[32] Volumetric data are calculated by the formula: $V = \Sigma_{i=1}^{n} A_i * H$, where V = volume; A = area of total vessel or lumen or plaque in a given cross-sectional ultrasound image; H = thickness of the coronary artery slice that is reported by this digitized cross-sectional IVUS image; and n = the number of digitized cross-sectional images encompassing the volume to be measured.[31] The residual plaque burden (%) on each cross section was calculated as total vessel area minus lumen area divided by the total vessel area. To assess the volume changes at 6-month follow-up, meticulous matching of the region of interest must be performed by comparing the longitudinal reconstruction to that after treatment. The feasibility and intra- and interobserver variability of our system have been previously reported.[33]

Interpretation of Intravascular Ultrasound Images

The tomographic capabilities of ultrasound imaging allow the display of cross-sectional, microanatomic images, somewhat similar to histologic cross sections. In muscular arteries (external iliac, femoral, renal, and coronary), a three-layered appearance is often observed with ultrasound examination, corresponding to the intima, media, and adventitia layers (Fig. 2a).[34] These are differentiated on the basis of their echogenicity (the local mean gray level on the ultrasound image). Typically, the echoes from the adventitia, rich in collagen, are used as a brightness reference. The media, rich in smooth muscle cells but with less collagen, is generally hypoechoic (darker) and the intima can be more or less echogenic than the media depending on its content of elastic and collagen fibers.[35] The intima, originally a monolayer lamina, thickens with age and is normally 200 to 300 microns thick by adulthood. Fibrous degeneration of the media may lead to ultrasonic homogeneity throughout the wall and poor delineation of the layers. Conversely, in elastic arteries (aorta, carotids, common iliac, and pulmonary), the media normally contains more collagen fibers than in muscular arteries and results in a similar echogenicity as the thickened intima and adventitia. Therefore, in elastic arteries the gray level of the wall is more homogenous throughout the cross section. In IVUS images, blood is characterized by the speckled pattern that changes randomly during real-time imaging, an

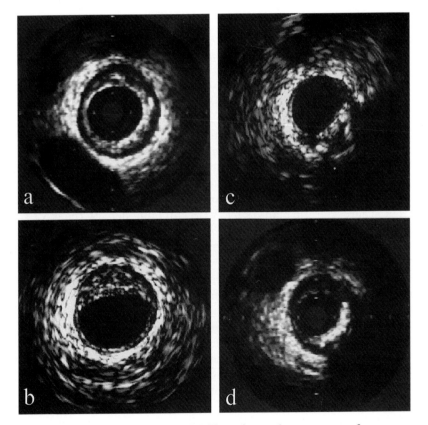

Figure 2. Characteristic IVUS images. **(a)** Three-layered appearance of a coronary artery with a thickened intima. The echolucent feature from 6 to 8 o'clock is a vein. Calibration is 1 mm. **(b)** IVUS of a coronary artery with an eccentric fibrofatty lesion from 10 to 2 o'clock. **(c)** IVUS of a coronary artery with a fibrous plaque between 3 and 6 o'clock. A side branch is apparent at 11 o'clock. **(d)** IVUS image of a coronary artery with 45 degrees of calcium in the second quadrant. A hypoechoic perivascular structure is visible at 10 o'clock.

identifiable feature that cannot be appreciated from single image frames. At 20 to 40 MHz, the echogenicity of blood is much higher than in transthoracic echocardiography (2.5 to 5 MHz).

IVUS detects the particular echo characteristics of different plaque types. Fibrofatty plaque has a relatively low echogenicity with respect to the adventitia, depending on fibrous and fatty content (Fig. 2b). Fibrous plaques result in bright echos due to a high content of collagen and elastic components and often attenuate the echo resulting in distal shadowing (Fig. 2c). The presence of calcium within the plaque is identified by bright echoes with strong shadowing (Fig. 2d). Shadowing and attenuation limit the ability to visualize vessel structures distal to the bright echoes from calcium or fibrous plaques. Lipid accumulations are generally markedly hypoechoic. However, there is presently controversy over the ultrasonic appearance of some arterial components.[36] We have recently described the possibility of assessing mechanical properties of the arterial wall by the processing of the IVUS radiofrequency signal.[37] This data could be useful in the field of vascular brachytherapy to improve tissue characterization and address the influence of the plaque composition on dosimetry attenuation observed, mainly for beta and low-energy gamma sources, by calcified plaques.[38]

Intravascular Ultrasound in Diagnosis and Intervention

The clinical use of IVUS has recently been reviewed by the study group of intracoronary imaging of the European Society of Cardiology.[29] The consensus is that the diagnostic advantage of IVUS over angiography is associated with a more accurate morphological assessment of the lumen, with additional characterization of vessel wall morphology and composition. IVUS also provides imaging of the dynamics of blood. Angiographically ambiguous situations that are commonly assessed proficiently by IVUS include ostial and main stem lesions, branching and tortuous vessels, focal vasospasm, and ruptured or dissected plaques.[39] Direct assessment of atherosclerotic plaques by IVUS can help identify the most adequate therapeutic intervention for the case at hand. For some investigators, modification of the interventional strategy occurred in up to 40% of the cases after IVUS assessment of the lesion.[40]

Conflicting data exist in the literature regarding the value of post-intervention IVUS parameters in predicting the restenosis rate after percutaneous transluminal coronary angioplasty (PTCA). It remains unclear whether or not IVUS guidance decreases in-stent restenosis and improves the event-free survival after an intervention.[41] Mintz et al found that the residual plaque burden after PTCA, measured with IVUS, was an independent predictor of restenosis.[9] This was not the case in the PICTURE Study in which 200 patients were enrolled.[42] The final report of the GUIDE Trial of the value of IVUS-measured plaque area and minimum lumen cross section as a predictor of patient outcome is still pending.[43] The MUSIC Trial demonstrated that IVUS guidance, during intervention, improved the minimum cross-sectional area in the stent. This was associated with a very low restenosis rate (9.7%).[44,45] However, two recent randomized trials (RESIST and OPTICUS) comparing IVUS versus angiographic guidance did not show a difference in clinical and angiographic outcome at 6-month follow-up.[46,47] It has been demonstrated that the rate of target vessel revascularization in the randomized

CRUISE Trial was reduced from 15.3% to 8.5% ($P<0.05$) in the arm with IVUS-guided stent implantation.[48] In AVID, a large multicentric and randomized study including 800 patients not yet published, IVUS has been used in one arm to document the results of a stent implantation, whereas in the other arm IVUS was used to guide optimal stent implantation. In the IVUS-guided arm, 42% of the patients required additional treatment. This led to a mean increase of the minimal lumen diameter of 0.3 mm and of the minimal cross-sectional area of 1.27 mm^2 (+20.3%). At 12-month follow-up, the target lesion revascularization (TLR) rates were 12.4% in the IVUS documented arm, and 8.4% in the IVUS-guided arm. This difference did not reach statistical significance ($P=0.08$); however in different subgroups, a strong benefit of IVUS guidance could be demonstrated, for example when treating saphenous bypass lesions (TLR 20.8% versus 5.1%, $P<0.01$). It is, however, beyond the scope of this chapter to review in depth the numerous studies of IVUS to guide interventional procedures.

The unique characteristics of IVUS during interventions[49] may be ideally suited to the field of brachytherapy. Indeed, with its tomographic imaging possibilities of the complete arterial wall and the quantification of different structures such as the volume of the plaque or the in-stent hyperplasia, IVUS might fill the gap between the experimental knowledge acquired from histology and the results of ongoing clinical studies.

Dosimetry Methods

The calculation of dose within a specified volume is a standard means used by radiation oncologists/radiation physicists for planning teletherapy (external) or brachytherapy treatments. Dose calculation methods can be grouped into Monte Carlo methods and semi-empirical methods. Monte Carlo dose calculation methods use physical interaction principles to calculate the dose distribution of an irradiated medium. Even though Monte Carlo can be very accurate, it is generally not used because the amount of time required to get an accurate answer is excessive. Instead, most dose calculation involves the use of tabulated data generated from dose measurements or Monte Carlo calculations to perform a very fast and generally accurate assessment of the dose distribution. To determine the dose rate at a specific point from a radioactive source, the physical location, activity of the source(s), and the 3-D coordinates of the specific point must be known. Calculation of the dose at distances of 5 mm or less from a radioactive source is difficult to model accurately. For vascular brachytherapy, the American Association of Physicists in Medicine (AAPM) Task Group No. 60 (TG-60) has presented a standardized method for calculating the submillimeter dose distribution around beta-emitting and gamma-emitting catheter-based systems (seeds and wires),[50] which is a modification of the AAPM TG-43 protocol for calculating the dose distribution around interstitial sources. The TG-43 method uses tabulated dose distribution data, which is collected via dose measurements or Monte Carlo modeling techniques. These measurements are used to develop various tables based on the position and orientation of the source to the point of calculation. The methods used to develop the dosimetry tables are very important and should be determined and validated for each delivery system. AAPM TG-60 recommends a reference distance of 2 mm for the reporting of the radial dose function. For beta-emitting sources, AAPM TG-60 recommends the dose at 2 mm in water be used as the reference point.

Dose Evaluation Methods

Spatial Dose Evaluation

Spatial dose evaluation methods consist of visualizing dose distributions from treatment delivery devices superimposed with patient anatomic data. In the field of radiation therapy, this type of display is often referred to as iso-dose lines or curves. IVUS automated pullbacks give the anatomic map of the artery. Once the anatomic data is obtained, the iso-doses can be calculated and mapped to the anatomy and displayed to the physician. Assuming that the catheter containing the radioactive source is lying in the same position as the IVUS catheter, it is possible to measure the distance from the source to any vascular structure and calculate the dose rate when the activity and physical characteristics of the source are known.[51] This is illustrated in Figure 3 for a ^{90}Y/Sr beta (right panel) and ^{192}Ir gamma source (left panel), for the same dose of 16 Gy prescribed at 2 mm from source axis.

This type of process may give the clinician an opportunity to retrospectively evaluate the influence of dose on the success or side effects of the treatment at a particular location. However, the evaluation of the overall dosimetry in the arterial wall from successive cross-sectional images is difficult. Dose-volume histograms (DVHs) have been introduced in radiotherapy to condense the large body of information of the complete 3-D dose distribution data into a plot summarizing graphically the radiation distribution throughout the target volume and the anatomic structures of interest.[52,53]

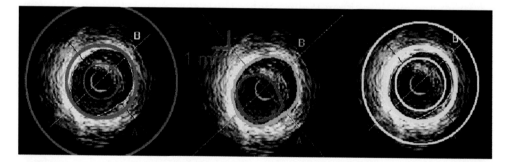

Figure 3. The middle panel demonstrates an IVUS cross-sectional image, with the catheter in the center, surrounded by blood. The catheter is against the lumen wall at 2 o'clock. The first detected contour that corresponds to the blood-vessel wall interface is highlighted. The second highlighted contour, more externally, corresponds to the media-adventitia interface (external elastic lamina), which encompasses the residual plaque lying between 11 and 4 o'clock. The iso-doses of 32, 16 (bold), and 8 Gy are superimposed on the left and right panels, corresponding respectively to a gamma ^{192}Ir (left) and a beta ^{90}Y/Sr (right) sources positioned at the IVUS catheter location, with a dose of 16 Gy prescribed at 2 mm from the center of the delivery catheter.

Quantitative Dose Evaluation

The use of quantitative dose evaluation methods such as DVHs and dose surface histograms (DSHs) will provide a snapshot view of the dose-volume relationship for a particular treated segment. DVHs have been proven to be a powerful
dose evaluation tool for the physician. DVHs summarize the dose distribution information for a region of interest and identify characteristics such as dose uniformity and hot or cold spots. To calculate a DVH, the dose distribution data must be
available for the region of interest. The histogram is a plot of the accumulated volume of those elements receiving a dose in a specified dose interval versus a set of
equal-spaced dose intervals. The *cumulative* DVH has been the most widely used
in radiation therapy. The cumulative DVH is displayed with each bin representing the volume that receives a dose greater than or equal to an indicated dose
level. In this chapter, DVH refers to the cumulative DVH. DSHs are computed for
the surface area of various target regions. The coronary segment corresponding to
the IVUS pullback is subdivided into small voxels, in which the dose is computed
(see Fig. 4). This methodology, reported in detail elsewhere,[54] has been useful to
understand the outcome of patients treated with brachytherapy after balloon angioplasty in our institution. However, we will first review the different applications of IVUS in the brachytherapy trials conducted so far, in which no DVHs have
been calculated.

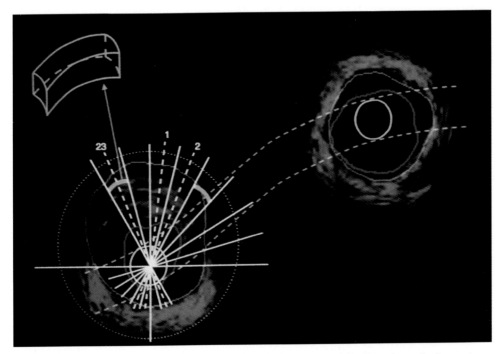

Figure 4. Dose-volume histograms are obtained by computing the dose in each elementary
voxel of the 3-D IVUS pullback corresponding to the irradiated coronary segment.

Overview of the Use of Intravascular Ultrasound in Clinical Brachytherapy Trials

The Venezuelan Experience

Condado et al explored the feasibility and safety of human coronary brachytherapy using a hand delivered ^{192}Ir wire into a noncentered closed-end lumen catheter in 22 lesions in 21 patients.[55] The doses were prescribed at 1.5 mm from the source (single doses of 18 Gy, n=1; 20 Gy, n=11; 25 Gy, n=9) using angiographic assessment. Although reported as positive, an unexplained early reduction of the minimal lumen diameter of 0.45 mm, on average, after only 24 hours might have blurred the real efficacy of the applied radiotherapy in these patients[49] who presented no additional loss in minimal lumen diameter between 24 hours and 6-month follow-up. It has been estimated that doses of up to 92.5 Gy could have been delivered to the lumen wall because of the eccentric source placement.[49] This dose may well be beyond vessel tolerance. Such a high dose could explain the occurrence of some adverse events: 2 patients experienced early total vessel occlusion, and 4 others developed an aneurysm at 2-year follow-up. IVUS guidance might have alerted the investigators to the potential overdoses.

The Geneva Trial

In Geneva, Verin et al investigated beta irradiation using a radioactive wire (^{90}Y) in a centering balloon device.[56] The dose prescribed was 18 Gy at the surface of the balloon corresponding to the vessel luminal surface. No IVUS assessment was performed. The findings were disappointing, with a restenosis rate of 40% among the 15 studied patients. A retrospective analysis of the dose prescribed revealed that at a depth of 2 mm in the vessel wall, the dose was only ~2.7 Gy, probably well below the nominal effective dose required to prevent cellular proliferation involved in the post-angioplasty restenosis process.[57]

The SCRIPPS Study

Teirstein et al set up the first randomized, placebo controlled study of gamma therapy to treat restenotic lesions. They demonstrated a substantial reduction of the angiographic restenosis rate (17% versus 54%) among 55 patients presenting with in-stent restenosis.[58] The recently published 2-year follow-up data demonstrate the long-term efficacy of this new therapeutic modality: the TLR was significantly lower in the ^{192}Ir group (15.4% versus 44.8%; $P<0.01$). The composite endpoint of death, myocardial infarction, or TLR was also significantly lower in ^{192}Ir-treated versus placebo-treated patients (23.1% versus 51.7%; $P=0.03$).[59]

A sealed [192]Ir g-source in a noncentered catheter was used (Best Medical/ Cordis Corp). This was the first study where dosimetry was based on IVUS measurements. The distance between the center of the ultrasound catheter (supposed equivalent to the source position) and the adventitial border (the target) was measured every 1 mm along the stented segment. As illustrated on Figure 5, the dwell time was optimized so that a dose of 8 Gy was administered to the target farthest

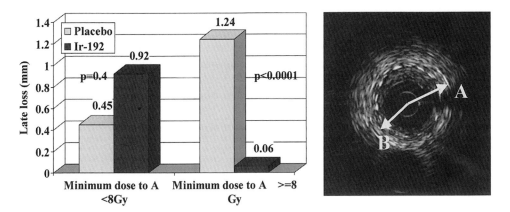

Figure 5. In the SCRIPPS prescription methodology the dwell time was adjusted in order to delivered 8 Gy to the furthest point of the external elastic lamina **(A)**. It was reduced when the closest point **(B)** would have received more than 30 Gy (right panel). A subgroup analysis (left panel) demonstrated that the patients with a minimum dose to A <8 Gy had a late loss which was not statistically significantly different than the placebo group. (Adapted from Reference 60.)

from the source (A), provided that no more than 30 Gy was delivered to the closest target (B). The importance of IVUS has been clearly demonstrated in a retrospective subgroup analysis[60]: late luminal loss and loss index were calculated for patients with diabetes, in-stent restenosis, or minimum dose exposure of the target to 8.00 Gy. Two-factor analysis of variance was used to test for an interaction between patient characteristics and treatment effect. In the treated group (^{192}Ir), late loss was particularly low in patients with diabetes (0.19 versus 0.46 mm), in-stent restenosis (0.17 versus 1.02 mm), and also in patients who received a minimum radiation dose to the entire adventitial border of at least 8.00 Gy (0.06 versus 0.92). The loss index in this subgroup was 0.03. The two-factor analysis of variance demonstrated a significant interaction between treatment effect (late loss) and the subgroup characteristic of receiving a minimum dose of 8.00 Gy to the adventitial border ($P=0.009$, Fig. 5, left panel). This illustrates the usefulness of IVUS to clarify the results of pioneering brachytherapy trials.

The WRIST Trials

The series of Washington Radiation for In-Stent Restenosis Trials (WRIST) have addressed a variety of patient and device issues such as: in-stent restenosis in native vessels or saphenous vein grafts, long lesions, and beta or gamma sources. They were initiated with a gamma ribbon source (^{192}Ir) or placebo ribbon. The prescribed dose was 15 Gy at 2 mm from the source in vessels 3.0 to 4.0 mm and at 2.4 mm for vessels greater than 4.0 mm in diameter. The data recently reported among 100 native coronaries and 30 saphenous vein grafts have demonstrated the efficacy of brachytherapy without the need for IVUS for dose prescription: incidence of major cardiac events was lower in the radiation group (29.2% versus 67.7% for placebo, $P<0.001$).[61] However, IVUS was performed systematically after irradiation and at 6-month follow-up for off-line analysis. From these measurements, it could be demonstrated that in 53.2% of the lesions from the irradiated group, there was an increase in luminal dimensions and a regression in the neointimal tissue at 6 months. None of the patients in the placebo group demonstrated a similar "melting" of the residual intimal hyperplasia left at the time of the procedure. IVUS was also necessary to estimate the minimum and maximum dose administered to the lumen border (7.3 and 45 Gy, respectively). The results of the Beta WRIST, investigating beta irradiation with a centered ^{90}Y source among 50 consecutive patients, demonstrated similarly favorable results with a major cardiac event rate of 34%.[62]

The BERT Trial

The Beta Energy Restenosis Trial (BERT) using a hand-held hydraulic delivery system employing ^{90}Sr/Y encapsulated sources in a 5.4 F catheter (Beta-Cath™, Novoste Corp., Norcross, GA) is extensively described elsewhere in this book. In the American arm (23 patients), there was neither IVUS guidance nor IVUS documentation. A late loss of 0.05 mm, a late loss index of 4%, and a restenosis rate of 15% were lower than in previous restenosis trials using similar angiographic methods.[63] In the Canadian arm initiated later, the 30 patients included were systematically documented by IVUS. Quantitative coronary angiography (QCA) data were similar, and the IVUS findings after 6-month follow-up showed[64] that there was no significant reduction in lumen area (from 5.7 ± 1.7 mm^2 post treatment to 6.0 ± 2.6 mm^2 at follow-up), with no significant change in external elastic lumina (EEL) area (13.7 ± 4.5 mm^2 post treatment to 14.2 ± 4.7 mm^2), suggesting that beta radiation inhibits neointima formation with no reduction of total vessel area at 6-month follow-up. Our findings, discussed in the following section, based on careful analysis of ECG triggered 3-D assessment of the treated area are more in favor of an adaptative remodeling with an increase of the vessel size (EEL) and plaque.[65]

More Recent Trials

Results of numerous other trials described in other chapters have been recently revealed or are still pending. Modalities of IVUS used in these trials have been very different.

In PREVENT, conducted with a ^{32}P beta source delivered with an automatic afterloader (Guidant Corp.), the radioactive wire was centered in the target lesion (de novo or in-stent restenosis) in a helical balloon which preserves distal perfusion.[66] The size of this balloon was based on the minimal lumen diameter derived from either QCA or IVUS measurements post-PTCA. Proximal and distal reference segments were measured to estimate the mean vessel diameter in order to prescribe a dose of 16, 20, or 24 Gy at 2 mm in the vessel wall.

In GAMMA-1,[93] a ^{192}Ir source or a placebo was manually delivered following successful treatment for in-stent restenosis in 252 patients. A dose greater than 8 Gy but less than 30 Gy was administered to the EEL, with similar IVUS guidance as used in the SCRIPPS Trial. However, the interpretation of the IVUS images may remain a challenge: as demonstrated by the core laboratroy of this study, 40% of the on-line EEL measurements were wrong.

In the ARREST Trial investigating the restenosis rate after PTCA and provisional stenting, a mechanical delivery of a ^{192}Ir source in a partial centering balloon (3.2 F) was used. A dose greater than 8 Gy but less than 30 Gy was prescribed to the adventitia based on IVUS measurements.

There are also numerous studies in which the dose is administered at a given distance from the source, without the use of IVUS: in the Beta-Cath Trial (^{90}Sr/Y source), it is 14 Gy in vessels greater than 2.7 mm and less than 3.35 mm, and 18 Gy in vessels greater than 3.35 mm and less than 4.0 mm; in SMART, which is designed for small vessels (<2.75 mm), it is 12 Gy to a distance of 2 mm from a ^{192}Ir source. In the ARTISTIC Trial investigating patients with instent restenosis, the same mechanical delivery system of a ^{192}Ir source as in ARREST is used, but a dose of 12, 15, or 18 Gy is prescribed at 2 mm from the source. In the CURE Study conducted with a balloon filled with ^{188}Re, a dose of 13 Gy at 0.5 mm from the surface of the balloon is prescribed. In the GAMMA-2 Trial, 14 Gy was prescribed at 2 mm from the center of the source and the restenosis rate and loss index were virtually identical to that of GAMMA-1.

The Schneider beta intracoronary irradiation Dose-Finding Study demonstrated for de novo lesion, as WRIST and GAMMA-2 for in-stent restenosis, that positive results can be obtained without using IVUS for dose prescription. With 9 to 18 Gy prescribed at 1 mm tissue depth, there was a significant dose-related inhibitory effect on restenosis after PTCA and a beneficial effect on remodeling.[67] The delivery of 18 Gy at 1-mm tissue depth resulted in a low overall restenosis rate of 15% and an even lower rate of 3.9% in those patients treated with balloon angioplasty and radiation alone. Measurements were based on QCA. However, dosimetry based on QCA measurements has limitations, as recently demonstrated by Russo et al, who have compared the method of dosage using IVUS during the SCRIPPS Trial to a method based on an angiographic model and a fixed-dose strategy.[68] From 119 IVUS pullbacks, the IVUS method would give mean minimum and maximum adventitial doses of 7.73±0.69 Gy and 25.81±5.26 Gy, and 10.9% of targets would receive less than 7 Gy, which is believed to be subtherapeutic. With the angiographic model, the mean minimal dose would be 7.51±1.44 Gy, but 38.7% of patients would receive a minimal adventitial dose less than 7 Gy. With a fixed-dose strategy of 15 Gy delivered at 2 mm from the source, the mean minimal dose would be 8.59±1.64 Gy, with 17.9% of patients receiving less than 7 Gy at the adventitia. However, with this strategy, 41.5% of targets would receive greater than 30 Gy. This demonstrates that IVUS permits the optimal dosimetry, adapted to the anatomy of the specific lesion of a patient.

Clinical Applications of Dose-Volume Histograms

One of the first IVUS scanners was developed in our institution.[69] We are systematically performing IVUS in studies evaluating new antirestenotic strategies, even when it is not mandatory for the trial. As experts in the field of interventional cardiology and quantitative angiography we have "refereed" the early developments performed by pioneers in intracoronary brachytherapy.[49,70] Later, we were the first center in Europe to develop a multidisciplinary and multi-tiered intracoronary brachytherapy program. Several findings of interest, recently reviewed,[71] came from carefully scrutinizing a cohort of more than 350 patients who have been already treated with brachytherapy in our institution. The following paragraphs summarize the correlation that we could derive between the late loss assessed by QCA, the changes in lumen, plaque, and vessel volumes, assessed by ECG-triggered IVUS, and the dose delivered in the arterial wall, estimated by DVHs.

Study Population

IVUS data acquired at our institution during the BERT Trial (1.5 arm) was studied. Thirty-one patients were enrolled, and twenty-three patients were studied who had an ECG-triggered pullback IVUS prior to stent implantation (18 male, 5 female, mean age 58±9 yr). The methodology of the BERT 1.5 Trial, the European arm of the feasibility study of coronary radiation therapy with the ^{90}Sr/Y Beta-Cath System, has been reported previously.[63]

Dose-Volume Histogram Methodology

Selection of the IVUS segment matching the irradiated site was based on anatomical landmarks such as side branches or bifurcations. An angiogram was performed after the placement of the delivery catheter to establish and document the relationship between the anatomic landmarks and the gold markers of the delivery catheter. The anatomic landmarks closest to either of the gold markers were used as reference points. This angiographic reference point was identified during a contrast injection with the IVUS imaging element at the same position as the gold marker. The image from the IVUS imaging element was recorded and the reference point was identified. During the subsequent pullback, this reference point was recognized and used for selecting the area subject to the analysis: 30 mm for the irradiated segment. The coordinate of the center of the IVUS catheter was used as a reference, and was considered at the same location as the center of the radiation train. This assumption is probably violated when looking at the differences in size of the IVUS and delivery catheters (2.9 F versus 5 F). However, the source does not occupy the center of the delivery catheter, and correction for this physical variability is difficult. The radius of the lumen and media-adventitia contours were calculated in 24 pie-slices (15°), in all the cross sections corresponding to the irradiated site (30 mm length of the train source, Fig. 4). The number of required slices was a function of their thickness, which was on average 0.2 mm.

Dose-volume histograms describe the cumulative distribution of dose over a specific volume, and summarize the dosimetry that would otherwise have to be interpreted from numerous IVUS cross sections with superimposed iso-doses plotted. Three volumes have been studied: the luminal surface, the adventitia volume, and the plaque and media volume. The level of the luminal surface was arbitrarily defined with a thickness of 0.1 mm from the automatically detected lumen contour. The adventitia volume was computed considering a thickness of 0.5 mm from the second contour detected, corresponding to the echogenic media-adventitia interface. The third volume, corresponding to the plaque and media structures, is encompassed between the two detected contours. The dose distribution over the total vessel wall was calculated with 0.1-mm spatial resolution. The DVH provided a tool for reporting the actual delivered dose in different arterial structures, or to detect excessive radiation at the luminal level. From the complete 3-D IVUS data set, simulations of DVH of alternative brachytherapy strategies such as the use of a gamma emitter or a centered radioactive source were tested.

Overview of Intravascular Ultrasound Data

The total number of analyzable patients treated with only PTCA and brachytherapy was limited to 23 due to stenting, the absence of an ECG-triggered pullback, or technical problems. For each patient, the minimal, mean, and maximal distance (~radius **r**) between the center of the IVUS catheter and the lumen or the media-adventitia interface were computed along the complete pullback. The minimal lumen **r** was 0.51±0.02 mm, the mean **r** was 1.42±0.25 mm and the maximal **r** was 3.36±0.70 mm. For the vessel (media-adventitia interface) minimal **r** was 0.88±0.17 mm, mean **r** was 2.07±0.25 mm, and maximal **r** was 3.80±0.63 mm. Computer simulation of the placement of the IVUS catheter in the center of the lumen in each cross section of the pullback demonstrated a significant increase of minimal **r** ($P<0.0001$): 0.67±0.17 mm and 1.23±0.25 mm, respectively, for the lumen and the vessel. Parallel to this, there was a significant decrease of maximal **r** ($P<0.0001$): 2.46±0.42 mm and 3.41±0.41 mm, respectively, for the lumen and the vessel.[72] Analysis of baseline and 6-month follow-up IVUS demonstrated that over the 30 mm of the irradiated segments, mean EEL and plaque volume increased significantly (451±128 mm³ to 490±159 mm³ and 201±59 mm³ to 242±74 mm³; $P=0.01$ and $P=0.001$, respectively), whereas luminal volume remained unchanged.[65] However, edges of the treated segments presented an increase in mean plaque volume with no net change in EEL, resulting in a decrease in mean luminal volume.

Dose-Volume Histogram Statistics

A typical DVH is given in Figure 6. On average, the minimal dose in 90% of the adventitial volume ($DV90_{EEL}$) was 37±16% of the prescribed dose (12, 14, or 16 Gy off source axis); the minimal dose in 90% of the plaque+media volume ($DV90_{P+M}$) was 58±24% and of the luminal surface volume ($DV90_{LUM}$) was 67±31%. The minimal dose in the 10% most exposed luminal surface volume ($DV10_{LUM}$) was 296±42%.[72]

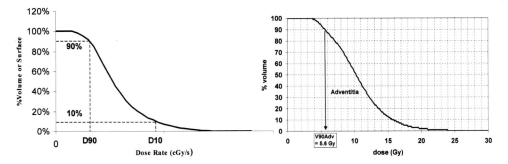

Figure 6. Dose-volume histogram (DVH) shows percentage of volume of vessel wall treated to a certain dose. D90 is the dose received by at least 90% of the volume/surface of tissue. D10 is the dose received by at least 10% of the volume/surface of tissue. The right panel demonstrates a typical DVH obtained in a patient included in the BERT study in our institution: the dose deposited in 90% of the predefined adventitial volume (see text) was at least 5.6 Gy.

Table 1

	Noncentered		Centered	
	DV90	DV10	DV90	DV10
Beta Source				
Lumen	0.67±0.31[#+]	2.96±0.42[#+]	1.06±0.31	2.03±0.49[+]
Plaque+media	0.58±0.24[#+]	2.16±0.32[#+]	0.73±0.20[+]	1.66±0.35[+]
Adventitia	0.37±0.16[#+]	1.33±0.19[#+]	0.49±0.14[+]	1.05±0.20
Gamma source				
Lumen	0.79±0.21[#]	2.34±0.31[#]	1.05±0.21	1.70±0.32
Plaque+media	0.72±0.17[#]	1.78±0.21[#]	0.83±0.13	1.45±0.23
Adventitia	0.58±0.12[#]	1.24±0.13[#]	0.67±0.09	1.05±0.13

[#]$P<0.001$, noncentered vs. centered; [+]$P<0.001$, beta vs. gamma source.

Simulation of the use of a gamma emitter were performed. As illustrated on Figure 6, the iso-doses corrresponding to the use of a ^{192}Ir ribbon positioned at the location of the IVUS catheter with the same dose of 16 Gy prescribed at 2 mm can be calculated, using the described depth dose curve of this emitter (Fig. 3).[51] Similarly, DVHs were computed for the 30-mm length of the available IVUS pullbacks. The use of a centered beta or gamma source could also be simulated by placing the source on each cross-sectional IVUS image in the center of gravity of the lumen. These simulations are summarized in Table 1. Figure 7 demonstrates the potential advantages related to the centering of the radioactive source, with a

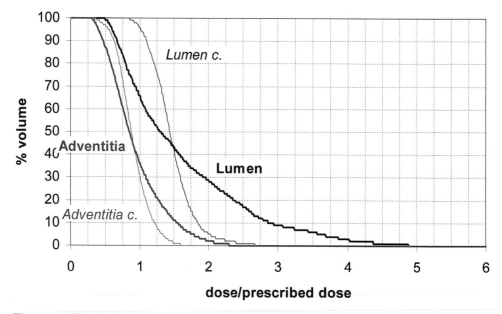

Figure 7. Illustration of the potential beneficial effect of centering the source on the homogeneity of the dose distribution. The dose-volume histogram curves for the centered position (Lumen c. and Adventitia c.) are steeper, with a DV10 for the lumen decreasing from 2.9 to 1.8. (Adapted from Reference 72.)

steeper DVH at the adventitial and luminal levels. Optimally, a DVH should demonstrate a right angle at the prescribed dose (x-axis=1, when the dose is given as dose/prescribed dose).

Dose-Volume Histogram to Predict 6-Month IVUS Outcome after Balloon Angioplasty and Beta Radiation Therapy

To establish the dose that could be predictive of efficacy in intracoronary brachytherapy, and to determine the IVUS predictors of the plaque volume at 6-month follow-up of coronary segments treated with balloon angioplasty followed by beta radiation therapy, irradiated segments were divided in 2-mm long subsegments. Since the irradiated segment measured 30 mm, 15 subsegments were defined per patient, each of them presenting 10 IVUS cross sections (0.2 mm/cross section). Two investigators, blinded to the dosimetry results, studied all individual cross sections. The type of plaque and the presence of dissection were qualitatively assessed. The type of plaque was defined in every cross section, as intimal thickening, soft, fibrous, mixed, and diffuse calcified according to the guidelines previously reported.[29] Intimal thickening was defined when the thickness of the intima-media complex was smaller than 0.3 mm. Soft tissue was defined when at least 80% of the cross-sectional area was constituted by material showing less echoreflectivity than the adventitia, with an arc of calcium less than 10°, fibrous plaque when the echoreflectivity of at least 80% of the material was as bright as or brighter than the adventitia without acoustic shadowing; diffuse calcified plaque when it contained material brighter than the adventitia showing acoustic shadowing in greater than 90°; and mixed, when the plaque did not match the 80% criterion. We categorized the 2-mm long subsegments as normal/intimal thickening, soft, hard (fibrous and mixed), and diffuse calcified, when at least 80% of the cross sections within the subsegment were of the same type. In those cross sections containing up to 90° of calcium arc, the contour of the external elastic membrane was imputed from noncalcified slices. Dissection of the vessel was defined as a tear parallel to the vessel wall. Changes in luminal, plaque, and total vessel volume between immediately post treatment and at follow-up were also computed per subsegment. Those subsegments in which the origin of side branches involved greater than 90° of the circumferential arc in more than 50% of the cross sections, or were defined as diffuse calcified, were excluded from the analysis.

Complete baseline and 6-month follow-up data were available in 18 patients successfully treated with balloon angioplasty alone followed by beta intracoronary brachytherapy.[73] Sixty-four subsegments were excluded from the final analysis due to either diffuse calcified plaque which precluded the quantification of the total vessel volume (n=30) or side branches which involved greater than 90° of the circumferential arc in more than 50% of the cross sections (n=34). Therefore, 206 irradiated subsegments were the subject of the study. Fifty-five subsegments (27%) were defined as soft, 129 (62%) as hard, and 22 (11%) as normal/intimal thickening. Dissection was observed in 34 subsegments (16.5%). Subsegments with hard tissue demonstrated a smaller increase in plaque resulting in an increase in luminal volume as compared to soft and normal/intimal thickening subsegments. Dissected subsegments demonstrated a trend towards a smaller increase in plaque as compared to nondissected subsegments.

The mean of the prescribed doses at 2 mm from the source was 14 ± 1.8 Gy. The calculated $DV90_{ADV}$ was 5.5 ± 2.5 Gy (range, 0.2 to 12.4). A wide range of dose distribution was observed in the irradiated coronary subsegments. The association between $DV90_{ADV}$ with the plaque volume at follow-up followed a polynomial equation with linear and nonlinear components. Nonlinear components described the increase in plaque volume at a lower dose, whereas the residual plaque volume post treatment accounted for the linear relationship of the curve. Changes in plaque volume appeared to decrease with dose. Four Gy was the minimum effective dose to be delivered to 90% of the adventitia since subsegments receiving at least this dose demonstrated a significantly smaller increase in plaque volume as compared to those receiving less than 4 Gy ($P<0.001$). As a result, luminal volume decreased significantly less in those subsegments receiving at least 4 Gy and even increased when the minimal dose to the adventitia was higher than 6 Gy (Fig. 8). Multivariable regression analyses identified plaque volume post treatment as a positive predictor of plaque volume at follow-up, whereas $DV90_{ADV}$ and type of plaque (hard) were negative predictors.

Dose-Volume Histogram to Predict 6-Month QCA Outcome after Balloon Angioplasty and Beta Radiation Therapy

During the past 10 years the efficacy of different techniques and medications in preventing restenosis after percutaneous interventions has been assessed by QCA. This technique has become the gold standard for the assessment of coronary angiograms in the context of scientific research due to a superior accuracy and ob-

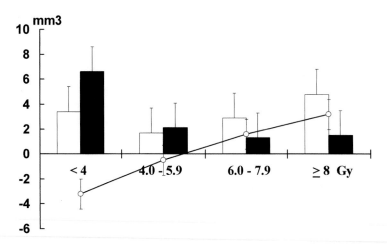

Figure 8. Changes in total vessel (white columns), plaque (black columns), and luminal volumes (open circles) regarding 5 ranges of doses as calculated by dose-volume histograms. For increasing doses deposited at the adventitial level, the vessel presents a remodeling (increase in TVV [total vessel volume]) higher than the increase in plaque, with a lumen at 6-month becoming bigger than in the baseline for doses ≥6 Gy. (Adapted from Reference 73.)

jectivity as compared to visual and hand-held caliper measurements, as well as a better inter- and intraobserver variability. Consequently, the percent diameter stenosis has become a usual output of this analysis and the value of 50% has gained widespread acceptance to define the presence of restenosis in the treated coronary segment. Although careful analysis with IVUS of 2-mm subsegments of coronary arteries treated by beta radiation could demonstrate a relationship between the dose deposited to the adventitial level and the volume of the plaque at 6 months, many patients included in brachytherapy trials are only assessed clinically and by angiography at 6 months. The major determinant of clinical recurrence of symptoms is the minimal luminal diameter at 6 months.[74,75] A recognized limitation of coronary brachytherapy is the development of new stenosis at the edges of the irradiated area, which has been associated with the radiation oncology concept of geographic miss, where the radiation field does not fully cover the target. Several brachytherapy trials have demonstrated that in a majority of patients the luminal diameter at the site of the treated lesion (target segment) may increase during the follow-up. This phenomenon is induced by positive remodeling of the vessel wall as demonstrated by IVUS.[65] Theoretically, if QCA analysis is restricted to the target segment, a region that was injured by the angioplasty balloon and that was fully covered by the radiation dosimetry, the results may demonstrate the selective efficacy of brachytherapy in optimal conditions. Therefore, we have investigated whether DVH could predict the angiographic outcome of the target segment in patients treated by brachytherapy after balloon angioplasty. In order to reach statistical significance, we have combined the DVH data derived from the IVUS pullbacks performed in the patients included in the BERT Trial in the Thoraxcenter (Rotterdam, The Netherlands) and in the Montreal Heart Institute.[64]

Angiograms were carried out before and after PTCA and at 6-month follow-up and were analyzed by the QCA core laboratory as previously described.[63] DVHs were computed retrospectively using an intracoronary treatment planning system (iPlan^{TM}, Atlanta, GA, US Patent 6,083,167) developed in Emory University. This therapy planning systems incorporates a dose calculation engine based on an AAPM TG-43 method using catheter-based delivery systems with the following radiation sources: ^{90}Sr/Y, ^{32}P, ^{125}I, and ^{192}Ir. For this study, the dosimetry used in iPlan was based on the method discussed by Soares et al for calibrating beta sources, and includes anisotropy factors to account for the dose fall-off on the end of the seeds on the transverse axis.[76] Validation of the iPlan dosimetry calculation has been reported previously.[77] iPlan has the following features: AAPM TG-43 dose engine, spatial dose evaluation, anatomic delineation, DVHs, dose surface histograms, statistical reporting, and documentation of the plan, on a PC-based platform. For each patient, a spatial dose distribution, cumulative dose surface histograms for the luminal (DSH$_{LUM}$) and adventitial (DSH$_{ADV}$) contours, and a cumulative DVH for the plaque+media (DVH$_{P+M}$) of the entire irradiated segment were calculated for the ^{90}Sr/Y source train. The maximum voxel dose, minimum voxel dose, and average voxel dose were recorded as well as two dose-volume measurements, D90 and D10. D90 is the dose received by at least 90% of the volume/surface of tissue. D10 is the dose received by at least 10% of the volume/surface of tissue (Fig. 6, left panel). Thus, the D90 and D10 doses represent a dose value based on a percentage of volume covered as opposed to the minimum and maximum doses which are the dose value given to a single voxel. Figure 9

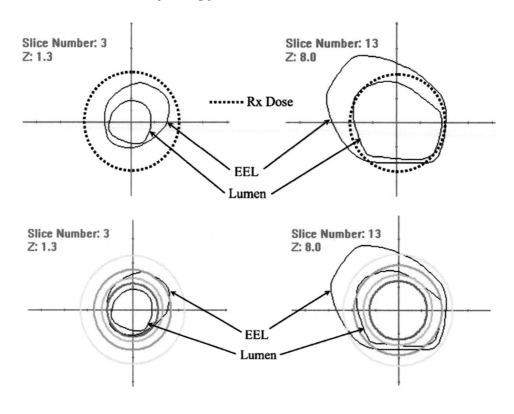

Figure 9. The two top drawings produced with the IVUS treatment planning software *i*Plan™ (Atlanta, GA) represent the segmented anatomy (shown in black) of a patient. The prescription dose line is drawn as a dotted line (16 Gy at 2 mm from the center of the source). Left and right panels show the variable size of the coronary anatomy within the irradiated vessel. The two lower panels show the coverage of the vessel wall by four iso-dose lines for the ^{90}Y/Sr Beta-Cath™ catheter, together with the patient's anatomy (lumen and external elastic [EEL] contours).

demonstrates a typical output of *i*Plan with the segmented coronary anatomy in two positions, the prescription dose line as a dotted line, and coverage of the vessel wall by four iso-dose lines.

The results are given in Table 2. In summary, at 6-month follow-up, the patients with a DS90$_{ADV}$ greater than or equal to 3.5 Gy (n=13) had a lower angiographic late lumen loss (−0.01 versus 0.31 mm, P=0.06, Mann-Whitney test). There was a trend for a lower late loss index that did not reach statistical significance (−3% versus 22%, P=0.1). This difference in outcome could not be predicted by post-intervention IVUS and angiographic data showing only that the vessel where a higher dose was deposited in the adventitia was, of course, smaller. However, it is not expected that these smaller vessels, which did not initially have a lower gain, could have demonstrated a smaller loss and loss index. Among the 13 patients with a DS90$_{ADV}$ greater than or equal to 3.5 Gy, the binary restenosis rate

Table 2

Quantitative Coronary Angiographic and Intravascular Ultrasound Results

DS90$_{ADV}$ < 3.5 Gy (n=27)	Pre Angioplasty	Post Irradiation	6-Month Follow-up
Reference vessel diameter (mm)	2.91±0.48	2.93±0.56	2.69±0.37
Minimal lumen diameter (mm)	0.89±0.29	2.06±0.40	1.75±0.66
Diameter stenosis (%)	69±10	29±12	35±22
Acute gain (mm)		1.17±0.49	
Late luminal loss (mm)			0.31±0.69
Loss index (%)			22±69
Binary restenosis N(%)			8 (30%)
MLCSA (mm²)		5.72±1.80	5.48±2.33
Vessel area (mm²)		15.38±4.17	15.86±4.31
Plaque area (mm²)		9.67±3.50	10.39±3.65

DS90$_{ADV}$ ≥3.5 Gy (n=13)	Pre Angioplasty	Post Irradiation	6-Month Follow-up
Reference vessel diameter (mm)	2.49±0.27**	2.51±0.29**	2.54±0.38
Minimal lumen diameter (mm)	0.63±0.23**	1.84±0.20+	1.85±0.48
Diameter stenosis (%)	74±9*	26±7	27±14
Acute gain (mm)		1.21±0.35	
Late luminal loss (mm)			−0.01±0.49+
Loss index (%)			−3±38
Binary restenosis (%)			1 (8%)
MLCSA (mm²)		4.01±1.10**	4.05±1.70
Vessel area (mm²)		10.52±3.81**	11.60±3.69**
Plaque area (mm²)		6.51±3.57**	7.55±2.89*

+P=0.06; *P<0.05; **P<0.01 by Mann-Whitney; DV90$_{ADV}$ < 3.5 vs. ≥ 3.5 Gy.

(diameter stenosis >50%) was only 8%, lower than the 43% observed in the 27 patients with a DV90$_{ADV}$ less than 3.5 Gy.[78]

Limitations of Dose-Volume Histograms

We assumed that the IVUS and the delivery catheters were lying in the same position in the treated coronary segment. The brachytherapy device (5 F) is larger than the IVUS catheter (2.9 F ≈1 mm) and is to some extent self-centering in the lumen. The potential advantages of centering a device, are demonstrated in Figure 7, by an increase of the DV90 and a decrease of the DV10 for the luminal, adventitial, and plaque+media volumes. In consequence, the homogeneity, which can be expressed as DV10-DV90, was improved for the lumen (0.97 versus 2.29), the adventitia (0.56 versus 0.96), and the plaque+media (0.93 versus 1.58), respectively, for a centered and a noncentered delivery system.72 However, one number such as DV10-DV90 cannot summarize a complete DVH curve. The complete shape of the curve is important (see Figs. 6 and 7). Several other parameters to assess dose homogeneity have been proposed,[79,80] but no definitive parameter has emerged as a gold standard. Looking at the slope of the DVH is a proposed option, but the slope will vary with the interval chosen to compute it. The DVHs presented in this report are cumulative plots: this integral format shows the fraction of volume receiving greater than or equal to a specific dose. Another format is the differential DVH constructed by dividing the range of dose values into equal intervals and accumulating partial volumes in those bins according to their dose values. Plots of dose-volume distributions have also been proposed.[81] We have stressed in the discussion of our study[72] that the true dose deposited in the vessel wall should lie between the data given in Table 1 for a centered and a noncentered position, since the true diameter of the Beta-Cath device is 1.7 mm. However, no easy correction can be applied since the source channel in this delivery catheter is not in the center of the catheter. Taking into account the true size of this catheter, Crocker et al have recently reported an analysis of centering the source among the patients included in the BERT Study in Montreal.[82] The reference vessel diameter was between 1.87 and 3.87 mm with an average residual stenosis of 26%. The minimum lumen diameter post angioplasty ranged from 1.40 to 3.07 mm with a mean of 2.06 mm, similar to other PTCA studies. Thus, on average, there was only 0.18 mm on each side of the Beta-Cath catheter, leaving little room for additional centering to take place. In these conditions, they did not find significant difference between the DVHs for centered and noncentered catheter positions, however a paired t-test was not applied.

When using a centering balloon for the source, such as in the PREVENT or the Schneider Dose-Finding studies, it is easy to calculate from the 3-D IVUS data set the center of gravity of the lumen of each slice and to position the source at this location. For a noncentered device, even with the use of brachytherapy and IVUS catheters of the same size, it is not certain that when advanced sequentially in the arterial lumen, they would occupy the same position. Although they should be on the shortest 3-D path in the lumen, coronary arteries have a complex curved geometry in space, and are partially deformed by the catheter lying in their lumen. Thus, catheters with differing rigidity will occupy different positions. It is important to keep in mind that the position of a catheter inside the arterial lumen is not fixed and will vary during the cardiac cycle.[28] These methodological limitations could be partially overcome with imaging wires, which could be introduced into the lumen of the irradiation delivery catheter itself.[83]

Animal studies showing the efficacy of intracoronary brachytherapy were followed immediately by human clinical trials. At the time that they were initiated there was little information available as to the mechanism of radiation in preventing restenosis. This situation continues today. Various opinions exist as to the target cell of radiation in preventing restenosis. Rubin et al have postulated the importance of the monocyte-macrophage in regulating the development of the proliferative neointima.[84,85] Robinson, Wilcox et al, and others have stressed the importance of the modified smooth muscle cell in the development of the restenotic lesion without invoking the monocyte-macrophage in the process.[86–88] The site of origin of these modified smooth muscle cells is, however, in dispute. Robinson[88] has proposed that these cells are most likely to originate in the torn edges of the media. Wilcox et al[86] have shown suggestive evidence that the proliferative activity in the vessel wall is seen first in the adventitia and only later in the media, suggesting that the neointimal cells may have migrated there from the adventitia. Thus, there remains debate as to how deep from the luminal surface the prescribed dose of radiation needs to be. There seems to be consensus that in animal models the proliferative cells forming the cellular neointima do not originate from the entire circumference of the vessel wall, but primarily from the site of damaged tunica media. The proliferation following PTCA in human coronary arteries seems to occur similarly in a focal manner. Recently, Mintz et al,[9] and others, have shown that shrinkage of the vessel (negative remodeling) may play the major role in late lumen loss following coronary intervention (atherectomy, PTCA). Waksman and Wilcox have shown that the adventitial myofibroblasts are responsible for this process, as a result of the contractile nature of these cells and their capacity to participate in a form of scar contraction of the arterial wall after angioplasty. This may present an additional reason to target dose to the tissues beyond the EEL.[89] One thing that is clear from the preclinical studies of restenosis is that a broad range of doses seems to be effective in preventing restenosis. Work carried out by the Emory group with gamma and beta sources has shown that doses of 3.5 to 56 Gy were all effective in reducing restenosis in comparison to controls.[15,90] However, the data of the subanalysis of the SCRIPPS Trial and of the recently presented Dose-Finding Study clearly demonstrated a dose-effect relationship in a narrower range of dose delivered to the vessel wall. In SCRIPPS, there was no difference between the placebo group and the patients who received less than 8 Gy to the most distant adventitia. In the Dose-Finding Study, for the patients treated by balloon angioplasty alone, the late lumen loss was 0.31 mm and the restenosis rate was 30.3% when 9 Gy was prescribed at 1 mm in the vessel wall, but, respectively, −0.04 mm and 3.9% when 18 Gy was prescribed.[67] These data support our findings of a significant relationship between the IVUS and QCA outcomes as a function of the dose deposited at the level of the adventitia, estimated by DVHs. However, these doses were not direct measurements. The theoretical value obtained at the level of the adventitia is derived from the fall-off of the isotope and the geometrical data obtained from the IVUS study. The influence of the attenuation of the radiation due to different tissue characteristics has not been taken into consideration so far, however this is likely to be significant and warrants further investigation.

We demonstrated a wide range of dose delivered to the vessel wall. This variation reflects the fact that the dose rate from a source falls off as a function of the square of the distance. Because of the need to administer the dose beyond the luminal surface of the vessel, portions of the vessel wall closer to the source will receive higher doses. These points may receive a dose in a single treatment that is greater than accepted tolerance doses for vascular tissues. It is important however to remember that the volume of tissue receiving higher doses is extremely small. Assuming a lumen diameter of 2 mm, a vessel wall diameter of 3.2 mm, and a 30-mm irradiated segment, the total volume of the irradiated media is 0.03 cc. This compares to volumes of 500 to 1500 cc, or volumes 30,000 times as large, for which conventional tolerance doses are quoted. It is well known that the tolerance doses for radiation injury are significantly higher when smaller volumes are treated. In general, the smaller the volume then the higher the dose that may be administered without complication. Powers et al demonstrated this point in intraoperative irradiations of the dog aorta.[91] In the clinical arena, we commonly observe minimal to no side effects of radiation when part of an organ is spared from the full dose. This is true for lung function, kidney function, and liver function, among other organs. The retrospective dosing analysis shows that some portion of the vessel wall receives a higher dose than what was prescribed. The fact that no aneurysms or perforations were observed support the safety associated with irradiating very small volumes with high doses.

A final limitation we face in our catheterization laboratory is that DVHs are not obtained on-line. Further implementations with faster processing of the 3-D IVUS data set for optimal automatic contour detection and the implementation of the dosimetry program on-line, in order to prescribe the radiation dose in a more refined fashion would be invaluable. A very interesting device, illustrated on Figure 10, has been recently developed. The unique characteristic of this catheter, designed for directional radiation (Brigade™, EndoSonics Corp., Rancho Cordova, CA), is the combination of a solid-state IVUS imaging array proximal to the source.[92] An on-line dosimetry program gives the actual dose at a point in any vascular structure. A second unique feature of this device is a gold attenuator asymmetrically surrounding the radioactive source, which preferentially directs radiation in eccentric plaques. The asymmetrical pattern of the iso-doses illustrated on the left side of Figure 10 were generated with our *i*Plan treatment planning software, in which the characteristics of this device could be implemented straightforwardly from the dosimetry data obtained by this company. The incorporation of on-line imaging allows for rotation of the system and conformal dose distribution with eccentric plaque. Phase I clinical trials will soon be launched, after the demonstration of the feasibility and safety of this new approach in an animal model.

In conclusion, we think that the body of additional information available from IVUS and derived dosimetry parameters like DVHs should improve our understanding of the mechanisms of action of brachytherapy and be helpful for the comparison of trials based on different dosimetry strategies. IVUS guidance and treatment planning may not be necessary for all patients and we are still investigating which patients will take advantage of this approach. However, we are convinced that at this level of development of this new method to prevent and treat restenosis, we must learn from each case, and in our center, we try to systematically interrogate the coronary lesions we treat by brachytherapy with IVUS.

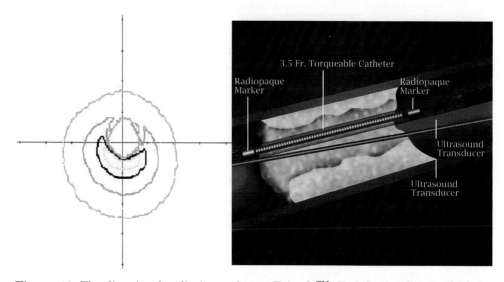

Figure 10. The directional radiation catheter (Brigade™, EndoSonics Corp.) which includes proximally an IVUS transducer. A gold attenuator partially surrounding the radioactive source gives an asymmetrical dose distribution, as demonstrated by the iso-doses shown in the left panel, generated with *i*Plan™.

Acknowledgments: We would like to thank Wendy Schumer for her critical review of this chapter and her numerous constructive comments, and the team of our catheterization laboratory and the radioncology department for their continuing support and cooperation in our endeavors to create a balance between clinical research and optimal patient care.

References

1. Grüntzig AR, Senning A, Siegenthaler WE. Nonoperative dilatation of coronary artery stenosis. N Engl J Med 1979;301:61–68.
2. Waller BF. Crackers, breakers, stretchers, drillers, scrapers, shavers, burners, welders and melters: The future treatment of atherosclerotic coronary artery disease. J Am Coll Cardiol 1989;13:969–987.
3. Topol EJ, Nissen SE. Our preoccupation with coronary luminology: The dissociation between clinical and angiographic findings in ischemic heart disease. Circulation 1995; 92:2333–2342.
4. Glagov S, Weisenberg E, Zarins CK. Compensatory enlargement of human atherosclerotic coronary arteries. N Engl J Med 1987;316:1371–1375.
5. Hodgson J, Reddy D, Suneja R, et al. Intracoronary ultrasound imaging: Correlation of plaque morphology with angiography, clinical syndrome and procedureal results in patients undergoing coronary angioplasty. J Am Coll Cardiol 1993;21:35–44.
6. Yock PG, Linker DT. Intravascular ultrasound: Looking below the surface of vascular disease. Circulation 1990;81:1715–1718.
7. Serruys PW, Luijten HE, Beatt KJ, et al. Incidence of restenosis after successful coronary angioplasty: A time-related phenomenon. A quantitative angiography study in 342 consecutive patients at 1, 2, 3 and 4 months. Circulation 1988;77:361–371.
8. Schwartz RS, Holmes DR, Topol EJ. The restenosis paradigm revisited: An alternative proposal for cellular mechanism. Am J Cardiol 1992;20:1284–1293.
9. Mintz GS, Popma JJ, Pichard AD, et al. Arterial remodeling after coronary angioplasty: A serial intravascular ultrasound study. Circulation 1996;94:35–43.
10. Hanke H, Kamenz J, Hassenstein S, et al. Prolonged proliferative response of smooth muscle cells after experimental intravascular stenting. Eur Heart J 1995;16:785–793.
11. van Beusekom HM, Whelan DM, Hofma SH, et al. Long-term endothelial dysfunction is more pronounced after stenting than after balloon angioplasty in porcine coronary arteries. J Am Coll Cardiol 1998;32:1109–1117.
12. Enhamre A, Hammar H. Treatment of keloids with excision and post-operative x-ray irradiation. Dermatologica 1983;167:90–93.
13. Bahrassa F, Datta R. Postoperative beta radiation treatment of pterygium. Int J Radiat Oncol Biol Phys 1983;9:679–684.
14. Wiedermann JG, Leavy JA, Amols H, et al. Effects of high-dose intracoronary irradiation on vasomotor function and smooth muscle histopathology. Am J Physiol 1994; 267:H125–H132.
15. Waksman R, Robinson KA, Crocker IR, et al. Endovascular low dose irradiation inhibits neointimal formation after coronary artery balloon injury in swine: A possible role for radiation therapy in restenosis prevention. Circulation 1995;91:1533–1539.
16. Mazur W, Ali MN, Khan MM, et al. High dose rate intracoronary radiation for inhibition of neointimal formation in the stented and balloon-injured porcine models of restenosis: Angiographic, morphometric, and histopathologic analyses. Int J Radiat Oncol Biol Phys 1996;36:777–788.
17. Waksman R, Robinson KA, Crocker IR, et al. Intracoronary low-dose beta-irradiation inhibits neointima formation after coronary artery balloon injury in the swine restenosis model. Circulation 1995;92:3025–3031.
18. Verin V, Popowski Y, Urban P, et al. Intra-arterial beta-irradiation prevents neointimal hyperplasia in a hypercholesterolemic rabbit restenosis model. Circulation 1995;92: 2284–2290.
19. Hehrlein C, Gollan C, Donges K, et al. Low-dose radioactive endovascular stents prevent smooth muscle cell proliferation and neointimal hyperplasia in rabbits. Circulation 1995;92:1570–1575.
20. Carter AJ, Laird JR, Bailey LR, et al. Effects of endovascular radiation from a beta par-

ticle emitting stent in a porcine coronary restenosis model. Circulation 1996;94:2364–2368.

21. Bom N, Carlier SG, van der Steen AF, et al. Intravascular scanners. Ultrasound Med Biol 2000;26(suppl 1):S6–S9.
22. Hausmann D, Erbel R, Alibelli-Chemarin MJ, et al. The safety of intracoronary ultrasound: A multicenter survey of 2207 examinations. Circulation 1995;91:623–630.
23. ten Hoff H, Korbijn A, Smit TH, et al. Imaging artifacts in mechanically driven ultrasound catheters. Int J Card Imaging 1989;4:195–199.
24. O'Donnell M, Shapo BM, Eberle MJ, et al. Experimental studies on an efficient catheter array imaging system. Ultrason Imaging 1995;17:83–94.
25. von Birgelen C, de Vrey EA, Mintz GS, et al. ECG-gated three-dimensional intravascular ultrasound: Feasibility and reproducibility of an automated analysis of coronary lumen and atherosclerotic plaque dimensions in humans. Circulation 1998;96:2944–2952.
26. Krams R, Wentzel JJ, Oomen JA, et al. Evaluation of endothelial shear stress and 3-D geometry as factors determining the development of atherosclerosis and remodeling in human coronary arteries in vivo: Combining 3-D reconstruction from angiography and IVUS (ANGUS) with computational fluid dynamics. Arterioscler Thromb Vasc Biol 1997;17:2061–2065.
27. Slager CJ, Wentzel JJ, Schuurbiers JC, et al. True 3-dimensional reconstruction of coronary arteries in patients by fusion of angiography and IVUS (ANGUS) and its quantitative validation. Circulation 2000;102:511–516.
28. Arbab-Zadeh A, DeMaria AN, Penny WF, et al. Axial movement of the intravascular ultrasound probe during the cardiac cycle: Implications for three-dimensional reconstruction and measurements of coronary dimensions. Am Heart J 1999;138:865–872.
29. Di Mario C, Görge G, Peters R, et al. Clinical application and image interpretation in intracoronary ultrasound. Study Group on Intracoronary Imaging of the Working Group of Coronary Circulation and of the Subgroup on Intravascular Ultrasound of the Working Group of Echocardiography of the European Society of Cardiology. Eur Heart J 1998;19:207–229.
30. Dijkstra J, Koning G, Reiber JH. Quantitative measurements in IVUS images. Int J Card Imaging 1999;15:513–522.
31. Li W, von Birgelen C, di Mario M, et al. Semi-automatic contour detection for volumetric quantification of intracoronary ultrasound. In: Computers in Cardiology 1994. Los Alamitos, CA: IEEE Computer Society Press; 1994:277–280.
32. von Birgelen C, di Mario C, Li W, et al. Morphometric analysis in three-dimensional intracoronary ultrasound: An in-vitro and in-vivo study performed with a novel system for the contour detection of lumen and plaque. Am Heart J 1996;132:516–527.
33. von Birgelen C, Mintz GS, Nicosia A, et al. Electrocardiogram-gated intravascular ultrasound image acquisition after coronary stent deployment facilitates on-line three-dimensional reconstruction and automated lumen quantification. J Am Coll Cardiol 1997;30:436–443.
34. Fitzgerald PJ, St. Goar RF, Connolly AJ, et al. Intravascular ultrasound imaging of coronary arteries: Is three layers the norm? Circulation 1992;86:154–158.
35. Porter TR, Radio SJ, Anderson JA, et al. Composition of coronary atherosclerotic plaque in the intima and media affects intravascular ultrasound measurement of intimal thickness. J Am Coll Cardiol 1994;23:1079–1084.
36. Hiro T, Leung CY, De Guzman S, et al. Are soft echoes really soft? Intravascular ultrasound assessment of mechanical properties in human atherosclerotic tissue. Am Heart J 1997;133:1–7.
37. de Korte CL, van der Steen AF, Cepedes EI, et al. Characterization of plaque components and vulnerability with intravascular ultrasound elastography. Phys Med Biol 2000;45:1465–1475.
38. Li XA, Wang R, Yu C, et al. Beta versus gamma for catheter-based intravascular brachytherapy: Dosimetric perspectives in the presence of metallic stents and calcified plaques. Int J Radiat Oncol Biol Phys 2000;46:1043–1049.
39. Erbel R, Roelandt JRTC, Ge J. Intravascular Ultrasound. London: Martin Dunitz; 1998.
40. Mintz GS, Pichard AD, Kovach JA, et al. Impact of preintervention intravascular ultrasound imaging on transcatheter treatment strategies in coronary artery disease. Am J Cardiol 1994;73:423–430.

41. Moussa I, Moses J, Di Mario C, et al. Does the specific intravascular ultrasound criterion used to optimize stent expansion have an impact on the probability of stent restenosis? Am J Cardiol 1999;83:1012–1017.
42. Peters RJG, Kok WEM, Di Mario C, et al. Prediction of restenosis after coronary balloon angioplasty: Results of PICTURE (Post-intracoronary Treatment Ultrasound Result Evaluation), a prospective multicenter intracoronary ultrasound imaging study. Circulation 1997;95:2254–2261.
43. The GUIDE Trial Investigators. IVUS-determined predictors of restenosis in PTCA and DCA: Final report from the GUIDE trial, phase II. J Am Coll Cardiol 1996;27(supplA):156A.
44. de Jaegere P, Mudra H, Figulla H, et al. Intravascular ultrasound-guided optimized stent deployment: Immediate and 6 months clinical and angiographic results from the Multicenter Ultrasound Stenting in Coronaries Study (MUSIC Study). Eur Heart J 1998;19:1214–1223.
45. Serruys PW, Deshpande NV. Is there MUSIC in IVUS guided stenting? Is this MUSIC going to be a MUST? Multicenter Ultrasound Stenting in Coronaries study. Eur Heart J 1998;19:1122–1124.
46. Schiele F, Meneveau N, Vuillemenot A, et al. Impact of intravascular ultrasound guidance in stent deployment on 6-month restenosis rate: A multicenter, randomized study comparing two strategies, with and without intravascular ultrasound guidance. RESIST Study Group. REStenosis after Ivus guided STenting. J Am Coll Cardiol 1998;32:320–328.
47. Mudra H, Macaya C, Zahn R, et al. Interim analysis of the "OPTimization with ICUS to reduce stent restenosis" (OPTICUS) trial. Circulation 1998;98:I–363.
48. Fitzgerald PJ, Oshima A, Hayase M, et al. Final results of the Can Routine Ultrasound Influence Stent Expansion (CRUISE) Study. Circulation 2000;102:523–530.
49. Serruys P, Levendag PC. Intracoronary brachytherapy: The death knell of restenosis or just another episode of a never-ending story? Circulation 1997;96:709–712.
50. Nath R, Amols H, Coffey C, et al. Intravascular brachytherapy physics: Report of the AAPM Radiation Therapy Committee Task Group no. 60. American Association of Physicists in Medicine. Med Phys 1999;26:119–152.
51. Amols HI, Zaider M, Weinberger J, et al. Dosimetric considerations for catheter-based beta and gamma emitters in the therapy of neointimal hyperplasia in human coronary arteries. Int J Radiat Oncol Biol Phys 1996;36:913–921.
52. Drzymala RE, Mohan R, Brewster L, et al. Dose-volume histograms. Int J Radiat Oncol Biol Phys 1991;21:71–78.
53. Fox T, Crocker I. Dosing in vascular radiotherapy. Vasc Radiother Monitor 1998;1:45–53.
54. Carlier SG, Marijnissen JPA, Coen VLMA, et al. Guidance of intracoronary radiation therapy based on dose-volume histogram derived from quantitative intravascular ultrasound. IEEE Trans Med Imag 1998;17:772–778.
55. Condado JA, Waksman R, Gurdiel O, et al. Long-term angiographic and clinical outcome after percutaneous transluminal coronary angioplasty and intracoronary radiation therapy in humans. Circulation 1997;96:727–732.
56. Verin V, Urban P, Popowski Y, et al. Feasibility of intracoronary beta-irradiation to reduce restenosis after balloon angioplasty. Circulation 1997;95:1138–1144.
57. Teirstein P. Beta-radiation to reduce restenosis: Too little, too soon ? Circulation 1997;95:1095–1097.
58. Teirstein PS, Massullo V, Jani S, et al. Catheter based radiotherapy to inhibit restenosis after coronary stenting. N Engl J Med 1997;336:1697–1703.
59. Teirstein PS, Massullo V, Jani S, et al. Two-year follow-up after catheter-based radiotherapy to inhibit coronary restenosis. Circulation 1999;99:243–247.
60. Teirstein PS, Massullo V, Jani S, et al. A subgroup analysis of the Scripps Coronary Radiation to Inhibit Proliferation Poststenting Trial. Int J Radiat Oncol Biol Phys 1998;42:1097–1104.
61. Waksman R, White RL, Chan RC, et al. Intracoronary gamma-radiation therapy after angioplasty inhibits recurrence in patients with in-stent restenosis. Circulation 2000;101:2165–2171.
62. Waksman R, Bhargava B, White L, et al. Intracoronary beta-radiation therapy inhibits recurrence of in-stent restenosis. Circulation 2000;101:1895–1898.

63. King SB, Williams DO, Chougule P, et al. Endovascular beta-radiation to reduce restenosis after coronary balloon angioplasty: Results of the Beta Energy Restenosis Trial (BERT). Circulation 1998;97:2025–2030.

64. Meerkin D, Tardif JC, Crocker IR, et al. Effects of intracoronary beta-radiation therapy after coronary angioplasty: An intravascular ultrasound study. Circulation 1999; 99:1660–1665.

65. Sabate M, Serruys PW, van der Giessen WJ, et al. Geometric vascular remodeling after balloon angioplasty and beta-radiation therapy: A three-dimensional intravascular ultrasound study. Circulation 1999;100:1182–1188.

66. Raizner AE, Oesterle SN, Waksman R, et al. Inhibition of restenosis with beta-emitting radiotherapy: Report of the proliferation reduction with vascular energy trial (PREVENT). Circulation 2000;102:951–958.

67. Verin V, Popowski Y, De Bruyne B, et al. Endoluminal beta-irradiation for the prevention of coronary restenosis after balloon angioplasty: The Dose-Finding Study Group. N Engl J Med 2001;344:243–249.

68. Russo R, Massullo V, Tripuraneni P, et al. Is intravascular ultrasound necessary for dose prescription during intracoronary radiation therapy? J Am Coll Cardiol 1999; 33:20A.

69. Bom N, Lancée CT, Van Egmond FC. An ultrasonic intracardiac scanner. Ultrasonics 1972:72–76.

70. van der Giessen WJ, Serruys PW. Beta-particle-emitting stents radiate enthusiasm in the search for effective prevention of restenosis. Circulation 1996;94:2358–2360.

71. Serruys PW, Carlier SG. Intracoronary brachytherapy: What have we learnt? Eur Heart J 2000;21:1994–1996.

72. Carlier SG, Marijnissen JPA, Coen VLMA, et al. Comparison of brachytherapy strategies based on dose-volume histograms derived from quantitative intravascular ultrasound. Cardiovasc Radiat Med 1999;1:115–124.

73. Sabate M, Marijnissen JPH, Carlier SG, et al. Residual plaque burden, delivered dose, and tissue composition predict 6-month outcome after balloon angioplasty and beta-radiation therapy. Circulation 2000;101:2472–2477.

74. Rensing BJ, Hermans WR, Deckers JW, et al. Which angiographic variable best describes functional status 6 months after successful single-vessel coronary balloon angioplasty? J Am Coll Cardiol 1993;21:317–324.

75. Serruys PW, Foley DP, Kirkeeide RL, et al. Restenosis revisited: Insights provided by quantitative coronary angiography. Am Heart J 1993;126:1243–1267.

76. Soares CG, Halpern DG, Wang CK. Calibration and characterization of beta-particle sources for intravascular brachytherapy. Med Phys 1998;25:339–346.

77. Fox T, Soares C, Crocker I, et al. Calculated dose distributions of beta-particles sources used for intravascular brachytherapy. Int J Radiat Oncol Biol Phys 1997;39:334.

78. Carlier SG, Crocker I, Sabate M, et al. Correlation between dose deposited to the vessel wall and outcomes following intracoronary beta-radiation. Circulation 1999;100: I–516.

79. Viggars DA, Shalev S, Stewart M, et al. The objective evaluation of alternative treatment plans III: The quantitative analysis of dose volume histograms. Int J Radiat Oncol Biol Phys 1992;23:419–427.

80. Panitsa E, Rosenwald JC, Kappas C. Developing a dose-volume histogram computation program for brachytherapy. Phys Med Biol 1998;43:2109–2121.

81. Niemierko A, Goitein M. Dose-volume distributions: A new approach to dose-volume histograms in three-dimensional treatment planning. Med Phys 1994;21:3–11.

82. Crocker I, Robinson K, Bonan R, et al. Active centering is not important for intracoronary radiation therapy. J Interv Cardiol 1999;12:247–253.

83. Di Mario C, Akiyama T, Moussa I, et al. First experience with imaging core wires. Semin Interv Cardiol 1997;2:69–73.

84. Rubin P, Williams JP, Riggs PN, et al. Cellular and molecular mechanisms of radiation inhibition of restenosis. Part I: Role of the macrophage and platelet-derived growth factor. Int J Radiat Oncol Biol Phys 1998;40:929–941.

85. Rubin P, Soni A, Williams JP. The molecular and cellular biologic basis for the radiation treatment of benign proliferative diseases. Semin Radiat Oncol 1999;9:203–214.

86. Wilcox JN, Waksman R, King SB, et al. The role of the adventitia in the arterial re-

sponse to angioplasty: The effect of intravascular radiation. Int J Radiat Oncol Biol Phys 1996;36:789–796.

87. Scott NA, Cipolla GD, Ross CE, et al. Identification of a potential role for the adventitia in vascular lesion formation after balloon overstretch injury of porcine coronary arteries. Circulation 1996;93:2178–2187.

88. Robinson KA. Animal models to study restenosis. In: Waksman R (ed): Vascular Brachytherapy. Armonk: Futura Publishing Company, Inc.; 1999:31–41.

89. Waksman R, Rodriguez JC, Robinson KA, et al. Effect of intravascular irradiation on cell proliferation, apoptosis, and vascular remodeling after balloon overstretch injury of porcine coronary arteries. Circulation 1997;96:1944–1952.

90. Waksman R, Robinson KA, Crocker IR, et al. Intracoronary radiation before stent implantation inhibits neointima formation in stented porcine coronary arteries. Circulation 1995;92:1383–1386.

91. Powers BE, Thames HD, Gillette EL. Long-term adverse effects of radiation inhibition of restenosis: Radiation injury to the aorta and branch arteries in a canine model [see comments]. Int J Radiat Oncol Biol Phys 1999;45:753–759.

92. Ciezki JP, Tuzcu EM, Lee EJ, et al. IVUS-directed conformal intravascular brachytherapy: The Navius system. Advances in Cardiovascular Radiation Therapy II, Proceedings. 1998:226.

93. Leon MB, Teirstein PS, Moses JW, et al. Localized intracoronary gamma-radiation therapy to inhibit he recurrence of restenosis after stenting. N Engl J Med 2001;344: 250–256.

## Chapter 47

"Geographic Miss" in Vascular Brachytherapy

Raoul Bonan, MD

The application of ionizing radiation as a therapeutic option for restenosis after vessel injury has recently generated much interest. Numerous methods have been developed in order to deliver an adequate radiation dose to the vessel wall. Low-activity sources rely on a platform, such as a stent, that is implanted in the vessel allowing dose delivery over a prolonged period up to several weeks. High-activity sources are used to deliver the desired dose during a single sitting, usually immediately following angioplasty. These sources include ribbons, seeds, and liquids and may be delivered by beta or gamma radiation. External beam radiation is also effective, but due to the constraints of the continuous motion of the coronary vessels, its application is currently limited to peripheral vessels. Each of the modalities and isotopes used differ to some degree in profile, and although each may successfully deliver the prescribed dose to a predetermined target, their complication and failure rates may vary due to these differences.

There is growing evidence that ionizing radiation is indeed effective in reducing neointimal formation and probably in preventing negative vessel remodeling, and hence, effective in reducing restenosis. Short-term experience with β- and γ-rays seems to indicate a wide therapeutic window in humans that needs to be confirmed over the long term.

Large ongoing trials using beta and gamma sources will bring new information during the next 2 years. Due to differing source profiles and the newly emerging problem of edge effect, dosimetric analysis and determination of vessel response to a spectrum of injury are assuming increasing importance. The adequate interpretation of these aspects requires the establishment of multidisciplinary teams to further explore this fascinating new application of an old therapy.

Angioplasty enlarges the vessel lumen principally through stretching the elastic components of the vessel wall. Inelastic portions of the wall and plaque tear or fracture resulting in focal arterial wall dissections.[1] The vessel wall's response to injury as a result of angioplasty follows a series of events much like that seen in generalized wound healing.

Three clear stages have been described.[2,3] During the initial thrombotic stage, platelet deposition occurs immediately on exposed lipid and collagen matrices. More platelets aggregate resulting in thrombus formation over the next several hours. This is followed by a granulation stage. Secondary to stimulation by cytokines and growth factors, normally quiescent vascular smooth muscle cells

From Waksman R (ed.). *Vascular Brachytherapy, Third Edition.* Armonk, NY: Futura Publishing Co., Inc.; © 2002.

(SMCs) undergo a change from a contractile to a mobile proliferative phenotype. Having migrated to the damaged areas, the SMCs proliferate and secrete extracellular matrix. The final stage is one of remodeling with the SMCs ceasing to proliferate but continuing to secrete and organize the extracellular matrix.

Restenosis has been demonstrated to be largely due to deleterious remodeling,[4] or to inadequate beneficial remodeling to accommodate the increased volume of neointima formed by SMC proliferation and matrix accumulation.[5]

Our ability to limit restenosis with the implantation of intracoronary stents has been due to the successful treatment of the remodeling stage. The stent props the vessel open and, regardless of the volume of neointima present, the lumen remains patent due to the larger initial vessel.[6,7] In spite of this, stents result in increased vessel wall damage and greater stimulus for neointimal formation. The limitation of this phase would further impair the restenotic process and potentially improve outcome.

Radiotherapy has been used in numerous benign proliferative states, such as heterotopic bone formation and pterygia, in an attempt to inhibit the growth of excessive tissue.[8] Keloid formation, a state of exaggerated wound healing in some ways akin to restenosis, has also been successfully treated with radiotherapy.[9,10]

Radiotherapy has been shown to inhibit neointimal formation in animal models.[11–18] Initial encouraging results were achieved following peripheral angioplasty, with a significant reduction of restenosis rate that has now been maintained for 6 years.[19] In addition, the restenosis rate and late luminal loss were significantly reduced in two randomized clinical trials to date using intracoronary gamma radiation.[20,21] These results were obtained after coronary stenting, in patients presenting with previous restenosis. Encouraging angiographic results have recently been reported with intracoronary beta radiation therapy after standard balloon angioplasty.[22,23]

At this pioneering stage of an extremely promising therapy, there are several issues that have not been entirely resolved. The delivered radiation dose at a set distance from the source center or surface can be measured, and usually accurately calculated, if the isotope, its activity, and the dwell time are known. The dose-rate gradient that occurs with distance can be determined based on the source. However, the distance between a given structure and the source is a variable that depends on the vessel size, eccentricity, plaque size, and position of the source (train, wire, fluid, gas) within the lumen as well as vessel tortuosity. Determination of these variables requires adequate visualization of the structures within the vessel and their relationship to the source.

Determination of doses delivered to these vessel wall layers, as well as length and the subsequent response to therapy, may contribute to the identification of which vessel layer should constitute the target site of action for brachytherapy and how much coverage of the injury is needed. A treatment that results in damage to the endothelium, intima, media, and adventitia may effect changes not only to the proliferative aspects of the restenotic process, but also to the geometric remodeling of the vessel.

Although vascular brachytherapy has been demonstrated to effectively prevent and treat restenosis, a technique-dependent issue, "geographic miss " (GM), has evolved as potentially causative in treatment failures. This issue may hinder the positive clinical outcomes of this new technology.[24]

In radiotherapy, GM represents an area planned in the treatment that has not received the prescribed dose, often related to inadequate margin, leading to local failure. GM is actively recognized in the treatment of different neoplasms, ie, breast, brain, cervix, prostate, and nasopharynx.[25–28]

In vascular brachytherapy, GM refers to an arterial portion, which has undergone injury during the interventional procedure but has not received the prescribed dose of radiation. This includes vessel zones receiving either no radiation or a dose less than that prescribed, and may be related to an inadequate radiation margin potentially leading to local failure.[25]

The vessel injury, created during percutaneous transluminal coronary angioplasty (PTCA) balloon inflations, stent deployment, or atherectomy procedures, initiates a physiological wound healing response, including cell proliferation and vascular remodeling, that is hypothesized to be a contributing factor to restenosis. Vascular brachytherapy, by its "killing effect," is hypothesized to inhibit cell proliferation and vascular remodeling, thereby reducing the incidence of restenosis following interventional revascularization procedures.[29] In practice, precise localization of the injury site may be difficult, particularly when each balloon inflation is often not routinely recorded.

Even when recording is meticulous, others factors can contribute to misjudgment of the injury length. Some balloons are longer than they appear, with long shoulders (from the marker to the balloon's tip) necessitating recorded images during both inflation and deflation to appreciate this issue. Radioactive source trains may move during the intravascular dwell time depending on patient compliance, respiration, and cardiac cycle. Sources comprising numerous seeds (to aid in ease of deployment) may separate if they are not tied or maintained together.

Due to the reduction of dose as an inverse relationship to the distance from the source, zones beyond the prescription point will receive diminishing doses. As line sources (such as ribbons or seed trains) are used, this phenomenon will be true both radially and longitudinally from the edge of the sources. This represents an important concept in radiation therapy, that of "dose fall-off," and must be accounted for when attempting to determine the delivered dose and vessel responses to injured areas (Figs. 1, 2, and 3). Application of this concept allows for the distinction between the length of vessel that received the prescribed dose (the prescribed dose length [PDL]) (Fig. 4), and zones that received doses less than those prescribed due to dose fall-off. Low-dose radiation associated with vascular injury has been reported to result in increased restenosis potentially due to gene stimulation through signal transduction with generation of cytokines and growth factors promoting proliferation, inflammation, extracellular matrix secretion, tissue repair, fibrosis, and negative vascular remodeling.

Finally, patient specificity (eg, diabetic, renal insufficiency) can also play a role in GM, or at least in the radial aspect of GM and as much as insufficient dosing.

Accurate evaluation of the respective sites of balloon and radiation injury will allow the detection of GM. This requires the performance of quantitative coronary angiography (QCA) with a view to these specific sites.

This form of QCA needs to assess the position of the different interventions relative to the baseline lesion over the length of the vessel. These intervention

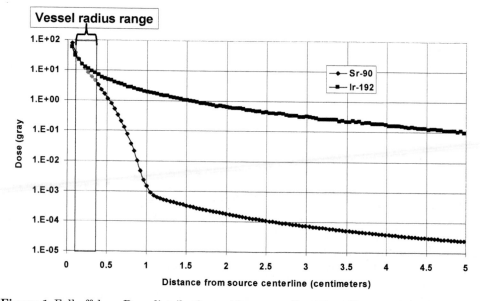

Figure 1. Fall-off dose. Dose distributions with gamma (Ir-192) and beta (Sr-90) line sources with a prescription point at 2 mm (0.2 cm). There is no significant difference at 3 mm.

sites can be projected on the follow-up angiograms allowing for subdivision into vessel zones based upon the types of injury to which they were exposed. Usually the segment to be analyzed will be long enough to include all the interventions that can be localized based on easily identifiable anatomic landmark, such as branches. Within this segment, the following zones can be identified and localized:

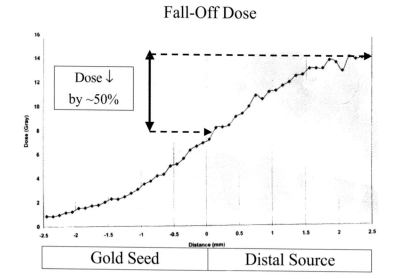

Figure 2. Longitudinal dose distribution. Effective measure of the delivered dose at the extremity of a Sr/Y line sources. There is no radiation at the end of the gold seed.

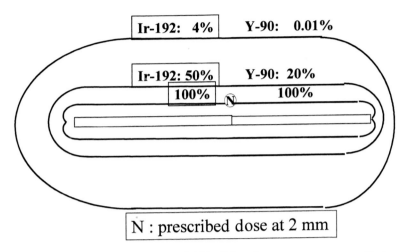

Figure 3. Comparison of the longitudinal fall-off dose between gamma and beta radiation with the same prescribed dose at 2 mm from the center of the source. Shown are 2-, 4-, and 8-mm radial iso-dose curves.

the original lesion with its minimum lumen diameter (MLD); the injury length (INL) representing the sum length of all the different interventions (balloon, laser, atherectomy, stent); and the irradiation length (IRL) with its subgroup of PDL (Figs. 5, 6, and 7). By assessing these different zones, it becomes easily apparent whether there was an adequate margin in the PDL to cover the injured zone (INL). When a portion of the injured zone is not included in the PDL, GM is determined to have occurred.

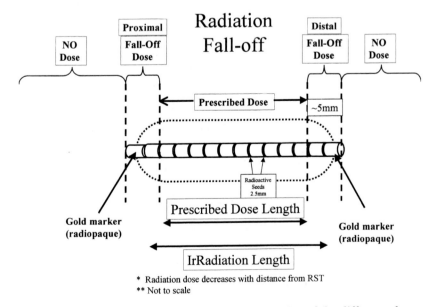

Figure 4. With the integration of the fall-off dose expression of the difference between the irradiation length and the prescribed dose length.

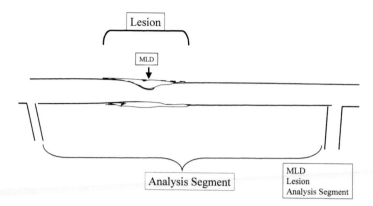

Figure 5. Quantitative coronary angiography (QCA) analysis. Schematic representation of the coronary artery with the lesion to be treated before intervention. MLD = minimal lumen diameter.

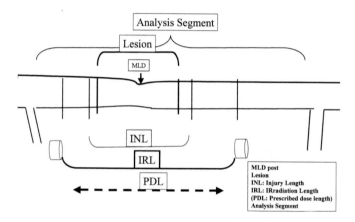

Figure 6. QCA analysis: post intervention. Schematic representation of the coronary artery with the lesion to be treated with the projection of the different interventions.

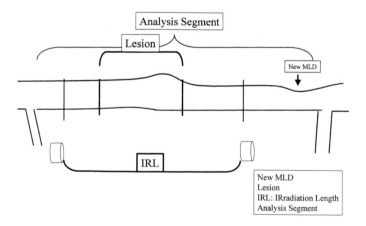

Figure 7. QCA analysis: follow-up. Schematic representation of the coronary artery at follow-up with the projection of the irradiation length. Note the displacement of the MLD: new MLD and the positive remodeling at the lesion site.

Case Examples

Two examples with baseline and follow-up QCA are illustrated in Figures 8 to 14 with evidence of MLD displacement and positive remodeling, the trademark of vascular brachytherapy.

Figure 15 depicts four different ways in which GM of radiation to the vessel injury length may occur. The first example describes a long balloon injury that extends to the "border" of the IRL. In this case, although the radiation covers the vessel injury length created by the balloon injury, there is no extension of radiation beyond the edge of the vessel injury. This situation, also termed "edge effect," is defined as a subset of GM where the proximal and distal ends of the vessel injury length receive less than the prescribed dose.

The second example highlights a "proximal" GM scenario. In this instance,

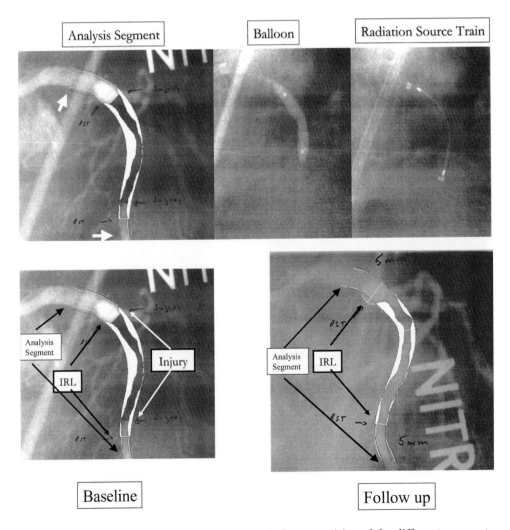

Figures 8 and 9. Authentic QCA analyses with the recognition of the different segments at baseline and at follow-up.

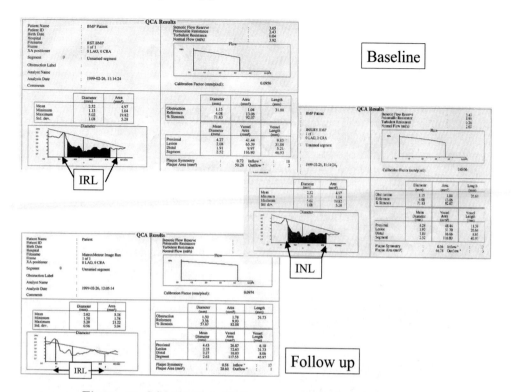

Figure 10. QCA results with the coronary measurement system.

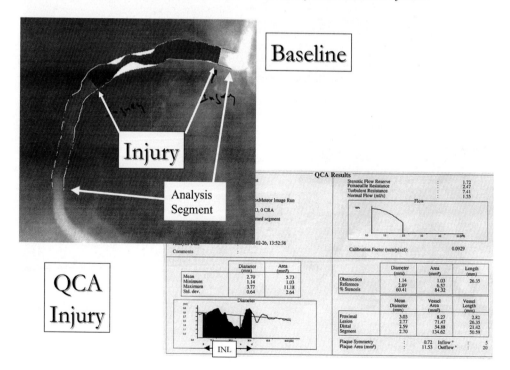

Figures 11, 12, 13, and 14. Authentic QCA analyses of the baseline and follow-up angiogram of a lesion treated on the right coronary artery.

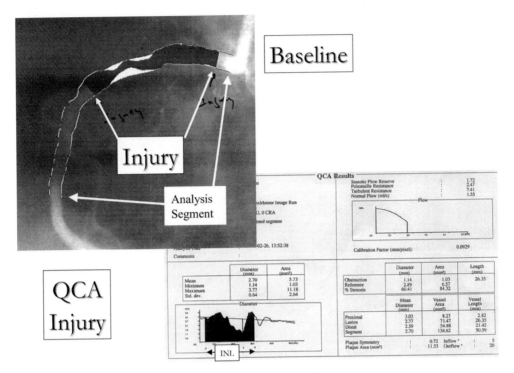

Figure 12 (continued).

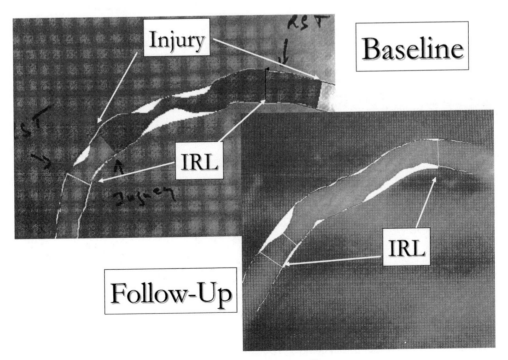

Figure 13 (continued).

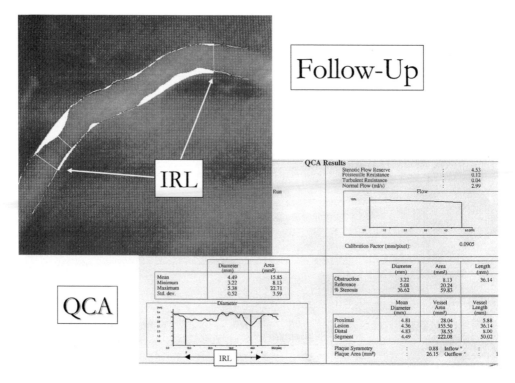

Figure 14 (continued).

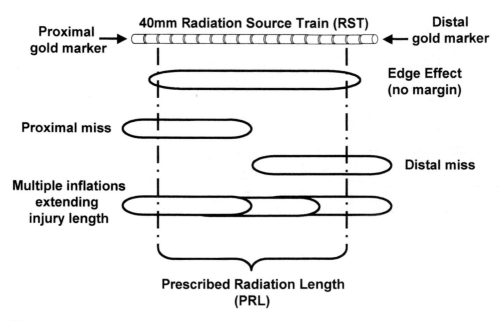

Figure 15. Schematic representation of the different possibilities of geographic miss (GM) of radiation to the vessel injury length. The edge effect is a GM.

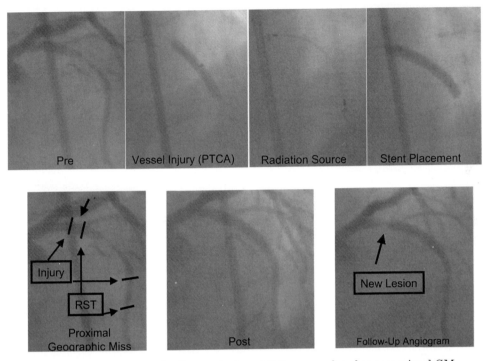

Figure 16. Case example of a new lesion at follow-up related to a proximal GM.

the radiation source is positioned beyond the proximal border of the vessel injury created by the balloon inflation, leaving the proximal zone of vessel injury unexposed to radiation treatment. This unexposed zone will clearly not benefit from the therapeutic effects of radiation. The third example demonstrates a similar situation, "distal" GM. This occurs when the radiation source is positioned short of the distal border of the vessel injury. The final example depicts a long vessel injury created by multiple inflations of the balloon, creating an extended vessel INL that is significantly longer than the effective radiation length (ERL). The result is that both the proximal and distal vessel injuries are left unexposed to the prescribed radiation dose.

A case example of proximal GM is shown in Figure 16. A lesion in the mid left anterior descending coronary artery underwent PTCA, followed by vascular brachytherapy. After radiation therapy, a stent was deployed. The proximal portion of the stent is noted to be proximal to the border of the ERL. Upon follow-up angiogram, a new lesion was found in the area of proximal vessel injury uncovered by radiation.

What is the clinical effect of GM? Although this has not been studied, it is hypothesized that, if GM occurs, the vessel injury will become restenotic at least at the same rate as if no radiation was applied (historical restenosis rates). Thus, the effectiveness of vascular brachytherapy in restenosis prevention may be influenced by the extent of GM. Table 1 describes the contribution of GM to the overall restenosis rate. This analysis concludes that, if 30% of vascular brachytherapy procedures have GM, this may contribute 10 percentage points to the restenosis

Table 1

Geographic Miss and Restenosis Rate

Total patients in trial	100
Geographic miss @ 30%	30 patients
Restenosis patients in "geographic miss" cohort @ 33% restenosis rate	10 patients
% Restenosis rate due to geographic miss	10%

Geographic miss may contribute to an increase in the restenosis rate by as much as 10%

rate outcome. It should be noted that vascular brachytherapy trial analyses suggest that a 30% GM rate may be a conservative estimate.

Conclusion

Geographic miss has emerged as a contributing factor that may have an impact on the clinical results with vascular brachytherapy. However, it can be eliminated through education, training, and awareness of:

1. Meticulous documentation of injury length (recording each step of the intervention);
2. Proper radiation source positioning; and
3. Availability of appropriate length radiation delivery devices (Table 2).

The successful mastery and application of vascular brachytherapy will be achieved by increased awareness of GM (Table 3). Radiation can work efficiently

Table 2

Training and Proper Recording to Prevent Geographic Miss and Edge Effect

- Record every interventional step to adequately assess injury area and proper radiation placement.
- Maintain an adequate margin of radiation coverage on both ends of injury area (>5 mm).
- Use "freeze frame/roadmapping" to assist with proper radiation source train placement.

Table 3

Evaluating the Results of Vascular Brachytherapy: Where Does the Minimum Lumen Diameter Appear on Follow-Up?

		Within the Injury Length (INL)?	
		Yes	**No**
Within the Prescribed Dose Length (PDL)?	**Yes**	Radiation Failed	? Radiation Related
	No	Geographic miss	Disease progression

only if the "injured area" is generously covered, necessitating exact determination of both injury and radiation margins. Elimination of GM is an important step toward optimization of the clinical outcomes with this new and exciting interventional technology.

References

1. Faxon DP, Coats W, Currier J. Remodeling of the coronary artery after vascular injury. Prog Cardiovasc Dis 1997;40:129–140.
2. Forrester JS, Fishbein M, Helfant R, et al. A paradigm for restenosis based on cell biology: Clues for the development of new preventive therapies. J Am Coll Cardiol 1991; 17:758–769.
3. Currier JW, Haudenschild C, Faxon DP. Pathophysiology of restenosis: Clinical implications. In: Ischinger T, Gohlke H, (eds.): Strategies in Primary and Secondary Prevention of Coronary Artery Disease. Berri, Germany: W. Zuckschwerdt Verlag; 1992: 182–187.
4. Mintz GS, Popma JJ, Pichard AD, et al. Arterial remodeling after coronary angioplasty: A serial intravascular ultrasound study. Circulation 1996;94:35–43.
5. Côté G, Tardif J-C, Lespérance J, et al. Effects of probucol on vascular remodeling and after coronary angioplasty. Circulation 1999;99:30–35.
6. Fischman DL, Leon MB, Baim DS, et al. A randomized comparison of coronary-stent placement and balloon angioplasty in the treatment of coronary artery disease. Stent Restenosis Study Investigators. N Engl J Med 1994;331:496–501.
7. Serruys PW, de Jaegere P, Kiemeneij F, et al. A comparison of balloon expandable-stent implantation with balloon angioplasty in patients with coronary artery disease. Benestent Study Group. N Engl J Med 1994;331:489–495.
8. Coventry MB, Scanlon PW. The use of radiation to discourage ectopic bone: A nine-year study in surgery about the hip. J Bone Joint Surg Am 1981;63:201–208.
9. Chaudry MR, Akhtar S, Duvalsaint F, et al. Ear love keloids, surgical excision followed by radiation therapy: A 10-year experience. Ear Nose Throat J 1994;73:779–781.
10. Kovalic JJ, Perez CA. Radiation therapy following keloidectomy: A 20-year experience. Int J Radiat Oncol Biol Phys 1989;17:77–80.
11. Waksman R, Robinson KA, Crocker IR, et al. Endovascular low-dose irradiation inhibits neointima formation after coronary artery balloon injury in swine. Circulation 1995;91:1533–1539.
12. Carter AJ, Laird JR, Bailey LR, et al. Effects of endovascular radiation from a beta particle emitting stent in a porcine coronary restenosis model. Circulation 1996;94: 2364–2368.
13. Laird JR, Carter AJ, Kufs WM, et al. Inhibition of neointimal proliferation with low-dose irradiation from a beta particle emitting stent. Circulation 1996;93:529–536.
14. Hehrlein C, Gollan C, Donges K, et al. Low-dose radioactive endovascular stents prevent smooth muscle cell proliferation and neointimal hyperplasia in rabbits. Circulation 1995;92:1570–1575.
15. Waksman R, Robinson KA, Crocker IR, et al. Intracoronary low-dose beta-irradiation inhibits neointima formation after coronary artery balloon injury in the swine restenosis model. Circulation 1995;92:3025–3031.
16. Verin V, Popowski Y, Belenger J, et al. Intra-arterial beta irradiation prevents neointimal hyperplasia in a hypercholesterolemic rabbit restenosis model. Circulation 1995;92:2284–2290.
17. Weiderman JG, Marboe CH, Amols H, et al. Intracoronary irradiation markedly reduces restenosis after balloon angioplasty in a porcine model. J Am Coll Cardiol 1994; 23:1491–1498.
18. Weiderman JG, Leavy JA, Amols H, et al. Effects of high dose intracoronary irradiation on vasomotor function and smooth muscle histopathology. Am J Physiol 1994;36: H125–H132.
19. Schopohl B, Liermann D, Pohlit LJ. [192]Ir endovascular radiation brachytherapy for avoidance of intimal hyperplasia after percutaneous transluminal angioplasty and

stent implantation in peripheral vellels: 6 years of experience. Int J Radiat Oncol Biol Phys 1996;36:835–840.

20. Teirstein PS, Massullo V, Jani S, et al. Catheter-based radiotherapy to inhibit restenosis after coronary stenting. N Engl J Med 1997;336:1697–1703.

21. Waksman R, White LR, Chan RC, et al. Intracoronary radiation therapy for patients with in-stent restenosis: 6 month follow of a randomized clinical trial [abstract]. Circulation 1998;98(suppl 1):I–651.

22. King SB III, Williams DO, Chougule P, et al. Endovascular beta radiation to reduce restenosis after coronary balloon angioplasty: Results of the Beta Energy Restenosis Trial (BERT). Circulation 1998;97:2025–2030.

23. Meerkin D, Bonan R, Crocker IR, et al. Efficacy of beta radiation inprevention of post-angioplasty restenosis: An interim report from the Beta Energy Restenosis Trial. Herz 1998;23:356–361.

24. Bonan, R. Radiation delivery and clinical effectiveness. In: Vascular Brachytherapy: State of the Art. London, UK: Remedica Publishing; 1999:4.

25. Kim RY, McGinnis LS, Spencer SA, et al. Conventional four-field pelvic radiotherapy technique without computed tomography–treatment planning in cancer of the cervix: potential geographic miss and its impact on pelvic control. Int J Radiat Oncol Biol Phys 1995;31:109–112.

26. Vijayakumar S, Low N, Chen GT, et al. Beams eye view-based photon radiotherapy I (comment). Int J Radiat Oncol Biol Phys 1992;22:1163–1164.

27. Fryer CJ. Advances in pediatric radiotherapy in the last ten years and future proposals. Cancer 1986;58(suppl):554–560.

28. Sedlmayer F, Rahim HB, Kogelnik HD, et al. Quality assurance in breast cancer brachytherapy: Geographic miss in the interstitial boost treatment of the tumor bed. Int J Radiat Oncol Biol Phys 1996;34:1133–1139.

29. Wilcox JN, Crocker IR, Scott NA, et al. Mechanisms by which radiation may prevent restenosis: Inhibition of cell proliferation and vascular remodeling. In: Waksman R (ed.): Vascular Brachytherapy, 2nd Edition. Armonk, New York: Futura Publishing Company; 1999:127–138.

Part VIII

Endovascular Radiation Clinical Trials in Coronary Arteries

Clinical Trials of Vascular Brachytherapy for In-Stent Restenosis: Update

Andrew E. Ajani, MD, Han-Soo Kim, MD,
and Ron Waksman, MD

Introduction

Coronary stents reduce angiographic and clinical restenosis compared to conventional balloon angioplasty in patients treated with percutaneous coronary interventions.[1,2] The rate of in-stent restenosis, although less frequent than post-angioplasty restenosis, is becoming increasingly prevalent due to the recent exponential increase in the use of intracoronary stents.

Annually, there are about 450,000 coronary angioplasties performed on de novo and restenotic lesions in the U.S. alone.[3] Approximately 70 to 80% of the patients who undergo angioplasty receive stents in an effort to reduce restenosis. Despite stent placement, 15 to 35% of these patients still develop restenosis, usually within 6 to 9 months after the procedure.[3] Although treatment of in-stent restenosis with conventional therapy is simple, the longevity of patent artery is short. Angiographic recurrences of in-stent restenosis are between 50 and 85% depending on the characteristics of the lesion, but are not influenced by the device.[4–8] Treatment of in-stent restenosis with balloon angioplasty results in high recurrence rates of greater than 50%. Ablative devices and techniques such as laser angioplasty and rotational atherectomy were successful in reducing the tissue volume, but did not alter the recurrence rate or the clinical course in these patients.[7,8] Additional stenting or re-stenting provides a larger and cleaner lumen immediately after the procedure, but with more exuberant tissue accumulation and with a higher recurrence rate at 6 months.[9]

Vascular brachytherapy is a promising technology with the potential to reduce the restenosis rate. Clinical trials to evaluate the effectiveness and safety of this technology are still ongoing with nearly 4000 patients enrolled in these trials. Some of these studies have recently reached 3-year clinical and angiographic follow-up. The 3-year follow-up data along with new data from larger trials demonstrate different levels of efficacy and raise questions regarding dosimetry perfection and its impact on related complications, such as edge effect, late thrombosis, and late restenosis.

From Waksman R (ed.). *Vascular Brachytherapy, Third Edition.* Armonk, NY: Futura Publishing Co., Inc.; © 2002.

Despite the differences in trial designs, more recent trials have focused on examining the use of vascular brachytherapy in preventing the recurrence of in-stent restenosis. Questions still remain, however, regarding whether beta emitters will be as effective as gamma emitters and whether centering delivery systems perform better than noncentering systems.

This chapter will provide an update of the current status of clinical trials utilizing vascular brachytherapy to prevent the recurrence of in-stent restenosis.

Gamma Radiation for In-Stent Restenosis

The only gamma emitter used in clinical trials for in-stent restenosis is ^{192}Ir. The efficacy of ^{192}Ir in reducing clinical and angiographic restenosis in patients with in-stent restenosis has been confirmed by a number of studies, including two single-center trials, SCRIPPS and WRIST, a multicenter trial, GAMMA-1, and a registry, GAMMA-2 (Table 1). All of these trials were performed using a manual delivery system with a noncentering catheter and either intravascular ultrasound (IVUS)-based or fixed depth dosimetry.

SCRIPPS (Scripps Coronary Radiation to Inhibit Proliferation Post Stenting) is the first randomized trial of the safety and efficacy of intracoronary gamma radiation given as adjunctive therapy to stents. In this study, 26 of 54 patients were randomized to receive ^{192}Ir (8 to 30 Gy, dosimetry guided by IVUS) utilizing a ribbon (19 to 35 mm) delivered in a noncentered, closed-end lumen catheter at the treatment site (dwell time, 20 to 45 min). Only 35 patients in this cohort were patients with in-stent restenosis. This study demonstrated that at 6-months the angiographic restenosis rate was reduced with radiation (17% versus 54%, $P<0.01$). At 3 years, these results remained consistent (33% versus 64.3%, respectively). Subanalysis of the lumen diameter for patients who did not have intervention demonstrated minimal reduction of the minimal lumen diameter (MLD) of the irradiated segments versus control at 3 years. There were no evident clinical complications resulting from the radiation treatment, and clinical benefits were maintained at 3 years with a significant reduction in the need for target lesion revascularization ($P=0.004$). A subgroup analysis for the 35 patients with in-stent restenosis has shown a 70% reduction of the recurrence rate in the irradiated group versus the placebo group.[9,10]

WRIST (Washington Radiation for In-Stent Restenosis Trial) is a series of studies that were designed to evaluate the effectiveness of radiation therapy for in-stent restenosis.[11] The gamma radiation in these studies is composed of ribbon with different trains of radioactive (^{192}Ir) seeds, which is inserted manually into a closed-end lumen catheter. In the initial study, 130 patients (100 patients with native coronaries and 30 patients with vein grafts) with in-stent restenosis lesions (up to 47 mm in length) were blindly randomized to treatment with either placebo or 15 Gy of ^{192}Ir at 2 mm from the source of the vessel wall. At 6 months, clinical and angiographic follow-up showed a dramatic reduction of the restenosis rate between the irradiated group and the control group, 19% versus 58%, respectively ($P=0.0001$). There was a 79% reduction in the need for revascularization and a 63% reduction in major adverse cardiac events ([MACE] ie, death, Q-wave myocardial infarction, or target vessel revascularization) in the irradiated group compared to control. IVUS subanalysis demonstrated that 53% of lesions from the irradiated group had increased luminal dimensions and regression of neointimal

Table 1

Clinical Trials for In-stent Restenosis Using Catheter-Based Systems with Gamma Radiation

Study Name	Design	Radiation System	Dose (Gy)	Results and Status
SCRIPPS	Single center, double-blind, randomized in 55 patients with restenosis.	Hand-delivered 0.030" nylon ribbon with seeds (Best Medical) into a noncentered closed-end lumen 4.5 F catheter (Navius).	≥8–<30 to media by IVUS	Completed. Showed reduction of restenosis in the irradiated group maintained at 3 years.
WRIST	Single center, double-blind, randomized in 130 patients with in-stent restenosis (100 natives, 30 vein grafts).	Hand-delivered 0.030" nylon ribbon with ^{192}Ir seeds (Best Medical) into a noncentered closed-end lumen 5.0 F catheter (Medtronic).	15 at 2.0 mm for vessels 3–4 mm. 18 for vessels >4mm	Completed. Showed reduction in restenosis (67%) and re-vascularization (63%). At 2 years, reduction in TLR and TVR <40%.
LONG WRIST	Two center, double-blind, randomized in 120 patients with in-stent restenosis lesions (36–80 mm).	Hand-delivered 0.030" nylon ribbon with seeds (Best Medical) into a noncentered closed-end lumen 5.0 F catheter (Medtronic).	15 at 2.0 mm for vessels 3–4 mm	Completed. At 6 months, restenosis rates were lower in irradiated group vs. control (32% vs. 71%, respectively).
LONG WRIST HD	Single center, registry in 120 patients with in-stent restenosis lesions (36–80 mm).	Hand-delivered 0.030" nylon ribbon with seeds (Best Medical) into a noncentered closed-end lumen 5.0 F catheter (Medtronic).	18 at 20 mm for vessels 3–4 mm	Enrollment completed. Initial results in 60 patients demonstrated further reduction of the restenosis rate compared to 15 Gy.
SVG WRIST	Multicenter, double-blind, randomized in 120 patients with in-stent restenosis.	Hand-delivered 0.030" nylon ribbon with seeds (Best Medical) into a noncentered closed-end lumen 5.0 F catheter (Medtronic).	15 at 2 mm for vessels <4.0 mm	Completed. At 6 months, irradiated patients had reduced restenosis (15% vs. 43%, $P=0.004$) and MACE (20% vs. 55%, $P<0.05$)
GAMMA-1	Multicenter, randomized double-blind study in 252 patients with in-stent restenosis.	Hand-delivered 0.030" nylon ribbon with seeds (Best Medical) into a noncentered closed-end lumen 4.0 F catheter (Cordis).	≥8–<30 to media by IVUS	Completed. Patients with radiation therapy had significant reduction of restenosis rate (22% vs. 52%), and clinical TLR at 9 months.

Table 1 (continued)

Clinical Trials for In-stent Restenosis Using Catheter-Based Systems with Gamma Radiation

Study Name	Design	Radiation System	Dose (Gy)	Results and Status
GAMMA-2	Multicenter, registry in 125 patients with in-stent restenosis.	Hand-delivered 0.030" nylon ribbon with seeds (Best Medical) into a noncentered closed-end lumen 4.0 F catheter (Cordis)	14 at 2 mm from the source	Completed. Similar to Gamma-1. MACE was reduced by 36% and TLR was reduced by 48% as compared to placebo.
ARTISTIC	Multicenter, double-blind, randomized in 110 patients with in-stent restenosis.	Mechanical delivery of 0.014" fixed wire 30 mm (Angiorad) into a monorail closed-end lumen with small balloon 3.2 F catheter.	12–15–18 at 2.0 mm from the source	Feasibility phase completed, with low restenosis rate. Pivotal study commenced.
PLAVIX WRIST	Registry of 120 patients with in-stent restenosis with 6 months of Plavix 75 mg/QD.	Hand-delivered 0.030" nylon ribbon with ^{192}Ir seeds into a noncentered closed-end lumen 4.0 F catheter (Cordis).	14 at 2mm distance from the source	Completed. Angiography at 6 months shows significant reduction of late total occlusion with 6 months of Plavix.
CURE	Registry of 120 patients with in-stent restenosis not considered good candidates for CABG or medical therapy.	Hand-delivered 0.030" nylon ribbon with ^{192}Ir seeds into closed-end lumen 4.0 F catheter (Cordis).	14 at 2mm from the source	Enrollment extended. Clinical follow-up available for initial 120 patients; 31% TVR and 33% MACE at 6 months.

SCRIPPS 2	Single center randomized study for patients with diffuse in-stent restenosis.	Hand delivered 0.030" nylon ribbon with Ir–192 seeds into a noncentered closed-end lumen 4.0F catheter (Cordis)	$\geq 8-<30$ to media by IVUS	Enrollment completed. Follow up will be available in the fall of 2000
SCRIPPS 3	Registry of 320 patients with in-stent restenosis with 6 months of Plavix.	Hand-delivered 0.030" nylon ribbon with ^{192}Ir seeds into a noncentered closed-end lumen 4.0 F catheter (Cordis).	14 at 2mm distance from the source	Enrollment completed. Clinical follow-up only available in 2001.
WRIST 12	Registry of 120 patients with in-stent restenosis with 12 months of Plavix and 15 months angiographic study.	Hand-delivered 0.030" nylon ribbon with ^{192}Ir seeds into a noncentered closed-end lumen 4.0F catheter (Cordis).	14 at 2mm distance from the source	Enrollment completed. Results available early 2002.
GAMMA-5	Multicenter registry in 600 patients with 12 months Plavix for new stent and 6 months for no new stent.	Hand-delivered 0.030" nylon ribbon with seeds (Best Medical) into a noncentered closed-end lumen 4.0 F catheter (Cordis).	14 at 2 mm from the source	Study initiated in the summer of 2000.
EDGE WRIST	Registry of 120 patients with in-stent restenosis with longer treatment margins.	Hand-delivered 0.030" nylon ribbon with ^{192}Ir seeds into closed-end lumen 4.0 F catheter (Cordis).	14 at 2mm from the source	Study initiated in the fall of 2000.
Integrilin WRIST	Randomized 300 patient trial: Radiation for in-stent restenosis $\pm$ Integrilin	Hand-delivered 0.030" nylon ribbon with ^{192}Ir seeds into closed-end lumen 4.0 F catheter (Cordis).	14 at 2mm from the source	Study initiated in 2000. Preliminary results available early 2002.

tissue at 6 months. At 1 year, the irradiated group had a 48% reduction in MACE compared to placebo. The WRIST Study is considered to be a landmark in establishing gamma radiation for the treatment of in-stent restenosis.

LONG WRIST is a randomized trial involving 120 symptomatic patients with diffuse in-stent restenotic lesions of 36 to 80 mm (mean stent length, 70 mm) who received either a ribbon bearing ^{192}Ir seeds or placebo seeds delivered to the target site via a noncentered, closed-lumen catheter. The radiation dose consisted of 14 to 15 Gy at a 2-mm distance from the center of the source. Quantitative coronary angiography at 6 months disclosed rates of restenosis within the stented segment of 32% in the irradiated group and 71% in the control group ($P=0.0002$). The rates of restenosis considering only the segment containing the lesion were 46% and 78%, respectively ($P=0.03$). The 6-month rates of MACE (death, nonfatal Q-wave or non-Q-wave myocardial infarction, target lesion revascularization) were 38.3% and 61.7%, respectively ($P=0.01$), with most of the significant difference accounted for by the target legion revascularization component, the rates for which were 30% and 60%, respectively ($P=0.001$). The combined rate of total target vessel occlusion or late thrombosis at any time during the follow-up was 15% of irradiated patients and 6.7% of controls.

LONG WRIST high dose is a registry of 60 patients with similar entry criteria to LONG WRIST. In comparison to LONG WRIST, a higher radiation dose was prescribed with 18 Gy delivered at a 2-mm distance from the center of the source. Baseline clinical and angiographic details were similar in both study groups. At 6-month follow-up, MACE (death, Q-wave myocardial infarction, or target vessel revascularization) were reduced by 39% in the high-dose group (23% versus 38%, $P=0.11$) compared to LONG WRIST. IVUS analysis of the high-dose group (18 Gy) showed increased minimal luminal area (4.0 versus 2.9 mm^2, $P<0.001$) and reduced change in intimal hyperplasia area (0.4 versus 2.4 mm^2, $P<0.001$) compared to LONG WRIST (15 Gy). A trend toward reduced in-stent late loss with quantitative coronary angiography (QCA) was also evident with the higher radiation dose (0.32 versus 0.65 mm, $P=0.054$). Diffuse lesions may require higher radiation doses to maintain the efficacy seen in focal lesions and minimize recurrent clinical events at 6 months.

The Washington Radiation for In-Stent Restenosis Trial for Saphenous Vein Grafts (SVG WRIST) is an FDA-approved double-blinded multicenter randomized trial in patients post coronary bypass surgery with diffuse in-stent restenosis in their saphenous vein grafts (SVG). SVG WRIST is the first study to examine the effects of gamma radiation therapy on patients with in-stent restenosis in bypass grafts. One hundred and twenty patients with diffuse in-stent restenosis in SVG underwent PTCA, laser ablation or rotational atherectomy, and/or additional stents. After the intervention, a noncentered closed-end lumen catheter was positioned at the treated site, and patients were randomly assigned to a ribbon either with ^{192}Ir or with nonradioactive seeds, both delivered by hand. Different ribbon lengths of 6, 10, and 14 seeds with a mean radiation length of 34 ± 22 mm were used to cover lesions less than 47 mm in length. The prescribed radiation doses were 14 or 15 Gy to a 2-mm radial distance from the center of the source for vessels with a diameter of 4 mm, and 15 Gy at 2.4 mm for vessels greater than 4 mm in diameter. The patients with restenosis at follow-up were eligible to receive radiation if they were initially randomized to placebo. The closed-end lumen catheter with either the active or the placebo seeds was delivered successfully to all patients. A mean dwell time of 21.1±4.8 minutes was well tolerated in irradiated patients. At 30 days, there were no adverse events related to the radiation therapy. At 6 months, the restenosis rate was significantly lower in the irradiated group compared to control (15% versus 43%, $P=0.004$). The need for repeat intervention at the treatment site was significantly reduced by 79% in the irradiated group compared to control (10% versus 48%, $P<0.001$), and the overall MACE were reduced in the irradiated group (20% versus 55%, $P<0.001$). The rate of late thrombosis in the irradiated group was 1.7% versus 6.7% in the control ($P=NS$), and there was no excess of edge effect in the irradiated group when compared to the control. Conventional treatment of in-stent restenosis in bypass grafts is associated with a high recurrence rate. The SVG WRIST Study demonstrated that catheter-based gamma radiation therapy for in-stent restenosis in bypass grafts is safe and effective in reducing the overall restenosis rate and the need for repeat revascularization.

PLAVIX WRIST is a registry of 120 patients with similar inclusion and exclusion criteria to the WRIST protocol, but with 6 months of clopidogrel 75 mg QD, to evaluate whether prolonged antiplatelet therapy results in a reduction of late thrombotic event rates.[12] The rate of target lesion revascularization was 21%, target vessel revascularization 23%, and cumulative MACE 23%, at 6 months. Eight patients (5.8%) had late total occlusion at 6-month follow-up, of which 3 patients (2.5%) developed late thrombosis. When the PLAVIX WRIST group was compared to irradiated patients in WRIST and LONG WRIST (1-month antiplatelet treatment), the strategy of prolonged antiplatelet therapy appears to reduce rates of thrombosis (2.5% versus 9.6%, $P=0.02$) to levels seen in nonirradiated controls. In 78 patients who stopped Plavix at 6 months with a mean follow-up of 90.4 days (range, 6 to 191 days) beyond this period, 2 patients (2.6%) had late total occlusions and myocardial infarction with an overall MACE rate of 6.4%. No events have been reported to date in 29 patients who continued taking Plavix. The optimal duration of Plavix therapy to prevent late total occlusion beyond 6 months is still unknown.

CURE (Compassionate Use Radiation Endovascular) WRIST is an FDA-approved open label registry in 120 patients with in-stent restenosis who had at least two episodes at the target lesion and are not considered good candidates for coronary bypass surgery or medical therapy. Patients with previous intracoronary stent implantation in native coronary arteries and saphenous vein grafts with vessel diameters between 2.5 to 5.0 mm and lesion length less than 80 mm were considered eligible after successful percutaneous transluminal coronary angiography (PTCA), atheroablation (laser or rotational atherectomy), or re-stenting (<30% residual stenosis). At 6 months, the rates of death (3.3%), Q-wave myocardial infarction (1.7%), target vessel revascularization (31%) and MACE (33%) in this high-risk population were similar to other radiation series. In 33 patients, two vessels were treated with gamma radiation, which appeared feasible and safe. Treatment of saphenous vein graft disease had comparable clinical benefit to native vessels with MACE rates at 6 months of 41% versus 30% ($P=0.25$).

GAMMA-1 is a multicenter, randomized, double-blind trial studying the effects of hand-delivered ^{192}Ir ribbon using IVUS to guide dosimetry (dose range, 8 to 30 Gy) in 252 patients with in-stent restenosis. Six-month angiographic results revealed significant reductions in the in-stent (21.6% versus 52%) and in-lesion

(33% versus 56%, $P=0.006$) angiographic restenosis rates of the radiation arm versus control (21.6% versus 52%). Subanalysis for lesion length demonstrated a 70% reduction in the angiographic restenosis rate for lesions less than 30 mm in length versus 48% for 30- to 45-mm lesions.[13] In addition, edge effect was noted in patients who did not have enough coverage of the lesion by the radioactive seeds. Clinical events demonstrated a reduction in the target legion revascularization rate from 42 to 24%. However, the rate of death (3% versus 0.8%) and the rate of acute myocardial infarction (12% versus 6%) were higher in the irradiated group versus control. These complications were related in part to the late thrombosis phenomenon.

GAMMA-2 is a registry of 125 patients who were treated for the same inclusion/exclusion criteria as GAMMA-1 but with a fixed dosimetry of 14 Gy at 2 mm from the center of the source. The treated lesions in Gamma-2 were more heavily calcified, whereby 45% of patients required rotablation in contrast to 26% of patients in GAMMA-1. Despite the differences in lesions, the results between GAMMA-1 and -2 were remarkably similar. Both studies had similar and infrequent in-hospital adverse clinical events (2%). GAMMA-2 patients had a lower post-procedural MLD; perhaps due to increased lesion complexity and the fact that fewer stents were placed in GAMMA-2 patients, as compared to GAMMA-1. Similar to GAMMA-1, there was a 52% in-stent and a 40% in-lesion reduction in restenosis frequency. Target legion revascularization was reduced by 48% and MACE was reduced by 36%. The late thrombosis rate was 4.0% at 270 days with only 8 weeks of antiplatelet therapy. It is believed that prolonged antiplatelet therapy will remedy the incidence of late thrombosis.

ARTISTIC (Angiorad Radiation Technology for In-Stent Restenosis Trial in Native Coronaries) is a blinded, randomized trial examining the benefits of using a flexible, 30-mm ^{192}Ir wire source in 300 patients with in-stent restenosis in native coronary arteries. The pilot phase of this study was recently completed and involved 26 patients at two centers, all of whom received radiation treatment. Inclusion criteria consisted of lesions less than 25 mm in length with a reference vessel diameter between 2.5 and 5.0 mm and a degree of stenosis between 50 and 99%. Radiation was successfully delivered to 25 of 26 patients. At 6-month angiographic follow-up, low binary restenosis rates of 14% were reported with a late loss index of 0.12, and a 15% rate of MACE.[14] A randomized study using the same system was halted after enrolling 110 patients. Preliminary results of this study demonstrated significant reduction in the angiographic restenosis rate in the irradiated arm. A pivotal trial with the Angiorad system is in progress.

New gamma studies for in-stent restenosis that have been initiated but have yet to be completed are SCRIPPS III, WRIST 12, and GAMMA-5. These studies are designed to address the issue of prolonged antiplatelet therapy and prevention of late thrombosis. Preliminary analysis of SCRIPPS III suggests no late thrombosis in 500 patients with 6 months of Plavix therapy after radiation. The preliminary results of WRIST 12 will be available in early 2002.

EDGE WRIST is a single center study that is designed to address the question of whether large margins from the injured segment will reduce the edge effect phenomenon. Integrilin WRIST is also a single center study and aims to assess the impact of glycoprotein IIBIIIA antagonists (integrilin) as adjunctive therapy to radiation for in-stent restenosis.

Beta Radiation for In-Stent Restenosis

With the encouraging results from the gamma trials for the treatment of patients with in-stent restenosis, studies have been initiated to test the effectiveness of beta radiation for the same indication. Initial clinical trials using beta emitters were designed to examine the effectiveness of beta radiation therapy for the prevention of restenosis in de novo lesions in native coronaries. Among these were the Geneva Trial[15] and the Dose-Finding Study which have used ^{90}Y, BERT (Beta Energy Restenosis Trial),[15] BRIE (Beta Radiation in Europe) and Beta-Cath which all used [90]S/Y, and the PREVENT (Proliferation REeduction with Vascular ENergy Trial)[16] and BETTER Trials which have used [32]P.

BETA WRIST was the first study to examine the efficacy of beta radiation for prevention of in-stent restenosis (Table 2). This registry included 50 patients who underwent treatment for in-stent restenosis in native coronaries and were treated with beta radiation using the ^{90}Y source, centering catheter, and an afterloader system. The clinical outcomes of these patients were compared to the control group of the original cohort of WRIST (randomized to either placebo or ^{192}Ir). The reported angiographic restenosis rate at 6 months in BETA WRIST was 22% with late total occlusion in 12% of the patients. The use of beta radiation for the treatment of in-stent restenosis demonstrated 58% reduction in the need for target lesion revascularization and a 53% reduction in the need for target vessel revascularization at 6 months compared to the historical control group of WRIST. No major differences were detected when comparing the outcome of the irradiated beta group with the gamma group of WRIST.[18] This benefit has been maintained at 2-year follow-up with beta radiation reducing target lesion revascularization (42% versus 66%, $P=0.016$), target vessel revascularization (46% versus 72%, $P=0.009$), and the composite clinical endpoint of death, Q-wave myocardial infarction or target vessel revascularization (46% versus 72%, $P=0.008$), compared to placebo. The efficacy of beta and gamma emitters for the treatment of in-stent restenosis appears similar at longer term follow-up.

START (STents And Radiation Therapy) is pivotal multicenter randomized trial involving 485 patients in over 55 centers in the U.S. and Europe, designed to determine the efficacy and safety of the Beta-Cath system for the treatment of in-stent restenosis. Patients eligible for the START Trial included those with native artery lesions less than 20 mm in length. On average, patients enrolled in the study had 16-mm long lesions in arteries 2.8 mm in diameter. Following angioplasty, these patients were treated with the Beta-Cath system containing [90]S/Y seeds that deliver beta radiation through a closed-end lumen catheter following angioplasty. Patients were randomized to either placebo or an active radiation train 30 mm in length. Depending on the diameter of the target vessel, a dose of either 16 or 20 Gy was administered at 2 mm from the center of the source. The antiplatelet therapy in this study consisted of at least 3 months of clopidogrel 75 mg/QD. At 8 months, angiographic restenosis rates in the irradiated segments were 29% versus 45% in the placebo group ($P=0.001$). Target legion revascularization was 16% in the irradiated group, as compared to 22% in control ($P=0.008$). Rates for target vessel revascularization were also similar (16% and 24%, respectively). Additionally, patients treated with radiation had a considerably lower rate of MACE than those in the placebo group (18% versus 26%). Importantly, there

Table 2

Clinical Trials for In-stent Restenosis Using Catheter-Based Systems with Beta Radiation

Study Name	Design	Radiation System	Isotope and Dose (Gy)	Results and Status
BETA WRIST	Registry for 50 patients with in-stent restenosis.	Schneider System ^{90}Y source centering balloon and an afterloader.	Dose 20.6 at 1 mm from the balloon surface	Completed. Restenosis rate of 22% at 6 months; MACE 46% at 2 years. Similar results to the gamma WRIST group.
INHIBIT	Multicenter, double-blind randomized for patients with in-stent restenosis (332 patients).	Automatic afterloader (Nucletron) 0.018" 27-mm fixed wire via a helical centering balloon.	^{32}P, dose 20 Gy at 1 mm into vessel wall	Completed. Demonstrated reduction of 50% in restenosis (analysis segment) and 55% in MACE.
START	Multicenter randomized double-blind design for 476 in-stent restenosis lesions (20 mm).	Beta-Cath system 30-mm source train.	^{90}Sr/Y, 18–20 Gy at 2 mm	Completed. Showed reduction in TLR, TVR, and MACE (35%) in the irradiated group. No late thrombosis.
START 40/20	A registry of 250 patients with in-stent restenosis.	Beta-Cath system 40 mm source train.	^{90}Sr/Y, 18–20 Gy at 2 mm	Completed. Results available December 2000.
BRITE	Feasibility study in patients with in-stent.	The Radiance system with a deployable ^{32}P balloon.	^{32}P, 20 Gy at 1.0 mm from the balloon	Enrollment completed. Demonstrated safety at 30 days and lower restenosis rates at 6 months.
R4	Registry in 50 patients with in-stent restenosis in South Korea.	Liquid-filled balloon, 36 mm in length.	^{188}Re, 15 Gy at 1 mm into the vessel wall	Showed that 6-month angiographic restenosis rate was 10.4%.
GALILEO™ INHIBIT	International multicenter registry in 120 patients with in-stent restenosis.	Automatic afterloader (Guidant GALILEO system) via a helical centering balloon.	^{32}P, 20 Gy at 1 mm into vessel wall	Enrollment completed in 2001.

were no events of late thrombosis and none of the patients developed acute myocardial infarction. Similar to the findings of BETA WRIST, results from the START Trial indicate the safety and effectiveness of using beta emitters for vascular brachytherapy.

INHIBIT, a multicenter randomized study involving 332 patients in 29 U.S. and international sites, examined the efficacy of the GALILEO system for the treatment of in-stent restenosis. The GALILEO system uses a ^{32}P source with a dose of 20 Gy at a depth of 1 mm into the vessel wall. The study mandated at least 3 months of antiplatelet therapy and 307 patients completed 9 months of clinical follow-up. The radiation was delivered successfully in 315 of the patients and tolerated well in all but two patients. At 30 days, 11 patients had clinical events (2 deaths; 2, Q-wave myocardial infarction; 3, non-Q-wave myocardial infarction; 3, PTCA; and 1 misadministration of the radiation dose). There were no adverse effects related to the radiation procedure. At 9 months, treatment with ^{32}P reduced the primary angiographic endpoint of binary restenosis by 66% (P=0.0001) in the stented segment, and by 50% (P=0.0003) in the analysis segment. There were no differences in the edge effect rates between the active and the control-treated groups. The radiated patients had improved MLD (1.52 versus 1.38 mm, P=0.01) and reduced late loss (0.4 versus 0.6 mm, P<0.001). ^{32}P significantly reduced rates of target legion revascularization (11% versus 29%, P<0.001) and MACE (14% versus 31%, P<0.001). Tandem positioning to cover diffuse lesions greater than 22 mm with 32P was feasible, safe, and effective. The results from INHIBIT demonstrate that beta radiation can be delivered safely and effectively to reduce the recurrence of restenosis following treatment of in-stent restenosis.

BRITE (Beta Radiation to Prevent In-sTent REstenosis) is a U.S. feasibility study to test the Radiance Radiation System which uses a balloon catheter encapsulating a ^{32}P radioactive sleeve for the treatment of in-stent restenosis. In the BRITE Trial, 30 patients were consented, 27 of whom were treated with PTCA (26 balloon, 1 rotoblator) for lesions less than 25 mm in length. Following intervention, the RDX catheter was successfully delivered in 26 of 27 attempts (one catheter did not reach the target location and was withdrawn after a 70-second attempt, delivering less than 1 Gy to adjacent tissue). The prescribed dose mean was 19.8±0.4 Gy at 1 mm from the inflated source surface and delivered in an average dwell time of 482±39 seconds. Seventy percent of the dose was administered when the balloon was inflated. The transit time was 8.5 seconds. None of the cases required interruption. The interventional procedure was predominately PTCA (24 of 27). All patients were prescribed 250 mg/QD ASA and 75 mg/QD clopidogrel for 3 months following the procedure. There were no procedural complications or MACE at 30-day clinical follow-up. It is anticipated that this pilot study will have low restenosis and revascularization rates. The randomized study with 500 patients was launched in late 2000.

R4 is a South Korean registry study to evaluate the feasibility and efficacy of beta radiation therapy with a ^{188}Re-MAG$_3$-filled balloon following rotational atherectomy for diffuse in-stent restenosis (length >10 mm). Fifty patients received the radiation dose of 15 Gy at 1.0 mm deep into the vessel wall. The radiation was delivered successfully to all patients, with a mean irradiation time of 201.8±61.7 seconds. No adverse events, including myocardial infarction, death, or stent thrombosis occurred during the follow-up period (mean 10.3±3.7

months), and nontarget vessel revascularization was needed in 1 patient. The 6-month binary angiographic restenosis rate was 10.4%.

Summary and Future Perspectives

Coronary radiation therapy trials using ^{192}Ir gamma source have demonstrated a significant reduction in clinical and angiographic restenosis in patients with in-stent restenosis. Trials using beta isotopes, such as ^{90}Sr/Y, ^{32}P, and ^{90}Y have also shown positive results for patients with in-stent restenosis. The positive results from these studies lead to the conclusion that beta emitters will be as effective as gamma emitters for the prevention of restenosis if the right dose is provided to the right target. Dosimetry still seems to play a major role in the success of the technology. Although not proven, head to head study of delivery systems with centering capability should allow researchers to determine a more homogenous dose to the target area.

Recently, two major complications have been identified in the clinical trials. The edge effect phenomenon, primarily seen with the radioactive stent, was also reported to occur with both beta and gamma catheter-based systems, especially when the treated area was not covered with wide enough margins.[19,20] Late thrombosis was reported in varying radiation trials with rates up to 10%. The phenomenon of late thrombosis was found to occur more with additional stent implantation, which is probably due to the delayed healing associated with radiation.[21,22] A potential solution to the late thrombosis phenomenon is prolonged antiplatelet therapy. The late thrombosis events were significantly reduced once prolonged antiplatelet therapy (3 months) was prescribed.[12] It is still unclear how long patients should be treated with antiplatelet therapy and whether patients who are undergoing additional stenting will require a longer course of treatment with antiplatelet therapy.

The encouraging results from the clinical trials are establishing vascular brachytherapy as a standard of care for patients with in-stent restenosis. Nevertheless, this technology requires further "fine-tuning" to achieve full optimization.

References

1. Fischman DL, Leon MB, Baim DS, et al. A randomized comparision of coronary stent placement and balloon angioplasty in the treatment of coronary artery disease. N Engl J Med 1994;331:496–501.
2. Serruys PW, de Jaegere P, Kiemeneij F, et al. A comparison of balloon-expandable-stent implantation with balloon angioplasty in patients with coronary artery disease. N Engl J Med 1994;331:489–495.
3. Casterella PJ, Teirstein PS. Prevention of coronary restensis. Cardiol Rev 1999;7:219–231.
4. Hoffmann R, Mintz GS, Dussailant GR, et al. Patterns and mechanisms of in-stent restenosis: A serial intravascular ultrasound study. Circulation 1996;94:1247–1254.
5. Baim DS, Levine MJ, Leon MB, et al. Management of restenosis within the Palmaz-Schatz coronary stent (the U.S. multicenter experience). Am J Cardiol 1993;71:364–366.
6. Reimers B, Moussa I, Akiyama T, et al. Long term clinical follow-up after successful repeat percutaneous intervention for stent stenosis. J Am Coll Cardiol 1997;30:186–192.
7. Goldberg SL, Shwal F, Buchbinder M, et al. Rotational atherectomy for in-stent restenosis: The BARASTER registry [abstract]. Circulation 1997;96(suppl I):I–80.

8. Mehran R, Mintz GW, Satler LF, et al. Treatment of in-stent restenosis with excimer laser coronary angioplasty: Mechanisms and results compared to PTCA alone. Circulation 1997;96:2183–2189.

9. Teirstein PS, Massullo V, Jani S, et al. Catheter-based radiotherapy to inhibit restenosis after coronary stenting. N Engl J Med 1997;336:1697–1703.

10. Teirstein PS, Massullo V, Jani S, et al. Two-year follow-up after catheter-based radiotherapy to inhibit coronary restenosis. Circulation 1999;99:243–247.

11. Waksman R, White RL, Chan RC, et al. Intracoronary radiation therapy after angioplasty inhibits recurrence in patients with in-stent restenosis. Circulation 2000;101:2165–2171.

12. Waksman R, Ajani AE, White RL, et al. Prolonged antiplatelet therapy to prevent late thrombosis after intracoronary gamma-radiation in patients with in-stent restenosis: Washington Radiation for In-Stent Restenosis Trial plus 6 months of clopidogrel (WRIST PLUS). Circulation 2001;103:2332–2335.

13. Leon MB, Teirstein PS, Lansky AJ, et al. Intracoronary gamma radiation to reduce in-stent restenosis: The multicenter GAMMA 1 randomized clinical trial. J Am Coll Cardiol 1999;33:56A.

14. Waksman R, Porrazzo MS, Chan RC, et al. Results from the ARTISTIC feasibility study of 192-iridium gamma radiation to prevent recurrence of in-stent restenosis. Circulation 1998;98:17, I–442:2327.

15. Verin V, Urban P, Popowski Y, et al. Feasibility of intracoronary beta-irradiation to reduce restenosis after balloon angioplasty: A clinical pilot study. Circulation 1997;95:1138–1144.

16. King SB III, Williams DO, Chougule P, et al. Endovascular beta-radiation to reduce restenosis after coronary balloon angioplasty: Results of the beta energy restenosis trial (BERT). Circulation 1998;97:2025–2030.

17. Raizner AE, Osterle SN, Waksman R, et al. Inhibition of restenosis with β-emitting radiotherapy report of the proliferation reduction with vascular energy trial (PREVENT). Circulation 2000;102:951–958.

18. Waksman R, White RL, Chan RC, et al. Intracoronary beta radiation therapy inhibits recurrence of in-stent restenosis. Circulation 2000;101:1895–1898.

19. Albiero R, Nishida T, Adamian M, et al. Edge restenosis after implantation of high activity (32)P radioactive beta-emitting stents. Circulation 2000;101:2454–2457.

20. Sabate M, Serruys PW, van der Giessen WJ, et al. Geometric vascular remodeling after balloon angioplasty and beta-radiation therapy: A three-dimensional intravascular ultrasound study. Circulation 1999;100:1182–1188.

21. Waksman R, Bhargava B, Mintz GS, et al. Late total occlusion after intracoronary brachytherapy for patients with in-stent restenosis. J Am Coll Cardiol 2000;36:65–68.

22. Costa MA, Sabat M, van der Giessen WJ, et al. Late coronary occlusion after intracoronary brachytherapy. Circulation 1999;100:789–792.

## Chapter 49

Intracoronary Gamma Radiation Following Balloon Angioplasty

The Venezuelan Experience

José A. Condado, MD, Ron Waksman, MD,
Orlando Gurdiel, MD, Harry Acquatella, MD,
Carlos Calderas, MD, Bogart Parra, MD,
Isabel Iturria, MD, and Jorge Saucedo, MD

Introduction

Despite dramatic improvements in equipment and the primary success of coronary angioplasty, restenosis after successful percutaneous transluminal coronary angioplasty (PTCA) remains the greatest challenge in interventional cardiology. A 30 to 60% restenosis rate is the major limitation to a full exploitation of revascularization procedures with the balloon and with other devices.[1]

Experimental and pathological studies have described restenosis as a healing response to vascular injury. Three fundamental mechanisms are thought to be involved in its development: elastic recoil, unfavorable remodeling, and a proliferative response to injury.[2-9]

The development of new recanalization procedures have widened the spectrum of vascular lesions that can be successfully treated, but has not reduced the restenosis rate. Only coronary stents, preventing early recoil and unfavorable remodeling have demonstrated a 30% reduction in the restenosis rate. However, stents may increase the proliferative response to injury.[10-12]

Ionizing radiation may affect cells mainly by damaging the nuclear structure of single and double strands of DNA. Its biological effects depend on the amount of energy delivered, which is a function of the distance to the source and the time of exposure.[13] It is well documented that ionizing radiation inhibits cell proliferation and formation of new tissue in certain clinical situations, including formation of keloids following surgery in the skin and reformation of pterygium following surgical removal.[14-19]

During the external radiation therapy for neoplastic disease, the blood vessels and the heart can suffer significant injury.[20-23] With experimental single radiation of 25 Gy, dogs may develop thrombosis and aneurysms in the aorta.[24] Increases in neointimal formation have been described after very low doses of external beam radiation were delivered to the atherosclerotic iliac arteries in rabbits.[25] External beam radiation delivered to the heart after stent implantation increased the restenosis rate in a porcine coronary model.[26]

The effective use of endovascular irradiation to prevent intimal proliferation in animal models of balloon arterial injury has been demonstrated in preclinical studies.[27–31] Endovascular irradiation with a high-energy gamma emitter (^{192}Ir), before or after overstrech balloon injury, significantly reduced neointimal formation when measured 2 to 4 weeks after injury.[28,29,31] This benefit was also seen with endovascular irradiation with a beta source using doses ranging from 14 to 25 Gy directed to the vessel wall,[30,32] and was sustained at 6-month follow-up.[33,34] Results of clinical studies with endovascular ^{192}Ir radiation in restenotic stented femoral arteries have indicated low restenosis rates in less than 6-year follow-up.[35,36] This study was designed to evaluate the feasibility and safety [38] as well as the middle- and long-term effects of human intracoronary gamma radiation therapy after coronary angioplasty.

According to standard protocols for evaluating restenosis, clinical and angiographic follow-up was performed at 6 months.[39,40] However, due to the potential effect of ionizing radiation on biological tissues that could manifest later in time, it was of invaluable interest to evaluate this group of patients as long as possible; thus clinical and angiographic follow-up was performed again after 2 and 3 years of the intracoronary radiation procedure.[41,42]

Methods

Between July 1994 and January 1995, intracoronary radiation therapy after PTCA was attempted in humans; all experimental protocols were approved by ethics and academic review boards of Miguel Perez Carreno and Centro Medico Hospital, Caracas, Venezuela. Informed consent was obtained in each case.

Patients and Lesion Characteristics

Patients suffering from symptomatic ischemic heart disease, the majority presenting with unstable angina (class II to IV) with at least one high-grade stenotic lesion in a native coronary artery that required PTCA, were included in the protocol. Twenty-one patients, 17 men and 4 women, with an average age of 52 years (34 to 73 years) were selected.

Twenty-two artery lesions were treated (1 patient had the procedure in both the left circumflex [LCX] artery and the right coronary artery [RCA]): 20 de novo lesions and 2 restenotic lesions (1 patient with PTCA restenosis and 1 patient with Palmaz-Schatz in-stent restenosis, both in the left anterior descending artery [LAD]); 11 in the LAD, 7 in the RCA, and 4 in the LCX. The majority of the lesions were type B (19 of 22; 86.4%), with 2 type A and 1 type C (total occlusion), according to the American Heart Association/American College of Cardiology (AHA/ACC) lesion classification.

Procedure

After analyzing the diagnostic angiograms, we performed all procedures with the use of an 8F guiding catheter system and a conventional balloon angioplasty technique (1 patient had rotational atherectomy ablation-PTCA technique). After the PTCA balloon was removed, the noncentered delivery catheter was inserted with the use of an angioplasty wire to fully cover the angioplasty site. To avoid extreme displacement of the source wire, we used a dummy wire following a nitroglycerin intracoronary bolus to check our ability to advance through narrow curves in the coronary arteries and to assure that the treatment segments to be irradiated did not show severely unfavorable conditions like tortuosities, narrow angulations, and spasm. The dummy wire was then removed, and the radioactive wire was positioned at the angioplasty site by both fluoroscopic control and distance measurement. After the radiation treatment, the radioactive wire was removed and placed in a shielded container. Intracoronary nitroglycerin was given and a final angiogram was taken immediately after the procedure. In the case of acute recoil, additional balloon angioplasty was performed. Control angiograms were performed after 24 hours. All patients were treated with heparin for 24 hours and discharged 48 to 72 hours after the procedure. After discharge, all patients were treated with aspirin and warfarin for a period of 3 months in order to reduce the risk of thrombosis that may occur due to the possibility of delayed reendothelialization.

Clinical and Angiographic Follow-Up

Clinical evaluation and careful angiographic follow-up was performed after 24 hours (18 patients), 1 to 2 months (12 patients), 1 year (20 patients), 2 years (19 patients), and 3 years (17 patients). Three patients who had total occlusion were excluded. All angiograms were obtained in the same projections and with identical angiographic technique.

Angiographic Analysis

All initial angiogram measurements of the reference vessel diameter and minimum lumen diameter (MLD) were performed with a careful manual caliper system over the 35-mm film to calculate the size of the angioplasty balloon and the radiation dose.

To evaluate the angiographic follow-up, quantitative coronary angiography (QCA) was read by independent observers according to a method validated in the core laboratory at the Washington Hospital Center, Washington, DC.

Radiation Delivery System

From a nickel-titanium alloy wire 0.57 mm in diameter with a 1-cm long ^{192}Ir active source sealed at the end of the wire that was used for brachytherapy in patients with lung cancer,[37] Liprie developed a wire 0.46 mm in diameter and with a 3-mm active length encapsulated iridium source that was suitable for porcine coronary arteries.[29] Following our recommendation, Liprie developed a source with diameters 0.018" and 0.014", both 30-mm active length, fixed to a wire of similar caliber. It was almost as flexible as a standard angioplasty coronary wire and was suitable for use in clinical research in human coronary arteries.

The delivery system consisted of a 4F noncentered, monorail polyethylene catheter (Fig. 1), sterilized as usual, that was resistant to damage caused by the

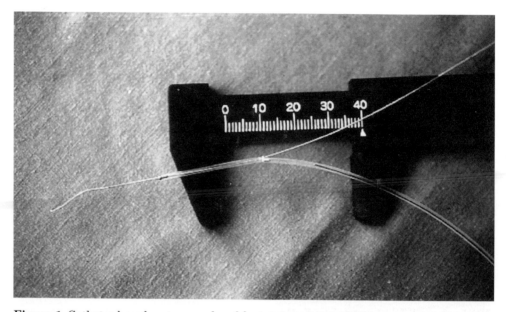

Figure 1. Catheter-based system employed for transportation of the source and testing wire.

source wire at any angle and allowed an easy introduction of the source into the catheter. The inner lumen was a closed channel with a radiopaque mark at the end that allowed visualization by fluoroscopy of the exact position of the source wire. The positioning procedure of the catheter was similar to the positioning of an intracoronary ultrasound transducer. The risk of placing the catheter was considered similar to that of the intracoronary placement of a standard angioplasty balloon or intracoronary ultrasound transducer, but less than that of a stent or rotational or directional atherectomy.

Dosimetry

The initial activity of the source was 1.2 and 1.5 Ci, estimated with the use of a well chamber calibrated for a ^{192}Ir wire. The dose rate at different depths was measured with the use of thermal luminescent dosimeter chips at various distances from the wire. When the treatment was initiated, the activity of the source was 529 to 982 mCi.

Taking into consideration that the target tissues received a very low dose (<10 Gy) with external beam irradiation, that brachytherapy resulted in increased hyperplasia,[25,26] that external beam radiation with doses higher than 25 Gy can be hazardous,[20,22,24] and that there were favorable effects on neointimal hyperplasia inhibition and minimal deleterious effects on the surrounding tissues with endovascular brachytherapy in the low dose range (10 to 20 Gy),[28,31,35] we decided to deliver a dose of 10 to 14 Gy to the target tissues, the adventitia and muscular layer, respectively, To achieve this dose (10 to 14 Gy), and considering that the coronary artery disease wall can be 0.5 to 2 mm thick and most plaques are eccentric, we calculated the time on the basis of the activity of the source and we prescribed a standard dose of 25 Gy to 1.5 mm depth using the 0.018" wire to the first group of 9 patients (10 arteries), so that if the reference vessel was 3.0-mm diameter, at 0.5 mm depth (the muscular layer) we delivered 14 Gy, and at 1.0 mm depth (adventitia) we delivered 10 Gy (Fig. 2). To reduce the risk of higher doses due to the use of a noncentered catheter, we used the 0.014" wire to prescribe a dose of 20 Gy adjusted to the radius of the reference vessel to the second group of 11 arteries (Fig.3). One patient received 18 Gy to the reference vessel radium.

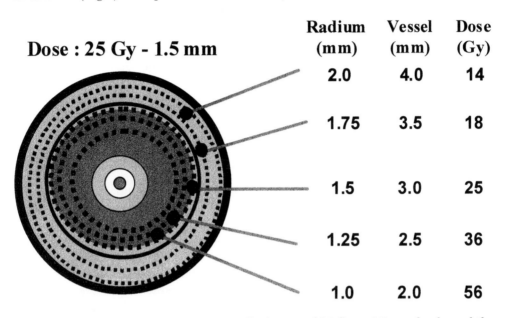

Dose : 25 Gy - 1.5 mm

Radium (mm)	Vessel (mm)	Dose (Gy)
2.0	4.0	14
1.75	3.5	18
1.5	3.0	25
1.25	2.5	36
1.0	2.0	56

Figure 2. Prescribed radiation treatment. Dosimetry of 25 Gy at 1.5 mm depths and the dose range at different distances from the gamma source (^{192}I).

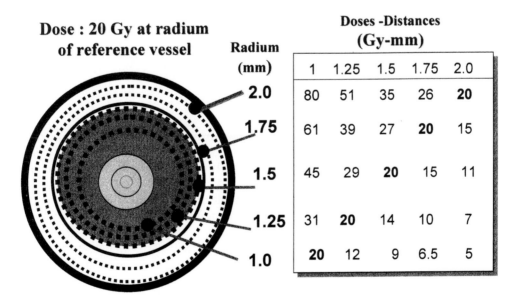

Dose : 20 Gy at radium of reference vessel

Doses -Distances (Gy-mm)

Radium (mm)	1	1.25	1.5	1.75	2.0
2.0	80	51	35	26	**20**
1.75	61	39	27	**20**	15
1.5	45	29	**20**	15	11
1.25	31	**20**	14	10	7
1.0	**20**	12	9	6.5	5

Figure 3. Prescribed radiation treatment. Dosimetry at different distances for a standard 20 Gy dose with a gamma source (^{192}I).

After determination by the core laboratory, based on QCA of the luminal diameters of the treated vessels, the actual dose delivered to the surface of the vessel was recalculated (assuming the catheter was positioned in the center of the artery) with the use of a standard, commercial treatment planning system. Because a noncentered system was used in this trial, it is likely that vessels that were treated with 25 Gy received even higher doses, up to a maximum of 92.5 Gy, when the catheter was lying against the vessel lumen surface, whereas the contralateral wall of those locations received a minimum dose of 7.2 Gy in large arteries.

Radiation Protection Considerations

Radiation safety was a major concern; thus, special safety precautions were taken during the procedure. The wire was the iridium source and the delivery catheter was a closed channel. The sources were transported in a shielded box and were manipulated only with the use of long forceps. Shielding included leaded glass goggles, two thyroid shields, and two fluoroscopy aprons. The handling of the source was shared among three operators. Total handling time of the radioactive wire was less than a minute per artery. Geiger count was used to check the radiation in patients during and at the end of the procedure, and also to check radiation inside and out of the laboratory. Three operators performed 22 radiation procedures. The radiation exposure of a single operator was calculated to be 2 mSv. The estimation of the maximal radiation dose delivered to an operator when the activity of the iridium sources was 1.5 Ci. In 10 minutes of exposure, it was: head (70 cm), 0.2 mSv/min; body (50 cm), 0.4 mSv/min; and hands (20 cm), 2.52 mSv/min – without considering the attenuation caused by proper operator shielding, the body of the patient, and the time-dependent radiation intensity reduction.

The estimation of the maximal radiation dose delivered to a patient was: to a distance of 1.5 mm, the maximal dose delivered was 25 Gy (coronary artery); to 50 cm, 0.02 Gy (abdomen); to 1 m, 0.005 Gy (groin); and to 1.5 m, 0.0025 Gy (foot). We registered 0.0006 Gy at 3 m away from the patient, and in the operator room, no radiation was detected.

Statistical Analysis

All data were recorded on a standardized form, entered into a computerized database, and expressed as proportions or as mean SD. Given the lack of a concurrent group of nonirradiated patients, the only comparison that was tested was the post-procedural MLD versus the MLD at 24 hours and at follow-up, for which the paired t-test was used. All tests of significance were tailed, and values of $P<0.05$ were considered to indicate statistical significance.

Results

From July 1994 to January 1995, 21 patients (22 arteries) were enrolled in the study. Angioplasty was successful (percent residual diameter stenosis <50%) in 19 of 22 sites (86.4%). However, intracoronary radiation therapy was successfully delivered to all treated sites. The time of treatment depended on the activity of the ^{192}Ir source and ranged from 164 to 929 seconds. The procedure was well tolerated and the patients presented no complications such ischemia, arrhythmia, or any other major complication. None of the radiation treatments were interrupted. One patient developed coronary spasm after the radiation treatment that was refractory to intracoronary nitroglycerin, but it resolved after prolonged balloon inflation.

The MLD of all lesions is shown in Table 1.The mean diameter of the reference vessel was 2.97 ± 0.49 mm (range, 1.8 to 4.0 mm), and the MLD before angioplasty was 0.98 ± 0.53 mm. The mean MLD after intervention was 1.98 ± 0.5 mm, and the mean MLD and the percent residual diameter stenosis after the procedure was $35\pm13\%$. All treated arteries undergoing 24-hour angiography were patent except one that sustained subacute thrombosis in a bifurcated site (without resulting in acute myocardial infarction or creatine phosphokinase elevation) (patient no. 12 in Table 1). This patient underwent successful angioplasty to both the thrombosed branch and the radiation-treated site. Early luminal loss was demonstrated in the treated arteries at 24 hours with a reduction of the MLD from 1.98 ± 0.5 to 1.54 ± 0.60 mm (early loss of 0.44 mm), leaving a mean percent residual diameter stenosis of $48\pm16\%$ ($P<0.001$) (Table 2). All patients were free from in-hospital major cardiac events such as myocardial infarction, bypass surgery, or death.

The first 9 patients (10 arteries) who were treated with a higher dose of 25 Gy had an angiogram between 30 and 60 days after the procedure. Two of these

Table 1

3-Year Follow-Up of Minimum Lumen Diameter after Gamma Intracoronary Radiation Therapy

	pre	PTCA	24 H	>6 M	2Y	3Y
1	0	2.04	1.81	0	0	0
2	0.98	1.75	1.62	1.47	1.97	2.04
3	0.68	1.78	1.36	0	0	0
4	0.7	1.43	1.37	1.78	2.38	2.05
5	0.83	2.24	1.75	2.53	2.38	2.14
6	1.42	1.95	1.78	2.55	2.38	2.22
7	1.35	2.27	2.17	2.55	2.7	5.3
8	0.64	1.99	2.13	2.78	2.52	3.58
9	0.45	1.47	0.94	2.07	1.16	2
10	0.77	1.27	1.23	1.21	1.57	1.65
11	1.29	1.23	1.11	1.32		
12	0.62	1.88	1.94	1.94	2.14	2.24
13	0.4	1.98	1.6	1.37	1.99	1.76
14	1.17	2.45	2.06	2.31	2.13	2.26
15	0.9	2.59	2.21	2.86	2.19	2.43
16	1.76	2.13	2.02	1.74	1.83	2.07
17	2.08	2.47	2.55	2.55	2.16	2.61
18	0.58	1.48	1.35	1.38	0.76	1.3
19	0.57	1.69	2.13	2.13	2.01	2.49
20	1.12	1.33	0.88	0.59	1.46	1.54
21	0.8	2.43	2.37	2.37		
22	1.74	2.8	1.06	1.06	0	0

Table 2

3-Year Follow-Up of Late Loss of Minimum Lumen Diameter

Patients	Artery	L loss Post 3Y	L loss 24h–3y	L Loss 6m–3y	L Loss 2y–3Y
1	RCA				
2	LAD	−0.29	−0.42	−0.57	−0.07
3	RM				
4	LAD	−0.62	−0.68	−0.27	0.33
5	RCA	0.10	−0.39	0.39	0.24
6	LAD	−0.27	−0.44	0.33	0.16
8	LCX	−3.03	−3.13	−2.75	−2.60
7	RCA	−1.59	−1.45	−0.80	−1.06
8	LCX	−0.53	−1.06	0.07	−0.84
9	LAD	−0.38	−0.42	−0.44	−0.08
10	RCA				
11	LAD	−0.36	−2.24	−0.30	−0.10
12	RCD	0.22	−0.16	−0.39	0.23
13	RCD	0.19	−0.20	0.05	−0.13
14	LCX	0.16	−0.22	0.43	−0.24
15	LAD	0.06	−0.05	−0.33	−0.24
16	RCA	−0.14	−2.61	−0.06	−0.45
17	LAD	0.18	0.05	0.08	−0.54
18	LAD	−0.80	−2.49	−0.36	−0.48
19	LAD	−0.21	−0.66	−0.95	−0.08
20	LAD,P				
21	LAD,P				
		−0.43	**−0.97**	**−0.35**	**−0.35**
		0.81	**1.02**	**0.73**	**0.69**

patients, although asymptomatic, had total occlusion at the treated site at 30 and 38 days (patients no. 1 and 3, respectively, in Table 1), without evidence of recent myocardial infarction on their electrocardiogram. One of these patients (patient no. 1) had a total occlusion before the initial angioplasty and radiation treatment. The other (patient no. 3) had severe dissection during the angioplasty procedure before the radiation treatment. One patient (patient no. 6) developed a small pseudoaneurysm appearance at the treatment site immediately after the angioplasty that was pronounced at 6 months. The 2- and 3-year angiograms showed no changes and the patient remains asymptomatic. Another patient (patient no. 2) who underwent uncomplicated PTCA to the proximal left anterior descending coronary artery, developed a pseudoaneurysm at the treatment site at 3 months, which was enlarged at 6 months (Fig 4). The pseudoaneurysm showed little increase at 2 years and no change after 3 years. This patient remained asymptomatic and refused bypass surgery. Angioplasty failed in patient no.10 because the balloon did not sufficiently dilate sequential severe calcificated lesions; however, radiation treatment was possible. The 2-year angiogram showed severe diffuse disease and occlusive lesion in the distal segment of the artery, not related to the irradiated site. The patient persisted with stable angina. Patient no. 19 experienced poor angioplasty results because there was no reflow with rotablator and dilatation was needed with a balloon in order to recover flow; the radiation treatment was possible without complications, but the patient presented with angina

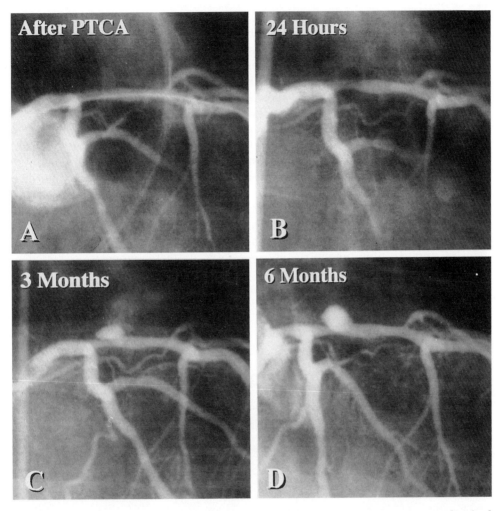

Figure 4. Pseudoaneurism development after 60 days post percutaneous transluminal coronary angioplasty and intracoronary radiation therapy in a proximal left anterior descending coronary artery.

and severe recoil that required new PTCA at 24 hours. This patient presented restenosis at 8 months and had a new PTCA without complications. The 2- and 3-year angiograms showed no restenosis and the patient remains asymptomatic. Immediately post PTCA, patients no. 20 and 21 presented severe acute recoil and patient no. 21 had acute occlusion with thrombus (bail-out situation); both received intracoronary radiation therapy, and Palmaz-Schatz and Gianturco-Roubin stents, respectively, were implanted. Patient no. 20 is asymptomatic with no restenosis at 2 and 3 years. Patient no. 21 presented in-stent restenosis and the vessel was occluded at 2 years. The patient has stable angina and refuses surgery.

The mean actual dose at the luminal surface of the treatment site was consistently higher than the prescribed dose and was calculated to be 35.6±11.1 Gy (range, 19.5 to 35 Gy for all arteries), whereas the mean dose at the reference vessel diameter was 23.3±7.3 Gy (range, 11.1 to 42.9 Gy). For patient no. 2, who developed a pseudoaneurysm at 60 days, the actual dose calculated was 38.5 Gy delivered to a distance of 1.5 mm from the source, and because the radiation was delivered by a noncentering deliver system, it is likely that the vessel wall at the treated site received up to 92 Gy. Two other vessels (the RCA and LCX) that were treated with 25 Gy (patient no. 7) showed vessel dilatation and irregular appearance at early (RCA) and late (LCX) follow-up.

The first angiographic follow-up was performed between 30 and 60 days in 12 patients and showed a mean luminal diameter of 1.63±0.89 mm, and a mean residual stenosis of 46±28%. The next angiographic control was performed in 20 arteries between 6 and 14 months (average 8±1.9 months). All were patent during the follow-up, with a mean luminal diameter of 1.94±0.62 mm and a mean residual stenosis of 41±24%, similar to the post-angioplasty results ($P=0.2$). The calculated late loss was 0.19±0.78 mm and the late loss index was 0.19±0.4. The MLD demonstrated negative late loss in 10 of the 22 arteries (Table 2). At 8±1.9 months, angiographic binary restenosis (>50% diameter stenosis) occurred in 27.3% of the arteries, including the 2 patients with early total occlusion. An example of a case with a negative late loss at 14 months with site dilatation is shown in Figure 5.

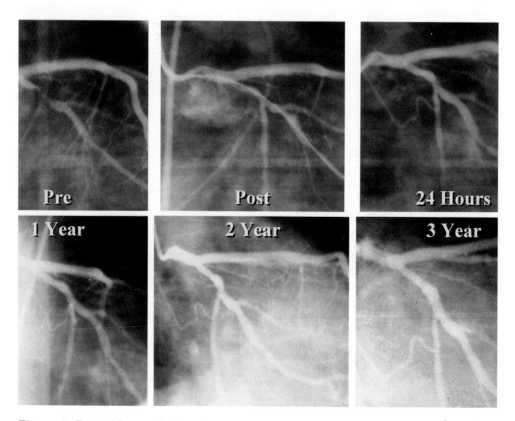

Figure 5. Favorable remodeling. Angiograms of a patient who was treated for a lesion of the left circumflex artery.

Two-year angiographic follow-up was performed in 19 treatment sites (1 patient refused because was he was completely asymptomatic). The MLD was 1.90±0.69 mm and the mean residual restenosis was 35±19%. Angiographic binary restenosis was present in 6 arteries (27.2%), including 1 patient that developed restenosis after 6 months and excluding 1 patient who had restenosis at 6-month follow-up with spontaneous regression at 2 years.

There were few changes in the 3-year angiographic follow-up. All arteries remained patent and there was no additional late loss. No adverse effect in adjacent segments and mild growth of the aneurysmal segments was observed.

The mean late loss between PTCA and 6 months was 0.20±0.59 mm, and 0.13±0.84 mm between 6 months and 2 years; the loss index was 0.26 and 0.33 at 2 and 3 years, respectively, in all patients, and 0.0 when the 3 patients with total occlusion at follow-up were excluded.

In the group of 4 patients with restenosis but patent arteries at 6 months, 2 had successful balloon angioplasty and at 2- and 3-year follow-up showed no new restenosis, 1 patient showed spontaneous regression, and 1 refused treatment and had a total occlusion at 2 years follow-up. One patient suffered septal myocardial infarction and developed post myocardial infarction angina, requiring new angioplasty 1 year after intracoronary radiation therapy and with no new restenosis at 2- and 3-year follow-up.

Four patients developed vessel ectasias at the treatment site, 2 early pseudoaneurysms (immediately and after 30 days) after PTCA-intracoronary radiation therapy that could be related to deep dissection during the angioplasty, and 2 late pseudoaneurysms that were observed at 6 months. The two pseudoaneurysms showed little increase at 2- and 3-year follow-up.

None of the patients or the medical personnel developed complications or illnesses that could be related to the effects of the radiation procedure.

Discussion

This study describes the first human intracoronary radiation therapy trial and is among the first to report clinical and angiographic follow-up of greater than 6 month's duration. The study demonstrates that intracoronary irradiation after standard balloon angioplasty using a catheter-based system is feasible and can be performed with a low and acceptable incidence of procedural or in-hospital adverse events.[38–40]

Freedom from myocardial infarction, bypass surgery, or revascularization of the target lesion at 1 year was 80.9%, similar to the value of 80.5% in the stent group at 6 months in the STRESS Trial[11] and higher than that reported in several other balloon angioplasty studies.[43,44] Furthermore, although our patients had a mean early loss of 0.45 mm at 24 hours, after 6 months the restenosis rate was 27% (Fig. 6). While Rodriguez et al,[45] using criteria of early loss at 24 hours of greater than 0.3 mm in MLD and/or greater than 10% increase in diameter stenosis, obtained a similar restenosis rate of 21% in the stent group, the non-stent group had a restenosis rate of 75.7% at 3-month follow-up. The very high early loss seen in this study could be related to a direct effect of radiation on tissues causing cellular edema, in addition to spasm, elastic recoil, dissection, and thrombosis.[46]

Although this study was not designed to evaluate restenosis, this finding sug-

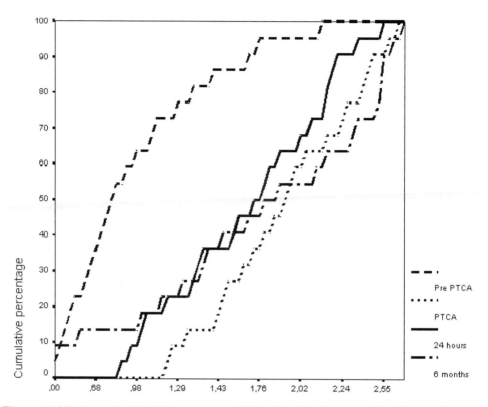

Figure 6. Minimum luminal diameter cumulative distribution curve of patients, showing the pre angioplasty, post angioplasty, 24 hours post angioplasty, and 6-month follow-up.

gested a beneficial effect of intracoronary radiation therapy in reducing the restenosis rate. Larger randomized studies have confirmed this finding.[49,50]

So far, none of the different revascularization device trials[10,11,45,47] have reported a negative late loss (late gain) after 24 hours to 6 to 8 months and that is maintained in the 2- and 3-year follow-up. Forty-five percent of patients in these reports (10 lesions) had an increase in lumen diameter during the follow-up period and mean late gain was 0.24±0.67 mm (Fig. 7). Radiation as an adjunct therapy to intracoronary stenting was suggested as an ideal combination because radiation has been shown to be very effective at suppressing the neointimal proliferation seen with stent placement, in which the stent prevents vessel contraction (unfavorable remodeling).[34,49] However, the results seen here with radiation alone showed a negative late loss in 10 arteries, and a late loss index of 0.19. This suggests that intracoronary radiation therapy could promote favorable remodeling after PTCA. This may be an alternative strategy for the routine need for intracoronary stenting after adequate balloon angioplasty for prevention of late constriction. Additionally, late thrombosis has been recently associated with coronary stenting and intracoronary radiation therapy.[51]

Another important observation is related to the favorable evolution of the group of patients that showed no restenosis at 6 months, which was maintained at 2- and 3-year follow-up. Additionally, 1 of the patients that showed restenosis at 6 months later became asymptomatic, showing no restenosis at 2 and 3 years. Also, we observed a favorable result in the 3 patients who had restenosis after un-

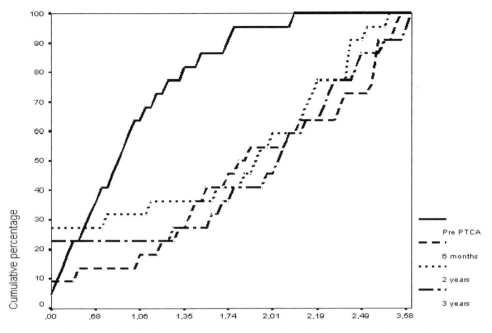

Figure 7. Minimum luminal diameter cumulative distribution curve, showing the results of pre angioplasty, 6-month follow-up, and late 2- and 3-year follow-up.

dergoing new single balloon angioplasty, which could be related to the radiation dose previously prescribed.

The lack of consistent effect after intracoronary radiation therapy, as well as other complications observed in the study may be related to the inhomogeneity of dosing because of the use of a noncentered system. Six of the 10 arteries that were treated with higher doses of 25 Gy developed angiographic complications (total occlusions in 2 and pseudoaneurysm and arterial dilatation in 4 vessels). It is possible that some areas of these vessels were exposed to 2 to 3 times the intended dose due to the noncentered catheter. Although the irregularity and pseudoaneurysm were seen immediately after the procedure in 2 of these patients, it is possible that irradiation and these high doses interfere with the wound healing process, and this could suggest an upper limit of vessel wall integrity and tolerance to likely toxic doses for this therapy after balloon angioplasty; in contrast, it is possible that the contralateral wall of larger arteries received lower doses than are required for therapy, which may explain the lack of consistency in the effectiveness of the treatment in the cohort.

The hand-loading delivery system used in this study is limited in the effective shielding of ^{192}Ir with standard lead aprons; thus, the medical personnel are exposed to additional radiation, especially when high activities are used. Additional studies can minimize this problem by using a remote afterloading device to deliver the source and a radiation shield to block exposure to personnel.

The importance of this trial primarily lies in demonstrating that intracoronary radiation therapy for prevention of restenosis is feasible, and free of any unexpected acute complications. In addition, this is the first method for preventing restenosis that has shown a negative late loss that is maintained in the very late 2- and 3-year angiographic follow-up.

References

1. Holmes DR Jr, Vliestra RE, Smith HC, et al. Restenosis after percutaneous transluminal coronary angioplasty (PTCA): A report from the PTCA Registry of the National Heart, Lung and Blood Institute. Am J Cardiol 1984;53(suppl):77C–81C.
2. Faxon DP, Samborn TA, Haudenschild CC. Mechanism of angioplasty and its relation to restenosis. Am J Cardiol 1987;60:5B–9B.
3. Liu MW, Roubin GS, King SB III. Restenosis after coronary angioplasty: Potential biologic determinants and role of intimal hyperplasia. Circulation 1989;79:1374–1387.
4. Austin GE, Ratlift MB, Hollman J. Intimal proliferation of smooth muscle cells as an explanation for recurrent coronary artery stenosis after percutaneous transluminal coronary angioplasty. J Am Coll Cardiol 1985;6:369–375.
5. Lafont A, Guzman LA, Whitlow PL, et al. Restenosis after experimental angioplasty: Intimal, medial and adventitial changes associated with constrictive remodeling. Circ Res 1995;76:996–1002.
6. Schwartz RS, Huber KC, Murphy JG, et al. Restenosis and the proportional neointimal response to coronary artery injury: Results in a porcine model. J Am Coll Cardiol 1992;19:267–274.
7. Glasgov S, Weisenberg E, Zarins CK, et al. Compensatory enlargement of human atherosclerotic coronary arteries. N Engl J Med 1987;316:1371–1375.
8. Scott NA, Cipolla GD, Ross CE, et al. Identification of a potencial role for adventitia in vascular lesion formation after balloon overstretch injury of porcine coronary arteries. Circulation 1996;93:2178–2187.
9. Schwartz RS, Holmes DR, Topol EJ. The restenosis paradigm revisited: An alternative proposal for cellular mechanisms. J Am Coll Cardiol 1992;20:1284–1293.
10. Serruys PW, de Jaegere P, Kiemeneij F, et al, for the BENESTENT Study Group. A comparison of balloon expandable stent implantation with balloon angioplasty in patient with coronary artery desease. N Engl J Med 1994;331:489–495.
11. Fishman DL, Leon MB, Baim B, et al, for the STRESS Trial Investigators. A randomized comparison of coronary-stent placement and balloon angioplasty in the treatment of coronary artery disease. N Engl J Med 1994;331:496–501.
12. Faxon DP. Mechanisms of Angioplasty and Pathophysiology of Restenosis: Practical Angioplasty. New York: Raven Press; 1994:5–12.
13. Kaplan HS. Biochemical basis of reproductive death in irradiated cells. Am J Roentgenol 1963;90:907–916.
14. Kovalic JJ, Perez CA. Radiation therapy following keloidectomy: A 20-year experience. Int J Radiat Oncol Biol Phys 1989;17:77–80.
15. Levy DS, Salter MM, Roth RE. Postoperative irradiation in the prevention of keloids. Am J Roentgenol 1976;127:509–510.
16. Enhamre A, Hammar H. Treatment of keloids with excision and postoperative x-ray irradiation. Dermatologica 1983;167:90–93.
17. Borok TL, Bray M, Sinclair I. Role of ionizing radiation for 393 keloids. Int J Radiat Oncol Biol Phys 1988;14:865–870.
18. Wilder RB, Buatt JM, Kittleson JM, et al. Pterygium treated with excision and postoperative beta irradiation. Int J Radiat Oncol Biol Phys 1992;23:533–537.
19. Ayers DC, Evarts CM, Parkinson JR. The prevention of heterotopic ossification in high-risk patients by low-dose radiation therapy after total hip arthroplasty. J Bone Joint Surg Am 1986;68:1423–1430.
20. Fajardo LF, Berthrong M. Vascular lesions following radiation. Pathol Ann 1988;23:297–330.
21. Hilaris BS, Martin N. Interstitial brachytherapy in cancer of the lung: 20 years experience. Int J Radiat Oncol Biol Phys 1979;5:1951–1956.
22. Boivin JF, Hutchison GB, Lubin JH, et al. Coronary artery disease mortality in patients treated for Hodgkin's disease. Cancer 1992;69:1241–1247.
23. Hancock SL, Tucker MA, Hoppe RT. Factors affecting late mortality from heart disease after treatment of Hodgkin's disease. JAMA 1993;270:1949–1955.
24. Guillete EL, Powers BE, McChesney SL, et al. Response of aorta and branch arteries to experimental intraoperative irradiation. Int J Radiat Oncol Biol Phys 1989;17:1247–1255.

25. Gellmam J, Healey G, Qingsheng, et al. The effect of very low dose irradiation on restenosis following balloon angioplasty: A study in the atherosclerotic rabbit. Circulation 1991;18:331A.

26. Schwartz RS, Koval TM, Edwards WD, et al. Effects of external beam irradiation on neointimal hyperplasia after experimental coronary artery injury. J Am Coll Cardiol 1992;19:1106–1113.

27. Shefer A, Eigler NI, Whiting JS, et al. Suppresion of intimal proliferation after balloon angioplasty with local beta irradiation in rabbits. J Am Coll Cardiol 1993;21:185.

28. Wiedermann JG, Marboe C, Schwartz A, et al. Intracoronary irradiation reduces restenosis after balloon angioplasty in a porcine model. J Am Coll Cardiol 1994;23:1491–1498.

29. Mazur W, Ali MN, Dabaghi SF, et al. High dose rate intracoronary radiation suppresses neointimal proliferation in the stented and ballooned model of porcine restenosis [abstract]. Circulation 1994;90:I-652.

30. Verin V, Popowski Y, Urban P, et al. Intraarterial beta irradiation prevents neointimal hyperplasia in a hypercholesterolemic rabbit restenosis model [abstract]. J Am Coll Cardiol 1995;25:2A–3A.

31. Waksman R, Robinson KA, Crocker IR, et al. Endovascular low dose irradiation inhibits neointima formation after coronary artery balloon injury in swine: A possible role for radiation therapy in restenosis prevention. Circulation 1995;91:1533–1539.

32. Waksman R, Robinson K, Crocker I, et al. Intracoronary low-dose β-irradiation inhibits neointima formation after coronary artery balloon injury in the swine restenosis model. Circulation 1995;92:3025–3031.

33. Wiedermann JG, Marboe C, Schwartz A, et al. Intracoronary irradiation markedly reduces neointimal proliferation after balloon angioplasty in swine: Persistent benefit at 6-month follow-up. J Am Coll Cardiol 1995;25:1451–1456.

34. Waksman R, Robinson K, Crocker I, et al. Intracoronary radiation prior to stent implantation inhibits neointima formation in stented porcine coronary arteries. Circulation 1995;92:1383–1386.

35. Liermann DD, Boettcher HD, Kollatch J, et al. Prophylactic endovascular radiotherapy to prevent intimal hyperplasia after stent implantation in femoro-popliteal arteries. Cardiovasc Intervent Radiol 1994;17:12–16.

36. Boettcher HD, Schopol B, Liermann DD, et al. Endovascular irradiation – a new method to avoid recurrent stenosis after stent implantation in peripheral arteries: Technique and preliminary results. Int J Radiat Oncol Biol Phys 1994;29:183–186.

37. Brach B, Buhler C, Hayman M, et al. Percutaneous computed tomography-guided fine needle brachytherapy of pulmonary malignancies. Chest 1994;106:268–274.

38. Condado JA, Gurdiel O, Espinoza R, et al. Percutaneous transluminal coronary angioplasty (PTCA) and intracoronary radiation therapy (ICRT): A possible new modality for the treatment of coronary restenosis: A preliminary report of the first 10 patients treated with intracoronary radiation therapy [abstract]. J Am Coll Cardiol 1994;288A.

39. Condado JA, Gurdiel O, Espinoza R, et al. Long term angiographic and clinical outcome after percutaneous transluminal coronary angioplasty and intracoronary radiation therapy in humans [abstract]. Circulation 1996;94:8,I–209:1218.

40. Condado JA, Waksman R, Gurdiel O, et al. Long-term angiographic and clinical outcome after percutaneous transluminal coronary angioplasty and intracoronary radiation therapy in humans. Circulation 1997;96:727–732.

41. Condado J, Saucedo J, Calderas C, et al. Two years angiographic evaluation after intracoronary 192 Iridium in humans [abstract]. Circulation 1997;96:I–20.

42. Condado J, Calderas C, Waksman R. Three years clinical and angiographic follow-up after intracoronary 192 iridium radiation therapy [abstract]. Circulation 1998;98:I–651.

43. Klein JL, Manoukian SV, Vogel RA, et al, for the Lovastatin Restenosis Trial Group. Computerized quantitative coronary arteriography: Performance standards and edge detection. Am J Cardiol 1996;77:815–822.

44. Weintraub WS, Boccuzzi SJ, Klein L, et al, and the Lovastatin Restenosis Trial Group. Local of effect of Lovastatin on restenosis after coronary angioplasty. N Engl J Med 1994;331:1331–1337.

45. Rodriguez A, Santaera O, Larriban M, et al. Coronary stenting decrease restenosis in

lesions with early loss in luminal diameter 24 hours after successful PTCA. Circulation 1995;91:1397–1402.

46. Weidermann JG, Leavy JA, Arnols H, et al. Effects of high dose intracoronary irradiation on vasomotor function and smooth muscle histopathology. Am J Physiol 1994;267:H125–H132.

47. Topol EJ, Leya F, Pikerton CA, et al, on behalf of the CAVEAT Study Group. A comparison of coronary angioplasty with directional atherectomy in patients with coronary artery disease. N Engl J Med 1993;329:221–227.

48. Fischell TA, Kharma BK, Fuschell DR, et al. Low dose β-particle emission from stent wire results in complete, localized inhibition of smooth muscle cell proliferation. Circulation 1994;90:2956–2963.

49. Teirstein P, Masullo V, Jani S, et al. Catheter-based radiotherapy to inhibit restenosis after coronary stenting. N Engl J Med 1997;336:1697–1703.

50. King SB III, Williams DO, Chougule P, et al. Endovascular β-radiation to reduce restenosis after coronary balloon angioplasty: Results of the Beta Energy Restenosis Trial (BERT). Circulation 1998;97:2025–2030.

51. Costa M, Sabate M, van der Giessen W, et al. Late coronary occlusion after intracoronary brachytherapy. Circulation 1999;100:789–792.

## Chapter 50

Clinical Restenosis Trials Using Beta Energy Radiation

Raoul Bonan, MD

Introduction

Restenosis following coronary interventions is the sum of three processes: (1) elastic recoil immediately following the procedure; (2) neointima formation; and (3) chronic constriction of the vessel. The initial recoil and the late chronic constriction are opposed by intracoronary stents, which were the first devices documented to reduce the restenosis process. Stenting, however, is not universally applicable and restenosis rates within stents have ranged from 10 to 40% in various subsets. Common to all forms of coronary interventions is the formation of neointima, which is composed of smooth-muscle-like cells in a collagen matrix. That process has histologic and pathophysiological similarities with wound healing of other tissues.

Ionizing radiation has been documented to inhibit cell proliferation and formation of new tissue in certain clinical situations, including formation of keloids following surgery on the skin and reformation of pterygium following surgical removal. Based on the assumption that the neointima formation found after injury to coronary arteries resembles wound healing, low-dose intracoronary radiation has been applied in an attempt to inhibit this phenomenon.

A trial of endovascular radiation by Liermann et al showed that, after refractory restenosis in femoropopliteal arteries undergoing angioplasty, brachytherapy resulted in long-lasting patency as assessed by noninvasive and invasive means.[1]

Animal studies have been carried out using the porcine coronary model. Studies at Emory University, Atlanta, GA,[2] and Columbia University, NY,[3] evaluated low-dose endovascular radiation on neointima formation in the porcine coronary model. Gamma radiation was initially tested and was found to inhibit neointima formation in a dose-related fashion. This effect was seen 2 weeks after vessel injury and was also seen to persist for 6 months.[4] Similar radiation experiments were performed with vessels that underwent intracoronary stenting, and a positive response was also noted. More recently, a system that has potential for clinical application was developed that delivers endovascular low-dose radiation using a beta source. Results of the experiments with this device show inhibitory effects similar to those seen earlier with gamma radiation.[5]

From Waksman R (ed.). *Vascular Brachytherapy, Third Edition.* Armonk, NY: Futura Publishing Co., Inc.; © 2002.

Clinical Trials

The availability of a clinically applicable catheter-based system sets the stage for human clinical trials. Since the catheter-based system can deliver beta radiation or no radiation in the same system, it is possible to conduct double-blind randomized trials with this device. This provides the first opportunity to perform device trials that will have similar blinding to drug trials.

Beta Energy Restenosis Trial (BERT)

The first trial that was initiated was the Beta Energy Restenosis Trial (BERT), a U.S. Food and Drug Administration (FDA)-approved feasibility clinical trial. The objectives of the trial were: (1) to evaluate the feasibility of the Novoste Beta-Cath™ System (Novoste Corporation, Norcross, GA) to deliver beta radiation sources to the appropriate coronary site in humans; (2) to confirm the operational specifications of the device delivery system; (3) to examine the safety of three different doses of radiation administered following angioplasty; and (4) to examine the incidence of restenosis following angioplasty and to compare this to similar historic control patients treated with angioplasty alone in the Lovastatin Restenosis Trial.

Patients in this trial were those planned for balloon angioplasty of a single lesion in a native coronary artery. In an effort to make some judgment on whether restenosis was being inhibited, quantitative angiography was conducted at 6 months to assess the minimal lumen diameter (MLD), the percent diameter stenosis, the initial gain, and late loss in lumen diameter. In addition, vessels were inspected for any alterations in healing pattern, and all clinical parameters were followed.

Procedures consisted of balloon angioplasty until the desired result was achieved, followed by delivery of the Beta-Cath System into the exact location of the injured lesion. The devices used were designed to allow an overlap so that the entire treated segment was radiated. The radiation dose delivered was based on the dwell time of the catheter; this was 2 minutes 20 seconds to 3 minutes 44 seconds.

The results of the first 20 patients in the feasibility study were published in 1998.[6] A total of 85 patients were recruited in the BERT Study: 15 from Emory University, Atlanta, GA, 8 from Brown University, Providence, RI, 30 from the Institut de Cardiologie de Montreal, Montreal, Quebec, 31 from ThoraxCenter, Rotterdam, The Netherlands, and 1 from the Scripps Clinic, La Jolla, CA.[7] Only 78 patients had their 6-month angiographic follow-up. The late lumen loss in those patients receiving beta radiation was negligible, 0.13±0.71 mm. Minimum lumen diameter before angioplasty was 0.75±0.26 mm, after angioplasty 2.05±0.41 mm, and, at 6-month follow-up, 1.93±0.74 mm. This translated to a diameter stenosis of 73% before angioplasty, 26% after angioplasty, and 30% at 6-month follow-up. Thirteen patients (16.7%) qualified as experiencing restenosis at the lesion site (20 mm centered by the MLD) by the 50% stenosis definition. In the intervention area (30-mm centered by the MLD), 6 new lesions appeared, revealing a new phenomena called "geographic miss," where the injury length was not covered by the prescribed radiation dose. This occurred in 11 patients, resulting in a target lesion revascularization rate of 14.1%.

These impressive results were obtained with doses of beta radiation given in 12-, 14-, and 16-Gy doses calculated at a radius of 2 mm from the source. Radiation levels measured were 2.1 mrem/h at the patient's chest and 0.3 mrem/h at the operator's position during the brief dwell time; dramatically lower than in studies of gamma radiation. This allowed the operators to remain with the patient during the procedure without any added shielding required.

An intravascular ultrasound (IVUS) study, conducted at the "Institut de Cardiologie de Montreal," demonstrated that the mechanism of action of post-PTCA beta radiation therapy appears to be the prevention of hyperplasic response and the inhibition of vascular remodeling.[8]

By measuring the distances between the center of the IVUS catheter (assuming it held the same position from the radiation catheter) and the different parts of the artery wall, minimum and maximum doses of radiation can be calculated. The average dose delivered to the nearest point (the luminal surface) and furthest point (the external elastic membrane) were calculated. These were, respectively, 23.5 to 9 Gy (distance: 1.4 to 2.6 mm; dose: 23.5 to 9.1 Gy).

Two-year angiographic follow-up has been completed at the Institut de Cardiologie de Montreal and showed that following a mean increase of vessel dimensions at the intervened segment (15-mm centered on the original lesion where balloon injury and radiation were applied) at 6 months, stability of mean vessel dimensions over the 2-year follow-up period was demonstrated with minimal late loss and no further vessel expansion as assessed by quantitative coronary angiography (QCA).[9]

Beta-Cath System Trial

The Beta-Cath System Trial, a prospective, randomized, placebo-controlled, triple-masked trial was designed to evaluate the safety and effectiveness of the Novoste Beta-Cath System in native coronary arteries with de novo or restenotic lesions. The objectives of the trial were to evaluate the safety and efficacy of the Beta-Cath System strontium 90 (^{90}Sr) source versus a placebo (passive control) in prevention of restenosis in de novo and restenotic lesions of native coronary arteries. The evaluation will examine the clinical event rates of approximately 1550 patients who undergo elective percutaneous transluminal coronary angioplasty (PTCA) or provisional stent placement (550 PTCA, 550 stent patients with short, conventional, antiplatelet therapy, and approximately 450 stent patients with at least 2- to 3-month antiplatelet therapy; 50% of each group will receive either active or passive treatment).

The primary endpoint is target vessel revascularization at 8 months. Safety endpoints include freedom from death, coronary artery bypass graft (CABG), myocardial infarction, target vessel revascularization, and coronary aneurysm (assessed by angiogram and IVUS) at 8 months (±1 month) and at 1 and 2 years post procedure. The incidence of late stent thrombosis (thrombosis occurring after the first month) will be compared between the two stent groups, potentially providing a solution to the higher than expected incidence of thrombosis seen when a new stent is implanted at the same time as radiation is administered. Follow-up angiograms will be obtained to evaluate lumen dimensions and the restenosis rates at 8 months (±1 month) after initial treatment.

Neointimal hyperplasia within the stent and PTCA segment will be estimated by IVUS for 200 consecutive patients (100 PTCA and 100 stent). The specified dose of radiation administered following balloon angioplasty or pre-stent implantation will be 14 Gy in vessels 2.7 to 3.35 mm in diameter or 18 Gy in vessels 3.35 to 4.0 mm in diameter. Finally, the technical specifications of the system will be evaluated and confirmed by documenting the ability to send, maintain, and retrieve the radiation source train as prescribed. Results of the trial were presented at the AHA meeting in March 2001.

Stents and Radiation Therapy Trial (START)

The Stents and Radiation Therapy Trial (START), a prospective, randomized, placebo-controlled, triple-masked trial, has been approved by the FDA to evaluate the safety and efficacy of the Novoste Beta-Cath System (encapsulated ^{90}Sr sources) in the treatment of in-stent restenosis of native coronary arteries.[10]

Between September 1998 and April 1999, 476 patients were enrolled into the START Trial at 50 clinical centers in North America and Europe. Patients were considered candidates for the trial if they were over 18-years old and had a single target site stent restenosis in a native vessel between 2.7 and 4.0 mm. Stent restenosis was defined as a visually determined diameter stenosis between 50 and 100% in the presence of objective evidence of myocardial ischemia, as manifested by symptoms or laboratory testing. A successful angiographic result (<30% residual stenosis by visual estimation) within the treated segment after conventional coronary intervention was required prior to randomization.

A 30-mm Beta-Cath System radiation source train was used for lesions treatable with a 20-mm balloon; a 40-mm source train was used for lesions treatable with up to a 30-mm balloon. Patients were excluded from the study if they required multivessel coronary intervention or had an unsuccessful treatment of the target lesion (>30% residual diameter stenosis), a recent (<72 hours) myocardial infarction, unprotected left main coronary artery disease, or a prior history of any chest radiotherapy. Patients were also excluded if they had angiographic findings that would preclude delivery of the Beta-Cath Delivery Catheter, including severe proximal tortuosity or vessel angulation. Informed consent approved by a local institutional review board was obtained before the procedure in all patients.

Patients were pre-treated with 325-mg aspirin prior to the procedure. Use of abciximab was discouraged. After successful treatment (<30% residual stenosis and no major coronary dissections) of stent restenosis using balloon angioplasty alone, or in combination with rotational or directional atherectomy or excimer laser angioplasty, patients were randomly assigned to treatment with ^{90}Sr/^{90}Y (N=244) or placebo (N=232). The use of additional stents was discouraged and reserved for "bail-out" indications, including a residual stenosis or major dissection.

The Beta-Cath System used in this study is composed of three main components, a portable transfer device that hydraulically delivers the radiation source train, a 30-mm ^{90}Sr/^{90}Y source train, and a 5F, over-the-wire, triple lumen catheter with a dedicated closed-end source delivery lumen. The Beta-Cath Delivery Catheter is advanced using an exchange wire to the target lesion so that the radiopaque marker bands on the delivery catheter were positioned on either side of the injured segment.

The ^{90}Sr/^{90}Y radioisotope used in this study has a 28.8-year half-life. The prescription point was 2 mm from the centerline of the axis of the radiation source train in water. The dose prescription was 18.4 Gy for reference vessel sizes greater than or equal to 2.7 mm and less than or equal to 3.35 mm and 23 Gy for reference vessel sizes greater than 3.35 mm and less than or equal to 4.0 mm, as determined by visual angiographic estimate. The treatment time ranged between 3 and 5 minutes.

Results

There were no significant differences in baseline demographics between the two groups (mean age ~61 years; ~63% male; ~31% diabetics and ~48% with prior myocardial infarction). The device success rate was similar (P=NS) in placebo-treated patients (~97%) and ^{90}Sr/^{90}Y-treated patients (~98%). The procedural success rate was also similar (~97%) in the two groups.

Debulking devices were used with similar frequency in the two groups: rotational atherectomy was used in ~40% of placebo-treated patients and ~44% of ^{90}Sr/^{90}Y-treated patients; excimer laser angioplasty was used in ~7% of placebo-treated patients and ~6% of ^{90}Sr/^{90}Y-treated patients; directional atherectomy was used in ~1% of placebo-treated patients and in none of the ^{90}Sr/^{90}Y-treated patients. New stents were placed with similar frequency in ~20% of placebo-treated patients and ~21% of ^{90}Sr/^{90}Y-treated patients.

The stented segment length was 22.7±10.7 mm, the injured segment length was 25.2±9.2 mm, the radiated segment length was 30.0±5.4 mm, and the analysis segment length was 40.8±9.4 mm.

The residual stenosis was similar in the two groups within the stented segment (22.9%) and within the analysis segment (30.7% in the placebo group and 31.4% in the ^{90}Sr/^{90}Y-treated patients).

At 240 days no difference was found between the 2 groups in clinical events: 1 death in the placebo-treated group versus 3 in the ^{90}Sr/^{90}Y-treated group; 7 non-Q-wave myocardial infarctions in the placebo-treated group versus 4 in the ^{90}Sr/^{90}Y-treated group.

The angiographic restenosis rate was stable in the placebo-treated group (41.2% in the stent segment to 45.2% in the analysis segment), while in the ^{90}Sr/^{90}Y-treated group there was a significantly lower restenosis rate in all measured parameters (14.2% in the stent segment to 28.8% in the analysis segment; P<0.001). This represents a reduction in restenosis rate of 66% in the stent segment and 36% in the analysis segment. Late loss in the placebo-treated group was 0.67 mm in the stent segment and 0.54 mm in the analysis segment; significantly higher than the late loss measured in the ^{90}Sr/^{90}Y-treated group (0.21 mm in the stent segment to 0.28 mm in the analysis segment; P<0.001). Total occlusion was found with similar frequency in 7 (3.7%) placebo-treated patients and 8 (4.0%) ^{90}Sr/^{90}Y-treated patients. There was no new aneurysm formation noted in either group.

The primary study endpoint, 8-month target vessel failure, defined as target vessel revascuariztion, myocardial infarction, or death attributed to the target vessel, was reduced by 31% in patients treated with ^{90}Sr/^{90}Y (25.9% versus 18%; P=0.039). Major adverse cardiac events (MACE) was reduced by 31% (25.9% versus 18%; P=0.039). Target vessel revascularization was reduced by 34% (24.1% versus 16%; P=0.028) and target lesion revascularization was reduced by 42% (22.4% versus 13.1%; P=0.008). There were no episodes of late clinical stent thrombosis in either group at 240 days. Freedom from target vessel failure, defined as target vessel revascularization, myocardial infarction, or death, at 8 months was 82% in the ^{90}Sr/^{90}Y group and 72% in the placebo group.

In addition to the START Trial, an additional study, the START 40 Trial, was subsequently initiated to obtain approval of a 40-mm radiation source train and to potentially help answer questions about the extent to which geographic miss may be avoided. A total of 200 patients will be treated following the START protocol; however all patients will be treated with an "active" 40-mm radiation source train and will be compared to the original START Study.

In the START 40, the patients were older, and had more unstable angina and more prior in-stent restenosis. The preliminary analysis (137 follow-up angiogram, 66% of the cohort) revealed similar reference vessel diameter and the lesion length; interestingly the balloon injury was a little shorter. Compared to placebo, treatment with ^{90}Sr using the 40-mm radiation source train reduced restenosis by 51% (versus 36% in ST30) in the entire analysis segment and by 61% (versus 66% in ST30) in the stent segment. Compared to START 30 patients the frequency of restenosis outside the stent (from the stent segment to the analysis segment) was reduced by 61% (5.7% versus 14.8%, $P<0.05$) while the stent segment restenosis remain unchanged. The reduction in restenosis outside the stent segment suggests that extension of the radiation treatment over the injury can further reduce overall restenosis.

Beta Radiation in Europe: The BRIE Trial

This study was designed to evaluate the safety and efficacy of the Beta-Cath System in patients with up to two discrete (treatable with a 20-mm balloon) de novo or restenotic lesions in different vessels who have undergone stand-alone PTCA or who are candidates for provisional stent placement.[11]

The evaluation was done on the clinical event rates, including freedom from death, CABG, myocardial infarction (Q-wave and non-Q-wave), and target lesion revascularization at 30 days, 6 months, and 1 year.

Lumen dimensions and angiographic restenosis rates at 6 months post procedure were estimated on the follow-up angiogram in all patients. Two doses of radiation were prescribed: 14 Gy at 2 mm in vessels 2.7 to 3.3 mm in reference vessel diameter, or 18 Gy at 2 mm in vessels 3.4 to 4.0 mm in reference vessel diameter. The radiation dose was administered following balloon angioplasty or before stent implantation.

One hundred and fifty patients were included in the BRIE Study. Six-month follow-up was completed by the end of 1999 in 149 patients with 175 lesions. Of these, 123 patients with a single lesion were treated, 59 in the stand-alone PTCA arm and 64 in the provisional stent arm. Of the 59 patients in the stand-alone PTCA arm, 11 patients underwent stent rescue with unplanned stent deployment after radiation treatment, leaving 48 unstented patients. Twenty-six patients with double vessel disease were included, with a total of 52 lesions. Sixteen lesions were enrolled in the stand-alone PTCA arm; two required subsequent stent rescue. The remaining 36 lesions were enrolled in the provisional stent arm of the study.

The radiation was well tolerated by the patients and no interruption of dose delivery was required. There were no acute radiation events. Three patients suffered Q-wave myocardial infarctions during their index hospitalization, one in the PTCA alone arm, and two in the stent arm. Three patients suffered non-Q-wave myocardial infarctions, two in the PTCA arm and one patient who had undergone double vessel treatment. There were no deaths, re-PTCAs, or CABG during the in-hospital period and 143 (96%) patients were free of MACE at discharge. At 30 days, one additional patient suffered a non-Q-wave myocardial infarction. Baseline QCA measurements revealed a mean reference vessel size of 3.06±0.50 mm. The mean lesion length was 11.1±3.9 mm, with an MLD of 1.01±0.31 mm representing a 67±10% diameter stenosis. The mean length of the entire vessel segment for analysis was 41.9±8.2 mm.

Clinical follow-up was obtained in 149 of the 150 patients at 6 months. Cumulative MACE to 6 months occurred in 52 patients representing 34% of the patient cohort. There were three deaths, eight Q-wave myocardial infarctions, and five non-Q-wave myocardial infarctions. Thirty-one patients underwent repeat PTCA and 4 patients underwent CABG.

QCA analysis demonstrated a small late loss with the results maintained within the initial lesion vessel subsegment. Total occlusions were detected in 7 of 88 vessels that had undergone stent deployment. This comprised 6 of 57 treated prior to January 1999 and 1 of 31 vessels treated after January 1999 with the longer antiplatelet regimen. This represents a 69% reduction in frequency of total vessel occlusion with this therapy.

Restenosis was found to be present in 12 of 152 (7.9%) lesions at the proximal edge of the radiation zone, 12 of 152 (7.9%) at the distal edge, and 30 of 152 (19.7%) entirely within the radiation zone. Of the 152 lesions analyzed, 37 were not interpretable for geographic miss, ie, injury by balloon or other device not covered by the prescribed dose of radiation, because of no correct matching of the views between radiation and dilation, not filming the inflations with contrast, no filming of the radiation; 37 show no geographic miss and 78 (51.4%) were recognized with geographic miss. Of these 78, 64 were proximal or distal and 14 were both, for a total of 92 of a potential 304 edges (152 lesions), or 30.3%. A correlation was found between the presence of inadequate radiation cover at the edges and the presence of edge restenosis. This was due to a trend present at the proximal edge and a strong correlation at the distal edge. This provides a relative risk ratio for stenosis at the proximal edge of 3.3 and 6.2 at the distal edge in the presence of inadequate radiation catheter coverage.

The Compassionate Use of Beta Radiation

The predefined enrollment criteria of ongoing randomized trials excluded many patients, but some of these patients were given access to vascular brachytherapy on a compassionate use basis.[12] All the patients reported were excluded for the concurrent Novoste clinical trials, which were limited to shorter native lesions and excluded a multivessel disease.

Ninety-six patients were recruited mostly in Europe (60%) and are included in this report. Eighty-seven percent were treated for in-stent restenosis almost exclusively in native coronary arteries; four stents in saphenous vein grafts were treated. The mean number of prior interventions was 2.4 and 25% of the patients had more than three interventions on the same lesion before this radiation treatment. The mean lesion length was 18±12.9 mm and the mean reference vessel diameter was 2.8±0.53 mm. Only 15.7% new stents were implanted and most patients were treated only with balloon angioplasty (rotablator 7.2%, DCA 1.2%, and laser 10.8%). The dosimetry prescribed in in-stent restenosis was at 2 mm from the source center and 16 and 20 Gy according to the reference vessel diameters (ie, less or greater than 3.35 mm).

The mean follow-up was 192.3±148.2 days, with almost 60% of the population having more than 5 months of follow-up. Total MACE was reported in 15 of the 96 patients (17.7%) with 3 deaths, 3 non-Q-wave myocardial infarctions, and 12 target vessel revascularizations (12.5%). The restenosis rate in the 46 patients who had a follow-up angiogram was at 31.9%, which can be related to the GAMMA-1 Trial (lesion <30 mm) with a 29% restenosis rate in the treated group versus 58% in the placebo.[13] Also, this restenosis rate of the compassionate use of strontium-yttrium beta radiation can be favorably compared to the in-stent trial of ARTIST (Angioplasty vs. Rotablation for the Treatment of diffuse In-STent restenosis) where the rotablator restenosis rate was 64.8% versus 51.2% in the PTCA group (similar population with the same lesion length).[14] In the subgroups of patients with a follow-up angiogram, 9.4% presented a total occlusion; in comparison, in the rotablator group of the ARTIST Trial, 6.6% were found to have total occlusion at 6 months versus only 1.4% in the balloon group.

In conclusion, this compassionate use registry of complex and difficult cases illustrates the high interest in utilizing vascular brachytherapy for in-stent restenosis. Beta radiation with the Beta-Cath System, however, appears feasible and safe in this high-risk population. These results offer promise to the cohort of patients with limited treatment options, particularly those patients with in-stent restenosis.

Proliferation Reduction with Vascular Energy Trial

The Proliferation Reduction with Vascular Energy Trial (PREVENT) is a prospective, randomized, sham-controlled study of intracoronary radiotherapy with a beta-emitting ^{32}P source wire, using a centering catheter and an automated source delivery unit from Guidant Vascular Intervention.[15]

A total of 105 patients with de novo (70%) or restenotic (30%) lesions who were treated by stenting (61%) or balloon angioplasty (39%) received 0 (control) 16, 20, or 24 Gy to a depth of 1 mm into the artery wall. Follow-up angiography at 6 months showed a restenosis rate at the target site that was significantly lower in radiotherapy patients (8% versus 39%; $P=0.012$) and at target site plus adjacent segments (22% versus 50%; $P=0.018$). Target lesion revascularization was needed in 5 radiotherapy patients (6%) and 6 controls (24%; $P<0.05$). Stenosis adjacent to the target site and late thrombotic events reduced the overall clinical benefit of radiotherapy.

Intracoronary Beta Irradiation Following PTCA for Reduction of Restenosis Using the Boston Scientific/Schneider System

This multicenter, prospective, randomized, dose-finding study was conducted between October 1997 and February 1999, and recruited 181 patients in five centers in Europe.[16] The primary objective was to determine the effect of 9, 12, 15, and 18 Gy of intracoronary beta radiation at 1-mm tissue depth on prevention of restenosis following angioplasty on de novo lesions (45 patients per dose group). The secondary objective was to determine the safety and efficacy of the procedure and technique of performance of the beta irradiation system. The lesion length needs to be less than 15 mm and the reference vessel diameter between 2.5 and 4.0 mm. The stent implantation was reserved only for suboptimal PTCA.

The restenosis rate was significantly different in the 9 Gy group versus the 18 Gy group with a restenosis rate of 27.5% in the 9 Gy group versus 8.3% in the 18 Gy group. This significant difference was also recognized at the level of the MLDs with 1.68 mm in the 9 Gy group versus 2.09 mm in the 18 Gy group. No significant difference was recognized between the 12, 15, and 18 Gy groups. In the 110 balloon patients, the difference was even more significant, with a restenosis rate of 4.2% in the 18 Gy group versus 26.1% in the 9 Gy group. No difference in restenosis was found between the different stent groups (25% in the 9 Gy stent group versus 16.7% in the 18 Gy stent group). It has to be noted that 4 occlusions were reported in the 110 PTCA patients and also 4 occlusions in the 38 stented patients at 6 months. Interestingly, 1 death and 4 myocardial infarctions were reported at 6-month follow-up, and a target lesion revascularization rate of only 8.3%, with no difference between groups.

The conclusion of this study was that intracoronary centred beta radiation produced a significant dose-dependent inhibitory effect on restenosis after PTCA and a beneficial effect on remodeling. The delivery of 18 Gy at 1-mm tissue depth results in low overall restenosis rate of 8.3% and even lower rate of 4.2% in patients with balloon angioplasty and radiation alone. The use of the Boston Scientific/Schneider intracoronary radiation system is associated with an excellent feasibility and a MACE-free rate at 6 months of 88.3%.

The Beta Washington Radiation for In-Stent Restenosis

The Beta Washington Radiation for In-Stent Restenosis Trial (WRIST) was designed to examine the safety and efficacy of the Boston Scientific/Schneider beta emitter ^{90}Y system for the prevention of recurrent of in-stent restenosis.[17] Fifty consecutive patients with in-stent restenosis in native coronaries underwent percutaneous coronary intervention. Following these interventions a segmented balloon catheter was positioned and automatically loaded with a ^{90}Y, 0.014-inch source that was 29 mm in length to deliver 20.6 Gy at 1 mm from the balloon surface. Manual stepping of the radiation catheter was necessary in 17 patients for lesions greater than 25 mm. The mean dwell time was 3.0 ± 0.4 minutes and fractionation of the radiation dose, due to ischemia, was required in 11 patients. At 6 months, the angiographic binary restenosis rate was 22%, and the target lesion revascularization rate was 26%, the target vessel revascularization rate was 34%; all rates were significantly lower than those of the placebo group of the gamma WRIST.

The Future

Although the trials of beta radiation on de novo lesions continues to be very encouraging, the value of adding radiation therapy to balloon angioplasty and stenting will only be established by the ongoing randomized trials. The randomized trials will also provide information that may lead to a reduction in stent use, if the provisional angioplasty results are excellent; this information may actually lead to an increase in stent use, if beta radiation proves to be effective in preventing in-stent restenosis. The randomized trials on in-stent restenosis have established radiation therapy as the treatment of choice for this serious disease.

References

1. Liermann D, Böttcher HD, Kollath J, et al. Prophylactic endovascular radiotherapy to prevent intimal hyperplasia after stent implantation in femoropopliteal arteries. Cardiovasc Intervent Radiol 1994;17:12–16.
2. Waksman R, Robinson KA, Crocker R, et al. Endovascular low dose irradiation inhibits neointima formation after coronary artery balloon injury in swine: A possible role for radiation therapy in restenosis prevention. Circulation 1995;91:1533–1539.
3. Wiedermann JG, Marboe C, Amols H, et al. Intracoronary irradiation markedly reduces restenosis after balloon angioplasty in a porcine model. J Am Coll Cardiol 1994; 23:1491–1498.
4. Wiedermann JG, Marboe C, Amols H, et al. Intracoronary irradiation markedly reduces neointimal proliferation after balloon angioplasty in swine: Persistent benefit at 6-month follow-up. J Am Coll Cardiol 1995;25:1451–1456.
5. Waksman R, Robinson KA, Crocker lR, et al. Intracoronary low-dose beta-irradiation inhibits neointima formation after coronary artery balloon injury in the swine restenosis model. Circulation 1995;92:3025–3031.
6. King SB III, Williams DO, Chougule P, et al. Endovascular β-radiation to reduce restenosis after coronary balloon angioplasty: Results of the Beta Energy Restenosis Trial (BERT). Circulation 1998;97:2025–2030.
7. Bonan R. Radioactive therapy to prevent in-stent restenosis. XXth Congress of the European Society of Cardiology, Vienna, Austria, Aug. 22–26, 1998.
8. Meerkin D, Tardif JC, Bonan R, et al. Effects of intracoronary β-radiation therapy after coronary angioplasty: An intravascular ultrasound study. Circulation 1999;99: 1660–1665.
9. Meerkin D, Joyal M, Bonan R, et al. Two year angiographic follow-up after β-radiation for restenosis prevention. AHA 72nd Scientific Sessions, Atlanta, GA, USA, Nov. 7–10, 1999. Circulation 1999;100(suppl I):I–517.
10. Popma J, et al. Late clinical and angiographic outcomes after the use of ^{90}strontium/^{90}yttrium beta radiation for the treatment of in-stent restenosis: Results from the Stents And Radiation Therapy (START) Trial, American College of Cardiology, 2000.
11. Serruys PW, et al. Safety and performance of 90 strontium for treatment of *de novo* and restenosic lesions: The BRIE (Beta Radiation In Europe). ESC 2000. Eur Heart J 2000; 21(suppl):398.
12. Urban P, et al, Intracoronary beta-radiation in compassionate use cases. AHA 72nd Scientific Sessions, Atlanta, GA, USA, Nov. 7–10, 1999. Circulation 1999;100(suppl I): I–75.
13. Leon M, et al. Intracoronary gamma radiation for the prevention of recurrent in-stent restenosis: Final results from the Gamma-1 Trial [abstract]. Circulation 1999;100:I–75.
14. von Dahl J, et al. Angioplasty versus rotational atherectomy for treatment of diffuse in-stent restenosis: Clinical and angiographic results from a randomized multicenter trial (ARTIST study) [abstract]. J Am Coll Cardiol 2000;35:7A.
15. Raizner AE, Osterle SN, Waksman R et al. Inhibition of restenosis with β-emitting radiotherapy: Report of the Proliferation Reduction with Vascular Energy Trial (PREVENT). Circulation 2000;102:951–958.
16. Verin V, et al. Intracoronary β-irradiation following PTCA for reduction of restenosis using the Boston Scientific / Schneider System: A multi-center, prospective, randomized, dose-finding study. ESC 1999.
17. Waksman R, Bhargava B, White L, et al. Intracoronary β-radiation therapy inhibits recurrence of in-stent restenosis. Circulation 2000;101:1895–1898.

Clinical Trials Using Beta Energy Radiation

Experimental and European Clinical Experience with Schneider-Sauerwein Intravascular Radiation System

Vitali Verin, MD, and Youri Popowski, MD

Introduction

Coronary artery disease remains a leading cause of morbidity and mortality in the industrialized world.[1] Percutaneous transluminal coronary angioplasty (PTCA), a technology allowing the reestablishment of normal coronary artery lumen dimension and blood flow, plays a leading role in the contemporary treatment of coronary disease and is annually performed in more than 900,000 patients worldwide.[2] Arterial renarrowing after PTCA, called restenosis, occurs in 30 to 40% of patients, leads to additional patient suffering, frustration among health professionals, and high costs, and represents a major limitation of this technique. Pharmacological approaches to restenosis prevention have so far been disappointing despite extensive theoretical and experimental rationales from a number of trials that have evaluated more then 20 candidate drugs. The advent of coronary stenting led to a significant (30 to 50%) decrease in the restenosis rate.[3–5] Conversely, a new entity of restenosis within stents (in-stent restenosis) emerged and a solution for this phenomenon has not yet been found.[6,7]

Several recent studies have shown the efficacy of intra-arterial gamma irradiation for prevention of relapses after PTCA of restenotic lesions in non-stented and stented arteries.[8–10] However, the wide-scale use of gamma radiation is hampered by significant difficulties related to the radioprotection measures that must be implemented in a conventional catheterization laboratory. Compared to gamma, beta radiation has the significant advantage of being compatible with the environment of an ordinary catheterization laboratory.[11,12] Several beta radiation techniques have been used as an approach for restenosis prevention after PTCA of primary (de novo) coronary lesions.[11–13] Drs. Verin and Popowski, together with Boston Scientific/ Schneider and Isotopen-Technik Dr. Sauerwein, developed a novel technique of endovascular beta irradiation using an endolumenally centered pure metallic yttrium 90 (^{90}Y) source.[14–18] This technique was the first beta radiation modality used in humans.[11]

From Waksman R (ed.). *Vascular Brachytherapy, Third Edition.* Armonk, NY: Futura Publishing Co., Inc.; © 2002.

Intravascular Radiation System

The intra-arterial beta radiation delivery system we described earlier[11,15,18,19] comprises three principal working elements: (1) ^{90}Y beta-emitting source (half-life: 64.1 hours; maximal energy 2.284 MeV); (2) centering balloon allowing homogeneous radiation dose distribution to the vessel wall (Schneider Worldwide, AG, Bülach, Switzerland); and (3) automated afterloader (Isotopen-Technik Dr. Sauerwein, GmbH, Haan, Germany).

The *radioactive source* consists of a 29-mm long flexible coil with an outer diameter of 0.34 mm (0.014") manufactured from titanium-coated pure yttrium wire of 0.1-mm diameter (Fig. 1A). It is secured at the end of a 0.014" thrust wire be-

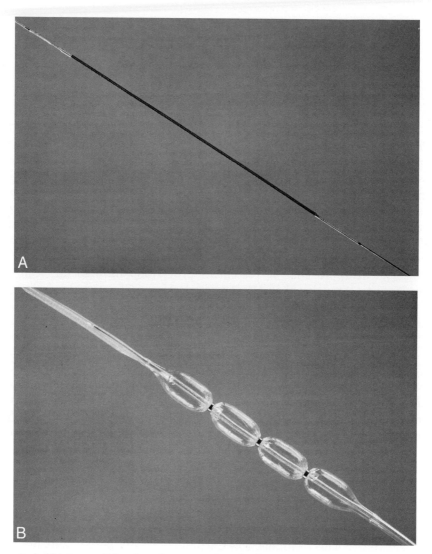

Figure 1. A. Yttrium coil fixed on the extremity of a thrust wire. The coil (arrows) is made of titanium-coated pure yttrium wire. **B.** Centering balloon. The four interconnecting chambers allow centering of the source lumen relative to the arterial lumen. Note the 20-mm-long distal tip of this device ensuring its "monorail" introduction and the three radiopaque tungsten markers situated at sites of balloon waists (arrows).

tween two (distal and proximal) radiopaque tungsten markers which allows for an excellent flexibility of the whole system, and permits precise localization of the source under fluoroscopy. Because the half-life of ^{90}Y is 64 hours, the useful clinical life of a source following activation is in the range of 1 week.

The *centering device* is designed to obtain a central position of the flexible ^{90}Y source inside the arterial lumen (Fig. 1B). It consists of a 30-mm long segmented balloon with four interconnected compartments mounted on a double lumen plastic shaft with an internal (source) blind lumen diameter of 0.40 mm (0.016"). The 20-mm long distal tip of this device enables its introduction in a monorail fashion over a conventional 0.014" angioplasty guidewire. Three radiopaque tungsten markers are located at the balloon waists and allow positioning of the device at the site of the previous angioplasty using fluoroscopy. A flexible stainless steel stylet is placed inside the source lumen of the centering device to optimize tracking of the system through the guiding catheter and the target coronary artery. It is withdrawn prior to source insertion.

The *automated afterloader* (Fig. 1C) makes dose delivery reliable, user-friendly,

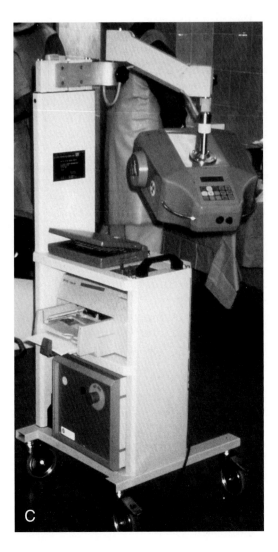

Figure 1. (continued). C. Afterloader.

and provides for an important degree of safety and radiation protection security. The distinguishing features of this device are:

- fully automated irradiation protocol
- automated advancement and positioning of the source
- dedicated dummy source to check friction and to determine exact position
- easy, quick, and safe exchange of the source
- automatic compensation for source decay

The recent evolution of the system consists of implementation of a [144]Ce/Pr beta source. The higher energy of this isotope (3.0 MeV) and longer half-life (285 days) will allow improvement in technical and clinical performances of the system.

Procedure

Interventions are done using local lidocaine 1% anesthesia, anticoagulation with heparin, aspirin, and sedation with benzodiazepines and morphine as needed, according to current practice. After an ordinary successful PTCA procedure through a 6 F or 7 F guiding catheter, a centering device with the same diameter as the balloon used for angioplasty is inserted in the lumen of the artery, and positioned to fully cover the PTCA segment length. After withdrawal of the stylet from the centering device source lumen, the centering balloon is connected to the afterloader and then inflated (Fig. 2) with contrast medium (Iohexol 518 mg/mL, Schering AG, Germany) or CO_2 at a pressure of 2 to 4 bar. Providing a dummy wire can be advanced into, and retrieved without difficulty, from the inflated centering balloon, the ^{90}Y source is then advanced into the centering device by pressing the corresponding afterloader button. The source is left in this position for the time necessary to apply the prescribed dose and then automatically withdrawn. Fluoroscopy is used to confirm the correct position of the dummy and the real sources inside the centering balloon (Fig. 2).

Experimental Study

Twenty-one hypercholesterolemic New Zealand white rabbits (19 females and 2 males) 4 to 5 months of age, were used in the study.

The impact of 6, 12, and 18 Gy radiation doses administered to the balloon-artery interface simultaneously with balloon dilatation was studied. One carotid and one iliac artery were used in each animal, forming four study groups: (1) control group, 11 arteries; (2) 6 Gy group, 11 arteries; (3) 12 Gy group, 10 arteries; (4) 18 Gy group, 10 arteries.

Ten animals were sacrificed at 8 days and 11 at 6 weeks after intervention. A minimum of 5 vessels (3 carotids and 2 iliacs or vice versa) was obtained for each study group at each study endpoint.

For all doses at 8 days compared to controls there was a significant decrease in labeled bromodeoxyuridine (245 ± 93 cell/cm in control, 42 ± 27 in 6 Gy, 72 ± 107 in 12 Gy, 2 ± 2 in 18 Gy groups; $P<0.001$) and in total neointimal cells (891 ± 415 cells/cm in control, 79 ± 43 cells/cm in 6 Gy, 192 ± 264 cells/cm in 12 Gy, and 22 ± 13

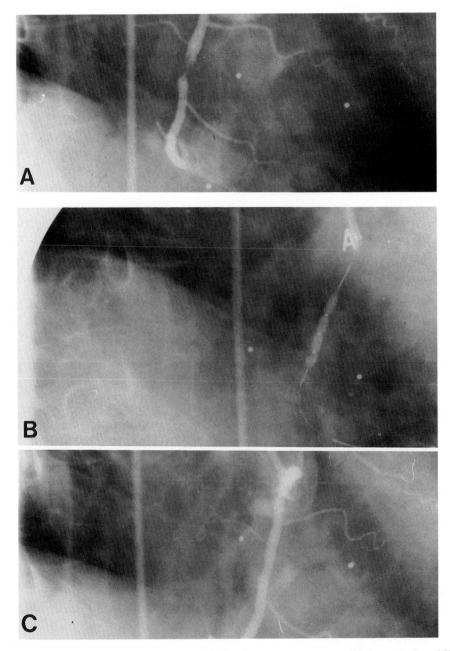

Figure 2. Endoluminal beta irradiation of right coronary artery. Right anterior oblique view. **A.** Tight right coronary artery stenosis. **B.** Intracoronary irradiation procedure. The four compartments of the centering balloon are inflated with contrast medium. The beta-emitting 90Y source is situated inside the centering balloon. Note that the length of the radioactive segment is delimited by two radiopaque tungsten markers (arrowheads). The centering balloon radiopaque waists (arrows) confirm the correct centering of 90Y source inside the artery. **C.** Good immediate angiographic result of PTCA-irradiation procedure.

cells/cm in 18 Gy groups; $P<0.0002$). At 6 weeks (Fig. 3), computer-derived histologic percent area stenosis was reduced from $26\pm10\%$ in the control group to $1\pm1.3\%$ in the 18 Gy group ($P<0.0001$), but lower doses had no significant effect. For arteries irradiated with 18 Gy, the neointimal formation was significantly reduced ($P<0.004$) in the area corresponding to the middle of the balloon as compared with areas corresponding to proximal and distal balloon borders. Further-

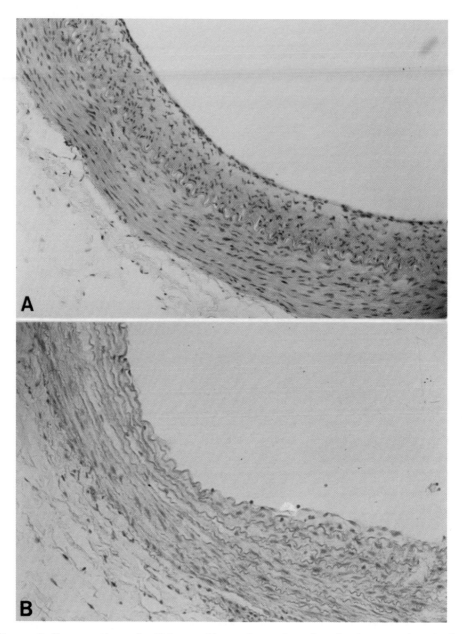

Figure 3. Cross-sections of rabbit carotid arteries at 6 weeks after intervention. **A.** Control artery (magnification ×200) **B.** Artery treated with 18 Gy (magnification ×200). Note near absent neointimal cell proliferation in the irradiated artery.

more, the regions corresponding to the distal and proximal extremities of the irradiated zone showed a trend toward a higher degree of percent area stenosis and an increased number of neointimal cell layers in comparison to the middle of the dilated region of control arteries.

We concluded that radiation doses between 6 and 18 Gy effectively inhibit neointimal smooth muscle cells proliferation as assessed at 8 days in a hypercholesterolemic rabbit model of post-angioplasty restenosis. This inhibitory effect is lost during the following post-treatment weeks in arteries having received radiation doses of 6 or 12 Gy. A radiation dose of 18 Gy effectively induces long-term inhibition of neointimal hyperplasia. The mild increase in neointimal proliferation in areas proximal and distal to the balloon suggest that the irradiated arterial segment should be at least as long as the injured (dilated) arterial segment, and perhaps even slightly longer.

Clinical Pilot Study

The purpose of the pilot study was to evaluate in a clinical setting: (1) the feasibility of intra-arterial beta radiation delivery, and (2) the safety of an 18 Gy beta radiation dose delivered to the inner arterial surface during a 6-month follow-up period.

Patients older than 64 years scheduled to undergo angioplasty of one of the native coronary arteries because of angina were eligible for the study. The target lesion was required to have a 50% or greater diameter stenosis by quantitative coronary angiography (QCA), to be less than 20-mm long, and to be located in a vessel with a 2.5-mm reference diameter or greater.

Between June 21 and November 15, 1995, 15 patients (6 women and 9 men, aged 71 ± 5 years) underwent intracoronary beta irradiation with an intra-arterially centered ^{90}Y source immediately after a conventional PTCA procedure.

In all, the PTCA-irradiation procedure was technically feasible and the delivery of the 18 Gy dose to the inner arterial surface was accomplished without any complication (Fig. 2).

Two cardiologists, one radiation oncologist, and one technician remained in the catheterization laboratory during the entire procedure. Only routine radioprotection measures were used. During intracoronary irradiation, the radiation dose in contact with the patient's right chest side was 24 ± 7 mSv/h (range, 15 to 30) and no radiation was detectable at the level of the operator's head. In comparison, during fluoroscopy in the same positions, the radiation doses were 45 ± 25 mSv/h (range, 30 to 100) and 20 ± 3 mSv/h (range, 15 to 25), respectively (Monitor 4, S.E. International, USA).

During the follow-up period of 178 ± 17 days (range, 150 to 225 days) at least one clinical event occurred in 5 of the 15 patients. Angiographic restenosis occurred in 6 patients (40%; 95% confidence interval 16 to 68%). The minimal luminal diameter, reference vessel diameter, nd percent diameter stenosis were 0.9 ± 0.4 mm, 2.8 ± 0.5 mm, and $68\pm12\%$ at baseline; 2.5 ± 0.6 mm, 2.7 ± 0.5 mm, and $11\pm8\%$ just after the procedure; and 1.7 ± 0.9 mm, 2.7 ± 0.7 mm, and $39\pm25\%$ at 6-month follow-up, respectively. In 4 patients with restenosis, repeat PTCA of the lesion treated with beta irradiation was performed. All PTCA procedures for restenosis performed in the irradiated arterial segments were uncomplicated and lead to good angiographic results.

Results of a Prospective, Randomized, Multicenter, European Dose-Finding Study

To establish the optimal therapeutic dose of the centered beta radiation with ^{90}Y de novo coronary lesions, a multicenter, prospective, randomized study was performed between October 1997 and August 1999.

Following successful angioplasty, 181 patients were randomly assigned to receive 9, 12, 15, or 18 Gy delivered by a ^{90}Y source through a centering balloon. Adjunctive stent implantation was required in 28% of patients. The primary endpoint was the difference in minimal lumen diameter (MLD) at 6 months between the dose groups, measured by QCA.

The 6-month QCA was available in 169 patients (93%) showing the MLD of 1.63, 1.76, 1.83, and 1.97 mm in the 9, 12, 15, and 18 Gy dose groups, respectively (P=0.036, 18 versus 9 Gy). This resulted in the corresponding restenosis rates of 30%, 21%, 16%, and 15% (P=0.12, 18 versus 9 Gy). In 120 patients treated with balloon angioplasty alone, the corresponding MLD was 1.62, 1.82, 1.80, and 2.1 mm (P=0.003, 18 versus 9 Gy) resulting in restenosis rates of 30%, 17%, 16%, and 4% (P=0.016, 18 versus 9 Gy). The corresponding absolute loss in lumen diameter from the post-procedural result to follow-up in these patients was 0.31, 0.12, 0.09, and – 0.04 mm which led to a dose-dependent lumen enlargement in 25%, 40%, 50%, and 62% of patients, respectively.

In 49 patients treated with stents, the corresponding MLD was 1.67, 1.62, 1.89, and 1.73 mm (P=NS) resulting in restenosis rates of 30%, 33%, 15%, and 36% (P=NS). The 4 acute and 3 chronic occlusions were mostly responsible for the restenosis in stented arteries.

The overall freedom from major adverse cardiac events was 85.6% and the target lesion revascularization rate was 10.5%.

Discussion

With the aim of reducing the development of atherosclerosis, the first in vivo use of intravascular radiotherapy was reported 32 years ago by Friedman et al.[20] The concept was then more recently revived by Liermann et al.[21] in order to modulate the post-angioplasty restenotic process, and a number of animal studies have documented the favorable impact of intraluminal gamma irradiation on the occurrence of neointimal hyperplasia in several animal models.[19,22–25] Liermann et al.[21,26] used a ^{192}Ir source for irradiation of femoropopliteal arterial segments after stent implantation. The use of a gamma source made it necessary to transport patients from the catheterization laboratory to a shielded afterloading room prior to radiation treatment. A dose of 12 Gy was prescribed at a 3-mm distance from the source, but no centering was used. Follow-up periods of up to 69 months in 29 patients suggest a favorable impact on restenosis and show excellent clinical tolerance, with no vascular or perivascular side effects.[27] Condado et al.[28] were the first to report the use of intracoronary gamma irradiation, also using a ^{192}Ir source. A dose of either 20 or 25 Gy was prescribed and no acute complications were noted.

To the best of our knowledge, our clinical pilot study represents the first report on the clinical use of endovascular beta irradiation. In a similar manner to gamma sources, endovascular beta irradiation is also remarkably effective in different animal models to prevent fibrointimal proliferation in response to vessel injury.[19] The use of beta sources has several advantages over gamma irradiation: (1) lower undue irradiation of surrounding periarterial structures, due to a steeper depth-dose fall-off curve; (2) fewer radioprotection problems, making it compatible with a conventional catheterization laboratory; and (3) ability to deliver a high focal dose over a short period of time.

The pilot study demonstrated feasibility and lack of medium term toxicity of an 18 Gy dose of beta irradiation delivered to the balloon-artery interface (9 Gy at 1-mm tissue depth). The steep dose fall-off also makes it important to center the source within the vascular lumen, and such centering is a distinguishing feature of our approach when compared to other systems. Centering of the source is intended to homogenize the radiation dose delivered to different points of the arterial wall within the treated segment. In the case of atherosclerotic human coronary arteries, the target smooth muscle cells are situated within a thin walled (0.3 to 2 mm thick) tubular structure. Endoluminal inflation of the centering balloon forces the target tissues to occupy a position as equidistant as possible in respect to the radiation source, thereby allowing good circumferential and axial dose distribution. The increased distance between the source and arterial wall induced by balloon inflation can be compensated for by an appropriately calculated exposure time. It is obvious that an eccentric intraluminal position of the source would result in areas of both relative under- and overdose with respect to the prescribed dose level. This could be clinically relevant, since it has been suggested that low radiation doses may stimulate rather than inhibit neointimal proliferation,[19,22] while higher doses (30 Gy or more) could lead to late vascular complications.[29,30] As discussed earlier, in the hypercholesterolemic rabbit model, the delivery of 9 Gy radiation dose at 1 mm of tissue depth demonstrated marked inhibition of neointimal hyperplasia. The same radiation dose used in the clinical pilot series, however, did not suggest any positive impact on restenosis. We hypothesized that higher radiation doses were necessary since the arterial wall in the human is thicker than in the rabbit. Thus, the primary objective of the European Dose-Finding study was to determine the effect of 9, 12, 15, and 18 Gy of beta irradiation at 1-mm tissue depth on prevention of restenosis following a first coronary angioplasty. The secondary objectives were to determine the safety of the procedure and the technical performance of the ^{90}Y intracoronary beta irradiation system.

In summary, the results of the European multicenter Dose-Finding Study indicate that a marked dose-dependent reduction in restenosis rate can be achieved with the help of intracoronary beta irradiation. In non-stented arteries, the greatest reduction in restenosis rate was achieved in the highest dose group (3.9% versus 30.3% in the 9 Gy group), likely due to a beneficial effect of radiation on remodeling and an inhibitory effect on neointima formation. These findings do not suggest any favorable impact of beta radiation on restenosis in stented arteries. There was an excess incidence of subacute thrombosis and late arterial occlusions in stented arteries compared with non-stented. These findings provide important insights into potential therapeutic applications of beta radiation immediately after PTCA.

The extremely low restenosis rate observed in the highest dose group of this study suggests that this technology could be considered a first-line adjunct to PTCA. No device or pharmaceutical approach to date has yielded similarly low restenosis rates. The lowest restenosis rate of 16% at 6 months has been reported with stents.[5] The effect of stents to almost halve restenosis rates led to a world-wide expansion of this technology and well over 60% of coronary interventions are now accomplished using stent implantation.[31] Our data indicate that, with the use of radiation, an incidence of relapses below 5% is achievable. These findings have important implications for the practice of interventional cardiology. First, these findings imply that radiation could replace stents in the prevention of restenosis. Indeed, if our findings are confirmed, patients with good angiographic results after PTCA alone (which represents at least 50% of patients) could benefit from adjunctive beta radiation without stenting. A primary virtue of stents is the prevention of acute occlusions occurring in 3 to 8% of patients after ordinary PTCA.[32] Clearly, intracoronary beta radiation cannot replace stents for this indication. However, our study strongly suggests that radiation is superior to a stent as far as restenosis prevention is concerned. Definitive proof will require a randomized trial comparing PTCA with adjunctive beta radiation therapy versus stenting.

Our data suggest that caution should be exercised at this point when combining radiation with stents. We observed more acute thrombosis and late vessel occlusions in stented arteries as compared with non-stented arteries and this finding is consistent with recent reports by others.[33,34] In the beginning of the stent era, in the late 1980s, the problem of acute stent thrombosis emerged. This complication occurred in about 25% of cases during the first 2 weeks after stenting.[35,36] The bulk of scientific evidence indicates that the presence of a highly thrombogenic metallic foreign body noncovered by the endothelium is the cause of thrombosis.[35,36] Interestingly, stent thrombosis very rarely occurs at later time points (after 2 weeks) when the stent is completely covered by ingrowing arterial wall tissue. It is well known that the introduction of antiplatelet treatment with a combination of aspirin and ticlopidine for 4 weeks following stenting decreased the incidence of subacute stent thrombosis to below 1%.[37] We believe that, in the case of the combination of beta radiation with stenting, the increase in the incidence of late stent thrombosis is related to delayed stent coverage by arterial wall tissue. In other words, the virtue of radiation, which is to limit the proliferation of arterial wall tissue necessary for prevention of restenosis, can lead to a longer persisting risk of stent thrombosis. A very logical solution for this problem is the prolongation of antiplatelet therapy for several additional months (4 weeks in our study). We believe that further studies addressing the issue of safety and efficacy of beta radiation in stented arteries using longer-term antiplatelet coverage are necessary.

The current study shows outstanding results with the 18 Gy dose delivered at 1 mm tissue depth with the Boston Scientific/Schneider System. It is difficult, however, to compare these results with those of gamma radiation trials because different patient populations were studied (in-stent restenosis in SCRIPPS, WRIST, and GAMMA-1 trials versus de novo lesions in our study). From the radiation biology standpoint beta radiation should be as effective as gamma providing similar doses are delivered to the target tissue. We believe that the radiation system we used, because of its virtue of homogeneous dose distribution due to centering, can be even more efficacious than currently available noncentered gamma radiation systems.

The results of ^{90}Y dosimetry and intraprocedural measurements indicate that patients and catheterization laboratory personnel receive very low exposure using beta radiation systems.[11,12] Thus, the additional radiation will not lead to an excess over authorized levels and will not necessitate changes in the radiation protection conditions of conventional catheterization laboratories. In this regard, the major advantage of beta irradiation in comparison with gamma is the possibility for the interventional cardiologist to remain at the patient's side during the whole irradiation procedure. Our experience demonstrates that the study technique is user-friendly and can easily be included in standard angioplasty procedures. In addition, in cases of proven efficacy, this treatment can prevent the need for 20 to 30% of patients to have subsequent irradiation because of additional diagnostic and interventional procedures related to relapses.

Future Perspectives

We believe that the main findings of the European Dose-Finding Study have important implications for the field of interventional cardiology. The current practice in interventional cardiology is characterized by the "bigger is better" paradigm. Thus, the "bigger" the lumen dimension achieved during a coronary intervention the "better" the long-term result.[4,38] Currently, the biggest arterial lumen can undoubtedly be obtained with the use of coronary stents.[4,38] In addition, stents are capable of eliminating a negative (unfavorable) remodeling of the artery related to excessive constriction of the healing arterial wall during the months following injury by PTCA. Stents, however, do not inhibit the proliferative component of restenosis.[4,38] Despite the fact that this cellular proliferation inside stents results in a systematic decrease in lumenal dimension during the months following the intervention, the final lumen is nevertheless larger than that achieved by ordinary PTCA.[3,4,38] We believe that intracoronary beta radiation has the potential to introduce a change in this paradigm because of its capacity to interfere not only with proliferation of arterial wall smooth muscles cells and fibroblasts, but also because of its favorable effect on the arterial wall healing process. Similar to its effect on the healing surgical wound,[39,40] beta irradiation decreases chronic arterial constriction leading to arterial dilation as seen at follow-up. Thus, should further randomized trials confirm the safety and efficacy of intracoronary beta irradiation, its use will likely be generalized, allowing interventional cardiology to achieve the same long-term event-free survival as has been achieved with coronary artery bypass surgery.[41]

Conclusion

Intracoronary centered beta irradiation produces a significant dose-dependent decrease in restenosis rate after balloon angioplasty. The 18 Gy dose not only prevents the renarrowing of the lumen typically observed following successful balloon angioplasty, but also induces vessel enlargement. The absence of a favorable impact of intracoronary beta radiation on restenosis in arteries stented during the procedure is related to an excess incidence of acute and chronic occlusions. Whether the long-term use of contemporary antiplatelet therapy will improve the results of combined treatment by stenting and beta radiation awaits further investigation.

Appendix

The participating centers and investigators of the Dose-Finding Study Group are listed, with the number of patients included in parentheses.

- University Hospital, Geneva, Switzerland (57): Vitali Verin, MD, Youri Popowski, MD, Patrice Delafontaine, MD, John Kurtz, MD, Igor Papirov, PhD, Airiian Sergey, MD, Philippe Debruyne, MD, Jose Ramos de Olival, MD.
- Cardiovascular Center, Onze-Lieve-Vrouw Ziekenhuis, Aalst, Belgium (54): William Wijns, MD (Principal Investigator), Bernard de Bruyne, MD, Guy Heyndrickx, MD, Luc Verbeke, MD, Marleen Piessens, PhD, Jo De Jans, MSc.
- University Hospital, Essen, Germany (26): Dietrich Baumgart, MD, Wolfgang Sauerwein, MD, Raimund Erbel, MD, Michael Haude, MD, Dirk Flühs, PhD, Ulrich Quast, PhD, Andrea Müller, MD, Katelin Hidgeghty, MD, Clemens von Birgelen, MD.
- University Hospital, Kiel, Germany (22): Markus Lins, MD, Ruediger Simon, MD, Gyorgy Kovacs, MD, Martin Thomas, MD, Gunhild Herrmann, MD, Roland Wilhelm, MD, Peter Kohl, MD.
- Kings College Hospital, London, United Kingdom (22): Martyn Thomas, MD, Francis Calman, MD, Niel Lewis, PhD.
- Study Coordination: Thomas Thaler, PhD (Boston Scientific)
- Critical Events Committee: Jaap Dekkers, MD, Patrick Serruys, MD.
- Angiographic Core-Laboratory and Data Analysis: Yvonne Teunissen, PhD (Clinical Trial Manager), Astrid Spierings, Connie van der Wiel, Gitte Kloek, MSc, Clemens Disco, PhD.

References

1. Kannel WB. Incidence, prevalence and mortality of coronary artery disease. In: Fuster V, Ross R, Topol EJ (eds.): Atherosclerosis and Coronary Artery Disease. Philadelphia: Lippincott-Raven; 1996:13–24.
2. Bittl JA. Advances in coronary angioplasty. N Engl J Med 1996;335:1290–1302.
3. Serruys P, de Jaegere P, Kiemeneij F, et al, for the Benestent Study Group. A comparison of balloon-expandable-stent implantation with balloon angioplasty in patients with coronary artery disease. N Engl J Med 1994;331:489–495.
4. Fischman DL, Leon MB, Baim DS, et al, for the Stent Research group. A randomized comparison of coronary-stent placement and balloon angioplasty in the treatment of coronary artery disease. N Engl J Med 1994;331:496–501.
5. Serruys PW, van Hout B, Bonnier H, et al. Randomized comparison of implantation of heparin-coated stents with balloon angioplasty in selected patients with coronary artery disease (Benestent II). Lancet 1998;352:673–681.
6. Eltchaninoff H, Koning R, Tron C, et al. Balloon angioplasty for the treatment of coronary in-stent restenosis: Immediate results and six-month angiographic recurrent restenosis rate. J Am Coll Cardiol 1998;32:980–984.
7. vom Dahl J, Radke PW, Haager PK, et al. Clinical and angiographic predictors of recurrent restenosis after percutaneous transluminal rotational atherectomy for treatment of diffuse in-stent restenosis. Am J Cardiol 1999;83:862–867.
8. Teirstein PS, Massullo V, Jani S, et al. Catheter-based radiotherapy to inhibit restenosis after coronary stenting. N Engl J Med 1997;336:1697–1703.
9. Waksman R, White RL, Chan RC, et al. Intracoronary gamma-radiation therapy after angioplasty inhibits recurrence in patients with in-stent restenosis. Circulation 2000; 101:2165–2171.
10. Leon MB, Teirstein PS, Lansky AJ. Intracoronary gamma radiation to reduce in-stent

restenosis: The multicenter randomized GAMMA-1 clinical trial [abstract]. J Am Coll Cardiol 1999;33:56A.

11. Verin V, Urban P, Popowski Y, et al. Feasibility of intracoronary beta irradiation to reduce restenosis after balloon angioplasty: A clinical pilot study. Circulation 1997;95: 1138–1144.

12. King SB III, Williams DO, Chougule P, et al. Endovascular β-radiation to reduce restenosis after coronary balloon angioplasty: Results of the Beta Energy Restenosis Trial (BERT). Circulation 1998;97:2025–2030.

13. Lee DP, Lo S, Forster KM, et al. Intracoronary radiation with a 32P source wire. Herz 1998;23:362–365.

14. Popowski Y, Verin V, Urban P, et al. Intra-arterial yttrium-90 brachytherapy for restenosis prevention. In: Mould GBRF (ed.): Freiburg Oncology Series, Brachytherapy Review, Vol. Monograph No. 1. Freiburg, Germany: Albert-Ludwigs-University; 1994: 163–165.

15. Popowski Y, Verin V, Papirov I, et al. High dose rate brachytherapy for prevention of restenosis after percutaneous transluminal coronary angioplasty: Preliminary dosimetric tests of a new source presentation. Int J Radiat Oncol Biol Phys 1995;33:211– 215.

16. Popowski Y, Verin V, Papirov I, et al. Intra-arterial 90-yttrium brachytherapy: Preliminary dosimetric study using a specially modified angioplasty balloon. Int J Radiat Oncol Biol Phys 1995;33:713–717.

17. Popowski Y, Verin V, Urban P. Endovascular beta-irradiation after percutaneous transluminal coronary balloon angioplasty. Int J Radiat Oncol Biol Phys 1996;36:841–845.

18. Popowski Y, Verin V, Schwager M, et al. A novel system for intracoronary β-irradiation: Description and dosimetric results. Int J Radiat Oncol Biol Phys 1996;36:923–931.

19. Verin V, Popowski Y, Urban P, et al. Intraarterial beta irradiation prevents neointimal hyperplasia in a hypercholesterolemic rabbit restenosis model. Circulation 1995;92: 2284–2290.

20. Friedman M, Felton L, Byers S. The antiatherogenic effect of iridium 192 upon the cholesterol-fed rabbit. J Clin Invest 1964;43:185–192.

21. Liermann D, Bottcher HD, Kollath J, et al. Prophylactic endovascular radiotherapy to prevent intimal hyperplasia after stent implantation in femoropopliteal arteries. Cardiovasc Intervent Radiol 1994;17:12–16.

22. Wiedermann JG, Marboe C, Amols H, et al. Intracoronary irradiation markedly reduces restenosis after balloon angioplasty in a porcine model. J Am Coll Cardiol 1994; 23:1491–1498.

23. Wiedermann JG, Marboe C, Amols H, et al. Intracoronary irradiation markedly reduces neointimal proliferation after balloon angioplasty in swine: Persistent benefit at six-month follow-up. J Am Coll Cardiol 1995;25:1451–1456.

24. Waksman R, Robinson KA, Crocker IR, et al. Endovascular low-dose irradiation inhibits neointima formation after coronary artery balloon injury in swine. Circulation 1995;91:1533–1539.

25. Waksman R, Rodriguez JC, Robinson KA, et al. Effect of intravascular irradiation on cell proliferation, apoptosis and vascular remodeling after balloon overstretch injury of porcine coronary arteries. Circulation 1997;96:1944–1952.

26. Bottcher HD, Schopohl B, Liermann D, et al. Endovascular irradiation: A new method to avoid recurrent stenosis after stent implantation in peripheral arteries: Technique and preliminary results. Int J Radiat Oncol Biol Phys 1994;29:183–186.

27. Schopohl B, Jüling-Pohlit L, Böttcher HD, et al. Endovascular irradiation for avoidance of recurrent stenosis after stent implantation in peripheral arteries: Five years followup. In: Discoveries in Radiation For Restenosis. Atlanta, GA: Emory University School of Medicine; 1996:89–92.

28. Condado JA, Gurdiel O, Espinoza R, et al. Percutaneous transluminal coronary angioplasty and intracoronary radiation therapy: A possible new modality for the treatment of coronary restenosis. A preliminary report of the first 10 patients treated with intracoronary radiation therapy. J Am Coll Cardiol 1995;(suppl[Feb]):288A.

29. Gillette EL, Powers BE, McChesney SL, Withrow SJ. Aortic wall injury following intraoperative irradiation. Int J Radiat Oncol Biol Phys 1988;15:1401–1406.

30. Gillette EL, Powers BE, McChesnay SL, et al. Response of aorta and branch arteries

to experimental intraoperative irradiation. Int J Radiat Oncol Biol Phys 1989;17: 1247–1255.

31. Topol EJ. Coronary-artery stents: Gauging, gorging and gouging. N Engl J Med 1998; 339:1702–1704.

32. Ryan TJ, Bauman WB, Kennedy JW, et al. ACC/AHA task force report: Guidelines for percutaneous transluminal coronary angioplasty. J Am Coll Cardiol 1993;22:2033–2054.

33. Costa MA, Sabaté M, Giessen WJ, et al. Late coronary occlusion after intracoronary brachytherapy. Circulation 1999;100:789–792.

34. Waksman R. Late thrombosis after radiation: Sitting on a time bomb. Circulation 1999; 100:780–782.

35. Goy JJ, Sigwart U, Vogt P, et al. Long-term follow-up of the first 56 patients treated with intracoronary self-expanding stents (the Lausanne Experience). Am J Cardiol 1991;67:569–572.

36. Serruys PW, Strauss BH, Beatt KJ, et al. Angiographic follow-up after placement of a self-expanding coronary-artery stent. N Engl J Med 1991;324:1595–1598.

37. Schomig A, Neumann FJ, Kastrati A, et al. A randomized comparison of antiplatelet and anticoagulant therapy after the placement of coronary-artery stents. N Engl J Med 1996;334:1084–1089.

38. Kuntz RE, Gibson CM, Nobuyoshi M, Baim DS. Generalized model of restenosis after conventional balloon angioplasty, stenting and directional atherectomy. J Am Coll Cardiol 1993;21:15–25.

39. Gorodetsky R, McBride WH, Withers HR. Assay of radiation effects in mouse skin as expressed in wound healing. Radiat Res 1988;116:135–144.

40. Vegesna V, Withers HR, Holly FE, McBride WH. The effect of local and systemic irradiation on impairment of wound healing in mice. Radiat Res 1993;135:431–433.

41. Solomon AJ, Gersh BJ. Management of chronic stable angina: Medical therapy, percutaneous transluminal coronary angioplasty and coronary artery bypass graft surgery. Lessons from the randomized trials. Ann Intern Med 1998;128:216–223.

Part IX

Systems for Endovascular Radiation Therapy

## Chapter 52

Cordis Checkmate™:

Manually Loaded Iridium 192 Ribbon

Shirish K. Jani, PhD, Guo Long Chu, PhD,
Gerard B. Huppe, BS, Vincent Massullo, MD,
Prabhakar Tripuraneni, MD, and Paul Teirstein, MD

Introduction

Radioactive iridium 192 (^{192}Ir) has been used for a long time in conventional brachytherapy for the treatment of cancer. The physical and radiation properties of ^{192}Ir are somewhat unique in qualifying its entry into vascular applications. Iridium has a very high specific activity and therefore a source small enough to traverse through narrow coronary lumen can possess high enough activity to deliver a decent dose to arterial wall within a reasonable time. Some of the earliest animal experiments in coronary irradiation were conducted with ^{192}Ir by Weidermann et al[1] and Waksman et al.[2] High intensity ^{192}Ir using a remotely loaded system was first used in human coronary artery by Condado et al[3] and in peripheral vessels by Böttcher et al.[4] The first randomized double-blind trial on radiotherapy for treating or preventing restenosis was initiated in March 1994 at the Scripps Clinic in La Jolla, CA. The Scripps Coronary Radiation to Inhibit Proliferation Post Stenting (SCRIPPS) Trial used radioactive ^{192}Ir seeds (manufactured by Best Medical International, Springfield, VA) embedded in a nylon ribbon to form arrays of various lengths. Although the number of patients enrolled was small (55), it showed a significant reduction in the rate of further narrowing of the lumen among patients with known restenosis.[5,6] The Washington Radiation for In-Stent Restenosis (WRIST) Trial demonstrated similar potential benefits of localized radiation using ^{192}Ir in treating coronary restenosis.[7] In mid-1997, Cordis Corporation (A Johnson and Johnson Company, Miami Lakes, FL) entered into a partnership with Best Medical International to guide and support all the subsequent multi-institutional human trials using the ^{192}Ir radioactive seeds. This chapter will describe the basic properties of the ^{192}Ir radioisotope, the evolution of the delivery device under the leadership of Cordis, and a brief summary of the clinical trials conducted so far. At the time of this writing, the Cordis ^{192}Ir system had gained the approval of the panel convened by the U.S. Food and Drug Administration (FDA) and FDA approval to market this product was expected in the near future.

From Waksman R (ed.). *Vascular Brachytherapy, Third Edition.* Armonk, NY: Futura Publishing Co., Inc.; © 2002.

The Iridium 192 Radioisotope

Iridium, a metal of the platinum family, is white, similar to platinum, but with a slight yellowish cast. It is very hard and the most corrosion-resistant metal known. The specific gravity (or commonly called density) of iridium is very close to that of osmium which is believed to be the heaviest known element in our universe. It is measured to be about 22.5 gm/cc. In comparison, water or soft tissue in the human body has a density of 1 gm/cc and lead, commonly used as shielding material in radiology, has a density of 11.4 gm/cc. The atomic number of iridium is 77. In nature, it occurs with two different atomic mass values, 191 with a natural abundance of 38.5% and 193 with a natural abundance of 193. Iridium with all other mass values is unstable and, hence, radioactive. Iridium 192 is formed in a nuclear reactor when stable [191]Ir absorbs a neutron. Shipment of ^{192}Ir seeds to users is usually delayed until about 2 weeks after the seeds are removed from the nuclear reactor. This is to ensure that the amount of [194]Ir produced by the activation of [193]Ir in the seed core is almost completely depleted (the half-life of [194]Ir is 18 hours).

Iridium 192 decays mostly via negative beta emission (95.6%) to [192]Pt (platinum, Z=78). The excited nuclei of platinum reach the stable state by emitting a number of gamma rays in the energy range of 0.136 to 1.06 MeV, the primary emission is in the 0.3 to 0.6 MeV range. The maximum energy of beta emission is 0.67 MeV. The average energy of gamma radiation is about 0.37 MeV. Iridium 192 decays with a half-life of 74.2 days. Its half-value layer in lead is about 3 mm.[8,9]

The Iridium192 Source Ribbon

An individual seed source of ^{192}Ir is very small in size (0.05 cm diameter × 0.3 cm length) and contains a mixture of iridium (30%) and platinum (70%) in a stainless steel housing.[10] Figure 1 shows a schematic drawing of an individual source. These sources are embedded in a nylon ribbon to achieve a linear source of 2- to 10-cm active length. The spacing between seed sources may vary depending upon the application. For coronary irradiation where target tissues may be just a few millimeters away, a spacing of no more than 1 mm between adjacent seeds is recommended. Figure 2 shows a schematic drawing of ^{192}Ir seed

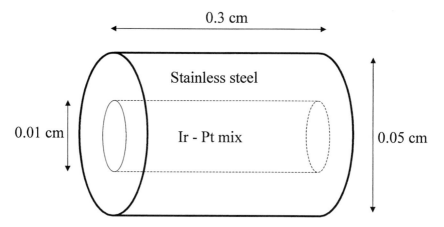

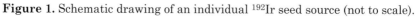

Figure 1. Schematic drawing of an individual ^{192}Ir seed source (not to scale).

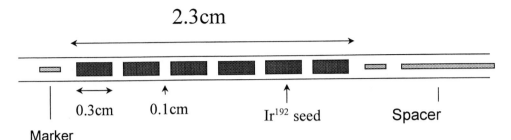

Figure 2. Schematic drawing of ^{192}Ir seed arrangement in nylon ribbon. These lengths of radioactive segment were initially chosen to match the required length of tissues to be irradiated around 1 or 2 Palmaz-Schatz stents. Figure is not drawn to scale.

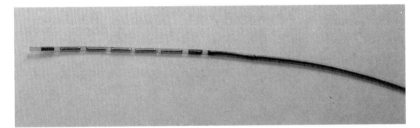

Figure 3. ^{192}Ir source ribbon manufactured by Best Medical International of Springfield, VA.

sources in nylon ribbon as used in the SCRIPPS and WRIST Trials. For irradiating peripheral arteries where arterial dimensions may be several millimeters, a seed spacing of greater than 1 mm may be acceptable. In any case, some amount of spacing between seeds is necessary to achieve flexibility of the active length to insert the ribbon to its target through a curved path. Figure 3 shows a photograph of a ^{192}Ir source ribbon manufactured by Best Medical International. The ribbon has an active tip that varies in length from ~3 to ~7 cm. The overall length of the nylon ribbon is 300 cm. It can be color-coded for sorting in clinical use.

The Iridium 192 Delivery Device

As stated earlier, ^{192}Ir emits gamma rays with moderately high energy. Therefore, the storage and transfer of the source ribbons require shielded containers in order to minimize exposure levels around them. Figure 4 shows a photograph of the original transfer container used in all the SCRIPPS, WRIST, and GAMMA Trials. It houses the radioactive ribbon at its center. The container has a sufficient amount of lead to stop most of the emitted gammas so that shipping and handling of the ribbons is safe. The container was designed and fabricated by Best Medical International for Cordis and it housed placebo ribbon during the randomized phase of the clinical trials.

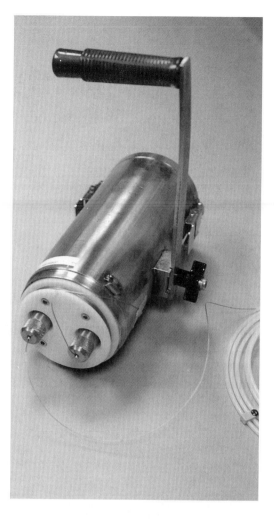

Figure 4. Transfer container for housing a ^{192}Ir ribbon, manufactured by Best Medical International of Springfield, VA, for Cordis Corporation.

Cordis has developed a new delivery system based on a hand-crank mechanism. The source ribbon, a delivery catheter, and its delivery system constitute the Cordis Checkmate system. Figures 5A through 5D show the delivery system and its components. At present, the system allows arrays of 6, 10, and 14 seeds with corresponding active lengths of 23, 39, and 55 mm. The system is intended for use in vessels 2.75 to 4.0 mm in diameter and for in-stent restenotic lesions of up to 45 mm in length.

The radiation delivery catheter (also called Checkmate Catheter) is a single lumen catheter with a distal rapid exchange tip which serves as a conduit for the nonradioactive dummy ribbon and the radioactive ^{192}Ir source ribbon. The catheter contains a single, closed-end source lumen that is isolated from the blood contact. The source lumen is accessed through a single port hub. A single radiopaque marker identifies the distal end of the source lumen and is located slightly proximal to the guidewire port.

To date, the hand-crank delivery device of the Cordis Checkmate System has been used only in Europe. Its use in the U.S. has not yet been initiated.

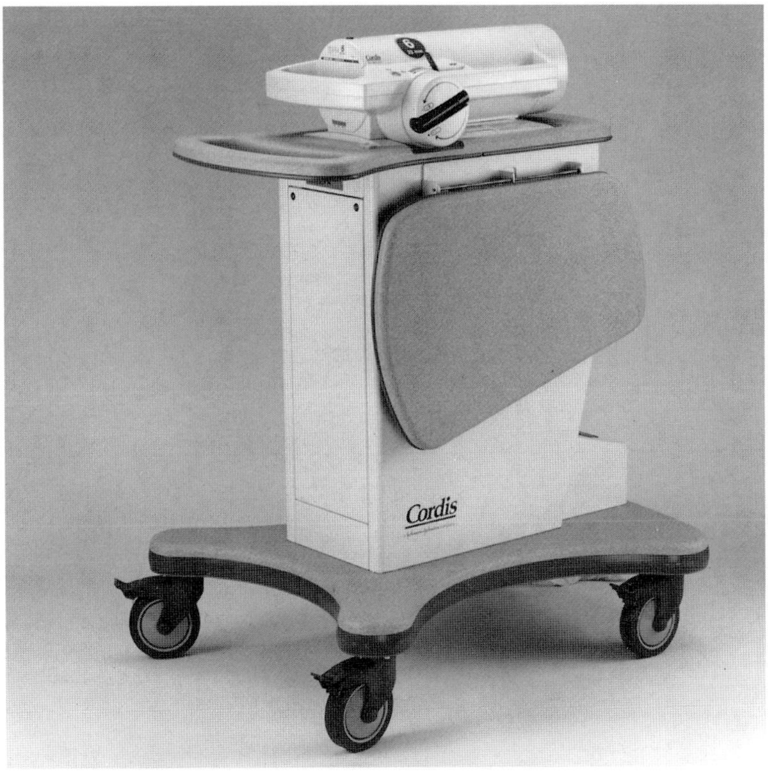

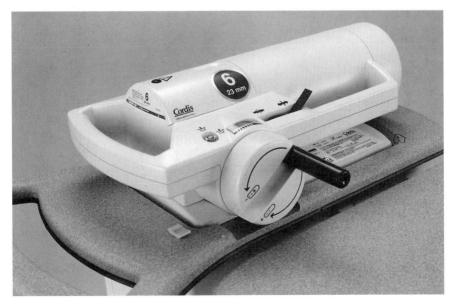

Figure 5A. Cordis Checkmate: radiation delivery system. The entire system is on a cart for easy transport.

Figure 5B. A side view of Cordis Checkmate source housing. It is marked clearly with number of seeds and radioactive length, and allows hand-crank delivery of source.

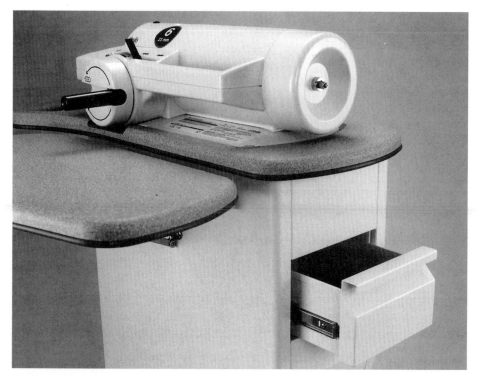

Figure 5C. A front view of Cordis Checkmate source housing showing connector to delivery catheter.

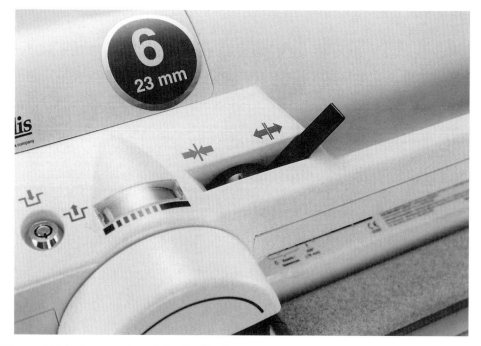

Figure 5D. A close-up view of Cordis Checkmate source housing showing continuous monitoring of source location.

Radiation Safety

Vascular brachytherapy brings the radioactive material, ie, ^{192}Ir, into the cardiac catheterization laboratory environment. This is a new practice, and thus raises a number of questions on the safety of personnel especially when a significant amount of ^{192}Ir activity is temporarily implanted in the patient. The area surrounding the procedure room may have radiation levels exceeding the value allowable by regulatory guidelines.[11] The subject of radiation protection and safety of personnel during catheter-based ^{192}Ir coronary brachytherapy has been fully evaluated by two studies, which were recently reported in the literature.[12,13] These two independent studies concluded that, with a prudent radiation protection program in place, the safety of personnel was easy to maintain.

Probably the highest amount of radiation is received by a medical physics staff who handles the radioactive ribbons during the QA procedure as well as during the actual treatment. The staff normally minimizes the whole body dose by using a lead shield specifically designed for protection during the handling of brachytherapy sources. Such a shield, commonly called L-block, is shown in Figure 6. Use of this block limits the exposed area to only the hands of the operator. Shields of these types were originally designed for handling the radium and cesium tube sources, both of which have gamma energy greater than that of [192]Ir. Use of radiation area monitors in the source storage room as well as the brachytherapy procedure room alerts the staff when the sources are out of the shielded container. During brachytherapy when the source ribbon is in the patient, the surrounding rooms, such as the control room, can be shielded from direct radiation by using a portable lead block. Figure 7 shows

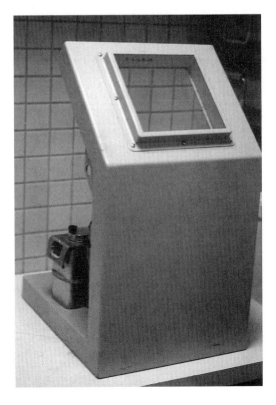

Figure 6. A typical L-shaped shielding block. It is used primarily to protect a radiation worker while handling high-energy gamma sources.

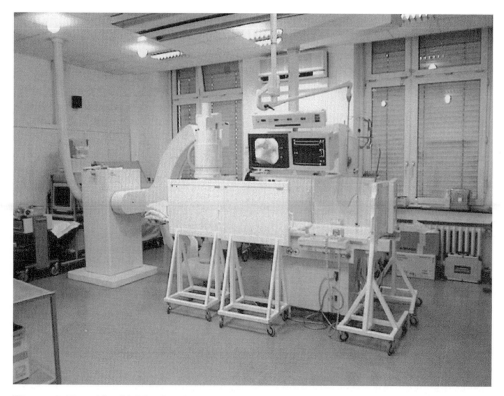

Figure 7. Portable shield to be placed near the patient during coronary Ir-192 brachytherapy. It contains 1-inch thick lead and provides greater than 99% attenuation of radiation.

the use of such portable shields at a facility in Europe. These shields have been commonly used in low dose rate brachytherapy for many decades.

Clinical Studies

SCRIPPS-I Trial

This single center, prospective, randomized trial at the Scripps Clinic enrolled 55 patients between March and December 1995. The patients studied had previously known restenosis in the native coronary or saphenous vein graft arteries. The ribbons used were 5 or 9 seeds in array and the dosimetry was intravascular ultrasound (IVUS) based. A dose of 800 to 3000 cGy was delivered to the farthest-closest portion of the leading edge of media as seen on ultrasound. This landmark trial's startlingly positive results fueled early enthusiasm in the field of vascular brachytherapy. The 3-year data show that ^{192}Ir still maintains its effectiveness.

GAMMA-I Trial

This multicenter, prospective, randomized trial with 252 patients follows the same approach as SCRIPPS-I Trial. The dosimetry was IVUS based with a range in dose of 800 to 3000 cGy. However, only the native coronary arteries were studied. It has also shown significant reduction in the rate of restenosis due to localized radiation from [192]Ir.

GAMMA-II Trial

This was a multicenter, prospective, nonrandomized study of patients with in-stent restenosis who were scheduled to undergo a current interventional procedure. Enrollment included 125 patients who, by visual assessment, had vessels of 2.75 to 4.00 mm in diameter and lesion length of 45 mm or less. The dosimetry was IVUS based with a range in dose of 800 to 3000 cGy. This trial has also shown significant reduction in the rate of restenosis due to localized radiation from [192]Ir.

WRIST Trial

This was a single center, prospective, randomized trial to investigate the safety and efficacy of localized gamma radiation after percutaneous treatment of in-stent restenosis. The design of the study and the source ribbons were the same as that of the SCRIPPS-I Trial. However, the dose delivered was prescribed at a fixed distance of 2 mm from the center of the noncentered source. A total of 130 patients with native coronary or saphenous vein graft restenosis were enrolled. The outcome was very similar to the SCRIPPS-I Trial; therefore, this trial was considered a very useful complement to the first SCRIPPS Trial.

European Studies

One of the earliest uses of ^{192}Ir-based brachytherapy using the Cordis C-snail (which is the delivery part of Checkmate system) in Europe was in Milan, Italy, in August 1999. The patients were enrolled in the Granite Trial, which is a registry in treating in-stent restenosis. The first use of the CE-marked Checkmate device under commercial status was in May 2000. The UMM Checkmate system is now in use in 13 centers throughout Europe.

Acknowledgments: The authors would like to acknowledge the help of K. Sudhandhiran and S. Ramaswami of Best Medical International, and Lars Janson of Cordis Corporation in obtaining valuable information on the source and delivery devices. The authors also wish to thank Marcia Straile of Scripps Clinic, and Ashish Jani and Shyam Jani for their help in preparing this manuscript.

References

1. Weidermann JG, Marboe C, Amols H, et al. Intracoronary irradiation markedly reduces restenosis after balloon angioplasty in a porcine model. J Am Coll Cardiol 1994;23:1491–1498.
2. Waksman R, Robinson KA, Crocker IR, et al. Endovascular low-dose irradiation inhibits neointima formation after coronary artery balloon injury in swine: A possible role for radiation therapy in restenosis prevention. Circulation 1995;91:1533–1539.
3. Condado JA, Waksman R, Gurdiel O, et al. Long-term angiographic and clinical outcome after percutaneous transluminal coronary angioplasty and intracoronary radiation therapy in humans. Circulation 1997;96:727–732.

4. Böttcher HD, Schopohl B, Liermann D, et al. Endovascular irradiation: A new method to avoid recurrent stenosis after stent implantation in peripheral arteries. Technique and preliminary results. Int J Radiat Oncol Biol Phys 1994;29:183–186.
5. Teirstein PS, Massullo V, Jani S, et al. Catheter-based radiotherapy to inhibit restenosis after coronary stenting. N Engl J Med 1997;336:1697–1703.
6. Teirstein PS, Massullo V, Jani S, et al. A subgroup analysis of the SCRIPPS coronary radiation to inhibit proliferation poststenting trial. Int J Radiat Oncol Biol Phys 1998;42:1097–1104.
7. Waksman R, Mehran R, Chan RC, et al. One-year follow-up after intracoronary gamma radiation therapy for in-stent restenosis: Results from a randomized clinical trial [abstract]. Circulation 1999;100:I–154.
8. Jani SK. Basic physics of gamma isotopes. In: Waksman R (ed.): Vascular Brachytherapy, 2nd Edition. Armonk, NY: Futura Publishing Company, Inc.; 1999:167–176.
9. Jani SK. Physics of vascular brachytherapy. J Invas Cardiol 1999;11:517–523.
10. Jani SK. Handbook of Dosimetry Data for Radiotherapy. Boca Raton, FL: CRC Press; 1993:137–167.
11. Jani SK, Massullo V, Steuterman S, et al. Physics and safety aspects of a coronary irradiation pilot study to inhibit restenosis using manually loaded ^{192}Ir ribbons. Semin Intervent Cardiol 1997;2:119–123.
12. Jani SK, Steuterman S, Huppe GB, et al. Radiation safety of personnel during catheter-based Ir-192 coronary brachytherapy. J Invas Cardiol 2000;12:286–290.
13. Balter S, Oetgen M, Hill A, et al. Personnel exposure during gamma endovascular brachytherapy. Health Phys 2000;79:136–146.

## Chapter 53

Novoste™ Beta-Cath™ System:

Intracoronary Radiation with Strontium 90

Kelly W. Elliott RN, MS, CCRN, Robert P. Walsh RN, MBA, and Richard diMonda, MS, MBA

Introduction

For many patients who suffer from coronary artery disease, percutaneous transluminal coronary angioplasty (PTCA) has long been regarded as a safe and effective alternative to coronary bypass surgery. When compared to coronary bypass surgery, patients opting for PTCA typically experience substantially less physical trauma, greatly reduced recovery time, and significantly less hospital costs. However, one significant drawback to PTCA continues to plague the long-term efficacy of this treatment. In 35 to 40% of all PTCA procedures performed, the dilated artery segment exhibits a significant reduction in luminal diameter within 4 to 6 months after the procedure. This luminal reduction, or restenosis, then requires additional percutaneous coronary intervention procedures in order to reopen the same lesion, thus negating many of the benefits anticipated from the initial PTCA.

It has been documented multiple times in the literature that stents have demonstrated a reduction in restenosis compared to PTCA alone. Stents are typically metallic, and most are expanded into place by use of a balloon catheter much like an angioplasty balloon. These devices have yielded varying degrees of success in addressing the late-stage geometric remodeling aspect of the restenosis problem, but have been less effective at preventing the proliferative smooth muscle response due to dilatation-induced vascular injury as well as the cellular response to a foreign implant. In many cases persistent restenosis ultimately leads to coronary bypass surgery. Intracoronary radiation with the Novoste™ Beta-Cath™ System (Novoste Corporation, Norcross, GA) is intended to be applied as an adjunct to PTCA or to other percutaneous coronary intervention.

Presently, in the U.S, the Novoste Beta-Cath System has Food and Drug Administration (FDA) approval for the treatment of in-stent restenosis. Outside the U.S., the Beta-Cath System is used for the prevention of restenosis in de novo lesions, restenotic lesions, saphenous vein grafts, and for treatment of in-stent restenosis.

From Waksman R (ed.). *Vascular Brachytherapy, Third Edition.* Armonk, NY: Futura Publishing Co., Inc.; © 2002.

The START Trial

Knowing the prevalence of in-stent restenosis, in September 1998, Novoste initiated the Stents and Radiation Therapy (START) Trial. This landmark trial showed a statistically significant reduction in in-stent restenosis compared to patients treated with percutaneous coronary intervention alone.

The START Trial enrollment was completed in April 1999. A total of 476 patients were enrolled at 50 clinical centers in North America and Europe. Patients were considered candidates for the trial if they were over 18-years old and had a single target site stent restenosis in a native vessel between 2.7 and 4.0 mm. Stent restenosis was defined as a visually determined diameter stenosis between 50 and 100% in the presence of objective evidence of myocardial ischemia, as manifested by symptoms or laboratory testing. A successful angiographic result (<30% residual stenosis by visual estimation) within the treated segment after conventional coronary intervention was required prior to randomization.

A 30-mm Beta-Cath System radiation source train was used for lesions treatable with up to a 20-mm balloon. Patients were excluded from the study if they required multivessel coronary intervention or had an unsuccessful treatment of the target lesion (>30% residual diameter stenosis), a recent (<72 hours) myocardial infarction, unprotected left main coronary artery disease, or a prior history of any chest radiotherapy. Patients were also excluded if they had angiographic findings that would preclude delivery of the Beta-Cath Delivery Catheter, including severe proximal tortuosity or vessel angulation. Informed consent approved by a local institutional review board was obtained before the procedure in all patients. Patients were pre-treated with 325-mg aspirin prior to the procedure. Use of abciximab was discouraged. After successful treatment (<30% residual stenosis and no major coronary dissections) of stent restenosis using balloon angioplasty alone, or in combination with rotational or directional atherectomy or excimer laser angioplasty, patients were randomly assigned to treatment with ^{90}Sr/^{90}Y (N=244) or placebo (N=232). The use of additional stents was discouraged and reserved for "bail-out" indications, including a residual stenosis or major dissection. The ^{90}Sr/^{90}Y radioisotope used in this study has a 28.8-year half-life. The prescription point was 2 mm from the centerline of the axis of the radiation source train in water. The dose prescription was 18.4 Gy for reference vessel sizes greater than or equal to 2.7 mm and less than or equal to 3.35 mm, and 23 Gy for reference vessel sizes greater than 3.35 mm and less than or equal to 4.0 mm, as determined by visual angiographic estimate. The treatment time ranged from 3 to 5 minutes.

Results

There were no significant differences in baseline demographics between the two groups (mean age ~61 years; ~63% male; ~31% diabetics and ~48% with prior myocardial infarction). The device success rate was similar (P=NS) in placebo-treated patients (~97%) and ^{90}Sr/^{90}Y-treated patients (~98%). The procedural success rate was also similar (˜7E97%) in the two groups. Debulking devices were used with similar frequency in the two groups: rotational atherectomy was used in ~40% of placebo-treated patients and ~44% of ^{90}Sr/^{90}Y-treated patients; excimer laser angioplasty was used in ~7% of placebo- treated patients and ~6% of ^{90}Sr/^{90}Y-treated patients; directional atherectomy was used in ~1% of placebo-treated patients and in none of the ^{90}Sr/^{90}Y-treated patients. New stents were placed with similar frequency in ~20% of placebo-treated patients and ~21% of ^{90}Sr/^{90}Y-treated patients. The stented segment length was 22.7+10.7 mm, the injured segment length was 25.2+9.2 mm, the radiated segment length was 30.0+5.4 mm, and the analysis segment length was 40.8+9.4 mm.

The residual stenosis was similar in the two groups within the stented segment (22.9%) and within the analysis segment (30.7% in the placebo group and 31.4% in the ^{90}Sr/^{90}Y-treated patients).

At 240 days, no difference was found between the two groups in clinical events: 1 death in the placebo-treated group versus 3 in the ^{90}Sr/^{90}Y-treated group, and 7 non-Q-wave myocardial infarctions in the placebo-treated group versus 4 in the ^{90}Sr/^{90}Y-treated group. The angiographic restenosis rate was stable in the placebo-treated group (41.2% in the stent segment to 45.2% in the analysis segment), while in the ^{90}Sr/^{90}Y-treated group there was a significantly lower restenosis rate in all measured parameters (14.2% in the stent segment to 28.8% in the analysis segment; $P<0.001$). This represents a reduction in the restenosis rate of 66% in the stent segment and 36% in the analysis segment. Late loss in the placebo-treated group was 0.67 mm in the stent segment and 0.54 mm in the analysis segment, significantly higher than the late loss measured in the ^{90}Sr/^{90}Y-treated group (0.21 mm in the stent segment to 0.28 mm in the analysis segment; $P<0.001$). Total occlusion was found with similar frequency in 7 (3.7%) placebo-treated patients and 8 (4.0%) ^{90}Sr/^{90}Y-treated patients. There was no new aneurysm formation noted in either group.

The primary study endpoint, 8-month target vessel failure, defined as target vessel revascularization, myocardial infarction, or death attributed to the target vessel, was reduced by 31% in patients treated with ^{90}Sr/^{90}Y (25.9% versus 18%; $P=0.039$). Major adverse cardiac events were reduced by 31% (25.9% versus 18%; $P=0.039$). Target vessel revascularization was reduced by 34% (24.1% versus 16%; $P=0.028$), and target lesion revascularization was reduced by 42% (22.4% versus 13.1%; $P=0.008$). There were no episodes of late clinical stent thrombosis in either group at 240 days. Freedom from target vessel failure, defined as target vessel revascularization, myocardial infarction, or death, at 8 months was 82% in the ^{90}Sr/^{90}Y group and 72% in the placebo group.

START Trial Long Lesion Subset Analysis

Not only did the START Trial show a statistically significant reduction in major adverse cardiac events, target vessel revascularization, target lesion revascularization, in-stent restenosis, and restenosis of the analysis segment compared to placebo, but an analysis of long lesions also showed similarly favorable results.

The mean lesion length in this subset was 21.8 mm (+5.3 mm). Compared to the placebo arm, the ^{90}Sr arm showed a 63% reduction in restenosis. The analysis segment showed a 45% reduction in restenosis compared to the placebo group. Most importantly, from a clinical perspective, the target vessel revascularization rate was reduced by 49% compared to the placebo arm.

START 40 Trial

The START 40 Trial was a registry trial that included 22 sites and 207 patients. The rationale for the START 40 Trial was to determine whether a 40-mm radiation source train would further reduce restenosis by providing more extensive margin coverage. The objective of the START 40 Trial was to investigate the relationship between radiation lengths by comparing patients in the START 30 Trial (30-mm radiation source train) to a similar cohort of START 40 patients treated with a longer 40-mm radiation source train. The differences between the START 30 and START 40 Trials were: (1) START 40 was a registry trial; (2) the 40-mm radiation source train was used to treat all patients; and (3) in START 40, there were longer radiation margins (+10 mm on each end).

The clinical outcomes analysis for START 40 showed the following: compared to the placebo arm in the randomized START Trial, the START 40 Trial revealed a 26% reduction in major adverse cardiac events, a 34% reduction in target vessel revascularization, and a 50% reduction in target lesion revascularization.

The angiographic outcomes analysis showed a 63% reduction in the stent segment restenosis rate, and a 44% reduction in the analysis segment restenosis rate.

A subset analysis of lesions greater than 20 mm from the START 30 and START 40 Trials combined showed highly positive results (Table 1). The START 40 Trial continues to support the efficacy of ^{90}Sr beta radiation for the treatment of in-stent restenosis. START 40 shows that there are no deleterious effects from adding 10 mm to the length of the source train, and supports the lack of relationship between geographic miss and clinical or angiographic outcomes for in-stent restenosis.

Table 1

START 30 and START 40 Subset Analysis: Lesions >20 mm

Baseline Data	Strontium 90	Placebo	P Value
Reference vessel diameter	2.7 mm	2.8 mm	NS
Mean lesion length	26.5 mm (±5.6)	25.7 mm (±4.6)	NS
8-Month Clinical Outcomes Analysis			
Any MACE	19.8%	33.3%	0.0416
Target vessel failure (Death, MI, TVR)	19.8%	33.3%	0.0416
Death	2.4%	1.6%	NS
Target lesion revascularization	11.9%	30.2%	0.0021
Target vessel revascularization	15.9%	21.2%	0.0118
Stent thrombosis (to 30 days)	0.0%	0.0%	—
Site thrombosis (31–240 days)	0.8%	0.5%	NS
8-Month Angiographic Outcomes			
In-stent restenosis rate	22.7%	52.0%	0.0003
Analysis segment restenosis rate	31.6%	54.9%	0.0059
Aneurysms	0.0%	0.0%	—

MACE = major adverse cardiac events; MI = myocardial infarction; TVR = target vessel revascularization.

System Configuration

The Novoste Beta-Cath System is a completely closed system designed specifically to be used in the cardiac catheterization laboratory (Fig. 1). The Beta-Cath System comprises four components: the transfer device, radiation source train, the delivery catheter, and the procedure accessory pack. The transfer device stores the ^{90}Sr radiation source train and allows for transport of the source train to and from the treatment zone. Outside the U.S., 30-mm, 40-mm, and 60-mm radiation source trains are available. Presently, 30-mm and 40-mm radiation source trains are FDA-approved in the U.S. The radiation oncologist or therapist has complete control over the delivery and return of the radiation source train.

The procedure accessory pack used with the Beta-Cath System enables the operator to bring the small portable device into the sterile field. To facilitate ease of use in the cardiac catheterization laboratory, the Beta-Cath™ catheter and the Beta-Rail™ catheter (outside the U.S.) were designed to exhibit performance characteristics similar to a standard angioplasty catheter. The Beta-Cath catheter is an "over-the-wire" catheter, meaning simply that the catheter is advanced into the target artery over a typical coronary guidewire used for the percutaneous coronary intervention.

After connection to the hand-held transfer device, the distal tip of the catheter is positioned at the treatment zone (Fig. 2). There are two radiopaque markers on the distal end of the catheter that indicate where to position the catheter.

The transfer device uses a 20-cc disposable syringe filled with sterile water for irrigation to deliver a "train" of beta-emitting sources to the distal end of the catheter. Since the delivery catheter together with the transfer device create a closed system, all of the sterile water used during this delivery process is returned to the transfer device via a return lumen in the catheter. At no time during the

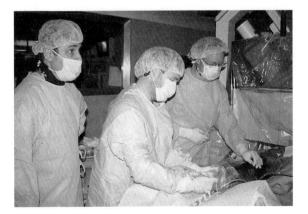

Figure 1. The Novoste™ Beta-Cath™ system is shown here delivering beta radiation to the coronary arteries of a patient undergoing balloon angioplasty at Emory University. Positioning of the ^{90}Sr beta source can be continuously confirmed on the fluoroscopic monitor. Catheterization laboratory personnel need no additional radiation shielding and are free to remain in close proximity to the patient throughout the approximately 3- to 4-minute dose-delivery period.

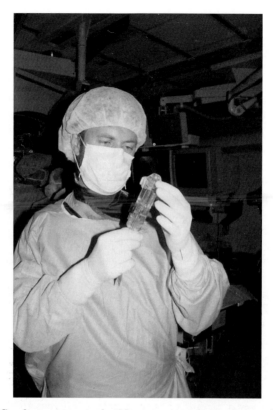

Figure 2. Dr. Ian Crocker prepares the Novoste transfer device model used during the BERT Trial for connection to the delivery catheter. This lightweight, hand-held device delivers and retrieves the radiation source train to and from the distal tip of the delivery catheter.

procedure is any delivery fluid injected into the patient's coronary arteries. This patented hydraulic system typically delivers the radiation source train to the treatment site in approximately 2 to 3 seconds. In addition to transporting and storing the sources, the transfer device also shields the operator from the beta radiation (Fig. 3).

The patented hydraulic system allows for positive pressure to deliver the sources, and positive pressure to return the sources to the transfer device. The proximal portion of the delivery catheter provides tactile feedback to the physician during the positioning of the distal tip under fluoroscopy. The catheter is responsive to the operator's manipulation and has a feel much like a PTCA balloon catheter. The distal tip of the catheter is highly flexible and conforms closely to the guidewire when negotiating tortuous anatomy (Fig. 4).

Positioning the beta source using the Novoste Beta-Cath System is done easily under conventional fluoroscopy. The physician has the ability to control the position of the radiation source train during the treatment. Due to the maneuverability of the highly flexible Beta-Cath System, the physician can easily position the delivery catheter precisely at the interventional injury site. There are two radiopaque markers near the distal tip of the catheter that define the treatment zone.

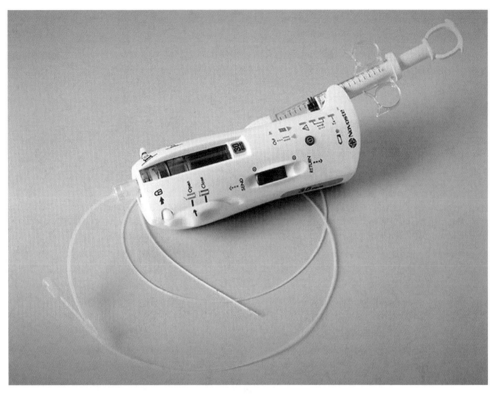

Figure 3. The Novoste Beta-Cath System with the delivery catheter attached.

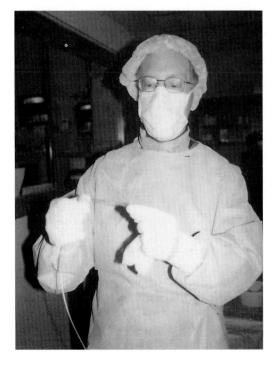

Figure 4. Dr. Spencer B. King III examines the distal tip of the Novoste Beta-Cath delivery catheter prior to placement in the patient's coronary artery. The catheter system is prepared for use in much the same fashion as a standard angioplasty balloon.

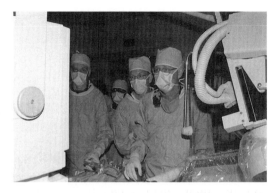

Figure 5. Physicians at Rhode Island Hospital (Providence, RI) use fluoroscopy to view the actual positioning of the distal tip of the delivery catheter as well as the ^{90}Sr source train during a coronary irradiation procedure. The beta-emitting isotope requires no special shielding, thus allowing the catheterization laboratory staff to remain at the patient's side throughout the procedure.

The positioning of the catheter takes place by the interventional cardiologist before the ^{90}Sr radiation source train is delivered to the treatment zone. The isotope is delivered to the treatment zone, which is defined as the interventional injury length, between the two markers. Using fluoroscopic guidance, the cardiologist advances the catheter so that the target segment of the artery is positioned between the two marker bands. The catheter position is verified prior to delivering the source train to the treatment zone (Fig. 5). The ^{90}Sr radiation source train is then delivered through the catheter to the distal tip, where it completely occupies the space between the radiopaque markers. When the treatment is complete and the source train is returned to the transfer device, the delivery catheter and transfer device can be removed from the procedural area, leaving the guidewire in place.

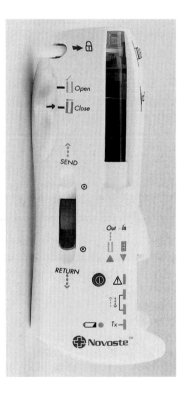

Figure 6. The Novoste Beta-Cath System incorporates a compact, lightweight, hand-held device, which allows the physician to position the ^{90}Sr beta sources using fluoroscopic guidance. This feature allows the physician to ensure that the source train is positioned precisely at the site of the percutaneous coronary intervention.

Source Selection

One of the most important considerations in selecting a system for intracoronary radiation delivery is the choice of radioactive isotope. The benefits of using a beta emitter, such as ^{90}Sr, instead of a gamma emitter, became evident early in the development of the Beta-Cath System. After our first few experiences in placing ^{192}Ir wire in the balloon injured coronary arteries of a domestic swine, it became obvious that we would face major difficulties incorporating a system using this gamma-emitting isotope in the cardiac catheterization laboratory. Not only did the ^{192}Ir tend to wash out the fluoroscopic image of the treatment area, making accurate positioning of the source nearly impossible, but the investigators had to leave the procedure room in order to reduce their personal radiation exposure levels to a safe limit. The lead aprons typically worn by catheterization laboratory personnel have little or no attenuating effect on gamma radiation of this intensity. After the cardiologist has placed the catheter correctly at the treatment zone, the radiation oncologist can then deliver the sources to the treatment zone.

There are three lengths of the radiation source train to choose from, based on the interventional injury length within the artery. These three lengths, 30, 40, and 60 mm, are currently available outside the U.S. In contrast to the challenges associated with shielding a gamma source, virtually all of the beta radiation is attenuated by the transfer device (Fig. 6). During the course of the treatment, almost all of the beta radiation is attenuated by the patient's body. This allows the cardiologist and the rest of the catheterization laboratory staff to continue performing their routine activities inside the catheterization laboratory. Additionally, the cardiologist is able to remain at the patient's side throughout the procedure to closely monitor the patient's condition and to provide reassurance whenever necessary. The type of physician/patient interaction during source delivery can only be achieved through the use of a beta-emitting isotope.

In addition to the advantages of beta emitters mentioned previously, there are specific advantages to the ^{90}Sr isotope. Strontium 90 has a half-life of 28.8 years. Because of the long half-life of the isotope, the radiation source train within the Beta-Cath System does not require routine dose decay calulations by the medical physicist. Additionally, the system is leak tested prior to shipping and returned to Novoste Corporation every 6 months or after 250 uses, whichever comes first. Because a leak test is only required every 6 momths, Novoste Corporation will leak test all radiation source trains and perform preventive maintenance on the transfer device upon receipt. Due to the long half-life, ^{90}Sr use results in no change in treatment time during the 6-month life of the device.

Isotope Half-Life Considerations

Several important considerations were examined in evaluating which isotope to use. Inventory planning was a major consideration with the shorter half-life sources. When a short half-life source is used, dosing also becomes a constant challenge. As the isotope decays, treatment times become longer. This additional treatment time could become cause for concern in a patient for whom prolonged radiation delivery may result in ischemia so severe as to warrant interruption of the procedure and a fractionated dose. When the isotope half-life is a matter of days, as with radioactive stents, inventory spoilage is also an important cost consideration.

In addition to the shelf life problems, short half-life isotopes are often as expensive to produce as their longer half-life counterparts. The ability to spread out the initial acquisition cost of a particular source over hundreds of patients may translate to a cost advantage in favor of a long half-life isotope, such as ^{90}Sr. In an age of health care cost containment, such considerations may have important implications.

Source Centering Issues

Because beta radiation is rapidly attenuated, concern has been expressed about the potential for target site under- or overdose. The very same reasons that make beta radiation ideal from a safety perspective give rise to questions concerning the ability of a selected beta isotope to deliver an effective dose inside a vessel lumen. The Novoste Beta-Cath System delivery catheter is appropriately proportioned to the artery size. Appropriate sizing should allow for adequate blood flow around the catheter, and will ensure that the isotope cannot be too close to the artery wall on one side, or too far away on the other.

An alternative to passive centering is the use of an active centering device such as a balloon. These devices often occlude blood flow to the distal segment of the artery, thus producing ischemia. Such an approach may result in the need to deflate the balloon to relieve patient pain, and a fractionated dose could then be required. This makes an otherwise straightforward procedure, with simple dose calculations, significantly more complex for the physician as well as for the patient. Novoste believes that a simple approach in this case is the best approach. It is better for the patient, more convenient for the physician, and should provide a similar clinical outcome.

Source Delivery Control Method

As mentioned previously, Novoste's approach allows the physician to control all aspects of source delivery, treatment positioning, and source return. When the radioactive source train is at the distal tip of the catheter, the physician is able to visualize the source position with regard to the target treatment site and make "real-time" adjustments as required. This user-friendly system provides visual and tactile positioning characteristics, allowing the cardiologist to navigate easily through tortuous anatomies. If an emergency arises, the physician simply removes the entire closed system, leaving the guidewire in place, and proceeds with any emergency intervention deemed necessary.

Vascular Brachytherapy in the Cardiac Catheterization Lab

A hospital interested in treating patients with the Beta-Cath System would benefit from establishing a vascular brachytherapy team. The team members consist of the interventional cardiologist, a radiation oncologist, a medical physicist, and a cardiac catheterizaton laboratory team member. The radiation oncologist is responsible for delivering the radioactive isotope to the treatment zone. The interventional cardiologist visually determines the reference vessel diameter and also manipulates and controls the catheter at all times. The medical physicist stores and transports the Beta-Cath System to and from the cardiac catheterization laboratory and is responsible for radiation safety. The cardiac catheterization team member may assist in gathering necessary equipment, coordinating the team members for the procedure, and caring for the patient during the interventional vascular brachytherapy procedure.

Conclusions

The Novoste approach to treating clinical restenosis represents a truly novel solution to a problem that has plagued PTCA and stenting since the inception of these procedures. The Beta-Cath System is compatible with most coronary interventions while still allowing last minute treatment decisions. The mechanism of restenosis so closely resembles other forms of runaway cell growth that have been effectively treated for many years with radiation therapy that we, as researchers and product developers, cannot ignore the exciting potential inherent in this approach. As with all new therapies, additional research is essential to fully understand and develop this treatment. Nevertheless, the results experienced thus far with the Beta-Cath System, indicate that intracoronary irradiation used as an adjunct with PTCA in the treatment of in-stent restenosis provides highly favorable outcomes.

References

1. King SB III, Williams DO, Chougle P, et al. Endovascular β-radiation to reduce restenosis after coronary balloon angioplasty: Results of the Beta Energy Restenosis Trial (BERT). Circulation 1998;97:2025–2030.
2. Hillstead RA, Johnson CR, Weldon TD. The Beta-Cath™ system. In: Waksman R, Serruys PW (eds.): The Handbook of Vascular Brachytherapy. London: Martin Dunitz Publishing Co.; 1998:41–51.
3. Hillstead RA. Novoste™ Beta-Cath™ intracoronary radiation system. In: Waksman R (ed.): Vascular Brachytherapy, Second Edition. Armonk, NY: Futura Publishing Co., Inc.; 1999.
4. Waksman R, Robinson KA, Crocker IR, et al. Intra-coronary low-dose beta irradiation inhibits neointima formation after coronary balloon injury in the swine model. Circulation 1995;92:3025–3031.
5. Fischell TA, Kharmea BK, Fuschell DR, et al. Low dose beta particle emission from stent wire results in complete, localized inhibition of smooth muscle cell proliferation. Circulation 1994;90:2956–2963.
6. Liu MW, Roubin GS, King SB III. Restenosis after coronary angioplasty: Potential biological determinants and role of intimal hyperplasia. Circulation 1989;79:1374–1387.
7. Gravanis MB, Robinson KA, Santoian EC, et al. The reparative phenomena at the site of balloon angioplasty in human and experimental models. Cardiovasc Pathol 1993;2: 263–273.
8. Wiedermann JG, Marboe C, Schwartz A, et al. Intracoronary irradiation markedly reduces neointimal proliferation after balloon angioplasty in swine: Persistent benefit after six-month follow-up. J Am Coll Cardiol 1995;25:1451–1456.
9. Liermann DD, Boettcher HD, Kollatch J, et al. Prophylactic endovascular radiotherapy to prevent intimal hyperplasia after sent implantation in femoropopliteal arteries. Cardiovasc Intervent Radiol 1994;17:12–16.
10. Hehrlein C, Zimmerman M, Metz J, et al. Radioactive stent implantation inhibits neointimal proliferation in nonarteriosclerotic rabbits [abstract]. Circulation 1993;88 (suppl I):I–65.

## Chapter 54

Peripheral Vascular Brachytherapy Using the Nucletron® PARIS® Catheter and the microSelectron-HDR Afterloader

Frits M. van Krieken, MSc, PhD,
and Edgar G. Löffler, PhD

Introduction

Brachytherapy using a vascular approach is not new; as early as 1958, Brasfield and Henschke[1] reported a mammary artery afterloading technique for the irradiation of the parasternal mammary lymph nodes in the treatment of breast cancer. In 1990, Androsov et al[2] reported a similar treatment using the Nucletron (Veenendaal, The Netherlands) microSelectron-LDR/MDR remote-controlled afterloader to safely handle the source. Early in the 1990s, two things motivated Böttcher, Schopohl, and Liermann[3] to start a peripheral artery brachytherapy program: the availability of the Nucletron microSelectron-HDR™ afterloader with its miniaturized ^{192}Ir source, and the successful experience with radiation treatment of keloids and hypertrophied scars to minimize pathological proliferation of connective tissue. These investigators treated patients following balloon angioplasty of narrowed stented femoral arteries.[4] On the basis of their favorable results, it was suggested that vascular brachytherapy for this application is safe and probably efficacious.[5] The encouraging result of this study has motivated other investigators[6] to conduct feasibility trials[7] in noncoronary vessels. It has also led Nucletron[8] to develop a dedicated centering catheter system in collaboration with Guidant Vascular Intervention (Santa Clara, CA). The resulting Nucletron® PARIS® centering catheter system is currently marketed outside the U.S. An ongoing multicenter trial for U.S. market approval, the Peripheral Artery Radiation Investigational Study (PARIS), is currently in its second, randomized phase.

The Peripheral System Approach

A brachytherapy system is used to bring a radioactive source close to the target tissue. It normally includes a source, an applicator or catheter that serves as

From Waksman R (ed.). *Vascular Brachytherapy, Third Edition.* Armonk, NY: Futura Publishing Co., Inc.; © 2002.

a channel towards the target tissue, and a device to store and deliver the source. The most advanced source delivery systems use a robotic device, called a remote afterloader. This device has a safe to store the source when it is not in use. The afterloader advances the source into the catheter for the duration of the treatment and automatically restores it afterwards. It then provides a complete and accurate record of the procedure.

The Nucletron approach to a peripheral vascular brachytherapy system[9] is based on two starting points:

- Optimization of dosage control in the larger peripheral lesions by the use of the Nucletron PARIS centering catheter in combination with a ^{192}Ir gamma stepping source. This allows for dose conformity and a sufficient radiation margin over a large range of target diameters and lengths.
- Promoting safe and reproducible delivery of radiation, using the proven and reliable microSelectron-HDR remote-controlled afterloader. Currently, more than 1000 of these devices are in clinical use worldwide.

The first system was developed for brachytherapy of superficial femoral and popliteal arteries in conjunction with angioplasty. The main elements of this system and its practical application are discussed below.

The ^{192}Ir Source

The diameters of peripheral arteries suitable for angioplasty vary widely but are typically larger than the diameters of coronary arteries. Femoral and popliteal artery diameters may range from 3 to 8 mm, and diameters of about 10 mm are reached in portoiliac and arteriovascular dialysis shunts. Also, wall thickness, and therefore the radius to the adventitial target cells, is usually larger than for coronary arteries. To provide a sufficient therapeutic dose at these treatment depths, beta radiation is not as useful or practical as it is for intracoronary applications. The preferred radioisotope for peripheral treatments is a gamma emitter.

The Nucletron Peripheral System uses a ^{192}Ir source that is well known in high dose rate cancer treatment. In order to limit treatment times in the large peripheral vessels to several minutes, the Nucletron ^{192}Ir source has a high nominal activity of 10 Ci. It is entirely sealed in a stainless steel capsule to prevent patient and catheter contamination. The capsule is laser welded to an ultra flexible distal part of a flexible cable (Fig. 1). The source is only 3.6 mm long and functions in practice as a point source.

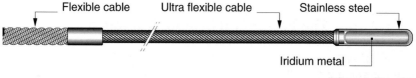

Figure 1. The miniaturized microSelectron-HDR™ ^{192}Ir source.

The microSelectron-HDR Afterloader

As with the treatment of cancer, essential radiation protection of the staff cannot be achieved with manually loaded sources, and therefore a remote-controlled afterloader is required to store, advance, and restore the source.

The central part of the Nucletron Peripheral System is the microSelectron-HDR afterloader (Fig. 2), designed to handle the ^{192}Ir source. The radiation dose to personnel is minimized by remotely initiating the automatic source advancement from outside the treatment room. By computer-controlled advancement of the source from the radiation storage safe into the treatment position, accurate delivery of radiation dose is possible without radiation hazard to the patient. The source moves to the treatment position within 3 seconds, minimizing radiation exposure during source transfer to a negligible level.

The use of a point source with an afterloader that allows for programmable stepped positioning and dwelling provides the freedom to shape the iso-dose in accordance with the target dimensions. For peripheral treatments, the afterloader can create a longitudinal dose field of virtually any desired length and diameter by moving the short source along the target length of the artery, in steps of 2.5 or 5 mm. Dwell times are optimized and therefore somewhat longer at the ends of the field, as illustrated by Figure 3. This helps to prevent edge underdosage and the resulting "candy wrapper" effect.

The afterloader is easy to program using integrated treatment libraries that can be prepared in advance. The afterloader has two wire drives. One drive advances an inactive check cable to detect catheter connection and any obstruction in the system. Only after verification of the patency of the source channel, does the other drive advance the source, and, after the treatment, it restores it into the

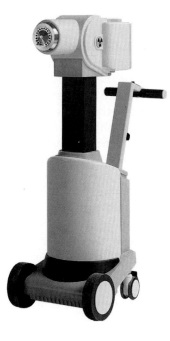

Figure 2. The microSelectron-HDR™ afterloader.

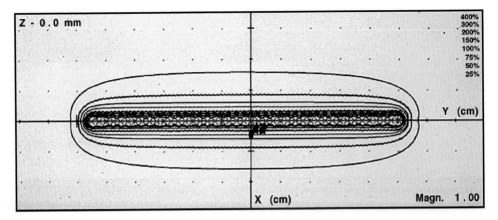

Figure 3. Example of an optimized iso-dose shape as used for endovascular radiation.

radiation-shielded safe. Treatment may be interrupted and resumed as needed since the device automatically stores and displays the remaining treatment time. For emergency interruption, an independent battery powered drive is integrated next to a manual retraction system.

The Nucletron PARIS Centering Catheter

For the PARIS Trial, a new radiation catheter system has been developed in association with Guidant (Fig. 4; see Table 1 for specification details). The Nucletron PARIS multiple balloon catheter system is specifically designed for endovascular radiation in the femoral and popliteal arteries following conventional angioplasty performed by the interventional radiologist or cardiologist. The bilumen catheter is introduced over a guidewire and positioned with its balloons spanning the target area. For optimal positioning of the catheter, a radiopaque marker is integrated that visualizes the most distal source position possible. Balloon inflation will center the catheter within the lumen of the artery, promoting uniform distribution of the dose in the vessel wall. An array of multiple balloons is used to keep the source in the center within curved arteries (Figs. 5 and 6). After balloon inflation, the guidewire is withdrawn and a closed-end radiation sheath is introduced into the guidewire lumen to serve as the channel that allows for safe transfer of the radiation source. After catheter fixation and patient transportation to the radiation suite, the proximal end of the radiation sheath is connected to the microSelectron-HDR afterloader for the actual radiation treatment. The target area includes the total lesion length *created* by the angioplasty, for example, the total balloon dilated length. The proposed target length is this lesion length plus 1-cm margin at each side. The stepping length of the source will, in practice, be the lesion length plus 3 cm, that is 1.5 cm at each side. Thus, a 20-cm balloon array will provide optimal centering for interventional lesions up to 17-cm lengths.

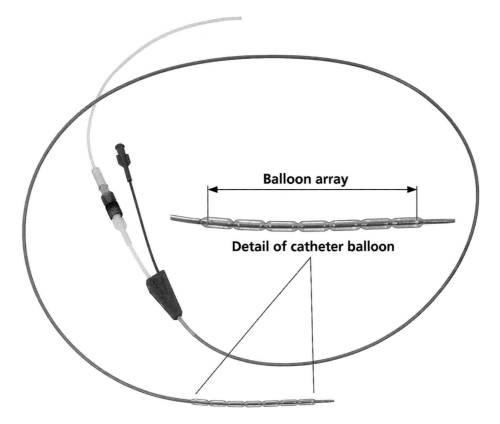

Figure 4. The Nucletron® PARIS® catheter.

Table 1

The Unique Features of the PARIS Catheter

Feature	Specification
Catheter parts	• Centering catheter with balloon array • Closed-end radiation sheath that fits in guidewire lumen • Polymer mandrel for stiffness
Centering balloon diameter	4, 5, 6, 7, or 8 mm
Centering balloon length	10 or 20 cm
Operating pressure	4 atm (4 bar, 60 PSI)
Insertion technique	over the wire
Recommended guidewire diameter	0.035″
Recommended introducer sheath size	8 F
Shaft diameter	7 F
Working length	1150 mm, allowing for cross-over insertion
Radiopaque marker	ring at 1500 mm reference position
Connection of radiation sheath and centering catheter	Luer lock for reproducible source location relative to the radiopaque marker
Connection to afterloader	6-F standard applicator adapter

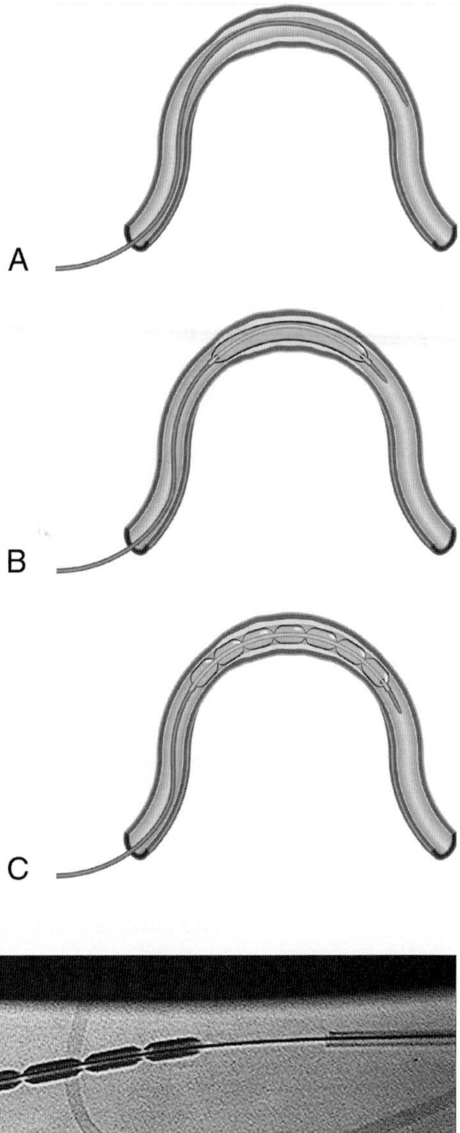

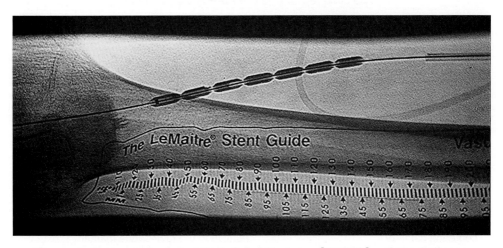

Figure 5. Diagram of a conventional brachytherapy catheter off center in a curved. vessel (**A**). Eccentricity occurs when the source is positioned in a single balloon catheter (**B**), as used for dilatation. Source forced into axial position using the multisegmented low-pressure Nucletron® PARIS® catheter balloons (**C**).

A

B

C

Figure 6. Fluoroscopic view of the inflated Nucletron® PARIS® catheter balloons.

Application Experience

The Nucletron PARIS system has European CE market approval and is in use in many countries around the world. For U.S. market approval, it is currently in use in the Food and Drug Administration-approved multicenter, double-blind PARIS Trial for treatment of femoral and popliteal arteries. This study is in its randomized second phase, involving 300 patients.

The 12-month clinical results of the earlier safety phase of the PARIS Study are reported elsewhere in this textbook. This phase included 40 patients who underwent radiation treatment with a dose of 14 Gy defined at 2 mm outside the balloon radius. At 6-month angiographic follow-up of 30 patients, only 4 patients (13%) had developed restenosis, 3 at the original lesion site. This result was maintained at 12-month clinical follow-up.

There is further interest in the use of the Nucletron PARIS system for reducing restenosis in Transjugular Intrahepatic Portosystemic Shunts (TIPS) and for treatment of arteriovenous dialysis shunts.

Conclusions

Nucletron's approach to peripheral artery brachytherapy is based on the unique Nucletron PARIS centering catheter system designed for safety and optimal dose distribution. It is used in combination with an afterloader and a short gamma radiation source that are well proven and widely distributed for radiation oncology. This same microSelectron-HDR afterloader was used in the study by Böttcher, Schopohl, Liermann,[4] who demonstrated the earliest promising results of peripheral endovascular radiation. The Nucletron PARIS system is in use worldwide and the first clinical results are positive.

References

1. Brasfield RD, Henschke UK. Treatment of internal mammary lymph nodes by implantation of radioisotopes into internal mammary artery. Radiology 1958;70:259.
2. Androsov NS, Nechuskin MI, Sushchikhina M. Treatment of parasternal nodes in patients with breast cancer. Activity 1990;4:24–25.
3. Liermann D, Böttcher HD, Kollath J, et al. Prophylactic endovascular radiotherapy to prevent intimal hyperplasia after stent implantation in femoropopliteal arteries. Cardiovasc Intervent Radiol 1994;17:12–16.
4. Böttcher HD, Schopohl B, Liermann D, et al. Endovascular irradiation—a new method to avoid recurrent stenosis after stent implantation in peripheral arteries: Technique and preliminary results. Int J Rad Oncol Biol Phys 1994;29:181–186.
5. Schopohl B, Liermann D, Jülling Pohlit, L, et al. ^{192}Ir endovascular brachytherapy for avoidance of intimal hyperplasia after percutaneous transluminal angioplasty and stent implantation in peripheral vessels: 6 years of experience. Int J Radiat Oncol Biol Phys 1996;36–44:835–840.
6. Steidle B. Präventive perkutane strahlentherapie zur vermeidung von intimahyperplasie nach angioplastie mit stentimplatation, strahlenther. Oncology 1994;170:151–154.
7. Waksman R, Crocker IA, Kikeri D, et al. Long term results of endovascular radiation therapy for prevention of restenosis in the peripheral vascular system. Circulation 1996;94:1745.

8. van t' Hooft E, Löffler EG, Schaart D, et al. Brachytherapy for prevention of restenosis—Afterloading requirements for endovascular use. In: Waksman R (ed.): Vascular Brachytherapy. Veenendaal, The Netherlands: Nucletron BV; 1996:318–325.
9. Waksman R. The Nucletron peripheral vascular brachytherapy system. In: Waksman R, Serruys P (eds.): Handbook of Vascular Brachytherapy. Armonk, NY: Futura Publishing Co; 1998:111–116.

## Chapter 55

The Guidant Coronary Source Wire System

Albert E. Raizner, MD, Grzegorz L. Kaluza, MD, PhD,
Richard V. Calfee, PhD, and Anthony J. Bradshaw, BS

Introduction

Restenosis remains a significant clinical challenge in interventional cardiology. While the introduction of stents has reduced the rates of restenosis following interventional procedures, restenosis continues to be a major problem. The use of radiotherapy in the treatment of various malignant and nonmalignant proliferative conditions has led several researchers to explore the use of radioisotopes to reduce the incidence of restenosis. Numerous animal studies and early clinical trials have demonstrated the potential of intravascular radiotherapy to reduce restenosis.[1]

The Guidant Coronary Source Wire System (Guidant, Santa Clara, CA) is the product of years of research and development efforts. The system consists of three elements: a beta-emitting (^{32}P) source wire (Fig. 1); a source delivery unit (Fig. 2); and a centering catheter (Fig. 3). It has been designed with three goals in mind: safety, simplicity, and precision.

The Guidant system takes advantage of significant medical device expertise. NeoCardia, which was acquired by Guidant in May 1997, was a pioneer in the field of intravascular radiotherapy, having conducted animal studies with investigators from Baylor College of Medicine as early as 1993. In addition, Guidant's Vascular Intervention Division brings years of experience developing innovative products in the field of interventional cardiology.

Furthermore, Guidant has formed two exclusive alliances with Nucletron (the worldwide leader in brachytherapy systems for oncology). As part of the first alliance, Guidant has developed a centering catheter (the PARIS® catheter) to be used with the Nucletron microSelectron-HDR afterloader (Nucletron, Veenendaal, The Netherlands) and iridium 192 (^{192}Ir) source (see Chapter 54).[2] Under the second alliance, Guidant and Nucletron have worked exclusively together to develop intravascular radiotherapy systems for coronary vessels and have used their combined expertise to develop, manufacture, and service coronary source wire systems. As a result, a specially modified version of the Nucletron microSelectron-HDR afterloader has been used in the first clinical trials. Further modifications resulting from animal and clinical research led to the construction of the

From Waksman R (ed.). *Vascular Brachytherapy, Third Edition.* Armonk, NY: Futura Publishing Co., Inc.; © 2002.

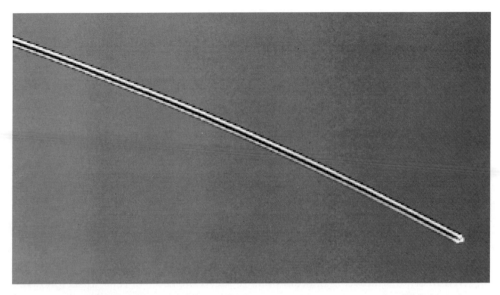

Figure 1. The Guidant intravascular radiotherapy coronary source wire. This is an investigational device limited by U.S. law to investigational use.

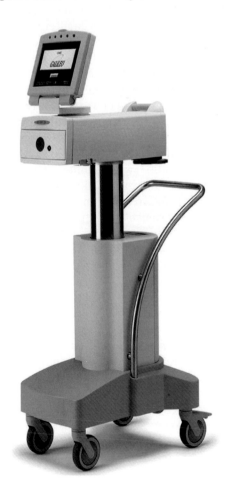

Figure 2. The Guidant Galileo™ intravascular radiotherapy source delivery unit. This is an investigational device that is limited by U.S. law to investigational use.

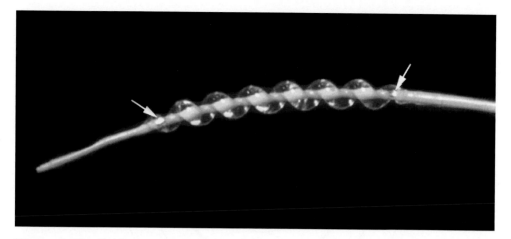

Figure 3. The Guidant intravascular radiotherapy centering catheter. This is an investigational device that is limited by U.S. law to investigational use.

second generation Galileo system, which has been launched in European markets and is currently being tested in the U.S. for clinical approval.

Overview of the Guidant Galileo Coronary Source Wire System

The Guidant Galileo Coronary Source Wire System consists of three components:

- A source wire containing phosphorus 32 (^{32}P), a pure beta-emitting isotope;
- A Source Delivery Unit, which stores and shields the source wire, calculates the dosimetry, and advances and retracts the wire;
- A centering catheter, which contains a dedicated, closed-end lumen through which the source wire travels, and also has a spiral balloon that centers the source wire within the artery and may allow for perfusion during the procedure.

These elements are discussed in detail below.

Source Wire

The Guidant coronary source wire is a flexible 0.018" nitinol wire with the beta isotope, ^{32}P, hermetically sealed within the distal tip. The source wire first approved for investigational use has an active length of 27 mm. Other lengths, however, will be available, by using a 20-mm stepping source within the centering catheter to provide a choice of 40- and 60-mm radioactive lengths. A pure beta emitter that is commonly used in medical and nonmedical applications, ^{32}P has a maximum energy of 1.71 MeV and a 14.3-day half-life. It features a rapid dose fall-off with the radial distance from the source,[3] which contributes favorably to its safety profile (Fig. 4). The source will be used for approximately two half-lives before being exchanged. Recent studies have shown that, to treat larger vessels and

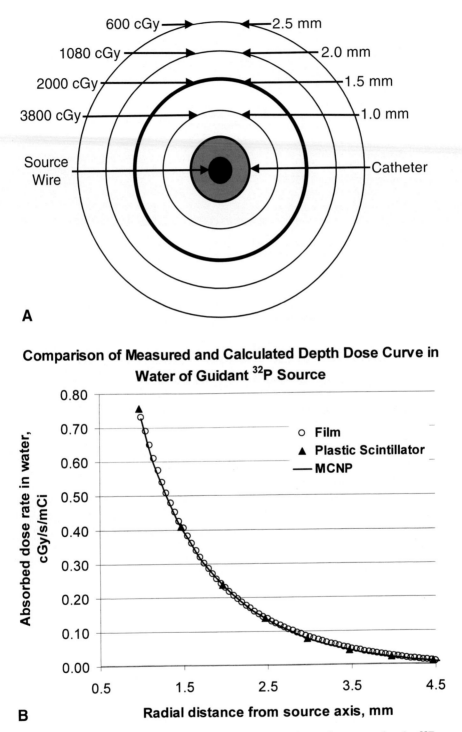

Figure 4. A. Dose fall-off with increasing distance away from the source for the ^{32}P source wire. Doses based on Monte Carlo calculations. **B.** Comparison of depth dose curve in water of the Guidant ^{32}P source measured with radiochromic film and plastic scintillator versus Monte Carlo calculation.

to extend the useful lifespan of the source wire, dose rates of up to 150 cGy/s (@ 0.5-mm tissue depth) may be safely used.[4,5] This development broadens the spectrum of treatable vessel sizes without prolonging radiation treatment time.

Source Delivery Unit

The source delivery unit serves several important functions.

- *Source storage and shielding:* The source delivery unit contains a safe that stores and completely shields the source wire when it is not in use.
- *Computer-aided dosimetry:* The source delivery unit contains a computer that assists the medical staff in performing the procedure. In order to complete the treatment, the physician enters the vessel diameter and the desired dose. The system then determines the current activity of the source at any moment and automatically calculates the treatment time required to deliver the desired dose.
- *Source delivery and retraction:* The source delivery unit also contains a drive mechanism to advance and retract the source wire. Once the treatment time has been determined, the system automatically advances to the treatment site a nonradioactive "dummy" or check wire. This nonradioactive wire, which has dimensions identical to the active wire, is advanced first in order to ensure that there are no kinks or obstructions in the catheter. Also, the physician uses this nonradioactive wire to conduct the final positioning under fluoroscopy. This wire is then retracted and the source wire is advanced.

Centering Catheter

The Guidant centering catheter is a low profile, rapid exchange catheter with a spiral balloon. The catheter has two radiopaque markers 27 mm apart to aid in the positioning of the source wire. (See Table 1 for additional technical specifications.)

There are three main purposes for the centering catheter.

- *Pathway for the source wire:* The centering catheter contains a dedicated, closed-end lumen for the source wire. During the procedure, the centering

Table 1

Centering Catheter Technical Specifications

Type	Rapid Exchange
Configuration	Spiral balloon
Catheter length	135 cm
Balloon/treatment length	27 mm
Shaft size	4.1 F
Balloon profile	<3.9 F
Balloon operating pressure	4 ATM
Balloon diameters	2.5, 3.0, 3.5 mm

catheter is connected to the source delivery unit and the source wire travels through this dedicated lumen. The fact that the source wire travels down this dedicated channel—never coming in contact with blood—allows the source wire to be used in multiple cases.

• *Centering:* Guidant believes that it is important to center the source wire within the artery (see centering discussion in "Precision" section, below). A traditional balloon catheter would not adequately center the wire (Fig. 5). The spiral balloon provides multiple points of contact with the vessel wall, achieving a greater degree of centering.

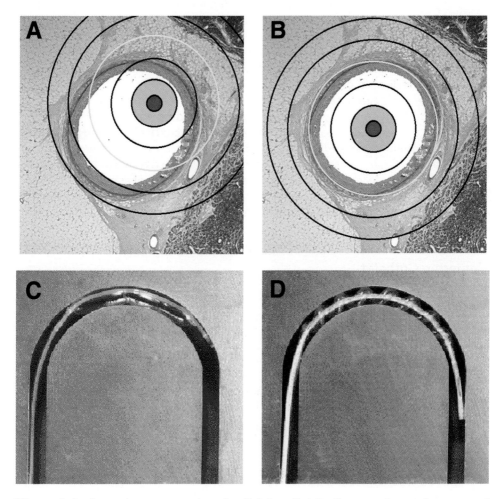

Figure 5. A schematic representation of radial dose distribution superimposed on a vessel cross section (**A, B**) and the difference between a conventional angioplasty balloon and the Guidant centering catheter (**C, D**). **A.** Asymmetric dose delivery to the structures of the arterial wall when the catheter (gray) containing the source (red) is not centered in the artery. **B.** In contrast, when the catheter (gray) containing the source (red) is centered in the artery, the radiation dose is more uniformly delivered to the vessel wall. **C.** A standard percutaneous transluminal coronary angioplasty catheter on a bend. **D.** The Guidant centering catheter on a bend. Note the constantly centered position of the lumen for the source wire (white). This is an investigational device that is limited by U.S. law to investigational use.

- *Perfusion:* Although the treatment times with Guidant's beta source are short (an average of <5 min in initial clinical studies), the ability to provide blood flow to the surrounding tissue will reduce the chances that the procedure must be stopped and the dose "fractionated" (delivered in two or more distinct fractions). The spiral balloon of Guidant's centering catheter may allow perfusion during the procedure. Blood moving around the catheter in a corkscrew fashion may provide for both side branch and distal perfusion (Fig. 6).

More recently, it has become evident that insufficient longitudinal radiation coverage at one or both ends of the intervention zone (commonly referred to as "geographic miss") may result from the dose fall-off at the ends of the source within an area of vascular injury.[6] This, in turn, may lead to the development of the "edge effect." The original centering balloon and source length were sufficient to appropriately cover the lesions whose interventional treatment length (balloon, stent) did not exceed 22 mm in length. Accordingly, longer balloons have

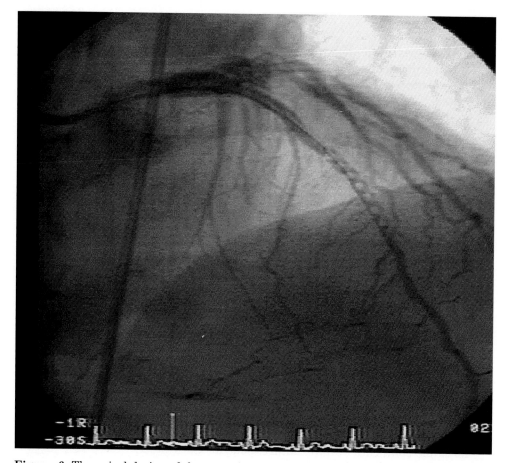

Figure 6. The spiral design of the centering catheter balloon enables perfusion to distal portion and the side branches of the irradiated vessel while ensuring the centering of the source wire. The angioplasty guidewire is apposed against the vessel wall.

been developed in conjunction with stepping the source within their length. Additionally, to minimize the chance of any vessel injury in the dose fall-off zone, the irradiated length was extended to 4 mm beyond the centering spiral balloon which has some potential for injury of the vessel wall by virtue of surface contact and inflation.

Another modification of the centering catheter currently under investigation is its adaptation for treatment of larger diameter vessels, including superficial femoral arteries.

Design Goals

The Guidant Coronary Source Wire System has been developed with three overlapping design goals in mind: safety, simplicity, and precision. Guidant believes that for any system to be used in a large number of catheterization laboratories worldwide, it must meet each of these three goals.

Safety

Guidant has attempted to develop a system that is as safe as possible—for the patient, the physician, and the catheterization laboratory personnel—by minimizing radiation exposure and designing multiple, redundant safety features into the system.

Minimal Radiation Exposure

- The use of ^{32}P, a pure beta-emitting isotope, minimizes both the total body dose of radiation to the patient and the radiation exposure to catheterization laboratory personnel. Compared to gamma radiation, beta radiation is more easily shielded. Less than 1 cm of acrylic substantially shields the source. In addition, when a beta source is inside the patient, the amount of radiation surrounding the patient is barely above background levels. With beta radiation, catheterization laboratory personnel can remain in the room during the delivery of radiation with minimal additional precautions.
- The Source Delivery Unit's touch screen display and drive mechanisms allow a completely hands-off delivery of radiation.

Multiple Redundant Safety Features

- The isotope is hermetically sealed within the source wire. A drive mechanism delivers this wire through a dedicated, sealed lumen in the centering catheter, providing double containment of the source. As a result, there is no single point catastrophic failure mode for the system.
- A nonradioactive "dummy" source wire is always advanced before the source wire in order to check the pathway for any kind or obstructions. Only

after the dummy wire has been successfully delivered and retracted will the source wire be advanced.

- The source delivery unit automatically calculates the correct treatment time, to reduce the possibility of human error. If the radiation dose must be fractionated, the computer stores the amount of radiation that has been delivered and automatically delivers only the remaining fraction.
- A force-sensing mechanism detects any obstructions as the source is delivered. If any obstructions are detected, the wire is automatically withdrawn.
- Once the total dose has been delivered, the source delivery unit automatically retracts the source wire, to prevent the delivery of any excess radiation.
- The physician can interrupt the treatment and automatically retract the source at any point by pressing an emergency "STOP" button.
- There are multiple fail-safe mechanisms in the system. The source delivery unit also has a back-up battery, which will automatically retract the source if power is lost. The unit also includes a back-up manual crank to retract the source in an emergency, as well as tools to remove the wire and a safe to store the source as a final back-up.
- The source delivery unit has password protection and keyed switches to prevent unauthorized use.

Simplicity

A primary design goal has been to develop a system that is as easy to use as possible. While drawing on the long history of afterloader and source wire systems in medical applications, the Guidant Galileo Coronary Source Wire System has been specifically designed for use in cardiac catheterization laboratories. A number of features have been developed in the Coronary Source Wire System to achieve that goal.

Ease of Operation

- The operation of the source delivery unit is conducted through a user-friendly touch-screen display (Fig. 7). The unit is positioned at catheterization laboratory table and can be controlled by the physician who is conducting the procedure.
- The centering catheter has a special "key" connector so that the source delivery unit can automatically determine the size of the catheter. The system uses this as the starting point to simplify the entry of the vessel lumen diameter.
- The system automatically determines the current activity of the source at any moment. The physician enters the vessel lumen diameter and the system automatically displays the desired dose and calculates the required radiation treatment time.

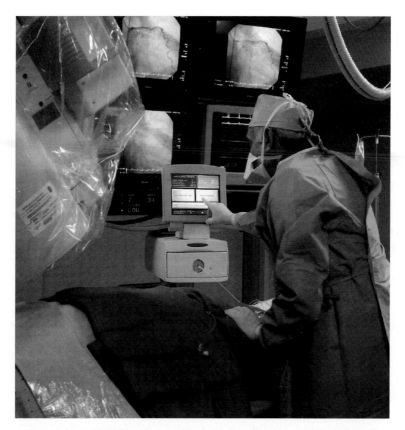

Figure 7. The Guidant Galileo™ intravascular radiotherapy source delivery unit is operated with a touch-screen display. This is an investigational device that is limited by U.S. law to investigational use.

Catheterization Laboratory Compatibility

- With the ^{32}P beta source, there is no need to add shielding to the catheterization laboratory or to modify the room in any way. Also, personnel are able to stay in the room during the radiation treatment. The total exposure from the beta radiation is significantly less than the exposure from fluoroscopy.
- Treatment times are short, averaging less than 5 minutes in initial clinical studies, preventing significant disruption to the catheterization laboratory schedule.
- After the procedure, the relevant information about the radiation treatment is displayed on the screen of the source delivery unit. This information can then be included in the patient's chart.
- The system is compatible with existing percutaneous transluminal coronary angioplasty (PTCA) products. The centering catheter is advanced over a 0.014" guidewire using standard rapid exchange techniques.
- The source delivery unit is portable; so one system can service multiple catheterization laboratories.
- There is no disposal of radioactive materials by the catheterization labora-

tory. After the case is completed, the centering catheter is disposed of as normal medical waste, since there is no radiation contamination of the catheter. The source wire is reused in multiple cases and is stored in the source delivery unit.

Precision

One of the main benefits of afterloading systems for oncology applications is the precision with which the dose can be delivered. These principles have been incorporated into Guidant's Coronary Source Wire System. In addition, Guidant believes that centering the beta source will allow for more precision in dosimetry. Recent evidence from human intravascular ultrasound data, which served to calculate the dose distribution in actual atherosclerotic vessels, suggests that guiding the prescription by the vessel size and source centering allow the most effective and uniform dose delivery to the adventitia (considered to be the target for vascular brachytherapy)[7] (see below).

Automated Source Delivery

- With the Guidant Coronary Source Wire System, the source wire is delivered and retracted automatically by a drive mechanism. This allows for precise delivery of the source to the treatment site. During the procedure, a nonradioactive "dummy" wire is first advanced. The physician can move this wire in 1-mm increments until it is precisely lined up with the radiopaque markers on the centering catheter. Once this has been done, the source wire can be delivered to exactly the same location.
- The source delivery unit also calculates the amount of time needed to deliver the correct dose, based on the reference vessel lumen diameter and the current activity of the source wire. As soon as the correct dose has been delivered, the wire is automatically retracted.
- If the treatment is interrupted at any point, the computer automatically records the data and calculates the remaining treatment time needed to complete the procedure.

Centering

- The rapid drop-off of radioactive sources over distance makes them ideally suited to intravascular applications. However, Guidant believes that this steep drop-off over distance results in the need to center the source within the artery.
- The Guidant centering catheter allows the physician to control the dose given to the artery walls. Noncentered systems could be lying at any point within the lumen of the artery, making it impossible to assess how much radiation the artery received. It is possible to determine the dosimetry with greater precision if the source is centered.
- In addition, centering can reduce the maximum dose received by the vessel wall, since the source is positioned in the center of the lumen. Similarly, cen-

tering can reduce the variability in dose received at various parts of the vessel.

Animal Study Results

The Guidant Coronary Source Wire System has undergone extensive animal studies. NeoCardia, in conjunction with the Baylor College of Medicine, performed its first animal study in 1993, using high dose rate ^{192}Ir delivered in the coronary arteries of Hanford minipigs. This study tested three doses of radiation and control, delivered through a noncentered catheter. The trial showed a dose-response effect in left anterior descending (LAD) and left circumflex (LCX) arteries. This effect was not seen in the right coronary artery (RCA), which led the investigators to hypothesize that the lack of centering in this curved vessel resulted in overdosing and underdosing, leading to the negative results.[8]

In 1994, NeoCardia and Baylor conducted a pilot animal study using a PTCA balloon filled with liquid ^{32}P. Substantial reduction in neointimal formation, normalized to the degree of injury, was observed at 30 Gy (at the lumen surface) versus control. In 1996, NeoCardia began conducting animal studies with a ^{32}P source wire system and a spiral centering catheter. A study of a 27-mm ^{32}P source was conducted in the coronary arteries of 76 pigs. Six doses, ranging from 7 to 36 Gy (measured 1 mm into the vessel wall) plus a control were studied in balloon-injured and stent-injured arteries. The study showed a significant reduction in neointimal area versus control. The most effective doses appeared to be from 14 to 26 Gy (Fig. 8). Notably, positive results with the centered system were seen in the RCA as well as in the LAD and LCX arteries[9–11] (Fig. 9).

Further research aimed at expanding the spectrum of applications by studying the effects of very high dose rates on the balloon-injured and stented arteries. Dose rates up to 150 cGy/s proved to be safe and effective in reducing neointimal formation. In balloon-injured arteries they induced positive remodeling proportionate to the dose rate used. A safety ceiling was suggested at the dose rate of 275 cGy/s which resulted in more adverse than favorable effects.[4,5,11] However, this observation was based on a very small sample size. More animals must be studied before such a ceiling can be verified.

Clinical Trials

Based on those results, Guidant began a clinical trial of the Coronary Source Wire System. This trial, called Proliferation REduction with Vascular ENergy Trial (PREVENT),[12] was a prospective, blinded, randomized trial designed to test the safety and performance of the Guidant system. Patients were randomized to receive placebo or doses of 16, 20, and 24 Gy (measured 1 mm into the vessel wall). The U.S. Food and Drug Administration approved Guidant's Investigational Device Exemption in September 1997, and the first patient was treated on October 28, 1997. The first PREVENT sites were:

- The Methodist Hospital, Houston, TX, USA
  Albert E. Raizner, MD, Principal Investigator
- Stanford University Medical Center, Stanford, CA, USA
  Stephen Oesterle, MD, Principal Investigator

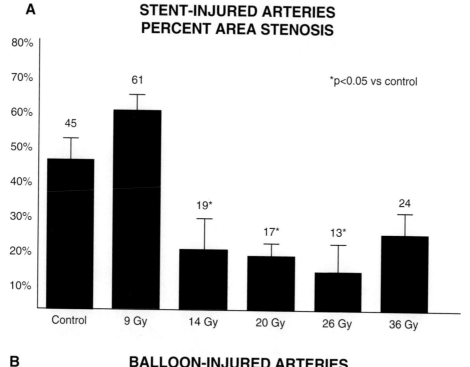

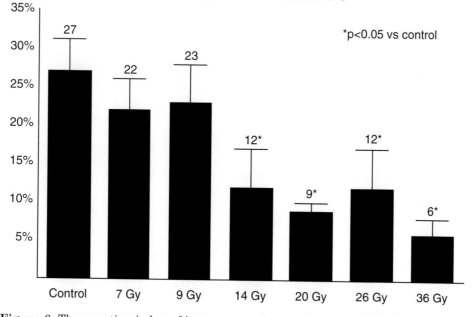

Figure 8. Therapeutic window of intracoronary beta radiation with the 27-mm centered ^{32}P source wire in a pig model of restenosis occurring 28 days after balloon or stent injury. Reduction in percent area stenosis with doses between 14 and 26 Gy to 1 mm beyond the lumen surface in stent (**A**) and balloon-injured arteries (**B**).

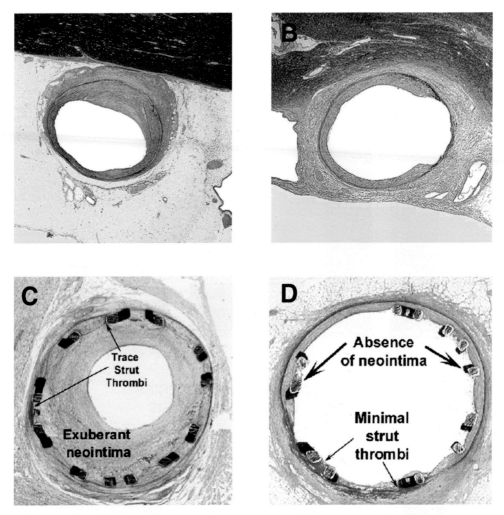

Figure 9. Histologic sections of the balloon-injured (**A, B**) and stent-injured (**C, D**) arteries at 4-week follow-up after injury and beta radiation from a centered ^{32}P source wire, magnification 20×. Optimal results of radiation. **A.** Control artery with abundant neointima. **B.** Artery irradiated with at 20 Gy to 1 mm depth of the vessel wall. Absence of neointima, some positive remodeling. **C.** Control stented artery with exuberant neointima. **D.** Artery irradiated after stent placement with 20 Gy to the adventitia. Inhibition of neointimal proliferation, minimal thrombi at the stent struts.

- Washington Hospital Center, Washington DC, USA
  Ron Waksman, MD, Principal Investigator
- Erasmus University-Thoraxcenter, Rotterdam, The Netherlands
  Patrick W. Serruys, MD, Principal Investigator
- Centro Cuore Columbus, Milan, Italy
  Antonio Colombo, MD, Principal Investigator
- National Heart Center, Singapore
  Yean-Leng Lim, MD, Principal Investigator

One hundred and five patients with de novo (70%) or restenotic (30%) lesions who were treated by stenting (61%) or balloon angioplasty (39%) received 0 (control), 16, 20, or 24 Gy to a depth of 1 mm into the artery wall. Angiography at 6 months showed a target site late loss index of $11\pm36\%$ in radiotherapy patients versus $55\pm30\%$ in controls ($P<0.0001$). A low late loss index was seen in stented and balloon-treated patients, and was similar across the 16-, 20-, and 24-Gy radiotherapy groups. Restenosis (defined as $\geq50\%$ diameter stenosis at follow-up angiography) rates were significantly lower in radiotherapy patients at the target site (8% versus 39%, $P=0.012$) and at the target site plus adjacent segments (22% versus 50%, $P=0.018$). Target site revascularization was needed in 5 radiotherapy patients (6%) and 6 controls (24%, $P<0.05$).

In summary, PREVENT showed that beta radiotherapy with a centered ^{32}P source proved to be safe and highly effective within a broad range of doses in inhibiting restenosis at the target site after stent or balloon angioplasty. However, stenosis adjacent to the target site and late thrombotic events reduced the overall clinical benefit of radiotherapy, similar to other early trials of beta and gamma radiation. Consequently, the technique has been modified to assure treatment of a 3- to 5-mm margin beyond the zone of injury in order to avoid "geographic miss." Also, to reduce late thrombotic events, treatment with antiplatelet drugs has been extended to 6 months. Preliminary data offer hope that these two measures may be effective in minimizing the observed adverse effects of intracoronary radiotherapy.

The INHIBIT trial studied the effectiveness of the Guidant System in 332 patients with in-stent restenosis randomized to receive 20 Gy 1 mm into the artery wall or a sham procedure. Restenosis rates were reduced by 67% (16 versus 48% in the stent segment), and 48% (26 versus 51% in the analysis segment. MACE at 9 months was reduced 56% (14 versus 31%) by radiotherapy. The incidence or late clinical thrombosis was only 1.8%, not significantly different than control.

The INHIBIT study demonstrated that radiotherapy with the Guidant system was safe and highly effective in reducing repeat restenosis in patients with in-stent restenosis.

References

1. Kuntz RE, Baim DS. Prevention of coronary restenosis: The evolving evidence base for radiation therapy. Circulation 2000;101:2130–2133.
2. Waksman R. The Nucletron peripheral vascular brachytherapy system. In: Waksman R, Serruys PW (eds.): Handbook of Vascular Brachytherapy. London: Martin Dunitz Ltd.; 2000:61–68.
3. Mourtada FA, Soares CG, Seltzer SM, et al. Dosimetry characterization of ^{32}P catheter-based vascular brachytherapy source wire. Med Phys 2000;27:1770–1778.
4. Kaluza GL, Raizner AE, Ali NM, et al. Dose rate mediated vascular remodeling of porcine coronary arteries following balloon injury and intracoronary β-radiation. Circulation 1999;100(suppl I):I–75.
5. Kaluza GL, Raizner AE, Ali NM, et al. High dose rates of intracoronary beta radiation in stented porcine coronary arteries: Efficacy for inhibition of restenosis. Am J Cardiol 1999;84:(suppl 6A):11.
6. Sabate M, Costa MA, Kozuma K, et al. Geographic miss: A cause of treatment failure in radio-oncology applied to intracoronary radiation therapy. Circulation 2000;101: 2467–2471.
7. Kaluza GL, Ali NM, Raizner AE, et al. Targeting the adventitia with intracoronary beta radiation: Comparison of two dose prescriptions with intravascular ultrasound. Circulation 1999;100(suppl I):I–516.
8. Mazur W, Ali MN, Raizner AE, et al. High dose rate intracoronary radiation for inhibition of neointimal formation in the stented and balloon-injured porcine models of

restenosis: Angiographic, morphometric, and histopathologic analyses. Int J Radiat Oncol Biol Phys 1996;36:777–788.

9. Ali NM, Buergler JM, Raizner AE. The effect of intracoronary β-radiation dose on neointimal formation and vascular remodeling after arterial injury in a porcine coronary restenosis model. Circulation 1998;98(suppl I):I–676.

10. Ali NM, Buergler JM, Raizner AE, et al. The effect of intracoronary β-radiation dose on neointimal formation and percent area stenosis in a stented porcine coronary restenosis model. Circulation 1998(suppl I):I-676.

11. Ali NM, Kaluza, Raizner AE, et al. The effect of intracoronary β-radiation dose on neointimal formation and vascular remodeling in balloon injured porcine coronary arteries: Effect of dose rate. J Interven Cardiol 1999;12:271–282.

12. Raizner AE, Oesterle SN, Waksman R, et al. Inhibition of restenosis with beta-emitting radiotherapy: Report of the Proliferation Reduction With Vascular Energy Trial (PREVENT). Circulation 2000;102:951–958.

Liquid-Filled Balloons for Coronary Brachytherapy

Judah Weinberger, MD, PhD,
and F.F. (Russ) Knapp, Jr., PhD

Introduction

The use of radiation delivered in sufficient dose to the vessel wall is a promising method – the only method to prevent restenosis after arterial angioplasty or stent implantment. Although the identity of the actual target cell(s) and mechanism of action are not well understood, use of radiation offers the promise of a simple method, and both gamma- and beta-particle-emitting radionuclides as well as x-ray sources are being evaluated for this application. Several vehicles for delivering the radioactive source are being actively pursued, including catheter-based systems for delivery of an acute dose in a short time period (ie, 3 to 20 min), and the use of radioactive metal stents for permanent placement, for delivery of a chronic dose over a much longer time period. Catheter-based systems that are currently being evaluated in both the preclinical phase and for clinical vessel irradiation after angioplasty include the use of radioactive wires and encapsulated linear trains or ribbons of radioactive sources. In addition, the use of radioactive solutions for balloon inflation for intravascular vessel irradiation is being evaluated.

An important issue is which type of radiation is most effective and most easily used for vessel irradiation. The relative merits and issues associated with the handling, safety, disposal, and use of gamma-emitting radioisotopes (ie, iridium 192) and beta-particle-emitting radioisotopes (strontium 90, rhenium 188, etc.) are also being widely discussed. In addition, it is not clear which radioisotope may be the most optimal for this unique application. While the solid sources do not inherently require special handling in terms of staff or patient contamination, liquids require a careful assessment of the best choice of chemical species. For the liquid-filled balloon approach, the patient safety issues in the event of balloon rupture, and the radiological issues associated with the handling and use of radioactive solutions for both the patient and catheterization laboratory staff, require careful consideration.

Research at Oak Ridge National Laboratory was sponsored by the Office of Biological and Environmental Research, U.S. Department of Energy, under contract AC05–96OR22464 with Lockheed Martin Energy Research Corporation.

From Waksman R (ed.). *Vascular Brachytherapy, Third Edition.* Armonk, NY: Futura Publishing Co., Inc.; © 2002.

The use of angioplasty balloons filled with radioisotope solutions inflated at low pressures offers an attractive alternative for coronary vessel wall irradiation for the inhibition of restenosis following percutaneous transluminal coronary angioplasty (PTCA) or stenting for both de novo and "in-stent" restenosis.[1] Although most catheter-based radioisotopic approaches utilize radioactive wires or wire coils attached to flexible guidewires or a linear array of radioactive seeds, the centering of the sources within the vessel lumen can often be a problem. Use of a radioactive solution uniformly fills the expanded balloon and provides the most uniform and homogeneous dose to the vessel wall. The liquid-filled balloon approach does not require any capital investment or special consumables, since standard equipment is used for low-pressure inflation with the radioactive solution. In this chapter, the requirements of radioisotope candidates for the liquid-filled balloon approach are discussed, and the use of rhenium 188 obtained from the tungsten 188/rhenium 188 generator for vessel irradiation is discussed in detail.

Technical Issues Associated with the Liquid-Filled Balloon Approach

Physical Requirements for Candidate Radioisotopes

Inflation of angioplasty balloons with radioactive liquids for intravascular brachytherapy requires that the chemical species of the radioisotope ensure rapid excretion via the urinary bladder in the unlikely event of balloon rupture. In addition, adequate procedures and safeguards must be available to minimize the possibility of contamination of the facilities. Special liquid-handling precautions, and physical separation from the other cath lab facilities, are important to minimize any likelihood of contamination.

Liquid-Filled Balloons with Beta-Emitters Versus Solid Sources

Although solid beta-emitting sources such as strontium 90/yttrium 90 are expected to have a long useful shelf life and can be used without the possible ramifications of balloon rupture, the practical issues associated with the handling and use of a highly penetrating, high-energy gamma-emitting radioisotope such as iridium 192 must be assessed, and the issues associated with nonuniform vessel wall irradiation resulting from noncentering may be very important because of the stimulation of neointimal growth from low dose irradiation. For the use of liquid-filled balloons, although the practical and radiological protection issues associated with filling the balloon with a radioactive solution are essentially the same for any radioisotope, an evaluation of the ramifications of the worst case scenario of balloon rupture and release of the radioactive contents into the circulation is probably the most important issue that must be addressed from a regulatory and safety perspective. It should be noted that balloon rupture or radioisotope release is expected to occur in less than 1 in 10,000 cases.

Liquid-Handling Issues

Handling of radioactive liquids in the catheterization laboratory requires an awareness of radiological protection issues and careful planning. For this approach, the radioactive species must be prepared in an approved facility, such as the radiopharmacy. Quality control includes sterility, pyrogenicity, rhenium 188 yield, tungsten 188 parent breakthrough, and alumina breakthrough testing. Dependent upon the radioisotope being used, concentration steps may be required to obtain the very high specific volumes (mCi/mL) required for balloon inflation such as with rhenium 188, or transformation of the lanthanide (+3) radioisotopes to stable chemical complexes that would have rapid excretion in the event of balloon rupture. After quality control, the final radioactive solution is then loaded into a sterile syringe enclosed in shielded delivery device ready for transfer to the catheterization laboratory. Since all radioisotopes evaluated to date for the liquid-filled balloon approach are high-energy beta emitters which emit only low-energy gamma photons in low abundance, Lucite is efficient for shielding. The shielded, loaded syringe is then transported to the catheterization laboratory. Since the only possibility of leakage is at the catheter attachment or via balloon rupture, we use a containment system that houses the shielded delivery device. Currently, this consists of a sterile plastic glove bag, and in other cases a sterile Lucite box.

Dosimetry of the Rhenium 188 Liquid-Filled System

Dosimetry issues include the uniformity of vessel wall irradiation from rhenium 188, definition of target tissue, and the ramifications on patient safety in the unlikely event of balloon rupture and release of the radioactive contents into the circulation. Another key issue is the acute and accumulative radiation dose to both the patient and staff from this procedure. A central issue of importance for use of the liquid-filled balloon approach for vascular therapy is the uniformity of vessel wall irradiation. Since one of the important requirements for this approach is to minimize dose to critical organs in the event of balloon rupture, it is important that any radioactive species released into the circulation exhibit rapid excretion, primarily via the urinary bladder.

Candidate Radioisotopes

Rhenium 188

In spite of the many advantages of using angioplasty balloons inflated at low pressure with radioactive solutions for vessel wall irradiation, only a limited number of reports have described this approach, which initially evaluated the use of rhenium 188.[2,3] We have proposed the use of liquid-filled balloons using rhenium 188 (16.9-hour half-life, 2.1 MeV maximal beta energy) as an excellent new candidate for use as an intravascular radiation source for uniform vessel wall irradiation. Rhenium 188 is an attractive therapeutic radioisotope conveniently obtained from the tungsten 188/rhenium 188 generator.[4–13] Because of the long useful generator shelf life (ie, 3 to 6 months), high daily elution yields (>60%), and chemistry similar to pertechnetate, rhenium 188 is a cost-effective radioisotope for restenosis therapy. The high beta energy, uniform dose delivery, and rapid urinary excretion, make rhenium 188-perrhenate an excellent new candidate for catheter-based vessel irradiation following PTCA. Swine studies using a coronary balloon overstretch model have validated the expected usefulness of rhenium 188 to inhibit coronary restenosis following balloon overstretch injury.[2] Descriptions of the tungsten 188/rhenium 188 generator system, the use of new systems for the concentration of rhenium 188-perrhenate to high specifc volumes, and the use of rhenium 188 for intravascular brachytherapy are described later in this chapter.

Rhenium 186

Other examples of radioactive solutions that are currently being evaluated for vessel irradiation include rhenium 186-perrhenate[14] and holmium 166,[15] presumably as the trivalent cation (Ho $^{+3}$). Rhenium 186 is a reactor-produced radioisotope with a 90-hour half-life (Table 1), which emits a 1.076 MeV beta particle accompanied by a 136 keV gamma photon (9% abundance). Rhenium 186-perrhenate has the same pharmacokinetic properties as rhenium188-perrhenate and is being evaluated in swine with a coronary balloon overstretch model and in an AV shunt model in sheep studies.[14] Although these limited reported results of coronary irradiation studies with rhenium 186 in the swine balloon overstretch model have shown a reduced incidence of restenosis in comparison with control overstretched arteries,[14] the ramifications of the much lower beta energy of rhenium 186 (1.076 MeV) versus rhenium 188 (2.12 MeV) on reducing restenosis in larger diameter coronary vessels, especially in the presence of eccentric or calcified plaque, remain to be seen. Since many investigators have identified the macrophage/monocyte cellular target present in the adventitia as an important target site in reducing restenosis, it would appear a priori because of the rapid drop-off of dose with radial distance (Fig. 1), that a beta energy higher than 2 MeV would be expected to be required to deliver an adequate dose (ie, 30 Gy at 0.5 mm) at the adventitia and still spare the surface dose (<60 Gy).

Another advantage of the use of rhenium 188 for vascular therapy in comparison with rhenium 186 is the availability of rhenium 188 from the tungsten

Table 1

Characteristics of Beta-Emitting Radioisotopes Used for Liquid-Filled Balloon Approach for Vascular Brachytherapy

Radioisotope	Half-life (Hours)	Beta Energy (Maximum, MeV)	Production Mode
Rhenium 188	16.9	2.12	Available on demand from in house tungsten 188/rhenium 188 generator system
Rhenium 186	90.6	1.09	Reactor-produced by irradiation of rhenium 185
Holmium 166	26.8	1.076	Reactor-produced by irradiation of holmium 165

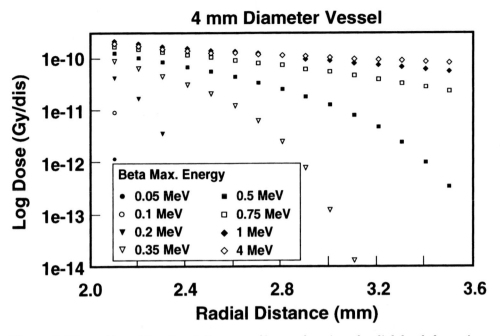

Figure 1. Illustration of the dose delivery profile as a function of radial depth for various maximal beta-article energies. Adapted with permission from Mike Stabin, PhD, Oak Ridge Associated Universities.

188/rhenium 188 generator system.[3–13] Since the generator provides high levels of rhenium 188 on a daily basis and has a useful shelf life of at least 2 to 3 months, the logistics of using rhenium 188 on an acute basis are simplified and use of rhenium 188 is expected to be very cost-effective because of its availability from the tungsten 188/rhenium 188 generator. In contrast, rhenium 186 is directly produced in a nuclear reactor by neutron irradiation of enriched rhenium 185 targets and is not available from an in-house generator. The 90-hour half-life would suggest that the logistics and costs of production, distribution, inventory, and scheduling for acute procedures would be challenging.

Holmium 166

More recently, the use of holmium 166 for intravascular brachytherapy in a swine coronary overstretch model has also been reported.[15] Holmium is a lanthanide (rare earth) element. Holmium 166 has a 26.8-hour half-life and decays with the emission of high-energy beta particles with energies of 1.77 MeV (48%) and 1.85 MeV (51%), and with emission of one gamma photon with an energy of 80.5 keV (6.2%). Holmium 166 can be produced either by neutron activation of holmium 165 with relatively high specific activity (8 to 9 Ci/mg at saturation at 2 $\times$ 10^{15} neutrons/cm^2/s) or by decay of reactor-produced dysprosium 166.[16] The production, distribution, inventory, and scheduling of studies with holmium 166, even from sites in proximity to a research reactor, would be expected to pose greater challenges than the use of rhenium 186. In addition, special considerations are required for the direct production of holmium 166 by irradiation of holmium 165, since a competing neutron capture process also produces the very long-lived metastable form, holmium 166*m* (half-life, 1200 years). Because of the possible release of radioactive balloon contents in the unlikely event of rupture, the presence of significant levels of long-lived contaminants such as holmium 166*m* cannot be tolerated. It is thus important that the irradiation conditions of the particular reactor used are carefully planned so that production of holmium 166 is optimized and the levels of holmium 166*m* impurity are minimized.

Holmium 166 is also formed via radioactive decay of dysprosium 166 parent, and can be obtained by separation from the dysprosium 166 parent (81.6-hour half-life). This would suggest that a type of radionuclide generator system for in-house separation of holmium 166 as required may be possible. Because of the close similarity in physical properties of Ho^{+3} and Dy^{+3}, even the most successful attempts to date[16] have only succeeded in systems in which both the dysprosium 166 parent and holmium 166 daughter radionuclides are separated but both are removed from the generator, requiring reprocessing of the dysprosium 166 and reloading on the generator system; this would be very impractical in a hospital-based radiopharmacy setting.

Another more ominous characteristic of holmium 166 and all lanthanide radioisotopes is the very efficient localization of the free +3 lanthanides in the cortical bone. This issue must be addressed and resolved before solutions of such radioisotopes would be acceptable for balloon inflation. Rupture of balloons containing the +3 radioisotopes would result in a dangerous radiological risk because of skeletal localization and marrow suppression. However, the possible complexation of lanthanides to chemical species which would not localize in the skeleton and which would show rapid urinary bladder excretion would be an interesting area of research.

Although it is not yet established which radioisotope and which irradiation method will be optimal and cost-effective, it is important to note that nearly all of the radioisotopes which have been proposed for vessel wall irradiation after PTCA are neutron-rich. Since they are usually reactor-produced, nuclear reactors in the U.S. will thus play a key role as this important new technology develops.

Samarium 153

Recently, the use of samarium 153 for intravascular brachytherapy in a rabbit iliac overstretch model has also been reported. Samarium is a lanthanide (rare earth) element and samarium 153 has a 46.3-hour half-life and decays with the emission of high-energy beta particles with energies of 0.802 MeV and with emission of one gamma photon with an energy of 103 keV (28%). Samarium 153 is produced by neutron activation of samarium 152 in large amounts with high specific activity even in moderate flux reactors. The accessibility of production and a somewhat longer half-life make commercialization of this isotope distinctly less complex than some of the shorter half-life isotopes. In contrast, the lower energy of beta emission will require either higher activities or longer radiation times for compararable target doses. In addition, near-field doses are higher with lower energy isotopes. This isotope is currently being developed for palliation of bone pain, and is used as a chelate of ethlenedaaminetrimethylene phosphonic (EDTMP) acid.

Use of the Tungsten 188/Rhenium 188 Generator as a Readily Available Source of Rhenium 188 for Liquid-Filled Angioplasty Balloons

The tungsten 188/rhenium 188 generator represents a cost-effective and reliable system for providing rhenium 188 as required for vascular therapy.[4–13] For therapeutic applications, the rhenium 188 radioisotope (half-life 16.9 hours; E_{max} 2.12 MeV; 15% gamma 155 keV) has many attractive properties, since it is obtained carrier-free from the reactor-produced tungsten 188 parent (half-life, 69 days) (Fig. 2). The tungsten 188/rhenium 188 generator is thus an attractive candidate for use in a clinical setting and especially in a centralized radiopharmacy. The generator system essentially represents an in-house production system and the advantage of such a system is that it can be eluted at any time required to provide the rhenium 188 daughter, although elution more than once a day would probably be impractical and is not required because of the 16.9-hour half-life of rhenium 188. From an operational standpoint, the generator has an indefinite useful shelf life and provides high yields of rhenium 188 for several months (Table 2). The useful shelf life is determined by the levels of rhenium 188 required when the generator is at equilibrium.

Tungsten 188 is produced[17–25] by irradiation of enriched tungsten 186 oxide targets in the Oak Ridge National Laboratory (ORNL; Oak Ridge, TN), High Flux Isotope Reactor (HFIR) at a thermal neutron flux of 2 to 2.5 × 10^{15} neutrons/cm²/s. The targets are processed by dissolution in dilute base in the presence of the hydrogen peroxide oxidizing agent. The specific activity of tungsten 188 averages 4 to 5 mCi/mg tungsten 186 for a one cycle, 24-day irradiation. Following dissolu-

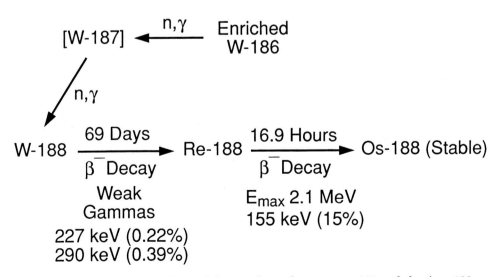

Figure 2. Nuclear production and decay scheme for tungsten 188 and rhenium 188.

Table 2

Characteristics of the ORNL Clinical-Scale Alumina-Based Tungsten
188/Rhenium 188 Generator System[¶]

Parameter	Typical Values
Clinical scale – mCi tungsten 188 loaded	1 Ci
Generator column adsorbent	10–12 ? gm aluminum oxide
Generator column dimensions (length × i.d.)	3 cm × 1.6 cm
Rhenium 188 elution yields (% of available)	75–85%/bolus
Equilibrium rhenium 188 elution yields (mCi)	750–850 mCi/bolus
Initial values before tungsten 188 decay	
Daily rhenium 188 elution yields (mCi)	500–550 mCi/bolus
24 hours between elutions (65% available)	
Tungsten 188 parent breakthrough	$<10^{-6}$ /bolus
Other radionuclide impurities[§]	Iridium 192 <5 μCi/bolus
	Osmium 191 <1 μCi/bolus
Initial bolus volume	12–15 mL
Concentrated bolus volume	<1 mL 0.9% NaCl
After tandem cation/anion column elution	
Shelf life	Unlimited, at least 6–8 mo

[¶]Data are based on experience with >twenty 500–1000 mCi generators.

[§]Iridium 192 and osmium 191 are formed by nuclear reactions during the irradiation of enriched tungsten 186 and are not formed by activation of impurities present in the target material. Impurities are essentially only detected in the initial eluant and are removed by subsequent passage through the cation/anion column system.

ORNL = Oak Ridge National Laboratory.

tion, the highly basic (pH >14) sodium tungstate solution was acidified to pH 2 to 3 with dilute HCl and then adsorbed on a column of acid-washed BioRad alumina housed in a lead shield. Generators are then conditioned by washing thoroughly with saline by slow elution and are ready for use. A photograph of the generator system housed in a lead shield is shown in Figure 3.

Because rhenium 188 is obtained from a generator, complex logistics are avoided which are associated with the repeated production, inventory, and scheduling of relatively short-lived beta-emitting radioisotopes that have been proposed for vascular therapy, such as rhenium 186 and holmium 166.

In order to minimize exposure, the tungsten 188/rhenium 188 system is used behind a leaded glass and/or Lucite shield. A short length of disposable extension tubing is attached to the lower Luer outlet connection of the generator. Inclusion of an in-line 0.22 μmol Millipore filter ensures trapping of any alumina fines or other particles that may be eluted from the generator.[4] The in-line alumina Sep-Pak® (Waters Corporation, Milford, MA) traps the low levels of tungsten 188 parent breakthrough.[26] The tandem cation/anion concentration system (Figs. 4 and 5) consists of a commercially available cation exchange cartridge with a capacity of 2 to 4 mEq attached to a three-way stopcock connected at the outlet to the QMA SepPak anion-exchange column. Another length of extension tubing then connects the outlet of the anion exchange column to the rhenium 188 collection vessel, which is housed in a lead or Lucite shield. With the stopcock open, the generator is eluted with 12 to15 mL of either saline or 0.15 M ammonium acetate solution

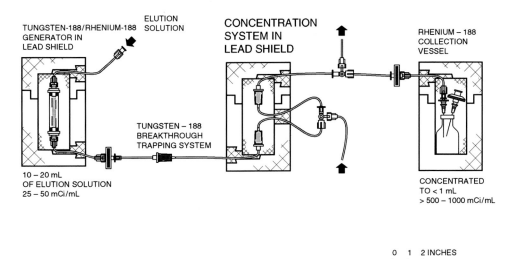

Figure 3. Schematic of the alumina-based tungsten 188/rhenium 188 generator system.

and the eluant collected from the QMA column contains only low levels of radioactivity and is discarded. The stopcock is then adjusted to permit elution of rhenium188 Na-perrhenate from the QMA anion trapping column with 0.9 mL of 0.9% saline.

We have demonstrated that clinical-scale generators loaded with levels of tungsten 188 greater than 200 mCi routinely provide reproducible high rhenium 188 yields of 75 to 85%/bolus and low tungsten 188 parent breakthrough ($<10^{-6}$)/bolus for periods of several months.[4] These studies have demonstrated that the costs of rhenium 188 will be very low on a bolus or unit dose basis.

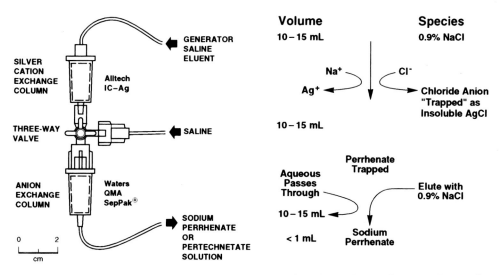

Figure 4. Tandem system using silver-impregnated cation/anion exchange columns for concentration of the rhenium-188 bolus obtained from generator elution to high specific volume.

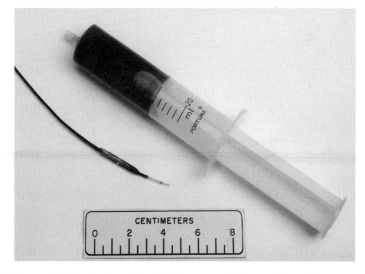

Figure 5. Photograph illustrating the effectiveness of the tandem column system for concentration of a 20 mL generator bolus to the small volume required for filling angioplasty balloon.

Concentration of Rhenium 188 Solution to High Specific Volume

Because tungsten 188 is produced[17–25] with relatively low specific activity in high flux research reactors (typically <5 mCi/mg [186]W), the large amounts of alumina required to bind the low specific activity tungsten 188 parent results in high elution volumes and low specific volume solutions of rhenium 188. Traditional chromatographic-type generators using an alumina adsorbant onto which reactor-produced tungsten 188 is adsorbed can initially provide for the first 1 to 2 weeks of use of rhenium 188 with the high specific volume (>80 mCi/mL) which is required for balloon inflation. As the tungsten 188 decays (half-life, 69 days), however, even the equilibrium levels of rhenium 188 that are obtained decrease to the level where the specific volume is significantly less than 80 mCi/mL. These dilute solutions result from the high volumes of eluant which are required to elute the bolus from the large generators required because of the low specific activity of the tungsten 188, which requires a large mass of the alumina adsorbant.

Simple effective methods are thus required for concentration of the generator eluant to the high specific volumes required for the special application of angioplasty balloon inflation for vascular therapy. Simple new methods have been developed using tandem cation/anion exchange column concentration systems[27–34] for the efficient concentration of rhenium 188-perrhenate. Use of these methods readily provides the high specific volume solutions of carrier-free rhenium 188 and extends the generator shelf life to several months. Our results have demonstrated that concentration is readily feasible for multiple elutions of clinical-scale tungsten 188/rhenium 188 (1 Ci) generators.

The bolus volume from a typical 1-Ci alumina-type tungsten 188/rhenium 188 generator is about 10 to 12 mL. Although the void volume can be discarded and the principal bolus peak collected, the initially high specific volume (60 to 80 mCi/mL) of eluant of course decreases with time as the tungsten 188 (69-day half-life) decays. Since the long useful shelf life is an important aspect for use of this generator system, the availability of simple, efficient methods for concentration of the generator eluant is very important. The technical problem involves development of methods required for separation of very low microscopic levels of per-rhenate anions in the generator eluant from large macroscopic levels of chloride anions.

The most obvious strategy for concentration involves "trapping" of the per-rhenate anion on a column from which it can then be retrieved by elution with saline. Since the traditional generator eluant is physiological saline (0.9% NaCl), the concentration of chloride anions far exceeds the concentration of the carrier-free perrhenate anions. Use of ion-exchange columns for eluant concentration thus faces the requirement of removal of the chloride anions prior to the specific trapping of perrhenate.

Efficient new methods have recently been developed using concentration of generator saline elute with a tandem silver cation/anion system,[27–29] and using the salt of a weak acid such as ammonium acetate for generator elution with subsequent concentration with a cation/anion system.[30–34] These simple methods using inexpensive, disposable concentrator components significantly increase the specific volume of the rhenium 188 solutions which increase the generator shelf life and permit the use of low-level generators for extended time periods. These methods involve the post-column elution concentration of the low specific volume solutions of rhenium 188 that are obtained from the chromatographic-type tungsten 188/rhenium 188 alumina generators.

Using these approaches, the high volumes required for generator elution do not represent a problem, because, subsequently, the solutions are easily and rapidly concentrated. The approaches are based on the selective anion trapping of the microscopic levels of the perrhenate anion following removal of the macroscopic levels of the anion of the generator salt eluant. These methods can also extend the useful shelf life of the generator, which can be as long as 1 year. The long useful shelf life of the generator is expected to provide rhenium 188 at very reasonable costs for routine use of the liquid-filled balloon approach for the inhibition of coronary restenosis after PTCA. The silver cation/anion tandem column concentration system used for post-elution rhenium 188 concentration is illustrated in Figure 5.

Consequences of Intravascular Rupture of Balloons Filled with Rhenium 188

An important consideration for the use of balloons filled with rhenium 188 for vessel wall irradiation is the consequence of balloon rupture; thus, studies have evaluated, in both animals[34] and human volunteers,[35,36] the pharmacokinetics of several chemical forms of rhenium 188, which include sodium perrhenate salts, the rhenium(V)-MAG$_3$complex,[34] and the rhenium-DTPA complex.[49] In the case of use of the perrhenate salt, concomitant administration of potassium perchlorate has been suggested to mitigate thyroid uptake in the event of balloon rupture.[47,48]

Animal Studies with Rhenium 188 for Inhibition of Coronary Restenosis

In an effort to deliver homogeneous, centered radiation fields in a technically straightforward fashion, the effects of a liquid radioisotope-filled balloon to deliver beta radiation at the time of coronary injury were studied. The first reported animal studies with rhenium 188 for vascular brachytherapy involved coronary vessel irradiation in juvenile swine (control, 11 Gy, or 25 Gy) to a segment of the left coronary system.[2] Radiation was delivered using a perfusion balloon inflated with a rhenium 188 solution. Subsequently, overdilatation PTCA was performed at the pre-treated segment. Analysis at 30 days revealed that balloon overdilatation was associated with significant vascular injury and marked neointimal proliferation in control arteries. High dose (25 Gy) radiation inhibited neointima formation compared to controls (Fig. 6). This effect was not observed with lower dose radiation (11 Gy). Thus, intracoronary radiation treatment using aqueous radioisotope sources was found to be straightforward and it effectively prevented restenosis in the porcine coronary overstretch model. Similar, more recent, studies have been reported following rhenium 188 liquid-balloon irradiation of swine arteries after coronary stent placement.[37,38]

A single-center study of the safety of intracornary beta radiation using rhenium 188-filled perfusion balloons to treat patients who have interventions in native coronary vessels has begun. In the Columbia University Restenosis Elimination (CURE) Study, 25 patients will receive open-label treatment with beta irradiation using a rhenium 188 solution to fill a perfusion balloon. These patients will be followed for 1 year, and angiographic follow-up will occur at 6 months. The data from this initial cohort of patients will provide initial insight into the relative safety of the liquid system, both in the patient and in the catheterization laboratory. This information will also lay the groundwork for a future multicenter efficacy trial.

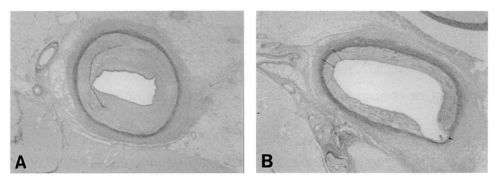

Figure 6. Illustration of the effectiveness of vessel wall irradiation with rhenium 188 liquid-filled balloon approach for the inhibition of neointimal hyperplasia in a swine coronary balloon overstretch injury model. **A.** Control artery 30 days after balloon overstretch injury. **B.** Injured artery 30 days following 25-Gy dose from rhenium 188. From Oak Ridge Associated Universities.

Dosimetry of Liquid-Filled Balloons

The use of angioplasty balloons filled with radioactive solutions of beta-emitting radioisotopes offers a unique opportunity for uniform dose delivery to the vessel wall. Several investigators have developed dosimetry models using both point kernel[39,40] and Monte Carlo code calculations[41,42] to estimate the vessel wall dose from rhenium 188 and other radioisotopes introduced as liquid sources into the balloons. In addition, the effects of stent structure on the delivery of radiation to the vessel wall using rhenium 188 liquid-filled balloons within a stented arterial segment have also been evaluated.[43,44] Finally, recent availability of rhenium 188 calibrated standards available from the National Institute of Standards and Technology (NIST) will now provide accurate calibration of dose calibrators used for determination of activity levels of rhenium 188.[45,46]

Clinical Results Using Liquid-Filled Balloons for Restenosis Therapy

As many as 30 centers care in the U.S., Europe, and Asia are currently utilizing rhenium 188-liquid coronary brachytherapy in various investigative protocols. The CURE Trial is a single center (Columbia University, NY) open-label safety trial rhenium 188-MAG$_3$ coronary brachytherapy in native coronary lesions (de novo or restenotic). Patients had clinical follow-up at 30 days and 12 months, and angiographic follow-up at 6 months. Twenty-five patients with an average of 2.5 previous interventions underwent percutaneous coronary intervention, followed by intravascular ultrasound (IVUS)-guided delivery of 13-Gy adventitial radiation from an ACS Rx Lifestream balloon inflated with the radioisotope solution. The average solution activity was 93±43 mCi/mL, and the average dwell time was 6.9±2.2 minutes. The average lesion length was 17.1 mm. There were no deaths, emergency revascularizations, or myocardial infarctions (CK >3 times control) among this group of patients. There was no intra-patient release of isotope. To date, there have been 2 "candy-wrapper" recurrences at the borders (within 4 mm) of the edge of the treatment zone. There were 4 target lesion revascularization events, and 3 patients underwent coronary artery bypass graft by 6 months. Kaplan-Meier analysis revealed a 12-month target lesion revascularization-free rate of 74.6%. It was concluded that coronary brachytherapy using a rhenium 188 solution for perfusion balloon inflation is feasible and can be performed safely.

Recently, Hoher and colleagues evaluated the feasibility and safety of intra-coronary irradiation with a balloon catheter filled with rhenium 188-perrhenate liquid. The dose given in this open-label study was 15 Gy at 0.5-mm tissue depth. Twenty-eight lesions were treated after balloon dilation (n=9) or stenting (n=19). Lesions included 19 de novo stenoses, 4 occlusions, and 5 restenoses. Irradiation time was 515±199 seconds in 1 to 4 fractions. No perfusion technology was utilized. There were no procedural complications. Quantitative coronary angiography (QCA) after intervention showed a reference diameter of 2.77±0.35 mm and a minimal lumen diameter of 2.36±0.43 mm. At 6-month follow-up, minimal lumen diameter was 1.45±0.88 mm (late loss index, 0.57). Target lesion restenosis rate (>50% in diameter) was low (12%; 3 of 26). Nine stenoses were observed at the edges of the irradiation zone. The total restenosis rate was 46% and was significantly lower (29% versus 70%, $P=0.042$) when the length of the irradiated segment was more than twice the lesion length. It was concluded that coronary irradiation with a rhenium 188-filled balloon was technically feasible and safe, requiring only standard PTCA techniques. The target lesion revascularization rate was low.[50]

Another ongoing trial, the Seoul National University Post Angioplasty Rhenium (SPARE) Trial, is a randomized, placebo-controlled study of rhenium 188-DTPA brachytherapy with a dose of 17.6 Gy at 1-mm tissue depth. Ninety-nine patients were enrolled in the study and 30 patients have completed the mandated 6-month angiographic follow-up. In the in-stent radiation group, there was no in-stent or in-lesion restenosis except in one patient who had 75% narrowing in the proximal segment of stent, which had residual dissection flap (type B) with good distal blood flow just after stenting. Final QCA and IVUS data is expected to be available in early 2001 (personal communication, In-Ho Chae, MD).

It is clear that radioactive liquid brachytherapy offers a practical, economical alternative to solid-source radiation delivery. The proof of the comparable efficacy of this approach to encapsulated source delivery awaits a sponsored randomized double-blind multicenter trial. In order to make this approach clinically viable, liquid handling technology needs to be developed, consensus must be reached on suitable isotope selection, and optimized distribution systems for isotope delivery must be put in place. These requirements are certainly achievable with incremental developments over existing technologies.

References

1. Amols H, Reinstein LE, Weinberger J. Dosimetry of a radioactive coronary balloon dilation catheter for treatment of neointimal hyperplasia [abstract]. Med Phys 1996;23:1080–1081.
2. Gledd KN, Amols H, Marboe C, et al. Effectiveness of beta-emitting liquid-filled perfusion balloon to prevent restenosis [abstract]. Circulation 1997;96:I–220.
3. Knapp Jr FF, Guhlke S, Beets AL, et al. Rhenium-188—Attractive properties for intravascular brachytherapy for inhibition of coronary restenosis after PTCA [abstract]. J Nucl Cardiol 1997;4:S–118.
4. Knapp FF Jr, Beets AL, Guhlke S, et al. Development of the alumina-based tungsten-188/rhenium-188 generator and use of rhenium-188-labeled radiopharmaceuticals for cancer treatment. Anticancer Res 1997;17:1783–1796.
5. Knapp Jr FF, Mirzadeh S, Beets AL, et al. Curie scale tungsten-188/rhenium-188 generators can cost-effectively provide carrier-free rhenium 188 for routine clinical applications. In: Nicolini M, Bandoli G, Mazzi U (eds.): Technetium in Chemistry and Nuclear Medicine. Padova: SG Editoriali; 1995:319–334.
6. Knapp FF Jr, Guhlke S, Weinberger J, et al. High specific volume rhenium-188: Clinical potential of a readily available therapeutic radioisotope [abstract]. Nuklearmedizin 1997;36:A38.
7. Knapp FF Jr, Guhlke S, Beets AL, et al. Intraarterial irradiation with rhenium-188 for inhibition of restenosis after PTCA: Strategy and evaluation of species for rapid urinary excretion [abstract]. J Nucl Med 1997;38:124P.
8. Knapp Jr FF, Mirzadeh S, Zamora P, et al. Rhenium-188 – Cost-effective therapeutic applications of a readily available generator-derived radioisotope [abstract]. Nucl Med Commun 1996;17:268.
9. Knapp FF Jr, Mirzadeh S, Beets AL, et al. Curie-scale tungsten-188/rhenium-188 generators provide carrier-free rhenium-188 for clinical applications. In: Nicolini M, Badoli G, Mazzi U (eds.): Fourth International Symposium on Technetium in Chemistry

and Nuclear Medicine. Bressanone, Italy, September 12–14, 1994. Padova, Italy: SG Editorali; 1995;3:319–324.

10. Knapp FF Jr, Lisic E, Mirzadeh S, et al. A new clinical prototype tungsten-188/ rhenium-188 generator to provide high levels of carrier-free rhenium-188 for radioimmunotherapy. In: Nuclear Medicine in Research and Practice. Stuutgart, Germany: Schattauer Verlag; 1992:183–186.

11. Callahan AP, Rice DE, Knapp FF Jr. Rhenium-188 for therapeutic applications from an alumina-based tungsten-188/rhenium-188 radionuclide generator. Nuc Compact 1989; 20:3–6.

12. Knapp FF Jr. Radionuclide generators in nuclear medicine: Present status and future perspectives. In: Proceedings, International Trends in Radiopharmaceuticals for Diagnosis and Therapy. Lisbon, Portugal: March 30–April 3, 1998; IAEA TECDOC-1029, 485–495.

13. Kamioki H, Mirzadeh S, Lambrecht RM, et al. Tungsten-188/rhenium-188 generator for biomedical applications. Radiochim Acta 1994;65:39–46.

14. Smith EF, Pipes D, Konijnenberg M, et al. Efficacy of a Re-186-filled PTCA balloon system to prevent restenosis of peripheral vessels in swine and A-V graphs in sheep [abstract]. In: Syllabus, Advances in Cardiovascular Radiation Therapy, Sponsored by the Cardiology Research Foundation. Washington, DC, February 20–21, 1997:20.

15. Kim H-S, Cho Y-H, Oh Y-T, et al. Effect of transcatheter endovascular holmium-166 irradiation on neointimal formation after balloon injury in porcine coronary artery [abstract]. J Am Coll Cardiol 1998;31(suppl A):277A.

16. Dadachova E, Mirzadeh S, Lambrecht RM, et al. Separation of carrier-free holmium-166 from neutron-irradiated dysprosium targets. Anal Chem 1994;66:4272–4277.

17. Knapp FF Jr, Callahan AP, Beets AL, et al. Processing of reactor-produced tungsten-188 for fabrication of clinical scale alumina-base tungsten-188/rhenium-188 generators. Appl Radiat Isot 1994;45:1123–1128.

18. Mirzadeh S, Knapp FF Jr, Lambrecht RM. Burn-up cross section of tungsten-188. Radiochemica Acta 1997:77:99–102.

19. Knapp FF Jr, Mirzadeh S, Beets AL. Reactor production and processing of therapeutic radioisotopes for applications in nuclear medicine. J Radioanalyt Nucl Chem Lett 1996;205:93–100.

20. Knapp FF Jr, Callahan AP, Beets AL, et al. Processing of reactor-produced tungsten-188 for fabrication of clinical scale alumina-based tungsten-188/rhenium-188 generators. Appl Rad Isot 1994;45:1123–1128.

21. Knapp FF Jr, Mirzadeh S. Reactor production of radionuclides for nuclear medicine. In: Wagner HN, Szabo Z (eds.): Principles of Nuclear Medicine, 2nd Edition. Philadelphia: WB Saunders, Co.; 1995:135–144.

22. Knapp FF Jr, Beets AL, Callahan AP, et al. Optimized processing of reactor-produced tungsten-188 for clinical-scale W-188/Re-188 generators [abstract]. Eur J Nucl Med 1994;21:S201.

23. Knapp FF Jr, Beets AL, Guhlke H-J, et al. Rhenium-188 liquid-filled balloons effectively inhibit restenosis in a swine coronary overstretch model: A simple new method bridging nuclear medicine and interventional cardiology. 45th Annual Meeting, Society of Nuclear Medicine, Toronto, Canada, June 7–11, 1998. J Nucl Med 1998;39:48P.

24. Callahan AP, Mirzadeh S, Knapp FF Jr. Large-scale production of tungsten-188. In: Proceedings of Symposium on Radionuclide Generator Systems for Medical Applications. Amer. Chem. Soc., Washington, DC, August 24–28, 1992. Radioact Radiochem 1992;3:46–48.

25. Mirzadeh S, Knapp FF JR, Callahan AP. Production of tungsten-188 and osmium-194 in a nuclear reactor for new clinical generators. In: Qaim SM (ed.): Proceedings of the International Conference on Nuclear Data for Science and Technology. New York: Springer-Verlag; 1992:595–597.

26. Callahan AP, Rice DE, McPherson DW, et al. The use of alumina "SepPaksR" as a simple method for the removal and determination of tungsten-188 breakthrough from tungsten-188/rhenium-188 generators. Appl Radiat Isot 1992;43:801–804.

27. Singh J, Reghebi K, Lazarus CR, et al. Studies on the preparation and isomeric composition of [186]Re- and [188]Re-pentavalent rhenium dimercaptosuccinic acid complex. Nucl Med Commun 1993;14:197–203.

28. Blower PJ. Extending the life of a Tc-99m-generator: A simple and convenient method for concentrating generator eluate for clinical use. Nucl Med Commun 1993;14:995–997.

29. Blower PJ, Lam A, Knapp FF Jr, et al. Preparation, biodistribution and dosimetry of Re-188(V)-DMSA in patients with disseminated bone metastases [abstract]. Nucl Med Commun 1996;17:258.

30. Guhlke S, Beets AL, Knapp FF Jr, et al. Elution of Re-188 from W-188/Re-188 generators with salts of weak acids permits efficient concentration to low volumes using a new tandem cation/anion exchange system [abstract]. J Nucl Med 1997;38:125P.

31. Guhlke S, Beets AL, Mirzadeh S, et al. Tandem cation/anion column treatment of ammonium acetate eluants of the alumina-based tungsten-188/rhenium-188 generator: A new simple method for effective concentration of rhenium-188 perrhenate solutions. J Nucl Med 2000;41:1271–1278.

32. Guhlke S, Beets AL, Biersack H-J, et al. Elution of Re-188 from W-188/Re-188 generators with salts of weak acids permits efficient concentration to low volumes using a new tandem cation/anion exchange system [abstract]. J Nucl Med 1997;38:125P.

33. Guhlke A, Beets AL, Oetjin K, et al. Convenient concentration of rhenium-188 and technetium-99m eluates from tungsten-188/rhenium-188 or (n,)-produced molybdenum-99/technetium-99m generators to high specific volumes. In: Proceedings, XII International Symposium on Radiopharmaceutical Chemistry. Uppsala, Sweden, June 15–19, 1997.

34. Knapp FF Jr, Guhlke S, Beets AL, et al. Endovascular beta irradiation for prevention of restenosis using solution radioisotopes: Pharmacologic and dosimetric propreties of rhenium-188 compounds. Cardiovasc Rad Med 1999;1:86–97.

35. Kotzerke J, Rentschler M, Glatting G, et al. Dosimetric fundamentals of endovascular brachytherapy using rhenium-188 to prevent restenosis after angioplasty. Nuklearmedizin 1998;37:68–72. (In German.)

36. Kotzerke J, Fenchel S, Guhlmann A, et al. Pharmacokinetics of Tc-99m-pertechnetate and Re-188-perrhenate after oral application of perchlorate: Option of subsequent care using liquid Re-188 in a balloon catheter. Nucl Med Comm 1998;19:795–801.

37. Eigler N, Whiting J, Chernomorsky A, et al. RADIANT™ liquid intravascular radiation therapy system [abstract]. In: Proceedings, Second Annual Symposium on Radiotherapy to Reduce Restenosis, Scripps Clinic and Research Foundation. La Jolla, CA, January 16–17, 1998.

38. Makkar R, Whiting J, Li A, Cordero H, et al. A beta-emitting liquid isotope-filled balloon markedly inhibits restenosis in stented porcine coronary arteries [abstract]. J Am Coll Cardiol 1998;31(suppl A):350A.

39. Fox RA. Dosimetry of beta-emitting radionuclides for use in balloon angioplasty. Austral Phys Eng Sci Med 1997;20:139–146.

40. Amols HI. Debate: The preferred isotope source—beta versus gamma? [abstract] In: Syllabus, Advances in Cardiovascular Radiation Therapy. Sponsored by the Cardiology Research Foundation, Washington, DC, February 20–21, 1997:64.

41. Stabin M, Konijnenberg M, Knapp FF Jr, et al. Interactive computer program for calculation of radiation dose to the walls of blood vessels in intravascular radiation therapy. In: Syllabus, Advances in Cardiovascular Radiation Therapy. Sponsored by the Cardiology Research Foundation, Washington, DC, March 8–10, 1998.

42. Whiting JS, Li AN, Litvack F, et al. Comparison of the 3-D dose distributions in the arterial media delivered by P-32 and V-48 stents, Re-188 and Re-186 liquid balloons, and Y-90 seeds using dose-volume histograms based on Monte Carlo simulations [abstract]. In: Syllabus, Advances in Cardiovascular Radiation Therapy. Sponsored by the Cardiology Research Foundation, Washington, DC, February 20–21; 1997:5.

43. Amols HI, Weinberger J, Mirzadeh S, et al. Beta irradiation for restenosis: Considerations for stent implantantation [abstract]. Circulation 1996;94(suppl I): I–210.

44. Weinberger J, Mirzadeh S, Knapp FF Jr, et al. Beta irradiation for restenosis after stent implantation: Dose variations among differing stents [abstract]. J Am Coll Cardiol 1997;29(suppl A):238A.

45. Li AN, Zimmerman BE, Knapp FF Jr, et al. Reconciliation of directly measured Re-188 balloon dosimetry with calculations based on new NIST Re-188 activity calibration [abstract]. In: Proceedings, Second Annual Symposium on Radiotherapy to Reduce

Restenosis, Scripps Clinic and Research Foundation. La Jolla, CA, January 16–17, 1998.

46. Whiting JS, Li AN, Zimmerman BE, et al. Reconciliation of directly measured Re-188 balloon dosimetry with calculations based on a new NIST Re-188 activity calibration [abstract]. In: Proceedings, Second Annual Symposium on Radiotherapy to Reduce Restenosis, Scripps Clinic and Research Foundation. La Jolla, CA, January 16–17, 1998.

47. Kotzerke J, Fenchel S, Guhlmann A, et al. Pharmacokinetics of 99Tcm-pertechnetate and 188Re-perrhenate after oral administration of perchlorate: Option for subsequent care after the use of liquid 188Re in a balloon catheter. Nucl Med Commun 1998;19: 795–801.

48. Lin WY, Hsieh JF, Tsai SC, et al. A comprehensive study on the blockage of thyroid and gastric uptakes of 188Re-perrhenate in endovascular irradiation using liquid-filled balloon to prevent restenosis. Nucl Med Biol 2000;27:83–87.

49. Lee J, Lee DS, Kim KM, et al. Dosimetry of rhenium-188 diethylene triamine penta-acetic acid for endovascular intra-balloon brachytherapy after coronary angioplasty. Eur J Nucl Med 2000;27:76–82.

50. Hoher M, Wohrle J, Wohlfrom M, et al. Intracoronary beta-irradiation with a liquid (188)Re-filled balloon: Six-month results from a clinical safety and feasibility study. Circulation 2000;101:2355–2360.

The Angiorad™ Gamma Wire System

Ron Waksman, MD, David P. Faxon, MD, and Samuel F. Liprie, PD (Nuc)

Introduction

The field of vascular brachytherapy has developed largely through the technical advances that have occurred over the last 10 years. The development of small, flexible source wires and catheters has allowed for applications in the cardiovascular system. Along with technological advances, the appreciation that restenosis may be a radiosensitive process similar to hypertrophic scars and the safe and effective use of low dose radiation in the treatment of keloids as well as other benign tumors, has led to considerable experimental literature that supports the current ongoing clinical investigation of intravascular radiation devices.

In 1995, Samuel Liprie, PD (Nuc) created a unique device that incorporates a 3-cm, iridium 192 (^{192}Ir) source within a 0.014" flexible nitinol wire. Liprie's invention evolved into the Angiorad™ Gamma Wire System, currently in development at the Vascular Therapies Division of United States Surgical Corporation (Norwalk, CT).

Background

The initial use of radiation to inhibit atherosclerosis was reported by Friedman et al[1] in 1964. With the use of a ^{192}Ir catheter placed in the aortas of atherosclerotic rabbits, significant inhibition of the growth of atherosclerosis was noted. Subsequently, Lamberts and De Boer[2] reported a significant decrease in atherosclerosis with external beam radiation, in doses ranging from 500 to 3000 R in an atherosclerotic rabbit model. Numerous experimental studies have followed over the last 35 years, with studies conducted in rat, rabbit, dog, and swine models, with use of both external and intravascular gamma and beta radiation.[3-9] In 1994, Wiedermann et al[6] reported the beneficial effects of 2000 cGy intracoronary radiation with use of a ^{192}Ir ribbon in 19 juvenile swine undergoing angioplasty. Further studies demonstrated a dose-response relationship with prolonged benefits seen up to 6 months following radiation. Subsequently, Waksman and colleagues[7] confirmed these findings and have shown benefit in a swine model undergoing balloon angioplasty as well as stent implantation. A similar study using beta radiation in a swine model was also reported by the same group. Fischell and colleagues have shown that a beta-emitting ^{32}P Palmaz-Schatz stent was also capable of re-

From Waksman R (ed.). *Vascular Brachytherapy, Third Edition.* Armonk, NY: Futura Publishing Co., Inc.; © 2002.

ducing restenosis in a swine model. In all of these studies, a dose-dependent relationship has been shown, with effective doses ranging from 1000 to 5000 cGy targeted between 1 and 2 mm from the source.

Clinical experience has also confirmed these observations in animals. Studies by Böttcher et al[10] in the superficial femoral artery (SFA) have demonstrated the benefit of ^{192}Ir intravascular radiation following stent placement for SFA restenosis. The study referenced has had the longest follow-up, with up to 8 years of clinical follow-up in 31 lesions in 28 patients. Condado et al[11] have also reported a 3-year follow-up with 21 patients who underwent intravascular brachytherapy using a ^{192}Ir source. The guidewire used in this study was an early prototype of the current Angiorad device. Teirstein and colleagues[12] reported a randomized trial comparing ^{192}Ir gamma radiation in patients with restenosis, either following stent placement or in whom the stent was used to treat the restenosis, with patients who received no radiation. In this study, an 82% reduction in restenosis was noted in the irradiated group. More recently, the BERT Pilot Trial was reported in 31 patients and, in a Canadian parallel study, in 30 patients. In both studies, an extremely low level of restenosis with a late loss index of less than 5% was noted.

These experimental and clinical studies strongly support the concept of intravascular brachytherapy for the prevention of restenosis. Given the more predictable dosimetry and the larger experimental experience with gamma radiation, Angiorad's system was developed in order to provide a safe, easy to use, and versatile brachytherapy method for intravascular radiation.

Description of the Device

The Angiorad system is composed of three components: a small flexible source wire, a delivery catheter, and a manual afterloader which stores, advances, and retracts the source wire (Fig. 1A).

The source wire is a 0.014" nitinol tube with a 4.5-cm core of ^{192}Ir at its tip (Fig. 1B). The source is entirely encapsulated and has passed all requirements for a radioactive encapsulated source. The flexibility of the wire allows for excellent trackability through the delivery catheter, permitting access to nearly all locations in the coronary vasculature.

The delivery catheter is a 3.5F catheter with a 1-cm monorail tip. A 4.5-cm spacing balloon is just proximal to the monorail and has two gold markers to identify the ends of the balloon, as well as the treatment site. The balloon comes in 1.6 mm in diameter at 6 atm of pressure. The balloon size allows perfusion around the balloon during inflation. The balloon is coated with tungsten to block the beta rays and to prevent administrating high doses to the vessel wall (Fig. 1C).

The afterloader (Fig. 1) is a portable unit that can be easily moved next to the angiographic table and the patient. The unit includes a high-density tungsten safe, in which the source wire is located. A wire spool and manual crank allow advancement and retraction of the wire. A clutch device stops wire motion just prior to the treatment site; when released, it allows delivery of the wire into the treatment area within the balloon segment of the delivery catheter. The wire can be delivered and retracted within 3 to 4 seconds. The afterloader also contains a test nonradioactive wire that is otherwise the same as the treatment wire, in order to test for safe passage for the treatment wire prior to initiating therapy. The next generation will be fully automated.

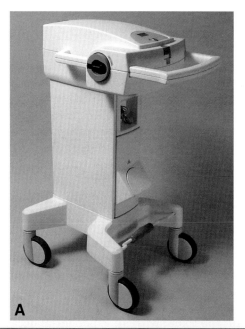

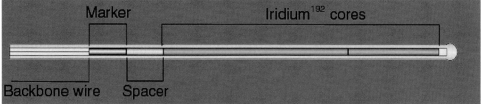

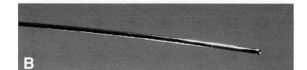

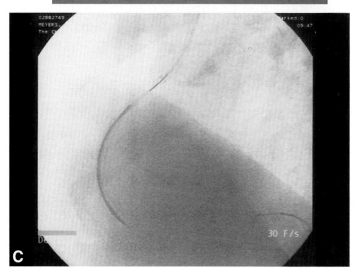

Figure 1. Components of the Angiorad System (see text for explanation).

Procedure

Following the successful angioplasty or stent placement, the delivery catheter is passed into the dilated area. The catheter is positioned in such a way that the markers, 4.5 cm apart, span the dilated area and extend beyond the dilated segment at both ends. The balloon is inflated to the desired pressure and perfusion is verified by angiography. The afterloader is connected to the hub of the center lumen of the catheter through an extension catheter. The test wire is then advanced under fluoroscopic guidance into the treatment area to verify safe passage. The wire is retracted and the treatment wire afterloader is connected to the catheter. The room is then cleared of all unnecessary personnel. The radioactive wire is advanced into the catheter and its location at the treatment site is verified by cineangiography. The treatment times are determined by the angiographic lumen diameter, with a goal of delivering approximately 18 Gy at 2 cm from the source. At the end of treatment, the wire is rapidly removed by withdrawal into the afterloader. Radiation exposure during treatment and immediately after is monitored by the radiation protection officer. Repeat coronary angiography is performed before and after guidewire removal.

While high radiation doses are present close to the patient, normal radiation exposure occurs within the room, with an exponential decay to a level that is tolerable for personnel who remain in the room 6 to 8 feet from the table. An example of radiation exposure on one patient is shown in Figure 2.

Preliminary Clinical Results

Two clinical trials evaluating the benefit of intravascular radiation are currently in progress: one study in patients with in-stent restenosis, and the other in patients with de novo or restenotic lesions undergoing balloon angioplasty with provisional stenting.

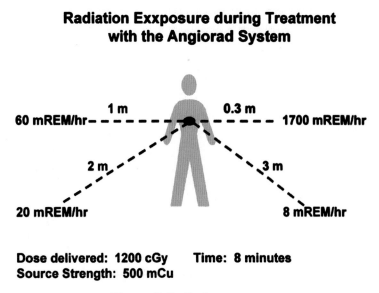

Radiation Exxposure during Treatment with the Angiorad System

1 m — 60 mREM/hr
0.3 m — 1700 mREM/hr
2 m — 20 mREM/hr
3 m — 8 mREM/hr

Dose delivered: 1200 cGy   Time: 8 minutes
Source Strength: 500 mCu

Figure 2. Radiation exposure.

Pilot studies with both protocols have been completed in 25 patients each. A dose of 12 Gy to the external elastic membrane, defined by intravascular ultrasound (IVUS), was used in both studies. The studies have shown that successful delivery of radiation to the vessel can be accomplished in 98% of the patients attempted. No in-hospital or 30-day complications have been noted, and in particular, no deaths, myocardial infarction (MI), need for bypass surgery, abrupt closure, or rehospitalization have been reported. An example of a representative cine is shown in Figure 3.

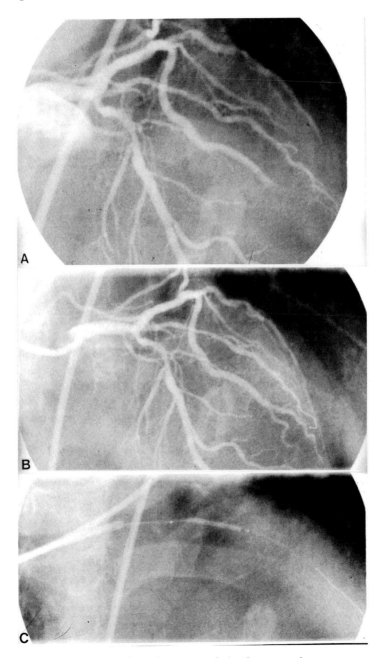

Figure 3. A patient example in three panels.

In the ARTISTIC feasibility study, 26 patients with in-stent restenosis underwent successful intervention and were treated with open-label ^{192}Ir using a high-activity line source. The specific activity of the source wire was 372 ± 51 mCi, and the dwell time was 10.8 ± 1.9 minutes. The primary endpoint was freedom from death, MI, and repeat target lesion revascularization (TLR) at 6 months. Secondary endpoints included angiographic restenosis and IVUS neointimal hyperplasia. Procedural success was high (96.2%), and in-hospital and 30-day complications were low with no deaths, MI, or requirement for repeat revascularization. At 6 months, event-free survival was 85%: 1 patient required repeat percutaneous transluminal coronary angiography (PTCA), 1 underwent bypass surgery, and 2 had an MI. Baseline lesion length measured 15.77.0 mm. Follow-up angiography was available in 21 of 25 (84%) patients. The binary restenosis rates were 19.0% (4 of 21) in-stent and 23.8% (5 of 21) in-lesion. Follow-up IVUS was available in 20 of 25 patients. There was no increase in intimal hyperplasia from post intervention to follow-up ($3.11.8$ mm^2 versus $3.41.8$ mm^2; $P=0.32$). Eight patients had a reduction of neointimal intimal tissue at follow-up. These results indicate that intracoronary gamma radiation with the Angiorad source wire is safe and effective in preventing in-stent restenosis.

A larger double-blind, multicenter, randomized trial is now under way. The in-stent restenosis study, called the ARTISTIC Trial, has two phases: in phase I, 110 patients were randomized to receive either radiation or placebo after intervention with doses varying from 12 to 18 Gy at 2 mm depending on the vessel size. In phase II, 180 patients are being enrolled as a registry and treated with a dose of 18 Gy at 2 mm for vessel sizes 2.5 to 4.0 mm. The primary endpoint of this study is also target vessel failure at 8 months. The trials are anticipated to be completed by the end of 2001.

Conclusion

The Angiorad Gamma Wire System has been shown to be easy to use and safe for intracoronary use. The small size and flexibility of the source wire permits access to all parts of the coronary circulation, with a balloon delivery catheter that permits positioning to more optimally deliver a more uniform radiation dose to the artery. The techniques used are similar to standard balloon angioplasty. While gamma sources have a significantly higher risk of radiation exposure to catheterization laboratory personnel, with the short treatment times and radiation monitoring, the technique is safe and easily applicable to nearly all clinical situations. Future studies will confirm whether this system, the currently selected dose, and the radiation source are effective in reducing restenosis following angioplasty.

References

1. Friedman M, Felton L, Byers S, with the technical assistance of Hayashi W, Omoto C, Tam A. The antiatherogenic effect of iridium upon the cholesterol-fed rabbit. J Clin Invest 1964;41:185–192.
2. Lamberts HB, DeBoer WG. Contributions to the study of immediate and early x-ray reactions with regard to chemoprotection. VII. X-ray-induced atheromatous lesions in the arterial wall of hypercholesterolemic rabbits. Int J Rad Biol 1963;6:343–350.
3. Gellman J, Healey G, et al. The effect of very low dose irradiation on restenosis fol-

lowing balloon angioplasty: A study in the atherosclerotic rabbit. Circulation 1991;84: 1146–1159.

4. Mayberg MR, Luo Z, London S, et al. Radiation inhibition of intimal hyperplasia after arterial injury. Radiat Res 1995;142:212–220.

5. Shimotakara S, Mayberg M. Gamma irradiation inhibits neointimal hyperplasia in rats after arterial injury. Stroke 1994;25:424–428.

6. Wiedermann JG, Marboe C, Amols H, et al. Intracoronary irradiation markedly reduces restenosis after balloon angioplasty in a porcine model. J Am Coll Cardiol 1994; 23:1491–1498.

7. Waksman R, Robinson KA, Crocker IR, et al. Endovascular low-dose irradiation inhibits neointimal formation after coronary artery balloon injury in swine: A possible role for radiation therapy in restenosis prevention. Circulation 1995;91:1533–1539.

8. Popowski Y, Verin V, Papirov I, et al. Intra-arterial ^{90}Y brachytherapy: Preliminary dosimetric study using a specially modified angioplasty balloon. Int J Radiat Oncol Biol Phys 1995;33:713–717.

9. Wiedermann JG, Marboe C, Amols H, et al. Intracoronary irradiation markedly reduces neointimal proliferation after balloon angioplasty in swine: Persistent benefit at 6-month follow-up. J Am Coll Cardiol 1995;25:1451–1456.

10. Böttcher I, Schopohl B, Liermann D, et al. Endovascular irradiation–a new method to avoid recurrent stenosis after stent implantation in peripheral vessels: Technique and preliminary results. Int J Radiat Oncol Biol Phys 1994;29:183–186.

11. Condado JA, Waksman R, Gurdiel O, et al. Long-term angiographic and clinical outcome after percutaneous transluminal coronary angioplasty and intracoronary radiation therapy in humans. Circulation 1997;96:727–732.

12. Teirstein PS, Massullo V, Jani S, et al. Catheter-based radiotherapy to inhibit restenosis after coronary stenting. N Engl J Med 1997;336:1697–1703.

## Chapter 58

Intravascular Soft X-Ray Therapy

Victor Chornenky, PhD

Introduction

Restenosis, which occurs in 25% to 45 % of patients, remains the major limitation of percutaneous transluminal coronary angioplasty. It is generally accepted that the most important contributors to restenosis are neointimal proliferation, which leads to thickening of the vessel wall, and unfavorable vascular remodeling, which causes contraction of the artery. It has been demonstrated that placing stents into stenotic arteries after balloon angioplasty successfully addresses remodeling and significantly reduces the restenosis rate.[1,2] At the same time, stents, as foreign objects in the body, increase cellular proliferation in surrounding tissue and make the neointimal component of restenosis even worse. Intravascular irradiation has been suggested as a means against this exuberant cellular proliferation and has proven to be efficient in reducing it.[3–6] These studies seem to suggest that intravascular irradiation is capable of reducing the restenosis rate to a one-digit level, a result that is hard to overestimate.

In spite of encouraging clinical data, there are a lot of questions about the healing mechanism of irradiated injured vessels and long-term side effects that limit the therapy that are not yet answered.

What is the safe therapeutic window for radiation dose for prevention of restenosis? It seems that the minimum dose is approximately 15 Gy; lower radiation doses have proven to be unable to significantly inhibit restenosis. But what is the maximum tolerable dose and what is the nature of the side effects that limit this dose? If a vascular fibrosis is the dominant long-term side effect of radiation overdose, at what level does it become symptomatic for cardiovascular patients, and when? How deep into the vessel wall should irradiation be extended? Where is the trade-off between the requirements of irradiation of the vessel wall and sparing the vasa vasorum, which probably, as with any small blood vessels, are especially vulnerable to the irradiation?

What is the nature of the most proliferating clone of cells? Do they come from intima or adventitia? What is the quantitative law of their migration? What is the mechanism of inhibition of the migration by radiation? How far beyond a lesion should irradiation be extended to avoid migration from uninjured adjacent parts of the vessel? These questions are a subject of basic science, but the answers will help to formulate scientific requirements of the vascular irradiation for prevention of restenosis.

From Waksman R (ed.). *Vascular Brachytherapy, Third Edition*. Armonk, NY: Futura Publishing Co., Inc.; © 2002.

What fraction of a vessel wall can be underirradiated, for example, behind a stent in the artery, or overirradiated at its inner surface, without causing consequent restenosis or any other serious side effects? What kind of response is expected for a local radiation overdose to the inner surface of the wall? In this regard, how important is the centering of the catheter in the vessel, and what is the correlation between the quality of centering and the long-term success of the radiation treatment?

All of these questions must be answered in order to provide a scientific foundation for the successful development of safe and efficacious radiation intravascular devices.

Devices for Intravascular Delivery of Ionizing Radiation

In order to be adequate for treatment against restenosis, the radiation catheters must meet the fundamental requirements imposed by the nature of the disease. Even though today not everything is known about restenosis, the radiation intravascular devices should be designed in such a way that they meet the requirements that are known, and they should be adaptable for future details. It is mandatory that these devices be safe for the patient, physician, and the catheterization laboratory staff during operation. Safe shipping, handling, and storage, as well as economics, are also issues. It is important and desirable for the catheter to be compatible with the existing catheterization laboratory environment and routine procedures. The catheter should not necessitate significant changes in the lab itself, such as installation of a radiation shielding; nor should it require changes in its procedures, such as leaving the patient in the lab alone during radiation treatment for the sake of safety of the physician and the catheterization laboratory staff.

What kind of radiation should be used: beta, gamma, or x-rays? From the point of view of radiobiology, they all have one feature in common: namely, they are ionizing radiation. Their fundamental biological action on a live tissue is basically the same—they damage cellular DNA directly by ionizing it, or indirectly by creating chemically active free radicals, which attack DNA. The equal doses of radiation prescribed with equal dose rates result in the same biological effect. In this regard, there is no difference between them. The inequality of particular sources appears in different tissue penetrations, activities, half-lives of the isotopes, methods of manufacturing and disposal, and designs of active elements of the catheters. These features affect their ability to perform adequate irradiation of the lesion, treatment time, handling, safety requirements, and, finally, the associated cost of the procedure.

The x-ray irradiation is a new modality of intravascular treatment for prevention of restenosis. The most important feature of the x-ray catheter, as with any other radiation catheter, is the irradiation pattern it can provide for the vessel. Ultimately, this feature will determine its therapeutic value and its ability to survive in competition with other devices for intravascular irradiation.

The nature of x-ray radiation is similar to that of gamma radiation. Both of them are electromagnetic radiation. Gamma radiation is emitted by atomic nuclei. It has very high energy and associated tissue penetration. X-ray radiation is emitted when energetic electrons bombard a metal target in a vacuum tube. The energy of the x-ray radiation depends on the voltage applied to the vacuum tube.

As x-ray radiation propagates in tissue, it is absorbed. The intensity of radiation decreases exponentially as a function of the distance passed by the radiation in tissue. Every time it passes the so-called half-value layer (HVL), its intensity drops in a half. The HVL depends on the nature of the tissue and the energy of the x-ray radiation. The function that describes dependence of the HVL for monoenergetic x-rays versus energy is a cubic parabola shown in Figure 1. As the energy increases by two times, the penetration becomes eight times deeper. Over the range of 10 to 20 keV, the HVL has values from 1.5 mm to 9 mm. It seems reasonable to suggest that the optimal HVL for intravascular irradiation lies between these two values. An x-ray emitter emits not monoenergetic radiation but a spectrum of energies. A typical spectrum is shown in Figure 2. It comprises two components: a smooth continuum of bremsstrahlung radiation extending from zero to a maximum energy, defined by applied voltage and sharp peaks of characteristic radiation imposed on it. The nature of these two components is different. The bremsstrahlung radiation is emitted by decelerating electrons as they bombard the target material, while the characteristic radiation is emitted by the atoms of target excited by collisions with electrons. The bremsstrahlung spectrum can be shifted to higher energy by filtration of the radiation with a layer of a metal that preferentially absorbs the low-energy radiation. The characteristic radiation is bound to the nature of atoms comprising the target and can be modified only by changing the target material. It should be mentioned that characteristic radiation for efficient emission requires 25% to 30% higher voltage than the emitted energy

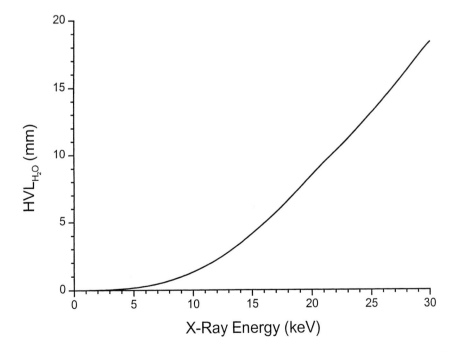

Figure 1. The half-value layer of x-rays in water versus energy. The penetration ability of x-rays in water is very close to that in blood and vascular tissue.

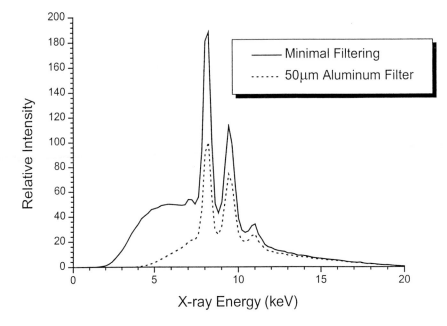

Figure 2. A typical soft x-ray spectrum with the anode voltage 20 kV.

measured in electron volts. For example, for generation of 15-KeV characteristic x-rays, the anode voltage should be approximately 20 kV or higher. Theoretical analysis suggests that at the anode voltage of 20 kV, special filtration and selection of the target material allow for the tailoring of the HVL of the intravascular x-ray radiation to different values between 1.5 and 5 mm. If the electric power dissipated at the emitter is 1 W and the lesion length is 3 mm, the treatment time is expected to be 3 to 10 minutes. In these calculations, the target tissue is assumed to be at a 2-mm distance from the center of a 3-mm-diameter vessel and the dose prescription is 15 Gy.

When an x-ray catheter is placed in a vessel and the x-ray radiation propagates in the radial direction, it diverges and is absorbed by the blood and vascular tissue. In Figure 3 the intensities of several sources of ionizing radiation are plotted as functions of radial distance from the center of the blood vessel. This graph takes into account both geometrical divergence and absorption of radiation into blood or tissue. The data on the radioactive sources are, in part, from a paper by Amols et al.[7] The x-ray data were calculated as the catheter moved along the axis of the blood vessel. As can be seen from the plot, the curves, which show penetration ability for the different x-ray energies, fall between the curves for a ^{32}P source and a ^{103}Pd gamma source. The penetration ability of the x-ray radiation can be close to or two to three times higher than that of the ^{90}St/^{90}Y source. To its great advantage, it is still much lower than that of the ^{192}Ir source. At these penetrations the x-ray radiation is safe for the physician and catheterization laboratory staff, because it is completely shielded by the patient's body.

A prototype of the soft x-ray system is shown schematically in the Figure 4.[8] The x-ray emitter, connected to the distal end of a coaxial cable, consists of an anode and cathode assembly mounted in a miniature vacuum tube. To activate the

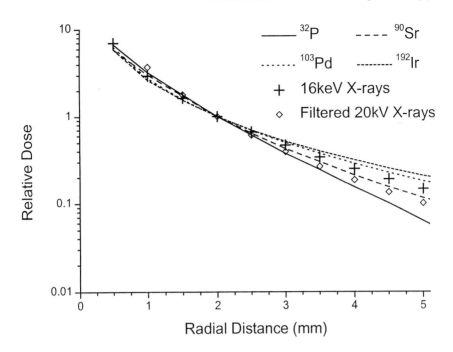

Figure 3. The relative radiation doses in tissue versus radial distance for different sources of ionizing radiation.

system, a high voltage (20 kV) is applied to the tube. Electrons emitted by the cathode are accelerated in the electrical field and strike the anode, radiating bremsstrahlung radiation as they stop, and exciting characteristic lines in the target material. A metal film deposited on the emitter's external wall provides filtration of the x-ray radiation. The HVL in the first prototype is 1.6 mm. This value

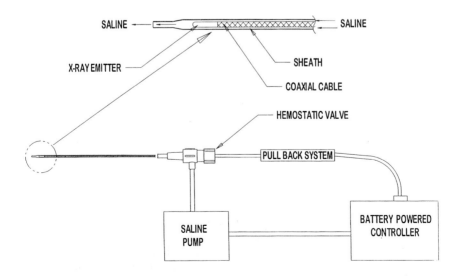

Figure 4. The soft x-ray system.

approximately matches the penetration ability of a $^{90}St/^{90}Y$ radioactive beta source. The x-ray emitter consumes 0.5- to 1.0-watt power. To provide necessary cooling, a saline solution is continuously pumped through the sheath at a flow rate of 10 to 15 cc/min. The proximal end of the coaxial cable is connected to a pullback device that moves the emitter along the sheath with a predetermined speed as the blood vessel is irradiated. The length of irradiation is programmable in the range of 0 to 100 mm.

The x-ray system is delivered over a previously positioned standard-length guidewire. There are marker bands located at the tip of the sheath and at both ends of the guidewire lumen. The emitter is also radio-opaque and is easily visible under fluoroscopy. The emitter and cable assembly are advanced to the treatment site, and the treatment is performed over a programmed length. As irradiation is completed, the emitter is repositioned back to the proximal position. If the guidewire is needed for further procedures, it can be easily repositioned to the treatment site. Otherwise, the entire assembly is removed.

Conclusions

Intravascular x-ray therapy is a feasible technique. Appropriately engineered x-ray catheter for coronary application can be safe and efficacious. The state-of-the-art coaxial cables allow for the safe delivery of a 20- to 25-kV battery-powered voltage to the emitter. The tissue penetration of the radiation can be tailored to 1.5 to 5.0 mm HVL, which is probably the optimal range for both coronary and peripheral applications. The pattern of the radiation generated by the x-ray emitter is adequate for the intravascular use. Thermal load on the x-ray catheter is approximately 0.5 to 1.0 W. With a forced saline cooling system, the temperature of the catheter can be kept at a safe level of 41° to 42°C. The treatment time for a 3-cm-long lesion is expected to be 3 to10 minutes.

Future animal and clinical trials will show how this new modality of intravascular radiation therapy performs in comparison with established beta and gamma emitters.

Acknowledgments: The author would like to express his acknowledgments to Dr. Mike Satteson for performing computer simulations and Dr. Neal Scott of Emory University for valuable discussions.

References

1. Investigators. A randomized comparison of coronary stent placement and balloon angioplasty in the treatment of coronary artery disease. N Engl J Med 1994;331:496–501.
2. Serruys PW, de Jaegere P, Kiemeneij F, et al, for the BENESTENT Study Group. A comparison of balloon-expandable stent implantation with balloon angioplasty in patients with coronary artery disease. N Engl J Med 1994;331:489–495.
3. Waksman R, Robinson KA, Crocker IR, et al. Endovascular low dose irradiation inhibits neointima formation after coronary artery balloon injury in swine. A possible role for radiation therapy in restenosis prevention. Circulation 1995;91:1533–1539.
4. Wiedermann JG, Marboe C, Amols H, et al. Intracoronary irradiation markedly reduces neointimal proliferation after balloon angioplasty in swine. J Am Coll Cardiol 1995;25:1451–1456.
5. Verin V, Popowski Y, Urban P, et al. Intra-arterial beta irradiation prevents neointimal

hyperplasia in a hypercholesterolemic rabbit restenosis model. Circulation 1995;92: 2284–2290.

6. Teirstein PS, Massullo V, Jani S, et al. Catheter-based radiation therapy to inhibit restenosis following coronary stenting [abstract]. Circulation 1995;92:543.

7. Amols HI, Zaider M, Weinberger J, et al. Dosimetric considerations for catheter-based beta and gamma emitters in the therapy of neointimal hyperplasia in human coronary arteries. Int J Radiat Oncol Biol Phys 1996;36:913–922.

8. Chornenky VI. The soft x-ray system. In: Handbook of Vascular Brachytherapy. London: Martin Dunitz Ltd; 1998.

Xenon 133 Gas-Filled Balloon

Marc Apple, MD, and Ron Waksman, MD

Ionizing radiation delivered via catheter-based systems has been shown to reduce neointima formation in animal models. Both beta and gamma emitters have
demonstrated effectiveness and safety in the porcine coronary model.[1–7] The majority of the catheter-based systems used in the animal models and in the feasibility clinical trials are based on a source wire or seeds delivered into a closed-end
lumen catheter, either centered or noncentered, with a manual or automatic afterloader. We propose a novel system for vascular brachytherapy that uses a ^{133}Xe
radioactive gas-filled balloon.

Benefits of an Inert Radiogas

Xenon 133 is one of the few radioisotopes of xenon (another is ^{127}Xe) with a
multidecade history of safe and routine clinical use. Typically, it has been applied
in gaseous form (mixed with 95% pure carbon dioxide) or partially solubilized in
saline for functional ventilation imaging or brain perfusion imaging, as used
throughout the world.

Xenon 133 has a physical half-life of 5.3 days and emits both beta particles
(360 keV max) and relatively low energy γ- and x-rays of 81 keV and 32 keV, respectively.[8–10] ^{133}Xe decays to a stable, nonradioactive isotope of cesium. It is produced in single-unit individualized dosing ampules (Dupont Inc.) or in bulk cylinders (Nordion Inc.).[11] Therefore, because of its clinical use history and high-volume
commercial radiopharmaceutical production, it is readily available, with flexible
dosing and quantity, as needed on a daily or weekly basis, fully dose-calibrated
and quality tested.

The inert chemical properties of this radioagent offer enormous safety and bio-
exposure benefits. In vivo, whether inhaled or injected, xenon is poorly solubilized
and is rapidly excreted via the lungs.[9,12] More than two thirds of the dose rapidly dis-
sipates in vivo with a biologic half-life of 23 seconds.[12–14] Ninety percent or more may
be exhaled upon first pass through the lungs. As such, it remains chemically unchanged and is not excreted through the genitourinary or gastrointestinal systems.
It therefore poses negligibly small routine dose exposure to any specific organs, and
residual circulating molecules are rapidly released from the lung unchanged.[15]

Any free ^{133}Xe gas may be readily and safely exhausted from a standard directional venting system. Rapid air dilution and low-energy emissions allow for
an excellent safety profile. Even in high activity concentrations or continuous low

From Waksman R (ed.). *Vascular Brachytherapy, Third Edition.* Armonk, NY: Futura Publishing Co., Inc.; © 2002.

Table 1

Comparison of Personnel Exposure at Bedside During Vascular Brachytherapy with ^{133}Xe and Other Applications with the use of Radionuclides

Application	Radiation Exposure
Xeron 133 Catheter (2.4 min)	<0.17 mR–0.24 mR
	Max 2–5 mCi average loss
Chest x-ray	20 mrem
CT head	4200 mrem
Single balloon angioplasty	300–350 mR
T1–201 Imaging study	0.5–4.5 mR/h (2 mR)
Iridium 192 for vascular brachytherapy	20 mR/hr
Iodine 131	17.5 rad/mCi in the adrenals,
	3.9 rad/mCi in the bladder

CT = computed tomography.

activity levels, personnel and patient dose exposure is far below safe allowances and comparatively less than most standard diagnostic procedures or other potential intravascular brachytherapy sources (Table 1). There are no current reports indicative of any known adverse reactions or toxic radiation incidents, despite tens to hundreds of thousands of patient administrations. As a gas, xenon can be rapidly and continuously "vacuumed" and exhausted safely out of a room or work area without additional clean-up equipment or personnel attentively performing assays. It is highly unlikely that an excessive leak or accident would obligate prolonged or risky room isolation or decontamination, with simple external venting, as might occur with other radiosources.[16]

Dosimetry

A radio-xenon–filled balloon-type catheter system can inherently provide self centering and homogeneous radiation delivery while accommodating to any vessel curvatures or lumen irregularity, and can ensure uniform dosing to the target area.

The combination of lower energy beta particles and γ-ray/x-ray emissions of ^{133}Xe allows for both high dose deposition and dose rates over the first 1 mm of tissue/balloon interface, with rapid dose fall-off and normal tissue sparing thereafter. Individual lesion and vessel sizes are readily accommodated by the choice of the physician by selecting the appropriate balloon length and the diameter for adequate proximal and distal coverage of the angioplastied segment. The dose is targeted to the adventitia of the vessel wall, which play an important role in the process of restenosis.[17] This can routinely be achieved without requirement of simulation or complex dosimetry because each balloon size has a relatively fixed volume and thickness when adequately inflated.[18,19] As such, since the area of primary vessel wall injury will be juxtaposed with the inflated balloon surface, it is therefore possible to ensure constant expected dosimetry and depth dose. By simply knowing or varying the activity of [133]Xe (in millicuries) injected into a precalibrated balloon catheter system, all that is then required is the prescribed dose. A treatment exposure time can then be calculated for a specific balloon size.

Example For a *dose* of 15 Gy at a 0.25-mm distance from the surface of the balloon, with *activity* of ^{133}Xe at 210 mCi at a *dose rate* of 3.5 cGy-mCi-min, the *treatment time* is 2.1 minutes.

Xenon 133 is delivered within 90% to 95% pure CO_2 as carrier gas. As such, unlike liquid sources, intrasource attenuation should be much less and the reference "center" of activity will be much closer to the tissue interface due to the lower density gas state. Decay emission energy will travel to the balloon wall with minimal attenuation (except if striking the central catheter wall) and therefore begin dose deposition at the first layer of tissue.

Available applicable evidence indicates that with the proportion of 95% CO_2 content and intended maximal volumes of 1.0 to 1.5 cc, balloon rupture would not demonstrate increased risk of intracoronary embolism.[20–22] The CO_2 is relatively quickly dissipated and/or metabolized, unlike known effects with air or nitrogen or volumes of greater than 10 to 15 cc of CO_2.[23,24]

Dosimetric Measurements

Prior to the initiation of animal studies, in vitro microdosimetry and safety studies were carried out. Multiple trial runs were performed with use of GrII balloon catheters by Cook Inc. (Bloomington IN), varying in size from 2.5 mm × 30 mm to 4.0 mm × 40 mm. Customized solid water phantoms were fashioned such that a tangential section of balloon wall was adequately exposed during inflation and upon which multiple layers of 0.125-mm to 0.250-mm–thick GafChromic film could be placed prior to inflation. At least 5 cm of Solid Water™ were placed above and below the piece containing the catheter to compensate for scattering and absorption.

Within an externally vented hood and with both a xenon alert and survey monitors in position, several timed xenon inflation experiments were carried out with controlled parameters including balloon size, amount of injected xenon activity, and exposure times. A guidewire was not present in the lumen during injection. Pre- and postinjection measurements were made of the ^{133}Xe vial contents, the "gas-tight" syringe (10 to 25 cc) (Hamilton Inc., Reno, NV), and the tested catheter. Quantified estimates of any free gas loss, residual catheter containment, and syringe residuals were all recorded in order to confirm assumed injected radio activity amounts, as well as to assess the incidental microleakage per exposure sample.

Exposure rates and cumulative levels were measured and documented at various distances from the catheter and within the room. Any radio-emitting materials were properly bagged and labeled and allowed to decay according to guidelines set forth by the Radiation Safety Committee. After 7 days, the GafChromic film layers, which had been stored away from light exposure, were measured for maximal exposure point readings as performed using a spot densitometer (MacBeth #TD 502 [Victoreen Inc., Carle Place, NY] with broadband spectrum).

Reference tissue depths were equivalent to film layer depths and each measured optical density was correlated to an equivalent total dose with use of a dose-response curve analysis published using [125]I (closest γ-ray/x-ray emission energy). The type of film used is known to require 800 to 1000 cGy in order to cause a measurable change in optical density.[25,26] In addition, sensitivity of the film can somewhat underestimate true administration of the dose because of different energy levels of decay emissions. This is why an ^{125}I reference dose for our type of densitometer was applied. The calculations of the dose rate as a function of distance from the balloon into the vessel wall are displayed in Table 2.

Table 2

Measurements of Radiation Dose Rate at Various Tissue Depths
from the Balloon Surface*

Tissue Depth from Balloon Surface	Dose Rate (cGy/mCi/h)
0.125 mm	880–920
0.250 mm	210–240
0.375 mm	132–150
0.500 mm	32–50
0.750 mm**	14–20
1.00 mm**	10–12

*Balloon wall thickness is 80 to 100 μm. *Range of gross injection activity of ^{133}Xe = approximately 50 to 200 mCi. *Percent balloon volume of total injected volume = 45% to 60%.
**Values for 0.75 to 1.00 mm may actually be greater, but undermeasured due to minimal exposure threshold requirements for film change of 800 to 1000 cGy.

Accumulated averages of film readings of dose response per depth are listed below. Results were also comparatively matched to preliminary standard Monte Carlo simulations. These include any related dose build-up secondary to bremsstrahlung or scatter radiation. Summarized results are with originally tested nonspecific catheters and do not represent modified xenon-specific balloon catheters subsequently manufactured and under evaluation.

Preclinical Studies

Xenon 133 in the Porcine Model

The overall objective for these studies was to determine whether a ^{133}Xe-filled balloon catheter can prevent intimal hyperplasia following balloon angioplasty in the porcine balloon overstretch model of restenosis. The hypothesis of the study was that intracoronary radiation using ^{133}Xe in doses of 7.5 to 30 Gy prescribed to the vessel wall delivered intraluminally is sufficient to prevent restenosis, safely and free from adverse effects.

Experimental Methods

Coronary overstretch injury was performed with an angioplasty balloon, 30% larger in size than the reference vessel diameter, that was positioned in the proximal segments of the left anterior descending (LAD) artery, the left circumflex (LCX) artery, and the right coronary artery (RCA), inflated to 10 atm three times for 30 seconds in each artery. Inflation periods were separated by 1-minute deflation periods to restore coronary perfusion. After the completion of the third inflation, the angioplasty balloon was withdrawn and additional nitroglycerin (200 μg) was administered to limit coronary spasm. Final angiography was then performed to assess vessel patency and degree of injury.

A delivery balloon catheter 2.5 or 3.0 mm in diameter (30 mm in length) was positioned over a flexible 0.014″ wire at the injured artery assigned to receive radiation treatment. The ^{133}Xe was inserted into the lumen of the radiation delivery catheter. Cinefluoroscopic visualization verified positioning of the delivery catheter and a gamma camera documented the source in the balloon catheter (Fig. 1). The source was left in the balloon for a period sufficient to deliver the assigned dose (7.5 Gy, 15 Gy, or 30 Gy). After irradiation, the delivery catheter and the guiding catheters were removed and the carotid cutdown repaired. Nitroglycerin ointment (1 inch) was administered topically and the animals were returned to routine care.

Animals were sacrificed 2 weeks following treatment. The arteries were perfusion fixed. The injured segments of the LAD, LCX, and RCA were located with the guidance of the coronary angiograms, then dissected free from the heart. Serial 2- to 3-mm transverse segments were processed and embedded in paraffin. Cross sections (4 μm) were stained with hematoxylin and eosin (H&E) and Verhoeff-van Gieson (VVG) elastin stain. An experienced observer blinded to the treatment group examined histology. Each specimen was evaluated for the presence of neointima formation, luminal encroachment, medial dissection, alteration of the internal and external elastic lamina, and morphological appearance of the cells within the media, adventitia, and neointima.

Histomorphometric analysis was performed on each segment with evidence of

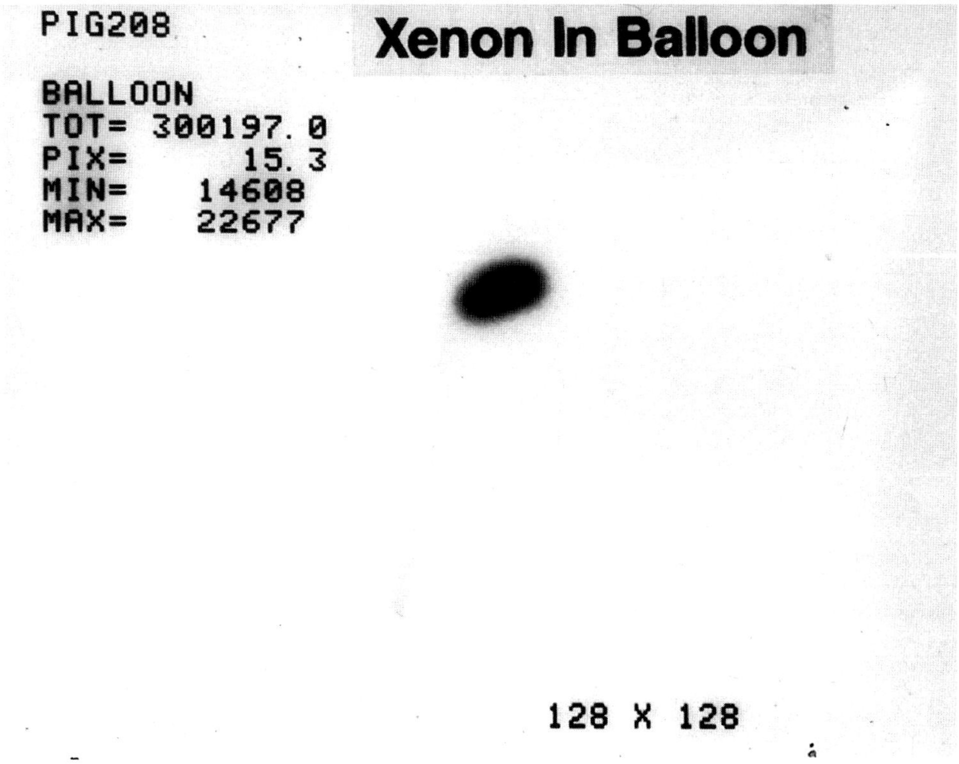

Figure 1. Xenon 133 in the inflated balloon in the coronary artery of the pig during treatment; detected by gamma camera.

medial fracture. The histopathological features were measured by use of a computerized PC-compatible image analysis program (Optimas 6, Optimas Inc., Bothell, WA). VVG-stained sections were magnified at 25×, digitized, and stored in a frame-grabberboard (DAGE-MTI, Michigan City, IN). The maximal intimal thickness (MIT) was determined by a radial line, drawn from the lumen to the external lamina at the point of greatest tissue growth. The arc length of the medial fracture (FL), traced through the neointima from one dissected medial end to the other, was used as a measure of the extent of injury. Area measurements were obtained by tracing the lumen perimeter (luminal area [LA] mm^2), neointima perimeter (intimal area [IA] mm^2, defined by the borders of the internal elastic lamina, lumen, media, and external elastic lamina), and external elastic lamina (vessel area [VA] mm^2). To correct for extent of injury, the ratio of intimal area to fracture length (IA/FL) was obtained. Measurements were cross checked for accuracy by random repetition of 25% of stenosis and determination of percentage variability.

Comparisons of LA, VA, IA, MIT, and IA/FL between control and irradiated arteries were made by use of either one-way analysis of variance (ANOVA) with the Bonferroni correction for groups whose standard deviation (SD) of the means was not statistically different ($P>0.05$ by Bartlett's test) or by the Kruskall-Wallis test for groups whose SD of the means was statistically different ($P<0.05$ by Bartlett's test). By this analysis, statistically significant differences between treatment groups were considered to be those with $P<0.05$.

Morphometric and Histology Results

The morphometric measurements of the treated groups are displayed in Table 3. Significant reduction of neointima formation, IA, IA/FL, and MIT was demonstrated across all ^{133}Xe-treated groups (7.515, and 30 Gy) when compared with control (Fig. 2). In the 15 Gy group there was further reduction in the adventitial area. A higher dose of 30 Gy was associated with excess of fibrin or thrombus compared with low doses or control. There was no additional significant reduction of neointima formation with 30 Gy. As shown before with other beta

Table 3

Morphometric Results Xenon 133 Studies

	IA (mm^2)	FL mm	IA/FL Ratio	MIT mm	AA (mm^2)	VA (mm^2)	LA (mm^2)
Control n = 8	1.51	2.04	0.76	0.50	5.1	5.96	3.2
7.5 Gy n = 9	0.32*	2.02	0.16*	0.23*	3.8*	6.08	3.9*
15 Gy n = 10	0.10*	2.14	0.04*	0.06*	3.0*	6.43	4.3*

*$P < 0.0001$ versus control. IA = intimal area; FL = fracture length; MIT = maximal intimal thickness; AA = adventitial area; VA = vessel area; LA = luminal area.

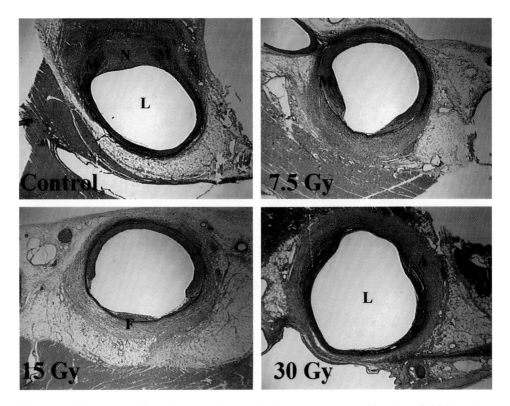

Figure 2. Representative micrographs at 40× instrument magnification of thick sections from injured pig coronary arteries, stained with Verhoeff-van Gieson elastin. Healing responses at 2 weeks in four treatment groups are compared. Samples are shown from the control group, 7.5-Gy–treated group, 15-Gy–treated group, and 30-Gy–treated group. A = adventitia; L = lumen; M = media; N = neointima.

isotopes, larger doses were associated with larger vessel area and suggested favorable remodeling of the vessel.

In general, the histology pattern of the treated vessels was similar to the findings with other isotopes, both beta and gamma emitters, described before in the pig model. There was no excess of fibrosis or necrosis in the ^{133}Xe-treated segments versus control injured vessels.

Experimental tests were performed to confirm the expected historical safety profile in the very rare potential event of the ^{133}Xe/CO_2 loss by catheter, in vivo. Animal results demonstrated excellent tolerance without morbid or mortal effects and with rapid, safe clearance of intentional in vivo coronary injection. Measurement parameters included blood pressure, pulse rate, real-time gamma camera imaging, and multi-interval blood activity assays (Fig. 3). In the circumstance of ^{133}Xe radiogas loss from balloon failure, no "hot spot" bolus effect was observed and the gas rapidly solubilized in blood and was rapidly excreted/diluted to baseline values in just 3 to 4 minutes. No radiation damage would be expected in tissue since the duration of exposure is far too short and remains in very diluted activity concentration (Fig. 4).

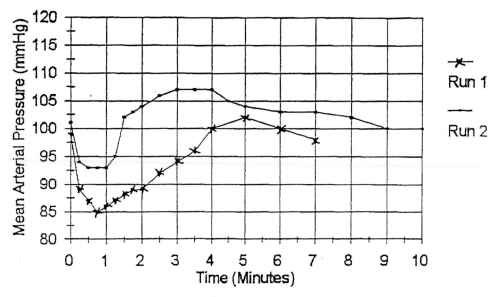

Figure 3. Mean arterial pressure measured at baseline and after injection of a 2 cc ¹³³Xe radiogas bolus. Injection occurred at time = 0.

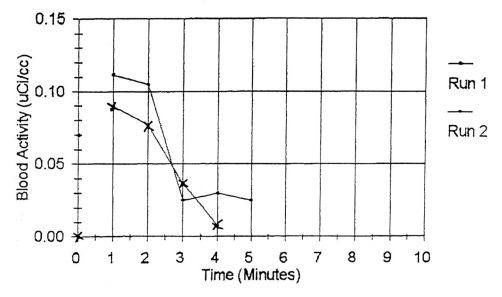

Figure 4. ¹³³Xe activity measured in the blood at baseline and after injection of a 2 cc ¹³³Xe radiogas bolus. Injection was administered at time = 0.

Radiation Exposure and Comparisons to Other Applications

The application of ¹³³Xe in a closed and retained intravascular delivery system portrays a uniquely safe radiation exposure profile for both the patient and health care personnel. The previously described properties of radioxenon, including its inert state, beta and gamma emission profile, and rapid dilution in air, if released, allow for extremely low radiation risks whether for routine treatment seepage or accidental complete loss in vivo.

Personnel, doing routine XenaCath treatments with an injection dose of 350 mCi and an average pass-through exposure of 2 to 5 mCi per procedure, would still only receive approximately 4.5 mrem/year for 1000 treatments (with standard protective apparel).[27] The Nuclear Regulatory Commission (NRC) shallow dose allowance (SDE) per year is 50 rem.[28] This represents only 1/11,000 of the allowed dose reached per year. Radiation exposure only exists during the injection time, as opposed to exposure that may occur with other systems during catheter placement or source transit time. According to data published by Landauer Inc.,[29] the internal dose for equivalent activity exposure per year is still only 0.004 to 0.4 mrem. Personnel dose from external, xenon-filled, catheter length during treatment is 2 to 4 mrem/h at 12 inches with proprietary catheter loading.

Standard exhaust venting and general temporary closure of the treatment suite during use would provide rapid elimination in equilibrium with any expected minor routine activity loss, and would quickly reduce unexpected accidental losses to safe concentrations of minimal derived air concentration levels (1.0 to 4.0 μCi/mL)[30] within 9 to 11 minutes (for assumed 350 mCi loss). Even with an initially perceived "high" activity loss, personnel exposure both with and without lead apron/glasses is still only 0.44 to 1.0 mrem and 44 to 100 mrem, respectively.

A report published by the Atomic Energy Control Board of Ottawa, Canada demonstrated that even under "worst conditions" (without a ventilation system), a workload loss of greater than 50 mCi per week (without a lead apron) still showed low skin exposure well below the maximum permissible limit. We recommend a very simple and inexpensive exhaust system for such applications. This can be done relatively quickly in most hospitals and suites.

Comparison of radiation exposure received to tissue (without protective wear) for other procedures is displayed in Table 1. For example, the exposure during angioplasty is 350 mrem, chest x-ray 20 mrem, mammogram 100 mrem, or computed tomography (CT) head 4200 mrem. The potential organ cumulative dose to patients/personnel from liquid sources such as ^{131}I, ^{32}P, or ^{188}Re are much higher when compared to the radiation exposure with ^{133}Xe, even in high concentrations, when used with standard venting and radiation apparel. It appears that from radiation protection and exposure for the patient and personnel, use of the ^{133}Xe system for vascular brachytherapy is safe. An abbreviated comparison of average body dose exposure to the patient from a 3-minute XenaCath treatment shows an average exposure dose of 7 to 10 mrem versus at least 20 rem from an angioplasty procedure. For comparison, consider that the average person in the U.S. receives an annual total effective dose of 360 mrem, primarily from background radiation and commercial products. Radiation exposure of 1000 XenaCath per year will be associated with radiation exposure for the operator of 4.5 mR if he or she uses protective apparel. Current annual maximal skin NRC SDE allowance for personnel is 50 rem. Additional computations based on NRC guidelines and xenon radiogas properties demonstrate that for the above-described routine procedural exhaust quantities, as well as with allowance for infrequent accidental losses, public exposure is still well within safe guidelines (which allow only 1 rem SDE per year-public).

Summary

A ^{133}Xe radiogas catheter delivery system offers a combination of advantages—in terms of radiation exposure, pragmatism, clinical effectiveness, and cost-effectiveness—that are equal to or surpass many other proposed systems. Thus far, for the parameters tested in the balloon overstretch porcine coronary model, the inhibition of neointimal hyperplasia and morphometric results on intimal area and IA/FL ratios have been similar to those described before with other beta and gamma emitters. Treatment time for delivered effective doses was completed, on average, in less than 2.25 minutes, with effective dose rates of greater than 4 to 5 Gy per minute.

This system provides a safe and inexpensive source, requiring minimal dosimetry efforts, and can routinely administer a consistent, homogeneous prescription dose to a predictable depth. Inventory of expensive or decay-wasted radiosources can be minimized, as ^{133}Xe can be delivered as needed for patient variable loads, and is good for a week.

Physicians and staff can remain at bedside throughout the intravascular brachytherapy procedure and any incidental gas loss is quickly "vacuumed" right out the venting system without any additional effort or cumulative contamination. Other potential applications, such as peripheral vascular disease, can be treated with this system due to the centering capability and proximity of the dose to the vessel wall.

Individual target lesions can be selectively covered by the simple selection of an appropriate balloon size and referral to a preprinted guide card as to the treatment time for an activity dose of ^{133}Xe.

Evolving systems are expected to allow for use of a premeasured dose of ^{133}Xe to be "dropped and loaded" into a placed catheter, with maximal seal, and treatment completion in 1.5 to 2.0 minutes. Disposal requires only standard decay bags, or the xenon may be safely reused for a limited number of additional treatments.

The feasibility clinical trials planned to start at the beginning of 1999 will determine the practicality of this system in the real world of interventional cardiology, and the pivotal trials will determine the future use of this system for the prevention of restenosis.

References

1. Waksman R, Robinson KA, Crocker IR, et al. Endovascular low dose irradiation inhibits neointima formation after coronary artery balloon injury in swine: A possible role for radiation therapy in restenosis prevention. Circulation 1995;91:1533–1539.
2. Wiedermann JG, Marboe C, Schwartz A, et al. Intracoronary irradiation reduces restenosis after balloon angioplasty in a porcine model. J Am Coll Cardiol 1994;23:1491–1498.
3. Mazur W, Ali MN, Dabaghi SF, et al. High dose rate intracoronary radiation suppresses neointimal proliferation in the stented and ballooned model of porcine restenosis. Int J Radiat Oncol Biol Phys 1996;36:777–788.
4. Verin V, Popowski Y, Urban P, et al. Intra-arterial beta irradiation prevents neointimal hyperplasia in a hypercholesterolemic rabbit restenosis model. Circulation 1995;92:2284–2290.
5. Waksman R, Robinson KA, Crocker IR, et al. Intracoronary low dose beta irradiation inhibits neointima formation after coronary artery balloon injury in the swine restenosis model. Circulation 1995;92:3025–3031.

6. Hehrlein C, Zimmerman M, Metz J, et al. Radioactive stent implantation inhibits neointimal proliferation in non-atherosclerotic rabbits. Circulation 1995;92:1570–1575.

7. Carter JC, Laird RJ, Bailey LR, et al. Effects of endovascular radiation from a b particle-emitting stent in a porcine coronary restenosis model: A dose-response study. Circulation 1996;94:2364–2368.

8. Thrall, JH, Ziessman, HA. Nuclear Medicine, The Requisites. St. Louis, MO: Mosby Press; 1995:129–132.

9. Kowalsky R, Perry JR. Radiopharmaceuticals in Nuclear Medicine Practice. Norwalk, CT: Appleton and Lange Press; 1987:249–258.

10. Kocher DC. Radioactive Decay Data Tables. DOE/TIC-11026; pp. 138–170.

11. Package Insert Label: Xenon-133 Gas. March 1994, Dupont/Merck, Inc., Radiopharmaceutical Division.

12. Susskind H, et al. Whole-body retention of radioxenon. J Nucl Med 1977;18:462.

13. Ponto RA, et al. Radioactive gases: Production, properties, handling and uses. In: Subramanian G, et al. (eds.): Radiopharmaceuticals. New York: Society of Nuclear Medicine; 296–300.

14. Goddard BA, Ackery DM. Xenon-133, Xe-127 and Xe-125 for lung function investigations. A dosimetric comparison. J Nucl Med 1975;16:780.

15. Atkins HL, Robertson JF, Croft BY, et al. Estimates of radiation absorbed doses from radioxenons in lung imaging. J Nucl Med 1980;21:459.

16. Deschamps U, et al. Occupational Exposure to Xenon-133 Among Hospital Workers. Research report; Ottawa, Canada: Atomic Energy Control Board; 1984.

17. Wilcox J, Waksman R, King SB, Scott NM. The role of the adventitia in the arterial response to angioplasty: The effect of intravascular radiation. Int J Radiat Oncol Biol Phys 1996;36:789–796.

18. Catheter-Balloon Specifications and Inserts as Published. Cook, Inc.; 1997 (Data on file).

19. Apple M. In Vitro Microdosimetry with Venous Catheter. Cook, Inc.; 1996 (Data on file).

20. Smits PC, Post MJ, Velema E, et al. Percutaneous coronary and peripheral angioscopy with saline solution and carbon dioxide gas in porcine and canine arteries. Am Heart J 1991;122:1315–1322.

21. Shifrin EG, Plich MB, Verstandig AG, Gomori M. Cerebral angiography with gaseous carbon dioxide CO_2. J Cardiovasc Surg 1990;31:603–606.

22. Lambert CR, de Marchena EJ, Bikkina M, Arcement BX. Effects of intracoronary carbon dioxide on left ventricular function in swine. Clin Cardiol 1996;19:461–465.

23. Kahn JK, Hartzler GO. The spectrum of symptomatic coronary air embolism during balloon angioplasty: Causes, consequences, and management. Am Heart J 1990;119:1374–1377.

24. Van Bankenstein JH, et al. Effect of Arterial Blood Pressure and Ventilation Gases on Cardiac Depression Induced by Coronary Air Embolism. American Physiological Society; 1994:1896–1902.

25. Chiu-Tsao ST, de la Zerda A, Lin J, Kim JH. High sensitivity GafChromic film dosimetry for 125I seed. Med Phys 1994;21:651–657.

26. Gatchromic Dosimetry Media, type MD-55, 1996. Data for MD-55–2, Dose Response Curves. Supplied by Nuclear Assoc., Inc.

27. Apple MG. XenaCath Dosimetry and Radio Safety Profile. Data and calculation on file: 1996–98. Cook, Inc.

28. United States Nuclear Regulatory Commission Regulatory Guidelines – Appendix D; Sections 0.1 and 0.2. Model Procedures for Calculating Worker Dose Concentrations of Gases/Aerosols in Work Areas.

29. Landauer, Inc. A Guide to Personnel Monitoring for Radiation in the Hospital Environment. Washington, DC: Library of Congress, 1993.

30. Kereiakas JG. Handbook of Radiation Doses in Nuclear Medicine and Diagnostic X-Ray. Boca Raton, FL: CRC Press; 1980.

## Chapter 60

RDX™ Coronary Radiation Delivery System: Balloon-Based Radiation Therapy

Maurice Buchbinder MD, Gary Strathearn PhD, and Brett Trauthen, MS

Introduction

Intravascular brachytherapy has become a promising technique for the treatment of restenosis, with two early devices potentially being approved by the U.S. Food and Drug Administration (FDA) in late 2000. Several studies have reported reductions in the restenosis rates to as low as 10 to 15%, even in lesion types prone to recurrence.[1,2,3,4] Animal investigations into the mechanism of this therapy have shown that ionizing radiation inhibits the formation of neointimal tissue in response to the injury following balloon angioplasty.[5]

The first studies of intracoronary brachytherapy adapted ^{192}Ir ribbons from radiation oncology for use in coronary arteries. The use of this high-energy gamma source presents several challenges to the physician. Depending on the activity of the source, protecting laboratory personnel from radiation requires over a centimeter of lead to effectively block the emissions while the source is in the patient. Hence, most studies utilizing this isotope require that the laboratory staff vacate the room during the radiation treatment, which can last over 15 minutes.

To address these issues, several systems have been proposed that utilize high-energy beta-emitting isotopes such as ^{90}Sr/Y, ^{32}P, and [188]Re[6]. Beta sources such as these can be shielded with plastics instead of lead, but the limited penetration depth of beta particles through the tissue make these sources very sensitive to position within the vessel, making source centering an important consideration for treatment, especially in larger vessels. Moreover, all of the systems proposed to date require calibration and the aid of a medical physicist for dosimetry calculations.

Overview of the Radiance RDX Coronary Radiation Delivery System

In a novel approach to intracoronary brachytherapy, the RDX Coronary Radiation Delivery System (Radiance Medical Systems, Irvine, CA) (Fig. 1) seeks to optimize dosimetry characteristics and simplify the use of radiation through a

From Waksman R (ed.). *Vascular Brachytherapy, Third Edition.* Armonk, NY: Futura Publishing Co., Inc.; © 2002.

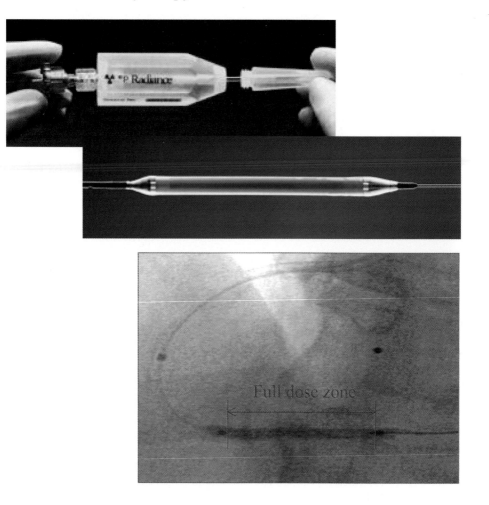

The radiopaque markers define the effective source length

Figure 1. Radiance RDX System, showing the source shield, balloon/source, and source-in-use. The radiopaque markers define the effective source length.

new source and delivery system design. The device was designed specifically for use in the cardiac catheterization laboratory, with delivery and operational techniques closely matching present techniques to simplify use and training. In addition, the system reduces the time required to perform the procedure, which should improve schedule coordination among the cardiologist, radiation oncologist, and radiation physicist.

Catheter Description

The RDX System incorporates the ^{32}P isotope directly into the balloon material (a tri-layer construction, with internal and external walls completely encapsulating the active source) of a percutaneous transluminal coronary angioplasty

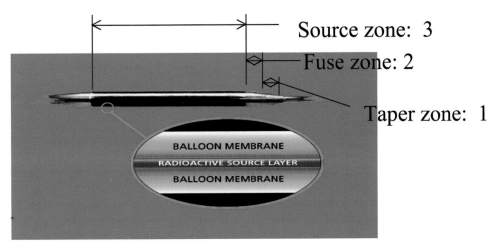

Source zone: 3

Fuse zone: 2

Taper zone: 1

BALLOON MEMBRANE
RADIOACTIVE SOURCE LAYER
BALLOON MEMBRANE

Figure 2. RDX System design showing the construction of the balloon section.

(PTCA)-type catheter as shown in Figure 2. This approach takes advantage of source apposition to the vessel wall, thereby simultaneously fully exploiting the beta characteristic of a short penetration depth providing centering for uniform dose distribution within the vessel wall. In addition, direct vessel apposition of the source reduces the activity required to deliver therapeutic doses to the target tissue, allowing simplistic shielding and a disposable device design. The disposable aspect eliminates the need for constant source recalibration and dosimetry calculation prior to each usage. Generally, the RDX System is a simple device to deliver since it utilizes the same delivery techniques as standard angioplasty.

Nuclide Selection and Activity

The first consideration for any brachytherapy system is the choice of isotope. With consideration of the advantages and limitations of both the gamma and beta isotopes mentioned earlier, the optimum source design is the use of a beta isotope characterized by a delivery system design providing proximity to the target tissue and concentricity with respect to the target tissue.

Generally speaking, particle energy, whether beta or gamma, dictates the suitability of an isotope for use in brachytherapy. Experiments and dosimetry models suggest that gamma emitters must have a minimum average emission energy of 20 to 30 keV, while beta emitters must have a minimum average energy of about 700 keV[7,8] to achieve adequate penetration into the vessel wall. A second important criterion for usage of a given isotope is its half-life. Although a longer half-life is desirable for a reusable source, a disposable device requires a shorter half-1ife in order to decrease the decay time prior to disposal. A 2- to 3-week shelf life is reasonable for a disposable system considering waste management issues.

Several isotopes meeting these criteria were considered for use in the RDX System, most notably ^{125}I and ^{103}Pd among gamma isotopes, and ^{32}P, ^{90}Sr/Y, and ^{188}W/Re among beta isotopes. Among these, ^{125}I and ^{90}Sr/Y activities were deemed too hazardous for a disposable system. ^{188}W/Re and ^{103}Pd were not readily available in a high specific activity and at a cost reasonable for a disposable system.

Given the requirements, P-32 appeared to be the best overall choice of isotope. Its half-life is close to ideal for a disposable product, and it is commonly available at high specific activities (>150,000 μCi/μg). Furthermore, ^{32}P is known by licensing agencies and its use is understood, enabling hospitals beyond those with large radiation staffs to license more easily.

Catheter Description

With selection of the isotope, a completely new source technology was developed specifically for the RDX System. The source was constructed using a proprietary "attachment" system that binds the isotope onto a substrate through a chemical reaction. This attachment technique can be performed on almost any surface. In the case of the RDX System, a thin plastic film was chosen as the substrate in order to minimize the balloon profile while providing support for a non-compliant balloon (see "Dosimetry" section below). In this particular case, sheets are customized and cut in length and width to match the final balloon size. The source sheets are then wrapped around the RDX balloon, and sealed within a secondary cover, forming a tri-layer system. Generally, the greatest concern for any thin film solid source had been the ability to attach enough activity to enable the delivery of an adequate dose with a maximum treatment time of 10 minutes. In the case of the RDX System, which uses ^{32}P, less than 1 μg of the isotope is required to achieve the necessary dose rate to the target tissue. This can be easily attached to even the smallest size (2.0-mm diameter by 33-mm long) active source.

The delivery system design for the RDX System is similar to that of a conventional balloon angioplasty catheter. It is a 0.014" wire compatible device constructed in over-the-wire or rapid-exchange configuration. Its profile and flexibility are similar to a stent delivery system. As mentioned earlier, the balloon itself has a unique tri-layer construction as shown in Figure 2. The encapsulation of the radiation source within the balloon layers seals it from direct contact from both the blood stream and the inflation fluid. The balloon membranes are constructed from a mixture of materials specifically designed for this purpose.

Shield and Packaging

The RDX System has a radiation shield as part of the unit, as seen in Figure 1. The shield was optimized to fully protect the staff exposed to the system while being easily handled in normal catheterization laboratory procedures. In use, the shield attached directly to the Touhy-borst valve of the guide and the balloon is introduced as per normal balloon catheters.

The RDX System is delivered in a standard catheter tray and sterile packaging within a box. The system is designed so that the source activity can be directly measured by insertion of the box into a National Institute of Science and Technology (NIST)-traceable activity meter, where the activity is directly read from the meter. With this process, it is possible to measure a week's supply of units in a few minutes. This verifies the dose prescription (see "Dosimetry" section below).

With simplicity and ease of use in mind, the dwell time for each RDX System is precalculated and listed on the package label (Fig. 3). This is possible because the balloon is noncompliant, and so the source diameter at inflation is consistent in all

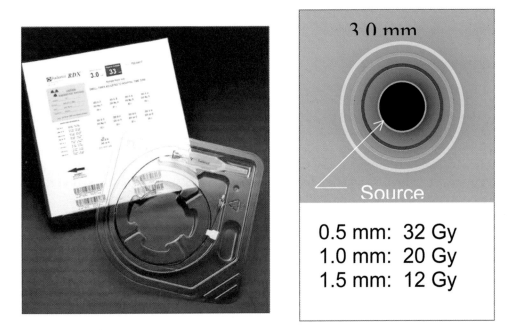

Figure 3. On the left, the packaging of the RDX, with the box showing the label including pre-calculated dwell times. The figure on the right shows the dosimetry associated with the RDX System.

balloons of the same model. The dose rate at the prescribed target (1 mm from the balloon surface) is thus dependent only upon the activity per unit area. Knowing the activity of the source enables the dose rate to be determined (see "Dosimetry" below), and from this, the total dwell time for a prescribed dose (20 Gy). The activity is determined by the manufacturer (traceable to NIST and PTB) and validated on site by the radiation physicist using equipment designed for this purpose. This enables the catheterization laboratory staff to use the source without lengthy calculations with the ever-present danger of calculation error while allowing the radiation oncologist and radiation physicist full control over the prescription dose.

Testing of the RDX System

The RDX System has undergone in vitro and in vivo testing. The balloon is designed to fully inflate at 2 atmospheres (atm) of pressure. This low operating pressure was intentionally chosen to minimize the potential for barotrauma to the vessel wall. The integrity of the source seal under cyclic conditions appears to be excellent. In qualification tests, each balloon underwent 120 inflation cycles at 3 atm (1 atm above the operating pressure) without damaging the balloon or compromising the source. The behavior of the RDX System under balloon burst conditions is an important design consideration. Using different compositions and dimensions for each layer of the balloon, the relative strength of each zone within the balloon can be varied (see Fig. 2). By making the single-layer "taper zone" the weakest, the failure mode of the balloon can be directed to this area. When the balloon breaks here, the source may not be compromised and only contrast media escapes into the bloodstream.

ISO/ANSI Testing

The RDX System has undergone ISO/ANSI testing for a sealed source. It has achieved a testing rating of ISO 2919–1999 & ANSI N542 77C23323. While no specific performance requirements have been set for intravascular brachytherapy, the RDX System passes the performance requirements for Medical: Interstitial and Intracavity Applications, the closest medical application, except for the temperature requirement. The RDX System has passed at the 80°C level of temperature, rather than the 600°C testing requirement, due to the source construction of plastic.

Nuclear Regulatory Commission Registration

The RDX System has been approved by the State of California (NRC Agreement State) as a Sealed Source and Device Registration.

Safety: Radiation Exposure to Staff

A major concern by both the NRC and the catheterization laboratory staffs is personnel exposure to radiation. Alarms have been given for the gamma systems, and although the doses to staff are significant, they are not a major health concern.[11] Radiance specified that one of its design goals be to reduce staff exposure to radiation. Two studies have been done by Radiance,[12] one using staff dosimeters during clinical trials and the other based on exposure levels from a source. In the former trial, no difference could be seen between staff exposed to the source and those not exposed. The dose to staff was less than 1% of the fluoroscopy dose. Calculations made from source data indicate that, at highest dose potential (the interventional cardiologist), the dose rates would be 0.2 μSv per case, as opposed to up to 95 μSv per case (radiation oncologist) from a gamma procedure.

RDX System Technology

Dosimetry

Dosimetry models and direct measurements have been undertaken at several laboratories, including the National Institute of Science and Technology (C. Soares) in Washington, DC, and Cedars-Sinai Medical Center (J. Whiting) in Los Angeles. These studies have been confirmed by work at clinical sites (M. Piessens, OLV Hospital, Aalst, Belgium, and D. Corletto, HSR Hospital, Milan, Italy). All of these studies found excellent correlation between the models (both Monte Carlo and PNK) with actual measurements (GAFChromic™ film).

The results of these studies showed remarkable dose rate efficiency of the RDX System source (Gy/mCi/min) compared to other source configurations using the same isotope. This result is due to the enhanced proximity of the source relative to the target tissue. The RDX System source requires significantly less activity to deliver a dose rate similar to other beta systems. For example, if one desires a prescription dose of 20 Gy given to a depth of 1 mm in 5 minutes to a 25-mm long lesion, a 0.5-mm wire source requires approximately 100 mCi of ^{32}P, a liquid-isotope-filled balloon requires 75 mCi, and the RDX System source requires 30 mCi. This reduction in activity translates to a lessened exposure risk to the patient and laboratory personnel.

The dosimetry characteristics of the RDX System were made using two different types of phantoms. As can be seen in Figure 4, both axial and linear images of the source were taken and analyzed. In all cases, calibrated GAFChromic film was used to record dose measurements. These images show the uniform penetration of the radiation around the surface of the balloon, and the uniformity of the radiation along the source surface.

Stenting is expected to be a common adjunctive procedure to radiation, so the effect of the stent on the dose was studied. The apposition of the RDX System source to the vessel wall appears to greatly reduce the impact of metal shielding. This rather unique property is illustrated in Figure 5, which shows a dosimetric

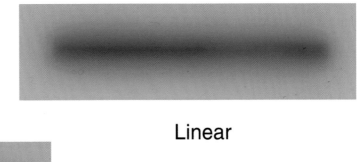

Linear

Axial

Figure 4. Axial and linear dosimetry of the RDX System.

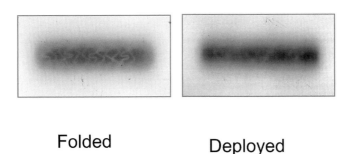

Folded source

Deployed source

Figure 5. Dosimetry measurements of the RDX System at 1 mm through a stent.

image of the RDX System within a stent in both a deflated and an inflated, or deployed, condition. As can be seen, the stent strut pattern is readily apparent due to the shielding effect (shadowing) of the metal strut on the beta particles in the deflated condition. In the inflated condition, the image of the stent is difficult to discern. The proximity of the source to the stent reduces the shielding effect of the stent on the delivery of radiation. This particular study verifies the concern that stents can indeed block some of the beta particles, and hence affect the uniformity of the dose. This is especially applicable to beta sources that are not in close proximity to the stent. In this study, metallic stents appear to reduce the overall dose rate to the surrounding tissue to between 10 and 12%.

A key aspect of the RDX System is the automatic centering of the source in the vessel. Figure 6 shows the effect of centering for beta systems. With the RDX System, a dose prescribed at 1 mm from the balloon surface will be consistently delivered. However, in a beta system that is not centered, the dose at 1 mm may vary from 12 Gy to 32 Gy for a 20 Gy prescription.

A second aspect seen in the dosimetry of the RDX System is the increased effective radiation length (ERL). This is the length of 90% prescribed dose at the target tissue. Figure 7 shows PNK modeling of various systems, indicating that the greatest ERL for commonly used beta systems is provided by the RDX System. This is due to the choice of ^{32}P as the nuclide and the proximity of the source to the target tissue.

Animal Studies

In preparation for clinical studies, the RDX System has been tested in over 40 animals. Using a classical porcine stent-injury model, the RDX System has been used to administer doses ranging from 10 to 40 Gy at a 1-mm depth. At 1 month, there is a significant reduction in neointimal formation within the treated segments compared to control vessels at doses over 15 Gy. These findings are consistent with similar reported studies using wire and seed sources.[9,10] An example of the radiation effect using the RDX is shown in Figure 8, where a dose of 20 Gy at a 1 mm depth was delivered, resulting in a total lack of neointimal formation. The control artery shows marked neointimal growth completely surrounding the stent and significantly reducing the lumen of the vessel.

These results are extremely encouraging. The performance of the RDX in the in vivo animal trials was most remarkable in its simplicity of use. Given its flexibility and trackability, the device was placed quickly and safely in all vessels. Although slightly larger than a standard balloon angioplasty catheter, the tip profile of the RDX remains very good, allowing for crossing of freshly implanted stents, even in small vessels.

Clinical Studies

The first human trial of the RDX System was started in September 1999 as part of an international multicenter feasibility study involving approximately 150 patients. In an open label prospective registry, the Beta Radiation Trial To Eliminate Restenosis Study (BETTER), the RDX System was evaluated in both de novo and restenotic lesions (stented and nonstented). The trial has completed enroll-

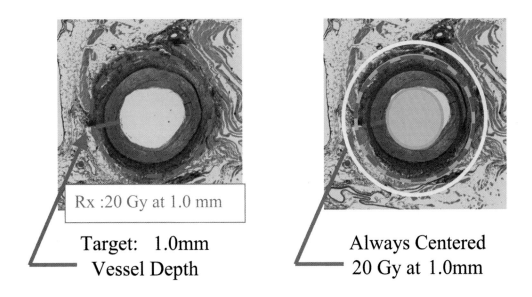

Target: 1.0mm
Vessel Depth

Rx :20 Gy at 1.0 mm

Always Centered
20 Gy at 1.0mm

0.5 mm: 32 Gy 1.0 mm: 20 Gy 1.5 mm: 12 Gy

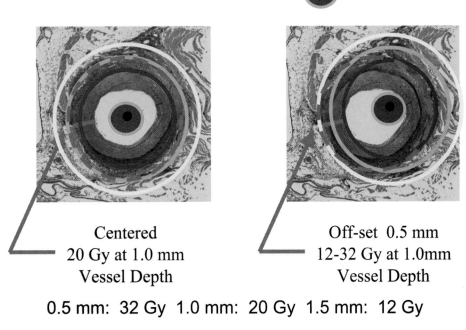

Centered
20 Gy at 1.0 mm
Vessel Depth

Off-set 0.5 mm
12-32 Gy at 1.0mm
Vessel Depth

0.5 mm: 32 Gy 1.0 mm: 20 Gy 1.5 mm: 12 Gy

Figure 6. Centered versus noncentered dosimetry of beta systems.

Dose Profiles

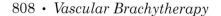

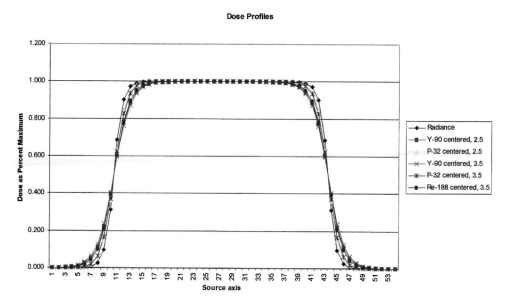

Figure 7. The Point Kernel Dosimetry Model showing the effective radiation lengths of centered versus Radiance RDX System for various vessel diameters. The effective radiation length (ERL) is increased in the RDX System due to a placement of the source at the vessel walls and the lower energy of the P-32 nuclide.

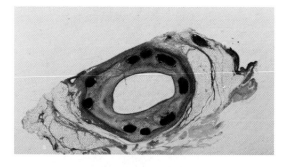

Control

Figure 8. Animal studies of the RDX System, showing comparison of irradiated versus control vessel segments.

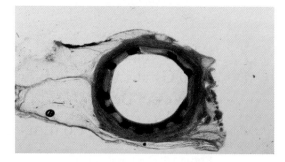

18 Gray at 1.0 mm

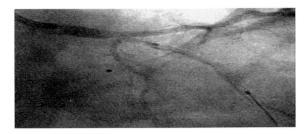

•RDX position with contrast injection

•RDX 3.0 x 33 mm inflated

•20 Gv @ 1.0 mm dose

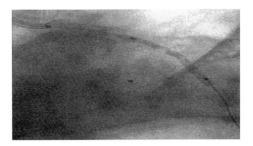

W. Wijns, OLV Hospital Aalst Belgium

Figure 9. Clinical studies showing the RDX in use.

ment; results from the trial are available in 2001. Figure 9 shows an example of a clinical case. Results of the trial are not available as of the date of writing.

Concurrently, the RDX System was evaluated in a randomized clinical trial testing its safety and efficacy for in-stent restenosis, the Beta Radiation to Reduce In-Stent Restenosis (BRITE) Study. This study was performed in the U.S. between February and April 2000. Results from the trial were available in late 2000.

Summary

The RDX System represents an exciting new generation radiation delivery system. The system design optimized dosimetry and simplifies the use of intracoronary brachytherapy in the catheterization laboratory setting. Utilizing the concept of "proximity" between radiation source and target tissue, the RDX System uses as little isotope as possible with uniform dosimetry, even in the presence of obstacles such as a stent.

In the course of developing this concept, an entirely novel radiation source technology was invented. Theoretical dosimetry models predicted an increase in dose delivery efficiency that has since been proven by quantitative studies showing superior treatment characteristics. The promise of the RDX System was validated in animal investigations; this system achieved a similar degree of neointimal inhibition as has been reported with other radioactive systems. Clinical results are to be released in the near future, and expectations for this system are high.

References

1. Tierstein P, et al. Catheter-based radiotherapy to inhibit restenosis after coronary stenting. N Engl J Med 1997;336:1697–1703.
2. King, SB III, et al. Endovascular β-radiation to reduce restenosis after coronary balloon angioplasty: Results of the Beta Energy Restenosis Trial (BERT). Circulation 1998;97:2025–2030.
3. Verin Y, et al. Feasibility of Intracoronary β-irradiation to reduce restenosis after balloon angioplasty. Circulation 1997;95:1138–1144.
4. Condado J, et al. Long-term angiographic and clinical outcome after percutaneous transluminal coronary angioplasty and intracoronary radiation therapy in humans. Circulation 1997;96:728–732.
5. Waksman R, et al. Intracoronary low dose β-irradiation inhibits neointima formation after coronary artery balloon injury in the swine restenosis model. Circulation 1995;92: 3025–3031.
6. Waksman R, et al. In: Waksman R, Serruys PW (eds.): Handbook of Vascular Brachytherapy. London: Martin Dunitz; 1998.
7. Amols H. Review of endovascular brachytherapy physics for prevention of restenosis. Cardiovasc Radiat Med 1999;1:64–71.
8. Nath R, et al. On the depth of penetration of photons and electrons for intravascular brachytherapy. Cardiovasc Radiat Med 1999;1:72–79.
9. Wiedermann JG, et al. Intracoronary irradiation markedly reduces restenosis after balloon angioplasty in a porcine model. J Am Coll Cardiol 1994;23:1491–1498.
10. Waksman R, et al. Intracoronary radiation before stent implantation inhibits neointima formation in stented porcine coronary arteries. Circulation 1995;92:1383–1386.
11. Balter S et al. Personnel exposure during gamma endovascular brachytherapy. Health Physics 2000;79:136–146.
12. Strathearn G, Fisher D, Rege S. Radiation safety issues associated with a plastic encapsulated intravascular brachytherapy source [abstract]. Health Physics Annual Meeting, 2000.

Balloon Catheters Impregnated with Radioisotopes for the Prevention of Restenosis

Christoph Hehrlein, MD, Adalbert Kovacs, MS,
Gerhard K. Wolf, PhD, Ning Yue, PhD,
and Ravinder Nath, PhD

Introduction

According to early clinical trials, vascular brachytherapy performed prior to or shortly after coronary angioplasty is very effective in lowering restenosis rates. However, some brachytherapy instruments do not allow centering of the source. Others, especially beta-particle emitters from wire sources, are equipped with centering balloons but cannot be used in arteries of large diameters. Moreover, balloons filled with radioactive liquids have a risk of balloon rupture or liquid leaking which may result in severe radioactive contamination of the environment. Radiation therapy using conventional afterloading technology after an angioplasty procedure may still be too time-consuming to be easily implemented on a routine basis in busy interventional catheterization laboratories. Balloon catheters impregnated with radioisotopes can be used to irradiate tissue prior to or post angioplasty only, but the most efficient way to use these instruments appears to be performing angioplasty and vessel irradiation simultaneously. In this chapter, we report early bench tests and animal results studying this novel concept for vascular brachytherapy.

Restenosis is a major problem after initially successful angioplasty procedures.[1-3] Recently, vascular brachytherapy with gamma and beta radiation sources has been shown to markedly reduce restenosis rates in animal models and in preliminary clinical trials.[4-6] Beta radiation offers the advantage of shorter irradiation periods and less radiation protection in the catheterization laboratory compared with gamma radiation.[7] In 1995, a procedure was developed to impregnate conventional balloon catheters with radioisotopes. This coating process minimizes the risk of radioisotope contamination. An angioplasty balloon impregnated with radioisotopes provides homogeneous vessel irradiation. The following is a report of early pre-clinical results evaluating this concept for vascular brachytherapy.

From Waksman R (ed.). *Vascular Brachytherapy, Third Edition.* Armonk, NY: Futura Publishing Co., Inc.; © 2002.

Materials and Methods

Ex Vivo Bench Testing of Angioplasty Catheter Impregnated with Radioisotopes

An impregnation process was developed resulting in thin films containing ^{32}P which tightly adhere to the surface of the balloon of a conventional angioplasty catheter. In brief, ^{32}P in solution was mixed with a polymer carrier which was attached homogeneously to the balloon surface. The ^{32}P impregnation process of the balloon was performed with and without a protective coating of the radioisotope film. The protective film was applied to seal off the radioisotope layer. The loss of ^{32}P from the catheter with and without protective film was measured after multiple balloon inflations and deflations using a beta-scintillation counter.

Dosimetry

Radiation doses were calculated using a Monte Carlo simulation model. At a given mean wall thickness of the rabbit iliac artery of 0.2 mm, the radiation dose penetrating to the adventitia was calculated for different balloon surface activities and periods of balloon expansion, ie, balloon surface contact with the arterial wall. The appropriate period of balloon inflation was chosen from the calculated dose charts according to the actual surface activity of the catheter. In the dosimetric calculation, it was assumed that the balloon is of the shape of a cylinder and the ^{32}P isotope is distributed uniformly on the curved surface of the balloon.

In the calculation, a first order approximation was made to neglect the self-absorption by the ^{32}P isotope itself. The point dose rate kernel of ^{32}P in water was obtained with Monte Carlo simulation. The Integrated TIGER Series (ITS) of Coupled Electron/Photon Monte Carlo Code System was used for kernel calculation. The ITS system was run on a DEC AlphaStation 200/66. The cutoff energy was 1 keV. The number of histories was 100,000. The energy spectrum of a beta particle emitted by ^{32}P source was computed based on the work by Prestwich et al.[8] The maximum beta energy used was 1.708 MeV. The ITS calculated dose corresponds to that deposited by a single beta particle emitted by a ^{32}P point source. The point dose rate kernel per unit ^{32}P activity (mCi) is obtained by multiplying the dose with a constant 3.7×10^7 s^{-1}.

Animal Experiments

Female New Zealand white rabbits weighing between 2.3 and 2.6 kg were studied. Anesthesia was performed with ketamine (35 mg/kg) and xylazine (5 mg/kg). Both femoral arteries were exposed and a 4 F pediatric sheath was inserted into each artery. Five-hundred units of heparin were given IA via the sheath. Retrograde angiograms were performed to determine the diameters in the iliac arteries. A ^{32}P-impregnated balloon with a total surface activity of 2 mCi was used for the study. The ^{32}P-impregnated angioplasty balloon catheter (3.0 mm diameter, 20 mm length) was advanced into the iliac artery of the rabbit. The balloon was inflated with physiologic saline solution to 6 atm and remained inflated for a period of 20 minutes. It was calculated to deliver a dose of 20 Gy to the adventitia of the rabbit arteries. The contralateral iliac artery of the rabbit was then dilated for another 20 minutes with a nonimpregnated conventional balloon angioplasty catheter (control). The rabbits were killed after 6 weeks for histologic analysis.

Tissue Collection and Fixation

The rabbits were sacrificed by a lethal dose of sodium pentobarbital (120 mg/kg). The abdominal aorta was canulated and the iliac arteries were flushed with physiological saline solution for 3 minutes. The iliac arteries were then removed and fixed according to standard protocols. The arterial specimens were dehydrated using graded alcohol solutions, and were then embedded in paraffin. The specimens were cut into serial 4- to 6-μm thick cross-sections at a rate of 20 cross-sections per artery.

Histomorphometry and Cell Counting

After staining the sections with hematoxylin-eosin, the neointimal cross-sectional areas were measured by a computer-assisted technique using a light microscope (Olympus) connected to a video camera (Sony) and a high-resolution digitizing image analyzer (Pavlov Inc., Heidelberg), as described previously.[9] Vessel perimeter, delineated by length of the external elastic lamina, and neointimal area were measured from each cross-section. Total cell numbers of the neointima in an area 0.05 mm^2 were counted and compared between the study groups by two independent observers.

Results

Ex Vivo Bench Testing

Figure 1 shows a schematic cross-section of a sealed source design of this technology. The manufacturing process for such a catheter has been reported previously.[10] The radioisotope loss from the impregnated catheter without a protective coating was 1% of the total activity. The loss was less than 0.1% with a protective film covering the impregnated balloon surface of the catheter (sealed source). Figure 2 shows a photograph from an impregnated balloon catheter at the bench site. Multiple balloon inflations and deflations of the balloon with a sealed source produced no detectable beta activity in the test medium blood, ie, the activity of the blood was below the detection limit of the scintillation counter.

Dosimetry Calculations

Three dimensional dosimetric distributions were calculated for ^{32}P-impregnated balloons of a length of 20 mm and diameters of 2.5, 3.0, and 3.5 mm. The dose is uniform, for the most part, along the longitudinal axis of the balloon, and drops off rapidly at both ends of the balloon. The dose increases with a decrease in balloon diameter. For this study, a balloon activity level of 2 mCi was chosen.

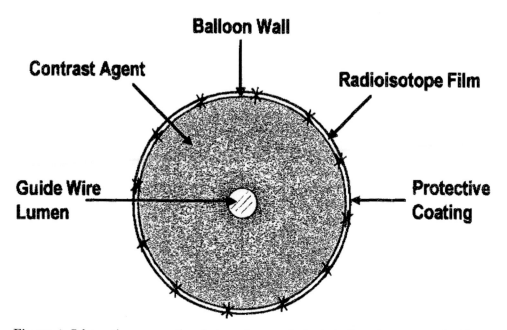

Figure 1. Schematic cross-sectional view of an angioplasty balloon impregnated with radioisotopes.

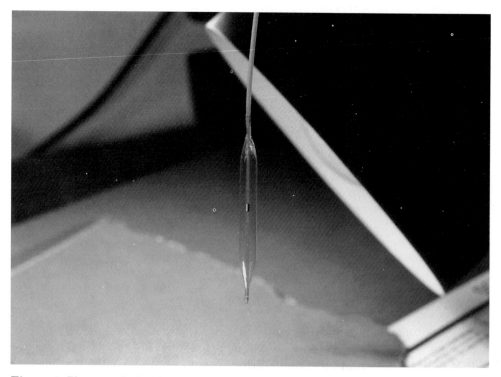

Figure 2. Photograph showing the angioplasty balloon covered with a translucent protective film after the impregnation process.

High source activities, ie, above 20 mCi, require only brief inflation periods to deliver a therapeutic dose of 20 Gy to the arterial wall. A detailed data dosimetry calculation for these radioactive balloons from a Monte Carlo simulation has been published previously.[11] If the radioactive balloon is inflated with the contrast agent Hypaque™ (composition, 7.88% of C, 7.42% of H, 22.73% of I, 67% of N, 58.92% of O, and 1.38% of Na; density 1.32 g/cm²), the overal effect of the contrast agent on the changes in dose is negligible with an uncertainty of ±5%.

Neointimal Formation

Neointimal areas in the arterial cross-sections obtained at 6 weeks after simultaneous dilatation and vessel irradiation was markedly smaller than after conventional balloon dilatation. The significant reduction of neointimal formation in the arteries after use of the ^{32}P-impregnated angioplasty catheter was observed in all dilated arteries. The cell number in the neointima after simultaneous balloon dilatation and vessel irradiation was markedly smaller at 6 weeks compared with the cell number in the neointima after conventional vessel dilatation.

Vascular Remodeling

Conventional balloon dilatation causes constrictive vascular remodeling in the rabbit. However, constrictive remodeling was abolished with irradiation of the arteries at the time of balloon dilatation. The vessel perimeter was significantly greater after simultaneous balloon dilatation and vascular irradiation compared with balloon dilatation alone at 6 weeks.

Discussion

Several studies have indicated that restenosis after angioplasty is due to neointimal hyperplasia and constrictive vascular remodeling.[12–14] Vascular brachytherapy has been shown to effectively reduce the restenosis rate in animal models and preliminary clinical trials.[4–6] This chapter reported on bench tests and animal results using a novel balloon angioplasty catheter impregnated with the radioisotope ^{32}P. The impregnated balloon is designed to perform simultaneous angioplasty and vessel irradiation to prevent restenosis; however, balloon inflation for brachytherapy only is another option. A radioisotope impregnation of the balloon centers the radiation source in the vessel, and allows homogeneous irradiation along the natural shape of the lumen during dilatation. Beta-particle emitters may be preferentially used for impregnation of balloon catheters since these radioisotopes have steeper dose fall-off characteristics than gamma emitters. In addition, when a beta source is in direct contact with the vessel wall instead of being centered in the vessel lumen, a steep dose gradient across the arterial wall is present. There was no radioisotope contamination after multiple balloon inflations and deflations with a protective film that seals off the radioisotope layer. Bench tests showed a very tight adherence of ^{32}P to the balloon even without a protective coating. Monte Carlo calculations showed that the radiation doses of this device delivered to the target area vary with balloon inflation diameter, balloon length, activity, and contact time at the arterial wall. However, radiation doses can be easily calculated if these parameters are known. Contrast agents in the balloon may not significantly change the dose delivered by balloons impregnated with ^{32}P.

The findings reported here, of a reduced neointimal hyperplasia and an increased vessel perimeter after radiation therapy using an angioplasty balloon impregnated with ^{32}P, are consistent with previous observations in animals studying other brachytherapy sources for the prevention of restenosis.[4,15,16]

A short inflation time of the radioisotope balloon resulting in a brief irradiation period eliminates the need for an autoperfusion system of this catheter if the catheter is going to be used in coronary arteries. In addition, the radioisotope balloon may be temporarily deflated to allow reperfusion of the coronary artery.[17] Cyclic inflations and deflations of the balloon may be used because approximately 80% of the total dose is delivered if the balloon is deflated. Further improvements of the radioisotope balloon technology include the local delivery of radiosensitizers to reduce cumulative radiation doses and potential radiotoxicity, and are considered to improve the long-term results of this treatment. An eluting radiosensitizer deployed by the balloon catheter may also further reduce the risk of edge restenosis at the dose fall-off zone of the balloon.

References

1. Block PC. Restenosis after percutaneous transluminal coronary angioplasty-anatomic and pathophysiological mechanisms: Strategies for prevention. Circulation 1990;81 (suppl IV):2–4.
2. Schwartz RS, Huber KC, Murphy JG, et al. Restenosis and the proportional neointimal response to coronary artery injury: Results in a porcine model. J Am Coll Cardiol 1992;19:267–274.
3. Serruys PW, Luijten HE, Geuskens BR, et al. Incidence of restenosis after successful coronary angioplasty: A time-related phenomenon. Circulation 1988;77:361–371.
4. Waksman R, Rodriguez JC, Robinson KA, et al. Effect of intravascular irradiation on cell proliferation, apoptosis, and vascular remodeling after balloon overstretch injury of porcine coronary arteries. Circulation 1997;96:1944–1952.
5. Teirstein PS, Massullo V, Popma JJ, et al. Catheter-based radiotherapy to inhibit restenosis after coronary stenting. N Engl J Med 1997;336:1697–1703.
6. Condado JA, Waksman R, Gurdiel O, et al. Long-term angiographic and clinical outcome after percutaneous transluminal coronary angioplasty and intracoronary radiation therapy in humans. Circulation 1997;96:727–732.
7. King III SB, Williams DO, Chougule P, et al. Endovascular beta-radiation to reduce restenosis after coronary angioplasty: Results of the beta energy restenosis trial (BERT). Circulation 1998;97:2025–2031.
8. Prestwich WV, Nunes J, Kwok CS. Beta dose point kernel for radionuclides of potential use in radioimmunotherapy. J Nucl Med 1989;30:1036–1046.
9. Hehrlein C, Gollan C, Dönges K, et al. Low-dose radioactive endovascular stents prevent smooth muscle cell proliferation and neointimal hyperplasia in rabbits. Circulation 1995;92:1570–1575.
10. Hehrlein C, Kovacs A, Löscher F, et al. Novel radioisotope coated angioplasty catheter to prevent restenosis: Initial bench test results. Am J Cardiol 1997;80(8A):26S.
11. Yue N, Nath R, Hehrlein C. Dosimetry calculation for a novel phosphorus-32 impregnated balloon angioplasty catheter for intravascular brachytherapy. Cardiovascular Radiat Med 1999;4:349–357.
12. Andersen HR, Maeng M, Thorwest M, et al. Remodeling rather than neointima formation explains luminal narrowing after deep vessel wall injury: Insights from a porcine coronary (re)stenosis model. Circulation 1996;93:1716–1724.
13. Luo H, Nishioka T, Eigler NL, et al. Coronary artery restenosis after balloon angio-

plasty in humans is associated with circumferential coronary constriction. Arteriosler Thromb Vasc Biol 1996;16:1393–1398.

14. Mintz GS, Popma JJ, Pichard AD, et al. Arterial remodeling after coronary angioplasty: A serial intravascular ultrasound study. Circulation 1996;94:35–43.

15. Wilcox JN, Waksman R, King SB, et al. The role of the adventitia in the arterial response to angioplasty: The effect of intravascular radiation. Int J Radiat Oncol Biol Phys 1996;36:789–796.

16. Crocker IR, Klein L, Williams DO, et al. Positive remodeling following intracoronary radiation therapy (ICRT): Results from the beta energy restenosis trial. Circulation 1998;98:652.

17. Hehrlein C, Kovacs A, Wolf GK et al. A novel balloon angioplasty catheter impregnated with beta-particle emitting radioisotopes for vascular brachytherapy to prevent restenosis: First in vivo results. Eur Heart J 2000;21:2056–2062.

## Chapter 62

The RadioVascular Systems Catheter

Neal A. Scott, MD, PhD, Janet Hampikian, PhD, and Jerome Segal, MD

Introduction

Despite the overwhelmingly positive results of trials using intracoronary radiation, the radiation catheters developed to date have many disadvantages. In an effort to develop a revolutionary radiation delivery catheter, RadioVascular Systems, Inc. (Washington, D.C.) has developed a radioactive coating technology for vascular applications and combined this technology with a unique catheter.

The FullFlow Catheter

Several years ago, Dr. Segal conceived of a novel approach to performing percutaneous transluminal coronary angioplasty (PTCA) procedures utilizing the FullFlow catheter. This device is a mechanical, non-balloon-based catheter that contains a radiopaque expandable spring mesh component, instead of a balloon, mounted at the distal end of the catheter (Fig. 1). When the mesh is expanded by use of an actuating handle at the proximal end of the catheter, a scaffold with multiple openings is formed which provides enough radial pressure (approximately 20 atm) to dilate an obstruction within a coronary vessel. Thus, a dilatation/perfusion system is created which allows physiological blood flow to occur through the mesh during vessel dilatation. Prolonged vessel dilatation may be performed without the risk of ischemia. Human trials of the nonradioactive FullFlow catheter system were initiated in Europe in May 1998 and in the U.S. in August 1999.

Although the clinical trials have not yet been completed, a representative case is shown below. It is clear that the FullFlow catheter will have its greatest utility in those patients who cannot tolerate any obstruction of blood flow caused by balloon inflation. It should be noted that, in an angioplasty procedure, the average time of balloon inflation is approximately 1 to 2 minutes. After this period of time, most patients develop chest pain from the obstruction to blood flow caused by the balloon. If prolonged inflation is necessary, the balloon is deflated to allow for the restoration of blood flow and then another inflation is performed. In some cases, a specially designed angioplasty balloon can be used for prolonged inflations. This device is known as a perfusion balloon. Perfusion balloons have small flow channels that allow some blood to flow past the balloon. However, perfusion

From Waksman R (ed.). *Vascular Brachytherapy, Third Edition.* Armonk, NY: Futura Publishing Co., Inc.; © 2002.

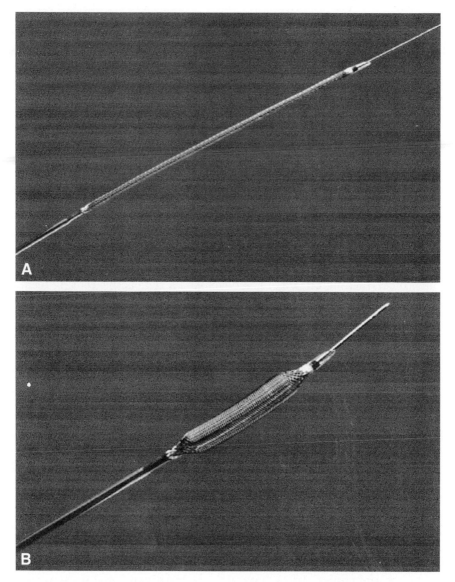

Figure 1. A. The FullFlow catheter in its contracted form. **B.** The FullFlow catheter in its expanded form.

balloons do not restore normal flow; they decrease flow by approximately 60% in vitro. The FullFlow device decreases flow by less than 20% in vitro. In an animal study, Segal et al have shown that, since the FullFlow dilates the artery in addition to providing flow, coronary artery flow actually *increases* when the device is expanded in vivo.[1]

Case Study

A 68-year-old man was admitted to the hospital with an episode of prolonged chest pain that was relieved only after the institution of maximal doses of oral and intravenous medications. On the morning of his procedure he experienced several episodes of chest pain. His coronary angiogram shows a very high-grade stenosis in the left anterior descending artery. The stenosis also involves a branch vessel (Fig. 2). A decision was made to perform angioplasty. During this procedure a tiny (0.014" diameter) guidewire is advanced through the stenosis. Equipment used to

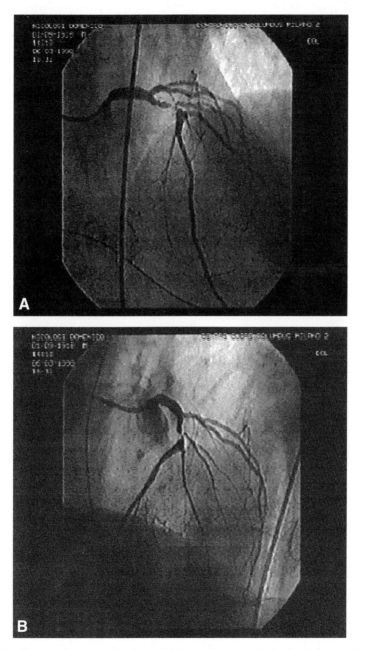

Figure 2. Baseline angiogram showing a high-grade stenosis in the left anterior descending artery (arrows). **A.** The view from the right anterior oblique position. **B.** The stenosis in the left anterior oblique view. All subsequent views are in the right anterior oblique position.

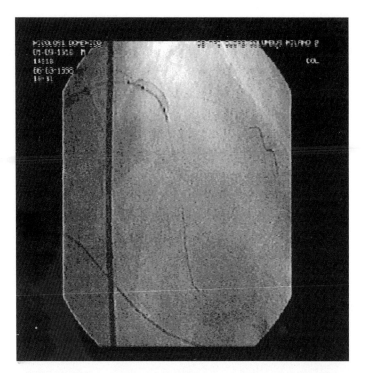

Figure 3. Expanded FullFlow device in the left anterior descending artery. Note how the device conforms with the tortuosity of the vessel.

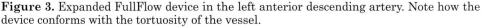

perform the angioplasty is then advanced over the guidewire. Since the guidewire has such a small cross-sectional area it usually does not impair blood flow through the stenosis. In this patient, however, when the guidewire was placed through the stenosis the patient experienced severe chest pain and had a decrease in blood pressure, consistent with the stenosis being so severe that the guidewire occluded flow. Also, it was immediately clear that this patient would not tolerate any occlusion of blood flow, no matter how brief. A FullFlow device was rapidly advanced over the guidewire and expanded at the stenosis (Fig. 3). The patient's chest pain completely resolved as soon as the FullFlow catheter was expanded. Figure 4 shows an angiogram with the FullFlow device in place and expanded, revealing excellent blood flow past the device and down the side branches. An excellent angiographic result was obtained after the FullFlow device was removed (Fig. 5).

The RadioVascular Systems Radiation Catheter

Using the proprietary RadioVascular Systems coating system (U.S. Patent Pending), a radioactive coating of ^{32}P can easily be placed on the surface of the dilating mesh of the fully assembled FullFlow catheter (Fig. 6). This process results in a coating of 1 to 5 microns in thickness (Fig. 6) that will provide up to 25 mCi of radiation on the surface of the mesh. This should result in more than enough radiation to be delivered to the adventitia to prevent restenosis. Proof of principle

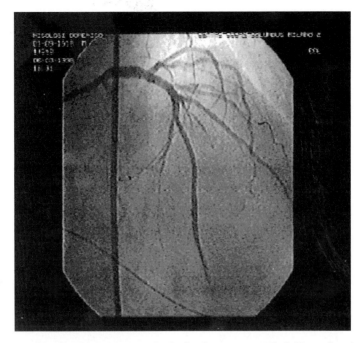

Figure 4. An angiogram of the artery *with the device expanded.* Note the abundant flow down the vessel and side branches.

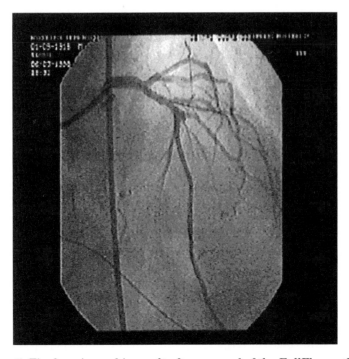

Figure 5. Final angiographic result after removal of the FullFlow catheter.

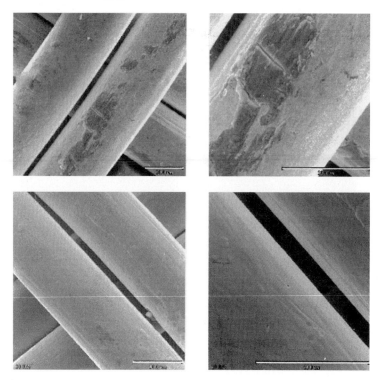

Figure 6. Scanning electron microscopy of the metal mesh of the FullFlow catheter. The mesh in the two top pictures is uncoated, while the mesh in the two bottom pictures has been coated with the proprietary coating that contains elemental phosphorus. Note that the surface of the coated catheter appears smoother.

was recently accomplished when a FullFlow catheter was coated with a layer of ^{32}P. The coatings are adherent and are deposited with a method that is usually used to confer corrosion resistance to metals.

Technical Advantages of the FullFlow

The FullFlow radiation catheter provides a unique platform for intravascular radiation delivery for coronary and peripheral arteries. In addition, it has a number of advantages over the current technology:

- The catheter, when deployed, is placed against the inner layer (lumen) of the artery. Therefore, proximity to the target tissue, the outer layer of the artery (adventitia), is maximized. Since radiation energy decreases by a factor of the square of the distance from the source, the amount of radiation needed to deliver the prescribed dose to the adventitia will be significantly lower than a source that is placed in the center of the artery (the current method of delivery for several beta sources). This should greatly increase safety for both the patient and the staff.
- Since the FullFlow radiation catheter provides physiological flow to the downstream coronary artery and side branches during dilatation and radiation, the radioactive mesh may be left in place for almost any length of time

necessary to deliver the required dose. Vessel ischemia during delivery is no longer a problem, as it is with centering balloon systems and systems that use a radioactive balloon or a balloon with a radioactive coating. Since blood flow is not impaired when the catheter is expanded, the catheter can be deployed in the artery for a longer period of time. As a result, the amount of radioactivity on the catheter can be lower than other catheters.

- A major advantage of this catheter is the ability to easily treat large arteries with beta radiation. Since the device is deployed against the artery wall, the device is one of the few catheters that can emit beta energy and effectively treat large vessels. The only other catheters that can accomplish this task are balloons that are filled with radioactive liquids or gases or balloons with a radioactive coating. In all of these competing devices, the time that the balloon can be left inflated is limited, since the balloon obstructs flow in the artery and the side branches. The FullFlow radiation catheter enables physiological flow to occur during its deployment. As a result, ischemia in the segment distal to the device or in the side branches does not occur.
- Radiation delivery will be uniform along the axial length of the artery. Since the catheter is deployed against the lumen of the artery, the delivery of radiation to the artery will be uniform even in kinked or tortuous segments.
- Since the radiation is delivered from the lumen, the dosing can be standardized so that the amount of radiation required can be delivered by expanding the mesh for a predetermined time, thus eliminating the need for complicated radiation physics calculations in the cardiac catheterization laboratory. In addition, the need for intravascular ultrasound is eliminated, since the catheter is placed adjacent to the lumen of the artery.
- Use of the catheter will require no additional training since physicians are already familiar with inflating and deflating angioplasty balloons. The method for deploying this catheter is very similar to inflating an angioplasty balloon. In addition, the nonradioactive version of the catheter should be approved and in use by the time the radioactive catheter is in clinical trials.
- Angioplasty and radiation delivery could be performed with the same device. The device can deliver more radial force (up to 25 atm) than most balloons and could be used to dilate and deliver radiation at the same time.
- Since the FullFlow radiation catheter can be left in place without causing ischemia, the shelf life for the catheter (^{32}P half-life = 14 days) would be significantly increased because the treatment times could be proportionally increased as needed without causing ischemia.

Conclusion

The RadioVascular Systems radioactive FullFlow catheter will provide beta radiation directly to the wall of the artery without occluding flow.

Reference

1. Segal J, Wolinsky SC, Sunew J, et al. Coronary angioplasty performed using the FullFlow mechanical dilatation-perfusion catheter: Initial animal experience. Cathet Cardiovasc Interv 2000;51:239–249.

Intravascular Ultrasound-Guided Catheter-Based System

Marco Roffi, MD, E. Murat Tuzcu, MD,
Patrick L. Whitlow, MD, Urs O. Häfeli, PhD,
and Jay P. Ciezki, MD

Introduction

Intravascular brachytherapy is a rapidly evolving therapeutic modality. Its efficacy in reducing restenosis after percutaneous coronary interventions (PCIs) has been demonstrated in randomized clinical trials mainly involving in-stent restenosis patients.[1–3] Despite some unresolved clinical issues, such as late total occlusion,[4] the marked benefits of intravascular brachytherapy over conventional PCI in the setting of in-stent restenosis has contributed to the enthusiasm characterizing this new brachytherapy application. The widespread use of these systems in the near future is likely to greatly benefit patients.

Our interest in intravascular brachytherapy is centered on the development of second-generation systems. The goals of our developmental work are increasing efficacy and decreasing toxicity by using a new guidance strategy that is attuned to the biology and anatomy of PCI procedures. We present an intravascular ultrasound (IVUS)-guided catheter-based system generated from cooperation between interventional cardiology and radiation oncology and sympathetic to the needs of both specialties.

Background

The first generation systems are varied in their design. On the surface there does not appear to be many shared qualities. These devices take many forms including afterloading catheters (with and without centering capability), stents, liquid-filled balloons, gas-filled balloons, and x-ray tubes mounted on catheters. The diverse embodiments of these devices belie their dosimetric similarities. All of them generate a radiation dose profile that is concentric perpendicular to the long axis of the delivery device. In contrast, the vessel wall is most often eccentrically narrowed by atherosclerosis. This dichotomy leads to a mismatch between the axial vascular anatomy and the radiation dose profile (Fig. 1). Both the radiation oncologist and the interventional cardiologist must try to solve this dosimetric prob-

From Waksman R (ed.). *Vascular Brachytherapy, Third Edition.* Armonk, NY: Futura Publishing Co., Inc.; © 2002.

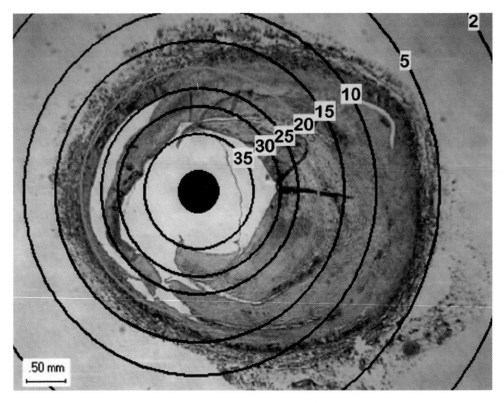

Figure 1. Axial image of a coronary artery ~24 hours after percutaneous coronary intervention. A radiation source (black dot) is centered in the lumen and 20 Gy is prescribed to a 1.5-mm radius. Note the inhomogeneity of dose to the adventitia.

lem by developing a second generation device that is more sensitive to the complex and variable anatomy of diseased vessels.

Our developmental goals center on the perceived need to match dosimetry with the complex anatomy of vascular lesions. Viewed in the axial plane, the anatomy may best be characterized as eccentric.[5,6] With interventions that target the lumen, such as balloon angioplasty, the axial anatomy is of little proven importance. However, the treatment targets for intravascular brachytherapy are likely to be located in the vascular wall.[7] There is also some evidence that the entire vascular wall, not just the periluminal portion, should be targeted.[6] Clinical correlations to these basic science observations are emerging. The efficacy of treatment with a ^{192}Ir-based system is closely linked to the minimum dose to the external elastic lamina (EEL) of the vessel as estimated from IVUS.[8,9] Although there is less direct evidence, the toxicity of intravascular brachytherapy may also be related to dose. For example, in the porcine animal model, a focal area of vascular wall necrosis, with or without overlying thrombus, was produced in a vessel 1 month after 15 to 25 Gy of ^{192}Ir was prescribed, to a 1.5 mm distance from the source.[10] The histologic pictures from that study look strikingly similar to the IVUS images of patients who developed delayed thrombosis in various clinical trials that predominately used beta emitters.[11] With these histologic and IVUS findings of focal vascular wall necrosis/thinning, one may hypothesize that late total occlusion after intravascular bracytherapy is the result of excessive dose from a catheter that lies too close to the vessel wall. Preventing focal areas of excessive dose, while ensuring that the remainder of the vessel wall gets adequate coverage, is the main goal of our development.

Three characteristics of an optimal device were ultimately decided upon. The first is the ability to conform the radiation dose to the vascular anatomy. This was the one quality of the device that could not be compromised because it alone would allow the dosimetric match with the vascular anatomy we sought. With the recognition that the axial anatomy of most vessels is eccentric, we investigated ways to create an eccentric radiation dose profile. The most reliable way of doing this is by partially shielding the circumference of the catheter segment containing the radiation source. The result is a radiation dose profile that resembles the vascular wall (Fig. 2). In our mind's eye we imagined the overlay of this dose profile on an axial section of a diseased vessel (Fig. 3) and thought that this is what we wanted to achieve. The second quality is the ability to image the axial anatomy of the vessel and know how this image relates to the radiation dose profile. Phased array IVUS is the most reasonable choice because it permits axial imaging, is small enough to be integrated into a catheter that can hold a radiation source, and has no moving

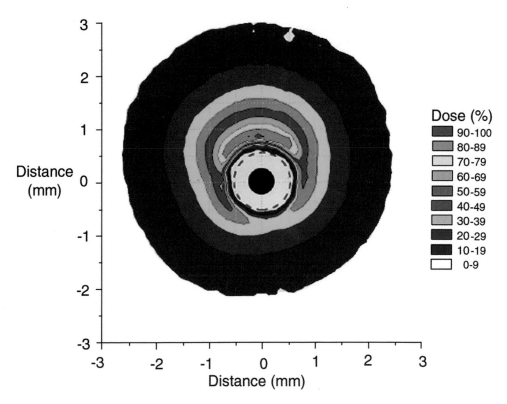

Figure 2. Axial image of a radiation dose profile from the Brigade catheter. The 10% of maximum iso-dose line is at about 3 mm from the center of the catheter (12 o'clock position) at the unshielded portion of the catheter, and at 2 mm from the center of the catheter (6 o'clock position) at the shielded portion of the catheter. The very intense areas of dose (red) are not present adjacent to the shielded portion of the catheter allowing it to lie against the vascular wall with impunity.

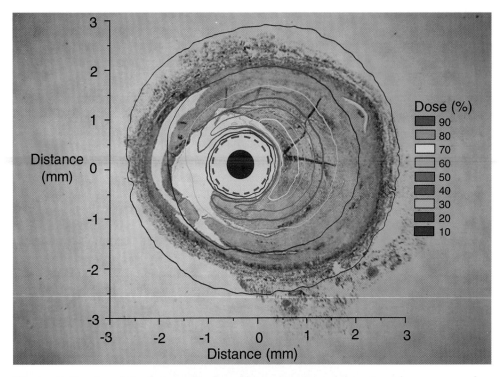

Figure 3. Overlay of the dose profile from Figure 2 on an axial section of a coronary after percutaneous coronary intervention. This orientation delivers a homogeneous dose to the adventitia.

parts so it can be linked with the radiation shield in a fixed orientation. The linking of the radiation dose profile and the vessel wall image is crucial because it allows the user see the best match between the dose profile and the image. The third characteristic enables the user to make the aforementioned match happen by mounting the radiation shield/IVUS combination on a torquable shaft.

After many iterations, we arrived at a design-freeze that captured all of the aforementioned elements (Fig. 4). The device is named the Brigade (Beta Radiation with IVUS Guidance and Directed Energy) catheter. This catheter-based system has a maximal outer diameter (OD) of 3.5 F. This occurs at the IVUS transducer. The shaft distal to the IVUS transducer has an OD of 2.5 F. This area contains the radiation shield and is where the radiation source dwells during use. The proximal shaft is 3.0 F and is composed of a combination of polymer and metal in order to transmit torque effectively while maintaining flexibility. The compromise between torque and flexibility was the developmental hurdle that took the most effort to overcome. The catheter travels over a 0.014" guidewire passed through a monorail system at the catheter's tip. A novel feature of this tip is the ability to rotate freely about the long axis of the catheter. This not only permits torque but also prevents guidewire prolapse because torque cannot build up as the catheter negotiates a curved pathway. The radiation source (OD of 0.45 mm) is passed into the catheter through the proximal port of the catheter. The central lumen of the catheter is closed to the patient.

The combination of the radiation shield, IVUS, and torque shaft suggests the method of use for this device. At the proper time during the intervention, the

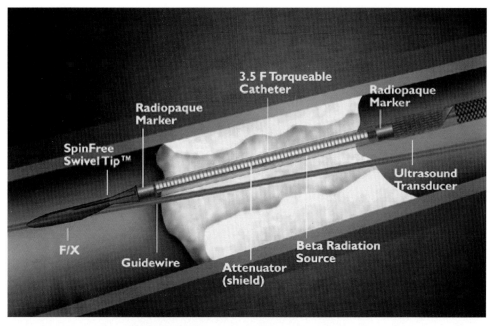

Figure 4. Schema of the Brigade Catheter.

catheter is inserted into the vessel and a survey of the vessel wall is done with the integrated IVUS. The orientation of the dose profile relative to the vessel's anatomy is noted. The dose profile is then altered to effect a match with the vascular anatomy by torquing the catheter (Fig. 5). The torquing is made easier by having real-time IVUS images of the vessel during manipulation.

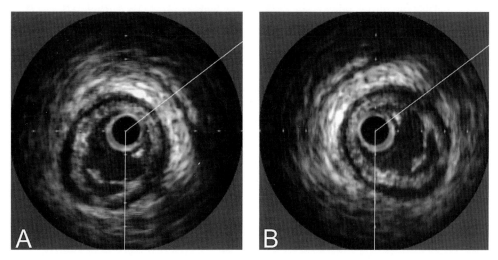

Figure 5. A. Intravascular ultrasound (IVUS) of a coronary artery with the Brigade catheter in situ prior to proper orientation. Cursors indicate the position of the shield (lower right is unshielded). **B.** IVUS of the same coronary artery with the Brigade catheter in situ after proper orientation. The unshielded portion of the dose profile is directed at the external elastic lamina furthest from the catheter.

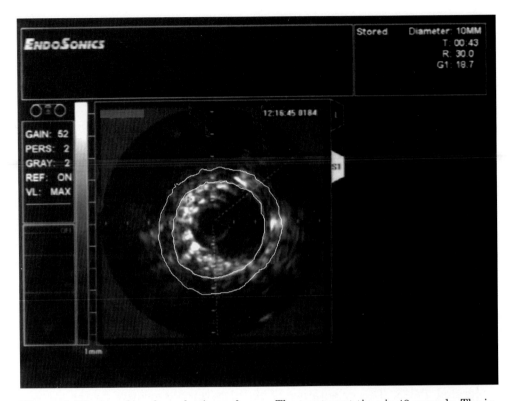

Figure 6. Display of iso-dose plotting software. The treatment time is 43 seconds. The inner iso-dose is the iso-dose line intersecting the normalization point (the external elastic lamina [EEL] nearest to the shielded portion of the catheter after positioning). 30 Gy is prescribed to this point. The outer iso-dose line intersects the far EEL. In this case, prescribing 30 Gy to the near EEL behind the shield gives 18.7 Gy to the far EEL. These three numbers are displayed in the upper right corner of the display (T: 00:43, R: 30.0, G1: 18.7 Gy).

The radiation oncologist is now able to prescribe a dose of radiation to the vessel wall that is relatively homogeneous. Software that is linked to the IVUS unit provides the computing power to generate a treatment plan in seconds by simply indicating a point on the image to use for dose normalization. Not only will the dose to various points of interest be listed, but the dwell time of the source will also be displayed (Fig. 6). The source is now loaded into the catheter for the length of the dwell time and removed at its completion. The source material chosen for the initial trials is ^{188}W/^{188}Re, a mixed beta and gamma emitter that can be used in activities yielding treatment times of ~2 minutes.[12] No additional shielding is necessary to protect the medical personnel.

Pre-Clinical Experimentation

The safety of this device was determined by experimentation in the porcine animal model of balloon overexpansion coronary injury. A group of 6 animals was sacrificed 3 days after treatment. Another group of 16 animals was sacrificed 6 months after treatment. The animals each received a balloon overexpansion injury of two coronary arteries. One of these injury sites received the brachytherapy catheter alone and one received the catheter and radiation (dose prescribed was 30 Gy to the EEL nearest the catheter). All animals survived the radiation procedure. Prior to sacrifice, all animals had an angiogram taken. After angiography, the animals were sacrificed and the hearts explanted and fixed under arterial pressure.

The primary endpoint of this series of experiments was safety. The assessment of safety was based on examination of the arterial segments by both light and electron microscopy. Under light microscopy there was no evidence of radiation necrosis or delayed thrombosis (Fig. 7). Electron microscopy of the

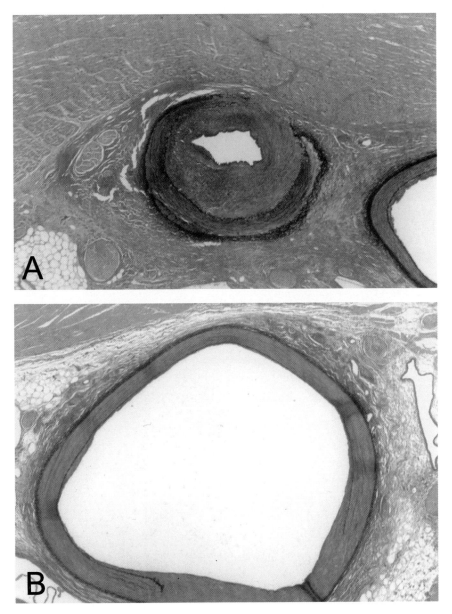

Figure 7. A. Coronary artery 6 months after balloon overstretch injury. Significant neointimal formation is present. **B.** Coronary artery 6 months after balloon overstretch injury and intravascular brachytherapy. Limited neointimal formation present and no evidence of radiation necrosis.

endothelium demonstrated complete endothelialization of all arterial segments (Fig. 8). Efficacy was superficially addressed by examining the angiographic restenosis (>50 % stenosis, angiographically) rate; in the 6-month group, it was 0% for the irradiated segments and 12% for the untreated segments.

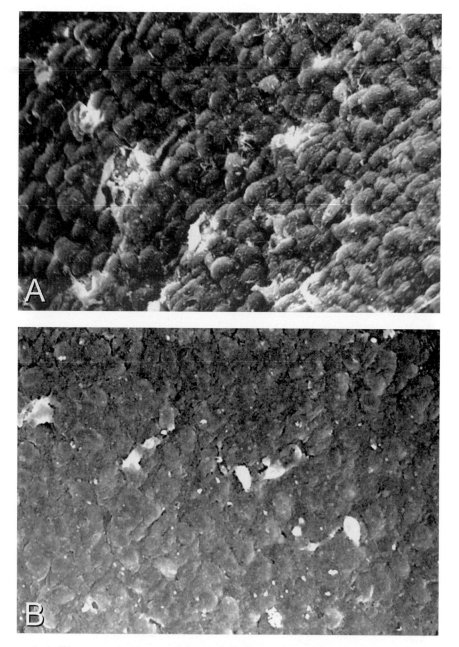

Figure 8. A. Electron microscopy of the endothelium of a coronary artery 6 months after balloon overstretch injury. Endothelialization is complete. **B.** Electron microscopy of the endothelium of a coronary artery 6 months after balloon overstretch injury and intravascular brachytherapy. Endothelialization is also complete.

Clinical Plan

The initial clinical investigation will consist of two phase I trials addressing the populations at high risk for restenosis after PCI, namely patients with in-stent restenosis and de novo lesions in diabetics. So far, most of the intravascular brachytherapy studies have involved patients with in-stent restenosis. However, diabetic patients may also have enhanced benefits from brachytherapy.[8] In fact, the pathophysiological mechanisms leading to restenosis in diabetics may partially differ from nondiabetics. Whereas, following balloon angioplasty in nondiabetics, negative remodeling leading to vessel shrinkage appears to be more important than neointimal proliferation in producing late lumen loss, the converse may be true in diabetics.[13] The predominant role of neointimal proliferation in restenosis makes this population, similarly to the in-stent restenosis population, particularly suitable for brachytherapy because of the ability of radiation to prevent neointimal formation.[14] Moreover, conventional percutaneous revascularization, including debulking devices, has shown limited efficacy in the treatment of both in-stent restenosis and lesions in diabetic patients.[15–20] Two phase I registries involving 30 in-stent restenosis patients and 30 diabetics are planned. The study summaries are reported in Table 1. The antiplatelet regimen consists of clopidogrel 75 mg daily for 6 months in addition to aspirin. Independent core laboratories will perform quantitative angiographic analysis and IVUS analysis at baseline and follow-up. Since late thrombosis following intravascular brachytherapy occurs more frequently after stenting than after balloon angioplasty,[4] the protocols favor provisional stenting, ie, stent deployment only for suboptimal balloon angioplasty results. In order to provide standard care and to minimize the

---

Table 1

Summary of Brigade In-Stent Restenosis Trial and Brigade Diabetic Trial

In-Stent Restenosis Trial

Objective	Safety and feasibility of IVUS-guided brachytherapy for in-stent restenosis.
Design	Prospective, nonrandomized trial.
Population	30 patients with in-stent restenosis.
Primary endpoints	30-day and 9-month composite endpoint of target vessel revascularization, death, and myocardial infarction.
Secondary endpoints	Angiographic restenosis (>50%) of the target vessel at 9-months Subacute/late thrombosis at 30 days and 9 months.

Diabetic Trial

Objective	Safety and feasibility of IVUS-guided brachytherapy in diabetics.
Design	Prospective, nonrandomized trial.
Population	30 diabetic patients with de novo or restenotic lesions ≥9 mm of length.
Primary endpoints	30-day and 9-month composite endpoint of target vessel revascularization, death, and myocardial infarction.
Secondary endpoints	Angiographic restenosis (>50%) of the target vessel at 9-months Subacute/late thrombosis at 30 days and 9 months.

risks of treatment effect based on different antithrombotic regimens, glycoprotein IIb/IIIa receptor inhibitors will be routinely administered, if no contraindications to the drugs are present.[21]

Conclusion

The Brigade system is a second generation brachytherapy system. It combines the input of both the interventional cardiologist and the radiation oncologist. Its design is intended to conform to the lesions treated so as to maximize efficacy and decrease toxicity. Based on the failure patterns of preexisting devices, this device seems poised to make improvements to the field of intravascular brachytherapy.

References

1. Teirstein P, Massullo V, Jani S, et al. Three-year clinical and angiographic follow-up after intracoronary radiation. Circulation 2000;101:360–365.
2. Waksman R, White R, Chan R, et al. Intracoronary γ-radiation therapy after angioplasty inhibits recurrence in patients with in-stent restenosis. Circulation 2000;101: 2165–2171.
3. Popma J. START Trial, American College of Cardiology 49th Annual Scientific Session. Anaheim, CA, March 12–15, 2000.
4. Waksman R, Bhargava B, Mintz G, et al. Late total occlusion after intracoronary brachytherapy for patients with in-stent restenosis. J Am Coll Cardiol 2000;36:65–68.
5. Berglund H, Luo H, Nishioka T, et al. Highly localized arterial remodeling in patients with coronary atherosclerosis. Circulation 1997;96:1470–1476.
6. Ciezki J, Hafeli U, Song P, et al. Parenchymal cell proliferation in coronary arteries after percutaneous transluminal coronary angioplasty: A human tissue bank study. Int J Radiat Oncol Biol Phys 1999;45:963–968.
7. Scott NA, Cipola GD, Ross CE, et al. Identification of a potential role for the adventitia in vascular lesion formation after balloon overstretch injury of porcine coronary arteries. Circulation 1996;93:2178–2187.
8. Teirstein P, Massullo V, Jani S, et al. A subgroup analysis of the Scripps coronary radiation to inhibit proliferation poststenting trial. Int J Radiat Oncol Biol Phys 1998;42: 1097–1104.
9. Tripuraneni P, Leon M, Kuntz R, et al. Gamma radiation to treat in-stent restenosis: A dose response relationship. Circulation 1999;100:I–308.
10. Mazur W, Ali M, Khan M, et al. High dose rate intracoronary radiation for inhibition of neointimal formation in the stented and balloon-injured porcine models of restenosis: Angiographic, morphometric, and histopathologic analysis. Int J Radiat Oncol Biol Phys 1996;36:777–788.
11. Costa M, Sabate M, van der Giessen W, et al. Late coronary occlusion after intracoronary brachytherapy. Circulation 1999;100:789–792.
12. Hafeli U, Roberts W, Meier D, et al. Dosimetry of a W-188/Re-188 beta line source for endovascular brachytherapy. Med Phys 2000;27:668–675.
13. Kornowski R, Mintz G, Kent K, et al. Increased restenosis in diabetes mellitus after coronary interventions is due to exaggerated intimal hyperplasia: A serial intravascular ultrasound study. Circulation 1997;95:1366–1369.
14. Waksman R, Robinson KA, Crocker IR, et al. Intracoronary radiation before stent implantation inhibits neointima formation in stented porcine coronary arteries. Circulation 1995;92:1383–1386.
15. Eltchaninoff H, Koning R, Tron C, Cribier A. Immediate and 6-month results of balloon angioplasty in the treatment of intra-stent restenosis in symptomatic patients. Arch Mal Coeur Vaiss 1998;91:1459–1463.

16. Mehran R, Mintz G, Popma J, et al. Mechanisms and results of balloon angioplasty for the treatment of in-stent restenosis. Am J Cardiol 1996;78:618–622.

17. Mehran R, Mintz G, Satler L, et al. Treatment of in-stent restenosis with excimer laser coronary angioplasty: Mechanisms and results compared with PTCA alone. Circulation 1997;96:2183–2189.

18. Van Belle E, Abolmaali K, Bauters C, et al. Restenosis, late vessel occlusion and left ventricular function six months after balloon angioplasty in diabetic patients. J Am Coll Cardiol 1999;34:476–473.

19. Gordon P, Gibson C, Cohen D, et al. Mechanisms of restenosis and reduction within coronary stents–quantitative angiographic assessment. J Am Coll Cardiol 1993;21: 1166–1174.

20. Koester R, Kaehler J, Terres W, et al. Six-month clinical and angiographic outcome after successful excimer laser angioplasty for in-stent restenosis. J Am Coll Cardiol 2000; 36:69–74.

21. Lincoff A, Topol E. Platelet glycoprotein IIb/IIIa inhibition during percutaneous coronary revascularization: What more needs to be proven? Eur Heart J 2000;21:863–867.

Part X

Regulatory and Health Care
Milieu Issues

Radiation Safety Requirements for Vascular Radiotherapy in the Catheterization Laboratory

Billy G. Bass, PhD, and Shashadhar Mohapatra, PhD

Introduction

The introduction of radioisotopes in the catheterization laboratory as brachytherapy sources for the treatment of coronary artery restenosis post percutaneous transluminal coronary angioplasty (PTCA) and other revascularization techniques has also introduced new safety concerns for the cath lab personnel. Typically, radioisotope sources can produce radiation exposures many times greater than those experienced with fluoroscopy systems. Additionally, the radioisotope sources produce radiation fields that continue as long as the source is in the patient, but the fluoroscopy system only produces a field when the system is activated by the operator. The usual protective devices used by cath lab personnel are minimally effective for the radioactive sources typically used in cardiovascular brachytherapy. Federal and state regulations place severe restrictions on who is authorized to administer radioactive material to humans for either diagnostic or therapeutic purposes.[1] These regulations specify the exposure levels that are permitted for the public as well as for occupationally exposed individuals. The regulations also specify safety procedures that must be followed in the handling and administration of radioactive materials to humans.[2] The goals of this chapter are to describe the regulatory and physical concerns relative to the safety of laboratory personnel during the treatment of coronary artery restenosis with radioactive sources and the recommended techniques for reducing the risks involved in their use.

Units and Terminology

Radioactivity is the characteristic of material that undergoes spontaneous transmutation from an excited nucleus to a stable one. Radioactive material is that which has been partially transformed to the excited state by one of several methods and is undergoing transformation to nonradioactive material by emitting either particulate or radiant energy. Elements can be either naturally radioactive or made artificially radioactive by absorbing neutrons from a nuclear reactor or neutron generator (sometimes with a cyclotron or linear accelerator). Radium is

From Waksman R (ed.). *Vascular Brachytherapy, Third Edition.* Armonk, NY: Futura Publishing Co., Inc.; © 2002.

a naturally radioactive element that has been used extensively in the past for brachytherapy. Radium is a product of uranium decay and exists in large quantities in mountainous regions of the world. Cesium 137 is a radioactive element that is the product of the fission of an isotope of uranium that undergoes spontaneous fission in a nuclear reactor and is used extensively now in various brachytherapy procedures. Radium and cesium are useful because they are long-lived and are relatively inexpensive. Radium has a half-life of 1600 years and cesium has a half-life of 30 years. Half-life is the time required for a radioactive material to decay to one half of its initial quantity. Radioactivity is expressed quantitatively in terms of the number of transformations that occurs per unit time (usually seconds). The term traditionally used to specify a quantity of radioactivity is the curie, which is equivalent to the decay of one gram of radium in equilibrium with its daughter products. Quantitatively, the curie (Ci) is equal to 3.7×10^{10} transformations per second. Subunits of the curie are the thousandth of a curie (millicurie or mCi) and the millionth (microcurie or μCi). Note that the curie designates the activity of the radioactive material. It does not describe any characteristic of the radioactivity other than the decay (transformation) rate. In recent years the radiation protection communities (international and national) have adopted a new unit called the becquerel (Bq) which is defined as exactly one transformation per second. Using that nomenclature, one curie equals 3.7×10^{10} Bq. All the regulatory bodies in the U.S. still require reports to use the curie or its subunits. International regulators use the Bq, and most of the radiation safety literature uses the Bq.

Radioactive material transforms to nonradioactive material by the emission of particles or photons. The particles are predominately beta particles, which are electrons ejected from excited nuclei that are neutron rich, ie, having more neutrons than their nonradioactive counterparts. In many cases the beta emission does not get rid of enough energy for the nucleus to reach ground potential or stable condition. In these cases the nuclei also emit a gamma ray, an electromagnetic parcel of energy that behaves physically like light but is invisible due to its very short wavelength. We have all heard our favorite radio station or television station give its call letter and a frequency over which it transmits its signals. That frequency is a specification of how fast the radiant energy is oscillating as it travels through the air at the speed of light. The wavelength is the distance between crests of the wave traveling through the air. Wavelength also relates to the electromagnetic energy (also includes light) that is corpuscular in nature. That means that the energy travels as packets or parcels of oscillating electric and magnetic energy, termed photons. As a result, gamma rays are called photons. X-rays are also called photons. The basic difference between the gamma ray photons and x-ray photons is their origin. Ultraviolet rays and the light that emanates from an incandescent lamp are also photonic in nature. Beta particles are not photons, but they do possess certain wavelike qualities as they traverse various materials. This will be discussed later in the chapter. There are several other emissions from radioactive materials such as positrons, protons, and alpha particles, but they have little to no application in cardiovascular radiation therapy and will not be discussed in this chapter.

The beta particles and gamma photons are ejected from the excited nuclei with kinetic energy or energy of motion. Most people are familiar with the velocity of a bullet that is ejected from the muzzle of a rifle. That velocity is the result of the energy given to the bullet from the explosion that takes place in the firing chamber of a bullet casing when the rifle trigger is pulled. Also familiar is the energy that is imparted to a baseball or football when the pitcher or quarterback throws it toward his target. In the real world, kinetic energy is expressed in joules (or ergs). That baseball thrown at 100 miles per hour has about 490 joules (4.9 billion ergs) of kinetic energy. The particles ejected from excited nuclei have kinetic energies expressed in electron volts. An electron volt is equivalent to about 1.6×10^{-19} joules. Typically, an electron ejected from the nucleus of an excited atom will have between 15,000 and 2,000,000 electron volts of kinetic energy. Most often, that energy is expressed in kiloelectron volts (keV) or megaelectron volts (MeV). For example, phosphorus 32, a beta emitter that is used in cardiovascular brachytherapy, ejects a beta particle that has 1.7 MeV maximum kinetic energy. Gamma photon energies are also expressed in electron volts.

When beta particles and gamma photons are ejected from radioactive materials, their energies are absorbed, either in the parent material (self absorption), in air (air KERMA), or in some target material. In the case of radiation protection, that target material is defined as human tissue. In brachytherapy, that energy inhibits neointimal growth. The exact mechanism is not known, but many theories abound. The field of radiobiology is extensive and well beyond the scope of this chapter. The energy deposited in material is expressed in terms of joules per kilogram (gray [Gy]). The energy deposited in tissue is expressed in joules per kilogram but is called the sievert (Sv) and is also known as the dose equivalent to take into account the complex biological interaction that living systems exhibit with radiation absorption. In much of the literature and even the regulations, these terms will be expressed differently but equivalently. The regulatory agencies have continued to use the older units. These units are the rad and rem for dose and dose equivalent, respectively. The differences are in magnitude mainly. The rad is defined as the amount of ionizing radiation that deposits 100 ergs of energy in 1 gram of any material. The rem is defined in practice as 100 ergs deposited in tissue. A more rigorous explanation of the rem is the deposition of 100 ergs in tissue multiplied by terms called quality factors. These quality factors take into consideration the effectiveness of the radiation compared to betas and gammas in producing a particular biological effect. These quality factors are normally applied to situations where more radiosensitive organs are irradiated by highly ionizing radiations such as high-energy protons, alpha particles, and fast neutrons. This chapter is only concerned with the effects of betas and gammas, therefore, the quality factors will not be considered.

Another unit of radiation is called the exposure unit. This unit, for the past 75 years, has been called the roentgen, which was named after the discoverer of x-rays and is a measure of the ionization caused by x-rays in air. The roentgen is still used extensively because almost all of the radiation survey meters are still calibrated in the unit. At this time there are few commercial units that measure coulombs per kilogram, which is the new unit of exposure. Likewise, there are no commercial survey meters that measure grays and sieverts. These new SI units must be inferred from the older units. One gray is equal to 100 rads. One sievert is equal to 100 rems. Most radiation measurements made in the catheterization laboratory are expressed in roentgens per hour. Some of the newer fluoroscopy units are calibrated in centigrays per second (cGy/s), but these measurements represent the intensity of the primary beam and do not represent the scatter component. In this chapter, radiation exposure units will be expressed as roentgens per hour (or milliroentgens per hour, mR/h).

Radiation Environment in the Catheterization Laboratory

In the U.S., the average person is exposed to about 360 mrem per year. This value is highly variable depending on geographical location, latitude, and lifestyle.[3] For example, a person living in Miami, FL, might receive about 300 mrem, while a person living in Butte, Montana, or Denver, Colorado, might receive close to 400 mrem because of the differences in radiation from uranium deposits and higher cosmic radiation at higher elevations. A person undergoing a chest x-ray might receive about 12 mrem for a two-film exposure. A person receiving a gastrointestinal exposure might receive several thousand mrems to the lower torso.[3] A person undergoing a complex cardiac catheterization or angioplasty might receive anywhere from several thousand mrem up to possibly 200,000 mrem of skin entrance exposure. A person working in the cath lab will not receive anywhere near those levels. For the patient, the exposures are to small areas of the body and the effective dose is much lower. The cath lab worker receives exposure from the scattered radiation from the patient. Typically, the exposure to the cardiologist from a modern fluoroscopy unit with no shielding around the patient might be several hundred mR per hour. These exposures vary significantly with position of the x-ray generator relative to the patient. Measurements by the authors have indicated levels of 200 mR/h at the right side of the patient for an RAO projection and 50 mR/h for an LAO projection. During a cine episode, the exposure level to that cardiologist can be as high as 800 to 1000 mR/h. Usually, the cine periods are very short (several seconds) and the total exposure will only be a fraction of that rate. The exposures to the technologist or fellow at the groin area might be about 10 mR/h for regular fluoroscopy and 50 to 100 mR/h for the cine episode. A number of investigators have reported doses to cardiac catheterization personnel.[4] These doses vary widely with location of the worker relative to the patient and are of the order of tens of millirem per case. In many cases, if the authors' experience is typical, the cardiologist can receive 500 to 600 mrem per month to the head and shoulders for a relatively busy schedule. When cardiologists and fellows adopted the appropriate shielding devices, used the fluoroscopy and cine prudently, and wore film badges correctly, the doses dropped dramatically to 50 to 100 mrem per month. Additionally, the cath lab personnel wear lead aprons and thyroid shields that provide some measure of protection from the scattered radiation. In most situations, a 0.25-mm lead equivalent apron is adequate to block over 80% of the radiation from scattered x-rays.

Radionuclides as Radiation Sources in the Catheterization Laboratory

In the authors' view, the planned use of radioisotopes as radiation sources for cardiovascular brachytherapy is expected to increase significantly in the near future. The U.S. Food and Drug Administration (FDA) has approved the use of the iridium 192 source supplied by the Cordis Company (A Johnson and Johnson Company, Miami Lakes, FL) the strontium 90/yttrium 90 source supplied by the Novoste Corporation (Norcross, GA). The recent successes in treating in-stent restenosis with radiation has generated a great deal of enthusiasm among invasive cardiologists,[5] so much so that many facilities appear to be rushing to set up radiation treatment centers in their cath labs. This enthusiasm presents the lab administrators and the radiation safety officers with a number of dilemmas in trying to support the clinical needs of the lab, while at the same time staying within the limits set by the regulations and good radiation safety practices. One example of this is that Regulation 10 CFR 35.940 is very explicit about the nature of the training a physician is required to have in order to be authorized to administer therapeutic amounts of radioactivity to humans. However, few cardiologists have this training. The radiation oncologists, who are trained in the therapeutic use of radiation and are authorized to administer radioactivity to humans, on the other hand, are not trained in the placement of the catheter-based sources in the appropriate lesion site. Additionally, neither of these professionals is qualified to perform dosimetry in the administration of the radiation. This requires certified radiation physicists. The procedure that has worked well in the authors' facility, and other facilities as well, is a collaborative effort involving four professionals. The fourth professional is the radiation safety physicist who is required to ensure compliance with appropriate safety regulations. The procedure is very expensive in terms of the human resources required. At some point in time, assuming the procedure is as effective as early results indicate, that cost will have to be allocated to the support of each of the four professionals. Another example is the time allocation between the four professionals. Typically, the cath lab cardiologists do not have a schedule per se. Patients are entered into a queue and alloted times for their angioplasties or other procedures, but those times do not always correspond to reality. Emergencies arise, such as difficulties with patients in early time slots, and determination that other forms of revascularization, ie, rotational atherectomy or laser ablation, are needed before continuing with the radiation treatment. Obviously, the oncologist, physicist, and radiation safety physicist cannot be idle while waiting for the cardiologist to finish the patient preparation. This was the case in many of the early trials at the Washington Hospital Center, and it created some difficult scheduling concerns. Eventually, better coordination through the efforts of the cath lab research nurse coordinators allowed the support groups to wait until the cardiologist had almost finished the patient preparation before going to the cath lab. This policy has worked quite well at the Washington Hospital Center in over 1200 treatments in patient trials. A better sense of cooperation has developed between the individuals involved and, in the authors' view, the patients have benefited as well. The wait time for the physicists and oncologists is about 15 minutes. This spirit of cooperation and collaboration will need to be adopted by any organization that becomes involved in the radiation treatment of cardiovascular radiotherapy in order for the method to evolve into an efficient and cost-effective treatment modality.

Beta Particle Cardiovascular Brachytherapy

Beta particles are free electrons that have been released in nuclear transitions and ejected from the nucleus of a radioactive material. High-energy betas can travel several meters in air but they penetrate through only a small thickness of solid materials. Typically, this thickness may be a few millimeters of soft tissue. Therefore, beta particles present special problems in their detection and measurement especially when they originate inside the body and a detector is located outside. The ranges of beta particles in different elements are different. There is an empirical formula that relates the range in water or soft tissue and the energy of beta particles. In water or soft tissue, this range is approximately 1 centimeter per 2 MeV of energy. For phosphorus 32, the maximum beta particle range is about 0.8 cm in water.

The radiation hazard from beta emitters is minimal as far as whole body exposure is concerned. Care must be exercised in handling of high-energy beta emitters, but the exposure is mostly to the hands (fingers). Film badges are not very useful for monitoring exposure from beta emitters. Thermoluminescent dosimeters (TLD) are usually inserted into plastic rings and the radiation worker wears these rings. These TLDs are usually given to the physicists and oncologist. The finger dosimeter for the oncologist can be omitted if the frequency of use does not exceed 2 or 3 times a week. For a facility that performs 5 to 10 treatments a week or more, the finger badge is a recommended practice. Beta particles interact with material to form electromagnetic photons called Bremsstrahlung radiation ("braking radiation"). Bremsstrahlung is like x-rays and is just as penetrating. Bremsstrahlung is produced most efficiently if the target material is very dense, like stainless steel, titanium, or lead. Beta emitters that are encapsulated in metal sheaths must also be treated as x-ray sources. The exposure levels at 1 foot from a catheter containing 60 mCi (2.2 GBq) of strontium 90/yttrium 90 is about 14 R/h. At 1 meter, this exposure is 480 mR/h. About two thirds of this exposure comes from the Bremsstrahlung and a third comes from the betas.

Beta particle brachytherapy has two basic modalities: permanent implants (low dose rate) and catheter-delivered (high dose rate) high-intensity sources for short time delivery of radiation energy. The permanent implants are cardiovascular stents that have had beta-emitting atoms implanted on the stent surface. The stent is implanted in the coronary artery at the lesion site and the radioactive atoms emit the betas that are absorbed by the neointimal tissue (and probably the adventitia as well) directly adjacent to the stent. Because of the limited range of the beta particle in tissue, only those tissues about 1 or 2 mm from the stent surface receive the major portion of the energy that is released. The radionuclide implanted on the stent surface is a short-lived nuclide such as phosphorus 32. The radiation dose is delivered over a period amounting to 6 or 7 half-lives of the radionuclide. As of this June 2001, phophorus 32-impregnated stents have received FDA approval to be used in clinical trials and implanted in patients. The stents contained about 0.75 microcurie (28 kBq) of radioactivity. The time required to deliver the desired dose (15 Gy or 1500 rads) is about 100 days.

The catheter-delivered high dose rate (HDR) high-intensity sources contain about 60 mCi (2.2 GBq) of high-energy beta radioactivity. The most advanced system in present clinical trials utilizes a strontium 90/yttrium 90 source to deliver the desired dose to the lesion area in 3 to 5 minutes.[6] The source contains strontium 90, but the strontium decays with the emission of a moderate energy beta (0.60 MeV) to yttrium 90, which decays with the emission of a high-energy (2.27 MeV) beta. The beta sources are contained in a transfer device that shields the user from the beta energy, but when the source train is moved from the transfer device into the catheter and to the treatment site, the operators (cardiologist, radiation oncologist, and physicists) may receive a low exposure during the transit. The level of exposure depends on the time the seeds are in transit. Under normal conditions, this time is a matter of fractions of a second. In several cases, the source string does not get into the patient. It gets stuck somewhere along the catheter between the delivery device and the patient entry point (femoral artery at groin area), exposing the operators with about 400 mR/h exposure rate. When the source is in the patient, the exposure to operators is negligible (a few mR/h at the patient's chest).

In summary, the radiation safety problems involved with beta-particle–emitting sources are readily solved with conventional health physics principles. The regulatory conditions can be met easily with appropriate operational constraints (as addressed later in this chapter).

Gamma Ray Cardiovascular Brachytherapy

There are several gamma ray sources that have been demonstrated as effective methods for delivering restenosis-inhibiting doses to the coronary arteries.[7,8] As of this writing, the most popular source in clinical trials is iridium 192. This radionuclide is contained in an enclosed catheter as seeds or as contiguous wire at the distal tip of the catheter, which is inserted via the catheter system to the lesion site. Iridium 192 emits a number of medium-energy gamma rays (0.296, 0.308, 0.317, 0.468, 0.589, 0.604, and 0.612 MeV).[9] Typically, one assumes the average energy to be 360 keV. This energy is about nine times the typical fluoroscopy x-ray energy (80 to 100 KVp). The x-rays are emitted as a spectrum of energies with the average being only about 40% of the maximum, whereas gamma rays are emitted with discrete characteristic energies which makes protective equipment designed for x-rays less effective against the gammas. For example, the "lightweight" lead aprons used in cardiac cath labs have 0.25- to 0.5-mm lead equivalent thickness in the material. This thickness of lead will absorb 80 to 85% of the typical fluoroscopic x-rays (personal measurement), while the same lead apron will absorb less than 10% of the gamma rays from iridium 192 (personal measurement). Another consideration is that x-rays are produced only when the fluoroscopy button or pedal is pushed, but gamma rays are emitted continuously from the source. The only way to reduce the gamma ray flux is to keep the source in a container (called a "pig") shielded with a dense material such as lead until it is ready to be inserted into the patient. As of June 2001, the method of source insertion of choice is by manually pushing the wire through the catheter until it is in position as verified by fluoroscopy. Several newer delivery devices have been evaluated at the Washington Hospital Center (a hand-cranked friction insertion device and a computer-controlled afterloader-type device), but the most reliable and easiest to operate is the more primitive hand insertion. The manual method does have problems, such as the crimping of the wire after a number of operations. We expect that the eventual device of choice will be a motor-driven friction mechanism that will minimize this crimping. We do not expect the radiation safety concerns to be affected by the more elaborate and sophisticated devices.

Radiation Safety Considerations

Safety considerations in the use of gamma-emitting brachytherapy sources are many and varied. The source intensities that are now in use produce exposure rates in the 400 to 1000 mR/h range at the side of the patient. Even at 1 meter from the patient, the exposure rates are 60 to 200 mR/h.[10] In earlier trials, source lengths of 6, 10, and 14 seeds were common. More recently, source lengths of 17, 19, and 23 seeds are being used. With an activity of 30 mCi per seed, the total activities of the longer source ribbons are 510, 570, and 690 mCi, respectively. The magnitude of the exposure rates varies with the location of the lesion and the size of the patient. Figure 1 shows the distribution of exposure around the patient for a 350-mCi activity in the right heart. Figure 2 shows the scatter radiation around the patient for a 362-mCi activity in the mid heart. Figure 3 shows the scatter around the patient for a 382-mCi activity in the left heart.[9]

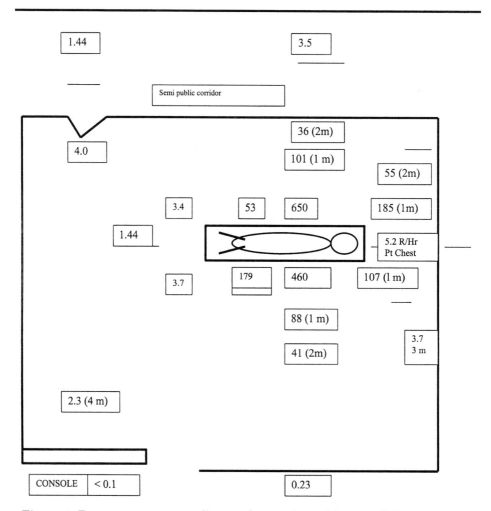

Figure 1. Exposure rates versus distance from patient with 350 mCi in right heart.

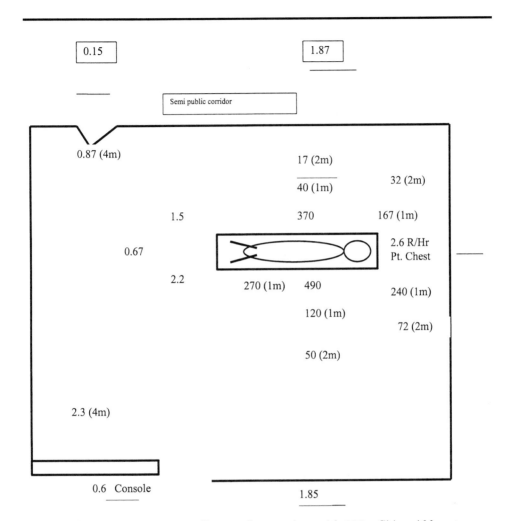

Figure 2. Exposure rates versus distance from patient with 362 mCi in mid heart.

The variation in the exposure levels with distance is due to the attenuation by the patient as well as that of the monitors and other equipment in the lab. The exposure rates are useful for evaluating the hazards to personnel who must go into the lab during the treatment, but a better way of looking at the radiation risks might be to plot the exposure per treatment. This is presented in Figures 4 and 5 for two different sources.

Another radiation concern involving the gamma sources is the exposure to personnel on the floors above and below the cath lab. This exposure is difficult to estimate using calculations alone. One of the problems is the unkown attenuation of the gamma rays by the patient. Measurements at the Washington Hospital Center have provided some insight into the problem. For several treatments, the exposure rates at 1 meter from either side and above the chest of the patient were made. Immediately after the treatment, the exposure rates at 1 meter from the bare source

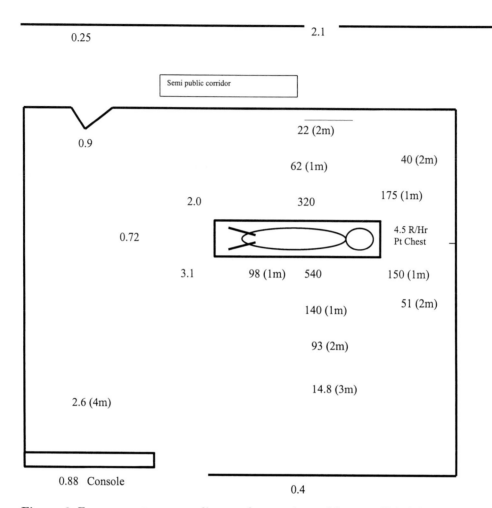

Figure 3. Exposure rates versus distance from patient with 382 mCi in left heart.

were made. The results of the measurements are shown in Table 1. One can see that the attenuation by the patient of the ^{192}Ir gamma rays can be substantial (>50%) in the lateral direction. This is explainable by the fact that the arms and shoulders present a greater distance through which the gamma rays pass. For the vertical direction, the attenuation is approximately 20%. This is again highly variable due to the different treatment locations and the thickness of the patient.

In Table 2, we tabulate the exposure levels to a person on the floor above or below the cath lab. Calculations were made from actual measurements at 1 meter above the patient with varying source strengths and applying the inverse square principle along with the attenuation characteristics of concrete. Measurements were made with a recently calibrated Victoreen 450 Ion Chamber Survey Meter. We kept the measurements in mR/h since that was how the instrument was calibrated. Rather than converting to the international units the traditional units are presented since the reader can readily convert the readings by multiplying by 100 to get mSv. The assumption is made that the conversion from air ex-

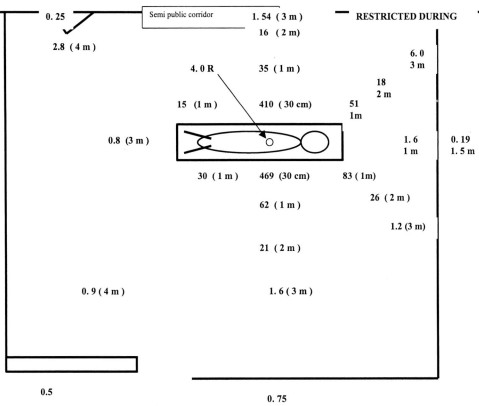

Figure 4. Exposure per treatment. Activity of 612.3 mCi, 23 seeds, treatment time, 18.5 minutes.

posure units to tissue dose is unity, which is a reasonable assumption for shielding comparisons. The assumption was made that the vertical distance from the patient to a person's waist in the room above or below the lab was 3.4 meters. This distance was measured at the Washington Hospital Center and may be different for other hospitals. Again, this measurement is adequate for evaluating the shielding capabilities of a floor.

In Table 2, we also tabulated the dose per treatment to a hypothetical person on the floor above the lab. This presents an index of allowable cases per week (or year) for the facility. In the Code of Federal Regulations, Title 10, Part 20, 1301 (a), the dose limit to a member of the public is specified. In this regulation, the limit for a member of the public is 1 mSv (100 mrem) per year. From Table 2, one can see that, using a very low-activity source (~ 230 mCi), a facility with a 6-inch concrete floor can safely perform nearly 300 procedures a year. However, if a 560-mCi source is used, only about half that number would be permitted by regulation. Note that thicker floors will allow more procedures. Recently, the authors learned that some newer hospitals are using a construction technique called the "waffle slab floor."[11] This structure contains only 3 inches of concrete and an 18-gauge steel sheet. Looking at Table 2, one can see that

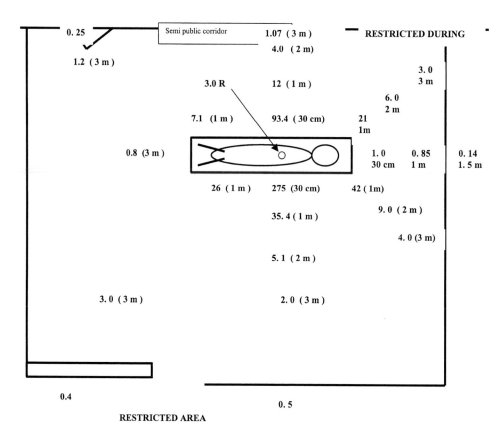

Figure 5. Exposure per treatment. Activity of 339 mCi, 10 seeds, treatment time, 17 minutes.

only two procedures a week could be performed using the low-activity sources. With the larger sources only one procedure per week would be allowable. Of course, this limitation assumes that the floor above is occupied and the occupancy factor would be 1. If the space above were unoccupied, for the most part, the occupancy factor could be one fourth, thereby increasing the allowable cases by a factor of 4.

Laboratory Personnel Exposures

Laboratory personnel could be subject to excess exposures from the high-intensity sources used for cardiovascular brachytherapy. Several mechanisms can be used to minimize these radiation exposures. These are the three basic principles in radiation protection. The first is distance. One can see from Figures 1 to 3 that the exposure rate from a patient undergoing radiation treatment decreases rapidly as you get farther away from the patient. The principle can also be understood by invoking the inverse square attenuation of radiant energy from a

Table 1

Measured Exposures with Source In-Patient Versus In-air Exposures at 1 Meter

Source Activity		Source in Patient	Source in Air	Calculated Exposure @ 1 m
(mCi)	(GBq)			
316	11.69	Over chest 141	154	152
		Left lat. 74	230	
322	11.9	Left lat. 76	190	154
		Right lat. 61	190	
		Diag. 100	190	
232	8.58	Over chest 127	164	111
		Left lat. 44	164	
		Right lat. 47	164	
350	12.95	Over chest 185	196	168
		Left lat. 57	180	
		Right lat. 83	180	
		Left diag. 110	180	
		Right diag. 126	180	
363	13.32	Left lat. 92	160	174
		Right lat. 67	160	
		Over chest 191	220	
394	14.6	Left lat. 102	220	189
		Right lat. 65	220	
		Diag. 174	220	
441	16.3	Over chest 199	250	207
		Left lat. 70	220	
		Right lat. 101	220	
563	20.7	Over chest 250	270	270
		Left lat. 91	260	
		Right lat. 113	260	
		Right diag. 150	260	

Measurements are in mR/h.

point source. To this end, cath lab procedures require personnel to vacate the lab during the treatment time. Only the radiation safety personnel are permitted in the lab to make measurements unless an emergency arises. The safety personnel wear double-thick lead aprons and are instructed to make measurements without receiving excess exposure. The one exception to this is one of the authors (BGB), who has made extensive exposure measurements over the past 3 years. During that time, over 1200 patients have been treated at the Washington Hospital Center, and the author has been involved in 98% of them. The author has accumulated a total whole body radiation dose of about 2000 mrem, or just under 2 mrem per procedure.

The second mechanism is time. The less time spent in the radiation field, the lower the dose received. Procedurally, this involves restricting the time the cardiologist and oncologist can stay close to the patient. On occasion, the need arises for adjustments of intravenous medication for the patient during the

Table 2

Shielding in Cardiovascular Brachytherapy

Source Activity		Exposure Rate @ 1 m Above Chest	Concrete Thickness (cm)	Exposure/ Treatment (mrem)
(mCi)	(GBq)			
232	8.58	127	7.6	1.03
			15.0	0.37
			20.3	0.17
			25.4	0.09
			30.0	0.03
350	12.95	185	7.6	1.5
			15.0	0.53
			20.3	0.24
			25.4	0.13
394	14.6	191	7.6	1.54
			15.0	0.55
			20.3	0.25
			25.4	0.13
441	16.3	199	7.6	1.6
			15.0	0.57
			20.3	0.26
			25.4	0.14
563	20.7	250	7.6	2.02
			15.0	0.7
			20.3	0.32
			25.4	0.17

treatment. This can be done under the supervision of the radiation safety person so that the staff person making the adjustment can be monitored and the stay can be minimized. Sometimes an emergency situation arises that requires the cardiologist's immediate attention. Again, the radiation safety person must be on hand to monitor the exposure levels at the patient's side where the cardiologist is required to be. In the event that the emergency will require more time than the radiation safety person feels is prudent, the treatment can be aborted or temporarily stopped until the emergency is evaluated. The source is removed from the patient and stored in the transfer device. If the emergency is treated successfully, the cardiologist and oncologist can determine if the treatment can be resumed.

The third mechanism for reduction of dose is shielding. Shielding is simply the placement of dense material (lead primarily) between the source and the operating personnel. Portable shields are available in different sizes and thicknesses. The primary problem with these portable shields, in the authors' opinion, is that they interfere with the placement of monitoring equipment (or, perhaps, it is the other way around—the monitoring equipment restricts the effective placement of the shields). To be maximally effective, the shields should be placed as close to the patient as possible. Unfortunately, the bulkiness of the shields presently available precludes them from being placed closer than about 1 meter from the patient. Most available shields are designed for cesium 137 and radium 226 and are about 2.5 cm thick. Iridium 192 gamma rays can be effectively reduced using 12- to 15-mm thick lead. This reduced thickness significantly reduces ($\sim \times \frac{1}{2}$) the weight and bulkiness of the shield, making it much easier to maneuver in the cath lab.

In an attempt to characterize the exposures of cath lab personnel to ionizing radiation, we have tabulated the film badge results for the 18 months (from June 2000) of all of the laboratory personnel who have been involved in the cardiovascular brachytherapy program. Of course, these persons have also been active in fluororadiography, which has contributed a substantial exposure to them. The attempt was to examine the exposures from brachytherapy in addition to the fluororadiograpy exposures. Table 3 lists the principal persons involved with brachytherapy as well as fluororadiography.

Eight cardiologists at the Washington Hospital Center have actively participated in the brachytherapy program. Only four radiation oncologists have participated along with twenty technologists, eleven nurses, two medical physicists, and two radiation safety persons. During this period, about 800 cardiovascular brachytherapy cases were performed. With the exceptions of the medical physicists and radiation physicists, there were no significant exposures to the lab personnel from the gamma radiation compared to the x-ray exposures. In the cases of the physicists, the exposures were almost totally from the gammas. The medical physicists received their exposures from handling the sources during calibration and transporting them to the labs for treatments. The radiation safety physicists received their exposures from frequent monitoring of exposure levels around the patient during the treatments. The exposures of the cardiologists and oncologists from brachytherapy treatments can be estimated by considering the average times spent near the patient and the average exposure rates as measured during the treatments. The average exposure per treatment at the cardiologist's typical

Table 3

Catheterization Laboratory Personnel Exposures

Personnel	Participation in Brachytherapy	
	Yes	No
Cardiologist	766 mrem (8) (120–2280)	569 mrem (30) (10–3340)
Radiation oncologists	92 mrem (4) (25–162)	
Technologists	202 mrem (20) (10 –1140)	412 mrem (6) (20–510)
Nurses	91 mrem (11) (10–520)	218 mrem (11) (10–540)
Medical physicists	615 mrem (2) 242–988	
Radiation safety staff	888 mrem (2) 81–1695	

location is 8 mrem. The average time the cardiologist spent at this location (based on the authors' measurements) is less than 3 minutes. This gives an exposure of less than 1.0 mrem per patient. For an average of 200 patients per year per cardiologist/oncologist, the expected exposure is no greater than 200 mrem per year. This level is consistent with the film badge records for the oncologists. The cardiologists, on the other hand, receive 700 to 800 mrem from fluororadiography for that number of patients. These measured and calculated exposures compare favorably with those of Balter et al.[12]

Federal and state regulations require facilities to limit public exposures to ionizing radiation to less than 1 mSv (100 mrem) per year. This means that exposure to both x-rays and gamma rays from the combined brachytherapy procedures must be less than 100 mrem per year. To evaluate exposures to the public, TLD monitors were installed outside the four cath labs that were used at the Washington Cardiology Center for the brachytherapy trials. These monitors have been in place for more than 3 years, since the center has been active in the brachytherapy programs. The monitors are replaced monthly and sent to the dosimetry contractor for reading. The exposures outside the cath labs for the 3-year monitoring period are shown in Table 4. During this monitoring period, more than 1200 patients were treated. As is apparent from the table, the exposures to public areas are well below the regulatory limits. It should also be noted that the Washington Hospital Center has a very active interventional cardiology practice, in addition to an extraordinary endovascular brachytherapy workload. The workload is about 400 cases a year over the past 2 and one half years, with about a 50 mrem per year dose to public areas for fluoroscopy and gamma brachytherapy combined.

Conclusions

Early concerns about radiation safety in cardiovascular brachytherapy have abated with recent experience. By exercising reasonable radiation safety precautions, the radiation exposures to operating personnel have been held to acceptable levels. Some of these precautions are listed below and represent what the authors believe to be the minimum operational measures that will ensure safe treatment of coronary artery in-stent restenosis.

- As long as the source is in the transport cask ("pig"), activities can be carried on as usual.

Table 4

Radiation Exposures to Public Areas Surrounding Brachytherapy Operations (mrem)

Monitor	1998	1999	2000	Total (~3 yrs)
1	40	53	12	105
2	40	65	34	139
3	30	64	28	132
4	40	53	12	105

- When the source has been inserted into the patient, all cath lab personnel must leave the treatment area and retire to the console area or to an area designated by the radiation safety officer as safe until the source has been transferred back into the pig.
- If an emergency arises, the radiation safety person will indicate the areas where patient care personnel can safely work. If the emergency appears to be a prolonged condition, the treatment may be aborted. If the cardiologist and oncologist agree to restart the treatment after the emergency condition has been taken care of satisfactorily, the treatment personnel will again vacate the lab and the source will be inserted into the patient for a time determined by the physicist and oncologist.
- When a treatment must be altered, such as adjustment of intravenous fluids, the person (nurse, technologist, or physicist) making the adjustment should approach the patient from the foot of the bed. The exposure levels are lowest in the direction of the feet and head of the patient. If the caregiver must get close to the patient, the time period must be short (<5 min) and under the supervision of the radiation safety person who will monitor the exposure levels during the incursion. The preferred side of the patient to be approached is the right side. This is the side normally occupied by the cardiologist and oncologist during the source insertion and it is the side having the most shielding devices. It **must** be remembered that the x-ray shields and the leaded aprons normally used for x-ray work have limited usefulness for the gamma radiation. These devices together only reduce the exposure levels by about 50%. The best safeguards are distance and time. Personnel should as far away from the patient as practical and spend as little time as possible to accomplish the caregiving activity.
- The radiation safety person will monitor the hallways and public access areas to ensure compliance with regulations, and will advise caregivers about access to the lab during treatments.

References

1. Title 10, Code of Federal Regulations, Part 20, 1997.
2. Title 10, Code of Federal Regulations, Part 35, 1991.
3. National Council on Radiation Protection and Measurements, Report No. 93, 1987.
4. Johnson LW, Moore RJ, Balter S. Review of radiation safety in the cardiac catheterization laboratory. Cathet Cardiovasc Diagn 1992;25:186–194.
5. Teirstein P, et al. Catheter-based radiotherapy to inhibit restenosis after coronary stenting. N Engl J Med 1997;336:1697–1703.
6. Hilstead RA, Weldon TD. Novoste® Intracoronary radiation system: A novel approach to preventing restenosis. In: Waksman R, King SB, Crocker IR, Mould RF (eds.): Vascular Brachytherapy. Veenendaal, The Netherlands: Nucletron BV; 1996:309–317.
7. Waksman R, et al. Intracoronary low dose irradiation inhibits neointima formation after coronary artery balloon injury in swine: A possible role for radiation therapy in restenosis prevention. Circulation 1995;91:1533–1539.
8. Waksman R, King SB, Crocker IR, Mould RF (eds.): Vascular Brachytherapy. Veenendaal, The Netherlands: Nucletron; 1996.
9. Nath R, Anderson, L, Luxton G, et al. Dosimetry of interstitial brachytherapy sources: Recommendations of the AAPM Radiation Therapy Task Group No. 43. Med Phys 1995; 22:209–234.

858 · *Vascular Brachytherapy*

10. Bass BG. Radiation safety requirements for vascular radiotherapy in the catheterization laboratory. In: Waksman R (ed.): Vascular Brahytherapy. Armonk, NY: Futura Publishing Co.; 1999:581–592.
11. Rickert K. Personal communication, Rickert Engineering.
12. Balter S, Oetgen M, Hill A, et al. Personnel exposure during gamma endovascular brachytherapy. Health Phys 2000;79:136–146.

Risks Associated with Exposure to Low Levels of Ionizing Radiation

Shirish K. Jani, PhD

Introduction

During vascular brachytherapy, a linear source is placed within the lumen at the sight of restenosis to deliver a therapeutic dose to the arterial wall. Radiation sources may be sealed sources or in liquid form, and may emit either gamma rays, x-rays, or beta particles.[1] Like most other brachytherapy procedures, vascular brachytherapy delivers a highly focal dose to tissues while sparing the rest of the patient's body from high levels of radiation. For gamma-emitting isotopes, the radiation levels in and around the procedure room may be significant and radiation safety precautions are required.[2,3] In general, the dose received by staff and the patient's body (other than the treatment site) during a vascular brachytherapy procedure is small compared with many diagnostic x-ray procedures. In this chapter, we discuss the risks to staff associated with exposure to very low levels of ionizing radiation. The risks to patients are generally compared to the direct benefit they derive from the therapy, and this issue is not discussed here.

The risks associated with exposure to low levels of ionizing radiation have been extensively studied and widely reported in the literature. The serious radiation-induced effects fall into two general categories: stochastic effects and somatic effects. These are both late effects of radiation.

Stochastic Effects

At low-level radiation, most of the exposed cells survive but some may be damaged and retain the legacy of radiation exposure. A damaged cell is changed in some way, and this change is passed on to the cell's offspring. When the radiation exposure damages a germ (reproductive) cell, the result may be a genetic mutation and expressed in future generation. If the cell damaged is a somatic (other than germ) cell, the consequence may be leukemia or cancer in the exposed individual. These two effects, genetic and carcinogenic, are late effects and are called stochastic. The stochastic effects are random and are considered the principal late effects that occur at low doses of radiation. A stochastic effect is statistical in nature and exhibits no threshold in dose. Its probability of occurrence, not severity, increases as the dose increases. A stochastic effect such as cancer is an all-or-none

From Waksman R (ed.). *Vascular Brachytherapy, Third Edition.* Armonk, NY: Futura Publishing Co., Inc.; © 2002.

response. The risk to an individual from stochastic effects depends on factors such as age, sex, etc. The stochastic effects are hard to distinguish from other effects. For example, a cancer resulting from an exposure to radiation is similar in all characteristics to that arising from other (natural) sources. Therefore, one can examine the magnitude of stochastic effects only by conducting large epidemiological studies on exposed and unexposed population. In any case, the stochastic effects are considered the principal late effects of low-level ionizing radiation. The probability of the associated risk is assumed to accumulate linearly with dose throughout the life span of an individual.

Deterministic Effects

A nonstochastic effect of radiation is a deterministic effect (somatic effect) where the severity of the effect increases with increased dose. Examples of deterministic effects are cataracts (lens opacification), organ atrophy, and fibrosis. These effects occur at relatively large doses and exhibit a threshold dose below which the probability of occurrence is almost zero. Early somatic effects are erythema and other skin damage and may occur in hours or days after exposure depending upon the exposure level. Late effects such as cataracts may occur years after the radiation exposure. Like stochastic effects, the probability of a deterministic effect and its associated risk increases with cumulative dose, but clearly shows threshold in dose.

Radiation Carcinogenesis

Radiation-induced cancer, even in populations exposed to relatively large doses, is a rare event. Nonetheless, it is the most important stochastic effect of low-level ionizing radiation. This subject has been studied extensively and conclusions are based on experience in humans rather than on animal data. There is a long history of a link between radiation exposure and an elevated incidence of cancer. Marie Curie and her daughter are thought to have died from leukemia as a result of the exposure to radiation from their experiments on isolating radium.[4] Skin cancer was common among x-ray workers before present-day radiation safety guidelines were implemented. Lung cancer was frequent among uranium miners who were exposed to intense alpha-particle radiation from radon gas and its daughter products. Bone tumors were observed in the radium dial painters who ingested radium that deposited on the growing bones and exposed them to alpha-particle radiation.

Carcinogenic effects of low levels of ionizing radiation were studied extensively by the Committee on the Biological Effects of Ionizing Radiation (BEIR) appointed by the National Research Council of the United States. The Committee's Report, BEIR V, outlines in detail the carcinogenic effects of radiation for various body organs.[5] The following paragraphs describe select cancers and their association with low-level ionizing radiation.

Leukemia

The induction of leukemia by ionizing radiation has been well documented in humans. Acute and myeloid leukemia are the types chiefly effected. The incidence of chronic lymphocytic leukemia does not appear to be affected by radiation. The most extensive human data on the dose-incidence relationship come from studies of the Japanese atomic bomb survivors and patients treated with x-rays for ankylosing spondylitis. Susceptibility to acute lymphatic leukemia seems to be higher for those exposed at a young age (<20 years) compared with those exposed at older ages. Increased death rate is estimated to be $15–25/10^6$/rem. Leukemia has the shortest latent period among all cancers. Excess leukemia began to appear in the survivors of Hiroshima and Nagasaki a few years after the radiation exposure, reached a peak at 7 to 12 years, and essentially disappeared by 20 years. By contrast, solid tumors show a mean latency of approximately 25 years. According to the United Nations Scientific Committee on the Effects of Atomic Radiation (UNSCEAR) report of 1988, the minimum latent period for the lifetime projection (ie, the beginning of the integration period for risk) was 10 years for most cancers, except leukemia (2 years) and thyroid cancer (5 years).[6] The risk of leukemia from radiation exposure seems to be higher for males than for females.

Breast Cancer

The sensitivity of the mammary gland to the carcinogenic effects of ionizing radiation has been well documented. The growth, development, and function of the normal mammary gland are dependent upon hormonal regulation. The data in humans lead to the conclusion that initiation of radiation-induced cancer is critically dependent upon the hormonal status of the cells over time. Conditions such as early and multiple pregnancies induce functional mammary differentiation, and hence, reduce the risk of breast cancer. Radiation-induced breast cancers are similar, in age distribution and histopathological types, to breast cancers resulting from other causes. Data show that induction of cancer does not depend on whether a single large dose is delivered or multiple small doses are received by the mammary gland. Age at exposure strongly influences susceptibility. Women who are irradiated at less than 20 years of age are at a higher relative risk for breast cancer than those who are irradiated later in life. Radiation-induced breast cancer does not seem to appear during the first 10 years following exposure. After this time, however, the incidence increases rapidly, reaching a peak at 15 to 20 years following exposure, and mortality approximately 5 years later. Increased death rate from radiation-induced breast cancer is estimated to be approximately $25/10^6$/rem.

Lung Cancer

Risks of radiation-induced lung cancer are similar for both sexes although baseline cancer risks are much higher for males than they are for females. Therefore, the excess relative risk for females is higher than for males. Age at the time for exposure does not influence the rate of induced cancer. Among women treated with radiotherapy for cancer of uterine cervix, the relative risk of lung cancer was observed to be increased.[7] The stray radiation dose from cervical radiotherapy was estimated to be approximately 35 cGy. There is a long list of carcinogens for lung cancer, including cigarette smoking, asbestos, chromium salts, radiation, and others. Therefore, isolating the carcinogenic effect of radiation, even among workers of uranium mines, is very difficult. Estimated risk for fatal lung cancer is approximately $20/10^6$/rem.

Thyroid Cancer

The thyroid gland is highly sensitive to radiation carcinogenesis. Cancer of the thyroid gland is well established as a late consequence of exposure to ionizing radiation from both external and internal sources. However, the malignant tumors of thyroid induced by radiation are well differentiated in their histology and they develop slowly. These tumors can be treated successfully with either surgery or radioactive ^{131}I therapy. Therefore, even though the incidence of radiation-induced cancer is high ($\sim$100/10^6/rem), the corresponding mortality rate is very low ($\sim$5/10^6/rem). Females are approximately three times more susceptible to radiation-induced cancer than males. However, the same is true for spontaneous thyroid cancer. Therefore, the relative risk estimates do not differ significantly by sex. Children are at greater risk for radiation-induced thyroid cancer than adults. It is estimated that this risk among children (<5 years of age) may be more than twice the risk among adults.

Radiation Mutagenesis

Genetic effects of radiation have been studied almost entirely through animal experimentation. The only human data with some significance were derived from following the offspring of the Japanese atomic bomb survivors. In this population, the average parental dose was 40 rem, delivered acutely from the neutron and gamma radiation spectrum of the bombs. No statistically significant increase in hereditary disease was detected in the first generation offspring of these survivors.[8]

Genetic mutations (ie, alterations) in humans occur from a variety of sources including natural background radiation. The fact that mutations produced by man-made radiation are similar in characteristics to the natural spontaneous mutations renders the study of them particularly difficult. We do know with reasonable certainty that radiation does not produce new, unique mutations but increases the incidence of the same mutations that occur spontaneously. It is estimated that a small fraction (<5%) of spontaneous mutations in humans may be a result of background radiation that is with us for many generations.

The natural or spontaneous incidence of diseases with a genetic component was estimated at 10% by the BEIR III report.[9] In other words, of every 1 million live-born human offspring, $\sim$107,000 would carry a spontaneous mutation of some sort, the majority of them from unrecognized sources. The BEIR V report has revised this estimate upward and included other disorders such as heart disease and cancer.[10] The genetic effect resulting from parental exposure of 1 rem dose-equivalent is 85 to 160 additional cases per 1 million live-born offspring.[11] In other words, the parental irradiation at 1 rem per 30-year generation results in 85 to 160 additional genetic disorders per million live-born children (first generation) as compared to a very large number of naturally occurring genetic defects.

It is important to emphasize that virtually all mutations have harmful effects. Some mutations have drastic effects that are expressed immediately, but then are not passed on to generations that follow. Other mutations have milder effects and persist for many generations. Since these long-term effects spanning many generations are hard to understand and estimate, the approach most commonly taken in radiation mutagenesis is to focus on and emphasize the effects on the first generation. At a chronic exposure of low levels of ionizing radiation (which is most common among occupationally exposed individuals), the genetic disorders are far fewer than those quoted for an acute exposure.

Radiation Teratogenesis

The developing embryo and fetus are very sensitive to radiation and even moderate doses can produce catastrophic effects. These effects depend on the stage of gestation, the amount of dose, and how fast it is delivered. Human gestation is divided into three stages: pre-implantation (0 to 9 days), organogenesis (~10 to 40 days), and fetal period (~6 weeks to birth). The main radiation-induced effects on the developing embryo and fetus are: (1) growth retardation; (2) embryonic or fetal death; and (3) congenital malformation.

Growth retardation is not observed when radiation exposure occurs during the pre-implantation phase. Exposure during early organogenesis may lead to temporary growth retardation. Irradiation during the fetal period leads to the greatest degree of permanent damage. The most frequently cited manifestation of growth retardation from radiation during gestation is microcephaly (abnormal smallness of the head).[12] This can occur at an air dose of 10 to 20 cGy. The principal effect of radiation during the pre-implantation phase is embryonic death. The radiation-induced death during organogenesis occurs at higher doses compared to the pre-implantation phase.

Radiation teratogenesis, or gross malformation, occurs most frequently when the fetus is irradiated during organogenesis. The most common malformation in humans is within the central nervous system. The best-documented central nervous system abnormality is mental retardation. Severe mental retardation is most radiosensitive at 8 to 15 weeks after conception and shows a linear relationship with dose. No threshold in dose is observed. Radiation-induced mental retardation has characteristics of both a stochastic and a deterministic effect. As discussed earlier in this chapter, a stochastic effect has no dose-threshold, and hence, mental retardation is a stochastic effect. On the other hand, the severity of mental retardation seems to depend upon the dose.[13,14] Thus, it also has characteristics of other deterministic effects. The dose required to render a normal person mentally retarded may be large, but an individual with a low IQ may be made retarded by a relatively small dose.

According to the BEIR V report, the risk of cancer in childhood following exposure in utero is approximately 200 to 250 excess cancer deaths/10^6/rem in the first 10 years of life. Approximately half of these malignancies are leukemia. Cancer in adults seems to be associated with radiation in utero, but its magnitude remains uncertain.

Risks associated with low levels of ionizing radiation to humans seem to be the most significant during gestation period. Therefore, the maximum permissible dose to the fetus (and thus, to a pregnant radiation worker) in the U.S. is kept at 50 mR/month during the entire gestation period.[15]

Assessment of Radiation Risk

Estimating the risk associated with low levels of ionizing radiation is a very complex issue. The availability of limited human data with many variables makes the risk estimates difficult and uncertain. For a population, a risk estimate is usually expressed as an absolute risk, which is the excess risk from radiation. It is the difference between the cancer risk in the exposed population and the corresponding risk in the unexposed (control) population. This excess risk, though small, continues to exist for a long time, typically 20 to 30 years. An absolute total risk to a *population* is expressed as: R = number of cases per 1 million exposed persons per rem.

For example, consider a population of 1 million people exposed uniformly to 1 rem of radiation and found to have an incidence of 1000 cases of certain cancer during a 20-year period after the exposure. A similar population over the same time period shows 990 cases of the same cancer without any radiation exposure. The excess risk is then calculated to be $10/10^6$/rem for that type of cancer.

The most reliable risk estimates for radiation-induced cancer relate to leukemia, thyroid, and breast cancer. Even for these frequently induced cancers, the risks are very small and the uncertainties are high.

Estimating *individual* risk from radiation-induced abnormality is rather difficult. Most of our current knowledge and estimates are based on the extrapolation from certain populations exposed to large as well as small acute exposures of radiation: for example, Japanese atomic bomb survivors. On the other hand, a patient undergoing a chest x-ray or inadvertent exposure to a brachytherapy source receives radiation to part of the body. A method needs to be developed to compare these nonuniform, partial body exposures to our estimates from uniform whole body exposures. The concept of effective dose was proposed as a solution to this problem in 1975 by Jacobi.[16] The International Commission on Radiation Protection (ICRP) adopted this concept in 1977, revised it in 1991, and reported its recommendations through the ICRP Publications.[17] The ICRP procedure of computing the effective dose is now widely accepted in dealing with radiation risk and protection.[18] The effective dose is defined as that dose which, if administered uniformly to the whole body, would carry the same risk of stochastic effect as the dose actually delivered to part of the body. It is computed by summing the dose to each sensitive organ or tissue, weighted by a factor equal to the relative contribution of stochastic effect from that organ. Mathematically, the effective dose for computing an individual risk is:

$$H_E = \Sigma \ W_T \cdot H_T$$

where H_E is the effective (whole body) dose, W_T is the weighting factor specific to an organ or tissue type T, and H_T is the radiation dose to that organ. The W_T is a dimensionless factor that accounts for the differences in the biological response of different tissues to radiation. The weighting factors for various organs (as recommended by ICRP-60 and NCRP-115) are listed below:

Gonads: 0.20
Bone marrow, lung, stomach, and colon: 0.12 each
Bladder, breast, liver, esophagus, and thyroid: 0.05 each
Skin, and bone surface: 0.01 each
Remainder: 0.05
Total : 1.00

For example, consider that the breast tissues of an individual are exposed to 100 mrem of radiation, and no other body parts are exposed. The weighting factor for breast tissues is 0.05. The whole body dose equivalent will be 0.05×100 mrem = 5 mrem. The stochastic effect of 100 mrem of breast irradiation would be equivalent to that from a whole body dose of 5 mrem. The risk associated with such an exposure is extremely small. This method of calculating the whole body dose equivalent and assessing its associated risk has its own uncertainties, but in absence of ideal methods available, it serves the purpose.

Summary

Low-level ionizing radiation refers to the exposure levels encountered by the majority of radiation workers in the U.S. from diagnostic and therapeutic radiographic procedures, including brachytherapy. At these levels of protracted radiation, the adverse effects are late and very rare, and predicting their probability of occurrence is very difficult. Most of our observations and learning has come from studying a few select populations such as survivors of Japanese atomic bombs. The late effects fall into two broad categories based on their distinct nature: stochastic effects and deterministic effects. Induction of cancer due to protracted radiation is considered to be a stochastic effect. A stochastic effect shows no threshold in dose and its severity is independent of dose level. These are principal effects at very low-level radiation. Induction of cataracts due to exposure to lens of the eye is considered to be a deterministic effect. For such an effect, the severity of the condition depends upon the amount of radiation dose. The deterministic effects show a dose threshold below which the probability of occurrence of that particular effect is close to zero.

Radiation carcinogenesis (induction of cancer) is very extensively studied and reported. Some of the more frequent cancers caused by radiation are leukemia, breast cancer, lung cancer, and thyroid cancer. Although these cancers have been observed as late effects of radiation in epidemiological studies, their rate of induction is very low. Moreover, the risk of induction for cancer is often estimated for a population exposed to a certain level of radiation rather than for an individual.

Radiation mutagenesis is the evaluation of genetic effects that are stochastic in nature. Genetic mutations (ie, alterations) in humans occur from a variety of sources, including radiation. Some mutations have drastic effects that are felt immediately, whereas other mild effects may be passed on to subsequent generations. The genetic effects of radiation are very rare and difficult to study in humans. Therefore, most of our learning on this effect has come from animal experiments.

Radiation teratogenesis is the study of radiation effects on the embryo and fetus. Studies indicate that the developing embryo and fetus are the most radiosensitive organs in human beings. In addition, the effects seem to be more severe for the unborn as compared to the effects after birth has occurred. Mental and growth retardations are some of the principal adverse effects of radiation. Growth retardation is most frequently observed in the form of microcephaly (abnormal smallness of the head). Because of the extreme sensitivity of the unborn to radiation, pregnant occupational workers are assigned lower exposure limits compared to others.

Assessment of risks associated with low levels of ionizing radiation is a complex issue and is discussed in detail throughout the literature. An absolute risk to a population is expressed in number of cases/10^6/rem. An individual risk from a partial body exposure (such as a computed tomography scan of a head or a chest x-ray) may be calculated by using a formalism that uses organ-weighting factors to account for the varying sensitivity of each tissue type.

In modern times, the radiation levels to occupational workers in medical facilities are very low. The radiation protection guidelines adopted and recommended by regulatory agencies have lowered occupational exposure. It is rare for a staff member to receive a whole body dose that is close to the established limits. The prestigious National Council on Radiation Protection and Measurements (NCRP) has recommended an occupational exposure limit of 5000 mrem/year for the whole body effective dose.[19] This limit of exposure to ionizing radiation was arrived at by comparing radiation risks to those associated with other safe industries. The radiation industry is considered a very safe working environment when these NCRP recommendations are adopted. It is very unusual for a staff member to receive whole body radiation, from a vascular brachytherapy procedure (even though high-energy gamma-emitting isotopes such as ^{192}Ir are used), that would exceed a few mrem.

The risks associated with low levels of ionizing radiation seem to be very low. Early detection of cancer and good record keeping will facilitate a further understanding of the late effects, which, at the present time, are difficult to predict.

Acknowledgments: The author wishes to thank Marcia Straile, Ashish Jani, and Shyam Jani for their invaluable help in preparing this manuscript.

References

1. Jani SK. Physics of vascular brachytherapy. J Invas Cardiol 1999;11:517–523.
2. Jani SK, Steuterman S, Huppe GB, et al. Radiation safety of personnel during catheter-based Ir-192 coronary brachytherapy. J Invas Cardiol 2000;12:286–290.
3. Balter S, Oetgen M, Hill A, et al. Personnel exposure during gamma endovascular brachytherapy. Health Phys 2000;79:136–146.
4. Hall EJ. Radiobiology for the Radiologist, 4th Edition. Philadelphia: J.B. Lippincott; 1994.
5. BEIR V. National Academy of Sciences/National Research Council, Committee on the Biological Effects of Ionizing Radiations. Health Effects of Exposure to Low Levels of Ionizing Radiation, BEIR V. Washington, DC: National Academy Press; 1990:242–351.
6. Annex F. Radiation carcinogenesis in man. In: Sources, Effects and Risks of Ionizing Radiation, Report to the General Assembly by the United Nations Scientific Committee on the Effects of Atomic Radiation (UNSCEAR). New York: United Nations; 1988: 405–543.
7. Boice JD, Day NE, Andersen A, et al. Second cancers following radiation treatment for cervical cancer: An international collaboration among cancer registries. J Natl Cancer Inst 1985;74:955–975.
8. Neel JV. Update on the genetic effects of ionizing radiation. JAMA 1991;266:698–701.
9. BEIR III. National Academy of Sciences/National Research Council, Committee on the Biological Effects of Ionizing Radiations. Health Effects of Exposure to Low Levels of Ionizing Radiation, BEIR III. Washington, DC: National Academy Press; 1980.
10. BEIR V. National Academy of Sciences/National Research Council, Committee on the Biological Effects of Ionizing Radiations. Health Effects of Exposure to Low Levels of Ionizing Radiation, BEIR V. Washington, DC: National Academy Press; 1990:70.
11. NCRP Report No. 115. Risk estimates for radiation protection. National Council on Radiation Protection and Measurements. Bethesda, MD, 1993:93.
12. Mettler FA Jr, Upton AC. Medical Effects of Ionizing Radiation, Second Edition. Philadelphia: WB Saunders; 1995.

13. Blot WJ, Miller RW. Mental retardation following in utero exposure to the atomic bombs of Hiroshima and Nagasaki. Radiology 1973;106:617–619.
14. Otake M, Yoshimaru H, Schull WJ. Severe mental retardation among the prenatally exposed survivors of the atomic bombing of Hiroshima and Nagasaki: A comparison of the T65DR and DS86 dosimetry systems. RERF Technical Report 16–87, Radiation Effects Research Foundation, Hiroshima, 1988.
15. NCRP Report No. 116. Limitation of exposure to ionizing radiation. National Council on Radiation Protection and Measurements. Bethesda, MD, 1993:37–39.
16. Jacobi W. The concept of effective dose: A proposal for the combination of organ doses. Radiat Environ Biophys 1975;12:101–109.
17. International Commission on Radiological Protection. ICRP Publication 26, Ann ICRP 1(3), 1977.
18. NCRP Report No. 115. Risk estimates for radiation protection. National Council on Radiation Protection and Measurements. Bethesda, MD, 1993:106–110.
19. NCRP Report No. 115. Risk estimates for radiation protection. National Council on Radiation Protection and Measurements. Bethesda, MD, 1993:4.

## Chapter 66

Regulatory Requirements for Approval of Vascular Radiation for Clinical Use in the United States

Tara A. Ryan, MS, MBA

Introduction

The U.S. Food and Drug Administration (FDA) of the Department of Health and Human Services (HHS) is a federal regulatory agency designed to protect the health of American public. All medical devices are regulated by the FDA's Center for Devices and Radiological Health (CDRH), which is responsible for ensuring that these devices are safe and effective.

As required by the Investigational Device Exemptions (IDE) regulations (21 CFR Part 812), a clinical investigation of vascular radiotherapy must be studied under an FDA-approved IDE application. In addition, approval from an institutional review board (IRB) must also be obtained. An IDE application must include information regarding the device description, prior investigations using the device, the complete investigational plan, a copy of the investigator agreement, manufacturing, and a copy of the patient informed consent form.

Although an approved IDE application exempts a device from certain provisions of the Food, Drug and Cosmetic Act, it does not exempt it from other federal, state, or local regulations. Investigational vascular radiotherapy devices are subject to radiological health regulation, including Nuclear Regulatory Commission (NRC) regulations and requirements.

Significant Risk Versus NonSignificant Risk

The question of whether some vascular radiotherapy studies—namely, studies in which external beam irradiation is used—should be considered nonsignificant risk, has been raised and carefully considered by the FDA. It is important that both investigators and IRBs have a clear understanding of what "significant risk" means in a regulatory context. Sherertz and Streed[1] report their experience with interpretation of this issue. Risk determination must be based on the proposed use of a device in an investigation, and not on the device alone.[2] A significant risk device study is defined [21 CFR 812.3(m)] as a study of a device that presents a potential for serious risk to the health, safety, or welfare of a subject

From Waksman R (ed.). *Vascular Brachytherapy, Third Edition.* Armonk, NY: Futura Publishing Co., Inc.; © 2002.

and: (1) is an implant; or (2) is used in supporting or sustaining human life; or (3) is of substantial importance in diagnosing, curing, mitigating, or treating disease, or otherwise prevents impairment of human health; or (4) otherwise presents a potential for serious risk to the health, safety, or welfare of a subject. Studies where the potential harm to subjects could be life-threatening, could result in permanent impairment of a body function or permanent damage to body structure, or could necessitate medical or surgical intervention to preclude impairment or damage should be considered significant risk. Also, if the patient must undergo a procedure as part of the investigational study, which in the case of external beam irradiation is a vascular intervention, then the potential harm that could be caused by the procedure in addition to the harm that could be caused by radiation must be considered. With this in mind, it becomes more clear that vascular radiation studies fall into the category of "significant risk," regardless of whether the radiation is delivered externally or intravascularly. Similarly, the site of application of the radiation does not eliminate the potential for serious risk to the subject.

Investigational Device Exemption Applications

Investigators who want to perform clinical studies at their institutions should either: (a) participate in an FDA-approved trial sponsored by a manufacturer or another investigator, or (b) obtain FDA approval for a single center study at their own institution. If the latter option is chosen, then the physician is considered the "sponsor-investigator," and, therefore, is required to meet all the obligations of both the investigator and sponsor of an IDE study.

What is involved in IDE application process? The term "application" is perhaps somewhat of a misnomer. There is no pre-clinical application or form that is required to be filled out. Rather, an IDE application is a summary of information. Within 30 days of submission of the IDE application, the FDA will make a final decision on whether to approve the application, approve the applications with conditions, or disapprove the application. Figure 1 is a schema of the major decisions in the IDE approval process.

The cover letter of the IDE application should specify the name and address of the sponsor, the centers that will be participating in the study, the radioactive isotope, the method that will be used to deliver the radiation, and the manufacturer(s) of the source and delivery system. If applicable, any pre-IDE meetings held with FDA review divisions (with meeting minutes attached) and/or pre-IDE applications submitted should also be documented in the cover letter. The specific information that is required to be submitted in the IDE is described below.

Reports of Prior Investigations

A report of prior investigations must include reports of all prior clinical, animal, and laboratory testing of the device. It should be comprehensive and adequate to justify the proposed investigation. A bibliography of all publications that are relevant to an evaluation of the safety and effectiveness of the device should be provided along with copies of all published and unpublished adverse information. Specific contents of the report must include the following.

Original IDE Application Review and Approval

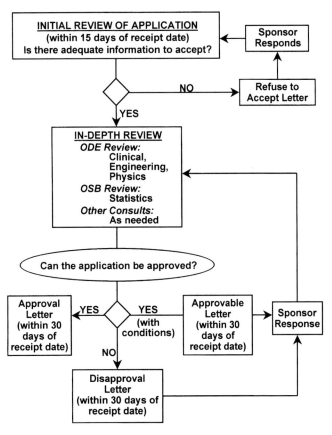

Figure 1

Bench Testing

Much of the bench testing may have already been conducted by the manufacturer. The types of bench testing appropriate to qualify vascular radiotherapy systems include: complete characterization of the radiation source, biocompatibility of blood-contacting materials used in the delivery system, mechanical integrity of the components used in the delivery system, electrical safety of all components, and sterility of the source and delivery system. Clinical investigators intending to submit a sponsor-investigator IDE should consult with the manufacturer to ensure that sufficient test data are available. The manufacturer may provide this information directly to the investigator for inclusion in the IDE application. Alternatively, the manufacturer may provide a letter to the investigator that references appropriate files within the agency where this bench testing is contained and provides the FDA with permission to review these data on behalf of the sponsor-investigator. This letter, which is then included in the IDE, should clearly specify the file numbers (or master file) and pages where these test data can be found.

Animal Testing

Any animal tests that have been conducted using the radiation source and delivery system proposed for use in the investigation should be described. The work of others may be referenced; however, differences in components and/or experimental methodologies must be noted or an explanation provided as to how such data are applicable to the study being proposed. This requires a careful analysis of the literature that is being referenced. Also, it should be specified whether the animal testing was done in compliance with Good Laboratory Practices (GLPs).[3]

Clinical Experience

All clinical data available using the radiation source and delivery system proposed for use in the investigation should be provided. Similar to the animal test results, work done by others may be referenced, but a justification is needed for how these data are applicable if the radiation source, delivery system, and/or methods used are not identical to those proposed in the study.

Investigational Plan

The investigational plan should include the following items:

1. A clear statement of the objectives of the proposed investigation.
2. A written protocol describing the methodology to be used and an analysis of the protocol demonstrating its scientific soundness, ie:
   (a) The study type (feasibility, concurrent control, randomized) and a specific identification of the control group;
   (b) Identification of the primary and (if applicable) the secondary endpoints;
   (c) Specification of all patient inclusion and exclusion criteria;
   (d) Specification of the study hypothesis;
   (e) Specification of the proposed sample size and statistical justification for such, given the study hypothesis;
   (f) A description of how patients will be assigned to the study and control groups and an explanation of how bias will be minimized;
   (g) A description of how (and when) the measures of the primary and secondary endpoints will be obtained; and
   (h) A complete list of all definitions (success, failure, complications, etc.).
3. A description and analysis of all increased risks to the research subjects, how these risks will be minimized, and a discussion of the benefits of using radiation in light of these risks.
4. A description of each important component, property, and principle of operation of the device and any anticipated changes in the device during the investigation.
5. A copy of all case report forms (these should reflect the type of data to be collected from each patient and must be consistent with the clinical protocol).
6. The patient informed consent form must comply with 21 CFR Part 50 including a clear explanation of treatment, all potential short- and long-term

complications, alternatives to treatment, the follow-up studies to be performed, and the time intervals involved.

7. A list of the centers/investigators participating in the study, noting the chairperson of the IRB at each participating center and a certification of any action taken by each IRB.
8. A draft of all device labeling, including the Instructions for Use.

Patients enrolled in vascular radiotherapy clinical trials should continue to be followed carefully for evaluation of the potential for unknown long-term effects of this treatment. In addition, the possibility that radiation simply shifts the maximal restenotic response time to a later time period must also be considered. At present, the FDA believes that patients undergoing this therapy should, at a minimum, have angiographic follow-up at 6 months and clinical follow-up at 9 to 12 months. In order to further characterize the long-term safety and effectiveness of a particular vascular radiotherapy system, post-approval studies may be required. Therefore, it is important that IDE sponsors make patients aware, in the informed consent form, that annual follow-up past 12 months will be required. Additional long-term studies performed for the suspicion of restenosis should be sent back to the core laboratory for review.

Dosimetry Issues

IDE and PMA (Pre-Market Approval) applications for vascular radiotherapy studies must specify the target tissue and dose that will be delivered to it. Accurate dosimetry and delivery of the expected dose to the target tissue are essential to confidently assess this treatment modality. For IDE applications, there are two major issues that must be considered: (1) the accuracy of the dose to the treatment volume required to validate the study hypothesis, and (2) how the dose at some point (or in some volume) is determined. To adequately address these questions, sponsors must carefully consider the different issues raised, depending on the radioisotope used, the method of radiation delivery, and the use of accessory components (eg, software to determine the dose or control the placement and/or delivery of the source).

For PMA applications, there must be sufficient information so that the user can fully assess the safety implications of using the device. At a minimum, the following information must be included: (1) A complete description of the dose rate along the perpendicular bisector of the source (train) axis per unit source output (eg, air kerma strength or contained activity). For photon sources, this information should be available from 0.5 to 10 mm from the source, and for beta sources, this information should be available from 0.5 mm to the end of the range of the maximum energy beta from the source; (2) A map of the dose (rate) along the source axis at equal contour lines should be shown for representative distances from the source axis. The anisotropic dose rate distribution at the ends of the source should be included; (3) The method used to achieve tractability to national standards maintained by the National Institute of Standards and Technology ([NIST]; air kerma strength, absorbed dose rate in water at 2 mm, or contained activity); and (4) The parameters of any model used to give the dose rate at various distances must be included and information must be provided on how the values were determined.

The FDA has prepared a draft guidance document entitled, *Vascular Radiotherapy—Guidance for Data to be Submitted in Support of Investigational Device Exception (IDE) Applications*. This document identifies the types of issues that should be addressed in the dosimetry of IDE application. The dosimetry part of this document is under revision so as to be applicable for PMA submissions. Until then, additional dosimetry information for photon sources can be found in *Guidance for the Submission of Premarket Notifications for Photon-Emitting Brachytherapy Sources*. It is recommended that the Good Guidance Document FDA website, http://www.fda.gov/cdrh/ggpmain.html#docs, be checked for the latest guidance document available.

Nuclear Regulatory Commission Requirements

The following description of requirements by the NRC for authorization (licensure) to participate in vascular radiotherapy investigational studies is excerpted from an outline presented at the "Advances in Cardiovascular Radiation Therapy"[5] symposium, Washington, D.C., March 8–10, 1998. Interested parties should contact the NRC directly to keep apprised of modifications in requirements.

The continued interest in investigating the applicability of the use of ionizing radiation therapy to reduce or eliminate restenosis in coronary and peripheral arteries after angioplasty has led to the continuing development of a varied number of innovative approaches. Most of these involve the use of by-product material(s) as the source of the ionizing radiation. As such, the use of these materials requires licensure by either the NRC or an Agreement State. As might be expected, the requirements for the NRC licensure for participation in these varied investigative studies of intravascular brachytherapy are, of necessity, being developed on a case-by-case basis as each of these evolving intravascular catheter-based systems often require unique radiation health and safety considerations. For example, for simple stent systems with microcurie quantities of implanted beta-particle emitters, the necessary radiation protection measures required to protect both the health care providers and the patient from unwarranted and potentially dangerous radiation exposures are quite basic and easily implemented. On the other hand, high dose rate afterloading systems, particularly those using sources emitting penetrating gamma radiation, can pose very serious radiation hazards not only to the patient and to health care providers, but also to the public if control of this source is lost for even a short time.

Despite the unique characteristics of each of these device-based protocols, which use sealed sources containing by-product materials, there are also several uniform requirements required by the NRC for authorization (licensure) to participate in these investigations. These are:

The requirements of 10 CFR 35.6, "Provisions for Research Involving Human Subjects," must be met (it is required by the FDA that U.S. patients be studied under an IDE application).

Only those physicians who meet the training and experience requirements set forth in 10 CFR 35.940, "Training For Use of Brachytherapy Sources," can be designated as authorized users for these procedures.

The radiation sources and/or devices used in the research must have undergone an appropriate sealed source and/or device review(s) and be listed in the Registry of Radioactive Sealed Sources and Devices as approved for use in intravascular radiotherapy.

If low activity unsealed sources (eg, implanted or plated stents) are used for intravascular brachytherapy procedures, then, at present, the training and experience requirements for designating the authorized user in item 2 (above) are those set forth in 10 CFR 35.930, "Training for Therapeutic Use of Unsealed By-Product Material," and the requirements in item 3 do not apply.

The other major consideration in NRC authorization (licensure) for participation in intravascular brachytherapy investigations is whether the licensee possesses a license of "Broad Scope" or a "Limited Specific" license. Generally, medical Broad Scope licensees can participate in these studies without any additional authorization by the NRC. Prior to doing so, however, it is incumbent upon such licensees to review their licenses and have one or more specific license conditions amended that would otherwise prohibit conduct of the protocol in question.

Limited Specific licensees must apply to the NRC for a license amendment authorizing each experimental study in which they wish to participate. This amendment request must contain the information set forth in the three aforementioned requirements (or the two alternate requirements stated for unsealed sources), and all necessary radiation protection and emergency response procedures. For Limited Specific licensees requesting authorization to participate in studies that use sealed sources of by-product material, such authorization cannot be granted unless the sealed source(s) and/or device(s) have been reviewed and approved for that use by the NRC or an Agreement State. For research and development purposes only, for unregistered sources, or for registered sealed sources not possessed and used in accordance with the registration, if the licensee is qualified by sufficient training and experience and has sufficient facilities and equipment to safely use and handle the requested quantity of radioactive material in unsealed form, an exemption to the registration requirement can be requested. This last condition could be best demonstrated if the licensee possesses, on their existing NRC license, a current authorization for the quantity of radioactive material in question.

Summary

The use of radiation to reduce restenosis has shown promise. Results reported in both single center and multicenter randomized trials have demonstrated a reduction in restenosis rates as compared to standard therapy. However, there are several important issues that should be investigated further to fully understand and optimize this treatment modality. These include issues such as the late effects of vascular irradiation, ideal therapeutic doses, appropriate adjunct therapy, and identification of the subgroup of patients that will benefit the most from this new technology. As the FDA continues to review submitted data, and as new devices undergo pre-market evaluation, the issues discussed in this chapter may be revised. The FDA encourages continued interaction with the scientific community and industry as the interdisciplinary field of vascular radiotherapy continues to advance.

References

1. Sheretz RJ, Streed SA. Medical devices: Significant risk vs. nonsignificant risk. JAMA 1994;272:955–956.
2. Less JR, Alpert S, Nightingale SL. Institutional review boards and medical devices. JAMA 1994;272:968–969.
3. 21 CFR part 58.
4. Intravascular Brachytherapy—Guidance for Data to be Submitted to the Food and Drug Administration in Support of Investigational Device Exemption (IDE) Applications. Interventional Cardiology Devices Branch, Division of Cardiovascular, Respiratory and Neurological Devices, Office of Device Evaluation, FDA, May 24, 1996.
5. Ayres RL. Regulatory and Health Care Millieu Issues—NRC Requirements [syllabus]. Advances in Cardiovascular Radiation Therapy Symposium. Washington D.C.; March 8–10, 1998.

## Chapter 67

The Economics of Restenosis:

Implications for Brachytherapy

William S. Weintraub, MD

Introduction

Brachytherapy is a promising new therapy that may prevent restenosis after coronary angioplasty,[1] a major limitation of angioplasty.[2,3] While restenosis results in recurrent angina as well as the need for additional procedures, it rarely results in acute myocardial infarction or death.[2] A successful therapy for restenosis that will prevent clinical recurrence will also have economic consequences.[4]

The costs of restenosis include both indirect and direct costs. The direct costs are any additional office visits, testing, hospitalizations, or procedures.[5] Indirect costs include time lost from work by patient and family, need for home health providers, and lost productivity.[5] Data from Emory University suggest that the cost of restenosis (diagnosed angiographically) is approximately $4000 to $7000 in direct costs for a first episode.[6] This may be an underestimation because there may be more than one episode of restenosis, indirect costs are unknown, and routine care may be more intense than would be needed if restenosis did not occur. If angiographically defined restenosis occurs somewhere between 30% and 45% of the time, then the cost of every angioplasty is probably raised on average by somewhere between $2000 and $5000 by restenosis. If there are 400,000 angioplasties performed annually, then the total societal costs of restenosis in the United States alone is somewhere between $800 million and $2 billion per year.[5]

When considering the place of an expensive new therapy to treat a condition that consumes considerable health care resources, it is appropriate to consider the economic consequences of the new therapy. This may be best approached through the methods of cost-effectiveness, in which the cost of therapy is evaluated per quality-adjusted life year (QALY) gained.[7] It is the purpose of the study discussed in this chapter to evaluate the cost-effectiveness of a new therapy to prevent restenosis after coronary angioplasty.

Methods

This study was performed as a simulation based on reference case methods as suggested by a United States Public Health Service publication.[7] A reference

From Waksman R (ed.). *Vascular Brachytherapy, Third Edition.* Armonk, NY: Futura Publishing Co., Inc.; © 2002.

case cost-effectiveness analysis permits comparison of the results, in principle at least, to all other therapies for other medical conditions that use similar methods. The data used in this study were gathered from the medical literature and from best possible estimates. The major estimates were varied between limits to permit a sensitivity analysis. The perspective of this study is that of society.

Outcome was measured in QALYs. The outcome of angioplasty was first assessed as a utility. The best outcome is assigned a utility of 1, and death a utility of 0. The impact of restenosis on utility was then assessed. The theoretical impact of restenosis on utility may be noted in Figure 1.[5] Two patients are displayed, one who suffers restenosis and one who does not. They start and end at the same place, but the patient who suffers restenosis has a noticeable dip in utility. The effect after 6 months was assumed to be no different between the treatment arms unless the patient died of restenosis. Thus, neither cost nor survival after 6 months were assessed and the data did not need to be discounted. Utility was converted to QALYs by estimating survival. The estimated survival was only relevant to determining the impact of mortality from restenosis on the QALYs in each arm, a small effect. The utility of each treatment arm may then be calculated using the decision tree and equations noted in Figure 2. Data for the nodes in the figure are shown in Table 1. The $12,000 cost of angioplasty is consistent with several reports in the medical literature,[8–10] as is the restenosis rate of 40%[11,12] and the use of repeat angioplasty in approximately 50% of those who suffer restenosis.[2] The mortality related to angioplasty is hard to determine, but an estimate of 1% is reasonable. The cost of a new therapy is unknown. Follow-up costs are an estimate. There are no data on the effect of restenosis on utility, or on the effect of increased surveillance and anxiety on utility, and these number are estimates. The expected

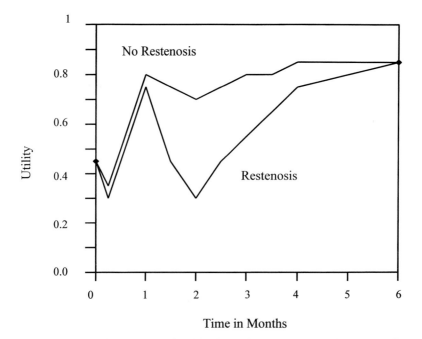

Figure 1. Theoretical time course of utility in patients who do and do not suffer restenosis after successful coronary angioplasty.

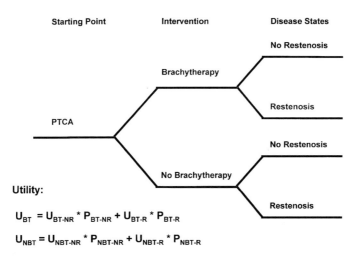

Figure 2. Decision tree evaluating the effect of a new therapy on restenosis for patients.

survival in QALYs in the absence of mortality is reasonably consistent with long-term outcome after angioplasty. By use of these estimates, the cost-effectiveness of a new therapy may be estimated from

$$\text{Cost-Effectiveness} = \frac{\text{Cost}_T - \text{Cost}_{NT}}{\text{QALYs}_T - \text{QALYs}_{NT}}$$

where T stands for therapy and NT for no therapy.

Results

The central assumptions lead to an estimated gain in QALYs of 0.0625 (3.25 weeks) for a therapy that decreased restenosis by 50%. This may at first seem a

Table 1

Central Assumptions for Cost Effectiveness Analysis

Variable	Assumption
Cost of angioplasty	$12000
Cost of therapy	$2500
Cost of 6 months of care	$600
Restenosis rate	40%
Re-PTCA rate	50% of restenosis rate
Effectiveness of therapy	50%
Effect of therapy on F/U costs	1/2 baseline effect
6-Month effect of restenosis on utility	30% of baseline utility
Mortality of restenosis	1%
Expected QALYs	10 years
Effect if surveillance	5% of baseline utility

bit disappointing, but it should not be. As restenosis rarely results in fatalities and the effect of restenosis is not likely to be very long lasting, this is quite a reasonable gain in QALYs. The 6-month cost of angioplasty without the new therapy is $15,000 and with the new therapy it is $16,400, assuming that the therapy costs $2500. It might be desirable to have the cost of the new therapy entirely offset by savings from the avoidance of additional medical care, but this as rarely achieved. This results in a cost-effectiveness ratio of $22,400 per QALY.

There is considerable uncertainty regarding many of the variables tested in this analysis. Thus, the results were tested in a series of sensitivity analyses. In the first analysis the cost of therapy was varied from 0 to $5000 per QALY (Fig. 3). The cost-effectiveness ratio may be noted to rise from −$20,000 to over $60,000 per QALY. A negative number for the ratio represents a savings. In the next analysis effectiveness was varied from 0.2 to 1 (Fig. 4). Thus, at 0.2 only 20% of restenosis was prevented, while at 1 all restenosis was prevented. The cost-effectiveness ratio was noted to decline as effectiveness increased from $60,000 to just under 0. Next, the probability of restenosis was varied from 0.20 to 0.50 (Fig. 5). As the probability of restenosis increased, the cost-effectiveness ratio declined from $50,000 to under $20,000 per QALY. Not surprisingly, it is less cost-effective to treat the problem as it becomes less frequent. The baseline analysis assumed a utility of 1, with a 30% effect of restenosis on this utility. As utility declined, the cost-effectiveness ratio rose from under $25,000 to $45,000 per QALY (Fig. 6). Thus, patients whose baseline condition is less than perfect health have less potential to benefit. In the next analysis the effect of restenosis on utility was assessed (Fig. 7). This is important, because the baseline analysis may have assumed too large an effect of restenosis on utility. The effect of restenosis was confined to 6 months. Thus, the effect of a 30% fall in utility due to restenosis was a fall in utility of 0.15. Thus, the scale is from 0.05, a 10% fall in utility over 6 months, to 0.20, a 40% fall in utility over 6 months. The cost-effectiveness ratio increases from under $20,000 to ap-

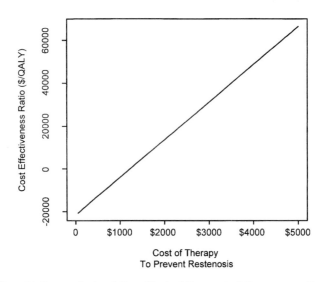

Figure 3. Sensitivity analysis of the effect of the cost of therapy on the cost-effectiveness of therapy to prevent restenosis.

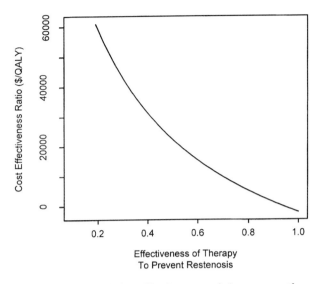

Figure 4. Sensitivity analysis of the effectiveness of therapy on the cost-effectiveness of therapy to prevent restenosis.

proximately $40,000 per QALY as the effect on utility declines from 40% to 10%. The effect of the cost of angioplasty is displayed in Figure 8. As the cost of angioplasty increases from $10,000 to $16,000, the cost-effectiveness ratio declines from over $25,000 to $16,000. Thus, if angioplasty is more expensive, it is more worthwhile to spend money to prevent additional angioplasty. The effect of mortality is shown in Figure 9. While mortality is unusual after angioplasty, this analysis is important because the effect of preventing even a few deaths may significantly im-

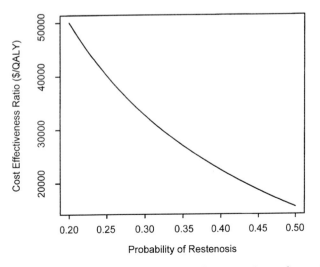

Figure 5. Sensitivity analysis of the probability of restenosis on the cost-effectiveness of therapy to prevent restenosis.

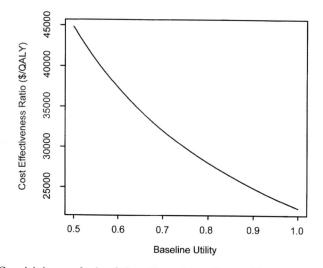

Figure 6. Sensitivity analysis of the effect of baseline utility on the cost-effectiveness of therapy to prevent restenosis.

pact overall outcome. Thus, as the probability of mortality rises from 0% to 3%, the cost-effectiveness ratio falls from over $30,000 to under $15,000.

Not surprisingly, the cost-effectiveness ratio was most sensitive to the variables "effectiveness of therapy" and "cost of therapy." This is explored in greater depth in the two-way sensitivity analysis presented in Figure 10. The effectiveness of therapy (X axis) was varied from 0.1 to 1.0. Cost-effectiveness varied from under −$20,000 to over $100,000 per QALY. Data are presented for cost from 0 on the bottom to $5000 on top in increments of $500. Thus, at any level of effective-

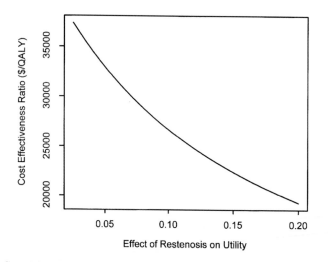

Figure 7. Sensitivity analysis of the impact of restenosis on utility on the cost-effectiveness of therapy to prevent restenosis.

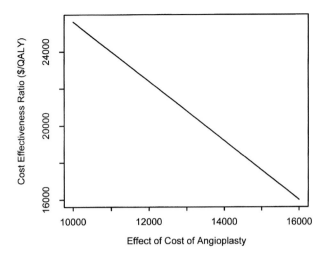

Figure 8. Sensitivity analysis of the cost of angioplasty on the cost-effectiveness of therapy to prevent restenosis.

ness, as therapy became more expensive, the cost-effectiveness ratio rose. Similarly, at any level of cost of therapy, as effectiveness rose, the cost-effectiveness ratio declined. Therapy that is free will always save money. Therapy that costs $1000 or less will be acceptably cost-effective at any level of efficacy above 10%. Thereafter, the issues become more difficult. Clearly, more expensive therapy at low levels of efficacy will have a high cost-effectiveness ratio. If the acceptable limit is $50,000 per QALY, a cost of therapy in excess of $3500 at 50% efficacy may start to approach the limit.

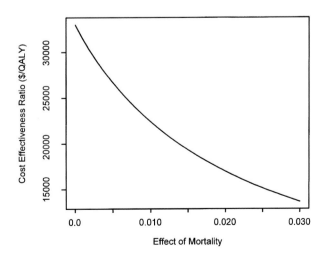

Figure 9. Sensitivity analysis of incidence of mortality on the cost-effectiveness of therapy to prevent restenosis.

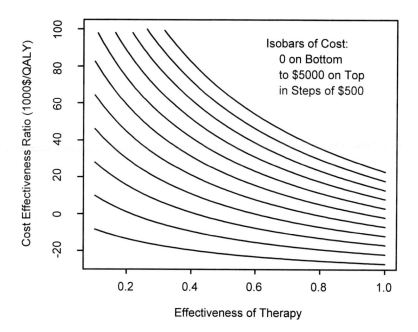

Figure 10. Two-way sensitivity analysis of the effect of the cost of therapy and effectiveness of therapy on the cost-effectiveness of therapy to prevent restenosis. Each line represents an isobar of cost from $0 to $5000 in steps of $500. Note the y scale is in $1000/quality-adjusted life year (QALY).

Discussion

The results of this study reveal that an effective therapy to prevent 50% of the incidence of restenosis after coronary angioplasty which costs $2500 will cost $22,400 per QALY gained, given the other central assumptions. This is in line with other accepted therapies such as t-PA compared to streptokinase[13] and ACE inhibition after myocardial infarction.[14] The cost-effectiveness of a therapy such as brachytherapy will be most sensitive to both its cost and its effectiveness (see Figs. 3, 4 and 10). Thus, the real place of brachytherapy will depend on how effective it is proven to be as clinical trial results become available and how expensive it turns out to be. While several other components of the model may be estimated from the literature, such as the cost of performing angioplasty or the incidence of restenosis, the effectiveness and cost of brachytherapy are yet to be determined. If brachytherapy turns out to be expensive and not very effective, it will not prove useful. On the contrary, if it is quite effective and reasonably priced, then it will be useful indeed.

Several other aspects of the sensitivity analyses are worthy of comment. As the probability of restenosis falls, the cost-effectiveness ratio rises. This is particularly important if there are therapies that otherwise seem to be complementary. Thus, if the use of stents in the community resembles the clinical trials[15,16] in which restenosis and additional procedures were decreased, then the cost-effectiveness ratio for brachytherapy in stented arteries may be correspondingly increased (see Fig. 5). In such a situation, brachytherapy might have to prove toward the upper end of the scale of effectiveness and/or be relatively inexpensive. The analyses presented here were all predicated on the notion that restenosis has a real impact on patients' quality of life (see Figs. 6 and 7). Should it turn out that restenosis is really only a minor problem with no demonstrable effect on quality of life, then a new therapy would have to be justified on the basis of cost alone. There are data that reveal that restenosis is usually accompanied with recurrent angina,[3] but there are essentially no data on the effect of restenosis on overall utility. There are multiple forces in society that are forcing down medical care costs—especially the payers. As the cost of angioplasty decreases (see Fig. 8), it will be increasingly difficult to justify an expensive new form of therapy aimed primarily at preventing angioplasty. Thus, brachytherapy may rapidly come under the kinds of pressure to keep costs to a minimum that have now become the norm in medical practice.

The presentation of the model and sensitivity analysis would seem to assume that brachytherapy would be used in all patients. This is not necessarily the case. The cost-effectiveness of brachytherapy can be improved by targeting therapy[17] to patients in whom it is shown to be most effective, perhaps by considering lesion characteristics. It can also be targeted to patients in whom the expected rate of restenosis[12] or clinical events is known to be higher.[18] Brachytherapy might be targeted to patients in whom restenosis is expected to have a significant effect on utility. For instance, if a patient is asymptomatic at the time of angioplasty, and is having the procedure in preparation for noncardiac surgery, then restenosis would probably not have an effect on utility. In such a patient brachytherapy might not be indicated. Thus, the issues concerning patient selection for therapy may be quite complicated, turning on several of the issues discussed above. However, the targeting of patients for therapy will require additional data.

The presentation of the model in this study is from the societal perspective, in accord with the reference case guidelines. However, no stakeholder in the medical care system actually takes a societal perspective. Consider the case of an effective therapy to prevent restenosis in 50% of patients that costs $1000 (Table 2).[4] Without therapy the cost of angioplasty will be $12,000 for the initial care plus $2400 for treatment of restenosis, under the central assumptions. With therapy the initial costs rises to $13,000 due to the additional cost of this therapy. However, follow-up cost falls to $1300 as the rate of angioplasty is decreased by 50%. The follow-up cost is $1300 instead of $1200 because the new therapy will be used on these repeat cases to prevent a second episode of restenosis. The total is then $14,300, a $100 savings or close to neutral for society. There are quite different economic consequences for payers and providers, which vary markedly with the payment scheme (Table 2). The following analysis assumes that the overall cost of society of varying the payment scheme is neutral. Under "fee for service," the risks are taken largely by the payer. Thus, the provider has an initial $100 savings or profit (plus signs mean net cost or loss; minus signs mean net savings or profit) due to ability to charge above the cost for the new therapy. In contrast, the payer loses $1100 due to the cost of therapy plus profit to the provider. At 6 months the provider has a cost of $110 and the payer a savings of $1210 as additional angioplasty has been decreased by 50%. The overall cost to society remains a $100 savings, because the provider has an overall cost of $10 ($100 profit initially and then a $110 cost over 6 months) and the payer has a $110 savings ($1100 cost ini-

Table 2

Provider and Payer Economic Consequences
By Type of Reimbursement, Central Assumptions

	Providers			Payers		
	Initial	6-Month Follow-up	Total	Initial	6-Month Follow-up	Total
Fee for service	−$100	+$10	$10	+$1100	−$1210	−$110
Package price	+$1000	+$200	$1220	0	−$1320	−$1320
Capitated	+$1000	−$100	−$100	0	0	0

signs: + cost or loss, − savings for profit

tially and a $1210 savings over follow-up). Under "package pricing" the provider has an initial $1000 loss and the payer no initial loss or gain, as the provider is paid a set amount and must pay for the new therapy completely. At 6 months, the provider has a further loss of $220, while the payer gains $1320 due to the reduction in additional angioplasty. Under "capitation" the provider has an initial cost of $1000 for the new therapy, but then gains $1100 due to less angioplasty, and thus has a small overall gain. The payer has no economic consequences, as risk lies entirely with the provider. For each scheme the overall societal impact remains a $100 decrease in cost. This analysis reveals that the economic impact of therapy on payers and providers cannot be ignored, even if the overall societal impact remains the most important issue.

The analyses presented in this chapter are all simulations. There is clearly a place for such analyses, as they bring into focus the issues that are faced in choosing therapy. While attempts were made to perform this analyses according to the reference case methods suggested by the United States Public Health Service Panel,[7] it is extremely difficult to be in full compliance with those recommendations, and this analysis can easily be criticized as being too simple to reflect the complex economic and clinical reality of patient recovery and potential for restenosis after angioplasty. Thus, there are very real limitations to what can be learned from simulations. Cost and cost-effectiveness analyses can be conducted as a part of clinical trials in which the costs and utility are actually measured with such tests as time trade-off or standard gamble.[7] Costs studies after angioplasty have been somewhat limited, as the costs need to be measured after the index hospitalization; this poses significant logistical problems. Difficulties notwithstanding, it will be essential for clinical trials of brachytherapy to have concurrent cost and utility assessment to establish the true place of the procedure.

Obviously cost and cost-effectiveness data on brachytherapy are still lacking. The present study should provide a perspective that will guide further research. The effectiveness and the cost of the therapy, in that order, will probably be the major determinants of how useful it proves to be. The perspective of society and that of each major stakeholder, payer, provider, and, most importantly, patient, must be considered. Nonetheless, there is clearly a place for an effective, moderately priced therapy to prevent restenosis after angioplasty.

References

1. Waksman R, King SB, Crocker IR, Mould RF (eds.): Vascular Brachytherapy. AX Veenendaal, The Netherlands: Nucletron BV; 1996.
2. Weintraub WS, Ghazzal ZMB, Douglas JS Jr, et al. Initial management and long term clinical outcome of restenosis after initially successful PTCA. Am J Cardiol 1992;70:47–55.
3. Weintraub WS, Ghazzal ZMB, Douglas JS Jr, et al. Long term clinical followup in patients with angiographic restudy after successful angioplasty. Circulation 1993;87:831–840.
4. Weintraub WS, Warner CD, Mauldin PD, et al. Economic winners and losers after introduction of an effective new therapy depend on the type of payment system. Am J Managed Care 1997;3:743–749.
5. Weintraub WS. Evaluating the cost of therapy for restenosis: Considerations for brachytherapy. Int J Radiat Oncol Biol Phys 1996;36:949–958.
6. Gilbert SP, Weintraub WS, Talley JD, Boccuzzi SJ, for the Lovastatin Restenosis Trial Group. The costs of restenosis (Lovastatin Restenosis Trial). Am J Cardiol 1996;77:196–199.
7. Gold MR, Siegel JE, Russell LB, Weinstein MC (eds.): Cost-Effectiveness in Health and Medicine. New York, Oxford: Oxford University Press; 1996.
8. Weintraub WS, Benard J, Mauldin PD, et al. Declining resource utilization in interventional cardiology? Am J Managed Care 1995;1:58–63.
9. Cohen DJ, Krumholz HM, Sukin CA, et al, for the Stent Restenosis Study Investigators. In-hospital and one-year economic outcomes after coronary stenting or balloon angioplasty: Results from a randomized clinical trial. Circulation 1995;92:2480–2487.
10. Ellis SG, Miller DP, Brown KJ, et al. In-hospital cost of percutaneous coronary revascularization: Critical determinants and implications. Circulation 1995;92:741–747.
11. Weintraub WS, Boccuzzi SJ, Klein JL, et al, and the Lovastatin Restenosis Trial Study Group. Lack of effect of lovastatin on restenosis after coronary angioplasty. N Engl J Med 1994;331:1331–1337.
12. Weintraub WS, Kosinski AS, Brown CL III, King SB III. Can restenosis be predicted after coronary angioplasty from clinical variables? J Am Coll Cardiol 1993;21:6–14.
13. Mark DB, Hlatky MA, Califf RM, et al. Cost effectiveness of thrombolytic therapy with tissue plasminogen activator as compared with streptokinase for acute myocardial infarction. N Engl J Med 1995;332:1418–1424.
14. Tsevat J, Duke D, Goldman L, et al. Cost-effectiveness of captopril therapy after myocardial infarction. J Am Coll Cardiol 1995;26:914–919.
15. Fischman DL, Leon MB, Baim DS, et al, for the Stent Restenosis Study Investigators. A randomized comparison of coronary-stent placement and balloon angioplasty in the treatment of coronary artery disease. N Engl J Med 1994;331:496–501.
16. Serruys PW, de Jaegere P, Kiemeneij F, et al, for the Benestent Study Group. A comparison of balloon-expandable stent implantation with balloon angioplasty in patients with coronary artery disease. N Engl J Med 1994;331:489–495.
17. Weintraub WS, Boccuzzi SJ, Shen Y, et al. Targeting patients for thrombus inhibition after angioplasty: Clinical and economic implications [abstract]. J Am Coll Cardiol 1997;29:500A.
18. Weintraub WS, Douglas JS, Ghazzal Z, Morris DC. Evaluation and prediction of clinical restenosis. Circulation 1996;94:I90.

Index